Neonatal Anesthesia

Jerrold Lerman
Editor

Neonatal Anesthesia

Springer

Editor
Jerrold Lerman, MD, FRCPC, FANZCA
Department of Anesthesia
Women and Children's Hospital of Buffalo
State University of New York at Buffalo
Buffalo, NY, USA

University of Rochester Medical Center
Rochester, NY, USA

ISBN 978-1-4939-4082-0 ISBN 978-1-4419-6041-2 (eBook)
DOI 10.1007/978-1-4419-6041-2
Springer New York Heidelberg Dordrecht London

Softcover reprint of the hardcover 1st edition 2015

Printed on acid-free paper

Springer is part of Springer Science+Business Media (www.springer.com)

Foreword

"The anesthesiologist…who has to spend more than a half hour in putting an infant to sleep because of unavoidable difficulties, and who during this time makes no excuses for his slowness and resorts to no drastic expedients to impress the onlookers or to console the impatient surgeon, is a gift beyond price to the welfare of children who are entrusted to his care in the operating room".

Willis J. Potts, *The Surgeon and the Child*, 1959

Those of us who have been privileged to practice neonatal anesthesia have indeed enjoyed a special relationship with our surgeons. We have also had to meet the challenges of working in one of the most demanding of the anesthesia subspecialties. The technical aspects of our practice require a level of precision and an attention to detail unparalleled in other areas of anesthesia practice. Successful perioperative management of the newborn requires obsessive monitoring and the potential for rapid and appropriate therapeutic responses based on a comprehensive knowledge of neonatal physiology and pharmacology. The neonatal anesthesiologist assumes a daunting responsibility—his patients are at a critical stage of development—and they are in the prelude to a potential lifetime of achievement.

Neonates have been given anesthetics since 1847, but the real history of neonatal anesthesia did not begin until halfway through the twentieth century. I started my training in pediatric anesthesia in 1967 at a world renowned Canadian children's hospital. One day I was assigned to assist with the anesthesia for a newborn with a pre-ductal coarctation of the aorta. I was told that the way to manage this patient was to give a large dose of d-tubocurarine and to ventilate with oxygen. My monitors were an esophageal stethoscope, an electrocardioscope, an oscillometer, and a rectal temperature probe. What a long way we have come in the past 40 or so years!

It is most appropriate that a comprehensive book devoted to neonatal anesthesia should be produced at this time. There has been a progressive accumulation of knowledge related to the subject over the past few decades. Well designed studies have been completed which now permit an evidence-based approach to neonatal anesthesia practice. In addition, simultaneous widespread advances in medical technology have presented us with efficient new means to improve all aspects of the care of small infants. All of this has resulted in a rapid evolution in our management strategies for the newborn. The neonatal anesthesiologist can now very safely apply a full range of modalities to prevent pain, to optimize the perioperative physiological status, and to contribute very significantly to the success of the surgery.

Dr. Lerman has very extensive personal experience as a clinical neonatal anesthesiologist, gained in the very busy neonatal surgical service at the Hospital for Sick Children, Toronto, and subsequently at the Buffalo Children's Hospital and the University of Rochester. As an investigator, he has contributed significantly to our knowledge. He has recruited an outstanding international team of contributors, each an expert in his field, to compile this source book for the practitioner.

BC, Canada

David J. Steward, MBBS, FRCPC

Acknowledgments

I wish to thank my wife, Robin, and my daughters, Ashley and Courtney, for their endless support and patience in undertaking this project.

I also wish to thank Dr. Robert E. Creighton and Dr. David J. Steward for their guidance and mentorship in shaping my academic career as a pediatric anesthesiologist.

Finally, not a day goes by that I do not reflect on the two anesthesiologists whose teaching, advice, influence, and mentoring set a trajectory for my academic career in pediatric anesthesia that would not have been possible otherwise: Drs. George Gregory and E.I. Eger II.

Thank you all.

Jerrold Lerman, MD, FRCPC, FANZCA

Contents

Contributors

Brian J. Anderson, PhD, FANZCA, FJFICM Department of Anaesthesiology, University of Auckland, Auckland, New Zealand

Adrian Bosenberg, MB, ChB, FFA (SA) Department Anesthesiology and Pain Management, Seattle Children's Hospital, University Washington, Seattle, WA, USA

Claire Brett, MD Department of Anesthesia and Perioperative Care, University of California, San Francisco, CA, USA

Jeffrey P. Burns, MD, MPH Division of Critical Care, Boston Children's Hospital, Boston, MA, USA

Susan M. Carden, MBBS, FRANZCO, FRACS, PhD Department of Paediatrics, University of Melbourne, Melbourne, VIC, Australia

Department of Ophthalmology, Royal Children's Hospital, Melbourne, VIC, Australia

Department of Ophthalmology, Royal Victorian Eye and Ear Hospital, Melbourne, VIC, Australia

Isabelle Constant, MD, PhD Department of Anesthesiology, Armand Trousseau Hospital, Paris, France

Kate Cross, FRACS Great Ormond Street Hospital NHS Trust, London, UK

Andrew J. Davidson, MBBS, MD, FANZCA Department of Anesthesia and Pain Management, Murdoch Children's Research Institute, Royal Children's Hospital, VIC, Australia

John E. Fiadjoe, MD University of Pennsylvania School of Medicine, The Children's Hospital of Pennsylvania, Philadelphia, PA, USA

Geoff Frawley, MBBS, FANZCA Department of Anaesthesia and Pain Management, Royal Children's Hospital, Parkville, VIC, Australia

Erin A. Gottlieb, MD Department of Pediatrics and Anesthesiology, Baylor College of Medicine, Texas Children's Hospital, Houston, TX, USA

Walid Habre, MD, PhD Paediatric Anesthesia Unit, Geneva Children's Hospital, Geneva, Switzerland

Christopher Heard, MD Department of Anesthesiology, Division of Pediatrics, Women and Children's Hospital of Buffalo, Buffalo, NY, USA

Richard F. Howard, BSc, MB, ChB, FRCA, FFPM Department of Anaesthesia and Pain Medicine, Great Ormond Street Hospital for Children, NHS Foundation Trust, London, UK

Pablo Ingelmo, MD Department of Anaesthesiology, Montreal Children's Hospital, Montreal, QC, Canada

Monica Kleinman, MD Department is Anesthesia, Perioperative and Pain Medicine, Division of Critical Care, Boston Children's Hospital, Boston, MA, USA

Pete G. Kovatsis, MD Department of Anesthesiology, Perioperative and Pain Medicine, The Division is Critical Care, Boston Children's Hospital, Boston, MA, USA

C. Dean Kurth, MD Cincinnati Children's Hospital Medical Center, University of Cincinnati College of Medicine, Cincinnati, OH, USA

Satyan Lakshminrusimha, MD Division of Neonatology, Department of Pediatrics, Women and Children's Hospital of Buffalo, Buffalo, NY, USA

Peter Larsson, MD Department of Physiology and Pharmacology, Section of Anaesthesiology and Intensive Care, Karolinska Institute, Solna, Sweden

Jerrold Lerman, MD, FRCPC, FANZCA Department of Anesthesia, Women and Children's Hospital of Buffalo, State University of New York at Buffalo, Buffalo, NY, USA

University of Rochester Medical Center, Rochester, NY, USA

Ronald S. Litman, DO University of Pennsylvania School of Medicine, The Children's Hospital of Pennsylvania, Philadelphia, PA, USA

Nicolas Louvet, MD Department of Anesthesiology, Armand Trousseau Hospital, Paris, France

Thomas J. Mancuso, MD Division of Critical Care, Boston Children's Hospital, Boston, MA, USA

John McAuliffe, MD Department of Anesthesiology, Division of Neurobiology, Cincinnati Children's Hospital Medical Center, University of Cincinnati College of Medicine, Cincinnati, OH, USA

Wanda C. Miller-Hance, MD Department of Pediatric Anesthesiology and Pediatric Cardiology, Baylor College of Medicine, Texas Children's Hospital, Houston, TX, USA

Pablo Motta, MD Department of Pediatric Anesthesiology, Baylor College of Medicine, Texas Children's Hospital, Houston, TX, USA

Reema Nandi, MBBS, MD, FRCA Royal Children's Hospital, Melbourne, VIC, Australia

Mario Patino, MD Cincinnati Children's Hospital Medical Center, University of Cincinnati College of Medicine, Cincinnati, OH, USA

David Robinowitz, MD UCSF Benioff Children's Hospital, San Francisco, CA, USA

Nada Sabourdin, MD Department of Anesthesiology, Armand Trousseau Hospital, Paris, France

Jonathan Smith, FRCA Great Ormond Street Hospital NHS Trust, London, UK

Portex Department of Paediatric Anaesthesia, Institute of Child Health, University College London, London, UK

David J. Steward, MBBS, FRCPC Department of Anaesthesia, University of British Columbia, Vancouver, BC, Canada

Paul A. Stricker, MD University of Pennsylvania School of Medicine, The Children's Hospital of Pennsylvania, Philadelphia, PA, USA

Isabeau A. Walker, FRCA Portex Department of Paediatric Anaesthesia, Great Ormond Street Hospital NHS Trust, Institute of Child Health, University College London, London, UK

The History of Neonatal Anesthesia

1

David J. Steward

Early Times

Diethyl ether was administered during operations by Crawford Long in 1842, but it was the demonstration by William G. Morton in 1846 at the Massachusetts General Hospital that led to the widespread introduction of general anesthesia. However the benefits of anesthesia during surgery were not immediately or universally applied. "They don't feel it like we do" was a saying held to be true by physicians and surgeons long after 1846 [1]. In 1847 one third of the surgical operations at the Massachusetts General Hospital, the site of Morton's demonstrations, were performed without anesthesia [1]. Anesthesia was selectively applied to those who it was judged felt pain more severely, i.e., white, wealthy, and especially female patients. Infants were considered incapable of perceiving pain; indeed Dr. Abel Pierson stated that "infants could sleep insensibly even while undergoing surgery" [1]. Henry J. Bigelow considered that like the lower animals, the very young lacked the mental capacity to suffer pain [2]. Indeed, in the case of the neonate, misunderstanding of their perception of pain persisted well into the twentieth century.[1]

During the second half of the nineteenth century and the early part of the twentieth century, the decision to administer anesthesia to a neonate to relieve the pain of surgery was inconsistent. This is perhaps not surprising given the primitive methods which were available to administer anesthesia, the rarity of neonatal surgery, and the fact that small infants could be quite easily restrained during an operation (in addition to the thought that they don't feel pain anyway!). Reports of operations on "impervious rectum," [4] strangulated inguinal hernia, and even meningomyelocele [5] without anesthesia can be found in medical journals of this era.

However reports from this time period can also be found describing anesthesia administered to infants in the first month of life. John Snow preferred chloroform and wrote in 1855 "*Chloroform may be given with propriety to patients of all ages. I have exhibited it to several infants aged from ten days to three weeks*" [6]. He went on to say "*Chloroform acts very favourably on infants and children. There has, I believe, been no death from chloroform under the age of fifteen years*." The most commonly described indication for elective surgery in neonates during these years was for correction of "harelip," an operation that was frequently performed "*at the earliest period of life.*".[2] On Saturday 4th of

D.J. Steward, MBBS, FRCPC (✉)
Department of Anaesthesia, University of British Columbia, Vancouver, BC, Canada, V6T 1Z1
e-mail: davidjsteward@comcast.net

[1]As recently as 1976, a technique of "anesthesia" for ductus arteriosus ligation in preterm infants, which was totally devoid of anesthetic or analgesic agents, was reported from a large American University Hospital in a widely respected British journal. The authors stated "*No premedication was given. Just before the procedure, if necessary, a paralysing dose of suxamethonium 1 mg/kg body wt. was given. No other anaesthetic agent was used…We have avoided the use of anesthetic or analgesic agents which in our opinion are unnecessary*" [3].

[2]Repair of cleft lip ("harelip") today conjures up thoughts of a delicate procedure with carefully planned and positioned skin flaps sutured using many fine sutures in a procedure lasting an hour or more. In the 1850s the repair would require 3–5 sutures and would occupy 3–5 min at most.

J. Lerman (ed.), *Neonatal Anesthesia*, DOI 10.1007/978-1-4419-6041-2_1,

July 1857, an entry in the case books of John Snow [7] reads *"Administered Chloroform at Kings College Hospital to an infant, 8 days old, previous to Mr Fergusson operating for hare-lip. The face piece was too large and the chloroform took very little effect."* Chloroform was administered on this occasion using Snow's inhaler with a small face piece; the latter however was still too large for a neonate. According to Snow, the use of the inhaler permitted *"a more gradual introduction of the agent than when administered on a sponge or handkerchief"* [6].

The alternative method was to administer chloroform to the infant using a sponge. *"Mr. Greenhalgh preferred a sponge to every other kind of apparatus. He had employed the chloroform in a great number of cases, and with success: one of the cases was an infant, three weeks old, for an operation for hare-lip"* [8].

During the second half of the nineteenth century, neonatal surgery was limited to superficial lesions. Abdominal surgery was largely confined to the emergency management of incarcerated inguinal hernia. Imperforate anus of the low type was relieved by incision, often without anesthesia. There were also reports of successful operations on neonates under chloroform for high imperforate anus. Thoracic surgery was certainly not attempted. However during these years, great progress was achieved in basic surgical techniques and the prevention of infection. The concepts of antisepsis and asepsis were recognized and applied. Many of the congenital lesions that would much later become the field of the neonatal surgeon were being recognized—though only as curiosities [9].

It is during this time that the first books on pediatric surgery were being published and special hospitals for children were being established. The Hospital for Sick Children at Great Ormond Street in London (GOS) opened in 1852, and in the USA, Boston Children's Hospital, which was modeled after GOS, opened in 1882 [9]. Other European and North American cities established children's hospitals at about this time. "Pediatric surgery" in these early years involved mainly orthopedic procedures, neonatal surgery was rarely performed, but the children's hospitals would serve as a site and a catalyst for the subsequent expansion of infant surgery.

In the late nineteenth century, progress was being made in the care of sick neonate and preterm infants. It was recognized that the survival of small preterm infants was improved if they could be kept warm. A warm-air heated incubator was developed by a French obstetrician, Stephane Tarnier, and installed at the Paris Maternity Hospital. This was based on a device for raising poultry, which Tarnier had seen at the zoological garden [10]. The design was improved by Pierre Budin, and his incubators were shown at the Berlin World Exhibition of 1896 by his associate Martin Couney, infants being provided by Dr. Czerny, who was the Professor of Pediatrics in the city. Couney later exhibited his incubators in London and at the Pan-American Exposition in Buffalo, New York. He also opened an exhibit at the Coney Island fairground in New York, which ran until 1943. Infants in incubators were also displayed at various other public exhibitions and fairgrounds. The public was invited to pay 25 cents to view these infants in incubators, an unlikely start for the specialty of neonatology. Once having been used in an exhibit, many incubators were later sold to hospitals.

The Twentieth Century

In 1905 ethyl chloride was being used for brief procedures in infants as young as five days of age. It was administered using an inhaler [9, 11, 12]:

> "A celluloid face-piece is generally preferable since it not only permits the anaesthetist to observe the patient more readily but also resists the action of the vapour better than rubber. For infants of a few days or a few weeks old I commence by spraying three cubic centimetres into the inhaler; for those of six months and upwards I give five cubic centimetres at once. The mask is then approached to the face but not pressed against it so that the baby has several breaths of air and vapour mixed; it is then more closely applied so as to exclude all air except that which is already in the bag, and in a few seconds the child becomes unconscious. When one is sure that the anaesthesia is deep and the surgeon has made his incision or begun the operation the mask should be removed from the face and a few breaths of air should be given. If it is desired to continue the period of narcosis for some time the mask should not be kept off for long but only raised occasionally for air. If the respiration indicates the lightening of the narcosis a few more cubic centimetres may be added to the bag; on these lines the anaesthesia may be indefinitely prolonged."

Abdominal surgery for infants became established around the turn of the twentieth century with the introduction of surgical procedures for the relief of pyloric stenosis. Originally managed by gastroenterostomy, the lesion was later corrected by pyloroplasty [13] and finally by Ramstedt's pyloromyotomy [14]. Though most patients were older, some neonates were operated upon for pyloric stenosis. Chloroform was preferred and the need for adequate and constant levels of anesthesia was recognized. Reporting success in their cases of pyloroplasty in the Lancet, Cautley, and Dent in 1902 state: *"Unless the patient is deeply under the influence of chloroform (which certainly appears to be the best anaesthetic) there is risk of protrusion of the intestine and rapidity of operating becomes a matter of great difficulty. On the other hand, in abdominal operations on very young children deep anaesthesia, unless most carefully induced and maintained, may lead to very sudden and alarming symptoms. Any interruption to the operative procedure while in progress would be a very serious matter, for if the patient is not deeply anaesthetised there is every likelihood of his recovering sufficiently to cry or to struggle. If any such event happens the intestines are likely to protrude at once with the most astonishing suddenness and force. In a case recorded by Stern; both of these troubles seem to have occurred. The child's breathing stopped just after the operation had begun ; the anaesthetic was so badly borne that it had to be discontinued while the operation was completed ; and the result was that the intestine protruded extensively, thus prolonging the operation and enormously increasing its severity"* [13]. There followed a much deserved tribute to the skill of their own anesthetists: *"The success of our cases was largely due to the extreme care and skill with which the anaesthetic was administered, in the first case by Dr. H. Menzies, and in the second by Dr. G. P. Shuter. The surgeon is too often inclined to absorb all the credit of a successful operation, when a great part of it is really due to the anaesthetist"* [13]. Anesthesia for infants was already recognized as requiring special attention to detail.

Monitoring during these early years depended on observation of the patient's color, the pattern of ventilation, and in older patients perhaps a finger on the pulse! Much skill must have been needed to maintain an airway without instrumentation, ensure a constant level of anesthesia, and avoid cardiorespiratory depression. It is not at all surprising that the mortality rate for infants was very high. However, some amazing successes were reported with what must have been very challenging clinical cases. One such was the resection of an extremely large teratoma from the neck of a child 3 weeks old [15]. Anesthesia was induced and maintained with chloroform on a sponge. *"The element of time was necessarily a most important point in the operation and it was hoped that as the cyst wall was well defined it might be possible to shell out the tumour throughout the greater part of its extent. This fortunately proved to be the case and the whole operation lasted only 12 minutes, notwithstanding the fact that the work had to be stopped every few seconds to allow the infant to breathe. In order to diminish the duration of the operation and the amount of shock a continuous catgut suture was used and no attempt was made to remove the superfluous skin"* [15].

These then were the early days of neonatal surgery. The treatment of major congenital anomalies would have to await further progress in the perioperative and anesthesia management of the infant. One major step forward was the introduction of endotracheal anesthesia and the associated potential for controlling ventilation.

Endotracheal Intubation of Neonates

MacEwen introduced the concept of passing tubes through the adult glottis into the trachea as an alternative to tracheotomy in 1880 [16]. Elsberg passed intratracheal catheters and used these to insufflate anesthetic gases describing his technique in 1909 [17]. When using an intratracheal insufflation technique, a small catheter was utilized so as to leave an adequate route for expired gases. Indeed common practice was to pass a second catheter through the glottis to provide a reliable route for expiration. This prompted C Langton Hewer, who a year later was to write the first British text on pediatric anesthesia, to state in 1924: *"Endo-tracheal anaesthesia is contra-indicated in the following class of case :— Babies below the age of one year. The lumen of the glottis is so small in babies that it is practically impossible to obtain a catheter of such size as will permit sufficient vapour to pass and yet leave an adequate return airway"* [18]. However also in 1924 Ivan Magill did describe an expiratory attachment for an intratracheal catheter which was available in five sizes—the smallest of which would attach to a 9 French catheter (i.e., a 3 mm external diameter catheter) [19]. The expiratory attachment was essentially a tapered metal tube, which could be sited at the level of the glottis and connected to a second catheter. He later reported that he had used this tube attachment in "children under 2 years."

In 1928 Magill was routinely using endotracheal tubes of sufficient caliber to permit to and fro ventilation, a method he preferred in small children and which he had first used in adults in 1920 [20]. Magill tubes were manufactured of red rubber and the smallest size was 00 which had an external diameter of 4 mm, similar to that of today's 3.5 mm ID plastic tube, though the internal diameter of the Magill 00 tube was only 3 mm.

Gillespie in 1939 described methods for the routine intubation of infants [21]. He stressed that though the advantages and safeguards of intubation were now universally accepted, the intubation itself was more difficult in infants and in inexperienced hands might endanger the patient. He favored a nitrous oxide/oxygen with ether anesthetic and added 5 % of pure carbon dioxide to induce hyperpnea and speed induction. When respiration was regular and automatic, the mandible relaxed, and no trace of glottic spasm evident, intubation could be attempted. (There were, of course, no relaxant drugs available at this time.) He had developed a modification of the smallest size Chevalier Jackson laryngoscope, which was marketed under the name "Shadwell" laryngoscope (Fig. 1.1). It was designed to be held with the fingers rather than in the palm of the hand *"to discourage the use of force."*

He noted that the epiglottis in the neonate was proportionally longer than in the adult and that with each breath, the larynx tended to move anteriorly and out of the field of vision; deepening the anesthetic to further relax the child tended to induce signs of impending cardiorespiratory failure. He stressed the need for gentleness and warned that any use of force might cause complications varying from a croupy cough to acute edema of the larynx. In his own reported series of 70 infants under the age of 2 years, he had remarkably few complications, especially in view of his

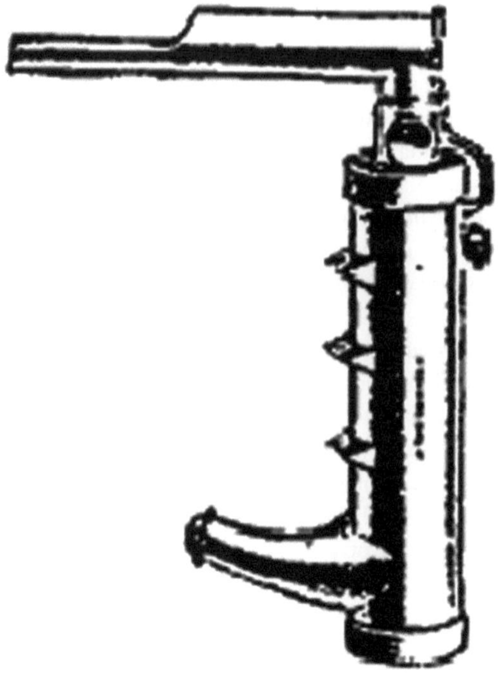

Fig. 1.1 The Shadwell laryngoscope

statement that the largest possible tube should be passed. He was concerned not to narrow the airway, as all his patients were breathing spontaneously. However, he did stress the need to attempt to pass the tube "gently."

The use of endotracheal intubation in infants was not without problems however, and cases of postoperative laryngeal edema and, more rarely, subglottic stenosis were reported. The need to use a tube, which passed easily through the glottis and subglottic space and allowed a slight leak on pressurization of the anesthesia circuit, was, in time, recognized by anesthesiologists. A classic paper by Eckenhoff [22] in 1951 described the anatomy and dimensions of the infant larynx and stressed the need to avoid injury to the mucosa in the region of the cricoid ring. The problems that sometimes followed intubation and the fear that these might adversely affect outcomes led many surgeons, particularly in USA, to oppose this practice in their patients. Anesthesia providers were directed to manage neonates for complex repairs, e.g., tracheoesophageal fistula or coarctation of the aorta, using mask anesthesia. However, the pioneers of pediatric anesthesia persisted, perfected safer methods, and thus facilitated acceptance of the need for endotracheal intubation, essential if progress in neonatal surgery was to continue.

Red rubber tubes were largely abandoned in favor of plastic tubes in the 1950s. However, early plastic tubes were also not without problems. Irritant chemical substances (Organotins) within the plastic material were found to be capable of stimulating local tissue reactions that could lead to fibrosis [23]. The establishment of routines for implantation testing of plastic material led to improvements in endotracheal tube composition and manufacture and a subsequent decrease in complications.

In 1945 Cole described a new endotracheal tube for infants. This tube had a wider proximal portion and a narrower distal segment to pass through the glottis, the rationale being that the wider portion would decrease the resistance to airflow. In addition, it was claimed that the shoulder of the tube would decrease the likelihood of the tube passing too far and entering a bronchus. In fact, the resistance of the Cole tube was found to be greater than that of a similar internal diameter parallel-sided tube [24]. This was attributed to turbulent flow within the Cole tube. More seriously, the shoulder on the tube was shown to cause laryngeal damage if advanced into the glottis [25]. The Cole tube was generally abandoned for use during anesthesia but remained in use for neonatal resuscitation in some centers, the claim being that it was easier for the less expert practitioner to insert.

The concept of prolonged endotracheal intubation as an alternative to tracheostomy was presented by Bernard Brandstater at the First European Congress of Anesthesiology in 1962 [26]. He reported his experience with seven patients ranging in age from the neonate to 4 years. Until that time it had been customary to perform a tracheostomy if infants required ventilator assistance [27]. The tracheostomy tubes in general use were uncuffed and the variable leak that occurred via the glottis made a constant level of ventilation difficult to attain—especially in patients with reduced pulmonary compliance. Fortunately the ventilators in common use in North America at this time were pressure cycled (the "Bird" mark VIII) and this reduced the problem to some extent. In the middle 1960s, the use of intermittent positive pressure ventilation (IPPV) in the therapy of newborn respiratory distress syndrome was becoming established as was the need to treat respiratory insufficiency in the postoperative cardiac patient [28]. In 1965 Reid and Tunstall reported a case of respiratory distress syndrome in a 1,800 g preterm infant successfully treated by IPPV via a 2.5 mm ID nasotracheal tube [29]. In the same year, McDonald and Stocks from the Royal Children's Hospital in Melbourne Australia reported a larger series of infants treated with prolonged nasotracheal intubation [30]. They described the complications, including post-intubation subglottic stenosis, and offered suggestions to minimize the incidence of this serious outcome. By the end of the 1960s, prolonged endotracheal intubation had superseded tracheostomy as the management of choice for infants requiring ventilatory assistance.

During the 1960s and 1970s, it was a very common, almost standard, practice to intubate the trachea while the infant was awake, before induction of anesthesia. This minimized the danger of regurgitation and aspiration and facilitated the rapid induction of anesthesia [31]. In addition, if tracheal intubation failed, there was little danger as the infant would usually maintain the airway and ventilation. Awake intubation of the neonate continued to be widely practiced until toward the end of the twentieth century when concerns that the physiological stress that might be imposed on the infant prompted further consideration [32]. In addition, it was demonstrated that intubation is much more likely to be successful with fewer attempts at and less time for successful intubation if performed in the anesthetized infant [33].

Having intubated the airway in the neonate, the scene was set to control ventilation during anesthesia. This would facilitate procedures to correct intrathoracic congenital defects. In addition, it would allow the administration of neuromuscular blocking drugs to provide optimal conditions for abdominal surgery and reduce the need for high concentrations of inhaled anesthetics.

Neuromuscular Blocking Drugs

d-Tubocurarine was introduced into anesthesia practice in the 1940s and succinylcholine became available in the 1950s. Both drugs were used in neonates soon after their introduction, but initially there was a lack of universal enthusiasm for using relaxant drugs in the neonate. In Europe a pioneering neonatal anesthetist, Dr. Jackson Rees, wrote in 1950 "*In the newborn, as has already been shown, control of the respiration is easily obtained at light levels of anaesthesia without the use of relaxants: muscle relaxation does not appear to be of major importance in the production of good operating conditions, and the usual untoward effects of endotracheal-tube induction are not seen.(sic) On these grounds it can be said that the use of relaxant drugs in anaesthesia is contra-indicated in the newborn patient, and I have abandoned these drugs in such cases* [34]."

In the USA, the study of Beecher and Todd published in 1954 [35] demonstrated an increased mortality associated with the use of relaxant drugs—especially in those in the early years of life. Postoperative respiratory difficulties were reported in infants given relaxants [36]. In 1955, Stead reported that the neonate was sensitive to the effects of non-depolarizing neuromuscular blocking drugs but was resistant to the effect of the depolarizing drug succinylcholine [37]. This further supported the impression that residual curarization was a problem in infants. However Rackow and Salanitre in New York reported their experience with relaxant drugs [38] and suggested that postoperative respiratory depression was seen only as a result of drug overdose or with hypothermia; the latter was not uncommon at that time in the smaller infants. Warming from hypothermia had been demonstrated to potentiate any residual block [39]—hence the infant placed in a heated isolette to rewarm after surgery was at risk! This observation encouraged efforts to maintain normothermia during neonatal surgery (see below).

In the 1960s, the use of neuromuscular blocking drugs in the neonate was widely accepted, and the use of heating blankets and overhead warmers to maintain normothermia became routine. Rees wrote "*Following intubation the child may be saturated with nitrous oxide as rapidly as possible by intermittent positive pressure ventilation, and the relaxant drug may then be administered. In this way perfect operating conditions are obtainable, and the more potent and, therefore more toxic agents are eliminated from the anesthetic technique*" [31]. This was the "Liverpool technique," which was widely used in Britain and elsewhere. For brief procedures, it was not uncommon to use repeated injections of succinylcholine as a relaxant.

The question of the sensitivity of the neonate to d-tubocurarine (dTc) was finally resolved by Fisher in 1982 [40]. The neonatal neuromuscular junction is indeed sensitive to the effects of dTc, but this is largely compensated by the increased volume of distribution of the drug in this age group [40].

Anesthesia Circuits and Controlled Ventilation

The T-piece system was considered by many to be the anesthesia circuit of choice for the neonate. It is lightweight and simple and has low dead space and resistance, and ventilation could be controlled simply by intermittently occluding the expiratory limb with the finger. Jackson Rees in Liverpool improved on this system by adding an open-ended bag to the end of the expiratory limb [34]. A vulcanite tap was inserted into the open end of the bag and adjusted to maintain the bag inflated but to allow escape of expired and excess gases. Manual controlled ventilation was readily applied with this system. However, a fresh gas flow of 2–2.5 times the minute ventilation was required to prevent rebreathing of expired gases. This was wasteful of anesthetic gases, which were cheap in those days, and potentially caused significant atmospheric pollution (not appreciated to be a problem until the 1970s). A modification to prevent rebreathing with lower fresh gas flows was to use a small-sized Waters soda lime canister on the expiratory limb for CO_2 absorption, but this was generally considered less easy to apply to the small infant. Indeed, Leigh and Belton writing in 1950 stated "*Use of absorption technic in the first few months of life is impracticable and affords no distinct benefits to patient, surgeon and anesthesiologist*" [41].

The pattern of ventilation chosen by the Liverpool group for infants is interesting. Dr. Jackson Rees always encouraged the use of rapid shallow ventilation for the neonate. He admitted that this often led to hyperventilation and hypocapnia but did not consider this to be a significant problem [34]. In later years, he would add small concentrations of carbon dioxide to the inspired gases when indicated to prevent hypocapnia (Rees GJ, Personal communication). The pattern of ventilation used, however, did tend to limit the duration of expiration and maintain a constant positive pressure—both of which acted to reverse the reduction in lung volumes that occurs during anesthesia and muscle paralysis and thus improve gas exchange. Dr. Rees was quite gratified to read much later of the clinical studies that defined adverse changes in pulmonary function which accompanied infant anesthesia, changes which his technique had tended to moderate.

As neonatal surgery became more complex and longer procedures were performed, the need to provide for mechanical ventilation during surgery was apparent. Fortunately by this time, progress in ventilator design made this possible. Quite simply, the Bird mark VIII ventilator or the Ohio Ventimeter Ventilator could be adjusted so that they would periodically serve to occlude the expired limb of a T-piece system.

As an alternative to the T-piece system, which required a fresh gas flow 2–3 times the minute ventilation to prevent rebreathing, some anesthesiologists preferred to use non-rebreathing valves. These required only a gas flow equal to the minute ventilation. Ronald Stephen and Harry Slater described their non-rebreathing valve in 1948. It incorporated 2 rubber valves and was described as having very low resistance to breathing and negligible dead space. Controlled ventilation could be delivered by compressing the exhalation valve with a finger while compressing the reservoir bag, and the authors claimed to have used this method in infants of 3 weeks for up to 90 min [42]. In 1948, Digby Leigh independently described a valve of very similar design, which could be used in infants [43]. George Lewis modified the Leigh valve to permit controlled ventilation without the need to digitally compress the exhalation valve. The Lewis/Leigh valve incorporated a flap that would close the exhalation port if the reservoir bag were compressed [44].

A problem with the T-Piece system and with non-rebreathing valves was that they delivered very dry gases to the airway. In the USA, this concern led to the development of circle systems modified for the neonate. The Bloomquist infant circle was marketed by the Foregger company and incorporated a soda lime canister. However, a laboratory study of the humidity output of this circuit concluded that it offered no advantage over a humidified T-piece system and was more cumbersome to use [45]. The Columbia Valve was developed to allow a modified adult circuit to be used for infants; the valve had low resistance and a very low dead space of 0.5 ml [46]. This valve was used in a circuit in which the fresh gases were passed through the soda lime canister together with the expired gases in an effort to maximize the level of humification (Rackow H, Personal communication). The T-piece and its variants were almost always used for the neonate in Britain and Canada; non-rebreathing valves and various circle absorber systems were more commonly used in the USA.

In later years, pediatric anesthesiologists adapted various neonatal ventilators for operating room use. Progressive improvements in anesthesia machine design eventually allowed small infants to be successfully managed simply by changing to a smaller diameter set of circuit tubing.

Monitoring

As has been stated previously, monitoring in the early days consisted of watching the chest movements, examining the color, and perhaps feeling the pulse. Indeed this situation persisted well into the twentieth century. Writing on anesthesia for neonatal chest surgery in 1965, Bell stated "A guide to the general clinical condition I find useful is this:

> baby pink and pulses palpable-condition good;
> baby pale, pulses palpable or baby pink, pulses not palpable-condition satisfactory, but check ventilation and blood balance;
> baby pale, pulses not palpable—condition serious.
> I do not think that cardiac stethoscopes (the heart action can be seen in thoracic operations), sphygmomanometers, pulse monitors or E.C.G. tracings contribute enough additional information about a baby's condition to merit their use; they may be distracting" [47].

I cannot say that this was the general attitude to monitoring in those years but it is a recorded opinion.

Accounts of neonatal anesthesia prior to 1960 make little or no mention of monitoring [31, 34, 36]. In fact the technology to satisfactorily monitor blood pressure in the neonate was not generally available until the late 1950s. Palpation or auscultation distal to a blood pressure cuff was noted to be very difficult in small infants. Oscillometry had been used but was not uniformly reliable. Hence, it was not common practice to monitor the blood pressure even in larger infants. Anesthesia records from this era commonly displayed only a heart rate. In an article on anesthesia for major surgery in 1950, CR Stephen displayed an anesthesia record for pyloromyotomy on which the only vital signs recorded were the heart rate and respiratory rate [48].

The optimal width of the blood pressure cuff (one inch) that was required for accurate measurement in the neonate was determined in 1939 by direct comparison with an intra-arterial needle [49]. However, as noted above, it was uncommonly used in anesthesia practice. Detection of pulsation distal to the cuff most often depended upon oscillometry. To detect the very small deflection of the oscillometer needle was frequently highly dependent upon "the eye of faith." This could be very worrying during thoracic surgery or indeed any other major procedure; this I remember well.

In 1969, the use of the Doppler flow meter to monitor flow in the radial artery distal to a blood pressure cuff and reliably measure intraoperative blood pressure in infants was reported [50]. The battery-operated "Parks Doppler Flowmeter" became widely available and took much of the worry out of neonatal anesthesia. It could be used to measure blood pressure and also served as a continuous audible monitor of the pulse volume, serving as an early warning of adverse changes.

Direct measurement of intra-arterial pressure in the neonate was initially performed via the umbilical artery; however this resulted in a relatively high incidence of serious complications (e.g., bowel infarction) and was only applicable in the immediate neonatal period. Percutaneous cannulation of the radial artery in neonates was described in 1975 as a safer alternative [51, 52]. The use of the temporal artery for monitoring was also suggested [53] but was later generally abandoned when it became known that retrograde cerebral embolism was associated with this technique [54]. Femoral artery lines were also used on occasion but, in the neonatal age group, the incidence of ischemic complications exceeded that with radial lines [55].

Monitoring the oxygen saturation of blood during anesthesia was described by a group from Montreal in 1950 [56]. They used an earpiece which had been developed during World War II for the purpose of studying pilots flying at various altitudes. The equipment they used was delicate however and required a dedicated technician to operate it. Continuous monitoring of transcutaneous oxygen tension ($TcpO_2$) in neonates was described in 1972 [57], but this was not introduced as a routine into the neonatal nursery for several years. Though $TcpO_2$ was capable of indicating trends, individual readings lacked precise accuracy especially with decreased skin blood flow [58]. Electrodes required frequent attention and had to be moved periodically to prevent burns. During anesthesia it was found that inhaled agents further interfered with the performance of the electrode and decreased accuracy, though not to a significant degree [59].

Pulse oximetry became available for clinical use in 1983 [60] and was rapidly adopted as a routine monitor during the surgery and acute care of neonates; it was far easier to apply than the TcpO2 electrode. It was now possible to continuously display the level of oxygenation throughout the perioperative period and immediately respond to any adverse changes. It was also quite possible to apply two probes: one in the preductal area and one in the postductal area. The question now arose as to the safe level of preductal oxygen saturation to maintain in the preterm infant at risk for retinopathy of prematurity (ROP). Surveys performed in recent years indicate that many units aim to maintain SpO_2 in the 85–93 % range [61] and that this does indeed decrease the incidence of serious ROP changes [62].

Monitoring of end-tidal carbon dioxide as a routine procedure in anesthesia care became commonplace during the 1980s. When applied to the neonate, it became apparent that both methods for CO_2 analysis, mainstream and sidestream, are problematic [63]. The increase in dead space with mainstream analysis may lead to rebreathing in small infants. During sidestream analysis the site of sampling, flow rate, and length of the sampling tube are critical factors in obtaining valid results.

Intraoperative Temperature Control

As more prolonged surgery was being performed in neonates, the problem of intraoperative hypothermia became recognized [64] and identified as a cause of increased morbidity and mortality [38, 65–67]. Two of five postoperative deaths in a series of twelve neonates were attributed to hypothermia [65]. In another series of 67 infants, 12 patients died; seven of these were judged due to postoperative hypothermia [67]. It was noted that the decrease in body temperature was directly related to the duration of surgery and that smaller infants suffered a greater decrease. The vulnerability of the small infant to heat loss as a result of the large body surface area to weight ratio was suggested [68]. At this time in the 1950s, little was done to keep the neonate normothermic during surgery and indeed intraoperative hypothermia was considered by some to be beneficial.

An improved understanding of the adverse physiological effects of hypothermia came in the early 1960s. It also became recognized that it was much easier to keep the patient warm during surgery than to resort to rewarming postoperatively. The adverse effects of cooling on oxygen consumption [69], catecholamine levels [70], and acid/base status [71] were identified. Oxygen consumption in the neonate was shown to correlate most closely with the skin to environment temperature gradient, hence the significance of the "neutral thermal environment." With this new understanding, efforts were made to maintain normothermia intraoperatively. Hot water bottles alongside the infant were recommended, but unfortunately this sometimes led to burns. Heating pads for the operating room table were described by Leigh and Belton in the second edition of their book on pediatric anesthesia published in 1960 [72]. Wrapping the limbs in cotton wadding and placing the infant on a warming blanket set at 40 °C was advocated by Smith in 1968. It was also found that heating blankets were more effective in maintaining normothermia in smaller infants—a beneficial effect of the large surface area to body mass ratio [73]. The addition of overhead radiant heaters during preparation for surgery and humidification of anesthetic gases provided for what was considered optimal patient management in the late 1960s and 1970s [74]. In the 1990s forced air warmers became generally available and proved very effective in maintaining normothermia [75].

Neonatal Anesthesia: Some Landmark Procedures and Their Development

Repair of Esophageal Atresia and Tracheoesophageal Fistula

The first operation for esophageal atresia was performed in London, England, by Charles Steele in 1888 [76]. The diagnosis was made when the infant became livid and had difficulty breathing "after the first nourishment"; a sound could not be passed by mouth for further than five inches. Surgery was performed the next day after "*the infant took chloroform well.*" The stomach was opened via an abdominal incision and an unsuccessful attempt was made to pass a gum elastic catheter retrograde up the esophagus, in the hope that a simple membrane could be perforated. The surgery was abandoned and the infant died 24 h later. At autopsy, the upper and lower esophagus ended blindly one and one half inches apart. There is no mention of an associated fistula.

The first successful ligation of a tracheoesophageal fistula with anastomosis of the associated esophageal atresia was reported by Haight in 1943 [77]. Local analgesia was used for the first part of the operation; open ether was added during the esophageal anastomosis in order to obtain optimal surgical conditions. Spontaneous ventilation was maintained throughout. In Britain, Franklin described two successful repairs of TEF with esophageal anastomosis in 1947 [78]; both of these procedures were performed using infiltration of local anesthetic (1 % procaine) to the chest wall incision line and no other anesthesia. During the operation "*the infant was secured prone over a rubber hot water bottle.*"

As has been previously stated, in early days, many surgeons opposed the use of endotracheal intubation for their patients. Swenson, a much respected pioneer pediatric surgeon, reported his experiences with TEF in 1943 and advocated the administration of cyclopropane via a tightly applied face mask [79]. Kennedy and Stoelting reported a series of 86 cases of TEF operated upon at Indiana University Hospital from 1940 until 1956 [80]. Before 1948, 17 cases were managed without intubation using a combination of local analgesia and open ether; the mortality rate was 88 %; two patients died during surgery. After 1948, all 69 neonates underwent tracheal intubation, none died during surgery, and the overall mortality rate was 42 %. Many factors were considered responsible for these improved results, but the role of endotracheal intubation and tracheobronchial toilet was considered to be very significant. General anesthesia methods reported by Zindler and Deming in 1953 [81] employed awake endotracheal intubation to administer cyclopropane via a non-rebreathing valve and controlled ventilation. They also stressed the need for frequent suctioning of the trachea.

Progressively improving results from the surgical and anesthesia management of TEF can be followed by examining the Toronto experience. A review of the results from 1959 to 1964 [82] shows an overall mortality rate of 36.5 %, with a rate of 57.5 % for the infants who were under 2,500 g body weight. The predictors of mortality were prematurity, the presence of associated congenital malformations (especially cardiac), and extensive pulmonary disease (i.e., delayed diagnosis). A subsequent review [83] of the years 1964–1968 noted an overall mortality rate of 22 %, and the mortality rate for those under 2,500 g had decreased to 40 %.

The problem of gastric distension due to gases passing through the fistula into the stomach was a concern for the anesthesiologist, especially as this has been reported to cause serious ventilatory embarrassment and cardiac arrest [84]. Some preferred to maintain spontaneous (perhaps gently assisted) ventilation until the fistula was ligated. Other suggestions to prevent this complication included performing a preliminary gastrostomy under local analgesia [85]; this was also favored by some surgeons as part of a two-stage repair, especially in critically ill infants. Passing an endotracheal tube (without a side hole) into the bronchus and withdrawing it until bilateral ventilation could be heard; then positioning the tube with the bevel facing anteriorly was also suggested [86]. This would direct ventilation to the lungs and protect the fistula with the longer side of the bevel. (However the fistula is occasionally at the level of the carina!) Some more complicated methods to position the tube and prevent gastric distension have also been described. If a gastrostomy was present, it was suggested that placing the gastrostomy tube under water in a beaker while advancing the endotracheal tube could indicate when the ETT was below the fistula [87], i.e., no more bubbles! The significance of leaks via the fistula increased as preterm infants with respiratory distress syndrome requiring greater airway pressures presented for surgery. Karl suggested that a balloon catheter should be inserted into the lower esophagus via the gastrostomy to control the leak [88]. Others suggested that a Fogarty or pulmonary artery catheter should be advanced via a bronchoscope directly into the fistula [89]. In many units, it became a routine to perform early ligation of the fistula in preterm infants, thus largely avoiding the problem.

Preoperative endoscopic examination of the fistula was introduced in the 1980s [90] and became routine in some centers [91]. It was suggested that an exact knowledge of the size and site of the fistula would improve results and in addition endoscopy permitted placement of balloon catheters to occlude the lumen. Others preferred to keep things simple and manage the airway without endoscopy [92].

Congenital Diaphragmatic Hernia

Congenital diaphragmatic hernia (CDH) was described in 1757 by a Society of Physicians in London following post-mortem examination of an infant who died under 2 h of age in respiratory distress [93]. Early reports of operations for CDH are found in the medical literature of the 1930s [94] and 1940s [95], but it is significant that the neonates were all more than 20 h of age, and some patients were much older, i.e., they had adequate pulmonary function to survive the immediate neonatal period. In 1946, Robert Gross reported seven cases that came to surgery with ages ranging from 22 h to 7 years; he also recorded his preferred anesthesia technique [95]:

> "The choice of anesthetic agent and the method of its administration are important considerations, particularly in the cases of patients in whom cyanosis and respiratory embarrassment are pronounced. Ether can be employed, and indeed may be given with an open mask. It is preferable to use a closed system, so that a higher percentage of oxygen can be supplied to the patient and so that collapse of both lungs can be prevented in those rare cases in which there is a free communication between the two pleural cavities. In all cases of the present series, cyclopropane was used and was eminently satisfactory. It is clear, however, that this choice depended on my good fortune in having an anesthetist who is expert in handling babies and who has had enough initiative to devise a homemade apparatus which is suitable for babies of the smallest size. It must be emphasized that cyanosis should not be a deterrent to operation, since the administration of a gas containing a high percentage of oxygen will improve the baby's color, and the operative removal of the abdominal viscera from the chest will also facilitate the child's breathing efforts. It is unnecessary to use an intratracheal tube ; indeed, this is apt to be followed by troublesome edema of the larynx in the ensuing twenty-four hours. Only a tightly fitting mask, without an intra-tracheal tube, was used for all of the patients reported on here." [95]

CDH was considered a surgical emergency [96] and immediate operation was recommended once the diagnosis had been made—especially if respiratory distress was present. A case report from 1950 [97] demonstrated the extent to which improvisation was employed to facilitate urgent surgery. The child was five days old and in considerable respiratory distress and required oxygen at all times—a decision was made to perform immediate surgery. "*Ether was the anesthetic agent of choice. The equipment at hand was a small open mask, an infant-sized metal oral pharyngeal airway, a rubber infant-sized mask from a Kreiselman resuscitator, a socket elbow, a short corrugated tube section, a Peterson ether drop cup, and for a breathing bag a toy red rubber balloon.*" During the procedure the two red rubber balloons that were available both disintegrated due to contact with liquid ether and were replaced by rubber condoms! To the credit of the team, the infant survived.[3]

In the 1950s, the association between pulmonary hypoplasia and CDH was reported [98]. At this time and into the 1960s, improvements in the care and transportation [99] of critically ill neonates resulted in more infants with CDH presenting for emergency surgery. Many of these who would have died without surgery now died postoperatively secondary to their pulmonary disease. The high mortality rates associated with repair CDH stimulated many investigators and clinicians and attention turned to means to optimize pulmonary function postoperatively. These means included various patterns of controlled ventilation and measures to reduce pulmonary vascular resistance (PVR) [100]. The thought developed that the cause of death in some cases was not simple hypoplasia but potentially reversible changes in PVR [100]. The standard approach to anesthesia for CDH at this time, no bag and mask ventilation, endotracheal intubation, avoidance of N_2O, and care to avoid large positive pressures, was augmented by steps to control PVR if required.

One problem that had complicated the management of the infant with CDH was that some experienced very few problems postoperatively while others were desperately ill. Hence, there was great interest in identifying those prognostic factors that determine which infants would require aggressive invasive measures. Raphaely and Downs in Philadelphia developed a scoring system based on the preoperative and postreduction alveolar/arterial oxygen tension gradient [101]. Desmond Bohn and his colleagues in Toronto suggested a system to predict the extent of pulmonary hypoplasia based on the preoperative arterial CO_2 tension and a ventilatory index (mean airway pressure x ventilatory rate) [102]. Bohn et al. also suggested that consideration should be given to an initial nonsurgical approach to CDH in the expectation that impaired pulmonary function not due to hypoplasia might improve [102]. In the same year, 1987, another study from Toronto had shown that surgical repair of CDH impaired rather than improved respiratory mechanics [103]. Thus CDH management evolved from a surgical emergency into a potential complex management problem for the neonatal intensivist, sometimes involving preoperative ECMO therapy. Surgery was now performed only when the respiratory status was improved.

Abdominal Wall Defects

Reports of exomphalos (omphalocele) are found in medical writings from the middle ages onwards, but the infants generally soon died—usually of peritonitis. There are a few instances where conservative treatment using antiseptic preparations applied to the lesion resulted in granulation tissue formation and epithelialization with survival. Operative treatment before the 1940s was usually fatal [104]. Successful surgical treatment was reported in 1948 [105], and in 1949 a further successful case was reported in which the anesthetic

[3] The other obvious question that this case raises is whether the reporting institution was the most appropriate place to be performing this surgery. However, in 1950, the concept of regionalization of pediatric and neonatal services was undeveloped even in Europe and was largely unrecognized in North America.

used "*was sugar and whisky administered on a small gauze nipple*" [106]. The postoperative course was complicated by peritonitis; however the patient recovered and was discharged on the 75th postoperative day. Much credit for the recovery was given to the use of prolonged intravenous fluid therapy. At this time, it was recognized that omphalocele was often associated with other significant congenital malformations. It was also noted that the immediate prognosis depended on whether the membrane covering the viscera was intact or ruptured; in the latter case, a fatal result was certain [107]. In 1953, a successful case is recorded in which open ether was administered for anesthesia: "*The bowels were returned to the abdominal cavity with difficulty, and the wound was closed in a single layer. The anaesthesia must be sufficiently deep to relax the abdominal muscles. This requires the services of a skilled anaesthetist*" [107]. It was suggested that a stomach tube should be in place to aspirate secretions as the bowel was reduced into the abdomen—obviously a serious concern when an open technique was used.

By the 1970s, the problems of heat conservation, fluid therapy, prevention of infection, and prolonged postoperative ileus were recognized and being managed [108]. Local analgesia infiltrated by the surgeon was still quite frequently utilized "with anesthesia standby." This led to cautions in the 1979 edition of the *Manual of Pediatric Anesthesia* [109]: first to monitor how much local analgesic the surgeon injected and second to consider intubating the airway—to protect it against aspiration of regurgitated stomach contents. The introduction of endotracheal intubation and controlled ventilation greatly facilitated general anesthesia management but introduced the problem of determining whether the infant could tolerate the increased intra-abdominal pressure (IAP) postoperatively. Controlled ventilation could be continued postoperatively, and simple closure of the skin only and delayed closure using Silon pouch were options. It was appreciated that increased IAP not only impaired ventilation and circulation but also severely compromised splanchnic and renal perfusion. In 1989, Yaster et al. suggested that the intragastric pressure (IGP) and/or central venous pressure (CVP) should be monitored during replacement of the viscera; IGP in excess of 20 mm/Hg or CVP increases of 4 mm/Hg are unlikely to be tolerated [110].

By the end of the twentieth century, prenatal diagnosis and progress in anesthesia management, critical care, and intravenous alimentation resulted in significantly reduced mortality and morbidity. The mortality rate for gastroschisis was under 10 % and the mortality in cases of omphalocele was largely dictated by the presence or absence of associated malformations.

Neonatal Cardiovascular Surgery

Surgery of the heart and great vessels was introduced in the 1940s and 1950s, but initially very few of the patients were neonates. Robert Gross ligated a persistent ductus arteriosus in a child in 1939 and launched pediatric cardiovascular surgery. Most of his early patients were older but he did describe division of vascular ring in patients that included a 3-week-old infant in 1951 [111]:

> "Anesthesia in all these subjects has been with a closed system, using ether or cyclopropane. In all cases, an intratracheal tube, preferably of soft polyethylene, has been employed. Such a tube is essential for the maintenance of an adequate airway, particularly in the first four types of anomalies just described, in each of which the trachea is markedly narrowed and an adequate exchange might not be obtained until a tube is passed down beyond the obstructed point." [111]

William Mustard in Toronto operated on neonates with preductal coarctation of the aorta in 1953 [112] with long-term success. The anesthetic regimen was: "*Induction is with pentothal 5 mg per pound and syncurine 0.01 mg per pound mixed together in the same syringe. Orotracheal intubation is performed after succinylcholine 1 mg per 5 pounds. The patient is maintained on a 50 to 75 % nitrous oxide with oxygen mixture, and control of ventilation is maintained by means of frequent small doses of succinylcholine*" [112]. The anesthetics were all administered by Dr. Code Smith who first described the esophageal stethoscope [113], developed in order to monitor heart and breath sounds reliably during thoracic surgery in small infants.

Open Heart Surgery

The use of open heart surgery with cardiopulmonary bypass (CPB) in neonates was initially associated with very high mortality rates. In 1963, it was stated "*It is apparent that perfusion can be performed on even the smallest infants. It is equally certain that present methods of perfusion in small infants are hazardous and should be applied only in extraordinary circumstances*" [114]. The authors reported a mortality rate of 66 % for infants of 0.2 sq M BSA. The mortality was considered related to the severity of the CHD and to postoperative complications related to the "*marginal status of the infant's cardiopulmonary system.*" There were, however, also frequent technical problems related to the small size of the patients. The problems of applying CPB to the smaller infants stimulated an interest in performing surgery under deep hypothermic circulatory arrest (18–20 °C) using only surface cooling and rewarming [115]. The technique originated in Japan but was adopted by several North American centers. Anesthesia was maintained using diethyl ether, which was considered to protect against ventricular fibrillation during the cooling phase [115]. Using this technique, an overall mortality rate of 42 % was reported [115]. As techniques for CPB rapidly evolved, and as flammable ether was considered an unacceptable hazard by many groups, cooling of neonates on bypass became more common.

Profoundly hypothermic circulatory arrest (PHCA) was commonly used in neonates during and after the 1960s. Intra-atrial repair was simplified in the absence of venous cannulae. However controversy soon emerged concerning the long-term safety of PHCA versus continued perfusion [116]. There was also much debate concerning the optimal management of the pH status and other variables (e.g., hematocrit) during cooling bypass [117].

Regional Analgesia

Bier popularized spinal analgesia in 1898, though Corning had successfully used the method 15 years earlier. The use of spinal analgesia in a neonate 24 h old with acute intestinal obstruction due to congenital hernia of the umbilical cord was described in 1912 [118]. The method used was that of Dr. Tyrell Gray, at that time medical superintendent at the Hospital for Sick Children, Great Ormond Street, who had written extensively on the subject of spinal anesthesia in infants and children [119]. The drug used was Stovaine (0.012G) with glucose. Stovaine (Amylocaine) was the first synthesized local anesthetic and was widely used for spinal anesthesia being less toxic than cocaine. The dose used would produce anesthesia for up to 1 h. Reports of the use of spinal analgesia for abdominal and perineal surgery in infants are found from several centers during the first half of the twentieth century.

In the 1960s, an interesting series of neonates with open myelomeningocele underwent corrective surgery after direct injection of local analgesic into the lesion by the surgeon [120]. A solution of 1 % lidocaine was used and produced anesthesia very adequate for the repair—which was always completed in less than one hour. No complications were noted and the decrease in blood pressure after the injection was small. The rationale for the use of this technique was that it was less hazardous than general anesthesia administered by an inexperienced anesthetist.

Spinal anesthesia for preterm neonates with inguinal hernia became popular late in the twentieth century when it was suggested that postoperative respiratory complications were less common than after general anesthesia [121]. Studies also confirmed that the effect of a spinal block on the blood pressure is relatively minor in small infants [122]. There was also renewed interest in some centers for the use of spinal anesthesia for abdominal and even thoracic surgery.

As has been mentioned throughout this chapter infiltration of local anesthetics was often employed for the neonate. In 1930, Denis Browne, the surgeon at Great Ormond Street Hospital, described a restraint for the small infant that could be used during local or general anesthesia (Fig. 1.2) [123]. This was widely used in England for many years, and he wrote of it: "*In operating on babies there are certain special difficulties. Owing to their light weight and powers of contortion they need careful holding for greater or less time, according to the type of anaesthetic, and their small size makes it difficult for the holder to avoid the operators. In work on these cases, both as operator and anaesthetist, I have found great help in a simple device which holds the child firmly, prevents chilling, and permits the use of local anaesthesia or the minimum of general. It is a " crucifix," the original model of which was a simple T of 2-inch wood, the cross limb 18 inches long and the main one 24 inches. As this was awkward to carry and had an inauspicious look about it when taken into a private house, I devised a collapsible model in duralumin, with a sponge rubber padding, and this has been very satisfactory*" [123].

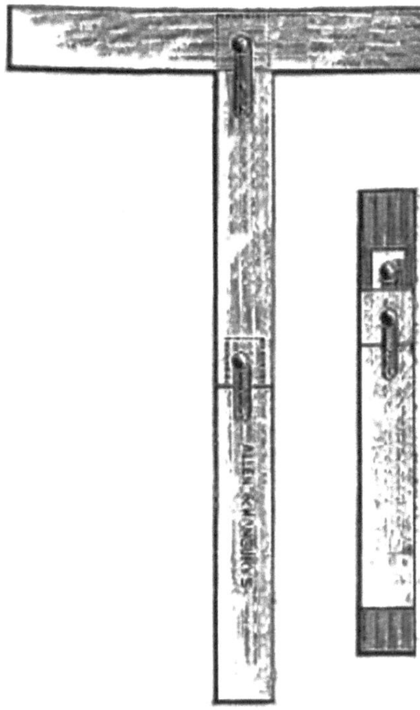

Fig. 1.2 The Denis Browne Crucifix

Regionalization of Neonatal Services

Progress in modern neonatal surgery commenced in 1945 after World War II. In 1949, there were 58 neonatal surgeries at the Hospital for Sick Children in London and 27 (46 %) of these infants died [124]. These results and similar figures from the Alder Hey Hospital in Liverpool led Peter Rickham to write "*If in this country we are to improve the chances of survival of children born with congenital malformations an efficient neonatal surgical service must be organized*" [124]. At this time, congenital malformations were listed as the third most common cause of neonatal death in the USA, but there were 3 centers (Boston, Philadelphia, Chicago) where Rickham observed very good results for neonatal surgery: "*Surgical management and technique differed very little. American neonatal anesthesia was definitely inferior to that in Liverpool, many operations being done under local or ether anesthesia. The important difference was the postoperative management. There were more highly trained medical personel and nurses in the American Hospitals providing a highly efficient round the clock service....*"

Mr. Rickham went on to act as a prime mover in the establishment of the "first neonatal unit in the world" which opened in 1953 at the Alder Hey Children's Hospital [125]. In the last half of the twentieth century, regionalization of neonatal services progressed steadily in Great Britain and in other European countries. The standards for the staffing and equipping of neonatal units and the organization for the transport of patients to these units are rigidly controlled. The concentration of patients in a few units ensured that the medical and nursing staff could gather the experience necessary to ensure optimal outcomes for their patients, while providing training for the next generation of care providers. In Canada, complex neonatal surgery has been largely concentrated within the children's hospitals which are situated in most provinces, and thus a similar regionalization has been achieved.

In the USA, regionalization of neonatal services and the establishment of units to serve all regions with an associated high volume of patients has been less consistent [126]. There are many geographic problems involved, and there has also been a desire by many smaller hospitals to have a neonatal unit and to provide pediatric surgical services. This has sometimes led to problems with providing an adequate pediatric case load for credentialing purposes [127] and might indeed sometimes compromise results. In many states, however, neonatal emergency transport systems have been effective in directing a high volume of patients to regional neonatal surgical units [128]. The American Academy of Pediatrics has formulated and published general guidelines for referral of patients with major congenital anomalies to pediatric surgical specialists [129].

Research in Neonatal Anesthesia

Before 1960 very little research was conducted, those anesthetizing infants were busy with their clinical work [126], and anesthesia methods were largely based on what had worked in the experience of the teachers and the practitioners. However, early investigations into the pharmacology of the anesthetic drugs in the neonate were commencing. Stead in 1955 reported the effects of neuromuscular blocking agents in the neonate [130]. Rackow and Salanitre studied the pharmacokinetics of the inhaled anesthetics in infants and reported these in 1969 [131]. The volatile anesthetic dose requirements for the neonate were the subject of some confusion until more precise studies in tightly controlled age groups were carried out in the 1980s [132]. Similar studies in preterm infants were conducted by Ledez and Lerman shortly thereafter [133]. As the numbers of pediatric anesthesia subspecialists swelled in the last decades of the twentieth century, there was a corresponding increase in research output and a more scientific approach to neonatal anesthesia became a reality. This did however require a closer evaluation of the ethics of performing studies in infants [134] and indeed the ethics of providing anesthesia for infants.

Ethical Considerations and Infant Anesthesia

The suggestion that the administration of anesthesia to infants might have long-term adverse consequences has been raised. In the 1970s it was suggested the incidence of asthma and respiratory allergies might be increased in children who were administered anesthesia in infancy [135]. A subsequent study failed to corroborate this association [136]. Late in the twentieth century, learning disabilities were described in children who had general anesthesia in infancy [137]. However, a study in more than 1,100 identical twins in the Netherlands demonstrated that in discordant twins (i.e., one had an anesthetic and the other did not), the IQ values in each pair were identical in a 10-year follow-up [138]. Concerns were also raised by numerous neonatal rodent and monkey studies that suggested that most general anesthetic agents are toxic to the developing brain [139], although neither surgery nor inflammatory pain was present in any of these studies. Interestingly, when ketamine was administered to randomly selected neonatal rodents stressed by having subcutaneous formalin injections, impaired cognition was attenuated in the ketamine-treated rodents [140]. Although evidence had emerged that anesthesia drugs are not completely innocuous to the neonate, this finding is offset in part by the knowledge that inadequately treated pain during infancy also results in both short-term and long-term adverse effects [141]. Currently, the preponderance of evidence supports the ethical path of administering anesthesia to prevent pain and modulate the physiological responses to surgery in neonates.

The future path for pediatric anesthesiology is to pursue the ideal of perfecting agents and techniques that will cause the least harm and ensure the greatest benefits for our precious neonatal patients. The full history of neonatal anesthesia cannot yet be written—the future may be just as exciting as was the past.

References

1. Pernick MS. "A calculus of suffering: pain, professionalism and anesthesia in 19th C. America. New York: Columbia University Press; 1985.
2. Bigelow HJ. Trans AMA. 1848; 1: 211
3. Lippmann M, Nelson RJ, Emmanouilides GC, Diskin J, Thibeault DW. Ligation of patent ductus arteriosus in premature infants. Br J Anaesth. 1976;48(4):365–9.
4. Pickop J. On an instance of impervious rectum in a newly born infant, successfully treated by operation. Lancet. 1850;55:146.
5. Odell R. A case of spinal meningo-myelocele in an infant aged 13 days; recovery. Lancet. 1902;160:508.
6. Snow J. On the employment of chloroform in surgical operations. Lancet. 1855;66:361–63.
7. Ellis RH. The case books of Dr John Snow, vol. Medical History Suppl#14. London: Wellcome Institute for the History of Medicine; 1994. p. 493.
8. Reports of Westminster Medical Society, Lancet. 1855: 312
9. Touloukian RJ. Pediatric surgery between 1860 and 1900. J Pediatr Surg. 1995;30:911–16.
10. Editorial. The use of incubators for infants. Lancet. 1897: 1490–91.
11. Kingsford AB. New inventions. Lancet. 1904: 837
12. Murray F. Ethyl chloride as an anaesthetic for infants. Lancet 1905; 1542
13. Cautley E, Dent CT. Congenital hypertrophic stenosis of the pylorus and its treatment by pyloroplasty. Lancet 1902: 1679–85
14. Rammstedt C. Zur Operation der angeborenen Pylorusstenose. Med Klin. 1912;8:1702–5.
15. McGregor AN, Workman C. A large teratoma of the neck successfully removed from an infant three weeks old. Lancet. 1906;167:433–35.
16. MacEwen W. Clinical observations on the introduction of tracheal tubes by the mouth instead of performing tracheotomy or laryngotomy. Br Med J. 1880;2:163–5.
17. Elsberg C. New York medical record; 1910
18. Hewer CL. The endotracheal administration of nitrous oxide-oxygen-ethanesal as the routine anaesthetic of choice for major surgery. Br J Anaesth. 1924;1:113–22.
19. Magill IW. An expiratory attachment for endotracheal catheters. Lancet. 1924: 1320
20. Magill IW. Endotracheal anaesthesia. Proc R Soc Med. 1928;22:83–8.
21. Gillespie NA. Endotracheal anaesthesia in infants. Br J Anaesth. 1939;12:2–12.
22. Eckenhoff JE. Some anatomic considerations of the infant larynx influencing endotracheal anesthesia. Anesthesiology. 1951;12:401–10.
23. Editorial. Toxic substances in endotracheal tubes. Br Med J. 1968:2;566–7.
24. Hatch DJ. Tracheal tubes and connectors used in neonates – Dimensions and resistance to breathing. Br J Anaesth. 1978; 50:959–64.
25. Mitchell MD, Bailey CM. Dangers of Neonatal intubation with the Cole tube. BMJ. 1990;301:602–3.
26. Brandstater B. Prolonged intubation: an alternative to tracheostomy in infants. In: Proc First Europ Congress Anaesth, Vienna, Paper 106. 1962.
27. Delivoria-Papadopoulos M, Swyer PR. Intermittent positive pressure respiration as a treatment in severe respiratory distress syndrome. Arch Dis Child. 1964;39:481.
28. Brown K, Johnston AE, Conn AW. Respiratory failure and its treatment following paediatric cardiovascular surgery. Can Anaesth Soc J. 1966;13:342–60.
29. Reid DHS, Tunstall ME. Treatment of respiratory distress syndrome of the newborn with nasotracheal intubation and intermittent positive pressure ventilation. Lancet. 1965;I:1196–7.
30. McDonald IH, Stocks JG. Prolonged nasotracheal intubation. A review of its development in a paediatric hospital. Br J Anaesth. 1965;37:161–72.
31. Rees JG. Neonatal anaesthesia. Br Med Bull. 1958;14:38–41.
32. Duncan HP, Zurick NJ, Wolf AR. Should we reconsider awake neonatal intubation? A review of the evidence and treatment strategies. Paediatr Anaesth. 2001;11:135–45.
33. Cook-Sather SD, Tulloch HV, Cnaan A, et al. A comparison of awake versus paralysed tracheal intubation for infants with pyloric stenosis. Anesth Analg. 1998;86:945–51.
34. Rees JG. Anaesthesia in the newborn. Br Med J. 1950;2:1419–22.
35. Beecher HK, Todd DP. A study of deaths associated with anesthesia and surgery based on a study of 599,548 anesthetics in 10 institutions. Ann Surg. 1954;140:2–34.
36. Wilton TNP. Anaesthesia and the neonate. Br J Anaesth. 1960;32:116–24.
37. Stead AL. Response of the newborn infant to muscle relaxants. Br J Anaesth. 1955;25:124.
38. Rackow H, Salanitre E. Respiratory complications associated with the use of muscle relaxants in young infants. Anesthesiology. 1961;12:194–8.
39. Zaimis E, Cannard TH, Price HL. Effects of lowered muscle temperature upon neuromuscular blockade in man. Science. 1958;128:34.
40. Fisher DM, O'Keeffe C, Stanski DR, Cronnelly R, Miller RD, Gregory GA. Pharmacokinetics and pharmacodynamics of d-tubocurarine in infants, children, and adults. Anesthesiology. 1982;57:203–8.
41. Leigh MD, Belton MK. Special considerations in the selection and employment of anesthetic agents and methods in infants and children. Anesthesiology. 1950;11:592–8.
42. Stephen CR, Slater H. A non-resisting, non-rebreathing valve. Anesthesiology. 1948;9:550–2.
43. Leigh MD, Kester HA. Endotracheal anesthesia for operations on cleft lip and cleft palate. Anesthesiology. 1948;9:32–41.
44. Cullen SC. Current comment and case reports. Anesthesiology. 1956;17:618–30.
45. Ramanathan S, Chalon J, Turndorf H. Humidity output of the Bloomquist Infant Circle. Anesthesiology. 1975;43:679–82.
46. Rackow H, Salanitre E. A new pediatric circle valve. Anesthesiology. 1965;29:833–4.
47. Bell HE. Neonates and chest surgery. Thorax. 1965;20:1–7.
48. Stephen CR. Anesthesia in Infants and young children for major surgical procedures. Arch Surg. 1950;60:1035–44.
49. Robinow M, Hamilton WF, Woodbury RA, Volpitto PP. Accuracy of clinical determinations of blood pressure in children: with values under normal and abnormal conditions. Am J Dis Child. 1939;58:102–18.
50. Kirby RW, Kemmerer WT, Morgan JL. Transcutaneous Doppler measurement of blood pressure. Anesthesiology. 1969;31:86.
51. Todres ID, Rogers MC, Shannon DC, Moylan FMB, Ryan JF. Percutaneous catheterization of the radial artery in the critically ill neonate. J Pediatr. 1975;87:273–75.
52. Adams JM, Rudolph AJ. The use of indwelling radial artery catheters in neonates. Pediatrics. 1975;55:261–65.
53. Gauderer M, Holgersen LO. Peripheral arterial line insertion in neonates and infants: a simplified method of temporal artery cannulation. J Pediatr Surg. 1974;9:875–7.

54. Prian GW, Wright GB, Rumac CM, et al. Apparent cerebral embolization after temporal artery catheterization. J Pediatr. 1978;93:115–6.
55. Glenski JA, Beynen FM, Brady J. A prospective evaluation of femoral artery monitoring in pediatric patients. Anesthesiology. 1987;66:227–9.
56. Johnson AL, Stephen CR, Sekelj P. Clinical use of the oximeter. Can Med Assoc J. 1950;63:552–5.
57. Huch R, Huch A, Lubbers DW. Transcutaneous measurement of blood Po2 (tcPo2) – Method and application in perinatal medicine. J Perinat Med. 1973;1:183–91.
58. Clarke T, Mannino F, Baird K, Gluck L. Experience and problems in the first six months of transcutaneous PO2 (tcPO2) monitoring in routine neonatal intensive care. Acta Anaesth Scand Suppl. 1978;68:83–7.
59. Tremper KK, Barker SJ, Blatt DH, Wender RH. Effects of anesthetic agents on the drift of a transcutaneous oxygen tension sensor. J Clin Monit. 1986;2:234–6.
60. Yelderman M, New Jr W. Evaluation of pulse oximetry. Anesthesiology. 1983;59:349–52.
61. Anderson CG, Benitz WE, Madan A. Retinopathy of prematurity and pulse oximetry: a national survey of recent practices. J Perinatol. 2004;24:164–8.
62. Vanderveen DK, Mansfield TA, Eichenwald EC. Lower oxygen saturation alarm limits decrease the severity of retinopathy of prematurity. J AAPOS. 2006;10:445–8.
63. Kirpalani H, Kechagias S, Lerman J. Technical and clinical aspects of capnography in neonates. J Med Eng Technol. 1991;15:154–61.
64. Bigler JA, McQuiston WO. Body temperatures during anesthesia in infants and children. JAMA. 1951;146:551–6.
65. France GG. Hypothermia in the newborn: Body temperatures following anaesthesia. Br J Anaesth. 1957;29:390–96.
66. Hercus V. Temperature changes during thoracotomy in children, infants and the newborn. Br J Anaesth. 1960;32:476–80.
67. Farman JV. Heat losses in infants undergoing surgery in air conditioned theatres. Br J Anaesth. 1962;34:543–57.
68. Bruck K. Temperature regulation in the newborn. Biol Neonat. 1961;3:65.
69. Adamsons K, Gandy GM, James L. The influence of thermal factors upon O2 consumption in the newborn. J Pediatr. 1965;66: 495–508.
70. Stern L, Lees MH, Leduc J. Environmental temperature, oxygen consumption, and catecholamine excretion in newborn infants. Pediatrics. 1965;36:367–73.
71. Schultz K, Soltesz G, Molnar D, Mestyan J. Effect of hypothermia on plasma metabolites in preterm newborn infants with particular references to plasma free amino acids. Biol Neonate. 1979;36: 220–4.
72. Leigh MD, Belton MK. Pediatric anesthesiology. New York: Macmillan; 1960. p. 433.
73. Goudsouzian NG, Morris RH, Ryan JF. The effects of a warming blanket on the maintenance of body temperatures in anesthetized infants and children. Anesthesiology. 1973;39:351–3.
74. Gauntlett I, Barnes J, Brown TC, Bell BJ. Temperature maintenance in infants undergoing anaesthesia and surgery. Anaesth Intensive Care. 1985;13:300–4.
75. Kurz A, Kurz M, Poeschl G, Faryniak B, Redl G, Hackl W. Forced-air warming maintains intraoperative normothermia better than circulating-water mattresses. Anesth Analg. 1993; 77:89–95.
76. Steele C (1888) Case of deficiency of oesophagus. Lancet II: 764
77. Haight C, Towsley HA. Congenital atresia of the esophagus with tracheo-esophageal fistula. Extrapleural ligation of fistula and end-to-end anastomosis of esophageal segments. Surg Gynecol Obstet. 1943;76:672–88.
78. Franklin RH. Congenital atresia of the oesophagus: Two cases successfully treated by anastomosis. Lancet. 1947;2:243–4.
79. Swenson O. The diagnosis and treatment of atresia of the esophagus and tracheoesophageal fistula. Pediatrics. 1948;1:195–204.
80. Kennedy RL, Stoelting VK. Anesthesia for surgical repair of oesophageal atresia and tracheoesophageal fistula. Can Anaesth Soc J. 1958;5:132–6.
81. Zindler M, Deming M. The anesthetic management of infants for the surgical repair of congenital atresia of the esophagus with trachea-esophageal fistula. Anesth Analg. 1953;32:180–90.
82. Johnston AE, Conn AW. The anaesthetic management of tracheo-oesophageal fistula: a review of five years' experience. Can Anaesth Soc J. 1966;13:28–39.
83. Calverley RK, Johnston AE. The anaesthetic management of tracheo-oesophageal fistula: a review of ten years' experience. Can Anaesth Soc J. 1972;19:270–8.
84. Baraka A, Slim M. Cardiac arrest during IPPV in a newborn with tracheoesophageal fistula. Anesthesiology. 1970;32:564–5.
85. Myers CR, Love JW. Gastrostomy as a gas vent in repair of tracheoesophageal fistula. Anesth Analg. 1968;47:119–21.
86. Salem MR, Wong AY, Lin YH, Firor HV, Bennett EJ. Prevention of gastric distention during anesthesia for newborns with tracheoesophageal fistulas. Anesthesiology. 1973;38:82–3.
87. Dierdorf SF, Krishna G. Anesthetic management of neonatal surgical emergencies. Anesth Analg. 1981;60:204–15.
88. Karl HW. Control of life threatening air leak after gastrostomy in an infant with respiratory distress syndrome and tracheoesophageal fistula. Anesthesiology. 1985;62:670–2.
89. Filston HC, Chitwood WR, Schkolne B, et al. The Fogarty balloon catheter as an aid to management of the infant with esophageal atresia and tracheoesophageal fistula complicated by severe RDS or pneumonia. J Pediatr Surg. 1982;17:149–51.
90. Filston HC, Rankin JS, Grimm JK. Esophageal atresia: prognostic factors and contribution of preoperative telescopic endoscopy. Ann Surg. 1984;199:532–37.
91. Reeves ST, Burt N, Smith CD. Is it time to reevaluate the airway management of tracheoesophageal fistula? Anesth Analg. 1995;81:866–9.
92. Diaz LK, Akpek EA, Dinavahi R, Andropoulos DB. Tracheoesophageal fistula and associated congenital heart disease: implications for anesthetic management and survival. Paediatr Anaesth. 2005;15:862–9.
93. Macaulay G. An account of a child whose abdominal viscera were chiefly found within the cavity of the thorax. Med Observ Inq. 1757;1(25).
94. Truesdale PE. Diaphragmatic Hernia in children with a report of thirteen operative cases. NEJM. 1935;213:1159.
95. Gross RE. Congenital hernia of the diaphragm. Am J Dis Child. 1947;74:370–1.
96. Baumgartner CJ, Scott RF. Surgical emergency of diaphragmatic hernia in infancy. Arch Surg. 1950;61:170–82.
97. Gardiner JMC. Repair of diaphragmatic hernia in an infant: a case report. Anesthesiology. 1950;11:377–8.
98. Campanale RP, Rowland RH. Hypoplasia of the lung associated with congenital diaphragmatic hernia. Ann Surg. 1955;142:176.
99. Eckstein HB, Glover WJ. Transport of neonatal emergencies. Lancet. 1964;1:427–8.
100. Collins DL, Pomerance JJ, Travis KW, Turner SW, Pappelbaum SJ. A new approach to congenital posterolateral diaphragmatic hernia. J Pediatr Surg. 1977;12:149–56.
101. Raphaely RC, Downes Jr JJ. Congenital diaphragmatic hernia: prediction of survival. J Pediatr Surg. 1973;8:815–23.
102. Bohn D, Tamura M, Perrin D, Barker G, Rabinovitch M. Ventilatory predictors of pulmonary hypoplasia in congenital diaphragmatic hernia, confirmed by morphologic assessment. J Pediatr. 1987;111:423–31.

103. Sakai H, Tamura M, Hosokawa Y, Bryan AC, Barker GA, Bohn DJ. Effect of surgical repair on respiratory mechanics in congenital diaphragmatic hernia. J Pediatr. 1987;111:432–8.
104. Bradshaw-Isherwood PA. Two cases of exomphalos. Lancet. 1896;148:748–9.
105. Adams FH. Omphalocele. J Pediatr. 1948;32:304–7.
106. Burgess CM, Palma J, Myers WA. Omphalocele. Pediatrics. 1951;7:627–31.
107. Smithells RW. Management of omphalocele. Lancet II. 1953: 431–2
108. Ryan DW. Anaesthesia for repair of exomphalos; Problems associated with immediate repair in the neonate. Anaesthesia. 1973;28:407–14.
109. Steward DJ. Manual of pediatric anesthesia. New York: Churchill Livingstone; 1979.
110. Yaster M, Scherer TLR, Stone MM, et al. Prediction of successful primary closure of congenital abdominal wall defects using intraoperative measurements. J Pediatr Surg. 1989;24:1217–20.
111. Gross RE, Neuhauser EBD. Compression of the trachea or esophagus by vascular anomalies. Pediatrics. 1951;7:69–88.
112. Mustard WT, Rowe RD, Keith JD, Sirek A. Coarctation of the aorta with special reference to the first year of life. Ann Surg. 1955;141:429–36.
113. Smith C. An endo-oesophageal stethoscope. Anesthesiology. 1954;15:566.
114. Baffes TG, Riker WL, DeBoer A. Open Heart Surgery for Infants and Small Children; Mortality and Morbidity. Arch Surg. 1964;88:675–80.
115. Wong KC, Mohri H, Dillard D, et al. Deep hypothermia and Diethyl ether anesthesia for open-heart surgery in infants. Anesth Analg. 1974;53:765–71.
116. Newburger JW, Jonas PA, Wernovsky G, et al. A comparison of the perioperative neurologic effects of hypothermic circulatory arrest versus low-flow cardiopulmonary bypass in infant cardiac surgery. NEJM. 1993;329:1057–64.
117. Amir G, Ramamoorthy C, Riemer RK, Reddy VM, Hanley FL. Neonatal brain protection and deep hypothermic circulatory arrest: pathophysiology of ischemic neuronal injury and protective strategies. Ann Thor Surg. 2005;80:1955–64.
118. Waugh GE. Enterectomy under spinal anaesthesia for acute intestinal obstruction in an infant 24 hours old; Survival for one month. Lancet. 1912;1:427–8.
119. Tyrrell GH. A study of spinal anaesthesia in children and infants. Lancet. 1909;2:913–7.
120. Calvert DG. Direct spinal anaesthesia for repair of myelomeningocele. Br Med J. 1966;2:86–7.
121. Welborn L, Rice LJ, Hannallah RS, et al. Postoperative apnea in former preterm infants: Prospective comparison of spinal and general anesthesia. Anesthesiology. 1990;72:838–42.
122. Dohi S, Naito H, Takahashi T. Age related changes in blood pressure and duration of motor block in spinal anesthesia. Anesthesiology. 1979;50:319–23.
123. Browne D. An aid to operations on babies. Lancet. 1930;1:624.
124. Rickham PP. Neonatal surgery: early treatment of congenital malformations. Lancet. 1952;1:333–9.
125. Rickham PP. Thoughts about the past and future of neonatal surgery. J Pediatr Surg. 1992;27:1–6.
126. Smith RM. The Pediatric Anesthetist 1950-1975. Anesthesiology. 1975;43:144–55.
127. Macario A, Hackel A, Gregory GA, Forseth D. The demographics of inpatient pediatric anesthesia: Implications for credentialing policy. J Clin Anesth. 1995;7:505–11.
128. Battaglia JD. Neonatal surgery: changing patterns 1972-1980. J Pediatr Surg. 1982;17:666–9.
129. Surgical Advisory Panel, American Academy of Pediatrics. Guidelines for referral to pediatric surgical specialists. Pediatrics. 2002;110:187–91.
130. Stead AL. The response of the newborn infant to muscle relaxants. Br J Anaesth. 1955;27:124–30.
131. Salanitre E, Rackow H. The pulmonary exchange of nitrous oxide and halothane in infants and children. Anesthesiology. 1969;30:388–94.
132. Lerman J, Robinson S, Willis MM, Gregory GA. Anesthetic requirements for halothane in young children 0-1 month and 1-6 months of age. Anesthesiology. 1983;59:421–4.
133. LeDez KM, Lerman J. The minimum alveolar concentration (MAC) of isoflurane in preterm neonates. Anesthesiology. 1987;67:301–7.
134. Anand KJ, Aranda JV, Berde CB, Buckman S, et al. Analgesia and anesthesia for neonates: study design and ethical issues. Clin Ther. 2005;27:814–43.
135. Johnstone DE, Roghmann KJ, Pless IB. Factors associated with the development of asthma and hay fever in children: the possible risks of hospitalization, surgery, and anesthesia. Pediatrics. 1975;56:398–403.
136. Jones A, Steward DJ, Donsky GJ, Orange RP, Milko T. Incidence of respiratory allergy not increased after anesthesia in infancy. Anesthesiology. 1976;45:29–30.
137. Wilder RT, Flick RP, Sprung J, et al. Early exposure to anesthesia and learning disabilities in a population based birth cohort. Anesthesiology. 2009;110:796–804.
138. Bartels M, Althoff RR, Boomsma DI. Anesthesia and cognitive performance in children: No evidence for a causal relationship. Twin Res Hum Genet. 2009;12:246–5.
139. Istaphanous GK, Loepke AW. General anesthetics and the developing brain. Curr Opin Anaesthesiol. 2009;22:368–73.
140. Rovnaghi CR, Garg S, Hall RW, Bhutta AT, Anand KJS. Ketamine analgesia for inflammatory pain in neonatal rats: a factorial randomized trial examining long term effects. Behav Brain Funct. 2008;4:35.
141. American Academy of Pediatrics. Prevention, management of pain, stress in the neonate. American Academy of Pediatrics Committee on fetus and newborn, Committee on drugs, Section on Anesthesiology, Section on Surgery, and Canadian Paediatric Society, Fetus and newborn committee. Pediatrics. 2000;105: 454–61.

Physiology and Development of the Term and Preterm Neonate

2

Claire Brett and David Robinowitz

Perinatal injury, prematurity, and/or congenital anomalies inflict profound long- and short-term physical, psychological, emotional, social, and financial stresses on survivors, their families, and society. Both the Annual Summary of Vital Statistics: 2007 [1] and the National Vital Statistics Reports (April 30, 2010) [2] list "disorders relating to short gestation and low birth weight" as the second leading cause (16–17 %) of infant death, second only to congenital malformations, deformations, and chromosomal abnormalities (19.7–21 %). However, for non-Hispanic black and Puerto Rican women, low birth weight was the leading cause [2]. In 2011, 11.7 % of the 3.95 million live births (or 462,570) were preterm (<37 weeks gestation), 8.1 % (320,241) were low birth weight (<2,500 g), and 1.44 % (56,932) were very low birth weight (<1,500 g) in the United States [3]. In that year, two-thirds of the 23,910 infants who died (infant mortality was 6.05 per 1,000 live births), died in the neonatal period, and 45 % died as a result of congenital or chromosomal abnormalities (21 %), preterm age or low birth weight (17 %), and sudden infant death syndrome (7 %). In 2006, 54 % of all infant deaths occurred in the ~2 % of infants born less than 32 weeks gestation; 36 % of infant deaths were "preterm related" [1].

Infant mortality for late preterm infants (34–36 weeks gestation) is threefold greater than for full-term infants, often related to a combination of intrapartum events (e.g., placental and umbilical cord injury) and postnatal complications (e.g., respiratory problems, sepsis, and metabolic instability such as hypoglycemia and hypothermia). The morbidity and mortality associated with late preterm infants are particularly stunning because of their large numbers (i.e., 9 % or 388,540) [1].

The outcome of the extremely low birth weight (ELBW) infant continues to receive intense scrutiny. A prediction model of survival using gestational age, birth weight, and gender in preterm infants showed increasing survival from 28 or 34 % at 23 weeks (for males and females) to >99 % at 32 weeks in the United Kingdom [4]. Although results vary, two reports noted that a decrease in short-term complications has lagged behind the improved survival of ELBW infants [5, 6]. Of importance, major morbidities (e.g., chronic lung disease, retinopathy of prematurity, brain injury (intraventricular hemorrhage, or periventricular leukomalacia) predict death or survival with significant neurodevelopmental impairment [7, 8]. The incidence of poor outcome at 18 months is doubled, tripled, or quintupled when 1, 2, or 3 of these morbidities, respectively, are encountered [8]. Infection (sepsis, meningitis) seems to inflict less of an impact on outcome than the three major morbidities. Intrauterine and early postnatal events impact long-term survival, health, and function. Developing strategies to prevent preterm birth and devising interventions to treat anomalies both in utero and postnatally remain strategic priorities.

Over the last 2 decades, a significant epidemiology-based literature has suggested the importance of the "developmental origins of health and disease." That is, an environmental insult (e.g., over- or undernutrition, infection, psychological stress) during a critical period of fetal or early postnatal development may "program" long-term physiologic changes that increase the risk for various diseases in adulthood. In his initial study, Barker correlated increased mortality from coronary disease with low birth weight in a cohort from Hertfordshire, United Kingdom [9]. His "thrifty phenotype hypothesis" (survival of the undernourished fetus demands that nutrition be directed to vital organs such as the brain, resulting in insulin resistance in other tissues such as the muscle and pancreas) [10, 11] provided a framework to suggest that an adverse fetal environment (e.g., chronic placental insufficiency) elicited an adaptive response to protect critical organs such as the brain and heart at the expense of other sites (e.g., kidney) that involve long-term physiologic

C. Brett, MD (✉) • D. Robinowitz, MD
Department of Anesthesia and Perioperative Care, UCSF School of Medicine, 521 Parnassus Ave, San Francisco, CA 94143, USA
e-mail: brettc@anesthesia.ucsf.edu; robinowitzd@anesthesia.ucsf.edu

J. Lerman (ed.), *Neonatal Anesthesia*, DOI 10.1007/978-1-4419-6041-2_2,

reprogramming associated with risk for hypertension, type II diabetes, and hyperlipidemia, which predispose to the metabolic syndrome and cardiovascular disease [12–15]. Of note, the most significant glucose intolerance has been correlated with low birth weight combined with rapid postnatal weight gain [16, 17]. In addition to these effects, restricted intrauterine growth has been associated with reduced number of nephrons, a recognized pathway to renal failure and hypertension. Similar to intrauterine growth retardation, preterm birth is also associated with an apparent arrest of nephron growth and later hypertension and insulin resistance [18, 19].

More recently, the "thrifty phenotype hypothesis" shifted to a "developmental plasticity" theory [20, 21], which captures the effects of a wider variety of early derangements on risk for diseases in adulthood, including small-for-gestational age [22], large-for-gestational age [23], and preterm infants [24–27]. Thus, the initial report from Barker has spawned an entire research focus and model, the "developmental origins of health and disease" [21, 28–30]. The full impact of and/or synergistic role of "the thrifty phenotype" and/or "developmental plasticity" on the well-established lifelong diagnoses associated with preterm birth and congenital anomalies remains to be defined.

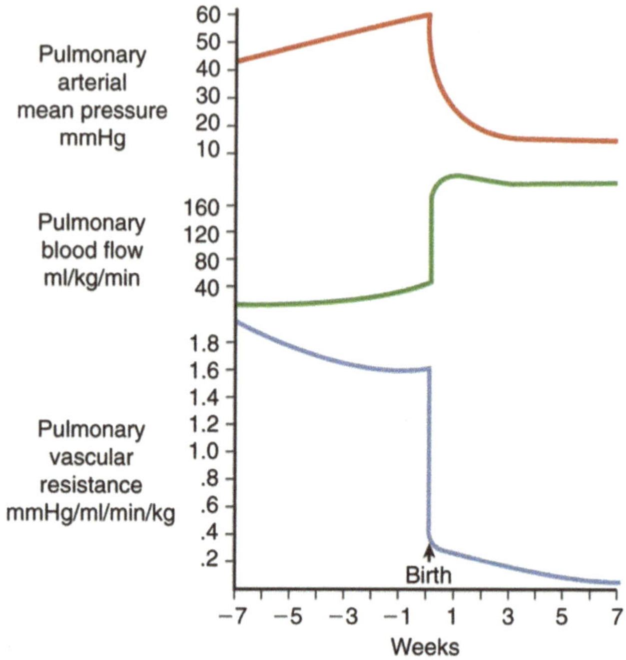

Fig. 2.1 The fetal circulation is characterized by high pulmonary arterial mean arterial pressure and pulmonary vascular resistance and low pulmonary blood flow. At birth, the dramatic decrease in pulmonary vascular resistance is accompanied by a parallel decrease in pulmonary arterial blood pressure and an increase in pulmonary blood flow. Of note, the pulmonary vascular resistance gradually decreases further over the first 6 weeks of life (from Rudolph [31])

Cardiovascular Function

The Transitional Circulation

The fetal circulation is characterized by increased pulmonary vascular resistance, decreased pulmonary blood flow (Fig. 2.1), decreased systemic vascular resistance, and right-to-left blood flow through the patent ductus arteriosus and the foramen ovale (Fig. 2.2). In the fetus, blood return to the heart is derived from both the body and the placenta. Similarly, blood distributed to organs and the placenta from the heart is derived from both ventricles. Thus, the fetal circulation is not in series as it is in the adult. Furthermore, in utero, volumetric outputs from the right and left ventricles differ. Therefore, cardiac output is expressed as the combined ventricular output, the total volume ejected by the two ventricles. For example, in fetal sheep, the right ventricle ejects 300 mL/min/kg (or 66 % of the combined ventricular output) compared with 150 mL/min/kg (or 33 % of the combined ventricular output) from the left ventricle. Based on ultrasound studies, the human fetus has a more closely matched output from the right (250 mL/min/kg) and left (200 mL/kg/min) ventricles [33].

The umbilical vein enters the hilum of the liver where it divides into three branches: vessels that provide flow directly to the left lobe, a large arcuate branch that joins the portal vein to supply the right lobe, and the ductus venosus that proceeds cephalad to join the inferior vena cava (Fig. 2.3). Umbilical venous blood flowing into the inferior vena cava is preferentially directed across the foramen ovale into the left atrium and then the left ventricle. Thus, highly oxygenated blood exits the placenta, bypasses the liver, and flows directly to the myocardium and brain. Desaturated blood from the superior vena cava and the abdominal vena cava enters the right atrium and ventricle and then returns to the placenta after crossing the ductus arteriosus. A variety of anatomic features of the atrial septum (e.g., crista dividens, eustachian valve) and the angle of entry of the ductus venosus into the inferior vena cava facilitate this preferential streaming [33].

Although reduced throughout gestation, pulmonary blood flow in the human fetus increases from ~13 % of the combined ventricular output at mid-gestation to 25 % at 30 weeks [35]. In addition, the pulmonary vascular resistance of human fetuses responds to maternal oxygen administration ($FIO_2=0.60$) after 31 weeks gestation [36]. Similar studies in fetal lambs documented that the fetal circulation is briskly responsive to both hyperoxia and hypoxia and that these responses are greater in late gestation (Fig. 2.4) [38]. Vasomotor control of the pulmonary circulation in utero, however, may be disturbed in the presence of a congenital heart defect in which oxygen delivery to the lungs may be abnormal (e.g., aortopulmonary transposition) thereby

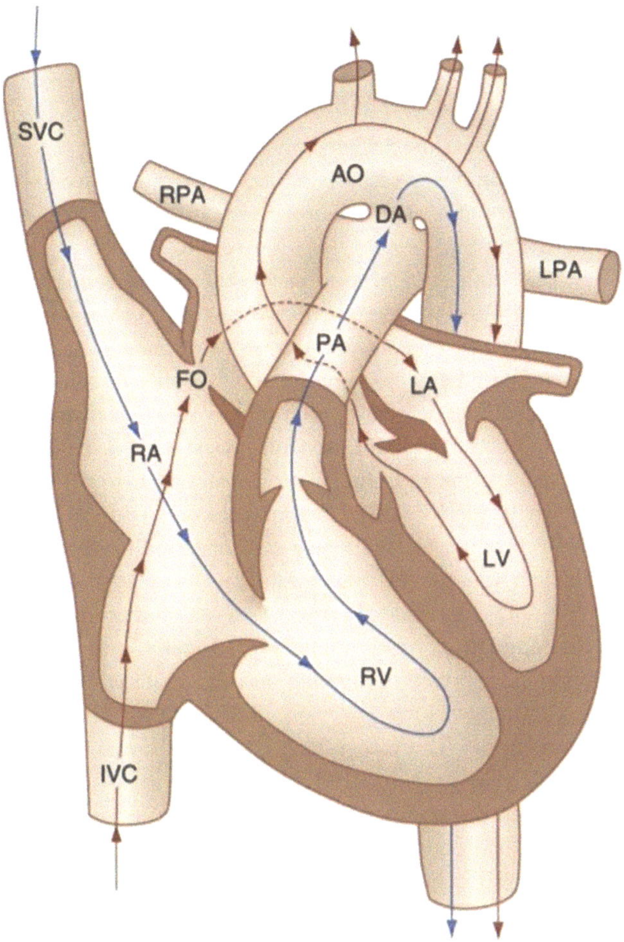

Fig. 2.2 The fetal circulation. Desaturated blood from the superior vena cava preferentially flows into the right ventricle, into the pulmonary artery, across the ductus arteriosus and to the descending aorta to the placenta. Relatively well-saturated blood from the ductus arteriosus enters the inferior vena cava and preferentially crosses the foramen ovale to the left atrium, the left ventricle, and to the cerebral circulation (from Marx [32])

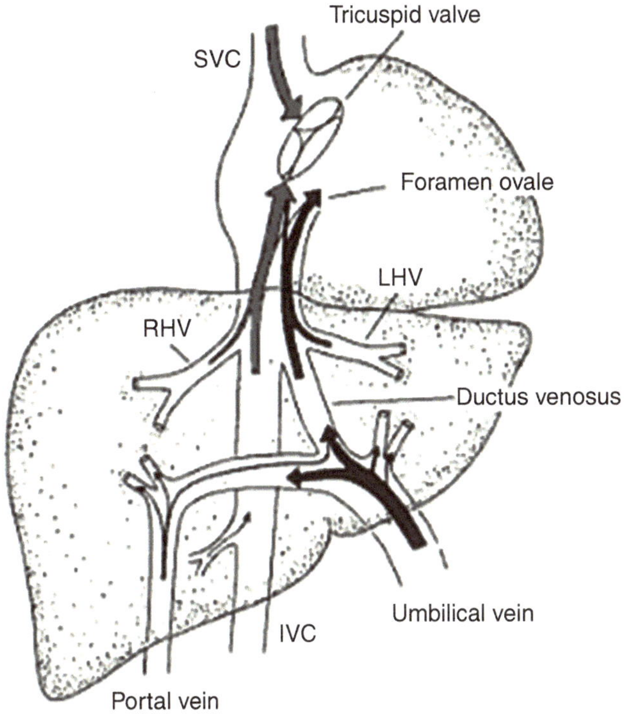

Fig. 2.3 The fetal circulation. The blood from the umbilical vein that enters the ductus venosus preferentially streams across the foramen ovale to enter the left atrium and ventricle and the cerebral circulation (from Rudolph [34])

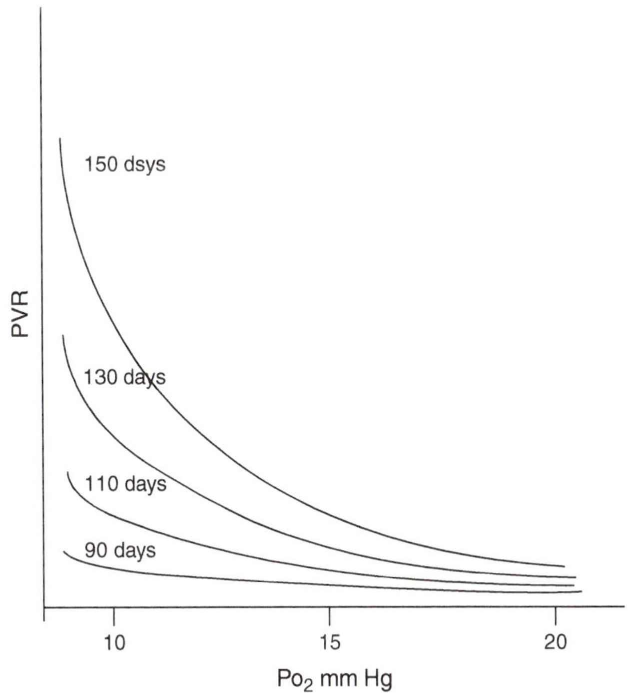

Fig. 2.4 Response of the fetal pulmonary circulation to hypoxia (fetal lamb). With advancing gestation, the response of the pulmonary circulation to decreasing oxygen saturation becomes more pronounced (from Rudolph [37])

dramatically affecting the development of vessel morphology [37]. At birth, when the placenta separates, pulmonary vascular resistance decreases dramatically, and pulmonary blood flow increases in response to the rapid increase in oxygen tension and the onset of alveolar ventilation (Fig. 2.1). Simultaneously, both systemic vascular resistance and left atrial pressure increase, eliminating the right-to-left shunting through the foramen ovale. However, bidirectional shunting through the ductus arteriosus may continue in the normal full-term infant during the first 48 h of life. With normal transition, the distinct, separate pulmonary and systemic circulations are established.

Postnatally, the marked vasoconstrictor responses of the pulmonary circulation to hypoxia persist, and pulmonary vascular resistance also responds significantly to changes in pH (Fig. 2.5) [39]. This may be due in part to the persistent

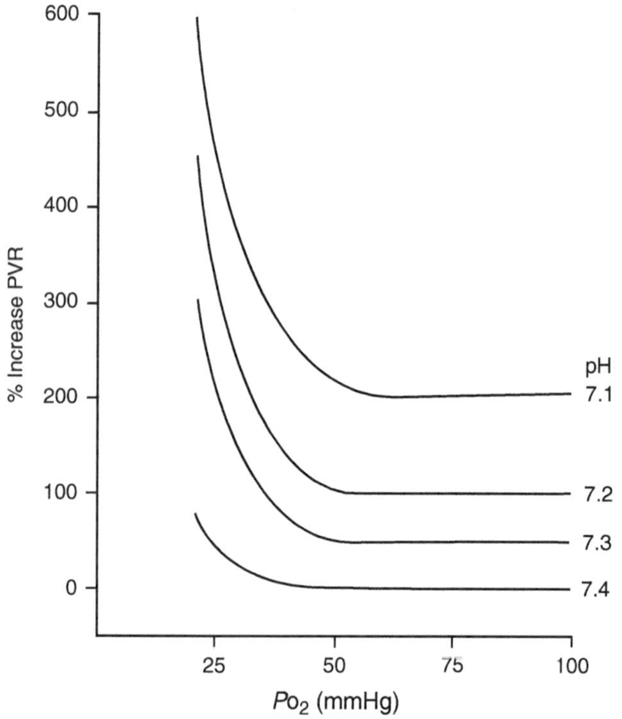

Fig. 2.5 Response of the neonatal pulmonary circulation to hypoxia and acidosis (lamb). The break point for marked increase in pulmonary vascular resistance in response to decreasing oxygen saturation is dramatically dependent on pH (used with permission from Rudolph and Yuan [39])

increase in pulmonary vascular resistance during the first few weeks of postnatal life and greater than that in the older infant despite decreasing dramatically at birth (Fig. 2.1). The reactivity of the pulmonary vasculature can be striking, and, in the neonate, arterial hypoxemia or acidosis can vasoconstrict the pulmonary arteries and induce pulmonary hypertension, thereby impeding forward blood flow and, by default, forcing right-to-left shunting through the foramen ovale and/or ductus arteriosus. This return to a fetal circulatory pattern, termed persistent fetal circulation or persistent pulmonary hypertension of the newborn (PPHN), further exacerbates the hypoxemia and acidosis. PPHN may be an isolated phenomenon or a part of various clinical scenarios including meconium aspiration, sepsis, polycythemia, and diaphragmatic hernia. An echocardiogram is routinely performed in infants manifesting signs and symptoms of persistent pulmonary hypertension to definitively exclude structural cyanotic heart disease [40].

Although the control of the pulmonary circulation, especially during the transition from fetal to postnatal life, is complex and depends on the interaction of a variety of mediators and factors, receptors, and neurologic, endocrine, and vascular control mechanisms, nitric oxide (NO) undoubtedly plays a critical role in mediating the vasodilating effect of oxygen [41], although other mechanisms contribute as well (e.g., oxygen-sensitive K^+ channels in pulmonary vascular smooth muscle) [42]. Despite the enormity of the research that has been focused on this topic, no single factor has yet been identified as the primary trigger responsible for the initiation of pulmonary vasodilatation at birth, nor do we know whether the endothelial cell or the smooth muscle cell is the prime target [43].

A wide range of therapies and agents (hyperventilation, vasoactive agents) have been investigated to treat PPHN, but the only selective vasodilator of the pulmonary circulation is NO. In many cases, inhaled NO induces a selective, rapid, and potent decrease in pulmonary vascular resistance without affecting systemic vascular resistance [43]. At low doses, toxicity is minimal. Unfortunately, up to 40 % of infants with PPHN do not respond to NO. The effects of NO on mortality, the incidence of bronchopulmonary dysplasia, and neurodevelopmental deficits have been conflicting [44, 45], as has its effects as an antioxidant and anti-inflammation (in animals) [46]. Finally, endogenous NO may have a role in alveolar and vascular development in the immature lung [47, 48]. Because production and metabolism of NO are regulated on several levels, it is not surprising that its clinical effectiveness in both term and preterm infants remains controversial. For example, NO production depends on endothelial nitric oxide synthetase activity (eNOS; lung eNOS is type III). eNOS has both reductase and oxygenase domains. When its substrate L-arginine is available, oxidation of NADPH and NO synthetase produces NO. On the other hand, when the concentration of substrates or cofactors (e.g., heat shock protein 90) is reduced, NOS is uncoupled, and reactive oxygen or nitrogen species such as peroxynitrite are produced instead of NO. In fact, oxidative stress may contribute to the development of PPHN [49]. Similarly, the activity of soluble guanylate cyclase and cGMP-specific phosphodiesterase (PDE5) on smooth muscle cells potentiates the effectiveness of NO in augmenting cGMP production. PDE5 hydrolyzes cGMP, which controls the duration and magnitude of cGMP's effect. Agents that inhibit PDE5, such as sildenafil, promote pulmonary vasodilatation and have been used extensively to treat pulmonary hypertension in adults, although there is less experience with this therapy for PPHN in neonates [50].

Myocardial Development

Myocytes: Fetal and adult myocardia contract and relax similarly. That is, with activation, the cytosolic calcium concentration increases, inducing force generation, and as the cytosolic calcium concentration decreases, relaxation ensues. At all stages of maturation, the ventricle develops force against a varying resistance or load (contraction/ejection) followed by a period of relaxation (filling). The membranes in the adult myocardium that control calcium flux and the contractile system that responds to calcium are present in the fetal heart; however, structures associated with the mechanics of force generation (sarcomere, myofibril), those correlated with controlling calcium flux (sarcoplasmic reticulum and other membrane components including receptors, channels, exchangers, transporters, and pumps), those related to myocardial compliance (extracellular matrix/cytoskeleton), and sympathetic innervation undergo qualitative and quantitative age-related changes. In part, age-related differences in cardiovascular function and responses to calcium and other pharmacologic agents can be attributed to the developmental state of these various components of myocardial anatomy and function.

During fetal and neonatal development, myocytes differentiate markedly and increase in number and size, which correlate with profound changes in mechanical properties and therefore contractility and performance. In the perinatal period, the myocytes complete "terminal differentiation" and lose their capacity to proliferate, as evidenced by their transition from mono- to binucleation (a final nuclear division without cellular division) [51]. Concurrently, the shape and size of myocytes change, gradually remodeling from a spherical to a more rectangular shape by adulthood. Since shortening typically occurs along the long axis, the adult myocyte (dimensions of the adult vs. neonate myocyte: 150 vs. 40 μm in length; 5 vs. 25 μm in width) generates a more rapid response and larger increase in amplitude than the neonatal myocyte [52].

Recent studies in both human [53] and animal [51] fetuses have documented that the late gestational exponential cardiac growth secondary to the increase in size and number of myocytes correlates with an increase in both left ventricular volume and active tension per unit of myocardial volume. Of possible importance in the setting of congenital heart disease (e.g., single ventricle associated with pulmonary or aortic atresia), marked differences between the development of the left and right ventricles have been noted, including fewer but larger myocytes in the right ventricle [51].

Subcellular Components: In addition to the increase in the number of myocytes, age-related changes in subcellular components also contribute to maturation in excitation-contraction and force development in the myocardium and, therefore, cardiovascular function. Not only does the number of myocytes per cross-sectional area increase, but the organization of the myofibrils also undergoes striking age-related changes [52]. In the immature myocardium, myofibrils appear in thin layers, and groups of nuclei and mitochondria congregate chaotically in the center of the cell. In contrast, in the mature myocardium in adults, long parallel rows of myofibrils alternate with rows of mitochondria (and sarcoplasmic reticulum). The chaotic arrangement of mitochondria and myofibrils in the immature myocardium contributes in part to the reduced contractility compared with the adult heart.

In addition to the effects of age-related changes in gross anatomy, changes in various membranes that control the regulation of calcium flux also exert substantial effects on the force of myocardial contraction. Both the cell membrane (sarcolemma) and the intracellular sarcoplasmic reticulum modulate the increase in cytosolic calcium that facilitates contraction and undergo developmental changes. In the adult, a small calcium influx via L-type calcium channels stimulates calcium release from the sarcoplasmic reticulum (calcium-induced calcium release, CICR). CICR depends on an intricate coupling of the C-type calcium channel, the ryanodine receptor, and t tubules (invaginations of the sarcolemma) [54, 55]. In spite of differences among various species, in general, CICR has been allocated a secondary role in the generation of a myocardial contraction in the immature myocardium because of limited sarcoplasmic reticulum and underdeveloped t tubules [56, 57]. Recently, attention has focused on a role that links the Na^+–Ca^+ exchanger with the ryanodine receptor to allow an age-defined reverse version of CICR [58, 59]. An L-type calcium current mediated by CICR is now recognized to play an increasingly critical role as the myocardium matures, although the details of the molecular mechanisms remain unclear.

Clinically relevant developmental changes are pervasive in the developing myocardium including the sarcoplasmic reticulum, t tubules, and various channels and regulatory proteins. That is, the volume of sarcoplasmic reticulum and its ability to pump calcium (uptake, longitudinal sarcoplasmic reticulum; storage and release, junctional sarcoplasmic reticulum) increase in utero and postnatally. Furthermore, the various subtypes of sarcoplasmic reticulum are less differentiated functionally in the immature heart. As a result, immature hearts are more sensitive to calcium channel antagonists [60], and maximal contractility depends to a greater extent on extracellular calcium that does the mature heart [61].

When compared with the adult myocyte, the reduced velocity and magnitude of sarcomere shortening in the immature myocyte may also be attributed to age-related changes in expression of various isoforms of contractile proteins such as troponins [62]. The troponin complex, which consists of 3 subunits (structural proteins: troponin C, I, and T) and binds to the thin filament of the myofibril, regulates the calcium-dependent activation of actin and myosin interaction that results in force generation. Both troponin I and T exist in multiple isoforms that are developmentally regulated.

For example, an isoform identical to that in slow skeletal muscle (ssTnI) is expressed in embryonic, fetal, and neonatal myocardium, whereas the cardiac isoform (cTnI) is expressed predominately in the adult myocardium. The myocardial expression of the slow skeletal muscle in terms of the cardiac isoforms of troponin I may be of particular importance in the immature myocardium since this has been correlated with the relative resistance of the immature heart to acidosis [63]. The response of the immature myocardium to sympathetic stimulation is similarly correlated with the expression of slow skeletal troponin I. Cardiac, but not slow skeletal muscle troponin, is phosphorylated in response to β-stimulation, which may correlate with the difference in diastolic function noted in the neonate [64]. This phosphorylation decreases the sensitivity to calcium, facilitating diastolic relaxation.

TnT isoforms vary among species and stages of development. The human cardiac muscle contains four isoforms of TnT (cTnT 1–4); cTnT1 expression peaks in the fetus, whereas only cTnT3 is expressed in the adult. Calcium sensitivity has been correlated with the shift in the expression of the troponin T isoform [62]. The expression of specific isoforms of troponin T has been correlated with the responsiveness of myofilaments to calcium.

Although cardiac troponins are routinely used to evaluate and monitor cardiac injury in children and adults, only recently has their importance in the intensive care nursery been recognized [65]. Troponins are typically bound to the thin filament of the myofibril, but with acute injury to the myocardium, bound troponin is released from damaged tissues, first appearing in blood after 2–4 h and persisting for up to 21 days. The range of normal concentrations of the isoforms of troponin in the neonate has been reported for both cTnT and cTnI. The concentrations of troponins in cord blood samples vary as a function of gender, mode of delivery, and assay. Both cTnT and cTnI increase after asphyxia-associated myocardial injury, although the variability in the responses among studies is notable. As in children and adults, laboratory evidence of injury is often an adjunct to other assessments (e.g., echocardiogram) of cardiac function. For example, asphyxiated neonates have greater concentrations of cTnT than normal-term infants that correlate with echocardiographic evidence of myocardial dysfunction. Nonetheless, in many cases, cardiac output is similar in asphyxiated and non-asphyxiated neonates. The concentrations of troponins are generally increased in preterm infants, although treatment with inotropes correlates with greater cTnT concentrations in both term and preterm neonates. Thus, although troponin concentrations in neonates are likely to become an integral segment of evaluating perinatal injury in both preterm and term infants, its specific prognostic and therapeutic roles have not been completely defined.

Myocardial Compliance: Extracellular Matrix/Cytoskeleton

The cytoskeleton includes the contractile proteins and titan (a large protein that extends over half the span of the sarcomere) as well as microfilaments, intermediate fibers, and microtubules. This intricate complex provides the structural framework for intracellular and extracellular communication that allows the contractile movement of the individual sarcomeres to be translated into effective systolic contraction and diastolic relaxation. That is, the cytoskeleton provides the system for mechanical signaling. Examining the general appearance of the immature sarcomere provides an overview of the dramatic changes in organization during early development. In the immature myocyte, A and I bands are more irregular, M bands are absent, and Z bands vary in width. Several of the proteins and microfilaments, intermediate fibers, and microtubules develop postnatally, which is critical in mediating a range of activities such as cell growth, migration, and adhesion as well as signaling for remodeling in response to adaptation of the transitional circulation at birth [33]. For example, desmin, a protein important that links Z bands of myofibrils, improves the connection of myofibrils with mitochondria facilitating the mechanics of contraction. The amount and types of collagen change their expression of various isoforms that improve resting load and passive state of the myocardium. For example, the type I isoform correlates more tightly with developing rigidity, whereas the type III isoform contributes to elasticity, and the relative proportion of these two correlates with myocardial compliance. As the collagen network becomes progressively more organized with maturation, the population of type III isoform increases, eventually equaling or exceeding that of type I [66]. That is, the ratio of types I–III isoforms is increased in preterm and term infants, a level that persists until at least age 6 years and decreases thereafter to ~0.5 by adulthood [66].

Sympathetic Innervation: The sympathetic nervous system modulates cell growth and differentiation, as well as the distribution of and sensitivity to calcium. For example, the increased concentration of α-adrenoreceptors in the early postnatal period may be critical in stimulating left ventricular growth [67]. Furthermore, the increase in the network of adrenergic fibers innervating the myocardium induces widespread development and expression of the various contractile systems (e.g., the expression of the contractile proteins, the efficiency of the calcium channel, expression of the myosin ATPase isoforms). Finally, the activity of adenylate cyclase, an important enzyme involved in the intracellular transmission of β-stimulation, increases in parallel with the increase in catecholamine concentrations [33].

The Preterm Infant

The typical changes of the transitional circulation are blurred in the setting of the very low birth weight (VLBW; <1,500 g) and extremely low birth weight (ELBW; <1,000 g) infant. At less than 30 weeks gestational age, the ductus arteriosus often fails to close, systemic and pulmonary vascular resistances are high relative to the placental circulation, and, often, cardiac output does not increase dramatically in the first 24 or more postnatal hours. Because of the unique physiology of the ELBW infant, measuring cardiac output and establishing "normal" values for systemic blood pressure and heart rate become complicated. As a result, defining hypotension becomes difficult (see below) [68]. Consequently, diagnostic and therapeutic regimens in the intensive care nursery cannot be established based on clear-cut, abundant, evidence-based data for these infants.

At any developmental stage, ventricular function is governed by the same factors: preload, afterload, contractility, and heart rate. However, the ability to compensate for perturbations in these factors is limited in the neonate, especially in ELBW infant. In the preterm infant (i.e., in some cases, a mid-gestation fetus), the immature myocardium and the peripheral circulation present significant disadvantages when, at birth, the low-resistance placenta is abruptly replaced with the greater resistances of the pulmonary and systemic vascular beds, and interventions such as positive pressure ventilation and inotropic support are introduced. Sensitivity to changes in heart rate is also more dramatic for the preterm infant. Marked variability in the quantity of blood flowing across the foramen ovale and ductus arteriosus adds to the complexity of monitoring the cardiovascular function of the premature infant.

The relationship between blood pressure, cardiac output, and systemic vascular resistance is constant throughout life: BP=CO X SVR. That is, pressure and flow are not equal but are related via resistance (or SVR). Thus, flow to an organ may increase, decrease, or remain constant over a wide range of blood pressures depending on changes in resistance. Although the normal ranges for blood pressure correlate with gestational age [69, 70], the definition of hypotension remains elusive. Because a mean arterial pressure <30 mmHg for more than 1 h (measured on the first day of life, beginning at 5 h) has been associated with intracranial lesions [71] or reduced cerebral blood flow [72], many set a break point for hypotension at 30 mmHg in preterm infants. However, there are those who hold that the normal mean arterial blood pressure is <30 mmHg in the most preterm infants during the first 3 postnatal days (Fig. 2.6) [73]. Others suggest that a mean blood pressure that is less than the gestational age correlates with the 10th percentile for blood pressure [74], and this constitutes a definition of hypotension. Although studies have reported an association between hypotension and intraventricular hemorrhage [75, 76], a clear cause-and-effect

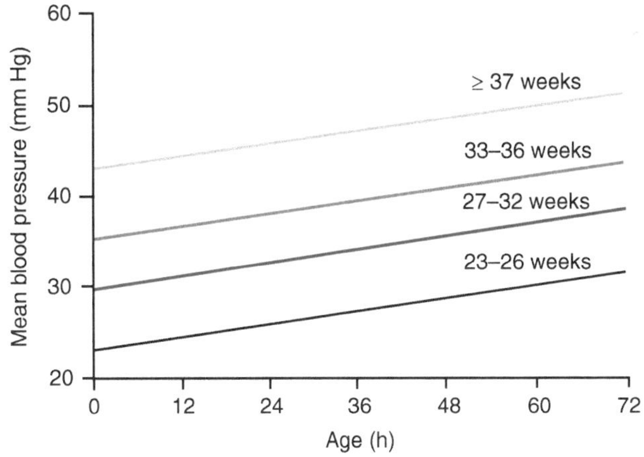

Fig. 2.6 Mean blood pressure in neonates predicted lower limit (initial 72 h of life) (from Nuntnarumit et al. [73])

relationship remains controversial. That is, aggressive treatment of "hypotension" has not been shown in prospective studies to affect morbidity or mortality [68] or long-term outcome [77]. And, unfortunately, identifying links between a specific inotropic agent, change in cerebral blood flow, and outcome remains at best an estimate. No study "has shown any improvement in any meaningful clinical outcome, short or long term, in response to a specific inotrope" [78].

Thus, the variability in "normal" for blood pressure and heart rate among infants of the same gestational and/or postnatal age creates a dilemma in the setting of clinical care, especially in the commonly unstable setting of the operating room. Furthermore, without access to reliable measures of perfusion to critical organs (i.e., the brain), devising precise guidelines for treating "hypotension" in the neonate is virtually impossible.

A number of investigators [79, 80] have proposed a novel next step to monitor cerebral blood flow in the setting of the transitional circulation of the preterm infant in the first few postnatal days. Recognizing that neither blood pressure [79, 80] nor capillary refill time [81] reliably correlates with left ventricular output in the preterm infant, the flow in the superior vena cava has been measured to estimate systemic blood flow to the brain (and upper body). Measuring blood flow of the superior vena cava eliminates the need to consider the influence of shunting via either the ductus arteriosus or the foramen ovale on the accuracy of their measurement [82]. In these studies, mean arterial pressure correlated poorly with superior vena cava flow (Fig. 2.7). Similarly, others noted that during the first 48 h of life, blood pressure did not correlate with the volume of blood flow in the descending aorta, superior vena cava, or left or right ventricle [80]. In fact, at some points, if any relationship between blood pressure and blood flow in the superior vena cava existed, it would most be accurately labeled as being "inverse," as reported in earlier studies [84]. Of interest, neither dopamine nor dobutamine

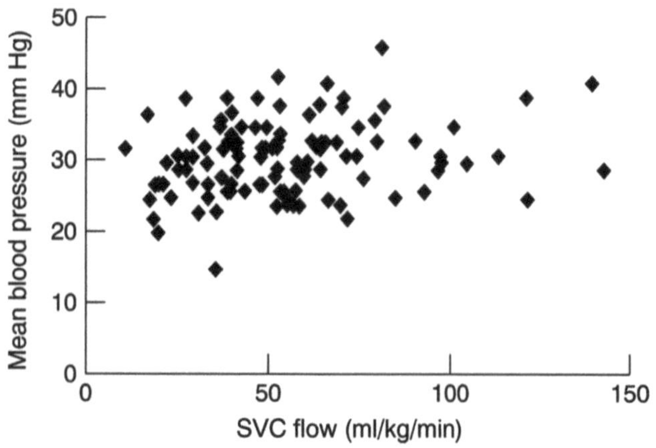

Fig. 2.7 Ultrasound measured flow in the superior vena cava has been validated as an estimate of cerebral blood flow. Notice the lack of correlation of SVC flow with simultaneously measured mean arterial blood flow (from Kluckow and Evans [83])

increased contractility when introduced in response to reduced superior vena cava blood flow [85].

Measuring superior vena cava flow (and other flows) may improve the accuracy of ensuring adequate oxygen and nutrient delivery, especially to the brain, and monitoring the effectiveness of therapy. For example, superior vena cava flow has been correlated with both the incidence of periventricular hemorrhage and neurodevelopmental outcomes [83, 86]. Unfortunately, "functional echocardiography" requires sophisticated equipment and experience precluding its use as a routine, bedside monitor.

Thus, given our inability to accurately measure the cardiac output and organ-specific blood flow (e.g., cerebral blood flow) in the neonate (Fig. 2.7), we are left with systemic blood pressure and heart rate and metabolic indices including blood gases/lactate/electrolytes and trends in clinical status to track cardiovascular homeostasis in the preterm infant. In fact, even investigators who have reported the relevance of superior vena cava flow have suggested a rational approach to clinical care based on commonly available cardiovascular indices as mentioned [78]. As always, a parameter such as blood pressure must be interpreted within the wider context of other clinical and diagnostic data. For example, even if superior vena cava flow were measured, these data might be correlated with MRI and near-infrared spectroscopy [see Section "Monitoring Cerebral Blood Blow: Near-Infrared Spectroscopy (NIRS)"] to establish rational therapies.

Clinical Significance and Summary

The neonate has the greatest cardiac output per body weight of all age groups (~300 cc/kg/min). The increased resting cardiac output of the neonates limits its ability to respond to an increased oxygen demand or to adapt to wide variations in preload or afterload. That is, the neonate cannot readily compensate for inadequate blood flow if the preload becomes inadequate or if the afterload, heart rate, or contractility wane. For example, the non-distensible heart has limited capacity to increase stroke volume to augment cardiac output in response to increasing preload [87, 88]. Although volume loading in the immature ventricle increases cardiac output, the effect is attenuated compared with the response at older ages. Similarly, the immature myocardium poorly tolerates increases in afterload compared with that at older ages. The increased content of collagen and high ratio of types I–III collagen may account for the relative noncompliance of the neonatal heart. These factors are all magnified in the case of the ELBW infant where marked variability exists for blood flow across the foramen ovale and ductus arteriosus. Finally, the normal heart rate in the neonate is quite rapid. Increasing the heart rate may not further increase the cardiac output, but decreasing the heart rate may dramatically decrease the cardiac output. Some propose that the resting myocardium in the neonate exists at a greater level of "β-adrenergic tone" than does the child and adult. As this β-adrenergic tone wanes over the first weeks to months after birth, adrenergic stimulation elicits a greater increase in cardiac performance [89].

The fetus (i.e., preterm baby) and neonate may have impaired ventricular function secondary to a decreased number of myofibrils, decreased sympathetic innervation, decreased β-adrenoceptor concentration, immaturity of the sarcoplasmic reticulum structurally and functionally, maturation-specific mechanisms for calcium uptake, release and storage, and a specific spectra of expression of various isoforms of contractile/noncontractile proteins, channels, exchangers, and enzymes. Over the first months of life, myocardial contractility gradually increases, which maintains cardiac output over wider ranges of preload and afterload. Similarly, the increase in contractile proteins and the shift in expression to various isoforms, the development of sarcoplasmic reticulum and t tubules, and adrenergic innervation all contribute to complex changes in force development, calcium recruitment, and transport that prime the myocardium for a more powerful response to stress and increased oxygen demands.

Central Nervous System Function

Discussing the central nervous system after cardiovascular function is intentional, since the physiologic vulnerability of the immature brain is inextricably linked to age-related hemodynamic function. Circulatory immaturity undoubtedly plays a fundamental role in perinatal brain injury. Hemodynamic instability is common in the neonatal period (especially in the preterm infant) and has been implicated in ischemic and hemorrhagic brain injury in both term and preterm infants. Unfortunately, cerebrovascular injury has been linked to life long dysfunction including motor disorders, learning/developmental delays, seizures, and secondary complications (e.g., from chronic lung disease secondary to recurrent aspiration pneumonia). Minimizing or preventing neurologic complications from perinatal injury requires a complete understanding of the cellular and molecular mechanisms of the responses of the developing brain to asphyxia, hypoxia, and/or inflammation. To date, such mechanisms have not been definitively mapped, and the extent and nature of the initial injury cannot clearly predict long-term outcomes.

The general pattern of injury to the developing brain involves an initial insult from hypoxia, inflammation, and/or ischemia followed by secondary damage from reperfusion that results in excitotoxicity and release of a host of cytokines [90]. Recently, Volpe introduced the concept of "panencephalopathy" [91] and "encephalopathy of prematurity" [92–94] to emphasize that the initial white and gray matter injury incurred by the preterm infant is manifested by more than a simple loss of tissue but also significantly impairs subsequent brain development. Volpe emphasizes that "neonatal brain injury and its subsequent clinical and anatomic consequences must be viewed as an amalgam of destructive and developmental disturbances." Kinney asserted that the term "encephalopathy of prematurity" emphasizes that "the constellation of cognitive, motor, and emotional impairment in long-term survivors of prematurity reflects the particular patterns of white and gray matter damage in combination with arrested developmental programs—patterns that depend upon the severity, timing, and chronicity of the injury as well as individual confounding factors" [95].

Normal Development of the Central Nervous System

The two primary structures of embryogenesis of the brain that develop early in gestation are the neural tube (future brain and spinal cord) by 3–4 weeks and the prosencephalon (future forebrain) by 2–3 months [96]. Early neural tube anomalies are dramatic and often fatal: anencephaly, craniorachischisis totalis, myeloschisis, and encephalocele. Similarly, severe prosencephalic anomalies (holoprosencephalies) are often fatal, especially when associated with chromosomal abnormalities (e.g., trisomy 13–15, trisomy/ring/deletion 18).

The less severe form of abnormal neural tube closure, lesions of spina bifida (incidence 3–7 per 10,000 births) are clinically important because affected infants frequently survive and have lifelong problems. The four primary types of spina bifida are categorized according to the severity of the defect [96]. In spina bifida occulta, the divided vertebral arch, the spinal cord, and the meninges are covered with skin. Hair often protrudes from the skin overlying the defect, forming a sacral dimple. In spina bifida cystica, neural tissue and its coverings protrude through the incompletely formed vertebral arch as a cystic-like structure. In meningocele, the neural tube lies in its normal position, but the meninges protrude through the defect; skin usually covers this lesion. In the fourth type, the myelomeningocele, both the spinal cord and the meninges protrude, often without skin. These lesions can occur at any level of the spine. Although commonly accompanying myelomeningocele (60 % in occipital, cervical, thoracic, or sacral lesions and about 90 % in thoracolumbar, lumbar, and/or lumbosacral lesions) [97], hydrocephalus often is not evident before the meningomyelocele is closed because cerebrospinal fluid leaks through the open lesion and decompresses the ventricles.

Arnold-Chiari malformation, an abnormality of the hindbrain, occurs in most patients with myelomeningocele. The medulla oblongata is flattened and elongated and, along with the fourth ventricle, protrudes into the spinal canal through the foramen magnum. The downward position of the medulla elongates the lower pons and upper medulla and may compress brainstem nuclei and cranial nerves. If the cerebellar tonsils are displaced through the foramen magnum, aqueductal stenosis and hydrocephalus can develop. Severe anomalies may cause apnea, vocal cord paralysis, and/or central and obstructive ventilatory disturbances and require early correction [98]. Of significance, as many as 20 % of infants with myelomeningocele have sleep-disordered breathing [99].

Agenesis of the corpus callosum and septum pellucidum are often associated with abnormal neuronal migration and significant clinical abnormalities. Agenesis of the corpus callosum is usually associated with a syndrome (e.g., Aicardi or Andermann syndrome) or a chromosomal [11, 14, 16, 18, 21] abnormality. As many as 80 % of patients without a corpus callosum have other brain anomalies, plus they have non-CNS malformations [100, 101]. Partial agenesis of the brain probably occurs later in development and is associated with clinical syndromes that have migrational and structural disorders. Agenesis of the septum pellucidum is never an isolated lesion and often occurs in conjunction with optic nerve hypoplasia (septo-optic dysplasia).

During the third trimester, cortical gray and white matter volumes increase four to fivefold [93, 94], secondary to growth and differentiation of dendrites and axons, proliferation of glia, synaptogenesis, and myelination (Fig. 2.8) [102]. The proliferation in the cerebellum is even more rapid than the cerebral cortex and is characterized by intense migration of various populations of cells (Fig. 2.9) [104–106]. In parallel with the intense growth of the parenchyma, the vascular network of the late gestation brain also develops rapidly. The long and short penetrators lengthen and arborize, decreasing border/end zone blood flow.

Age-Related Patterns of Injury

In addition to the overall intense growth of the brain in late gestation, specific transient cell types define the unique susceptibility of the preterm brain to ischemia, inflammation, excitotoxicity, and free radical injury. That is, various populations of cells are critical in forming cerebral pathways and, at the same time, are exquisitely sensitive to injury. This selective vulnerability of specific populations of cells at different developmental stages (24–28 weeks vs. 28–32 weeks vs. 32–37 weeks vs. term) leads to predictable patterns of pathology. Three examples have received prominent attention by experts in neonatal neuropathology (see Section "Vulnerable Cell Populations").

In general, the preterm infant is regarded as most vulnerable to white matter injury, whereas the term infant is regarded as vulnerable to injury in the deep gray nuclei (e.g., basal ganglia and thalamus). Emerging evidence suggests that periventricular white matter in premature infants is selectively vulnerable to ischemia during hypotension [107]. The pattern of clinical deficits in survivors of hypoxic-ischemic perinatal brain injury also differs between term and preterm infants. Recent evidence suggests that the new knowledge about brain development acquired from advanced MRI imaging (e.g., high-resolution MRI, spectroscopic imaging, diffusion tensor imaging) has produced a "blurring of the 'gray-white' dichotomy" [108]. Increasingly, white matter injury has been recognized in term infants, and gray matter injury has been identified in preterm infants. In addition, the detailed anatomy of injury identified via MRI imaging may be combined with the known selective vulnerability of various cell populations to estimate, first, the patterns of defective "connectivity" in brain development that develop subsequent to the injury and, second, to correlate these patterns with the clinical outcome identified during long-term follow-up.

Although glutamate plays a critical role in the proliferation, differentiation, and migration of developing cells, its excessive release in the setting of a hypoxic-ischemic injury contributes to a state of "excitotoxicity" that is associated with cell death. When glutamate receptors (NMDA, *N*-methyl-D-aspartic acid; AMPA, alpha-3-amino-hydroxy-5methyl-4-isoxazole propionic acid; kainate) are excessively stimulated (especially certain subtypes), intracellular calcium accumulates and activates caspase-3, which leads to abnormal apoptosis. The NMDA receptor predominantly mediates this activity, and one subunit (NR2B) that predominates early in gestation mediates slower deactivation, resulting in prolonged action compared with other subunits [109].

In addition to excitotoxicity, oxidative stress seems to be fundamental to neonatal brain injury. Of interest, areas of the brain expressing NMDA receptors also express neuronal (nNOS) and inducible nitric oxide synthase (iNOS) [110]. While endothelial nitric oxide (eNOS) mediates cerebral vasodilatation, excessive nitric oxide mediated by iNOS in response to hypoxia-ischemia generates reactive nitrogen species (free radicals). The excess oxygen and nitrogen free radicals generated in response to hypoxia-ischemia or to free iron (Fenton reaction generates the hydroxyl radical when hydrogen peroxide encounters free iron) [111, 112] associated with hemorrhage deplete endogenous antioxidant systems, damaging cell membranes and resulting in cell death. Oxidative stress seems to enhance excitotoxicity via regulatory effects on glutamate receptors [113]. Of note, antioxidant systems (e.g., Mg and Cu superoxide dismutase, catalase, vitamin A, and C) are also underdeveloped in the neonatal brain [109].

Vulnerable Cell Populations. The Preterm Infant: Two unique cell types (subplate neurons and pre-oligodendrocytes) with marked sensitivity to hypoxia-ischemia populate the white matter of mid-gestation fetuses and express glutamate receptors. The subplate neurons located in subcortical white matter first appear at ~10 weeks gestation and peak in number between 24 and 32 weeks [109, 114], when the subplate zone is 4–5 times thicker than the cortical plate. The subplate serves as a waiting zone for cells and thalamocortical axons, until their final ultimate location in the cortex is defined [115]. By expressing various neurotransmitters and growth

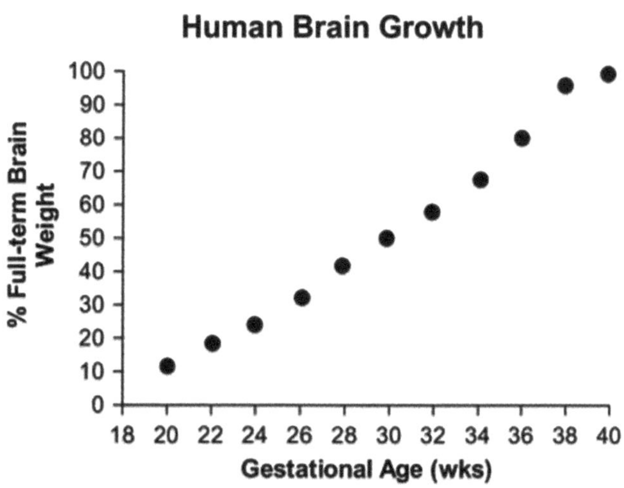

Fig. 2.8 Growth of the human brain over the second half of gestation as a function of % of the weight for the full-term infant. The 34-week gestation brain is only 65 % of its weight at term (from Kinney [102], Fig. 1, p. 82)

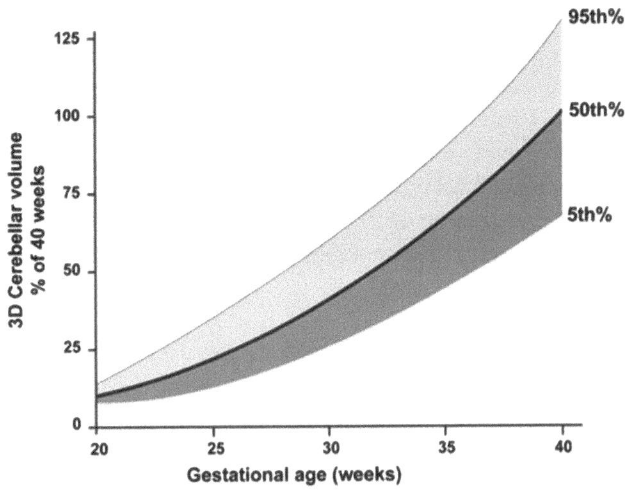

Fig. 2.9 Growth of the human cerebellum (5th, 50th, 95th percentile) during the last half of gestation as a function of % of the volume for the full-term infant. The 34-week gestation brain is only 65 % of its volume at term (from Volpe [103], Fig. 1, p. 1086)

factors, this site orchestrates the migration of cells from the germinal neuroepithelium to distant sites (e.g., corpus callosum, basal ganglia, thalamus) and initiates formation of synapses. These neurons have abundant receptors for excitatory amino acids (e.g., glutamate) that are critical modulators for normal development, but hypoxia-ischemia may stimulate excessive release of these modulators, excitotoxicity, and white matter injury. Recent in vitro studies documented the relative sensitivity of subplate neurons to glutamate compared with other cortical cells [116]. Damage to the subplate may disrupt axon development in vital sites such as thalamocortical areas, impeding critical innervation and interaction, interrupting feedback between the cortex and thalamus, and leading to long-term functional consequences. The connectivity among various distant structures during a period of critical brain development has been postulated to correlate with deficits identified in the ex-premature in the specific areas of behavior, cognition, and other complicated higher cortical functions (e.g., executive function) [105, 117–120]. In humans, the subplate gradually involutes during the third trimester and disappears by 6 months after birth. Thus, the subplate neurons are a transient cell population that mediates essential thalamocortical development.

Before myelination and during the time of peak vulnerability to periventricular leukomalacia (PVL) (23–32 weeks) (see Section "Cerebral White Matter Injury"), the late oligodendrocyte progenitors (pre-oligodendrocytes) are the predominant cells that populate the subcortical white matter. While mature oligodendrocytes are relatively resistant, pre-oligodendrocytes are especially susceptible to injury from oxidative and excitotoxic stress and, when injured, fail to reach full maturation, resulting in diffuse hypomyelination and axonal disruption. Thus, injury to progenitors inhibits their maturation, allowing the persistence of a population of cells that exhibit excitotoxicity as well as fail to generate mature oligodendrocytes that are capable of myelination [121].

Finally, microglia are unique macrophages that are initially identified in normal brain myelination development. They are concentrated in the cortical white matter during the third trimester, but decline rapidly after 37 weeks of gestation [122]. Although microglia are critical during normal development (apoptosis, axonal development, vascular development), their abnormal activation secondary to infection/inflammation precipitates cytokine and glutamate release that result in reactive oxygen and nitrogen species [112].

Thus, after the neural tube and the prosencephalon are established, the central nervous system primarily develops by proliferation and migration. Neurons proliferate from ventricular and subventricular regions at every level of the developing nervous system. From the second to the fourth month of gestation, most proliferating cells are neurons. From the fifth month of gestation into adulthood, glia are primarily proliferating. Interruption of migration (e.g., from the subplate), abnormal activation (e.g., microglia), and/or failure of proliferation/maturation (e.g., pre-oligodendrocytes) are key factors underlying the pathophysiology of injury to the immature brain.

The risk of white matter injury and the associated neurodevelopmental abnormalities increase with systemic illness such as chronic lung disease [123] and necrotizing enterocolitis [124]. In addition, the critical care of neonates is complex with their pharmacologic therapy, ventilatory support, infections, seizures, and hemodynamic instability all interacting to produce a final outcome.

Vulnerable Cell Populations. The Term Infant: The term infant experiences hypoxia-ischemia from several clinical sources [placental injury (e.g., abruption, infarct), birth trauma, umbilical cord prolapse/compression] that are distinct from those that commonly injure the preterm infant and others who are similar (e.g., infection/inflammation). In general, hypoxic-ischemic encephalopathy in the term infant primarily targets the deep gray nuclei, especially the basal ganglia. As in the preterm infant, the selective vulnerability is linked to overexpression of certain glutamate receptors (especially NMDA) and various subunits (e.g., NR2B > NR2A). In the basal ganglia, these receptors coexist with an abundant population of neurons that express nNOS, thus creating a site of increased susceptibility to injury. Additionally, free radicals generated from hypoxia-ischemia as well as from reactions with free iron (Fenton reaction produces the hydroxyl radical when hydrogen peroxide reacts with free iron) generated after hemorrhage may lead to oxidative damage [125].

Contrary to the traditional belief that injury at term is commonly associated with chronic in utero events (e.g., infection/inflammation), most encephalopathy at this developmental stage seems to be secondary to insults at or near birth [126–128] and evolves over the first few weeks (or months) of life. Since injury is relatively acute and evolves over time, neuroprotective therapy may be critically relevant for improving long-term outcome. For example, hypothermia has moved into the realm of standard therapy for the term infant with moderate to severe encephalopathy secondary to hypoxia-ischemia [129]. However, in spite of some evidence for its effectiveness, hypothermia is unlikely to be a panacea for preventing long-term complications associated with neonatal encephalopathy. Rather than relying on a single modality, many suggest that a multipronged approach to perinatal neuroprotection/rescue will be essential to improving outcome [111].

Advanced MRI techniques have identified two primary patterns of injury in the term infant [93, 108, 125]. First, a watershed pattern involves the vascular border/end end zones of the white matter that may extend into cortical gray matter after a severe insult. In general, watershed lesions are more often associated with cognitive than motor disorders. Second, the basal nuclei (basal ganglia/thalamus) pattern involves the deep gray nuclei that may extend throughout the cortex after a severe insult. That is, this pattern often includes diffuse cortical injury. At presentation, these neonates have had more severe clinical abnormalities including intensive resuscitation, severe encephalopathy, and seizures. In general, these lesions are typically associated with more severe cognitive and motor disabilities than in the watershed pattern. However, even when one pattern predominates, less severe damage is common in the other domain [127]. Thus, the spectrum of deficits on follow-up correlates with the pattern of injury on MRI, rather than simply the severity of the lesion.

Congenital Heart Disease: For more than a decade, we have known that more than 50 % of newborns with congenital heart disease have microcephaly and neurologic deficits that correlate with later neurodevelopmental abnormalities [130]. More recently, impaired brain development and metabolism that resemble the pattern of the preterm infant have been identified preoperatively in full-term infants with congenital heart disease, especially complex cyanotic lesions (hypoplastic left heart syndrome/single ventricle and aortopulmonary transposition). This delayed development may predispose these infants to similar vulnerability to white matter injury as that seen in the preterm infant [131–134]. Their outcomes reflect a complex interaction between a focal brain injury (e.g., white matter injury) and its profound effects on subsequent brain development. Although the specific mechanism for the in utero delay in development is unclear, disturbances in the fetal circulation with decreased delivery of oxygen and other metabolites to the brain may play a fundamental role [33, 135]. Although complex cyanotic heart disease confers a particularly high risk of developmental delay, delay is also common in children with either acyanotic or cyanotic lesions, especially those who undergo surgical intervention in the first few days of life [136].

Summary: That the brain of the 34-week gestation human weighs only 65 % of that of a term infant (Fig. 2.8) [102] implies dramatic development during the last month of normal fetal life. Overlap in the pathophysiology of lesions common in the preterm [periventricular leukomalacia (PVL) and germinal matrix-intraventricular hemorrhage (GM-IVH)] with those most common in the term infant (hypoxic-ischemic encephalopathy, arterial stroke) is not surprising. In part, the overlap can be explained by responses to injury in the setting of selective vulnerability of the immature/newborn brain coupled with disturbances in regulation of cerebral blood flow.

Autoregulation of Cerebral Blood Flow: Cerebral autoregulation accounts for a constant cerebral blood flow over a wide range of systemic blood pressure (in adults, between mean arterial pressures 60 and 150 mmHg) [137]. Such a phenomenon implies that vasoconstriction and vasodilation occur in response to changes in perfusion pressure to maintain a stable blood flow. Various vasoactive factors have been linked to local regulation of cerebral blood flow (e.g., hydrogen ions, potassium, adenosine, prostaglandins, osmolarity, and calcium) [111]. The term "pressure passive" refers to the disruption of this phenomenon so that changes in blood pressure alter cerebral blood flow. Pressure passive cerebral blood flow has been proposed as a critical risk factor for central nervous system injury in neonates and the subsequent adverse neurodevelopment, especially the preterm infant. Although autoregulation is intact in normal fetal/preterm and term animals and humans, the autoregulatory range is narrower in this age group compared with their more mature counterparts. Normal blood pressure increases markedly during the third trimester, but the upper limit of autoregulation does not. As gestational age decreases, the normal blood pressure in preterm infants is close to the lower limit of autoregulation [138–140]. Rapid increases in arterial blood pressure can rupture the fragile vessels in the immature brain (see Section "Germinal Matrix-Intraventricular Hemorrhage"), whereas hypotension and low perfusion pressure can cause ischemia. Thus, the cerebral blood flow of the preterm infant seems to be vulnerable to both hypo- and hypertension.

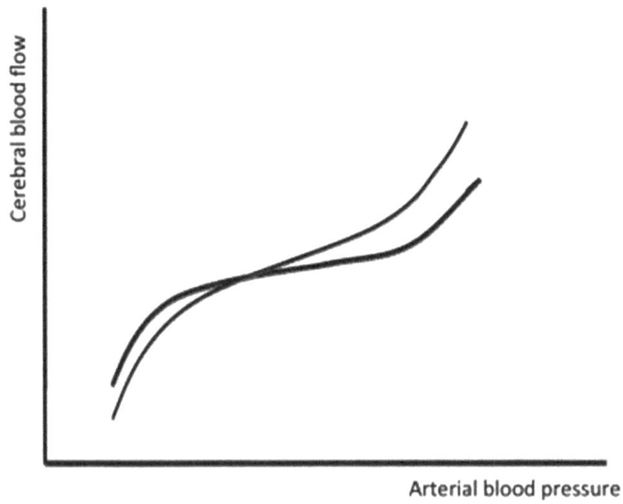

Fig. 2.10 Theoretical concept of autoregulation in the neonate. The flat section of the heavy line represents intact autoregulation, where cerebral blood flow changes minimally over a range of arterial blood pressure. Below the knee of this curve, cerebral blood flow decreases as blood pressure decreases. Similarly, above the flat part of the curve, cerebral blood flow increases as blood pressure increases. Greisen suggests that the flat part of the autoregulatory plateau may never be horizontal and the shape of the curve may change in various clinical scenarios. The degree of the tilt may be the critical clinical factor. He suggests that autoregulation should not be simply considered "present" or "absent" but instead should be approached as quantifiable (from Greisen [141], Fig. 6, p. 213)

Greisen posited that in critically ill neonates, cerebral autoregulation should be presumed to be "imperfect," not simply present or absent or "all or nothing." That is, the flat part of the autoregulatory plateau is not horizontal but upward sloping. The slope of this part of the curve defines the degree of disturbance in the autoregulation (Fig. 2.10) [141]. Although the limits of the autoregulatory plateau have not been defined with certainty, the range in the term infant is 25–50 mmHg (mean arterial pressure), whereas in the preterm infant, it is less and narrower. Similarly, postnatal age and other factors affect the range and the limits of autoregulation [111]. To complicate matters, metabolic abnormalities common in the neonate (e.g., hypoxia, hypercarbia) impact on cerebral autoregulation [139, 142–144]. For example, the series of reports by Lou documented reduced cerebral blood flow in the neonate (i.e., 20 mL/100 g/min) and, in various clinical settings, cerebral flow changed in response to blood pressure (i.e., disturbed autoregulation) [139, 143].

In the immature human (spontaneously breathing or after 48 h in the mechanically ventilated), with intact autoregulation, the response of cerebral blood flow to changes in carbon dioxide (4 % change for each 1 mmHg in $PaCO_2$) is more robust than to changes in blood pressure (1 % change for each 1 mmHg in pressure) [145, 146]. However, such responses are not predictable when autoregulation is markedly impaired, such as in severely asphyxiated infants [147], in response to seizures [148], and, to a less degree, in mechanically ventilated preterm infants especially in the first day of life [149, 150]. Thus, although impossible to accurately predict and although responses to changes in $PaCO_2$ vary with gestational and postnatal age, neurologic injury, systemic illness, and metabolic derangement, both hypo- and hypercarbia should be considered to have potential dramatic effects on cerebral blood flow [151]. In fact, in the neonate, both hypercarbia and hypocarbia have been associated with severe neurologic insults [152, 153]. In addition, hypercarbia has been shown to directly inhibit cerebral autoregulation in preterm infants (500–1,500 g) [152]. Similarly, within various developmentally distinct ranges, both hypoxemia and hypoglycemia directly increase cerebral blood flow [154].

Thus, common therapeutic maneuvers (mechanical ventilation, airway suctioning), metabolic derangements (hypoglycemia, hypercarbia, hypocarbia, hypoxia, hypo-/hypernatremia, and hypocalcemia), presence of a patent ductus arteriosus, and other insults (seizures, sepsis) may dramatically affect the neonate's ability to compensate for derangements in either hemodynamic or cerebrovascular status.

Monitoring Cerebral Blood Flow

Near-Infrared Spectroscopy (NIRS): NIRS is a noninvasive monitor that measures regional cerebral oxygen saturation. In preterm neonates (<32 weeks gestation) and term neonates, cerebral oxygen saturation is stable, reliable, and relatively unchanged among regions of the brain, although the measurements varied up to 18 % [155].

No bedside technique allows continuous monitoring of cerebral blood flow, and a "normal" blood pressure does not reliably reflect adequate cerebral perfusion (Fig. 2.7) (see Section "Cardiovascular Function") [79, 156]. Recently, some have proposed that NIRS reflects cerebral oxygenation and hemodynamics [157, 158]. NIRS takes advantage of the difference in absorption of infrared light by oxygenated and deoxygenated hemoglobin (HbD) to derive changes in cerebral blood flow. However, cerebral blood volume, systemic oxygen saturation, and cerebral metabolic rate also affect HbD. Thus, although in many cases, the difference in HbD trends with changes in cerebral blood flow, other derived parameters [tissue oxygenation index (TOI), regional cerebral oxygenation saturation ($rScO_2$), and cerebral fractional tissue oxygen extraction (cFTOE)] have been proposed to increase the accuracy of NIRS as a measure of cerebral blood flow.

Alternatively, several experts have combined continuous, simultaneous arterial pressure and NIRS data to quantify "cerebral pressure passivity" [159]. The loss of autoregulation was defined when changes in HbD correlated directly with changes in blood pressure. In this study of infants <1,500 g between the first 12 h after birth and day 5 of life, cerebral perfusion was pressure passive on average 20 % of the time, but up to 50 % of the time in some ELBW infants. Similarly, hypotension was most common (exceeding 80 % in some) in the ELBW. Because the monitoring was continuous, the authors documented the fluctuant nature of the pressure-passive cerebral flow, noting that arterial hypotension was not invariably associated with a pressure-passive state (and vice versa). That is, blood pressure and cerebral pressure passivity were not consistently related; the absolute value of blood pressure did not predict passivity. In contrast, others suggest a relationship between hypotension and loss of autoregulation [160]. Although cerebral pressure passivity did not correlate with the incidence of germinal matrix and/or intraventricular hemorrhage (GM-IVH), a subsequent study incorporated a complicated "coherence and transfer functional analysis" of HbD data that demonstrated a correlation between "high MAP-HbD gain" and the incidence of GM-IVH [161]. Using a sophisticated system of interrelating blood pressure and cerebral pressure passivity, the investigators generated a measure of the magnitude of pressure passivity that predicted GM-IVH (imaged on cranial ultrasound).

Thus, although this monitor has advanced the process of monitoring cerebral perfusion, NIRS currently is appropriately labeled "semiquantitative" and has been recognized as a trend monitor, but has not yet achieved a status of a "robust quantitative variable" [162]. For example, since movement artifacts interfere with continuous, long-term measurement of HbD, other analyses such as TOI or $rScO_2$ or other complicated derivations such as those of O'Leary [161] may be more reliable [163, 164]. Most agree that a reliable, easy-to-use, portable monitor of cerebral blood flow would contribute to rational care both in the intensive care nursery and the operating room.

Cerebral White Matter Injury

Periventricular leukomalacia (PVL) can have focal (cystic) and non-cystic components; [112] the incidence correlates inversely with gestational age. The focal lesion typically develops in the deep, periventricular white matter, consists of macroscopic necrosis, eventually evolves into cysts that are easily imaged on cranial ultrasound, and in the last decade, only develops in <5 % of VLBW infants. The diffuse, non-cystic component of PVL is generally identified in the more central white matter; preferentially involves the pre-oligodendrocytes; includes areas of astrogliosis and microgliosis; consists of focal, microscopic necrosis; is not readily identified on cranial ultrasound; and currently accounts for most of the cerebral white matter injury of the preterm brain [112, 165, 166]. With advanced MRI imaging techniques, white matter injury has been identified in as many as 50 % of ELBW infants [165]. Furthermore, the incidence of diffuse white matter abnormalities increases with postnatal age, for example, from 21 %, to 53 %, and 79 % between the first postnatal week and term equivalent [167].

Although white matter injury has been identified in premature infants for decades, associated gray matter developmental abnormalities have been increasingly recognized only over the last decade as quantitative MRI techniques have evolved. Volumetric analyses have documented neuronal/axonal disease most commonly in the thalamus, basal ganglia, cerebral cortex, and cerebellum. These lesions appear on MRIs performed as early as term–equivalent and persist to adulthood [91, 118]. Although the focal, cystic, necrotic lesions of PVL seem to correlate with motor deficits, only a more extensive insult can account for the widespread neurologic insults of the ex-ELBW infant. The non-cystic component of white matter injury of PVL may account for the cognitive deficits of ex-premature infants, although the attention deficits and behavior/socialization abnormalities are more likely related to the associated axonal/gray matter injury. Volpe emphasizes that the ultimate clinical outcome from this "panencephalopathy of prematurity" (i.e., white and gray matter injury) evolves not only from the primary injury (e.g., white matter injury) but possibly more importantly from the profound abnormalities in subsequent development [93, 94].

The vulnerability of the immature brain to white matter injury is attributed to a combination of insults: ischemia/disturbed autoregulation and/or infection/inflammation. The border/end zones of the immature cerebral circulation, with incomplete development of both long and short penetrators into the white matter, are inherently at risk for ischemia [168]. In fact, the deep focal necrotic lesions of PVL are identified in the end zones of the long penetrating vessels from the middle cerebral artery. In addition, the extremely low blood flow in the white matter especially in the first 1–2 days of life adds to the vulnerability [169]. Global cerebral blood flow is ~15 mL/100 g/min (compared with the human adult, 45–50 mL/100 g/min). Of importance, flow to white and gray matter can vary significantly. In one study, blood flow to white matter was only 17 % of that to the basal ganglia/thalamus [169]. Specifically, blood flow to the white matter is ~25 % of that to the cortex, ranging between 1.6 and 3.0 mL/100 g/min [112]. In the newborn puppy, the decrease in cerebral blood flow as a result of hypotension differed among various regions of the brain, but the white matter was most vulnerable [170].

In addition to the substantial incidence of hypotension in the premature infant in the setting of the transitional circulation during the first 48 h after birth, disturbed autoregulation (see Section "Autoregulation of Cerebral Blood Flow") augments the risk for injury from either over- or underperfusion.

Although hypoxia and/or ischemia stimulates the release of proinflammatory cytokines, a robust relationship between infection (e.g., production of cytokines/free radicals) and PVL remains elusive. Nonetheless, a clear-cut maturation-dependent susceptibility of pre-oligodendrocytes to free radical injury (both reactive oxygen species and reactive nitrogen species) in the presence of iron and decreased antioxidant mechanisms has been documented (see Section, Vulnerable Cell Populations: the Preterm Infant) [112]. Thus, the development of PVL seems to be multifactorial, involving complex interactions of immature cardiovascular, neurologic, and immunologic (and other) factors often in the presence of infection (e.g., neonatal sepsis) or chronic inflammation (e.g., chorioamnionitis).

Germinal Matrix-Intraventricular Hemorrhage

The etiologies of intracranial hemorrhage in the term infant generally include trauma, coagulation abnormalities, anatomic anomalies (aneurysm, arteriovenous malformation), and perinatal asphyxia. However, the most common intraventricular hemorrhage, the germinal matrix-intraventricular hemorrhage (GM-IVH), predominantly occurs in the preterm infant, with incidence and severity increasing with decreasing gestational age.

GM-IVH has been divided into categories that correlate with the severity and extent of the initial injury and with the clinical outcome. GM-IVH has been classified based on data from computerized tomography [171]. Grade I is a subependymal hemorrhage with minimal or no IVH (i.e., restricted to the germinal matrix). Grade II is an IVH into a lateral ventricle without distention. Grade III is IVH with enlargement of the ventricles by intraventricular blood. In that classification, a Grade IV hemorrhage includes ventricular dilatation and hemorrhage into the parenchyma of the brain.

This grading system was revised after correlating the severity of the GM-IVH with the severity of hemorrhage in the lateral ventricle on the parasagittal cranial ultrasound. In Grade I, the hemorrhage is limited to the germinal matrix, and ventricular enlargement is less than 10 %. In Grade II, 10–50 % of the ventricle is filled with blood. In Grade III, more than 50 % of the ventricle is involved, usually with enlargement of the lateral ventricles. Grade IV was eliminated, and, instead, an echo density of the periventricular parenchyma secondary to hemorrhage, a periventricular hemorrhagic infarction (PVHI), was included [172] to distinguish the lesion from GM-IVH. Thus, intraparenchymal lesions were labeled Grade IV GM-IVH, hypothesizing that the IVH had extended from the ventricle laterally into the white matter. The latter classification emphasizes that the pathophysiology of PVHI is a hemorrhagic venous infarction (see below), not simply a massive GM-IVH. This classification further stratifies PVHI according to severity based on three factors: size (localized vs. extensive), unilateral versus bilateral, and evidence of midline shift [172, 173].

GM-IVH has an overall incidence of 7–23 % [174] but may be as great as 30 % (750–1,000 g) to 40 % (501–750 g) in the ELBW infants [5]. In this same large cohort of the NICHD Neonatal Research Network, the incidence of severe IVH [Grade III and (PVHI)] (in 2000–2002) was 16 % and 24 %, respectively. In a small cohort, the overall incidence of GM-IVH decreased from 42 % in two earlier groups (1982–1989 and 1990–1999) to 22 % in the time frame (2000–2002). The incidence of severe GM-IVH also decreased from 15 to 2 % [175].

Although mortality is substantial in infants with PVHI (~50 %), it is not increased in those with Grades I–II bleeds [176]. Even though less significant neurodevelopmental delay occurs in near-term infants with uncomplicated Grade I or II IVH, they are reported to have reduced developmental functioning [173], and gray matter volumes are 16 % less than predicted based on MRI [177]. While Grades I and II IVH are not associated with severe neurologic sequelae, PVHI can be a devastating lesion. In a recent report, two-thirds of survivors of PVHI had motor delays, and one-half had cognitive impairment, with visual field abnormalities in one-third and epilepsy in 20 %. Ninety percent of PVHI have poor neurodevelopmental outcomes [178]. Furthermore, posthemorrhagic hydrocephalus (another complication of IVH) severe enough to require a ventricular-peritoneal shunt has the highest incidence of severe neurocognitive impairment in early childhood (78 % in the group with Grade III lesions and 92 % in those with a PVHI) [174].

The pathophysiology of GM-IVH is, at least in part, related to the structure of the immature brain. The specific vulnerability of the immature neurovasculature to GM-IVH correlates with the delayed development of the venous drainage compared with the arterial system. The immature veins are thin walled and their branching pattern predisposed to collapse. Because of underdevelopment of the superficial veins, most cerebral venous drainage depends on the deep venous system that drains the germinal matrix and most of the white matter.

The anatomy of the germinal matrix, the site of bleeding in this lesion (usually between the caudate nucleus and the thalamus at the level of the foramen of Monro) [172], also contributes to the greater risk for hemorrhage in the premature. Proliferating ventricular and subventricular areas of the germinal matrix produce neuroblasts (cerebral precursors for both gray and white matter) and glioblasts between 10 and 20 weeks that are densely cellular and vascularized, but gelatinous, providing poor support for the vascular network.

The gelatinous nature of the area gradually decreases with increasing age, being barely present in term infants. This dense vascular network arises from the middle and anterior cerebral and anterior choroidal arteries that enter into a bed of immature, large, irregular capillary-like vessels and eventually drain into the deep venous system from the brain. The veins become the terminal vein, which makes a "U-turn" near the head of the caudate nucleus to join the vein of Galen. Thus, the "terminal vein" courses within the germinal matrix and makes an abrupt change in course at the common site of GM-IVH. Because of this unique anatomy, a large GM-IVH may obstruct the terminal vein, leading to venous distension, ischemia, and rupture, producing a PVHI. Thus, PVHI either accompanies or follows but never precedes a large GM-IVH, and, if the GM-IVH is bilateral, the PVHI is always ipsilateral to the side of the larger hemorrhage [172].

The primary site of bleeding in the premature brain is the junction of the veins and capillaries, rather than at the junction of the arteries/arterioles and capillaries. Between 24 and 28 weeks gestation, the germinal matrix is most prominent at the body of the caudate nucleus and between 28 and 32 weeks resides at the level of the head of the caudate, involuting by ~36 weeks gestation [172, 179]. When hemorrhage extends from the germinal matrix into the ventricles, blood spreads throughout the ventricular system possibly causing arachnoiditis and obstructive hydrocephalus. The free iron that is released from hemoglobin may produce hydroxyl free radicals (Fenton reaction, see Section, Age-Related Patterns of Injury) [125], in addition to other free radicals that are generated during hypoxic-ischemic injury. Ideally, antioxidant systems (e.g., superoxide dismutase; glutathione peroxidase; catalase; vitamins A, C, and E; beta carotenes; glutathione) are robust and redundant to effectively scavenge free radicals. However, when excess free radicals are generated, stores of antioxidants are depleted. In that setting, the downstream effect is cell membrane damage, increased intracellular calcium, and eventually cell death. The neonatal brain encounters increased risk for injury secondary to the combination of high oxygen consumption coupled with a reduced concentration of antioxidant systems [180]. Coincident with the often-tumultuous events characterizing the transitional circulation including the high incidence of hemodynamic instability over the first few days of life, 50 % of GM-IVHs are diagnosed by day 1 and 90 % on day 4 [179]. In fact, the high incidence of pressure-passive cerebral blood flow correlates with the presence of GM-IVH (see Section "Autoregulation of Cerebral Blood Flow") [161]. In the presence of pressure-passive flow and because both the periventricular white matter and the germinal matrix lie within arterial end zones, both areas are at high risk for ischemia during periods of decreased cerebral perfusion and for rupture during periods of increased flow. Reperfusion after ischemia may contribute to excitotoxic injury [181].

Thus, in the presence of disturbed autoregulation, noxious stimuli (e.g., airway suctioning, painful procedures such as surgery), a rapid delivery of intravenous fluids, metabolic disturbances (e.g., hypoglycemia), and hypercarbia [144] may precipitate an acute increase in arterial and/or venous pressures that may contribute to a GM-ICH. In the opposite direction, hypotension from a variety of insults (e.g., asphyxia, anesthetic agents, sepsis, hypocarbia) may cause alternating cycles of decreased cerebral blood flow and reperfusion. Positive pressure ventilation or pneumothorax can abruptly increase central venous pressure, impeding cerebral venous drainage, possibly increasing the risk for venous hemorrhage.

Thus, although PVL (e.g., nonhemorrhagic, symmetrical) and GM-IVH (hemorrhagic, nonsymmetrical) are characterized by distinct pathophysiology, their underlying etiologies overlap and are related to the combination of immature cardio- and cerebrovascular function in the presence of vulnerable anatomy and age-specific metabolic requirements. Not surprising, PVL and GM-IVH are commonly identified on the same MRI.

Cerebellar Injury

In addition to the pervasive neuronal/axonal disturbances involving the cerebral cortex, thalamus, and basal ganglia of newborns secondary to PVL and GM-ICH, the cerebellum has recently been identified as a very vulnerable site for injury. "From 24 weeks to 40 weeks of gestation, the cerebellum undergoes a rate of growth nearly unparalleled elsewhere in the brain" (Fig. 2.9). The surface area of the cerebellar cortex increases more than 30-fold during this time period [103]. Of particular relevance to the preterm infant, cerebellar development accelerates between 20 and 30 weeks of gestation.

As with other neurologic injuries in the neonate, the incidence of insults to the cerebellum is inversely related to gestational age and can be attributed to two etiologies: destructive (hemorrhage/infarction) and impaired development. As in the case of GM-IVH, cerebellar hemorrhage is usually unilateral, with 77 % associated with supratentorial lesions (mostly white matter injury) [103]. Impaired cerebrovascular autoregulation predictably contributes to the pathogenesis. For example, in a group of ex-ELBW infants with cerebral palsy, 64 % (32/50 patients) had parenchymal cerebellar loss which coexisted with cystic PVL and/or cerebral white matter loss, suggesting a common etiology (i.e., ischemia, infection/inflammation) [182]. Destructive lesions can be confined to the cerebellum, and infants can be asymptomatic until delayed development is noted months to years after birth [183]. In those with severe destructive injuries, the impact on function can be significant, including spastic-ataxic-dyskinetic cerebral palsy, severe cognitive deficits, microcephaly, and epilepsy [184].

In other cases, MRIs reveal cerebellar underdevelopment (unilateral or bilateral symmetric deficits in cerebellar volumes) without destructive lesions [185] but in association with supratentorial lesions (i.e., PVL and/or GM-IVH). Injury to granular cells (e.g., secondary to injury from free iron after hemorrhage) [185] is significant not only because of decreasing this population of cells but also because of disturbing the excitatory input to other cells (e.g., Purkinje cells) that disrupts development of the intricate cerebellar circuitry [103]. The association of cerebellar underdevelopment with supratentorial lesions suggests the role of "multiple remote tropic transneuronal interactions" [103]. For example, unilateral PVHI may be associated not only with an expected loss of ipsilateral cerebral volume but also with loss of contralateral cerebellar volume; similarly, unilateral cerebellar hemorrhage is associated not only with decreased ipsilateral cerebellar volume but also with decreased contralateral cerebral volumes. Bilateral primary injury in the cerebrum is associated with secondary bilateral injury in the cerebellum and vice versa. Volpe suggests, "an intact reverberating circuit between cerebrum and cerebellum and vice versa may be especially critical for normal growth during this critical phase of development" [103]. In those with impaired cerebellar development, long-term outcome includes deficits in executive, visual-spatial functions, and language [186]. Others have disturbances of language and socialization [187].

Thus, cerebellar injury is associated with significant neuromotor and intellectual deficits, as well as learning, language. and social behavior deficits. That is, cerebellar injury can result in cognitive and affective disturbances, including socialization difficulties and some positive autism findings [188]. Finally, a "cognitive-affective disorder" (executive, visual-spatial, linguistic, affective deficits) has been described in older children and adults with cerebellar injury [189]. Thus, abnormalities in cerebellar developmental may cause cognitive, language, and socio-affective abnormalities in the ex-premature infant.

Clinical Significance and Summary

Many characteristics of the immature neurologic system predispose the neonate to injury in the predictably labile intraoperative period. Disturbed autoregulation combined with vulnerable populations of cells in the setting of labile hemodynamic and respiratory status in the perinatal period without a reliable system for monitoring cerebral perfusion demands that the neonatal anesthesiologist focus on defining "normal" preoperatively for each infant and attempting to maintain that status intraoperatively. Although easy to recommend, avoiding wide fluctuations in blood pressure, $PaCO_2$, and PaO_2 is frequently difficult but critical to achieve, especially in the intraoperative setting when cardiorespiratory instability is common. Hemorrhage often requires rapid infusions of crystalloid and colloid, which can clearly inflict neurologic injury. NIRS may be of value as a trend monitor, but artifacts are notoriously common.

The Pulmonary System

The transition from fetal to postnatal life requires dramatic adaptation in the physiology of respiration from complete dependency on the placenta to gas exchange via air-filled, perfused lungs within seconds after birth. For premature or asphyxiated infants or in the setting of anomalies associated with cardiorespiratory dysfunction (e.g., congenital diaphragmatic hernia, tracheoesophageal fistula, some types of congenital heart disease), the superimposed effects of surgery, inhalational anesthetics and other medications, positive pressure ventilation, and infection add to the critical short-term challenge of maintaining physiologic stability while minimizing long-term morbidity.

Embryology

The development of the pulmonary system has been divided into five stages (embryonic, pseudoglandular, canalicular, saccular, alveolar) based on morphology [190] (Fig. 2.11). Knowledge of the sequence of developmental events can inform estimates of the timing of congenital malformations [192] associated with fetal-maternal factors (e.g., oligohydramnios), genetic factors, or developmental insults [191].

The Embryonic Stage (0–7 Weeks Gestational Age): At 3–4 weeks gestational age, the laryngotracheal grove first appears as a ventral diverticulum from the primitive foregut, lined by epithelial cells of endodermal origin [192]. During the embryonic stage, the large airways first appear as epithelial cells from the foregut that eventually invade the mesenchyme to form the trachea. This structure then undergoes a series of branching events [193], requiring interaction of epithelial and mesenchymal cells [194]. By the fifth week of gestation, the branching has advanced to the level of lobar and segmental bronchi [193], so that five pulmonary lobes have been formed. By the end of the embryonic stage, the 18 major lobules are easily recognized [195]. Although the airway epithelium resembles that of the esophagus at this stage, over the course of development, differentiation and maturation of the primitive endodermal cells produce the population of epithelial cells that characterize the adult lung [193]. During the embryonic stage, the pulmonary

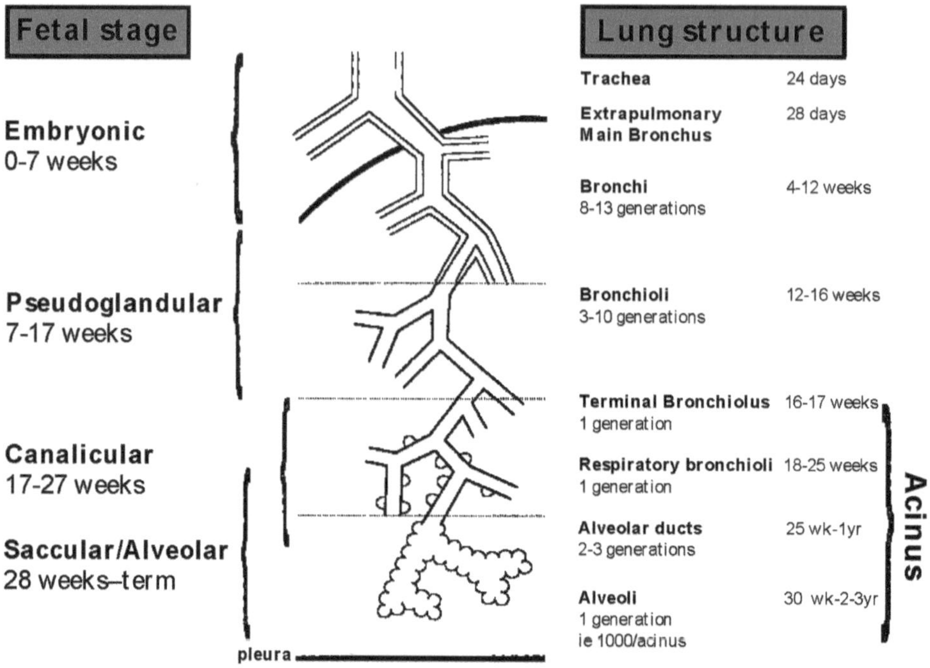

Fig. 2.11 Stages of normal lung development with the airway structure developing within each stage (from Kotecha [191])

vasculature develops in parallel with the airways. At 4 weeks gestational age, endothelial cell precursors around the developing lung bud eventually form endothelial tubes that continuously coalesce to form the intrapulmonary arteries [196]. Congenital malformations associated with events during the embryonic stage involve the large airways and/or whole sections of lung and include pulmonary agenesis, ectopic lobes, lobar cysts, agenesis, malformation, stenosis, or malacia and vascular malformations [192].

Pseudoglandular Stage (7–17 Weeks Gestational Age): The most rapid branching of the airways occurs during the pseudoglandular stage. As the epithelial cells divide, the surrounding mass of gland-like mesenchyme [191, 193] regulates the branching. The mesenchyme inhibits branching in the trachea but induces branching in bronchi [197]. By 14 weeks gestational age, 70 % of the airways present at birth have formed, and by 17 weeks, the conducting airways, terminal bronchioles, and primitive acini are completely established [191]. In parallel with the development of the airways during the pseudoglandular stage, the vascular structures branch rapidly leading to the formation of the pulmonary arteries and veins, which, along with the airways are derived from mesenchymal tissue [192, 196]. Further differentiation of the pseudostratified epithelium of the airway involves its progressive replacement with columnar cells proximally and cuboidal cells distally. Between 11 and 16 weeks gestation, ciliated epithelium appears and airway mucus is first synthesized [193]. The cuboidal cells eventually mature into type II pneumocytes. Insults during this stage of lung growth can alter bronchial growth patterns, producing lesions characterized by poor lung growth (pulmonary hypoplasia), sequestration lesions, and cystic adenomatoid malformations [192].

During this critical period of lung growth, the musculotendinous, dome-shaped diaphragm develops, which, in addition to becoming the primary muscle of respiration, serves to separate the pleural and peritoneal cavities and promote pulmonary growth [198]. At the end of the third week of gestation, the diaphragm consists of a collection of mesodermal tissue, the septum transversum, which separates the pleural-pericardial cavity from the peritoneal cavity. Of note, pleural-peritoneal canals allow limited but persistent communication between these two cavities [198, 199]. The septum transversum migrates downward from the level of the occipital and upper cervical somites (C3) to the level of the thoracic somites by the sixth week of gestation and to the level of L1 by the eighth week [198]. During the descent, the neural tissue of C3–C5 origin penetrates the mesoderm and eventually develops into the phrenic nerve. At approximately this time, the right and left pleuroperitoneal membranes close the communication between pleural and peritoneal cavities [198]. As elucidated in murine models, muscle precursor cells migrate laterally to form the lip of the primitive diaphragm and then radiate throughout the developing diaphragm accompanied by new phrenic nerve branches [199].

Congenital diaphragmatic hernia (CDH) results from failure of complete separation of the pleural and peritoneal cavities. At 10–12 weeks gestation, before the bowel returns to the abdominal cavity from the amnion (where it resides in early gestation), closure of diaphragm is complete. If the separation of the two body cavities is incomplete, the bowel enters the chest, the path of least resistance. However, bowel then occupies space needed for lung growth. A posterolateral CDH (Bochdalek hernia) results from failure of closure of the pleural-peritoneal membranes, accounts for 95 % of diaphragmatic hernias (approximately 1/2,000–1/4,000 live births) [200, 201], and is usually unilateral (78 % on left, 20 % on right, 2 % bilateral) [200] but often is associated with significant ipsilateral pulmonary hypoplasia as well as abnormal development of the contralateral lung [202]. In addition to abnormal lung development, other anomalies not directly related to the hernia often accompany this lesion (e.g., congenital heart disease, central nervous system anomalies) [200]. The etiology of CDH is not completely understood, but genetic associations have been noted (e.g., chromosomal aneuploidy) [203] (for a review, see [204]).

Intrauterine exposure to teratogens affecting the retinoic acid enzyme pathway induces CDH through malformation of the primordial nonmuscular diaphragmatic tissue as early as the fifth to seventh weeks of gestation via a cascade of events that leads to failure of closure of the posterolateral walls in later gestation [199, 205]. Of note, experiments in transgenic mice have induced absence of lung development without CDH, implying that CDH is a primary event [206, 207].

Canalicular Stage (17–27 Weeks): During the canalicular stage, the distal airways develop into primary acini, consisting of respiratory bronchioles, alveolar ducts, and rudimentary alveoli. The surrounding capillaries develop in parallel [195]. These represent the first units of gas exchange.

Epithelial cells differentiate into types I and II pneumocytes, with type I cells incorporated into the first alveolar-capillary barrier. Surfactant can be detected at approximately 24 weeks with active production beginning at 26–28 weeks. After 26 weeks gestation, respiratory saccules lie in close contact with pulmonary capillaries, increasing the likelihood of adequate gas exchange essential for extrauterine viability. Before this developmental age, gas exchange may be compromised because of inadequate surface area and function of the lung parenchyma and/or vasculature [190]. For example, survival after birth during the canalicular stage, in part, is determined by surfactant deficiency (respiratory distress syndrome) (see Respiratory Distress Syndrome, below). Although delivery of exogenous surfactant can improve neonatal lung function, subsequent insults associated with supportive care of the premature infant (e.g., supplemental oxygen, mechanical ventilation, infection) often result in pulmonary hypoplasia or acinar dysplasia [192] and later bronchopulmonary dysplasia.

Saccular Phase (28–36 Weeks Gestation): An increase in the surface area of gas exchange is the major feature of the saccular phase of lung growth [192]. The peripheral areas of the lung enlarge, as the acini dilate and the acinar walls thin. Gas exchange is further facilitated as type II pneumocytes increasingly differentiate into type I cells and capillaries develop in close approximation [195].

Alveolar Phase (36 Weeks Gestation Until ~2–3 Years): During the alveolar phase, the surface area for gas exchange increases as alveoli septate and increase in number, a process that continues through the third year of life [191, 196]. Type II pneumocytes proliferate and become prominent after 34–36 weeks of gestation. The key feature of type II pneumocytes is eosinophilic lamellar bodies, specialized vesicles that store and release surfactant lipids and proteins [208]. At term, the total number of alveoli in the healthy infant is only 20–50 million [195], increasing to adult numbers of more than 300 million per lung, by 2–3 years of age [209, 210]. Developmental abnormalities during the alveolar phase can result in respiratory distress syndrome, chronic lung disease (see below), and dysplasia of the acini or alveolar capillaries [192]. Although rare, several genetic disorders can also adversely affect lung development, such as mutations in the surfactant protein system [195].

The molecular basis of the control of lung development is incompletely understood, but involves many transcription and growth factors in critical roles [192]. In addition, the surrounding mesenchyme appears to direct the developing epithelial cells, and the mesenchymal-epithelium interactions seem to be essential for normal development [195]. A variety of mechanical factors affect lung growth in utero and postnatally [192]. For example, in animal models, inadequate fetal lung fluid secondary to a deficiency of amniotic fluid can induce pulmonary hypoplasia [211, 212]. In humans, pulmonary hypoplasia is prominent in the oligohydramnios sequence ("Potter's syndrome") associated with low urine output secondary to renal dysgenesis [213]. Similarly, oligohydramnios secondary to chronic leakage of amniotic fluid can interfere with lung development [214]. Finally, the role of maintaining adequate lung volume with fluid in promoting lung growth and development during the canalicular and saccular stages is the basis of various fetal therapeutic interventions (e.g., in utero tracheal occlusion) intended to induce lung growth in the presence of CDH [192, 215].

Fetal breathing may contribute to maintaining sufficient lung volume and, therefore, growth of the lung, possibly by activating stretch-mediated release of growth factors [192]. When fetal breathing is ablated in animals, lung growth decreases [216]. Decreased fetal breathing movements may underlie the pulmonary hypoplasia associated with some neurologic disorders, abdominal wall defects, and in utero exposure to certain substances (e.g., chronic exposure to diazepam and possibly maternal smoking) [217]. Although lesions occupying the intrathoracic space (e.g., CDH, congenital cystic adenoid malformations) and skeletal defects involving the thorax can impede lung development secondary to obvious mechanical effects, these anomalies may also impair fetal breathing, which may exacerbate the primary effect of the space-occupying lesion [217].

Postnatal Development of the Lung

Postnatal development of the lung includes the completion of the alveolar stage [218] to achieve airway and microvascular maturation (birth to 2–3 years). That is, alveolar-capillary microarchitecture is transformed from double to single capillary networks [219]. Postnatal therapy with corticosteroids may impair lung growth by arresting this process [192]. Beyond the first two years of life and until late adolescence, the lungs continue to grow via increase in size of both bronchioles and alveoli [220]. Whether late alveolarization continues after the toddler years (and beyond), and by what mechanism, remains controversial [219].

Premature birth and/or infection can severely impact growth of the lung, especially alveolarization [191]. For example, in utero infection (e.g., chorioamnionitis) and markers of lung inflammation have been associated with an increased incidence of chronic lung disease characterized by poor lung development [221, 222]. In addition, the lifesaving supportive therapies (e.g., mechanical ventilation, supplemental oxygen) commonly delivered to the premature infant have been reported to impair normal lung development, resulting in abnormal alveolarization [223]. Specifically, oxidative stress has also been implicated in disorders of lung growth (see Oxygen Therapy, below). Other physiologic events associated with prematurity, such as patent ductus arteriosus and immune dysfunction, are also associated with growth disorders [191]. Similar to the close relationship of the parenchyma and vasculature during normal development, the pulmonary vasculature is co-injured secondary to prematurity and associated treatment. For example, preterm infants with chronic lung disease have increased pulmonary arterial and venous smooth muscle, and infants born before 27 weeks gestation age often develop hypoplasia and dysplasia of the alveolar capillaries [196]. Thus, research in neonatal clinical care is currently focused on minimizing the long-term morbidity of lung injury while providing critical therapies, such as mechanical ventilation and supplemental oxygen [224].

Poor nutrition and environmental exposures such as maternal smoking during pregnancy have been associated with generalized poor growth and risk for prematurity. In addition, maternal smoking has been linked to long-standing respiratory disorders during infancy. These respiratory problems may improve in later childhood, but also are likely to persist into adulthood, becoming apparent as normal aging decreases lung function [225–227]. Both prenatal and postnatal secondhand smoke exposures are linked to structural changes in the developing lung, with altered airway geometry and size, increased wheezing with respiratory infections, as well as variable decreases in forced expiratory flows, possible increases in airway responsiveness and bronchospasm, and increased airway resistance (see [225] for a review).

Airway Anatomy

Neonatal airway anatomy differs from that of adult with significant implications for the anesthesiologist (see Chap. 5, Airway Management). With a relatively large head and prominent occiput, both flexion and hyperextension of the neck may obstruct the small, compliant airway (i.e., easily compressible) [228]. Because of the small diameter of the airways, flow may encounter greater resistance based on the presence of turbulent flow in the upper airways ($R \propto 1/r^5$) and laminar flow in the lower airways (beyond the fifth bronchial division) according to Poiseuille's law: $R \propto (\eta L)/r^4$, where R is airway resistance to flow; η is viscosity; L is length; and r is airway radius. That is, airway resistance varies inversely in proportion to the radius of the airway to the fifth or fourth power in different sections of the tracheobronchial tree. Notably, in the cricoid ring region of the upper airway, a 50 % decrease in the radius of the airway (e.g., airway edema with infection or trauma) increases the airway resistance and the work of breathing to the fifth power or by 36-fold.

Infants have traditionally been described as "obligate nasal breathers" because they often have difficulty maintaining adequate ventilation when the nasal passageways are obstructed secondary to congenital anomalies (e.g., bilateral choanal atresia), with inflammation or infection of the airways, which produce mucosal edema or secretions, and after certain therapeutic maneuvers (e.g., placement of an NG-tube). An alternative descriptor, "preferential nasal breathers," has been proposed, since many neonates with obstructed nasal passages can transition to oral breathing, a process involving activation of the levator veli palatini and musculus uvulae [229]. Nonetheless, in the setting of nasal airway obstruction, oxygen desaturation may occur, and—even after a successful transition to mouth-breathing—respiratory failure due to fatigue may follow [230].

The laryngeal structures of the neonate differ from those of children and adults. Based on observations of castings of cadaveric airways, the shape of the newborn larynx has been traditionally referred to as "funnel shaped," becoming more cylindrical (i.e., adultlike) with growth. However, recent reports of in vivo imaging have noted that the neonatal larynx is in fact cylindrical, similar to those of adults [231–233]. In sedated infants, the glottic opening appears to be the narrowest part of the juvenile upper airway, but the cricoid remains *functionally* the narrowest part of the airway. The confusion may be related to the failure to gate the MRI to respiratory phase when the glottis was filmed. While the rigid ring of cricoid cartilage is unyielding, the vocal cords can be opened gently, from the at-rest position, to accommodate rigid structures, like a tracheal tube [231]. In the neonate, the anterior larynx is more caudal than the posterior larynx, resulting in an elliptical shape, more narrow in the transverse plane than in the anterior–posterior dimension [232, 233]. Forcing a tight-fitting, circular tracheal tube through the subglottis can lead to excessive pressure in the anterior–posterior axis, resulting in mucosal ischemia, subglottic edema, short- or long-term stridor, and airway scarring or stenosis [231].

Other characteristics of the neonatal airway must be considered during endotracheal intubation [234]. The neonate's neck is relatively short and the larynx located more cephalad (C3–C4) (of note, the larynx is more superior, not more "anterior") compared with that in the adult (C4–C6). The narrow epiglottis may be omega or U-shaped and difficult to elevate directly with a laryngoscope blade. The relatively large tongue, soft submandibular structures that are prone to compression by a ventilator's fingers, or cricoid pressure predisposes the neonate to upper airway obstruction. With less cartilage, smooth muscle, and contractile elements, the trachea is more compliant but with greater resistance to flow [235]. Because of a lack of development of the fascia that stabilizes the neck and immaturity of control of the upper airway muscles that stabilize the pharynx, the upper airway of the premature is especially prone to collapse [236].

As in the case of the upper airway, the lower airways are very compliant and readily collapsible, decreasing peak flows and increasing airway resistance and work of breathing. Wheezing may be audible but may or may not be associated with actual bronchospasm. Not surprising, since wheezing is associated with many etiologies other than bronchospasm in the neonate, response to bronchodilators is unpredictable [237].

Anatomy of Chest Wall and Mechanics of Breathing

The chest wall—consisting of the rib cage, abdomen (despite the term "*chest* wall"), and associated musculature—functions both as the respiratory pump and framework for the respiratory system. When compared with older children and adults, the respiratory pump is less efficient in the neonate due to anatomic, mechanical, and histologic factors [238]. The geometry of the pliable rib cage in the neonate is more horizontal compared with the angulated structure in the adult, potentially limiting the outward and cephalad expansion of the thoracic cavity during inspiration [239] (Fig. 2.12).

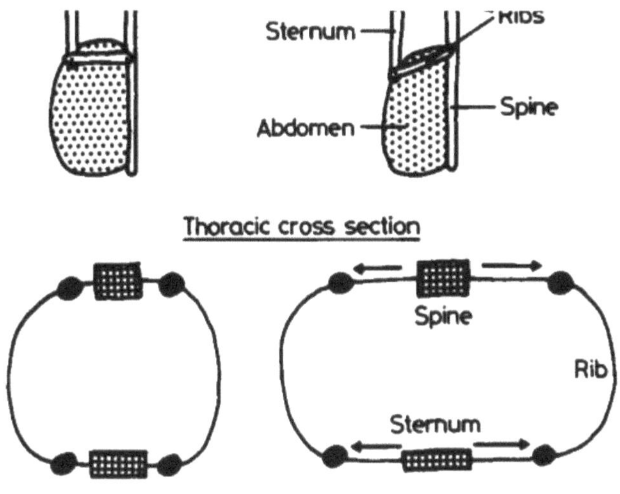

Fig. 2.12 Observed changes in configuration and cross-sectional shape of the thorax from infancy to early childhood. *Upper panel*: infantile and adult rib cage configurations. *Lower panel*: how rib growth at costochondral junctions and posterior rib angles could explain the observed changes in cross-sectional shape of the thorax (from Openshaw et al. [239])

The compliance (C_{CW}) of the cartilaginous chest wall is much greater than lung compliance (C_L) [240]. Although the pliable nature of the chest wall is advantageous during birth, in the postnatal period, this same characteristic introduces several disadvantages. Although C_L primarily determines the compliance of the entire respiratory system (C_{RS}) [241–243], the large C_{CW}:C_L ratio predisposes the neonate to a small resting lung volume [243]. Further, the compliant chest wall deforms inward during spontaneous inspiration, creating inefficient chest wall motion, significantly decreasing the mechanical efficiency of inspiration. That is, distortion of the chest wall wastes energy [240, 244, 245]. As the chest wall matures and stiffens (contemporaneously with the onset of the demands of upright posture), C_{CW} decreases to approximately C_L [240], perhaps mediated through mineralization of the rib cage and/or increased chest wall muscle tone, as suggested by studies in lambs [242, 246].

The respiratory muscles change in conformation, molecular biology, and function during development. During gestation, the respiratory muscles are trained by fetal breathing, so that at the time of term birth, they are ready to power respiration, although with a limited effort reserve [247]. The respiratory pump in the neonate does not tolerate a large respiratory load compared with the adult, and thus it is predisposed to failure [238, 239]. As with other muscle systems, the respiratory muscles, principally the diaphragm, can be characterized in terms of preload, afterload, and intrinsic properties of the fibers. The susceptibility of the neonatal diaphragm and intercostal muscles to respiratory fatigue often is logically attributed to the relative paucity of type I cells [248], p. 203]. That is, type I muscle cells are characterized by slow cycling, aerobic metabolism, resistance to fatigue, and seem well suited for respiratory cycling. The premature infant diaphragm may have less than 10 % type I cells; by term, the proportion increases to ~25–30 %, and through late infancy, the population of type I cells increases to the adult proportion of ~55 % [248], p. 203]. However, when other aspects of structure (e.g., myosin heavy chain isoform (MHC) expression, MHC protein content) and specific function (e.g., maximum specific force, twitch contraction times) were considered, the neonatal diaphragm was actually considered to be more resistant to fatigue [249, pp. 3159–239]. Developmental expression of distinct myosin heavy chain isoforms with less energy demands may actually protect the neonatal diaphragm from fatigue by decreasing energy demands ([249, pp. 3159–239], [250, pp. 3160–240]). Similarly, in a recent study of the diaphragm of the lamb over an extended developmental time period (mid-gestation to 2 months postnatal), the susceptibility to fatigue decreased in late fetal life but was highest at approximately 1 week after full-term delivery [251]. The susceptibility then decreased with increasing postnatal age. Of note, specific force increased twofold during the last 2 weeks before term and correlated with onset of fetal breathing movements. The improved maximum specific force correlated with the rise in MHC content. Similar to earlier studies, the increase in MHC 1 content correlated with increase in oxidative capacity. On the other hand, the in vitro changes in resistance to fatigue must be considered along with the intrinsic properties of the developing diaphragm, including decreased diaphragmatic thickness and less effective force-frequency length-tension, force-velocity functions [252, pp. 3166–241] that may increase the risk of respiratory failure [249, pp. 3159–239]. Clearly, the concept of susceptibility to diaphragmatic fatigue is complex and, in addition to developmental effects on maturation of this muscle, may be affected by the physiologic environment, including hormonal influence (e.g., cortisol, thyroid) and oxidative state (e.g., nutritional status, sepsis, acidosis). The respiratory pump may fail to produce sufficient work to maintain homeostasis, secondary to the intrinsic properties of the muscles of respiration or from unfavorable alterations in preload or afterload [253]. Conditions that affect intrinsic muscle function include metabolic derangements (e.g., electrolyte disturbances), hypoxemia, and shock [253]. Hyper-expansion of the lungs due to air trapping alters preload. Inherent inefficient chest wall mechanics (see above), increased upper airway resistance (due to airway size and propensity to collapse), and changes in lung compliance due to respiratory distress syndrome, pulmonary edema, and other lung disease increase afterload (i.e., work of breathing). The central and peripheral nervous system components that control the respiratory pump can also contribute to respiratory failure (see Control of Respiration, below). Respiratory failure in the neonate can present with respiratory distress (e.g., tachypnea, retractions, use of accessory muscles), hypercapnia/respiratory acidosis, hypoxemia, and/or apnea. In addition to appropriate interventions (e.g., supplemental oxygen, mechanical ventilatory support including continuous positive airway pressure, nutrition), methylxanthines, such as theophylline, are sometimes introduced to improve diaphragmatic function [254, 255].

Functional Residual Capacity

The quantity of gas remaining in the lungs in passive (i.e., with no activity of respiratory muscles) conditions is termed the functional residual capacity (FRC). The magnitude of the FRC results from the net effect of the competing forces of inward lung recoil and outward chest wall elasticity. In neonates, the transpulmonary (intrapleural) pressure at rest is 0 cmH_2O, compared with −5 cmH_2O in adults [256]. With a compliant chest wall, lung volumes at end-expiration during tidal breathing in the neonate approach FRC, creating a significant risk of small airway collapse [257], atelectasis, ventilation-perfusion mismatch, and hypoxemia. To compensate and to preserve FRC dynamically, neonates use several strategies: shortening exhalation via rapid respiratory rates [258], [259], "laryngeal braking" (auto-PEEP mediated by dynamic partial closure of the glottis) [247, 258], tonic activity of intercostal muscles to stabilize the chest wall [247], and, when lung volumes are reduced, grunting [260].

With limited respiratory reserve and a dependance on these dynamic alterations of exhalation to expand the end-expiratory volume above FRC, the neonate is at risk for ventilatory failure from conditions that increase respiratory work or impair neural control of respiration. Such conditions include general anesthesia (with or without neuromuscular blockade), REM (rapid eye movement) sleep [238, 261, 262], systemic infection, and shock. In addition to its effects on intercostal muscle function that contribute to paradoxical, inefficient respiratory movement, central nervous depression relaxes the muscles of the upper airway increasing airway resistance and respiratory work. Decreased FRC and the ensuing atelectasis inflict further demands on the diaphragm, as the reduced lung compliance increases the work of breathing, and energy is required to re-recruit alveoli [243]. Acute lung disease with decreased lung compliance, increased airway resistance (e.g., from airway edema), or decreased diaphragmatic function can exacerbate the effects of anesthesia, sleep, and various neonatal disorders (e.g., infection) and anomalies (e.g., pulmonary hypoplasia). Continuous airway distending pressure (e.g., CPAP) [263] will maintain FRC and mechanical efficiency during anesthesia and sleep in the setting of lung or other disease, including prematurity. Positive pressure ventilation can maintain and restore FRC, especially with PEEP (see Chap. 9, Neonatal Ventilation). A technique rarely used today is application of external negative extrathoracic pressure (−14 to −18 cmH_2O), which increases FRC in premature neonates [264].

Pulmonary Function Testing

Some techniques for pulmonary function testing (PFT) in adults have been adapted to neonates and young infants. Equipment to measure PFTs in neonates must address the smaller tidal volumes and dead space without sacrificing precision or increasing resistance to airflow. Additional challenges include the need to sedate the infants and a paucity of normal reference data as a function of age (Table 2.1) and for various disease states. The techniques adapted to neonates and young infants include whole body plethysmography, gas dilution and occlusion techniques, esophageal manometry, weighted spirometry, and interrupter techniques (for reviews, see [265–268]). Because nasal airway resistance contributes as much as 50 % of total airway resistance, obstruction of the nasal passage by a nasogastric tube can increase airway resistance by 50 %. Therefore, during studies of pulmonary function, tubes should be placed in the smaller nostril to permit maximum flow via the larger passageway [269].

Static volumes and capacities [e.g., FRC and tidal volume (V_t)] are generally similar to adult values when normalized for body mass. Anatomic dead space as a proportion of tidal volume is similar in the neonate and adult (i.e., about 25 % of V_t). Although the additional dead space introduced by airway devices (e.g., LMA) may be negligible in the adult, it is more significant in the neonate, given their smaller anatomic dead space. Closing capacity in the infant (~35 mL/kg) can exceed FRC (~30 mL/kg), leading to airway closure.

Alveolar surface area (VA) is 2.8 m^2 at birth, increasing to 75 m^2 in adults. This increase is related linearly to body surface area [270]. However, since the metabolic rate and consumption of oxygen (VO_2) per body mass is greater in the infant compared with the adult, the ratio of VA to VO_2 is reduced, increasing the infant's risk for impaired gas exchange, especially in the setting of underlying disorders that limit VA, such as pulmonary hypoplasia. Ventilation–perfusion (V–Q) mismatch (i.e., alveolar collapse leading to intrapulmonary shunting) commonly causes hypoxia and shunting that can be quantified by noting the difference between alveolar and arterial oxygen tension (which can also reflect diffusion failure).

V–Q mismatching is exaggerated in infants with lung disease [271]. The increased alveolar ventilation (V-dot A) in neonates (~136–168 mL/kg/min) is approximately 2–3 times that of adults (~60 mL/kg/min) [272–274] reflecting the greater metabolic demand for oxygen (VO_2) (6–10 mL/kg/min vs. ~3.5 mL/kg/min for the resting adult) and greater production of CO_2. Increased oxygen demand coupled with atelectasis and intrapulmonary shunting causes the rapid development of hypoxemia when apnea occurs (within ~30 s) [275], a finding with significant implications for induction of anesthesia (e.g., rapid sequence induction in the presence of a "full stomach").

Minute ventilation increases with either a greater V_t or respiratory frequency (f) or both. For a given alveolar ventilation, the optimal f and V_t minimizes the expenditure of energy [276, 277]. Although V_t per body mass in the neonate approximates that of adults, the normal respiratory rate is greater in the neonate (30–60 breaths/min) compared with the adult (18–22 breaths/min). That is, the work of breathing to achieve adequate minute ventilation in the healthy neonate is minimized at this increased respiratory rate [256, 278, 279]. Despite this strategy, the neonate (especially the premature infant) expends a larger portion of total body oxygen consumption on ventilation (i.e., the oxygen cost of breathing) than does the adult. This phenomenon is exaggerated in the setting of lung disease [280, 281].

Table 2.1 Typical values of lung function in healthy individuals

Parameter	Preterm	Newborn	1 year	7 year	Adult
Body weight (kg)	1	3	10	25	70
Crown-heel length (cm)	35	50	75	120	175
Respiratory rate (min^{-1})	60	45	30	20	15
Tidal volume (mL)	7	21	70	180	500
Anatomic dead space (mL)	3	6	20	50	150
Maximal flow at FRC (mL s^{-1})	80	150	300	–	–
FRC (mL)	25	85	250	750	2,100
Lung compliance (mL kPa^{-1})	15	50	150	500	2,100
Airway resistance (kPa L^{-1} s)	8	4	1.5	0.4	0.2
Specific compliance (kPa^{-1})	0.6	0.6	0.6	0.7	0.8
Specific conductance (s^{-1} kPa^{-1})	5	2.9	2.7	2.7	2.3

Divide compliance, and specific compliance by 10 to obtain values in cmH_2O, multiply resistance by 10 to obtain values as $cmH_2O\ L^{-1}$ s; divide specific conductance by 10 to obtain values in s^{-1} cmH_2O^{-1}

In the neonate, increased alveolar ventilation and constant FRC compared with adults lead to a smaller FRC "buffer" [282]. However, changes in inspiratory gas composition (e.g., oxygen, anesthetic gases) will be reflected in changes in the alveolar and plasma gas concentrations more rapidly.

Pulmonary Surfactant

Endogenous pulmonary surface-active agent, or "pulmonary surfactant," maintains lung volumes. This foamy, bubble-producing substance is a complex aggregation of macromolecules that reduces alveolar surface tension, decreases the tendency of alveolar units to become atelectatic, and increases pulmonary compliance [283, 284]. At approximately 20 weeks gestation, mechanical forces related to fetal breathing stimulate expression of genes that code for the expression of surfactant [285]. However, the quantity of surfactant is reliably sufficient to support spontaneous ventilation only after 32 weeks gestation, without medical intervention. In some premature infants (most commonly, <32 weeks gestational age), inadequate surfactant production manifests as respiratory distress syndrome (see below). Fetal lung maturity is estimated by the ratio of the lecithin to sphingomyelin surfactant components, in amniotic fluid (the L:S ratio). This ratio provides prognostic information of the neonate's expected pulmonary status. An L:S ratio >2.0 is associated with a reduced risk of RDS, whereas a ratio <2.0 is associated with an increased risk of RDS [286]. Hereditary defects in surfactant structure or the surfactant metabolism cycle can cause fatal (e.g., hereditary SP-B deficiency) or chronic lung disease, such as protein alveolar proteinosis [208]. Surfactant impairment has been implicated in a number of lung diseases beyond the neonatal period, including the adult respiratory distress syndrome.

Type II pneumocytes serve several critical functions in alveoli including as the progenitors of type I pneumocytes (the major population of the alveolar epithelium) to repair the epithelium after injury and to produce and secrete surfactant [208]. Surfactant is stored within characteristic organelles termed lamellar bodies, which are released by merocrine secretion, eventually forming a monolayer over the alveolar surface, reducing surface tension at the alveolar air-water interface [287]. Various configurations of surfactant are observed, such as tubular myelin, droplets, and the monolayer film, each serving to support specific functions including spreading throughout the alveoli, forming a monolayer, acting as reserve surfactant when the monolayer is disrupted (e.g., by oxidation), resisting compression during exhalation, and rapid reabsorption [288]. The local environment (such as the changing physical forces during the respiratory cycle and calcium concentration) and the composition of various phospholipids and surfactant-associated proteins (SPs) that compose a particular surfactant molecule [208, 287] influence the phases of surfactant. Thus, a complex pathway of highly regulated recycling or degradation (by alveolar macrophages) has evolved to allow for the energy and substrate intensive activity of this critical molecule [208]. Approximately 85 % of the components of surfactant are recycled via reuptake into type II pneumocytes [289–292].

Surfactant is an emulsion of lipids (~90 %), proteins (~10 %), and carbohydrates [293]. Most lipids are phospholipids (PLs) including the phosphatidylcholines (PCs) such as dipalmitoylphosphatidylcholine (DPPC), which comprises 40–45 % (by mass) of mammalian surfactant [287]. A heterogeneous mixture of lipids is necessary to convey the necessary properties of rapid spreading over the alveolar (water phase) surface and resistance to compression [294]. A variety of functions have been identified for the surfactant proteins (SP-A, SP-B, SP-C, and SP-D) [295]. SP-B and SP-C are small, hydrophobic proteins that interact closely with the surfactant lipids to reduce surface tension and stabilize surfactant when exposed to the changing mechanical forces of the respiratory cycle [296]. SP-A and SP-D are larger proteins, members of the Collectins family that bind infectious particles in the lung, facilitating immune cell recognition and clearance of pulmonary pathogens. Not only are these proteins important for the innate immune system of the lung, but in mouse models, they modulate alveolar macrophage activity. SP-A and SP-D may regulate surfactant uptake, but the precise roles of these proteins in this capacity are still being elucidated [293, 297].

Surface tension as modeled as a sphere is described by Laplace's law $P = 2\gamma/r$, where P is the intra-alveolar pressure or "collapse pressure" of the alveolus (i.e., the pressure necessary to counteract the contracting molecular forces produced at the air/fluid interface—the inward force acting to shorten the radius of the sphere, promoting collapse) [298]. This law states that the distending pressure is proportional to surface tension (γ) and inversely related the radius of the alveolus (r). During inspiration, alveolar radii generally increase due to forces generated by the respiratory pump, and therefore collapse pressure tends to decrease. At the end of expiration, significant distending pressure would be needed to prevent alveolar collapse without the effects of surfactant. In films lining the alveolus, surfactant can produce large surface pressures, decreasing the contracting force of surface tension. When alveoli are large, the surfactant monolayer is spread thinly over the alveolus, and because of the large radius, the effect of surfactant is not critical [299]. When alveoli are small (e.g., during exhalation), surfactant is compressed, further reducing surface tension in the setting of a small radius. Thus, surfactant acts to buffer surface tension over a large range of alveolar sizes.

However, alveoli do not operate in isolation and, instead, are organized into groups of acini [300]. The lung parenchyma, including the alveoli themselves, directly influences adjacent airways through traction [301]. At large lung volumes, such as those induced by positive pressure ventilation, the alveolar surface area to lung volume ratio is independent of surface tension (dependent instead on tissue interactions) [302]. In this case, 876, the beneficial effect of surfactant therapy may be masked by the artificially augmented lung volumes [287]. In the macro perspective, alveolar and airway collapse are counteracted by the outwardly acting elastic recoil of the lung and chest wall, as well as the active respiratory control mechanisms described above.

Respiratory Distress Syndrome

Neonatal respiratory distress syndrome (RDS), also known as hyaline membrane disease, results from insufficient surfactant production most often associated with prematurity, but can occur when surfactant release or synthesis is delayed, as with infants of diabetic mothers, or with secondary inactivation of surfactant, as in meconium aspiration syndrome. The clinical features of untreated RDS result from poor lung compliance, increased work of breathing, loss of FRC, V–Q mismatch, poor gas exchange, right-left shunting via the ductus arteriosus and/or patent foramen ovale, and lung injury from barotrauma and volumetric trauma, oxidative injury, and inflammation [303]. The presentation of RDS includes tachypnea or apnea, retractions, grunting, hypoxemia, and respiratory and metabolic acidosis. The typical appearance of RDS on chest radiograph is a diffuse pattern of reticulogranular, or ground glass, opacities and air bronchograms representing air-filled large airways surrounded by atelectatic alveoli [304]. Symptoms tend to worsen for several days after birth, followed by improved respiratory function as endogenous surfactant production increases. The infant with RDS is at risk of serious complications associated with positive pressure ventilation (e.g., chronic lung disease, pneumothorax, infection), comorbidities (such as sepsis), and prematurity [e.g., injuries to other organ systems including the brain (see Section "CNS")]. Neonates may present in the immediate postpartum period, since effective surfactant function is critical to establishing a gas-filled FRC during the first few breaths after birth.

The severity of pulmonary complications associated with RDS, such as chronic lung disease, has been reduced by exogenous surfactant, either synthetic or animal derived, delivered via a tracheal tube [305]. Commonly, transient hypoxemia may follow bolus delivery of surfactant. Obstruction of the tracheal tube, pulmonary hemorrhage, and inadvertent volutrauma (after compliance has improved) rarely complicates surfactant administration [306]. Symptoms and radiographic findings generally improve within hours [304]. The optimal dosing regimen (e.g., prophylactic vs. early rescue therapy; number and timing of doses) has yet to be confirmed [306]. Currently, the standard regimen consists of two doses of betamethasone 24 h apart, within 7 days prior to delivery, for fetuses 24–34 weeks gestational age [307]. Other treatment protocols for RDS include early introduction of nasal CPAP (nCPAP) in the delivery room in an effort to avoid intubation and the potentially injurious effects of positive pressure ventilation [308].

Treating the preterm fetus in utero via maternally administered steroids (betamethasone) accelerates lung maturation and increases the production and release of surfactant [309]. Of note, administering antenatal steroids provides an additive effect to that of exogenous surfactant in reducing the pulmonary sequelae associated with RDS, as compared with surfactant administration alone. In addition, a reduced incidence of IVH seems to be associated with the combination [305].

Despite advances in nursery care over the past several decades, approximately 20 % of infants with RDS will develop chronic lung disease, specifically bronchopulmonary dysplasia (BPD), characterized by persistent need for oxygen at 28 days of life [310], with grading of BPD at 36 weeks of gestation (for infants born <32 weeks gestation). BPD in the age of surfactant therapy differs from classic or "old" BPD, which was common in relatively mature premature infants who had been subjected to high levels of positive pressure ventilation and oxygen therapy [311]. Old BPD is characterized by alternating sites of hyperinflation (presumably areas of lung with normal compliance exposed to positive pressure ventilation) and atelectasis, extensive fibrotic areas, and severe epithelial and endothelial lesions [312]. "New" BPD develops in infants treated with modern RDS therapy (e.g., "gentle ventilation"), is most commonly seen in ELBW infants, and has different pathologic findings including enlarged, simplified alveoli, with some interstitial thickening [313]. New BPD appears to be a developmental disorder that results from disruptions in lung growth caused by factors other than a deficiency of surfactant [314]. Although neonates with the new BPD may have a more benign pulmonary presentation in the nursery, many develop a non-asthmatic obstructive airway disease as infants or children which has the potential to complicate ventilatory support, anesthetic care, and the postoperative course [311]. Although the long-term prognosis of new BPD has not been completely defined, the early disruption in normal lung growth and development may predispose to decreased respiratory reserve that may lie dormant until later life, becoming apparent when added to the expected decline in lung function associated with the aging process, smoking, or other respiratory insult [315].

Oxygen Toxicity

Although an essential metabolic substrate for human life, oxygen can also be toxic to the neonate through the creation of reactive oxygen species (ROS) [316]. ROS act as second messengers, and transcription factors important in growth and development are critical for immune function and regulate vascular beds including the ductus arteriosus [317]. However, exposure to ROS can also be harmful, leading to the release of mitochondrial cytochrome C and other apoptotic factors, degrading signal transduction, directly altering proteins and impairing protein synthesis, modifying nucleic acids including DNA base and strand injury, and affecting cell growth and development. Several mechanisms (thiol compounds such as thioredoxin and glutathione, uric acid, bilirubin, anti-oxyenzymes) maintain reduction-oxidation homeostasis [316, 317].

Eukaryotic life has evolved mechanisms to manage hypoxic environments, but not hyperoxia, as the atmospheric concentration of oxygen throughout evolution has been similar to or less than the current concentration [318]. In addition, during normal fetal development in utero, the expected environment is one of physiologic hypoxia compared with postnatal life, including the nearly anoxic conditions of the zygote, to late gestation, in which the PaO_2 reaches only 20–30 mmHg. Humans have evolved mechanisms to tightly regulate oxygen levels, both at the macro level (carotid body reflexes) and at the cellular/mitochondrial level, likely involving the hypoxia-inducible factor 1 (HIF-1) [318]. This protein complex interacts with erythropoietin and governs a range of responses to hypoxia including the shift from aerobic to anaerobic metabolism [319, 320]. Animal studies have demonstrated a role for HIF-1 in the activation of gene products important for angiogenesis (via VEGF), stem cells proliferation, and CNS and pulmonary alveolar development (via the related HIF-2α) [318]. Exposure to oxygen decreases HIF activity, affecting developmental signaling, and, in that way, impacting the growth trajectory of the premature neonate developing ex utero [318]. At birth, the infant's oxygen tension rapidly increases and may reach extreme levels if the FIO_2 is greater than 0.21. That is, the increase in pO_2 arrives during a period of critical growth for the premature infant, who, if developing in utero would be in a "hypoxic" milieu.

The effect of oxygen in the pathogenesis of retinopathy of prematurity (ROP) has long been recognized secondary to the obvious impairment of visual acuity. Although factors other than hyperoxia contribute to both the development and severity of ROP, the role of oxygen has been linked to the effects of changes induced in VEGF levels in the developing retina. In addition to toxicity in the retina, recent research has highlighted the potentially deleterious effects of oxygen on other organ systems after only a brief exposure (e.g., during neonatal resuscitation). In multiple systematic reviews, resuscitation with 100 % oxygen caused oxidative stress in animals [321–324] and humans [325]; neurologic injury in animals [326] and humans [327]; inflammation in the lung, heart, and brain in animals [328–330]; increased pulmonary vascular resistance and smooth muscle reactivity in animals [331]; kidney and cardiac cellular injury in humans [332]; and increased neonatal mortality [327, 333, 334].

Clinical guidelines for neonatal resuscitation have changed radically over the past decade as international and national associations have reacted to the mounting evidence of toxicity associated with excessive oxygen administration. Recommendations for resuscitation now include using preductal pulse oximetry to guide the administration of oxygen, recognizing the critical role of establishing adequate ventilation, not hyperoxia, in the transition to extrauterine life [335, 336]. For the first 5–10 min of life, the hemoglobin oxygen saturation of the healthy term neonate is frequently <90 % (Fig. 2.13). For this reason, if an infant responds to the initial ventilatory support, 100 % oxygen is best avoided. In most studies, premature infants who receive supplemental oxygen titrated to achieve oxygen saturations <93 % SpO_2 have a reduced incidence of ROP and lung injury compared with those maintained at excessive oxygen saturations (e.g., 95–98 %) [338, 339]. Still, the optimal targets for SpO_2 during long-term nursery care have yet to be clarified. Although the toxic effects of hyperoxia are now widely recognized, an ongoing study has suggested that the mortality in extremely premature infants is increased when the targeted SpO_2 is 85–89 % versus 91–95 % [340].

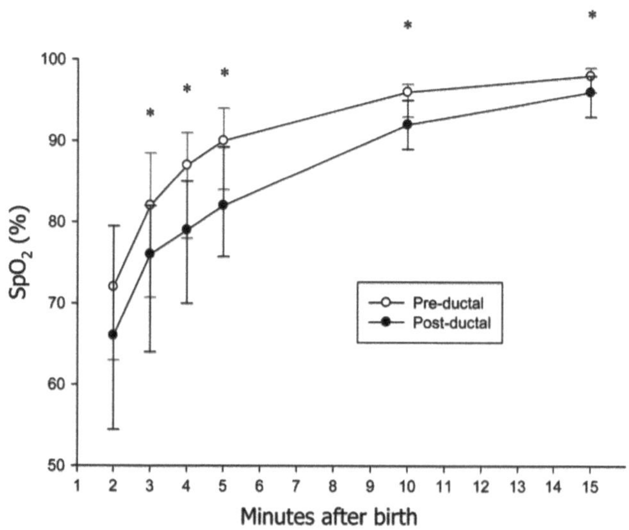

Fig. 2.13 Pre- and post-ductal SpO_2 levels in healthy term infants during the first 15 min after birth (median; IQR) Post-ductal SpO_2 levels were significantly lower than pre-ductal SpO_2 levels at 3, 4, 5, 10, and 15 min. $*P \leq 0.05$. Pre-ductal SpO_2 measured on right hand; post-ductal on one foot (from Mariani et al. [337]) lung early SpO_2

Control of Ventilation

Immature central nervous system control of ventilation may play a role in neonatal apnea and bradycardia [341] as well as postoperative apnea [342]. The process of maturation of the respiratory control responses begins in fetal life but continues after birth. For example, as discussed above, fetal breathing plays a critical role in lung growth and training of the respiratory pump. Although some aspects of fetal respiratory behavior persist postnatally, the responses of the healthy term neonate to hypoxia and hypercarbia and other respiratory stimuli are more appropriate [343]. In early gestation, fetal breathing is continuous and apparently under control of the spinal cord; as development progresses, fetal breathing is controlled more centrally and, by the third trimester, is a complex behavior that varies with sleep stage (e.g., in fetal lambs, breathing is inhibited during non-REM sleep by brainstem inhibitory nuclei) [343, 344]. In animals, hypercapnia stimulates the depth of fetal breathing [345–348]. Similar responses are present in the human fetus after 24 weeks gestation [348]. As is the case in adults, reduced CO_2 tension decreases fetal breathing. In contrast, hypoxemia also decreases fetal breathing. One hypothesis suggests that in the setting of limited access to oxygen, the fetus eliminates respiratory effort to decrease oxygen consumption when "breathing" does not contribute to gas exchange [343]. Both decreasing fetal breathing and gasping are signs of fetal distress, are a component of the obstetrical "biophysical profile," and correlate with abnormal fetal well-being [349–351]. After delivery, inhibition of breathing movements is life-threatening and must be reversed as the neonate now depends on pulmonary gas exchange for survival. The exact mechanism by which these pathways are reversed is unknown [343].

Although more mature than in utero, the neonate's responses to hypercapnia, hypoxemia, and afferent stimulation remain impaired, especially for preterm infants. The immature, central-chemoreceptor-mediated hypercapnic ventilatory response has a relatively flat slope in the neonatal period; with increased postnatal and gestational age, the slope increases toward adult values [352]. In animal studies, the immature ventilatory response to CO_2 is reflected in the failure to increase respiratory rate, although both immature and mature animals increase tidal volume in response to hypercarbia [353] (see Fig. 2.14). The origin of the diminished response to hypercapnia in the premature infant has been attributed to dysfunction of the central nervous system [343]. However, premature infants with a history of apnea exhibit a blunted ventilatory response curve to CO_2 with a slope that is even less than that exhibited by similar preterm infants without apnea [354–356].

The ventilatory response to hypoxia is also immature in the preterm infant. Hypoxic preterm infants and term babies less than 1 week of age respond to hypoxia with 1–2 min of increased ventilation. However, unlike adults and most term infants older than a few weeks who sustain this response, the ventilatory effort of premature infants and term infants during the first week of life then wanes to less than baseline, a phenomenon termed "hypoxic ventilatory depression" (HVD) [343, 357, 358]. The first phase of the response to hypoxia is likely mediated by peripheral chemoreceptor located in the carotid body as denervation of the carotid bodies in animals abolishes this reflex [358]. In animal studies, the initial increase in ventilation is characterized by an increase in tidal volume with a gradual decrease in respiratory rate. In the second phase, HVD, the increased tidal volume is preserved, but the respiratory rate continues to decrease, resulting in a net decrease in minute ventilation [359].

The mechanism of HVD is not fully elucidated [360] but is thought to be related to CNS descending inhibitory tracts as suggested by animal studies in which lesions in the pons resulted in less depression [361]. Many neurotransmitters have been implicated in this central response to hypoxia, including adenosine, endorphins, GABA, and an imbalance between neurokinin-1 and mu-opioid receptors, as pharmacologic modulation of these substances also resolves HVD [343, 362]. Further support for the central origin of HVD includes the finding that hypoxia, in near-term infants, shifts the CO_2 response curve to the right and decreases the slope (i.e., hypoxia blunts the CNS response to hypercapnia) [363].

Reflexes mediated by afferents in the airway, lungs, and chest wall that regulate ventilation are also immature in the preterm and young infant. For example, in preterm infants, mechanical or chemical stimulation of the larynx decreases ventilation and, in extreme cases, produces apnea [364]. Based on data from animals, the mechanism is associated with superior laryngeal nerve inhibitory stimulation leading to either decreased respiratory center activity or enhancement of CNS inhibition/expiratory pathways [365, 366].

The Hering–Breuer *inflation* reflex, a respiratory control mechanism observed in neonates, especially the preterm [367] that consists of inhibition of ventilation by lung *inflation*, is mediated by the slowly adapting pulmonary stretch receptors (SARs), disappears during REM sleep, and fades during the first few weeks of life. The Hering–Breuer reflex may stabilize ventilation in face of changing elastic loads [368].

A closely related phenomenon, the paradoxical reflex of Head, occurs when lung inflation triggers a large inspiratory effort resulting in a large lung volume and provides a rare example of a physiologic positive feedback mechanism. The reflex is accompanied by tonic inspiratory contractions [369, 370], which can be elicited in neonates via a forced inhalational maneuver with positive pressure [371], and is mediated by the rapid adapting stretch receptors (RARs) (also responsible for so-called Hering–Breuer *deflation* reflex in which rapid *deflation* of the lungs stimulates inspiration). The paradoxical reflex of Head may play a role in establishing the FRC during the transition from fetal life [371] and/or maintaining the lung volume in the setting of the compliant chest wall of the neonate [372].

Apnea of the Newborn

The immaturity of respiratory control and the mechanical properties of the preterm infant's respiratory system predispose to disorders of breathing, such as neonatal apnea. The definition of apnea of prematurity varies, but one common description is a pause in breathing for greater than 20 s or shorter pauses accompanied by clinical evidence of hypoxia such as cyanosis or bradycardia [373]. However, apneic events <20 s in duration can lead to clinical signs of hypoxia; conversely apneic events up to 30 s may be observed in healthy term babies. Apnea in neonates is classified according to the mechanism of dysfunction: *obstructive*, *central* (without respiratory drive), and—the most common—*mixed* apnea, with features of both obstruction and pauses in respiratory effort [365].

Apnea may be accompanied by bradycardia (so-called As and Bs)—with or without hemoglobin desaturation, suggesting that a common pathway (e.g., vagal inhibition) may contribute to both phenomena [365]. With hemoglobin desaturation, direct carotid body effects may lead to further bradycardia; the net result is decreased oxygen delivery (Fig. 2.15).

Apnea of the newborn, especially the premature infant, accompanies a wide variety of abnormalities such as sepsis, intracerebral hemorrhage, anemia, patent ductus arteriosus, neurologic abnormalities, airway anomalies, or other systemic illness. Standard therapy for apnea of prematurity includes caffeine—likely through direct CNS stimulation via blockade of inhibitory neurons—and continuous positive airway pressure that is often achieved using high flow nasal cannula [341]. Although a Cochrane review reported that caffeine significantly reduced the risk of postanesthetic apnea, the number of patients studied was small, and the report lacked detailed information about the severity of apneic events. Thus, caffeine is not routinely recommended for growing preterm infants without significant apnea [374].

Apnea due to immaturity should be differentiated from other breathing patterns of the neonate. For example, periodic breathing is a common, physiologic pattern that includes short pauses in respiration interspersed with high frequency ventilation attributed to discoordination in the feedback control mechanisms of the respiratory control center and generally resolving by one month of age in the term neonate [375, 376]. Apnea is associated with anesthesia and surgery in the preterm, term, and ex-premature infant, with the risk in ex-preterm infants from 5 to 49 % [342, 377–379]. Apnea secondary to anesthesia may be related to inhibition of central respiratory centers, decreased respiratory pump efficiency, and impaired V–Q matching. Factors associated with the risk for postoperative apnea include postconceptional and gestational age, history of apnea, anemia (commonly seen in the former preterm infant), neurologic disease (e.g., history of intraventricular hemorrhage), chronic lung disease, and requirement for oxygen [380]. Postanesthetic apnea has been commonly evaluated in the setting of inguinal herniorrhaphy, since inguinal hernias are more common in preterm infants and are commonly repaired before hospital discharge to avoid the risk of incarceration [377]. Although the use of regional and neuraxial anesthetics in this population has been proposed to obviate postoperative apnea [380], a Cochrane review in 2003 found insufficient evidence to recommend regional anesthetics in place of general anesthesia [381]. Preventing postanesthetic apnea depends on identifying who should be monitored postoperatively;

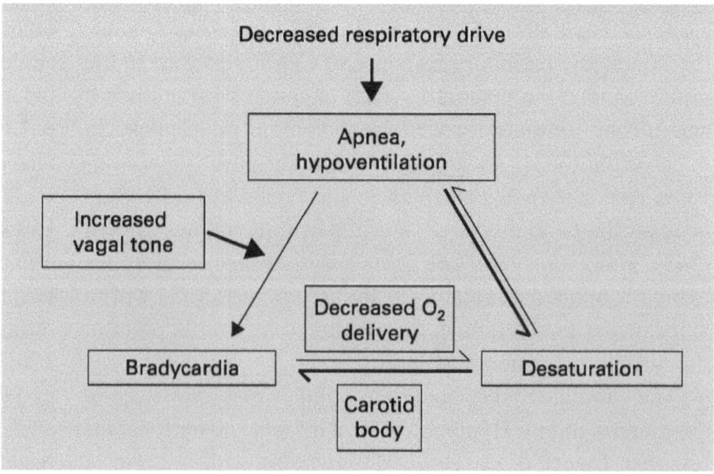

Fig. 2.15 A schematic representation of the sequence of events whereby apnea (or hypoventilation) results in various combinations of desaturation and bradycardia (from Martin and Abu-Shaweesh [365])

ex-premature infants <60 weeks postconceptional age should be monitored for respiration and hemodynamics after anesthesia until they are at least 12 h apnea free (see [380] for proposed algorithms).

Hepatic Function

Although the liver plays a critical role in fetal metabolism, the placenta and maternal liver manage a significant proportion of hepatic function in utero. However, shortly after birth, the neonatal liver must assume the same metabolic roles performed by the adult liver, a process largely completed within hours. Understanding the differences between fetal and neonatal versus adult hepatic physiology is a requisite for the provision of optimal care to the neonate.

Anatomy

The liver's unique architecture and cellular composition reflects its central role in metabolism, as well as hemostasis, hormonal regulation, biosynthesis, and clearance. In postnatal life, the liver has dual blood supplies. The hepatic artery carries richly oxygenated, arterial blood to the liver. The portal vein delivers a variety of substances from the digestive tract, including digested food products (e.g., free fatty acids, amino acids, glucose), as well as large proteins, gut-derived hormones (e.g., glucagon), microorganisms, and immune cells and signaling molecules [382]. The canaliculi are a network of tubules, joined by tight junctions, that coalesce to form ducts, through which bile is actively secreted and, under positive pressure, flows from the biliary tree into the small intestines [383]. Because of their unique anatomy, hepatocytes simultaneously communicate with the blood (hepatic artery/portal vein) and gut (canaliculi). Thus, these cells function as intermediaries between the gut, placenta, and bloodstream. Hepatocytes process absorbed nutrients, respond to gut hormones, and clear endogenous (e.g., damaged hemoglobin) and exogenous substances (e.g., drugs) from the blood, sometimes via the biliary tree. Disruption of these activities (e.g., with sepsis) can lead to cholestasis, hepatocyte injury, and giant cell hepatitis [382].

In Utero Development

The characteristic histologic features of the heterogenous liver parenchyma—including sinusoids and canaliculi secured by tight junctions with hepatocytes straddling the spaces between—are formed by a set of complex processes, including apoptosis, morphogenic signaling, proliferation, and polarization of hepatocytes, involving cells from many embryologic tissue types [382]. At approximately the third to fourth week of gestation, the hepatic diverticulum arises from endodermal epithelia of the posterior foregut. These primitive pre-hepatocytes fold into mesodermal mesenchymal cells of the diaphragm forming a mixed population of cells of endodermal and mesodermal origin [384]. Under the control of a host of transcription factors, endodermal stem cells differentiate into progenitor cells which then are committed to become either bile ducts or hepatocytes [382, 385, 386], while mesodermal cells form blood vessels, Kupffer cells, sinusoidal endothelium, and fibrous, connective tissue. Meanwhile, the precursors of the hepatic and portal venous systems are formed from the yolk sack [387]. Populations of cholangiocytes further differentiate into the intrahepatic and extrahepatic portions of the biliary tree. A variety of transcription factors have been identified in the morphogenesis pathway of the biliary tree [385, 386].

The common bile duct first appears as a connection between the hepatic bud and duodenum, and the gallbladder and cystic duct emerge as outgrowths. For the first three months of gestation, the extrahepatic bile ducts are occluded with endodermal cells. Biliary atresia can develop if these ducts do not recannulate, sometimes leading to liver failure as early as in the first months of life (see biliary atresia, below). Similarly, interrupting the formation of patent intrahepatic bile ducts also can present as liver failure during infancy. For example, Alagille syndrome is characterized by a paucity of intralobular bile ducts as well as cardiovascular, ocular, vascular, and vertebral anomalies [388]. A genetic association in Alagille syndrome involves Jag-1 and the NOTCH signaling pathway, which has been found to regulate the formation of intrahepatic ducts in mice [389–392]. Disruption of other signaling pathways have been associated with a variety of hepatic disorders such as alpha-1 antitrypsin deficiency, cystic fibrosis, Gilbert's disease, Dubin-Johnson syndrome, and Zellweger syndrome [382].

In the human, bilirubin can be detected by approximately 14 weeks gestational age. In contrast to postnatal life, the placenta removes most bilirubin in utero, with fetal hepatic-biliary pathways eliminating only a small amount (see Jaundice and Hyperbilirubinemia below). The human placenta permits bidirectional transit of unconjugated bilirubin [393]. In animal models, the placenta efficiently clears bilirubin from the umbilical artery [394] and from the amniotic fluid [395].

By end of the first month of gestation in the human, primitive hepatocyte function (protein synthesis and secretion) can be detected [396, 397]. In early fetal life, the major circulating protein is α-fetoprotein. Beginning at 5–6 weeks of gestation and through the second trimester, the liver enlarges 40-fold to assume the primary role of hematopoiesis [398]. In early gestation, the liver contains more hematopoietic cells than hepatocytes. By the third trimester, the bone marrow becomes the principle site of blood cell production, but extramedullary hematopoiesis continues in the liver until after birth [398].

At approximately two to three months of gestation, albumin synthesis begins, and adult serum concentrations are achieved by term. Glycogen synthesis starts by the tenth week of gestation, and by 12 weeks, bile is secreted at a rate to approximately 50–60 % of the level of adults [382].

Early Postnatal Hepatic Function: Anatomy

Throughout gestation, the fetus receives nutrients from the placenta via the umbilical vein, regulated by complex active and selective transport mechanisms for sugars, amino acids, fats, and molecules [399]. Before birth, the liver receives approximately 50 % of umbilical venous blood, with the remainder shunting through the ductus venous, flowing directly into the inferior vena cava and the right atrium. This shunt serves to stream oxygen-rich blood from the right atrium through the foramen ovale into the left-sided circulation and brain and may increase during periods of hypoxemia [400]. The liver receives variable amounts of the oxygen-rich blood flow, with most of the blood flow directed to the left lobe, but 50 % of that to the right lobe is also supplied by the umbilical vein. The remainder of blood supply to the right lobe is primarily derived from the portal circulation [401] (Fig. 2.3).

When the umbilical cord is clamped, the liver no longer receives nutrient and oxygen-rich blood from the placenta. Instead, the portal vein becomes the primary source for nutrients from the gut, and the hepatic artery provides arterial blood with significantly greater oxygen content. After meals, the portal venous flow increases, providing twice the blood flow of the hepatic artery. The ductus venous functionally closes over the first two postnatal weeks [402]. One-quarter of the neonate's cardiac output is directed to the liver. The liver in the neonate comprises 4 % of the body weight compared with only 2 % in the adult, reflecting its critical function in the former [382].

Early Postnatal Hepatic Function: Synthesis

Without a continuous supply of maternal substrates from the umbilical vein, the neonate must maintain glucose homeostasis from sources of digested food, glycogenolysis, and gluconeogenesis. Until feeding is established, glycogen that has been stored mainly in the liver and heart during the third trimester is broken down into glucose under the hormonal regulation of glucagon and catecholamines. Stress during delivery or due to illness can accelerate depletion of glycogen stores, which may lead to hypoglycemia. Of note, because they are deprived of glycogen that is synthesized and stored during late gestation, premature infants are particularly predisposed to hypoglycemia. In addition, glucose consumption per body mass is greater in the premature infant compared with the term, primarily secondary to greater metabolic requirements, primarily by the brain [403]. Although key enzymes are expressed in the fetus, gluconeogenesis may not be active during fetal life. However, within 4–6 h of birth, gluconeogenesis plays an important role in glucose homeostasis [404] even in premature infants [405].

Neonates who cannot tolerate adequate enteral caloric substrates must receive exogenous glucose support, usually intravenously, to prevent hypoglycemia (serum glucose of 40–90 mg/dL) (see Chap. 8). The neonate including the premature infant responds to increased concentrations of circulating glucose by producing insulin, which promotes the uptake of glucose either for immediate energy or for storage (as triglycerides or glycogen). Of importance, abruptly decreasing or discontinuing an exogenous source of glucose (e.g., discontinuing intravenous alimentation, separation from the placental delivery of high glucose concentrations during gestational diabetes, prolonged *NPO* period without an intravenous source of glucose) increases the risk for hypoglycemia. Other risk factors for hypoglycemia include liver dysfunction (e.g., shock or sepsis) and inborn errors of metabolism.

Amino acids via the portal circulation and plasma proteins via the hepatic artery are transported to the liver to be either degraded via the urea cycle or used as substrate for liver-derived plasma proteins. These liver-derived proteins include most circulating proteins with the major exception of immunoglobulin [382]. Malnutrition or liver disease may be manifested by reduced concentrations of circulating proteins (e.g., albumin or ceruloplasmin). Conversely, acute inflammation decreases the efficiency of hepatic update and metabolism of proteins that lead to increased concentrations of certain circulating proteins (e.g., fibrinogen, an *acute phase reactant*). Healthy premature infants often have a relative hypoalbuminemia, which results from decreased amino acid intake or albumin losses [renal, gut, or increased permeability (*third spacing*)], rather than an inability of the liver to synthesize large amounts of albumin [399]. Abnormal hypoalbuminemia can lead to or result from edema (i.e., *third spacing*), ascites, and congestive heart failure.

After a meal (or during parenteral nutrition), the hepatocytes regulate the metabolism of free fatty acids allowing their deposition as triglycerides in the liver or as adipose tissue. During fasting, these energy-rich molecules are converted to ketones and used for energy by neurons and other cells. A lack of ketone production is associated with a potentially fatal defect in metabolic pathways (e.g., deficiency of *long-chain 3-hydroxyacyl dehydrogenase*, an enzyme important in fat oxidation) [406, 407].

Early Postnatal Hepatic Function: Metabolism

The bile transport enzymatic system is also activated when the liver transitions to the primary organ for bile elimination. Bile includes bilirubin (the end product of heme degradation) and the detergent-like bile acids (amphipathic sterol molecules synthesized from cholesterol). In addition to serving as important molecular building blocks for a variety of synthetic pathways, bile acids play an essential role in lipid digestion by emulsifying partially digested fat droplets, adsorbing lipid-soluble vitamins (A, D, E, and K), and activating key endogenous digestive enzymes as well as breast milk lipase (also known as bile salt stimulated lipase) [408].

The enterohepatic circulation provides a critical mechanism for conserving bile. Approximately 95 % of bile acids secreted into the intestine are reabsorbed via the portal venous circulation and taken up by hepatocytes via a number of specific bile acid transporter proteins [409]. Although bile acid production may be detected as early as 14 weeks of gestation [410], production is immature in the neonate and the premature infant, increasing their risk for bile-deficiency associated steatorrhea ("diarrhea of infancy"), vitamin deficiency, and caloric malnutrition (see, Jaundice and Hyperbilirubinemia, below).

After birth, hepatic enzyme activity increases rapidly. For example, while levels in cord blood [411] and in neonates are normally increased (mean values, 3.8–4.6 mmol/L) [412, 413], the concentration of lactate typically decreases to near adult values within 24 h postnatally (mean 2.08 vs. 1.8 upper limit adult norm) [413]. Persistently increased serum lactate concentrations suggest increased production (poor perfusion and anaerobic metabolism), hepatic dysfunction, or mitochondrial metabolic defect [414].

The liver also plays key roles in biotransformation and detoxification of exogenous substances and xenobiotics (e.g., medications) via phase I (oxidation-reduction reactions and hydrolysis), phase II (conjugation with glucuronic acid and other substances), and phase III (excretion from the liver/biliary system) reactions (see Chap. 3, Anesthesia and Ancillary drugs in the Neonate). The cytochrome P450 system mediates phase I reactions and is variably induced at birth [415]. Fifty percent of medications are metabolized by the CYP3A subfamily. Of importance, the genes regulating the production of these proteins undergo developmental expression [416–418]. For example, CYP3A7 activity is very active in utero but decreases to negligible activity by birth. In contrast, CYP3A4 is expressed minimally in utero, but expression increases to approximately 50 % of adult levels by six months of age. Phase II reactions also follow age-related patterns. For example, glucuronidation of morphine does not reach adult rates until 2–6 months of age [418]. The immaturity of these pathways is associated with two clinically significant phenomena. First, the developing liver may be exposed to toxic effects of large concentrations of compounds that cannot be excreted [419]. Second, age-related dosing may be required for drugs that are inefficiently cleared by the immature liver to avoid side effects of large serum concentrations (e.g., certain muscle relaxants and narcotics [420–423], caffeine and theophylline [424], and propofol [425]).

Early Postnatal Hepatic Function: Common Neonatal Hepatic Disorders and Hemorrhagic Disease of the Neonate

At birth, the liver rapidly increases production of circulating proteins of the coagulation cascade (except factor VIII, which achieves adult levels within a few days). Although synthesized in the hepatocytes, the vitamin K (*koagulation*) carboxylation-dependent factors (II, VII, IX, and X) depend on maturation of the digestive system to achieve normal function. The first enteral feedings are accompanied by colonization of the intestines with bacteria that are an important source of vitamin K. Until the microflora is mature and absorption of fat-soluble vitamins is robust, quantities of vitamin K may be insufficient to prevent pathologic bleeding (e.g., intracranial hemorrhage) [426]. For this reason, current guidelines (in the United States) recommend that healthy neonates receive 0.5–1 mg of parenteral (intramuscular) vitamin K shortly after birth, which significantly decreases the risk of both early and late bleeding secondary to vitamin K deficiency [427]. Otherwise, healthy infants do not require further supplementation, and vitamin K deficiency after 6 weeks is rare [382] in the absence of conditions that impact its synthesis (such as antibiotic therapy affecting gut flora) or absorption of fat-soluble vitamins (such as liver disease, including hepatitis and alpha-1-antitrypsin deficiency) [428, 429].

Early Postnatal Hepatic Function: Common Neonatal Hepatic Disorders, Jaundice, and Hyperbilirubinemia

Neonatal jaundice refers to the easily visible cutaneous yellow-orange color that accompanies excess bilirubin deposits in the skin [total serum bilirubin levels >~5 mg/dL (85 micromol/L)] [430]. Increased serum concentrations of unconjugated bilirubin (which indirectly reacts with diazo reagents in the laboratory and therefore termed *indirect*) that is visually detectable occurs in approximately 65 % of all normal infants during the first week of life as a normal and transient phenomenon [431]. Cephalocaudal progression of jaundice is associated with, but is not a reliable measure of, absolute bilirubin levels. For example, when the bilirubin concentrations are <5 mg/dL, jaundice is generally most apparent in the face, but as the serum concentrations increase, jaundice appears in the skin of the thorax and abdomen, but in a quantitatively unpredictable manner. However, if there is no jaundice at all, pathologically increased concentrations of bilirubin can be excluded [432, 433].

The so-called physiologic jaundice of the neonate (generally less than 12 mg/dL) is associated with the normal hepatic immaturity combined with the transition from fetal to extrauterine life. Of primary significance, neonates encounter a large burden of bilirubin secondary to the breakdown of fetal erythrocytes because fetuses have a relatively large red blood cell (RBC) mass and a shortened erythrocyte life associated with fetal hemoglobin. Further, the large quantity of bilirubin stored in meconium may be a reabsorbed into the portal circulation (i.e., enterohepatic circulation) and hepatocytes, especially if elimination of stool is limited secondary to intestinal anomalies (e.g., bowel atresia and/or obstruction) or dysfunction (e.g., ileus with sepsis or necrotizing enterocolitis) [434, 435].

Finally, immature processes in the liver contribute to the substantive risk for indirect hyperbilirubinemia in the neonate. Uptake of bilirubin into the liver is less efficient, in part due to low levels of ligandin, a hepatocyte cytosol binding protein [436]. In the hepatocyte, lipophilic bilirubin is transformed into a polar, water-soluble substance suitable for excretion into urine (conjugated or *direct* bilirubin) by conjugation with one or two glucuronic acid molecules, a reaction catalyzed by uridine diphosphate glucuronyl transferase. The activity of this enzyme is diminished in neonates, increasing to adult levels by 1–2 months of age [437]. The sterile gut of the neonate lacks the bacteria-mediated conversion of bilirubin to urobilogen. As a result, conjugated bilirubin remains in the lumen, where it can be de-conjugated, in a reaction catalyzed by the enzyme beta-glucuronidase. This unconjugated bilirubin can be reabsorbed via the enterohepatic circulation, further decreasing the efficiency of bilirubin excretion.

The expected postnatal increase in bilirubin levels is termed "physiologic jaundice." The enterohepatic system in the neonate should "catch up" with the increased load of bilirubin and decreased clearance within the first 2 weeks after birth. Serum bilirubin concentrations should decrease to adult values by that time. Differentiating physiologic from pathologic concentrations of bilirubin presents a challenge as the range of "normal" varies among racial groups, with breast-feeding versus bottle-feeding, and other epidemiologic factors. Bilirubin concentrations are dynamic, and there is no absolute blood concentration that differentiates physiologic from pathologic [438]. Mechanisms for the production of and a differential diagnosis of neonatal hyperbilirubinemia are shown in Table 2.2. Because the placenta efficiently clears bilirubin, the neonate with conditions that are associated with pathologic jaundice, such as hemolysis, may not be immediately jaundiced at birth. However, postnatally, severely or persistently increased concentrations of bilirubin may develop.

Jaundice associated with breast-feeding (*breast milk jaundice*) is a benign, self-limited condition. Although a single specific cause has not been identified, substances in mature breast milk that promote enterohepatic uptake of bilirubin have been implicated [439–441]. This entity must be distinguished from jaundice due to "not enough breast-feeding," which is defined by poor feeding, infrequent stools, and poor weight gain. Although a similar pattern of inadequate oral intake can develop during feeding with formula, its association with breast-feeding requires careful assessment

Table 2.2 Mechanisms of newborn jaundice

Physiologic jaundice in the newborn
Catabolism of heme
From breakdown of fetal erythrocytes
From myoglobin, cytochromes, catalase
Decreased uptake into and excretion from liver cells
Low neonatal concentration of ligandin, the intracellular-binding protein
Low neonatal activity of uridine diphosphate glucuronyl transferase (UD-PGT)
Nonphysiologic jaundice
Increased heme catabolism
Congenital hemolytic anemias (e.g., glucose-6-phosphate dehydrogenease deficiency, spherocytosis)
Immunologically mediated hemolysis (e.g., rhesus and ABO incompatibility)
Extravasation of blood (bruising, fractures, intracranial hemorrhages)
Decreased bilirubin conjugation and excretion
Genetic defects in UDGPT (e.g., Crigler-Najjar, Arias type 2, Gilbert)
Hepatic and biliary disease (e.g., neonatal hepatitis, intra- and extrahepatic biliary atresia)
Increased enterohepatic circulation of bilirubin
Decreased bowel passage (e.g., intestinal atresias, necrotizing enterocolitis, fasting, inadequate nutrition [breast-feeding jaundice])
Increased deconjugation of bilirubin in the bowel (e.g., breast milk jaundice)

of maternal factors and techniques of feeding. To avoid dehydration and worsening of hyperbilirubinemia, adequate enteral feeding must be established or alternative hydration delivered (e.g., intravenous fluid) until the cause of inadequate oral intake is identified and eliminated [442].

Abnormalities in the enzymes of conjugation, anatomic malformations of the biliary system (e.g., biliary atresia), and obstructive processes (e.g., neonatal obstructive fibrosclerosing cholangiopathy) [443, 444] impair biliary function, often leading to jaundice in the first months of life. Prolonged (e.g., 2–3 weeks) and/or severe hyperbilirubinemia, development of progressive *direct* hyperbilirubinemia, and/or other signs of hepatic dysfunction (e.g., hepatomegaly, acholic stools, failure to thrive) demand meticulous evaluation to establish a definitive diagnosis. For example, without surgical intervention for biliary atresia (the *Kasai procedure*: resection of fibrotic extrahepatic biliary system and creation of a hepatoportoenterostomy) within several months after diagnosis dramatically increases the likelihood for infantile liver transplantation [445]. Of note, even after a timely Kasai, end-stage biliary cirrhosis eventually develops in 70–80 % of patients, so that biliary atresia remains the most common cause of chronic end-stage liver in liver disease in children [443, 446]. Thus, jaundice at the one-month pediatric evaluation should prompt consideration of hepatic disease, including biliary atresia and other cholangiopathies, and possibly referral to a pediatric gastroenterologist and/or surgeon.

Liver dysfunction (e.g., conjugated (direct) hyperbilirubinemia) or injury frequently accompanies hemodynamic insults associated with hypoxia, ischemia, sepsis, or primary liver infection. In such cases, increased serum concentrations of liver enzymes reflect hepatocyte injury. Of importance, hepatocyte injury impairs synthetic function, manifested by reduced serum albumin concentration and/or abnormal coagulation function (i.e., prolonged prothrombin time, decreased fibrinogen levels) [447–450]. Fulminant liver failure may result from gram-negative (e.g., Escherichia coli) or meningococcal bacteremia or viral infections (e.g., herpes simplex, adenovirus, or echovirus) [451, 452]. With prompt restoration of perfusion or effective treatment of infection, transaminase levels (so-called liver function tests) usually decrease, but hyperbilirubinemia may persist for weeks [382].

Liver injury during parenteral nutrition is a common neonatal cause of cholestasis, and, in this setting, elevated conjugated bilirubin is associated with significant morbidity [453, 454]. Premature infants are more vulnerable to liver injuries for a multitude of reasons, including a greater incidence of episodes of ischemia and hypoxia, of gastrointestinal and systemic infections due to immaturity of the gut epithelium, and of requiring parenteral nutrition [382, 455]. Exaggerated immune responses to inflammatory triggers such as lipopolysaccharide associated with decreased T-cell-mediated immune modulation may also predispose the neonate to hepatic injury during systemic infection [456].

In addition to its roles as a marker of liver disease, hyperbilirubinemia can directly injure neural tissue, resulting in a neuropathologic syndrome known as *kernicterus*, the pathologic term that describes the autopsy finding of yellow-stained deep brain nuclei. Kernicterus [(bilirubin-induced neurologic dysfunction (BIND)] includes an acute encephalopathy with nonspecific signs (lethargy, poor feeding, abnormal tone, retrocollis, a high pitched cry), changes in EEG and auditory brainstem responses, MRI abnormalities in the globus pallidus and subthalamic nuclei, and death [457, 458]. Chronic bilirubin encephalopathy (classic kernicterus) is characterized by a tetrad of clinical signs of varying severity: movement disorders (athetosis, dystonia, spasticity, and hypotonia), auditory neuropathy, oculomotor impairments, and dental enamel hypoplasia of the permanent teeth [457].

The blood–brain barrier prevents entry of water-soluble, conjugated bilirubin as well as bilirubin that is bound to albumin [459, 460]. Therefore, in addition to increased concentrations of bilirubin (i.e., unconjugated, lipophilic form), hypoalbuminemia increases the risk of kernicterus. Furthermore, insults that impair the function of the blood–brain barrier (e.g., hypoxia, respiratory acidosis, hypothermia, sepsis, trauma, and prematurity) predispose to primary central nervous system injury from hyperbilirubinemia because of increased access of bilirubin to the brain [461–464].

Various genetic enzyme deficiencies are also associated with neonatal hyperbilirubinemia by increasing risk of hemolysis (e.g., glucose-6-phosphate dehydrogenase deficiency, a hereditary condition prevalent in African Americans [465]). Reduced UDP-glucuronosyltransferase (UD-PGT) activity can also increase the concentration of unconjugated bilirubin, especially in the setting of prematurity, sepsis, or in certain defects in hemoglobin and biliary metabolism. With an incidence of ~1 %, Gilbert disease is characterized by slightly decreased activity of UD-PGT, but with activity markedly impaired during physiologic stress such as infection or neonatal asphyxia [466]. In contrast, Crigler-Najjar syndrome has decreased (type II) or absent (type I) UD-PGT activity secondary to a variety of mutations [467, 468], which, if untreated, leads to unconjugated hyperbilirubinemia and irreversible neurologic injury [469]. Other genetic and environmental factors (such as UDP-GT1A1 polymorphisms) may either increase the risk of kernicterus in the presence of relatively low bilirubin concentrations or protect from kernicterus despite hyperbilirubinemia [470–473, 474]. The guidelines from the American Academy of Pediatrics for management of hyperbilirubinemia in the term and near-term neonate stress prevention of kernicterus through primary prevention (i.e., establishing appropriate nutrition to decrease enterohepatic recirculation of bilirubin), secondary prevention (i.e., early detection of high-risk infants including screening of bilirubin levels) (see Fig. 2.16), and following

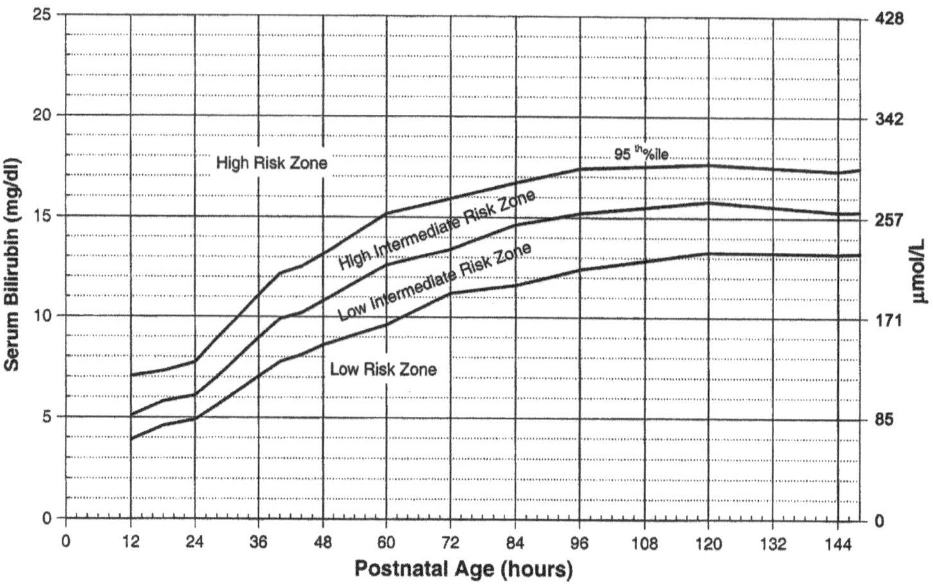

Fig. 2.16 Nomogram used for designation of risk in 2,840 well neonates at 36 or more weeks gestational age with birth weight of 2,000 g or more or 35 or more weeks' gestational age and birth weight of 2,500 g or more based on the hour-specific serum bilirubin values. Note that this nomogram is for predicting likelihood of a subsequent bilirubin level exceeding the 95th percentile—NOT to represent the natural history of neonatal hyperbilirubinemia (from [475]; citing Bhutani et al. [476])

specific protocols to initiate therapies such as phototherapy and exchange transfusion [475, 477].

Phototherapy was first demonstrated to attenuate the serum concentration of bilirubin in 1958 [478] and then became an accepted treatment in the United States in the late 1960s [479]. Phototherapy effectively decreases the serum concentration of bilirubin by converting lipophilic bilirubin to more soluble, structural isomers (lumirubin) or configurational isomers, facilitating the excretion in a non-conjugation-dependent process [462, 480–483]. Because it rapidly converts bilirubin to the more polar photo isomers, phototherapy may decrease bilirubin-associated central nervous system injury. That is, phototherapy may be effective because it produces photo isomers that inflict less direct neural toxicity, decreases the transit of the more polar bilirubin photoproducts across the blood–brain barrier, or changes the proportion of free bilirubin to total bilirubin [484, 485]. In lieu of exposure to sunlight, artificial light of modern phototherapy is designed to expose the infant to light of 450 nm wavelength (blue) to avoid overheating and permit detecting cyanosis clinically (i.e., less important in the era of pulse oximetry) [486]. Overall, the goal is to reduce the risk of kernicterus by decreasing the total concentration of bilirubin to less than that historically associated with kernicterus (~20 mg/dL (340 micromol/L) for healthy term babies). Compared with term infants, preterm and near-term infants are at greater risk of kernicterus, even at reduced concentrations of hyperbilirubinemia [487, 488]. Treatment protocols (i.e., when to initiate phototherapy, how long to continue, indications for exchange transfusion) should be based on several variables including the trend in the absolute concentration, the rapidity of the increase in bilirubin concentration (trend in the concentration from hour-to-hour), and the predicted risk (e.g., gestational and postnatal age, ongoing hemolysis, current medical status (acidosis, sepsis)) to allow more accurate and effective treatment [475]. Phototherapy may also be used as a bridging therapy to liver transplantation in Crigler-Najjar type I [489]. Finally, phenobarbital can be used to induce UD-PGT activity when it is insufficient (e.g., in Crigler-Najjar type II).

With the improvements in phototherapy, the need for exchange transfusion for neonatal jaundice (first found to be effective in 1951) [490] has all but disappeared [462, 491]. If an exchange transfusion is required, one or two central venous catheters are placed, and small aliquots of blood are removed and then replaced with a mixture of donor (and bilirubin-free) RBCs and plasma (or albumin). Infusion of albumin before the exchange transfusion may increase the amount of bilirubin removed during the procedure [492]. In addition to decreasing the bilirubin concentrations, exchange transfusion may reduce the circulating antibody concentrations during ongoing hemolysis. Severe complications in approximately 2 % of patients undergoing exchange transfusion [493] include problems associated with central line placement (thrombosis and necrotizing enterocolitis [494]), electrolyte disturbances, and thrombocytopenia. Currently, exchange transfusions are recommended only to treat acute bilirubin encephalopathy or hyperbilirubinemia resistant to phototherapy. Levels of total serum bilirubin at which exchange is recommended vary with associated risk factors (e.g., isoimmune hemolytic disease, G6PD deficiency, signs of sepsis or asphyxia, gestational and postnatal age, and the bilirubin-albumin ratio) [475].

Clinical Significance and Summary

Immature and/or abnormal hepatic function in the neonate presents several challenges in the setting of anesthesia and surgery. Some medications (e.g., ceftriaxone, furosemide, and oxacillin, but not methicillin) compete with bilirubin for albumin-binding sites. If displaced from albumin, the proportion of unbound or "free" bilirubin concentration increases, exaggerating the risk for neurotoxicity from this molecule crossing the blood–brain barrier [495, 496]. Of note, in some cases, a preservative or other additive to a pharmacologic preparation rather than the drug itself may displace bilirubin from albumin (the sodium benzoate in intravenous diazepam) [497].

Acidemia exaggerates bilirubin neurotoxicity primarily by its effects on bilirubin solubility and the decreased binding of protonated bilirubin to albumin [461, 462, 498]. In addition, neurologic injury associated with a given level of bilirubin may vary as a function of effectiveness of protective mechanisms that determine the relative transport into and out of the brain. That is, the active transport of bilirubin from the brain into the blood may diminish injury, but acidemia may inhibit this activity [498]. Similarly, the severity of injury depends on both the duration and concentration of unbound bilirubin in the vulnerable developing brain, since the immature brain may be particularly at risk for apoptosis and necrosis, especially in the presence of infection or other stressors [457].

Thus, the neonatal anesthesiologist must appreciate that the critically ill neonate who is a greater risk for hemodynamic and respiratory instability and associated respiratory or metabolic acidosis, hypoalbuminemia, and liver dysfunction may also be at increased risk for bilirubin neurotoxicity. In addition, hepatic dysfunction and immaturity may disrupt the normal metabolism of drugs including commonly used anesthetic agents (e.g., muscle relaxants). Finally, hemostasis must be meticulously evaluated preoperatively and aggressively monitored and treated intraoperatively.

Renal Function

In utero, the placenta maintains fetal metabolic and electrolyte homeostasis. Permanent kidneys appear during the fifth week of gestation and nephrons during the eighth week, initially in the juxtamedullary region and cortex. A complex interaction of genes [e.g., Wilms' tumor gene 1(WT1) and growth factors (neurotrophic factor (GDNF))] orchestrates this process [499, 500]. By 20 weeks gestation, one-third of the full complement of nephrons has developed [501]. By 35–36 weeks gestation, the number of nephrons equals that of the normal young adult [502]. Infants born prematurely develop new nephrons until about 34–35 weeks postconceptional age. When the full complement of nephrons has developed, the kidneys mature by increasing both glomerular and tubular size. Vascular growth and development parallel nephrogenesis.

Nonetheless, the number of nephrons varies by up to fivefold among mature healthy term infants [503]. Both genetic and environmental factors explain the reduced number of nephrons [18, 19, 504]. For example, a polymorphism of the RET gene is associated with a decreased number of nephrons [505] and a common variant of another gene, PAX2, with smaller kidneys at birth [506]. Of note, prematurity and intrauterine growth retardation both have negative effects on postnatal renal growth [18, 19, 507]. Finally, oxidative injury during the neonatal period has been associated with decreased capillary density and fewer nephrons in adult rats [508].

Urine is first formed by 10 weeks gestation, and production increases from about 2–5 mL/h at 20 weeks gestation to 10–12 mL/h at 30 weeks, 12–16 mL/h at 35 weeks, and 35–50 mL/h at 40 weeks gestation [509]. The fetal kidneys produce large volumes of hypotonic urine essential to maintain normal amniotic fluid volumes, especially after 18 weeks gestation. In turn, large volumes of fetal urine are necessary for normal pulmonary development. For example, oliguria results in oligohydramnios, which is associated with a specific facies, clubfeet, limb contractures, and, in severe cases, pulmonary hypoplasia (Potters sequence/oligohydramnios sequence).

Developmental Changes in Distribution of Total Body Water

At 16 weeks gestation, the total body water accounts for 94 % of the fetus' weight; at 32 weeks gestation, 82 %; and at term, approximately 75 %. The size of the extracellular compartment decreases from 65 % at 16 weeks to about 60 % at 24–25 weeks gestation and then to about 50 % at term. At the same time the intracellular compartment increases from 34 % in early gestation to 50 % at term [510, 511]. During the first 3–7 days of extrauterine life, healthy term infants lose about 5–10 % of their body weight, primarily through contraction of the extracellular water space. Transepidermal fluid loss is related to gestational age and can be as much as 60–100 mL/kg/day in ELBW infants. Over the first 5 days of life, fluid losses decrease dramatically (from 45 to about 19 g/m^2/h) in 25–27 week gestation infants [512]. During the first few postnatal days, naked preterm infants lose up to 15 times more water through evaporation than naked term infants [513]. Naked VLBW infants may lose up to 10 % of their body weight through evaporation during the first 24 h of life.

Renal Function

GFR and Blood Flow: Fetal and neonatal renal function is characterized by reduced renal blood flow, glomerular filtration rate (GFR), solid excretion, and concentrating capacity. In part, renal blood flow is reduced in utero because of increased renal vascular resistance. After birth, renal blood flow increases markedly due to an increase in the arterial blood pressure and a decrease in renal vascular resistance, which allow more of the cardiac output to flow to the kidneys (2–4 % in utero, 10 % at 1 week of age, 25 % in the adult). Renal blood flow is about 20 mL/min/1.73 m^2 at 30 weeks, 45 mL/min/1.73 m^2 at 35 weeks, about 80 mL/kg/1.73 m^2 at term, 250 mL/min/1.73 m^2 at 8 days, and 770 mL/min/1.73 m^2 at 5 months of age [514]. Similarly, GFR increases rapidly in utero as the number of nephrons increases. Because fetal kidney growth begins deep in the medulla, the juxtamedullary nephrons are more mature than other nephrons at birth and have greater tubular length than outer and inner cortical nephrons. Since the glomeruli are distributed uniformly, a "tubular-glomerular" imbalance, which allows less efficient reabsorption of substrates presented to the proximal tubules of neonates.

The GFR in preterm infants is a function of both gestational and postnatal age. During the first 24 h of extrauterine life, the GFR of infants born before 25 weeks gestation may be as low as 2 mL/min/1.73 m^2. Infants born between 25 and 28 weeks gestation have a GFR of 10–13 mL/min/1.73 m^2 and those born after 34 weeks gestation, 20–25 mL/min/1.73 m^2, which is similar to that of full-term infants [515]. Although GFR increases at a slower rate in ELBW infants, all neonates without acquired renal insufficiency double their GFR by two weeks of age and triple it by 3 months of age. Thereafter, GFR increases more slowly. A multicenter study from France reported GFR measurements obtained in 27–31 week gestation infants over the first month of life [516]. Although the precise values in GFR (mL/min/1.73 m^2) varied from previous studies, the general trend for increase is similar and reflects an approximate doubling over the first month, between day 7 and day 28 of life (day 7, 18.5 ± 12.6; day 14, 20.6 ± 13.1; day 21, 22.2 ± 11.7; day 28, 26.2 ± 19.6). The increase was inversely correlated with gestational age.

Adult values for GFR are reached by 12 to 24 months of age. Due to rapid renal maturation after birth, a 3-week-old, ex-27 week gestation infant may have significantly more mature renal function than a normal 6-h-old term infant. Renal maturation apparently occurs in response to "demand" (separation from the placenta plus solute exposure). Renal filtration and concentrating ability increase when the kidneys are exposed to substrate [517].

At birth, serum creatinine reflects maternal values (since placental not fetal renal function predominates in maintaining metabolic stability) and is greater than that of normal 1–2-week-old term neonates (0.4 mg/dL). For the first 4 weeks of life, the serum creatinine concentration of preterm infants exceeds that of term infants [518]. Interestingly, the serum creatinine concentration was the same at birth in infants born before 27 weeks compared with those born at 31–32 weeks gestation, increased in all groups over the first 3 days of life and then gradually decreased to <0.5 mg/dL [519]. However, the maximum creatinine concentration reported was greater and occurred later (day 3.5 vs. day 1) in the most immature neonates. Creatinine clearance increased in all groups but increased more slowly in the <27-week gestation infants. The variability in GFR and creatinine clearance, as a function of gestational and postnatal age, implies that drugs that depend on the kidneys for elimination may have a variable half-life in the neonates during the first weeks to months of postnatal life.

Renal Tubular Function: Extracellular fluid volume, water balance, and sodium and other electrolyte concentrations are interrelated and undergo significant change postnatally. In addition to the dramatic development in the number of nephrons, glomerular function, and renal blood flow, the renal tubules mature throughout fetal and postnatal life. Of note, tubular immaturity accounts for inefficient salvage of essential substrates (e.g., glucose, amino acids). The metabolic demands of rapid growth and/or illnesses coupled with neonatal renal function complicate managing fluids and providing nutritional support.

Renal tubular cells are polarized, just as other epithelia are. That is, specific, unique channels, transporters, and other proteins populate the apical (facing the urine) versus the basolateral membrane (facing the blood), which provides the mechanism for net movement of solutes both from lumen to capillary (reabsorption) and from capillary to lumen (secretion). This distribution of proteins to each membrane defines the anatomically and functionally distinct sections of the renal tubules and allows the kidney to salvage most substrates from the glomerular filtrate in the proximal tubule and fine-tune water and solute content in the more distal segments. For example, although sodium is absorbed along the entire system, the proximal tubules reabsorb 60–80 % of filtered sodium and water. In addition, glucose, phosphate, and most amino acids are salvaged primarily along the proximal tubule. The loops of Henle, the distal tubules, and the collecting tubules concentrate urine and secrete potassium.

An additional 10–15 % of filtered sodium is absorbed in the distal (aldosterone responsive) and collecting tubules (antidiuretic hormone determines water permeability). The amount of sodium in fluid presented to the distal tubules depends, in part, on the efficiency of the transport mechanisms of the proximal tubule.

The membrane proteins (transporters) that salvage amino acids, glucose, bicarbonate, and phosphate from the glomerular filtrate are located on the apical membrane of the proximal tubule and are "active" transporters (i.e., requiring energy to move substrates across the membrane against their concentration gradient). The simultaneous movement of sodium down its electrochemical gradient generates the energy for the transport of the substrate against its concentration gradient. For example, glucose and amino acids are cotransported with sodium across the apical membrane. Other substrates are counter-transported (e.g., H^+ and sodium) with sodium moving the opposite direction than that of the substrate (i.e., exchange mechanism). The sodium gradient then must be reestablished, which is mediated by the activity of the Na^+–K^+-ATPase pump. This metabolic role of the Na^+–K^+-ATPase pump in maintaining the sodium gradient for all eukaryotic cells is critical. Located on the basolateral membrane, the activity of this enzyme accounts for approximately 70 % of renal oxygen consumption.

Development of Sodium-Driven Transport Function: After birth, resorption of sodium in the proximal tubules increases 5–10-fold in response to increased Na^+–K^+-ATPase activity [520], in part secondary to developmental changes in its regulatory β subunit. That is, the fetal β2 isoform (which is present in both the apical and the basolateral membranes) is downregulated after birth, and β1 is upregulated and targeted only to the basolateral membrane [521]. The functional, mature enzyme consists of a heterodimer of α1 and β1 subunits. Glucocorticoid hormones increase mRNA for both subunits of this enzyme, and prenatal administration of betamethasone to the mother in preterm labor to induce maturation of the lungs may also mature renal function.

The proximal tubule increases its capacity for absorption with advancing gestational age. Five percent of the filtered sodium is excreted in the urine of <30-week gestation infants, but only 0.2 % is excreted in term infants [522]. Hypoxia, respiratory distress, and hyperbilirubinemia may increase fractional sodium excretion. Similarly, neonates concentrate urine to more limited degree than adults (245–450 mOsm/l in preterm infants vs. 600–800 mOsm/L in term infants vs. 1,200–1,400 mOsm/l in adults). In contrast, neonates >35 weeks gestation can dilute their urine to adult levels (~50 mOsm/l) and infants <35 weeks gestation to about 70 mOsm/l [523], but neither can excrete a water load as rapidly as the older child. That is, the maximum urinary osmolality attained after a dose of DDAVP was only ~520 mOsm/kg in 30–35-week gestation infants and 570 mOsm/kg in 4–6-week-old infants born at term. A 6-month-old child concentrates his urine to 1,300–1,400 mOsm/kg after a dose of DDAVP [515]. The majority of infants remain unable to maximally concentrate their urine at 6–12 months of life.

The limit in concentrating capacity of the immature kidney is not related to absence of arginine vasopressin [antidiuretic hormone (ADH)]. In fact, ADH levels are increased in both preterm and term infants, but decrease rapidly postnatally (see Section "Renin-Angiotensin System") [524]. The immature corticomedullary osmotic gradient and low GFR may contribute to the limited ability to both maximally dilute and concentrate urine.

The concentration of serum electrolytes in the neonate, especially the preterm, reflects renal tubular immaturity. For example, the reduced serum concentration of bicarbonate in the neonate (12–16 mEq/l in ELBW infants, 18–20 mEq/l in 30–35 week gestation infants compared with 20–22 mEq/l in term infants, and 25–28 mEq/l in adults) [525] develops secondary to the urinary loss of bicarbonate, which leads to urine with an alkaline pH and a mild serum metabolic acidosis. The Na^+/H^+ antiporter (NHE) plays a major role in secreting protons in exchange for bicarbonate and undergoes dramatic developmental changes. Although at least 6 different isoforms have been identified, NHE-3 (present in the proximal tubule and the thick ascending loop) is responsible for ~90 % of bicarbonate reabsorption as renal function matures postnatally, compared with ~60 % in the perinatal period [526]. Both glucocorticoids [527] and thyroid hormone [528] facilitate maturation of this transporter. Age-related differences in NHE may contribute to differences in acid–base balance among neonates and older children/adults. Hydrogen is actively secreted, and the secreted hydrogen reacts with bicarbonate to produce carbonic acid and carbon dioxide. These substances enter the tubular cells through the action of carbonic anhydrase. In addition to age-related dysfunction of NHE, carbonic anhydrase function may also be immature.

Glucose is reabsorbed in the proximal tubule via the sodium-glucose cotransporter (SGLT-2), and, similar to other carrier-mediated transporters, developmental changes have been documented [529]. In premature infants, tubular reabsorption is decreased so that glucosuria is common. The tubular reabsorption of glucose and the transport maximum (T_m) are both decreased in the neonate (150 mg/dL in term neonates compared with 180 mg/dL in older children and adults). Premature infants less than 34 weeks gestation have a greater fractional excretion of glucose and a lesser maximal reabsorption than full-term infants [530]. Finally, calcium absorption occurs in the proximal tubules of the kidneys, primarily by passive diffusion, but the large renal sodium losses increase calcium excretion.

Sick neonates, especially premature neonates, require supplemental intravenous calcium to maintain normal ionized calcium concentrations.

Serum potassium concentrations that exceed 5.0 mmol/l are relatively common in neonates, particularly in premature infants with a mild metabolic acidosis. Nonoliguric hyperkalemia (serum potassium >6.5 mmol/l in the absence of renal failure) is characterized by a rapid rise of serum potassium during the first one to three days of life and develops frequently in ELBW infants. In contrast to older infants, children, and adults, this hyperkalemia is not secondary to abnormal potassium excretion or excessive intake, but instead seems to result from rapid shifts of potassium from intra- to extracellular compartments [531, 532] and is associated with abnormal Na^+–K^+-ATPase activity in erythrocytes [533]. As in older children and adults, treatment of hyperkalemia includes insulin/glucose, calcium/bicarbonate, diuretics, albuterol, peritoneal dialysis, and binding resins. In neonates, exchange transfusion should also be considered [532].

Renin-Angiotensin System

Hormonal control of neonatal fluid and electrolyte homeostasis is complex and, in some ways, unique compared with the older child and adult. The renin-angiotensin system plays an especially critical role. Renin has been identified as early as 17 weeks gestation, and plasma renin activity (PRA) is inversely correlated with gestational age (60 mg/mL/h at 30 weeks; 10–20 ng/mL/h at term) [534] but remains at least threefold greater in the neonate than in the adult [535, 536]. The substantial PRA is associated with increased serum aldosterone compared with adults [537]. In addition, hypoxia [538] and hypovolemia [539] increase renin and angiotensin II levels. Although the specific role of the plasma renin activity in the perinatal period is unclear, it seems to be critical since administering angiotensin-converting enzyme (ACE) inhibitors to mothers has been associated with anuria-oligohydramnios, pulmonary hypoplasia, growth retardation, and renal tubular dysplasia in the fetus [540].

Prostaglandins play a role in maintaining GFR and renal blood flow, primarily by counterbalancing the vasoconstrictive effects of the renin-angiotensin system. The excretion of PGE_2 and prostacyclin metabolites is fivefold greater in the premature compared with the term infant and 20-fold greater than that of the older child [541]. Of importance, the renal failure associated with indomethacin given to close a patent ductus arteriosus has been correlated with the vasoconstriction induced by these hormones.

Plasma vasopressin [antidiuretic hormone (ADH)] concentrations are greater in neonates than later in life, especially after vaginal delivery [542], and are thought to be responsible, at least in part, for the reduced urine output during the first 24 h of life. In part, vasopressin may lead to the contraction of the extracellular volume immediately after birth and may contribute to the indomethacin-induced renal failure in premature infants. Hypoxia, atelectasis, intraventricular hemorrhage, and BPD increase urine ADH concentrations in both preterm and term infants [543].

Clinical Significance and Summary

Managing fluids and electrolytes in the neonates requires consideration of renal developmental physiology, especially related to sodium and water excretion and glucose homeostasis. Analyzing ongoing requirements for sodium, potassium, calcium, and glucose is essential preoperatively to estimate maintenance delivery and the need for monitoring laboratory values intraoperatively. In the setting of cardiorespiratory and central nervous system immaturity and vulnerability, normalizing intravascular volume and serum electrolytes preoperatively may enhance intraoperative stability. Although intraoperative events often demand rapid infusion of crystalloid and/or colloid, maximizing preoperative stability can only contribute to minimizing wide fluctuations in blood pressure perioperatively.

Providing a warm, humidified environment and inspired gases intraoperatively and minimizing transepidermal fluid loss during transport (i.e., plastic shields, head covers), especially in the ELBW infant, are essential aspects of fluid and electrolyte therapy.

References

1. Heron M, Sutton PD, Xu J, et al. Annual summary of vital statistics: 2007. Pediatrics. 2010;125(1):4–15.
2. Mathews TJ, MacDorman MF. Infant mortality statistics from the 2006 period linked birth/infant death data set. Natl Vital Stat Rep. 2010;58(17):1–31.
3. Hamilton BE, Hoyert DL, Martin JA, et al. Annual summary of vital statistics: 2010-2011. Pediatrics. 2013;131(3):548–58.
4. Manktelow BN, Seaton SE, Field DJ, et al. Population-based estimates of in-unit survival for very preterm infants. Pediatrics. 2013;131(2):e425–432.
5. Fanaroff AA, Stoll BJ, Wright LL, et al. Trends in neonatal morbidity and mortality for very low birthweight infants. Am J Obstet Gynecol. 2007;196(2):147e1-8.
6. Eichenwald EC, Stark AR. Management and outcomes of very low birth weight. N Engl J Med. 2008;358(16):1700–11.
7. Bassler D, Stoll BJ, Schmidt B, et al. Using a count of neonatal morbidities to predict poor outcome in extremely low birth weight infants: added role of neonatal infection. Pediatrics. 2009;123(1):313–8.
8. Horbar JD, Carpenter JH, Badger GJ, et al. Mortality and neonatal morbidity among infants 501 to 1500 grams from 2000 to 2009. Pediatrics. 2012;129(6):1019–26.
9. Barker DJ, Osmond C. Infant mortality, childhood nutrition, and ischaemic heart disease in England and Wales. Lancet. 1986;1(8489):1077–81.

10. Hales CN, Barker DJ. The thrifty phenotype hypothesis. Br Med Bull. 2001;60:5–20.
11. Hales CN, Barker DJ, Clark PM, et al. Fetal and infant growth and impaired glucose tolerance at age 64. BMJ. 1991;303(6809): 1019–22.
12. Barker DJ, Osmond C, Forsen TJ, et al. Trajectories of growth among children who have coronary events as adults. N Engl J Med. 2005;353(17):1802–9.
13. Ravelli AC, van der Meulen JH, Michels RP, et al. Glucose tolerance in adults after prenatal exposure to famine. Lancet. 1998;351(9097):173–7.
14. Singhal A, Lucas A. Early origins of cardiovascular disease: is there a unifying hypothesis? Lancet. 2004;363(9421):1642–5.
15. Singhal A, Fewtrell M, Cole TJ, et al. Low nutrient intake and early growth for later insulin resistance in adolescents born preterm. Lancet. 2003;361(9363):1089–97.
16. Forsen T, Eriksson J, Tuomilehto J, et al. The fetal and childhood growth of persons who develop type 2 diabetes. Ann Intern Med. 2000;133(3):176–82.
17. Singhal A, Cole TJ, Fewtrell M, et al. Promotion of faster weight gain in infants born small for gestational age: is there an adverse effect on later blood pressure? Circulation. 2007;115(2): 213–20.
18. Rakow A, Johansson S, Legnevall L, et al. Renal volume and function in school-age children born preterm or small for gestational age. Pediatr Nephrol. 2008;23(8):1309–15.
19. Huang HP, Tsai IJ, Lai YC, et al. Early postnatal renal growth in premature infants. Nephrology (Carlton). 2007;12(6):572–5.
20. McMillen IC, Robinson JS. Developmental origins of the metabolic syndrome: prediction, plasticity, and programming. Physiol Rev. 2005;85(2):571–633.
21. Gluckman PD, Hanson MA, Pinal C. The developmental origins of adult disease. Matern Child Nutr. 2005;1(3):130–41.
22. Modi N, Thomas EL, Harrington TA, et al. Determinants of adiposity during preweaning postnatal growth in appropriately grown and growth-restricted term infants. Pediatr Res. 2006;60(3):345–8.
23. Catalano PM, Kirwan JP, Haugel-de Mouzon S, et al. Gestational diabetes and insulin resistance: role in short- and long-term implications for mother and fetus. J Nutr. 2003;133(5 Suppl 2):1674S–83S.
24. Uthaya S, Thomas EL, Hamilton G, et al. Altered adiposity after extremely preterm birth. Pediatr Res. 2005;57(2):211–5.
25. Hofman PL, Regan F, Harris M, et al. The metabolic consequences of prematurity. Growth Horm IGF Res. 2004;14(Suppl A):S136–9.
26. Hofman PL, Regan F, Jackson WE, et al. Premature birth and later insulin resistance. N Engl J Med. 2004;351(21):2179–86.
27. Mikkola K, Leipala J, Boldt T, et al. Fetal growth restriction in preterm infants and cardiovascular function at five years of age. J Pediatr. 2007;151(5):494–9, e491–2.
28. Silveira PP, Portella AK, Goldani MZ, et al. Developmental origins of health and disease (DOHaD). J Pediatr (Rio J). 2007;83(6):494–504.
29. Gillman MW, Barker D, Bier D, et al. Meeting report on the 3rd International Congress on Developmental Origins of Health and Disease (DOHaD). Pediatr Res. 2007;61(5 Pt 1):625–9.
30. Warner MJ, Ozanne SE. Mechanisms involved in the developmental programming of adulthood disease. Biochem J. 2010;427(3):333–47.
31. Rudolph AM. Prenatal and postnatal pulmonary circulation. In: Rudolph AM, editor. Congenital diseases of the heart, clinical-physiological considerations. West Sussex: Wiley-Blackwell; 2009. p. 89.
32. Marx JA. Rosen's emergency medicine. Philadelphia: Mosby/Elsevier; 2010.
33. Rudolph AM. The fetal circulation. In: Rudolph AM, editor. Congenital diseases of the heart, clinical-physiological considerations. West Sussex: Wiley-Blackwell; 2009. p. 1–24.
34. Rudolph AM. The fetal circulation. In: Rudolph AM, editor. Congenital diseases of the heart, clinical-physiological considerations. West Sussex: Wiley-Blackwell; 2009. p. 2.
35. Rasanen J, Wood DC, Weiner S, et al. Role of the pulmonary circulation in the distribution of human fetal cardiac output during the second half of pregnancy. Circulation. 1996;94(5):1068–73.
36. Rasanen J, Wood DC, Debbs RH, et al. Reactivity of the human fetal pulmonary circulation to maternal hyperoxygenation increases during the second half of pregnancy: a randomized study. Circulation. 1998;97(3):257–62.
37. Rudolph AM. Congenital cardiovascular malformations and the fetal circulation. Arch Dis Child Fetal Neonatal Ed. 2010;95(2):F132–136.
38. Lewis AB, Heymann MA, Rudolph AM. Gestational changes in pulmonary vascular responses in fetal lambs in utero. Circ Res. 1976;39(4):536–41.
39. Rudolph AM, Yuan S. Response of the pulmonary vasculature to hypoxia and H+ ion concentration changes. J Clin Invest. 1966;45(3):399–411.
40. Peckham GJ, Fox WW. Physiologic factors affecting pulmonary artery pressure in infants with persistent pulmonary hypertension. J Pediatr. 1978;93(6):1005–10.
41. Moore P, Velvis H, Fineman JR, et al. EDRF inhibition attenuates the increase in pulmonary blood flow due to oxygen ventilation in fetal lambs. J Appl Physiol. 1992;73(5):2151–7.
42. Post JM, Hume JR, Archer SL, et al. Direct role for potassium channel inhibition in hypoxic pulmonary vasoconstriction. Am J Physiol. 1992;262(4 Pt 1):C882–890.
43. Kinsella JP, Neish SR, Ivy DD, et al. Clinical responses to prolonged treatment of persistent pulmonary hypertension of the newborn with low doses of inhaled nitric oxide. J Pediatr. 1993;123(1):103–8.
44. Steinhorn RH. Nitric oxide and beyond: new insights and therapies for pulmonary hypertension. J Perinatol. 2008;28 Suppl 3:S67–71.
45. Inhaled nitric oxide in term and near-term infants: neurodevelopmental follow-up of the neonatal inhaled nitric oxide study group (NINOS). J Pediatr. 2000;136(5):611–7.
46. Issa A, Lappalainen U, Kleinman M, et al. Inhaled nitric oxide decreases hyperoxia-induced surfactant abnormality in preterm rabbits. Pediatr Res. 1999;45(2):247–54.
47. McCurnin DC, Pierce RA, Chang LY, et al. Inhaled NO improves early pulmonary function and modifies lung growth and elastin deposition in a baboon model of neonatal chronic lung disease. Am J Physiol Lung Cell Mol Physiol. 2005;288(3):L450–459.
48. Ballard PL, Merrill JD, Truog WE, et al. Surfactant function and composition in premature infants treated with inhaled nitric oxide. Pediatrics. 2007;120(2):346–53.
49. Brennan LA, Steinhorn RH, Wedgwood S, et al. Increased superoxide generation is associated with pulmonary hypertension in fetal lambs: a role for NADPH oxidase. Circ Res. 2003;92(6):683–91.
50. Barrington KJ, Finer NN. Inhaled nitric oxide for respiratory failure in preterm infants. Cochrane Database Syst Rev. 2007;(3):CD000509.
51. Jonker SS, Zhang L, Louey S, et al. Myocyte enlargement, differentiation, and proliferation kinetics in the fetal sheep heart. J Appl Physiol. 2007;102(3):1130–42.
52. Nassar R, Reedy MC, Anderson PA. Developmental changes in the ultrastructure and sarcomere shortening of the isolated rabbit ventricular myocyte. Circ Res. 1987;61(3):465–83.
53. Pena E, Tracqui P, Azancot A, et al. Unraveling changes in myocardial contractility during human fetal growth: a finite element

analysis based on in vivo ultrasound measurements. Ann Biomed Eng. 2010;38(8):2702–15.
54. Fabiato A. Calcium-induced release of calcium from the cardiac sarcoplasmic reticulum. Am J Physiol. 1983;245(1):C1–14.
55. Gyorke S, Gyorke I, Lukyanenko V, et al. Regulation of sarcoplasmic reticulum calcium release by luminal calcium in cardiac muscle. Front Biosci. 2002;7:d1454–1463.
56. Klitzner TS. Maturational changes in excitation-contraction coupling in mammalian myocardium. J Am Coll Cardiol. 1991;17(1):218–25.
57. Nakanishi T, Seguchi M, Takao A. Development of the myocardial contractile system. Experientia. 1988;44(11–12):936–44.
58. Huang J, Hove-Madsen L, Tibbits GF. Ontogeny of Ca2+-induced Ca2+ release in rabbit ventricular myocytes. Am J Physiol Cell Physiol. 2008;294(2):C516–525.
59. Huang J, Hove-Madsen L, Tibbits GF. Na+/Ca2+ exchange activity in neonatal rabbit ventricular myocytes. Am J Physiol Cell Physiol. 2005;288(1):C195–203.
60. Boucek Jr RJ, Shelton M, Artman M, et al. Comparative effects of verapamil, nifedipine, and diltiazem on contractile function in the isolated immature and adult rabbit heart. Pediatr Res. 1984;18(10):948–52.
61. Jarmakani JM, Nakanishi T, George BL, et al. Effect of extracellular calcium on myocardial mechanical function in the neonatal rabbit. Dev Pharmacol Ther. 1982;5(1–2):1–13.
62. McCall SJ, Nassar R, Malouf NN, et al. Development and cardiac contractility: cardiac troponin T isoforms and cytosolic calcium in rabbit. Pediatr Res. 2006;60(3):276–81.
63. Solaro RJ, Lee JA, Kentish JC, et al. Effects of acidosis on ventricular muscle from adult and neonatal rats. Circ Res. 1988;63(4):779–87.
64. Noland Jr TA, Guo X, Raynor RL, et al. Cardiac troponin I mutants. Phosphorylation by protein kinases C and A and regulation of Ca(2+)-stimulated MgATPase of reconstituted actomyosin S-1. J Biol Chem. 1995;270(43):25445–54.
65. El-Khuffash AF, Molloy EJ. Serum troponin in neonatal intensive care. Neonatology. 2008;94(1):1–7.
66. Marijianowski MM, van der Loos CM, Mohrschladt MF, et al. The neonatal heart has a relatively high content of total collagen and type I collagen, a condition that may explain the less compliant state. J Am Coll Cardiol. 1994;23(5):1204–8.
67. Robinson RB. Autonomic receptor–effector coupling during postnatal development. Cardiovasc Res. 1996;31(Spec No): E68–76.
68. Short BL, Van Meurs K, Evans JR. Summary proceedings from the cardiology group on cardiovascular instability in preterm infants. Pediatrics. 2006;117(3 Pt 2):S34–39.
69. Hegyi T, Anwar M, Carbone MT, et al. Blood pressure ranges in premature infants: II. The first week of life. Pediatrics. 1996;97(3):336–42.
70. Hegyi T, Carbone MT, Anwar M, et al. Blood pressure ranges in premature infants. I. The first hours of life. J Pediatr. 1994;124(4):627–33.
71. Miall-Allen VM, de Vries LS, Whitelaw AG. Mean arterial blood pressure and neonatal cerebral lesions. Arch Dis Child. 1987;62(10):1068–9.
72. Miranda P. Intraventricular hemorrhage and posthemorrhagic hydrocephalus in the preterm infant. Minerva Pediatr. 2010;62(1):79–89.
73. Nuntnarumit P, Yang W, Bada-Ellzey HS. Blood pressure measurements in the newborn. Clin Perinatol. 1999;26(4):981–96.
74. Development of audit measures and guidelines for good practice in the management of neonatal respiratory distress syndrome. Report of a Joint Working Group of the British Association of Perinatal Medicine and the Research Unit of the Royal College of Physicians. Arch Dis Child. 1992;67(10 Spec No):1221–7.
75. Bada HS, Korones SB, Perry EH, et al. Mean arterial blood pressure changes in premature infants and those at risk for intraventricular hemorrhage. J Pediatr. 1990;117(4):607–14.
76. Watkins AM, West CR, Cooke RW. Blood pressure and cerebral haemorrhage and ischaemia in very low birthweight infants. Early Hum Dev. 1989;19(2):103–10.
77. Cayabyab R, McLean CW, Seri I. Definition of hypotension and assessment of hemodynamics in the preterm neonate. J Perinatol. 2009;29 Suppl 2:S58–62.
78. Evans N. Which inotrope for which baby? Arch Dis Child Fetal Neonatal Ed. 2006;91(3):F213–220.
79. Kluckow M, Evans N. Relationship between blood pressure and cardiac output in preterm infants requiring mechanical ventilation. J Pediatr. 1996;129(4):506–12.
80. Groves AM, Kuschel CA, Knight DB, et al. Relationship between blood pressure and blood flow in newborn preterm infants. Arch Dis Child Fetal Neonatal Ed. 2008;93(1):F29–32.
81. Osborn DA, Evans N, Kluckow M. Clinical detection of low upper body blood flow in very premature infants using blood pressure, capillary refill time, and central-peripheral temperature difference. Arch Dis Child Fetal Neonatal Ed. 2004;89(2): F168–173.
82. Kluckow M, Evans N. Superior vena cava flow in newborn infants: a novel marker of systemic blood flow. Arch Dis Child Fetal Neonatal Ed. 2000;82(3):F182–187.
83. Kluckow M, Evans N. Low superior vena cava flow and intraventricular haemorrhage in preterm infants. Arch Dis Child Fetal Neonatal Ed. 2000;82(3):F188–194.
84. Pladys P, Wodey E, Beuchee A, et al. Left ventricle output and mean arterial blood pressure in preterm infants during the 1st day of life. Eur J Pediatr. 1999;158(10):817–24.
85. Osborn D, Evans N, Kluckow M. Randomized trial of dobutamine versus dopamine in preterm infants with low systemic blood flow. J Pediatr. 2002;140(2):183–91.
86. Hunt RW, Evans N, Rieger I, et al. Low superior vena cava flow and neurodevelopment at 3 years in very preterm infants. J Pediatr. 2004;145(5):588–92.
87. Thornburg KL, Morton MJ. Filling and arterial pressures as determinants of left ventricular stroke volume in fetal lambs. Am J Physiol. 1986;251(5 Pt 2):H961–968.
88. Klopfenstein HS, Rudolph AM. Postnatal changes in the circulation and responses to volume loading in sheep. Circ Res. 1978;42(6):839–45.
89. Teitel DF, Sidi D, Chin T, et al. Developmental changes in myocardial contractile reserve in the lamb. Pediatr Res. 1985;19(9):948–55.
90. Perlman JM. Intervention strategies for neonatal hypoxic-ischemic cerebral injury. Clin Ther. 2006;28(9):1353–65.
91. Pierson CR, Folkerth RD, Billiards SS, et al. Gray matter injury associated with periventricular leukomalacia in the premature infant. Acta Neuropathol. 2007;114(6):619–31.
92. Volpe JJ. Encephalopathy of prematurity includes neuronal abnormalities. Pediatrics. 2005;116(1):221–5.
93. Volpe JJ. Brain injury in premature infants: a complex amalgam of destructive and developmental disturbances. Lancet Neurol. 2009;8(1):110–24.
94. Volpe JJ. The encephalopathy of prematurity–brain injury and impaired brain development inextricably intertwined. Semin Pediatr Neurol. 2009;16(4):167–78.
95. Kinney HC. The encephalopathy of prematurity: one pediatric neuropathologist's perspective. Semin Pediatr Neurol. 2009;16(4):179–90.
96. Volpe JJ. Neural tube formation and prosencephalic development. In: Volpe JJ, editor. Neurology of the newborn. Philadelphia, PA: Saunders/Elsevier; 2008. p. 3–50.

97. Lorber J. Systematic ventriculographic studies in infants born with meningomyelocele and encephalocele. The incidence and development of hydrocephalus. Arch Dis Child. 1961;36:381–9.
98. Kirk VG, Morielli A, Brouillette RT. Sleep-disordered breathing in patients with myelomeningocele: the missed diagnosis. Dev Med Child Neurol. 1999;41(1):40–3.
99. Kirk VG, Morielli A, Gozal D, et al. Treatment of sleep-disordered breathing in children with myelomeningocele. Pediatr Pulmonol. 2000;30(6):445–52.
100. Parrish ML, Roessmann U, Levinsohn MW. Agenesis of the corpus callosum: a study of the frequency of associated malformations. Ann Neurol. 1979;6(4):349–54.
101. Jeret JS, Serur D, Wisniewski KE, et al. Clinicopathological findings associated with agenesis of the corpus callosum. Brain Dev. 1987;9(3):255–64.
102. Kinney HC. The near-term (late preterm) human brain and risk for periventricular leukomalacia: a review. Semin Perinatol. 2006; 30(2):81–8.
103. Volpe JJ. Cerebellum of the premature infant: rapidly developing, vulnerable, clinically important. J Child Neurol. 2009;24(9): 1085–104.
104. Limperopoulos C, Soul JS, Gauvreau K, et al. Late gestation cerebellar growth is rapid and impeded by premature birth. Pediatrics. 2005;115(3):688–95.
105. Limperopoulos C, Soul JS, Haidar H, et al. Impaired trophic interactions between the cerebellum and the cerebrum among preterm infants. Pediatrics. 2005;116(4):844–50.
106. Limperopoulos C, du Plessis AJ. Disorders of cerebellar growth and development. Curr Opin Pediatr. 2006;18(6):621–7.
107. Borch K, Lou HC, Greisen G. Cerebral white matter blood flow and arterial blood pressure in preterm infants. Acta Paediatr. 2010;99(10):1489–92.
108. Miller SP, Ferriero DM. From selective vulnerability to connectivity: insights from newborn brain imaging. Trends Neurosci. 2009;32(9):496–505.
109. McQuillen PS, Ferriero DM. Perinatal subplate neuron injury: implications for cortical development and plasticity. Brain Pathol. 2005;15(3):250–60.
110. Ferriero DM, Holtzman DM, Black SM, et al. Neonatal mice lacking neuronal nitric oxide synthase are less vulnerable to hypoxic-ischemic injury. Neurobiol Dis. 1996;3(1):64–71.
111. Volpe JJ. Hypoxic-ischemic encephalopathy: biochemical and physiological aspects. In: Volpe JJ, editor. Neurology of the newborn. Philadelphia, PA: Saunders/Elsevier; 2008. p. 247–324.
112. Khwaja O, Volpe JJ. Pathogenesis of cerebral white matter injury of prematurity. Arch Dis Child Fetal Neonatal Ed. 2008;93(2):F153–161.
113. Gonzalez FF, Ferriero DM. Neuroprotection in the newborn infant. Clin Perinatol. 2009;36(4):859–80. vii.
114. Kostovic I, Jovanov-Milosevic N. The development of cerebral connections during the first 20-45 weeks' gestation. Semin Fetal Neonatal Med. 2006;11(6):415–22.
115. Leviton A, Gressens P. Neuronal damage accompanies perinatal white-matter damage. Trends Neurosci. 2007;30(9):473–8.
116. Nguyen V, McQuillen PS. AMPA and metabotropic excitoxicity explain subplate neuron vulnerability. Neurobiol Dis. 2010;37(1):195–207.
117. Kapellou O, Counsell SJ, Kennea N, et al. Abnormal cortical development after premature birth shown by altered allometric scaling of brain growth. PLoS Med. 2006;3(8):e265.
118. Boardman JP, Counsell SJ, Rueckert D, et al. Abnormal deep grey matter development following preterm birth detected using deformation-based morphometry. Neuroimage. 2006;32(1):70–8.
119. Counsell SJ, Dyet LE, Larkman DJ, et al. Thalamo-cortical connectivity in children born preterm mapped using probabilistic magnetic resonance tractography. Neuroimage. 2007;34(3):896–904.
120. Dudink J, Kerr JL, Paterson K, et al. Connecting the developing preterm brain. Early Hum Dev. 2008;84(12):777–82.
121. Karadottir R, Attwell D. Neurotransmitter receptors in the life and death of oligodendrocytes. Neuroscience. 2007;145(4):1426–38.
122. Billiards SS, Haynes RL, Folkerth RD, et al. Development of microglia in the cerebral white matter of the human fetus and infant. J Comp Neurol. 2006;497(2):199–208.
123. Anjari M, Counsell SJ, Srinivasan L, et al. The association of lung disease with cerebral white matter abnormalities in preterm infants. Pediatrics. 2009;124(1):268–76.
124. Shah DK, Doyle LW, Anderson PJ, et al. Adverse neurodevelopment in preterm infants with postnatal sepsis or necrotizing enterocolitis is mediated by white matter abnormalities on magnetic resonance imaging at term. J Pediatr. 2008;153(2):170–5, e171.
125. Volpe JJ. Hypoxic-ischemic encephalopathy: neuropathology and pathogenesis. In: Volpe JJ, editor. Neurology of the newborn. Philadelphia, PA: Saunders/Elsevier; 2008. p. 347–99.
126. Chau V, Poskitt KJ, Miller SP. Advanced neuroimaging techniques for the term newborn with encephalopathy. Pediatr Neurol. 2009;40(3):181–8.
127. Miller SP, Ramaswamy V, Michelson D, et al. Patterns of brain injury in term neonatal encephalopathy. J Pediatr. 2005;146(4):453–60.
128. Cowan F, Rutherford M, Groenendaal F, et al. Origin and timing of brain lesions in term infants with neonatal encephalopathy. Lancet. 2003;361(9359):736–42.
129. Edwards AD, Brocklehurst P, Gunn AJ, et al. Neurological outcomes at 18 months of age after moderate hypothermia for perinatal hypoxic ischaemic encephalopathy: synthesis and meta-analysis of trial data. BMJ. 2010;340:c363.
130. Limperopoulos C, Majnemer A, Shevell MI, et al. Neurologic status of newborns with congenital heart defects before open heart surgery. Pediatrics. 1999;103(2):402–8.
131. Miller SP, McQuillen PS, Hamrick S, et al. Abnormal brain development in newborns with congenital heart disease. N Engl J Med. 2007;357(19):1928–38.
132. Licht DJ, Shera DM, Clancy RR, et al. Brain maturation is delayed in infants with complex congenital heart defects. J Thorac Cardiovasc Surg. 2009;137(3):529–36. discussion 536–7.
133. Miller SP, McQuillen PS. Neurology of congenital heart disease: insight from brain imaging. Arch Dis Child Fetal Neonatal Ed. 2007;92(6):F435–437.
134. Limperopoulos C, Tworetzky W, McElhinney DB, et al. Brain volume and metabolism in fetuses with congenital heart disease: evaluation with quantitative magnetic resonance imaging and spectroscopy. Circulation. 2010;121(1):26–33.
135. McQuillen PS, Miller SP. Congenital heart disease and brain development. Ann NY Acad Sci. 2010;1184:68–86.
136. Majnemer A, Limperopoulos C, Shevell MI, et al. A new look at outcomes of infants with congenital heart disease. Pediatr Neurol. 2009;40(3):197–204.
137. Paulson OB, Strandgaard S, Edvinsson L. Cerebral autoregulation. Cerebrovasc Brain Metab Rev. 1990;2(2):161–92.
138. Versmold HT, Kitterman JA, Phibbs RH, et al. Aortic blood pressure during the first 12 hours of life in infants with birth weight 610 to 4,220 grams. Pediatrics. 1981;67(5):607–13.
139. Lou HC, Lassen NA, Friis-Hansen B. Impaired autoregulation of cerebral blood flow in the distressed newborn infant. J Pediatr. 1979;94(1):118–21.
140. Lou HC. Autoregulation of cerebral blood flow and brain lesions in newborn infants. Lancet. 1998;352(9138):1406.
141. Greisen G. To autoregulate or not to autoregulate–that is no longer the question. Semin Pediatr Neurol. 2009;16(4):207–15.
142. Tweed A, Cote J, Lou H, et al. Impairment of cerebral blood flow autoregulation in the newborn lamb by hypoxia. Pediatr Res. 1986;20(6):516–9.

143. Lou HC, Lassen NA, Friis-Hansen B. Low cerebral blood flow in hypotensive perinatal distress. Acta Neurol Scand. 1977;56(4): 343–52.
144. Kaiser JR, Gauss CH, Williams DK. The effects of hypercapnia on cerebral autoregulation in ventilated very low birth weight infants. Pediatr Res. 2005;58(5):931–5.
145. Noori S, Stavroudis TA, Seri I. Systemic and cerebral hemodynamics during the transitional period after premature birth. Clin Perinatol. 2009;36(4):723–36. v.
146. Greisen G. Autoregulation of cerebral blood flow in newborn babies. Early Hum Dev. 2005;81(5):423–8.
147. Pryds O, Greisen G, Lou H, et al. Vasoparalysis associated with brain damage in asphyxiated term infants. J Pediatr. 1990;117(1 Pt 1):119–25.
148. Boylan GB, Young K, Panerai RB, et al. Dynamic cerebral autoregulation in sick newborn infants. Pediatr Res. 2000;48(1):12–7.
149. Pryds O. Control of cerebral circulation in the high-risk neonate. Ann Neurol. 1991;30(3):321–9.
150. Pryds O, Greisen G, Lou H, et al. Heterogeneity of cerebral vasoreactivity in preterm infants supported by mechanical ventilation. J Pediatr. 1989;115(4):638–45.
151. Wyatt JS, Edwards AD, Cope M, et al. Response of cerebral blood volume to changes in arterial carbon dioxide tension in preterm and term infants. Pediatr Res. 1991;29(6):553–7.
152. Kaiser JR, Gauss CH, Pont MM, et al. Hypercapnia during the first 3 days of life is associated with severe intraventricular hemorrhage in very low birth weight infants. J Perinatol. 2006;26(5): 279–85.
153. Fujimoto S, Togari H, Yamaguchi N, et al. Hypocarbia and cystic periventricular leukomalacia in premature infants. Arch Dis Child. 1994;71(2):F107–110.
154. Liem KD, Greisen G. Monitoring of cerebral haemodynamics in newborn infants. Early Hum Dev. 2010;86(3):155–8.
155. Wijbenga RG, Lemmers PM, van Bel F. Cerebral oxygenation during the first days of life in preterm and term neonates: differences between different brain regions. Pediatr Res. 2011;70(4):389–94.
156. Limperopoulos C, Bassan H, Kalish LA, et al. Current definitions of hypotension do not predict abnormal cranial ultrasound findings in preterm infants. Pediatrics. 2007;120(5):966–77.
157. Tsuji M, Saul JP, du Plessis A, et al. Cerebral intravascular oxygenation correlates with mean arterial pressure in critically ill premature infants. Pediatrics. 2000;106(4):625–32.
158. Soul JS, Taylor GA, Wypij D, et al. Noninvasive detection of changes in cerebral blood flow by near-infrared spectroscopy in a piglet model of hydrocephalus. Pediatr Res. 2000;48(4):445–9.
159. Soul JS, Hammer PE, Tsuji M, et al. Fluctuating pressure-passivity is common in the cerebral circulation of sick premature infants. Pediatr Res. 2007;61(4):467–73.
160. Gilmore MM, Stone BS, Shepard JA, et al. Relationship between cerebrovascular dysautoregulation and arterial blood pressure in the premature infant. J Perinatol. 2011;31(11):722–9.
161. O'Leary H, Gregas MC, Limperopoulos C, et al. Elevated cerebral pressure passivity is associated with prematurity-related intracranial hemorrhage. Pediatrics. 2009;124(1):302–9.
162. van Bel F, Lemmers P, Naulaers G. Monitoring neonatal regional cerebral oxygen saturation in clinical practice: value and pitfalls. Neonatology. 2008;94(4):237–44.
163. De Smet D, Jacobs J, Ameye L, et al. The partial coherence method for assessment of impaired cerebral autoregulation using near-infrared spectroscopy: potential and limitations. Adv Exp Med Biol. 2010;662:219–24.
164. Wong FY, Silas R, Hew S, et al. Cerebral oxygenation is highly sensitive to blood pressure variability in sick preterm infants. PLoS One. 2012;7(8):e43165.
165. Volpe JJ. Cerebral white matter injury of the premature infant - more common than you think. Pediatrics. 2003;112(1 Pt 1): 176–80.
166. Dyet LE, Kennea N, Counsell SJ, et al. Natural history of brain lesions in extremely preterm infants studied with serial magnetic resonance imaging from birth and neurodevelopmental assessment. Pediatrics. 2006;118(2):536–48.
167. Maalouf EF, Duggan PJ, Rutherford MA, et al. Magnetic resonance imaging of the brain in a cohort of extremely preterm infants. J Pediatr. 1999;135(3):351–7.
168. Rorke LB. Anatomical features of the developing brain implicated in pathogenesis of hypoxic-ischemic injury. Brain Pathol. 1992;2(3):211–21.
169. Greisen G, Borch K. White matter injury in the preterm neonate: the role of perfusion. Dev Neurosci. 2001;23(3):209–12.
170. Young RS, Hernandez MJ, Yagel SK. Selective reduction of blood flow to white matter during hypotension in newborn dogs: a possible mechanism of periventricular leukomalacia. Ann Neurol. 1982;12(5):445–8.
171. Papile LA, Burstein J, Burstein R, et al. Incidence and evolution of subependymal and intraventricular hemorrhage: a study of infants with birth weights less than 1,500 gm. J Pediatr. 1978;92(4):529–34.
172. Volpe JJ. Germinal matrix-intraventricular hemorrhage of the premature infant. In: Volpe JJ, editor. Neurology of the newborn. Philadelphia, PA: Saunders/Elsevier; 2008. p. 517–88.
173. Bassan H, Limperopoulos C, Visconti K, et al. Neurodevelopmental outcome in survivors of periventricular hemorrhagic infarction. Pediatrics. 2007;120(4):785–92.
174. Adams-Chapman I, Hansen NI, Stoll BJ, et al. Neurodevelopmental outcome of extremely low birth weight infants with posthemorrhagic hydrocephalus requiring shunt insertion. Pediatrics. 2008;121(5):e1167–1177.
175. Wilson-Costello D, Friedman H, Minich N, et al. Improved neurodevelopmental outcomes for extremely low birth weight infants in 2000-2002. Pediatrics. 2007;119(1):37–45.
176. Vohr BR, Wright LL, Dusick AM, et al. Neurodevelopmental and functional outcomes of extremely low birth weight infants in the National Institute of Child Health and Human Development Neonatal Research Network, 1993-1994. Pediatrics. 2000;105(6): 1216–26.
177. Patra K, Wilson-Costello D, Taylor HG, et al. Grades I-II intraventricular hemorrhage in extremely low birth weight infants: effects on neurodevelopment. J Pediatr. 2006;149(2):169–73.
178. Vasileiadis GT, Gelman N, Han VK, et al. Uncomplicated intraventricular hemorrhage is followed by reduced cortical volume at near-term age. Pediatrics. 2004;114(3):e367–372.
179. Bassan H. Intracranial hemorrhage in the preterm infant: understanding it, preventing it. Clin Perinatol. 2009;36(4):737–62. v.
180. Gonzalez FF, Ferriero DM. Neuroprotection in the newborn infant. Clin Perinatol. 2009;36(4):859–80. vii.
181. Perlman JM. The relationship between systemic hemodynamic perturbations and periventricular-intraventricular hemorrhage–a historical perspective. Semin Pediatr Neurol. 2009;16(4):191–9.
182. Bodensteiner JB, Johnsen SD. Magnetic resonance imaging (MRI) findings in children surviving extremely premature delivery and extremely low birthweight with cerebral palsy. J Child Neurol. 2006;21(9):743–7.
183. Limperopoulos C, Benson CB, Bassan H, et al. Cerebellar hemorrhage in the preterm infant: ultrasonographic findings and risk factors. Pediatrics. 2005;116(3):717–24.
184. Messerschmidt A, Fuiko R, Prayer D, et al. Disrupted cerebellar development in preterm infants is associated with impaired neurodevelopmental outcome. Eur J Pediatr. 2008;167(10): 1141–7.

185. Messerschmidt A, Prayer D, Brugger PC, et al. Preterm birth and disruptive cerebellar development: assessment of perinatal risk factors. Eur J Paediatr Neurol. 2008;12(6):455–60.
186. Allin M, Matsumoto H, Santhouse AM, et al. Cognitive and motor function and the size of the cerebellum in adolescents born very pre-term. Brain. 2001;124(Pt 1):60–6.
187. Limperopoulos C, Bassan H, Gauvreau K, et al. Does cerebellar injury in premature infants contribute to the high prevalence of long-term cognitive, learning, and behavioral disability in survivors? Pediatrics. 2007;120(3):584–93.
188. Limperopoulos C. Extreme prematurity, cerebellar injury, and autism. Semin Pediatr Neurol. 2010;17(1):25–9.
189. Schmahmann JD. Disorders of the cerebellum: ataxia, dysmetria of thought, and the cerebellar cognitive affective syndrome. J Neuropsychiatry Clin Neurosci. 2004;16(3):367–78.
190. Langston C, Kida K, Reed M, et al. Human lung growth in late gestation and in the neonate. Am Rev Respir Dis. 1984; 129(4):607–13.
191. Kotecha S. Lung growth for beginners. Paediatr Respir Rev. 2000;1(4):308–13.
192. Joshi S, Kotecha S. Lung growth and development. Early Hum Dev. 2007;83(12):789–94.
193. Jeffrey PK. The development of large and small airways. Am J Respir Crit Care Med. 1998;157(5 Pt 2):S174–180.
194. Masters JR. Epithelial-mesenchymal interaction during lung development: the effect of mesenchymal mass. Dev Biol. 1976;51(1):98–108.
195. Kotecha S. Lung growth: implications for the newborn infant. Arch Dis Child Fetal Neonatal Ed. 2000;82(1):F69–74.
196. Hislop AA, Pierce CM. Growth of the vascular tree. Paediatr Respir Rev. 2000;1(4):321–7.
197. Merkus PJ, ten Have-Opbroek AA, Quanjer PH. Human lung growth: a review. Pediatr Pulmonol. 1996;21(6):383–97.
198. Schumpelick V, Steinau G, Schluper I, et al. Surgical embryology and anatomy of the diaphragm with surgical applications. Surg Clin North Am. 2000;80(1):213–39. xi.
199. Clugston RD, Greer JJ. Diaphragm development and congenital diaphragmatic hernia. Semin Pediatr Surg. 2007;16(2):94–100.
200. Yang W, Carmichael SL, Harris JA, et al. Epidemiologic characteristics of congenital diaphragmatic hernia among 2.5 million California births, 1989-1997. Birth Defects Res A Clin Mol Teratol. 2006;76(3):170–4.
201. Torfs CP, Curry CJ, Bateson TF, et al. A population-based study of congenital diaphragmatic hernia. Teratology. 1992;46(6):555–65.
202. Areechon W, Eid L. Hypoplasia of lung with congenital diaphragmatic hernia. Br Med J. 1963;1(5325):230–3.
203. Slavotinek AM. The genetics of congenital diaphragmatic hernia. Semin Perinatol. 2005;29(2):77–85.
204. Scott DA. Genetics of congenital diaphragmatic hernia. Semin Pediatr Surg. 2007;16(2):88–93.
205. Meyer CH, Sel S, Horle S, et al. Rosai-Dorfman disease with bilateral serous retinal detachment. Arch Ophthalmol. 2003;121(5):733–5.
206. Babiuk RP, Greer JJ. Diaphragm defects occur in a CDH hernia model independently of myogenesis and lung formation. Am J Physiol Lung Cell Mol Physiol. 2002;283(6):L1310–1314.
207. Arkovitz MS, Hyatt BA, Shannon JM. Lung development is not necessary for diaphragm development in mice. J Pediatr Surg. 2005;40(9):1390–4.
208. Whitsett JA, Wert SE, Weaver TE. Alveolar surfactant homeostasis and the pathogenesis of pulmonary disease. Annu Rev Med. 2010;61:105–19.
209. Ochs M, Nyengaard JR, Jung A, et al. The number of alveoli in the human lung. Am J Respir Crit Care Med. 2004;169(1):120–4.
210. Thurlbeck WM. Postnatal human lung growth. Thorax. 1982;37(8):564–71.
211. Moessinger AC, Harding R, Adamson TM, et al. Role of lung fluid volume in growth and maturation of the fetal sheep lung. J Clin Invest. 1990;86(4):1270–7.
212. Kitterman JA, Chapin CJ, Vanderbilt JN, et al. Effects of oligohydramnios on lung growth and maturation in the fetal rat. Am J Physiol Lung Cell Mol Physiol. 2002;282(3):L431–439.
213. Thomas IT, Smith DW. Oligohydramnios, cause of the nonrenal features of Potter's syndrome, including pulmonary hypoplasia. J Pediatr. 1974;84(6):811–5.
214. Fantel AG, Shepard TH. Potter syndrome. Nonrenal features induced by oligoamnios. Am J Dis Child. 1975;129(11):1346–7.
215. Khan PA, Cloutier M, Piedboeuf B. Tracheal occlusion: a review of obstructing fetal lungs to make them grow and mature. Am J Med Genet C Semin Med Genet. 2007;145C(2):125–38.
216. Wigglesworth JS, Desai R. Is fetal respiratory function a major determinant of perinatal survival? Lancet. 1982;1(8266):264–7.
217. Greenough A. Factors adversely affecting lung growth. Paediatr Respir Rev. 2000;1(4):314–20.
218. Zeltner TB, Burri PH. The postnatal development and growth of the human lung. II. Morphology. Respir Physiol. 1987; 67(3):269–82.
219. Burri PH. Structural aspects of postnatal lung development - alveolar formation and growth. Biol Neonate. 2006;89(4):313–22.
220. Zeman KL, Bennett WD. Growth of the small airways and alveoli from childhood to the adult lung measured by aerosol-derived airway morphometry. J Appl Physiol. 2006;100(3):965–71.
221. Watterberg KL, Demers LM, Scott SM, et al. Chorioamnionitis and early lung inflammation in infants in whom bronchopulmonary dysplasia develops. Pediatrics. 1996;97(2):210–5.
222. Speer CP. Chorioamnionitis, postnatal factors and proinflammatory response in the pathogenetic sequence of bronchopulmonary dysplasia. Neonatology. 2009;95(4):353–61.
223. Hislop AA, Wigglesworth JS, Desai R, et al. The effects of preterm delivery and mechanical ventilation on human lung growth. Early Hum Dev. 1987;15(3):147–64.
224. Van Marter LJ. Strategies for preventing bronchopulmonary dysplasia. Curr Opin Pediatr. 2005;17(2):174–80.
225. Stocks J, Dezateux C. The effect of parental smoking on lung function and development during infancy. Respirology. 2003;8(3):266–85.
226. Blair PS, Fleming PJ, Bensley D, et al. Smoking and the sudden infant death syndrome: results from 1993-5 case-control study for confidential inquiry into stillbirths and deaths in infancy. Confidential Enquiry into Stillbirths and Deaths Regional Coordinators and Researchers. BMJ. 1996;313(7051):195–8.
227. Cunningham J, Dockery DW, Speizer FE. Maternal smoking during pregnancy as a predictor of lung function in children. Am J Epidemiol. 1994;139(12):1139–52.
228. Reiterer F, Abbasi S, Bhutani VK. Influence of head-neck posture on airflow and pulmonary mechanics in preterm neonates. Pediatr Pulmonol. 1994;17(3):149–54.
229. Rodenstein DO, Perlmutter N, Stanescu DC. Infants are not obligatory nasal breathers. Am Rev Respir Dis. 1985;131(3):343–7.
230. Bergeson PS, Shaw JC. Are infants really obligatory nasal breathers? Clin Pediatr (Phila). 2001;40(10):567–9.
231. Motoyama EK. The shape of the pediatric larynx: cylindrical or funnel shaped? Anesth Analg. 2009;108(5):1379–81.
232. Dalal PG, Murray D, Messner AH, et al. Pediatric laryngeal dimensions: an age-based analysis. Anesth Analg. 2009;108(5):1475–9.
233. Litman RS, Weissend EE, Shibata D, et al. Developmental changes of laryngeal dimensions in unparalyzed, sedated children. Anesthesiology. 2003;98(1):41–5.
234. Dickison AE. The normal and abnormal pediatric upper airway. Recognition and management of obstruction. Clin Chest Med. 1987;8(4):583–96.

235. Cullen AB, Wolfson MR, Shaffer TH. The maturation of airway structure and function. Neoreviews. 2002;3(7):e125–130.
236. Morley C. Continuous distending pressure. Arch Dis Child Fetal Neonatal Ed. 1999;81(2):F152–156.
237. Stocks J. Respiratory physiology during early life. Monaldi Arch Chest Dis. 1999;54(4):358–64.
238. Muller NL, Bryan AC. Chest wall mechanics and respiratory muscles in infants. Pediatr Clin North Am. 1979;26(3):503–16.
239. Openshaw P, Edwards S, Helms P. Changes in rib cage geometry during childhood. Thorax. 1984;39(8):624–7.
240. Papastamelos C, Panitch HB, England SE, et al. Developmental changes in chest wall compliance in infancy and early childhood. J Appl Physiol. 1995;78(1):179–84.
241. Fisher JT, Mortola JP. Statics of the respiratory system in newborn mammals. Respir Physiol. 1980;41(2):155–72.
242. Mortola JP, Piazza T. Breathing pattern in rats with chronic section of the superior laryngeal nerves. Respir Physiol. 1987;70(1):51–62.
243. Frappell PB, MacFarlane PM. Development of mechanics and pulmonary reflexes. Respir Physiol Neurobiol. 2005;149(1–3):143–54.
244. Knill R, Andrews W, Bryan AC, et al. Respiratory load compensation in infants. J Appl Physiol. 1976;40(3):357–61.
245. Anthonisen NR, Engel L, Grassino A, et al. The clinical significance of measurements of closing volume. Scand J Respir Dis Suppl. 1974;85:245–50.
246. Davey MG, Johns DP, Harding R. Postnatal development of respiratory function in lambs studied serially between birth and 8 weeks. Respir Physiol. 1998;113(1):83–93.
247. Davis GM, Bureau MA. Pulmonary and chest wall mechanics in the control of respiration in the newborn. Clin Perinatol. 1987;14(3):551–79.
248. Keens TG, Bryan AC, Levison H, et al. Developmental pattern of muscle fiber types in human ventilatory muscles. J Appl Physiol. 1978;44(6):909–13.
249. Watchko JF, Sieck GC. Respiratory muscle fatigue resistance relates to myosin phenotype and SDH activity during development. J Appl Physiol. 1993;75(3):1341–7.
250. Zhan WZ, Watchko JF, Prakash YS, et al. Isotonic contractile and fatigue properties of developing rat diaphragm muscle. J Appl Physiol. 1998;84(4):1260–8.
251. Lavin T, Song Y, Bakker AJ, et al. Developmental changes in diaphragm muscle function in the preterm and postnatal lamb. Pediatr Pulmonol. 2013;48(7):640–8.
252. Watchko JF, Mayock DE, Standaert TA, et al. Postnatal changes in transdiaphragmatic pressure in piglets. Pediatr Res. 1986;20(7):658–61.
253. Nichols DG. Respiratory muscle performance in infants and children. J Pediatr. 1991;118(4 Pt 1):493–502.
254. Mayock DE, Standaert TA, Woodrum DE. Effect of methylxanthines on diaphragmatic fatigue in the piglet. Pediatr Res. 1992;32(5):580–4.
255. Aubier M. Effect of theophylline on diaphragmatic muscle function. Chest. 1987;92(1 Suppl):27S–31S.
256. Mortola JP. Dynamics of breathing in newborn mammals. Physiol Rev. 1987;67(1):187–243.
257. Williams JV, Tierney DF, Parker HR. Surface forces in the lung, atelectasis, and transpulmonary pressure. J Appl Physiol. 1966;21(3):819–27.
258. Kosch PC, Stark AR. Dynamic maintenance of end-expiratory lung volume in full-term infants. J Appl Physiol. 1984;57(4):1126–33.
259. Martin RJ, Okken A, Katona PG, et al. Effect of lung volume on expiratory time in the newborn infant. J Appl Physiol. 1978;45(1):18–23.
260. Harrison VC, Heese Hde V, Klein M. The significance of grunting in hyaline membrane disease. Pediatrics. 1968;41(3):549–59.
261. Gaultier C, Praud JP, Canet E, et al. Paradoxical inward rib cage motion during rapid eye movement sleep in infants and young children. J Dev Physiol. 1987;9(5):391–7.
262. Stark AR, Cohlan BA, Waggener TB, et al. Regulation of end-expiratory lung volume during sleep in premature infants. J Appl Physiol (1985). 1987;62(3):1117–23.
263. Gregory GA, Edmunds Jr LH, Kitterman JA, et al. Continuous positive airway pressure and pulmonary and circulatory function after cardiac surgery in infants less than three months of age. Anesthesiology. 1975;43(4):426–31.
264. Thibeault DW, Poblete E, Auld PA. Alevolar-arterial O2 and CO2 differences and their relation to lung volume in the newborn. Pediatrics. 1968;41(3):574–87.
265. Merkus PJFM, de Jongste JC, Stocks J. Respiratory function measurements in infants and children. Eur Respir Mon. 2005;31:166–94.
266. Hulskamp G, Pillow JJ, Stocks J. Lung function testing in acute neonatal respiratory disorders and chronic lung disease of infancy: a review series. Pediatr Pulmonol. 2005;40(6):467–70.
267. Stocks J. Lung function testing in infants. Pediatr Pulmonol Suppl. 1999;18:14–20.
268. Gappa M, Pillow JJ, Allen J, et al. Lung function tests in neonates and infants with chronic lung disease: lung and chest-wall mechanics. Pediatr Pulmonol. 2006;41(4):291–317.
269. Stocks J. Effect of nasogastric tubes on nasal resistance during infancy. Arch Dis Child. 1980;55(1):17–21.
270. Dunnill MS. Postnatal growth of the lung. Thorax. 1962;17:329–33.
271. Hand IL, Shepard EK, Krauss AN, et al. Ventilation-perfusion abnormalities in the preterm infant with hyaline membrane disease: a two-compartment model of the neonatal lung. Pediatr Pulmonol. 1990;9(4):206–13.
272. Evans JM, Hogg MI, Rosen M. Measurement of carbon dioxide output, alveolar carbon dioxide concentration and alveolar ventilation in the neonate. Br J Anaesth. 1977;49(5):453–6.
273. Cook CD, Cherry RB, O'Brien D, et al. Studies of respiratory physiology in the newborn infant. I. Observations on normal premature and full-term infants. J Clin Invest. 1955;34(7, Part 1):975–82.
274. Nelson NM, Prod'Hom LS, Cherry RB, et al. Pulmonary function in the newborn infant. I. Methods: ventilation and gaseous metabolism. Pediatrics. 1962;30:963–74.
275. Garcia-Fernandez J, Castro L, Belda J. Ventilating the newborn and child. Curr Anaesth Crit Care. 2010;21(5–6):262–8.
276. Otis AB, Fenn WO, Rahn H. Mechanics of breathing in man. J Appl Physiol. 1950;2(11):592–607.
277. Crosfill ML, Widdicombe JG. Physical characteristics of the chest and lungs and the work of breathing in different mammalian species. J Physiol. 1961;158:1–14.
278. Gagliardi L, Rusconi F. Respiratory rate and body mass in the first three years of life. The working party on respiratory rate. Arch Dis Child. 1997;76(2):151–4.
279. Mortola JP. Some functional mechanical implications of the structural design of the respiratory system in newborn mammals. Am Rev Respir Dis. 1983;128(2 Pt 2):S69–72.
280. Thibeault DW, Clutario B, Awld PA. The oxygen cost of breathing in the premature infant. Pediatrics. 1966;37(6):954–9.
281. Roze JC, Chambille B, Fleury MA, et al. Oxygen cost of breathing in newborn infants with long-term ventilatory support. J Pediatr. 1995;127(6):984–7.
282. Hansen T, Corbet A. Pulmonary physiology of the Newborn. In: Taeusch HW, Ballard RA, Gleason CA, Avery ME, editors. Avery's diseases of the newborn. Philadephia, PA: Elsevier; 2005.

283. Clements JA, Hustead RF, Johnson RP, et al. Pulmonary surface tension and alveolar stability. J Appl Physiol. 1961;16:444–50.
284. Klaus MH, Clements JA, Havel RJ. Composition of surface-active material isolated from beef lung. Proc Natl Acad Sci USA. 1961;47:1858–9.
285. Liu M, Post M. Invited review: Mechanochemical signal transduction in the fetal lung. J Appl Physiol. 2000;89(5):2078–84.
286. ACOG educational bulletin. Assessment of fetal lung maturity. Number 230, November 1996. Committee on Educational Bulletins of the American College of Obstetricians and Gynecologists. Int J Gynaecol Obstet 1997;56(2):191–8.
287. Parmigiani S, Solari E, Bevilacqua G. Current concepts on the pulmonary surfactant in infants. J Matern Fetal Neonatal Med. 2005;18(6):369–80.
288. Piknova B, Schram V, Hall SB. Pulmonary surfactant: phase behavior and function. Curr Opin Struct Biol. 2002;12(4): 487–94.
289. Jobe AH, Jacobs. Catabolism of pulmonary surfactant. In: Robertson B, editor. Pulmonary surfactant. Amsterdam: Elsevier Science; 1984. p. 271–93.
290. Stern N, Riklis S, Kalina M, et al. The catabolism of lung surfactant by alveolar macrophages. Biochim Biophys Acta. 1986;877(3):323–33.
291. Jacobs H, Jobe A, Ikegami M, et al. The significance of reutilization of surfactant phosphatidylcholine. J Biol Chem. 1983; 258(7):4159–65.
292. Ikegami M. Surfactant catabolism. Respirology. 2006;11(Suppl): S24–27.
293. Hawgood S, Poulain FR. The pulmonary collectins and surfactant metabolism. Annu Rev Physiol. 2001;63:495–519.
294. Bangham AD. Lung surfactant: how it does and does not work. Lung. 1987;165(1):17–25.
295. Possmayer F. A proposed nomenclature for pulmonary surfactant-associated proteins. Am Rev Respir Dis. 1988;138(4):990–8.
296. Whitsett JA, Weaver TE. Hydrophobic surfactant proteins in lung function and disease. N Engl J Med. 2002;347(26):2141–8.
297. Kingma PS, Whitsett JA. In defense of the lung: surfactant protein A and surfactant protein D. Curr Opin Pharmacol. 2006;6(3): 277–83.
298. Sanderson RJ, Paul GW, Vatter AE, et al. Morphological and physical basis for lung surfactant action. Respir Physiol. 1976;27(3):379–92.
299. Clements JA. Surface phenomena in relation to pulmonary function. Physiologist. 1962;5:11–28.
300. Bachofen H, Schurch S, Urbinelli M. Surfactant and alveolar micromechanics. In: von Wichen P, Miller B, editors. Basic research on lung surfactant. Basel: Karger; 1990. p. 158–67.
301. Takishima T, Mead J. Tests of a model of pulmonary elasticity. J Appl Physiol. 1972;33(5):576–81.
302. Davis JM, Veness-Meehan K, Notter RH, et al. Changes in pulmonary mechanics after the administration of surfactant to infants with respiratory distress syndrome. N Engl J Med. 1988;319(8):476–9.
303. Peterson SW. Understanding the sequence of pulmonary injury in the extremely low birth weight, surfactant-deficient infant. Neonatal Netw. 2009;28(4):221–9. quiz 255-228.
304. Agrons GA, Courtney SE, Stocker JT, et al. From the archives of the AFIP: Lung disease in premature neonates: radiologic-pathologic correlation. Radiographics. 2005;25(4):1047–73.
305. Engle WA, American Academy of Pediatrics Committee on, F and Newborn. Surfactant-replacement therapy for respiratory distress in the preterm and term neonate. Pediatrics. 2008;121(2):419–32.
306. Stevens TP, Sinkin RA. Surfactant replacement therapy. Chest. 2007;131(5):1577–82.
307. Jobe AH. Prenatal corticosteroids: a neonatologist's perspective. Neoreviews. 2006;7(5):e259–67.
308. Davis PG, Morley CJ, Owen LS. Non-invasive respiratory support of preterm neonates with respiratory distress: continuous positive airway pressure and nasal intermittent positive pressure ventilation. Semin Fetal Neonatal Med. 2009;14(1):14–20.
309. Liggins GC, Howie RN. A controlled trial of antepartum glucocorticoid treatment for prevention of the respiratory distress syndrome in premature infants. Pediatrics. 1972;50(4):515–25.
310. Bancalari E, del Moral T. Bronchopulmonary dysplasia and surfactant. Biol Neonate. 2001;80 Suppl 1:7–13.
311. Baraldi E, Filippone M. Chronic lung disease after premature birth. N Engl J Med. 2007;357(19):1946–55.
312. Bonikos DS, Bensch KG, Northway Jr WH, et al. Bronchopulmonary dysplasia: the pulmonary pathologic sequel of necrotizing bronchiolitis and pulmonary fibrosis. Hum Pathol. 1976;7(6):643–66.
313. Coalson JJ. Pathology of bronchopulmonary dysplasia. Semin Perinatol. 2006;30(4):179–84.
314. Bancalari E. Changes in the pathogenesis and prevention of chronic lung disease of prematurity. Am J Perinatol. 2001;18(1):1–9.
315. Bhandari A, Panitch HB. Pulmonary outcomes in bronchopulmonary dysplasia. Semin Perinatol. 2006;30(4):219–26.
316. Sola A, Rogido MR, Deulofeut R. Oxygen as a neonatal health hazard: call for detente in clinical practice. Acta Paediatr. 2007;96(6):801–12.
317. Saugstad OD. Oxidative stress in the newborn–a 30-year perspective. Biol Neonate. 2005;88(3):228–36.
318. Maltepe E, Saugstad OD. Oxygen in health and disease: regulation of oxygen homeostasis–clinical implications. Pediatr Res. 2009;65(3):261–8.
319. Semenza GL. Hypoxia-inducible factor 1: master regulator of O2 homeostasis. Curr Opin Genet Dev. 1998;8(5):588–94.
320. Wang GL, Semenza GL. Purification and characterization of hypoxia-inducible factor 1. J Biol Chem. 1995;270(3):1230–7.
321. Kondo M, Itoh S, Isobe K, et al. Chemiluminescence because of the production of reactive oxygen species in the lungs of newborn piglets during resuscitation periods after asphyxiation load. Pediatr Res. 2000;47(4 Pt 1):524–7.
322. Kutzsche S, Ilves P, Kirkeby OJ, et al. Hydrogen peroxide production in leukocytes during cerebral hypoxia and reoxygenation with 100 % or 21 % oxygen in newborn piglets. Pediatr Res. 2001;49(6):834–42.
323. Stevens JP, Churchill T, Fokkelman K, et al. Oxidative stress and matrix metalloproteinase-9 activity in the liver after hypoxia and reoxygenation with 21 % or 100 % oxygen in newborn piglets. Eur J Pharmacol. 2008;580(3):385–93.
324. Haase E, Bigam DL, Nakonechny QB, et al. Resuscitation with 100 % oxygen causes intestinal glutathione oxidation and reoxygenation injury in asphyxiated newborn piglets. Ann Surg. 2004;240(2):364–73.
325. Vento M, Asensi M, Sastre J, et al. Oxidative stress in asphyxiated term infants resuscitated with 100 % oxygen. J Pediatr. 2003;142(3):240–6.
326. Temesvari P, Karg E, Bodi I, et al. Impaired early neurologic outcome in newborn piglets reoxygenated with 100 % oxygen compared with room air after pneumothorax-induced asphyxia. Pediatr Res. 2001;49(6):812–9.
327. Saugstad OD, Ramji S, Soll RF, et al. Resuscitation of newborn infants with 21 % or 100 % oxygen: an updated systematic review and meta-analysis. Neonatology. 2008;94(3):176–82.
328. Borke WB, Munkeby BH, Halvorsen B, et al. Increased myocardial matrix metalloproteinases in hypoxic newborn pigs during resuscitation: effects of oxygen and carbon dioxide. Eur J Clin Invest. 2004;34(7):459–66.
329. Haase E, Bigam DL, Nakonechny QB, et al. Cardiac function, myocardial glutathione, and matrix metalloproteinase-2 levels in

hypoxic newborn pigs reoxygenated by 21 %, 50 %, or 100 % oxygen. Shock. 2005;23(4):383–9.
330. Munkeby BH, Borke WB, Bjornland K, et al. Resuscitation of hypoxic piglets with 100 % O2 increases pulmonary metalloproteinases and IL-8. Pediatr Res. 2005;58(3):542–8.
331. Lakshminrusimha S, Russell JA, Steinhorn RH, et al. Pulmonary arterial contractility in neonatal lambs increases with 100 % oxygen resuscitation. Pediatr Res. 2006;59(1):137–41.
332. Vento M, Sastre J, Asensi MA, et al. Room-air resuscitation causes less damage to heart and kidney than 100 % oxygen. Am J Respir Crit Care Med. 2005;172(11):1393–8.
333. Tan A, Schulze A, O'Donnell CP, et al. Air versus oxygen for resuscitation of infants at birth. Cochrane Database Syst Rev. 2005(2):CD002273.
334. Rabi Y, Rabi D, Yee W. Room air resuscitation of the depressed newborn: a systematic review and meta-analysis. Resuscitation. 2007;72(3):353–63.
335. Kattwinkel J, Perlman JM, Aziz K, et al. Neonatal resuscitation: 2010 American Heart Association Guidelines for Cardiopulmonary Resuscitation and Emergency Cardiovascular Care. Pediatrics. 2010;126(5):e1400–1413.
336. Morley C. New Australian neonatal resuscitation guidelines. J Paediatr Child Health. 2007;43(1–2):6–8.
337. Mariani G, Dik PB, Ezquer A, et al. Pre-ductal and post-ductal O2 saturation in healthy term neonates after birth. J Pediatr. 2007;150(4):418–21.
338. Tin W, Milligan DW, Pennefather P, et al. Pulse oximetry, severe retinopathy, and outcome at one year in babies of less than 28 weeks gestation. Arch Dis Child Fetal Neonatal Ed. 2001;84(2):F106–110.
339. Deulofeut R, Critz A, Adams-Chapman I, et al. Avoiding hyperoxia in infants < or = 1250 g is associated with improved short- and long-term outcomes. J Perinatol. 2006;26(11):700–5.
340. Network, SSGotEKSNNR, Carlo WA, Finer NN, et al. Target ranges of oxygen saturation in extremely preterm infants. N Engl J Med. 2010;362(21):1959–69.
341. Abu-Shaweesh JM, Martin RJ. Neonatal apnea: what's new? Pediatr Pulmonol. 2008;43(10):937–44.
342. Cote CJ, Zaslavsky A, Downes JJ, et al. Postoperative apnea in former preterm infants after inguinal herniorrhaphy. A combined analysis. Anesthesiology. 1995;82(4):809–22.
343. Abu-Shaweesh JM. Maturation of respiratory reflex responses in the fetus and neonate. Semin Neonatol. 2004;9(3):169–80.
344. Johnston BM, Gluckman PD. Lateral pontine lesions affect central chemosensitivity in unanesthetized fetal lambs. J Appl Physiol (1985). 1989;67(3):1113–8.
345. Dawes GS, Gardner WN, Johnston BM, et al. Effects of hypercapnia on tracheal pressure, diaphragm and intercostal electromyograms in unanaesthetized fetal lambs. J Physiol. 1982;326: 461–74.
346. Jansen AH, Ioffe S, Russell BJ, et al. Influence of sleep state on the response to hypercapnia in fetal lambs. Respir Physiol. 1982;48(1):125–42.
347. Ioffe S, Jansen AH, Chernick V. Maturation of spontaneous fetal diaphragmatic activity and fetal response to hypercapnia and hypoxemia. J Appl Physiol (1985). 1987;63(2):609–22.
348. Connors G, Hunse C, Carmichael L, et al. Control of fetal breathing in the human fetus between 24 and 34 weeks' gestation. Am J Obstet Gynecol. 1989;160(4):932–8.
349. Manning FA, Platt LD, Sipos L, et al. Fetal breathing movements and the nonstress test in high-risk pregnancies. Am J Obstet Gynecol. 1979;135(4):511–5.
350. Manning FA, Platt LD, Sipos L. Antepartum fetal evaluation: development of a fetal biophysical profile. Am J Obstet Gynecol. 1980;136(6):787–95.
351. Manning FA. Antepartum fetal testing: a critical appraisal. Curr Opin Obstet Gynecol. 2009;21(4):348–52.
352. Frantz 3rd ID, Adler SM, Thach BT, et al. Maturational effects on respiratory responses to carbon dioxide in premature infants. J Appl Physiol. 1976;41(1):41–5.
353. Abu-Shaweesh JM, Dreshaj IA, Thomas AJ, et al. Changes in respiratory timing induced by hypercapnia in maturing rats. J Appl Physiol (1985). 1999;87(2):484–90.
354. Gerhardt T, Bancalari E. Apnea of prematurity: I. Lung function and regulation of breathing. Pediatrics. 1984;74(1):58–62.
355. Rigatto H, Brady JP. Periodic breathing and apnea in preterm infants. I. Evidence for hypoventilation possibly due to central respiratory depression. Pediatrics. 1972;50(2):202–18.
356. Rigatto H, Brady JP, de la Torre Verduzco R. Chemoreceptor reflexes in preterm infants: II. The effect of gestational and postnatal age on the ventilatory response to inhaled carbon dioxide. Pediatrics. 1975;55(5):614–20.
357. Dripps RD, Comroe JH. The effect of inhalation of high and of low oxygen concentration upon human respiration and circulation. Am J Med Sci. 1947;213(2):248.
358. Rigatto H, Brady JP, de la Torre Verduzco R. Chemoreceptor reflexes in preterm infants: I. The effect of gestational and postnatal age on the ventilatory response to inhalation of 100 % and 15 % oxygen. Pediatrics. 1975;55(5):604–13.
359. Martin RJ, DiFiore JM, Jana L, et al. Persistence of the biphasic ventilatory response to hypoxia in preterm infants. J Pediatr. 1998;132(6):960–4.
360. Bissonnette JM. Mechanisms regulating hypoxic respiratory depression during fetal and postnatal life. Am J Physiol Regul Integr Comp Physiol. 2000;278(6):R1391–1400.
361. Gluckman PD, Johnston BM. Lesions in the upper lateral pons abolish the hypoxic depression of breathing in unanaesthetized fetal lambs in utero. J Physiol. 1987;382:373–83.
362. Moss IR, Laferriere A. Central neuropeptide systems and respiratory control during development. Respir Physiol Neurobiol. 2002;131(1–2):15–27.
363. Rigatto H, De La Torre Verduzco R, Gates DB. Effects of O2 on the ventilatory response to CO2 in preterm infants. J Appl Physiol. 1975;39(6):896–9.
364. Pickens DL, Schefft G, Thach BT. Prolonged apnea associated with upper airway protective reflexes in apnea of prematurity. Am Rev Respir Dis. 1988;137(1):113–8.
365. Martin RJ, Abu-Shaweesh JM. Control of breathing and neonatal apnea. Biol Neonate. 2005;87(4):288–95.
366. Abu-Shaweesh JM. Activation of central adenosine A(2A) receptors enhances superior laryngeal nerve stimulation-induced apnea in piglets via a GABAergic pathway. J Appl Physiol (1985). 2007;103(4):1205–11.
367. Breuer J. Self-steering of respiration through the nerves vagus. In: Porter R, editor. Breathing: Hering-Breuer Centenary Symposium. London: Churchill; 1868. p. 365–94.
368. McClelland AR, Sproule BJ, Lynne-Davies P. Functional importance of the Breuer-Hering reflex. Respir Physiol. 1972;15(1): 125–39.
369. Head H. On the regulation of respiration: Part I. Experimental. J Physiol. 1889;10(1–2):152–3.
370. Head H. On the regulation of respiration: Part II. Theoretical. J Physiol. 1889;10(4):279–90.
371. Cross KW. Head's paradoxical reflex. Brain. 1961;84:529–34.
372. Davies A, Roumy M. The effect of transient stimulation of lung irritant receptors on the pattern of breathing in rabbits. J Physiol. 1982;324:389–401.
373. Baird TM. Clinical correlates, natural history and outcome of neonatal apnoea. Semin Neonatol. 2004;9(3):205–11.
374. Henderson-Smart DJ, Steer P. Prophylactic caffeine to prevent postoperative apnea following general anesthesia in preterm infants. Cochrane Database Syst Rev. 2001;(4):CD000048.
375. Hoppenbrouwers T, Hodgman JE, Harper RM, et al. Polygraphic studies of normal infants during the first six months of life: III.

Incidence of apnea and periodic breathing. Pediatrics. 1977; 60(4):418–25.
376. Waite SP, Thoman EB. Periodic apnea in the full-term infant: individual consistency, sex differences, and state specificity. Pediatrics. 1982;70(1):79–86.
377. Murphy JJ, Swanson T, Ansermino M, et al. The frequency of apneas in premature infants after inguinal hernia repair: do they need overnight monitoring in the intensive care unit? J Pediatr Surg. 2008;43(5):865–8.
378. Welborn LG, Hannallah RS, Luban NL, et al. Anemia and postoperative apnea in former preterm infants. Anesthesiology. 1991;74(6):1003–6.
379. Malviya S, Swartz J, Lerman J. Are all preterm infants younger than 60 weeks postconceptual age at risk for postanesthetic apnea? Anesthesiology. 1993;78(6):1076–81.
380. Walther-Larsen S, Rasmussen LS. The former preterm infant and risk of post-operative apnoea: recommendations for management. Acta Anaesthesiol Scand. 2006;50(7):888–93.
381. Craven PD, Badawi N, Henderson-Smart DJ, et al. Regional (spinal, epidural, caudal) versus general anaesthesia in preterm infants undergoing inguinal herniorrhaphy in early infancy. Cochrane Database Syst Rev. 2003;(3):CD003669.
382. Beath SV. Hepatic function and physiology in the newborn. Semin Neonatol. 2003;8(5):337–46.
383. Meier PJ. Canalicular bile formation: beyond single transporter functions. J Hepatol. 2002;37(2):272–3.
384. Andres JM, Mathis RK, Walker WA. Liver disease in infants. Part I: Developmental hepatology and mechanisms of liver dysfunction. J Pediatr. 1977;90(5):686–97.
385. Tiao G, Warner BW. Transcription factors and cholangiocyte development. Gastroenterology. 2003;124(1):263–4.
386. Clotman F, Lannoy VJ, Reber M, et al. The onecut transcription factor HNF6 is required for normal development of the biliary tract. Development. 2002;129(8):1819–28.
387. Mitchell B, Sharma R. Embryology: an illustrated colour text. Philadelphia: Elsevier; 2009.
388. Alagille D, Odievre M, Gautier M, et al. Hepatic ductular hypoplasia associated with characteristic facies, vertebral malformations, retarded physical, mental, and sexual development, and cardiac murmur. J Pediatr. 1975;86(1):63–71.
389. Loomes KM, Taichman DB, Glover CL, et al. Characterization of Notch receptor expression in the developing mammalian heart and liver. Am J Med Genet. 2002;112(2):181–9.
390. Li L, Krantz ID, Deng Y, et al. Alagille syndrome is caused by mutations in human Jagged1, which encodes a ligand for Notch1. Nat Genet. 1997;16(3):243–51.
391. McDaniell R, Warthen DM, Sanchez-Lara PA, et al. NOTCH2 mutations cause Alagille syndrome, a heterogeneous disorder of the notch signaling pathway. Am J Hum Genet. 2006; 79(1):169–73.
392. Sparks EE, Huppert KA, Brown MA, et al. Notch signaling regulates formation of the three-dimensional architecture of intrahepatic bile ducts in mice. Hepatology. 2010;51(4): 1391–400.
393. McDonagh AF. Movement of bilirubin and bilirubin conjugates across the placenta. Pediatrics. 2007;119(5):1032–3. author reply 1033.
394. McDonagh AF. Controversies in bilirubin biochemistry and their clinical relevance. Semin Fetal Neonatal Med. 2010;15(3):141–7.
395. Bernstein RB, Novy MJ, Piasecki GJ, et al. Bilirubin metabolism in the fetus. J Clin Invest. 1969;48(9):1678–88.
396. Diehl-Jones WL, Askin DF. The neonatal liver. Part 1: embryology, anatomy, and physiology. Neonatal Netw. 2002;21(2):5–12.
397. Jones CT, Rolph TP. Metabolism during fetal life: a functional assessment of metabolic development. Physiol Rev. 1985;65(2):357–430.
398. Thomas DB, Yoffey JM. Human foetal haematopoiesis. II. Hepatic haematopoiesis in the human foetus. Br J Haematol. 1964; 10:193–7.
399. Van den Akker CH, Van Goudoever JB. Recent advances in our understanding of protein and amino acid metabolism in the human fetus. Curr Opin Clin Nutr Metab Care. 2010;13(1):75–80.
400. Rudolph AM. Hepatic and ductus venosus blood flows during fetal life. Hepatology. 1983;3(2):254–8.
401. Haugen G, Kiserud T, Godfrey K, et al. Portal and umbilical venous blood supply to the liver in the human fetus near term. Ultrasound Obstet Gynecol. 2004;24(6):599–605.
402. Lind J. Changes in the liver circulation at birth. Ann NY Acad Sci. 1963;111:110–20.
403. Hay Jr WW. Strategies for feeding the preterm infant. Neonatology. 2008;94(4):245–54.
404. Kalhan SC, Parimi P, Van Beek R, et al. Estimation of gluconeogenesis in newborn infants. Am J Physiol Endocrinol Metab. 2001;281(5):E991–997.
405. Chacko SK, Sunehag AL. Gluconeogenesis continues in premature infants receiving total parenteral nutrition. Arch Dis Child Fetal Neonatal Ed. 2010;95(6):F413–8.
406. den Boer ME, Wanders RJ, Morris AA, et al. Long-chain 3-hydroxyacyl-CoA dehydrogenase deficiency: clinical presentation and follow-up of 50 patients. Pediatrics. 2002;109(1): 99–104.
407. Saudubray JM, Martin D, de Lonlay P, et al. Recognition and management of fatty acid oxidation defects: a series of 107 patients. J Inherit Metab Dis. 1999;22(4):488–502.
408. Manson WG, Weaver LT. Fat digestion in the neonate. Arch Dis Child Fetal Neonatal Ed. 1997;76(3):F206–211.
409. Alrefai WA, Gill RK. Bile acid transporters: structure, function, regulation and pathophysiological implications. Pharm Res. 2007;24(10):1803–23.
410. Bile acid metabolism during development. In: Polin R, Fox W, editors. Fetal and neonatal physiology. Vol 1. Philadelphia: Saunders; 1998.
411. Dessolle L, Lebrec J, Darai E. Impact of delayed arterial cord blood sampling for lactate assay: a prospective observational study. Neonatology. 2009;95(3):224–9.
412. Groenendaal F, Lindemans C, Uiterwaal CS, et al. Early arterial lactate and prediction of outcome in preterm neonates admitted to a neonatal intensive care unit. Biol Neonate. 2003;83(3):171–6.
413. Nadeem M, Clarke A, Dempsey EM. Day 1 serum lactate values in preterm infants less than 32 weeks gestation. Eur J Pediatr. 2010;169(6):667–70.
414. Durand P, Debray D, Mandel R, et al. Acute liver failure in infancy: a 14-year experience of a pediatric liver transplantation center. J Pediatr. 2001;139(6):871–6.
415. Bars RG, Bell DR, Elcombe CR. Induction of cytochrome P450 and peroxisomal enzymes by clofibric acid in vivo and in vitro. Biochem Pharmacol. 1993;45(10):2045–53.
416. Hines RN, McCarver DG. The ontogeny of human drug-metabolizing enzymes: phase I oxidative enzymes. J Pharmacol Exp Ther. 2002;300(2):355–60.
417. Kearns GL, Abdel-Rahman SM, Alander SW, et al. Developmental pharmacology–drug disposition, action, and therapy in infants and children. N Engl J Med. 2003;349(12):1157–67.
418. de Wildt SN, Kearns GL, Leeder JS, et al. Cytochrome P450 3A: ontogeny and drug disposition. Clin Pharmacokinet. 1999;37(6):485–505.
419. McCarver DG, Hines RN. The ontogeny of human drug-metabolizing enzymes: phase II conjugation enzymes and regulatory mechanisms. J Pharmacol Exp Ther. 2002;300(2):361–6.
420. Fisher DM, O'Keeffe C, Stanski DR, et al. Pharmacokinetics and pharmacodynamics of d-tubocurarine in infants, children, and adults. Anesthesiology. 1982;57(3):203–8.

421. Fisher DM, Canfell PC, Spellman MJ, et al. Pharmacokinetics and pharmacodynamics of atracurium in infants and children. Anesthesiology. 1990;73(1):33–7.
422. Cook DR. Muscle relaxants in infants and children. Anesth Analg. 1981;60(5):335–43.
423. Gauntlett IS, Fisher DM, Hertzka RE, et al. Pharmacokinetics of fentanyl in neonatal humans and lambs: effects of age. Anesthesiology. 1988;69(5):683–7.
424. Hakkola J, Pasanen M, Purkunen R, et al. Expression of xenobiotic-metabolizing cytochrome P450 forms in human adult and fetal liver. Biochem Pharmacol. 1994;48(1):59–64.
425. Allegaert K, Peeters MY, Verbesselt R, et al. Inter-individual variability in propofol pharmacokinetics in preterm and term neonates. Br J Anaesth. 2007;99(6):864–70.
426. Saxonhouse MA, Manco-Johnson MJ. The evaluation and management of neonatal coagulation disorders. Semin Perinatol. 2009;33(1):52–65.
427. Controversies concerning vitamin K and the newborn. American Academy of Pediatrics Committee on Fetus and Newborn. Pediatrics. 2003;112(1 Pt 1):191–2.
428. Hope PL, Hall MA, Millward-Sadler GH, et al. Alpha-1-antitrypsin deficiency presenting as a bleeding diathesis in the newborn. Arch Dis Child. 1982;57(1):68–70.
429. Hussain M, Mieli-Vergani G, Mowat AP. Alpha 1-antitrypsin deficiency and liver disease: clinical presentation, diagnosis and treatment. J Inherit Metab Dis. 1991;14(4):497–511.
430. Hansen TWR. Core concepts: bilirubin metabolism. Neoreviews. 2010;11(6):e316–322.
431. Maisels MJ. Jaundice in healthy newborns-redefining physiologic jaundice. West J Med. 1988;149(4):451.
432. Knudsen A, Ebbesen F. Cephalocaudal progression of jaundice in newborns admitted to neonatal intensive care units. Biol Neonate. 1997;71(6):357–61.
433. Keren R, Tremont K, Luan X, et al. Visual assessment of jaundice in term and late preterm infants. Arch Dis Child Fetal Neonatal Ed. 2009;94(5):F317–322.
434. Stevenson DK, Bartoletti AL, Ostrander CR, et al. Pulmonary excretion of carbon monoxide in the human infant as an index of bilirubin production. II. Infants of diabetic mothers. J Pediatr. 1979;94(6):956–8.
435. Levi AJ, Gatmaitan Z, Arias IM. Deficiency of hepatic organic anion-binding protein, impaired organic amnion uptake by liver and physiologic jaundice in newborn monkeys. N Engl J Med. 1970;283(21):1136–9.
436. Wolkoff AW, Goresky CA, Sellin J, et al. Role of ligandin in transfer of bilirubin from plasma into liver. Am J Physiol. 1979;236(6):E638–648.
437. Kawade N, Onishi S. The prenatal and postnatal development of UDP-glucuronyltransferase activity towards bilirubin and the effect of premature birth on this activity in the human liver. Biochem J. 1981;196(1):257–60.
438. Maisels MJ. What's in a name? Physiologic and pathologic jaundice: the conundrum of defining normal bilirubin levels in the newborn. Pediatrics. 2006;118(2):805–7.
439. Alonso EM, Whitington PF, Whitington SH, et al. Enterohepatic circulation of nonconjugated bilirubin in rats fed with human milk. J Pediatr. 1991;118(3):425–30.
440. Gartner LM, Lee KS, Moscioni AD. Effect of milk feeding on intestinal bilirubin absorption in the rat. J Pediatr. 1983;103(3):464–71.
441. Kumral A, Ozkan H, Duman N, et al. Breast milk jaundice correlates with high levels of epidermal growth factor. Pediatr Res. 2009;66(2):218–21.
442. Preer GL, Philipp BL. Understanding and managing breast milk jaundice. Arch Dis Child Fetal Neonatal Ed. 2011;96(6):F461–6.
443. Schreiber RA, Kleinman RE. Biliary atresia. J Pediatr Gastroenterol Nutr. 2002;35 Suppl 1:S11–16.
444. Balistreri WF, Grand R, Hoofnagle JH, et al. Biliary atresia: current concepts and research directions. Summary of a symposium. Hepatology. 1996;23(6):1682–92.
445. Adkins Jr RB, Chapman WC, Reddy VS. Embryology, anatomy, and surgical applications of the extrahepatic biliary system. Surg Clin North Am. 2000;80(1):363–79.
446. Laurent J, Gauthier F, Bernard O, et al. Long-term outcome after surgery for biliary atresia. Study of 40 patients surviving for more than 10 years. Gastroenterology. 1990;99(6):1793–7.
447. Popovici RM, Lu M, Bhatia S, et al. Hypoxia regulates insulin-like growth factor-binding protein 1 in human fetal hepatocytes in primary culture: suggestive molecular mechanisms for in utero fetal growth restriction caused by uteroplacental insufficiency. J Clin Endocrinol Metab. 2001;86(6):2653–9.
448. Lackmann GM, Tollner U, Mader R. Serum enzyme activities in full-term asphyxiated and healthy newborns: enzyme kinetics during the first 144 hours of life. Enzyme Protein. 1993;47(3):160–72.
449. Shamir R, Maayan-Metzger A, Bujanover Y, et al. Liver enzyme abnormalities in gram-negative bacteremia of premature infants. Pediatr Infect Dis J. 2000;19(6):495–8.
450. Rosenthal P. Assessing liver function and hyperbilirubinemia in the newborn. National Academy of Clinical Biochemistry. Clin Chem. 1997;43(1):228–34.
451. Verboon-Maciolek MA, Swanink CM, Krediet TG, et al. Severe neonatal echovirus 20 infection characterized by hepatic failure. Pediatr Infect Dis J. 1997;16(5):524–7.
452. Lee WS, Kelly DA, Tanner MS, et al. Neonatal liver transplantation for fulminant hepatitis caused by herpes simplex virus type 2. J Pediatr Gastroenterol Nutr. 2002;35(2):220–3.
453. Whitington PF. Cholestasis associated with total parenteral nutrition in infants. Hepatology. 1985;5(4):693–6.
454. Willis TC, Carter BA, Rogers SP, et al. High rates of mortality and morbidity occur in infants with parenteral nutrition-associated cholestasis. JPEN J Parenter Enteral Nutr. 2010;34(1):32–7.
455. Owings E, Georgeson K. Management of cholestasis in infants with very low birth weight. Semin Pediatr Surg. 2000;9(2):96–102.
456. Zhao J, Kim KD, Yang X, et al. Hyper innate responses in neonates lead to increased morbidity and mortality after infection. Proc Natl Acad Sci USA. 2008;105(21):7528–33.
457. Shapiro SM. Definition of the clinical spectrum of kernicterus and bilirubin-induced neurologic dysfunction (BIND). J Perinatol. 2005;25(1):54–9.
458. Volpe JJ. Bilirubin and brain injury. In: Volpe JJ, editor. Neurology of the newborn. Philadelphia: Saunders; 2001. p. 490–514.
459. Ahlfors CE, Wennberg RP, Ostrow JD, et al. Unbound (free) bilirubin: improving the paradigm for evaluating neonatal jaundice. Clin Chem. 2009;55(7):1288–99.
460. Ahlfors CE, Wennberg RP. Bilirubin-albumin binding and neonatal jaundice. Semin Perinatol. 2004;28(5):334–9.
461. Wennberg RP. The blood-brain barrier and bilirubin encephalopathy. Cell Mol Neurobiol. 2000;20(1):97–109.
462. Dennery PA, Seidman DS, Stevenson DK. Neonatal hyperbilirubinemia. N Engl J Med. 2001;344(8):581–90.
463. Ahlfors CE, Herbsman O. Unbound bilirubin in a term newborn with kernicterus. Pediatrics. 2003;111(5 Pt 1):1110–2.
464. Ahlfors CE. Unbound bilirubin associated with kernicterus: a historical approach. J Pediatr. 2000;137(4):540–4.
465. Kaplan M, Herschel M, Hammerman C, et al. Hyperbilirubinemia among African American, glucose-6-phosphate dehydrogenase-deficient neonates. Pediatrics. 2004;114(2):e213–219.
466. Bancroft JD, Kreamer B, Gourley GR. Gilbert syndrome accelerates development of neonatal jaundice. J Pediatr. 1998;132(4):656–60.
467. Kadakol A, Ghosh SS, Sappal BS, et al. Genetic lesions of bilirubin uridine-diphosphoglucuronate glucuronosyltransferase

(UGT1A1) causing Crigler-Najjar and Gilbert syndromes: correlation of genotype to phenotype. Hum Mutat. 2000;16(4):297–306.
468. Sneitz N, Bakker CT, de Knegt RJ, et al. Crigler-Najjar syndrome in The Netherlands: identification of four novel UGT1A1 alleles, genotype-phenotype correlation, and functional analysis of 10 missense mutants. Hum Mutat. 2010;31(1):52–9.
469. Crigler Jr JF, Najjar VA. Congenital familial nonhemolytic jaundice with kernicterus; a new clinical entity. AMA Am J Dis Child. 1952;83(2):259–60.
470. Watchko JF. Vigintiphobia revisited. Pediatrics. 2005; 115(6):1747–53.
471. Watchko JF. Genetics and the risk of neonatal hyperbilirubinemia: commentary on the article by Huang et al. on page 682. Pediatr Res. 2004;56(5):677–8.
472. Kaplan M, Hammerman C, Maisels MJ. Bilirubin genetics for the nongeneticist: hereditary defects of neonatal bilirubin conjugation. Pediatrics. 2003;111(4 Pt 1):886–93.
473. Watchko JF, Daood MJ, Biniwale M. Understanding neonatal hyperbilirubinaemia in the era of genomics. Semin Neonatol. 2002;7(2):143–52.
474. Alencastro de Azevedo L, Reverbel da Silveira T, Carvalho CG, et al. UGT1A1, SLCO1B1, and SLCO1B3 polymorphisms vs. neonatal hyperbilirubinemia: is there an association? Pediatr Res. 2012;72(2):169–73.
475. Management of hyperbilirubinemia in the newborn infant 35 or more weeks of gestation. Pediatrics. 2004;114(1):297–316.
476. Bhutani VK, Johnson L, Sivieri EM. Predictive ability of a predischarge hour-specific serum bilirubin for subsequent significant hyperbilirubinemia in healthy term and near-term newborns. Pediatrics. 1999;103(1):6–14.
477. Maisels MJ, Bhutani VK, Bogen D, et al. Hyperbilirubinemia in the newborn infant > or =35 weeks' gestation: an update with clarifications. Pediatrics. 2009;124(4):1193–8.
478. Cremer RJ, Perryman PW, Richards DH. Influence of light on the hyperbilirubinaemia of infants. Lancet. 1958;1(7030):1094–7.
479. Lucey J, Ferriero M, Hewitt J. Prevention of hyperbilirubinemia of prematurity by phototherapy. Pediatrics. 1968;41(6):1047–54.
480. Lightner DA, McDonagh AF. Molecular mechanisms of phototherapy for neonatal jaundice. Acc Chem Res. 1984;17:417–24.
481. Lamola AA, Blumberg WE, McClead R, et al. Photoisomerized bilirubin in blood from infants receiving phototherapy. Proc Natl Acad Sci USA. 1981;78(3):1882–6.
482. Onishi S, Isobe K, Itoh S, et al. Demonstration of a geometric isomer of bilirubin-IX alpha in the serum of a hyperbilirubinaemic newborn infant and the mechanism of jaundice phototherapy. Biochem J. 1980;190(3):533–6.
483. Onishi S, Kawade N, Itoh S, et al. Kinetics of biliary excretion of the main two bilirubin photoproducts after injection into Gunn rats. Biochem J. 1981;198(1):107–12.
484. Ruud Hansen TW. Phototherapy for neonatal jaundice–therapeutic effects on more than one level? Semin Perinatol. 2010;34(3):231–4.
485. Mreihil K, McDonagh AF, Nakstad B, et al. Early isomerization of bilirubin in phototherapy of neonatal jaundice. Pediatr Res. 2010;67(6):656–9.
486. Maisels MJ, McDonagh AF. Phototherapy for neonatal jaundice. N Engl J Med. 2008;358(9):920–8.
487. Okumura A, Kidokoro H, Shoji H, et al. Kernicterus in preterm infants. Pediatrics. 2009;123(6):e1052–1058.
488. Sarici SU, Serdar MA, Korkmaz A, et al. Incidence, course, and prediction of hyperbilirubinemia in near-term and term newborns. Pediatrics. 2004;113(4):775–80.
489. van der Veere CN, Sinaasappel M, McDonagh AF, et al. Current therapy for Crigler-Najjar syndrome type 1: report of a world registry. Hepatology. 1996;24(2):311–5.
490. Diamond LK, Allen Jr FH, Thomas Jr WO. Erythroblastosis fetalis. VII. Treatment with exchange transfusion. N Engl J Med. 1951;244(2):39–49.
491. Hansen TW. Acute management of extreme neonatal jaundice–the potential benefits of intensified phototherapy and interruption of enterohepatic bilirubin circulation. Acta Paediatr. 1997;86(8):843–6.
492. Odell GB, Cohen SN, Gordes EH. Administration of albumin in the management of hyperbilirubinemia by exchange transfusions. Pediatrics. 1962;30:613–21.
493. Jackson JC. Adverse events associated with exchange transfusion in healthy and ill newborns. Pediatrics. 1997;99(5):E7.
494. Livaditis A, Wallgren G, Faxelius G. Necrotizing enterocolitis after catheterization of the umbilical vessels. Acta Paediatr Scand. 1974;63(2):277–82.
495. Stern L. Drug interactions. II. Drugs, the newborn infant, and the binding of bilirubin to albumin. Pediatrics. 1972;49(6):916–8.
496. Soligard HT, Nilsen OG, Bratlid D. Displacement of bilirubin from albumin by ibuprofen in vitro. Pediatr Res. 2010; 67(6):614–8.
497. Schiff D, Chan G, Stern L. Fixed drug combinations and the displacement of bilirubin from albumin. Pediatrics. 1971;48(1):139–41.
498. Ostrow JD, Pascolo L, Shapiro SM, et al. New concepts in bilirubin encephalopathy. Eur J Clin Invest. 2003;33(11):988–97.
499. Taeusch HW, Ballard RA, Gleason CA. Avery's disease of the newborn. Philadelphia, PA: Saunders/Elsevier; 2004.
500. Dziarmaga A, Quinlan J, Goodyer P. Renal hypoplasia: lessons from Pax2. Pediatr Nephrol. 2006;21(1):26–31.
501. Quigley R. Developmental changes in renal function. Curr Opin Pediatr. 2012;24(2):184–90.
502. Macdonald MS, Emery JL. The late intrauterine and postnatal development of human renal glomeruli. J Anat. 1959;93(pt. 3):331–40.
503. Merlet-Benichou C, Gilbert T, Vilar J, et al. Nephron number: variability is the rule. Causes and consequences. Lab Invest. 1999;79(5):515–27.
504. Lelievre-Pegorier M, Merlet-Benichou C. The number of nephrons in the mammalian kidney: environmental influences play a determining role. Exp Nephrol. 2000;8(2):63–5.
505. Zhang Z, Quinlan J, Hoy W, et al. A common RET variant is associated with reduced newborn kidney size and function. J Am Soc Nephrol. 2008;19(10):2027–34.
506. Quinlan J, Lemire M, Hudson T, et al. A common variant of the PAX2 gene is associated with reduced newborn kidney size. J Am Soc Nephrol. 2007;18(6):1915–21.
507. Keijzer-Veen MG, Devos AS, Meradji M, et al. Reduced renal length and volume 20 years after very preterm birth. Pediatr Nephrol. 2010;25(3):499–507.
508. Yzydorczyk C, Comte B, Cambonie G, et al. Neonatal oxygen exposure in rats leads to cardiovascular and renal alterations in adulthood. Hypertension. 2008;52(5):889–95.
509. Rabinowitz R, Peters MT, Vyas S, et al. Measurement of fetal urine production in normal pregnancy by real-time ultrasonography. Am J Obstet Gynecol. 1989;161(5):1264–6.
510. Friis-Hansen B. Water distribution in the foetus and newborn infant. Acta Paediatr Scand Suppl. 1983;305:7–11.
511. Brans YW. Body fluid compartments in neonates weighing 1000 grams or less. Clin Perinatol. 1986;13(2):403–17.
512. Sedin G, Hammarlund K, Stromberg B. Transepidermal water loss in full-term and pre-term infants. Acta Paediatr Scand Suppl. 1983;305:27–31.
513. Hammarlund K, Sedin G, Stromberg B. Transepidermal water loss in newborn infants. VIII. Relation to gestational age and post-natal age in appropriate and small for gestational age infants. Acta Paediatr Scand. 1983;72(5):721–8.

514. Heisler D. Pediatric renal function. Int Anesthesiol Clin. 1993;31(1):103–7.
515. Svenningsen NW, Aronson AS. Postnatal development of renal concentration capacity as estimated by DDAVP-test in normal and asphyxiated neonates. Biol Neonate. 1974;25(3–4):230–41.
516. Vieux R, Hascoet JM, Merdariu D, et al. Glomerular filtration rate reference values in very preterm infants. Pediatrics. 2010;125(5):e1186–1192.
517. Jose PA, Fildes RD, Gomez RA, et al. Neonatal renal function and physiology. Curr Opin Pediatr. 1994;6(2):172–7.
518. Bueva A, Guignard JP. Renal function in preterm neonates. Pediatr Res. 1994;36(5):572–7.
519. Gallini F, Maggio L, Romagnoli C, et al. Progression of renal function in preterm neonates with gestational age < or = 32 weeks. Pediatr Nephrol. 2000;15(1–2):119–24.
520. Holtback U, Aperia AC. Molecular determinants of sodium and water balance during early human development. Semin Neonatol. 2003;8(4):291–9.
521. Burrow CR, Devuyst O, Li X, et al. Expression of the beta2-subunit and apical localization of Na+-K+-ATPase in metanephric kidney. Am J Physiol. 1999;277(3 Pt 2):F391–403.
522. Vanpee M, Herin P, Zetterstrom R, et al. Postnatal development of renal function in very low birthweight infants. Acta Paediatr Scand. 1988;77(2):191–7.
523. Rodriquez-Soriano J, Vallo A, Castillo G, et al. Renal handling of water and sodium in children with proximal and distal renal tubular acidosis. Nephron. 1980;25(4):193–8.
524. Rees L, Forsling ML, Brook CG. Vasopressin concentrations in the neonatal period. Clin Endocrinol (Oxf). 1980;12(4): 357–62.
525. Schwartz GJ, Haycock GB, Edelmann Jr CM, et al. Late metabolic acidosis: a reassessment of the definition. J Pediatr. 1979;95(1):102–7.
526. Beck JC, Lipkowitz MS, Abramson RG. Ontogeny of Na/H antiporter activity in rabbit renal brush border membrane vesicles. J Clin Invest. 1991;87(6):2067–76.
527. Bobulescu IA, Dwarakanath V, Zou L, et al. Glucocorticoids acutely increase cell surface Na+/H+ exchanger-3 (NHE3) by activation of NHE3 exocytosis. Am J Physiol Renal Physiol. 2005;289(4):F685–691.
528. Gupta N, Dwarakanath V, Baum M. Maturation of the Na+/H+ antiporter (NHE3) in the proximal tubule of the hypothyroid adrenalectomized rat. Am J Physiol Renal Physiol. 2004; 287(3):F521–527.
529. You G, Lee WS, Barros EJ, et al. Molecular characteristics of Na(+)-coupled glucose transporters in adult and embryonic rat kidney. J Biol Chem. 1995;270(49):29365–71.
530. Arant Jr BS, Edelmann Jr CM, Nash MA. The renal reabsorption of glucose in the developing canine kidney: a study of glomerulotubular balance. Pediatr Res. 1974;8(6):638–46.
531. Mildenberger E, Oels K, Bauer K, et al. Digoxin-like immunoreactive substance in nonoliguric hyperkalemia of the premature infant. Biol Neonate. 2003;83(3):182–7.
532. Vemgal P, Ohlsson A. Interventions for non-oliguric hyperkalaemia in preterm neonates. Cochrane Database Syst Rev. 2007;(1):CD005257.
533. Stefano JL, Norman ME, Morales MC, et al. Decreased erythrocyte Na+, K(+)-ATPase activity associated with cellular potassium loss in extremely low birth weight infants with nonoliguric hyperkalemia. J Pediatr. 1993;122(2):276–84.
534. Richer C, Hornych H, Amiel-Tison C, et al. Plasma renin activity and its postnatal development in preterm infants. Preliminary report. Biol Neonate. 1977;31(5–6):301–4.
535. Van Acker KJ, Scharpe SL, Deprettere AJ, et al. Renin-angiotensin-aldosterone system in the healthy infant and child. Kidney Int. 1979;16(2):196–203.
536. Robillard JE, Nakamura KT. Hormonal regulation of renal function during development. Biol Neonate. 1988;53(4):201–11.
537. Sulyok E, Nemeth M, Tenyi I, et al. Relationship between maturity, electrolyte balance and the function of the renin-angiotensin-aldosterone system in newborn infants. Biol Neonate. 1979;35(1–2):60–5.
538. Nakamura KT, Ayres NA, Gomez RA, et al. Renal responses to hypoxemia during renin-angiotensin system inhibition in fetal lambs. Am J Physiol. 1985;249(1 Pt 2):R116–124.
539. Gomez RA, Meernik JG, Kuehl WD, et al. Developmental aspects of the renal response to hemorrhage during fetal life. Pediatr Res. 1984;18(1):40–6.
540. Pryde PG, Sedman AB, Nugent CE, et al. Angiotensin-converting enzyme inhibitor fetopathy. J Am Soc Nephrol. 1993;3(9):1575–82.
541. Arant Jr BS. Postnatal development of renal function during the first year of life. Pediatr Nephrol. 1987;1(3):308–13.
542. Pohjavuori M, Fyhrquist F. Hemodynamic significance of vasopressin in the newborn infant. J Pediatr. 1980;97(3):462–5.
543. Wiriyathian S, Rosenfeld CR, Arant Jr BS, et al. Urinary arginine vasopressin: pattern of excretion in the neonatal period. Pediatr Res. 1986;20(2):103–8.

Anesthesia and Ancillary Drugs and the Neonate

3

Brian J. Anderson, Peter Larsson, and Jerrold Lerman

Introduction

Neonates are a heterogeneous population characterized by a limited weight or size range. They are the group of children from birth up to the age of 28 days of life and include both preterm (i.e., born before 37 weeks of gestation) and term neonates. In practice, the word "neonate" extends to former preterm neonates. Consequently, postmenstrual age (PMA) may range from extreme preterm birth at 22 weeks to 50 weeks PMA, while weight commonly ranges from 0.5 to 5 kg, an entire order of magnitude. Age, size, comorbidity, coadministration of drugs and genetic polymorphisms contribute to the extensive interindividual pharmacokinetic (PK) and pharmacodynamic (PD) variability in this population. These phenomena distinguish neonates as a specific population with major pharmacological differences from their older counterparts. Although the general principles of clinical pharmacology also apply to neonates, their characteristics warrant a tailored approach. History provides us with evidence of the deleterious effects of drugs in this age group including chloramphenicol (grey baby syndrome) and benzyl alcohol (gasping syndrome) in neonates. Neonatal bupivacaine toxicity in those receiving long-term infusion [1] and acute fentanyl tolerance [2] are two recent anesthesia examples.

B.J. Anderson, PhD, FANZCA, FJFICM (✉)
Department of Anaesthesiology, University of Auckland, Auckland, New Zealand
e-mail: briana@adhb.govt.nz

P. Larsson, MD
Department of Physiology and Pharmacology, Section of Anaesthesiology and Intensive Care, Karolinska Institute, Solna, Sweden
e-mail: peter.larsson@karolinska.se

J. Lerman, MD, FRCPC, FANZCA
Department of Anesthesia, Women and Children's Hospital of Buffalo, State University of New York, Buffalo, USA

University of Rochester Medical Center, Rochester, NY, USA
e-mail: jerrold.lerman@gmail.com

Effective and safe pharmacotherapy depends upon an understanding of the clinical PK and PD properties of the drugs employed. Besides age-dependent differences in PK and PD, differences in adverse effects should also be considered. Although the available data on drug disposition and its effects in the neonate have increased considerably in the last few years, PK–PD interactions for many drugs remain poorly understood. Clinical studies in neonates encompass multiple challenges and difficulties, of which ethical issues, the perceived high vulnerability, technical difficulties, lack of self-assessment, immaturity and the need for specific formulations are salient examples. However, in recent years, important progress has been made that has improved the feasibility and the clinical relevance of such studies in neonates. Models have been developed to handle extensive interindividual variability in PK and PD parameter estimates and to formulate dose estimation [3]. Population-based modeling tools have helped to quantify the pharmacodynamics [4].

Two major considerations that influence drug action in children that are not important in adults are growth and maturation. How these factors interact is not necessarily transparent from simple clinical observations because they correlate very closely. Drug elimination may increase with weight, height, age, body surface area, and creatinine clearance. One approach is to standardize for size before incorporating a factor for maturation and organ function [5]. By adopting such an approach, one may directly compare pharmacokinetic variables in neonates with those in older children and adults to determine appropriate drug dosing.

Disentangling Pharmacokinetic Covariates in Neonates

Size

Allometry is a term used to describe the nonlinear relationship between size and function. This nonlinear relationship is expressed as

J. Lerman (ed.), *Neonatal Anesthesia*, DOI 10.1007/978-1-4419-6041-2_3,

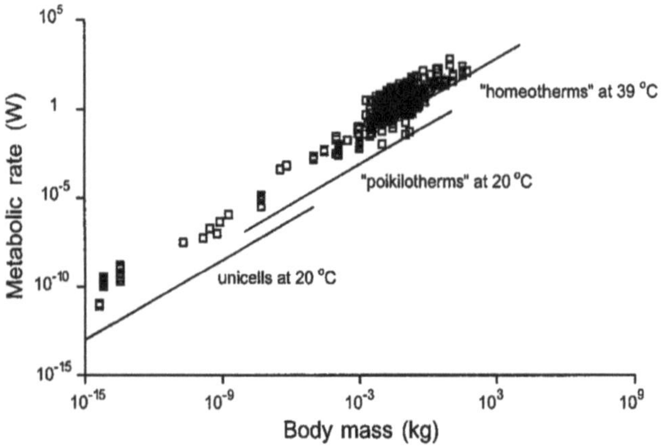

Fig. 3.1 A comparison of the temperature- standardized relation for whole-organism metabolic rate as a function of body mass. The "allometric ¾ power model" fits for unicells, poikilotherms, and homeotherms, uncorrected for temperature, are also shown. From Gillooly JF et al. Effects of size and temperature on metabolic rate. Science 2001; 293: 2248–2251, with permission

$$y = a \cdot \text{BodyMass}^{\text{PWR}},$$

where y is the variable of interest (e.g., basal metabolic rate), a is the allometric coefficient, and PWR is the allometric exponent. The value of the PWR has been the subject of much debate. Basal metabolic rate (BMR) is the most common physiological variable investigated, although camps are divided over its PWR value, 2/3 (i.e., body surface area) or ¾.

In all species including humans, the log of basal metabolic rate (BMR) plotted against the log of body weight produces a straight line with a slope of ¾ (Fig. 3.1). Fractal geometry is used to mathematically explain this phenomenon [6, 7].

The ¾ power law for metabolic rates was derived from a general model that describes how essential materials are transported through space-filled fractal networks of branching tubes. A great many physiological, structural, and time-related variables scale predictably within and between species with weight (W) exponents (PWR) of ¾, 1, and ¼, respectively [8]. These exponents have applicability to pharmacokinetic parameters such as clearance (CL), volume (V) and half-time [8]. The factor for size (*Fsize*) for total drug clearance, standardized to a 70 kg person, may be expected to scale with a power of ¾:

$$Fsize = \left(W/70 \right)^{3/4}.$$

Maturation

Allometry alone is insufficient to predict the clearance of drugs in neonates and infants from adult estimates [9–11]. The addition of a model describing maturation is required. The sigmoid hyperbolic or Hill model [12] is useful for describing this maturation process (MF):

$$\text{MF} = \frac{\text{PMA}^{\text{Hill}}}{\text{TM}_{50}^{\text{Hill}} + \text{PMA}^{\text{Hill}}}.$$

The TM_{50} describes the maturation half-time, and the Hill coefficient relates to the slope of this maturation profile. It is possible that there is asymmetry about the point of inflecion and the addition of an extra parameter describing this asymmetry can be used to provide extra flexibility for this empirical function [13].

Maturation of clearance begins before birth, suggesting that PMA would be a better predictor of drug elimination than postnatal age (PNA). The fetus is capable of metabolizing drugs. There are distinct patterns associated with isoform-specific developmental expression of the cytochrome P450 (CYP) enzymes. For example, CYP2D6 has been detected in preterm neonates as young as 25 weeks' PMA [14].

Organ Function

Changes associated with normal growth and development can be distinguished from pathological changes in organ function (OF) [5]. Pharmacokinetic parameters (P) can be described in an individual as the product of size (*Fsize*), maturation (MF) and organ function (OF) influences where *Pstd* is the value in a standard size adult without pathological changes in organ function [5].

$$P = Pstd \cdot Fsize \cdot \text{MF} \cdot \text{OF}.$$

Organ function is typically decreased in the presence of disease. However, it may also be increased by drugs. Phenobarbitone, a drug commonly given to neonates with seizures, can induce enzyme activity of a number of enzyme systems responsible for clearance [15] such as CYP1A2, CYP2C9, CYP2C19, CYP3A4, and UDP-glucuronosyltransferase (UGT) [16–18]. Phenobarbitone can increase bilirubin clearance in neonates through UGT induction [15]. Although an effect on the response to ketamine has been demonstrated in older children [19], there are no comparable examples in neonates to date.

Neonatal Pharmacokinetic Differences

Absorption

Anesthetic drugs are primarily administered via the intravenous and inhalational routes, although premedication and postoperative pain relief may be administered enterally. Drug absorption after oral administration is slower in

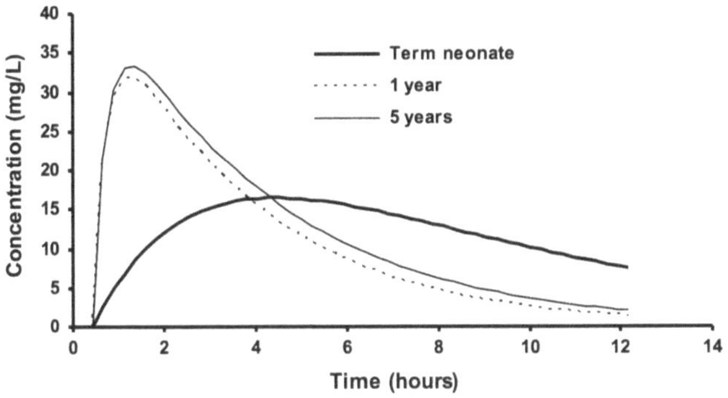

Fig. 3.2 Simulated mean predicted time-concentration profiles for a term neonate, a 1-year-old, infant and a 5-year-old child given paracetamol elixir. The time to peak concentration is delayed in neonates due to slow gastric emptying and reduced clearance (from Anderson BJ et al. Anesthesiology 2002; 96:1336–45)

neonates than in children due to delayed gastric emptying (Fig. 3.2). Adult absorption rates may not be reached until 6–8 months of PNA [20–22]. Congenital malformations (e.g., duodenal atresia), coadministration of drugs (e.g., opioids) or disease characteristics (e.g., necrotizing enterocolitis) may further affect the variability in absorption. Delayed gastric emptying and reduced clearance may dictate reduced doses and frequency of repeated drug administration. For example, a mean steady state target paracetamol concentration greater than 10 mg/L at trough can be achieved by an oral dose of 25 mg/kg/day in preterm neonates at 30 weeks, 45 mg/kg/day at 34 weeks and 60 mg/kg/day at 40 weeks' PMA [23]. Because gastric emptying is slow in preterm neonates, dosing may only be required twice a day [23]. In contrast, the rectal administration of some drugs (e.g., thiopental, methohexital) is more rapid in neonates than adults undergoing cardiac catheter study or radiological sedation. However, the interindividual absorption and relative bioavailability variability may be more extensive compared to oral administration, making rectal administration less suitable for repeated administration [24].

The larger relative skin surface area, increased cutaneous perfusion and thinner stratum corneum in neonates increase systemic exposure of topical drugs (e.g., corticosteroids, local anesthetic creams, antiseptics). Neonates have a greater tendency to form methemoglobin because of reduced methemoglobin reductase activity compared with older children. Furthermore, fetal hemoglobin is more readily oxidized compared with adult hemoglobin. Combined with an increased transcutaneous absorption, these have resulted in reluctance to apply repeat topical local anesthetics such as EMLA® (lidocaine-prilocaine) cream in this age group [25]. Similarly, cutaneous application of iodine antiseptics in neonates may result in transient hypothyroidism.

Inhalational anesthetic delivery is determined largely by alveolar ventilation and functional residual capacity (FRC). Neonates have increased alveolar ventilation to FRC ratio compared with adults, primarily the result of an increased metabolic demand for oxygen, which drives an increase in alveolar ventilation. Consequently, the alveolar to inspired fractions and therefore the blood to inspired partial pressure of anesthetics reach equilibration more rapidly in neonates than in children and adults [26]. The greater cardiac output and greater fraction of the cardiac output distributed to vessel-rich tissues (i.e., a clearance factor) and the lower tissue/blood solubilities (i.e., a volume factor) further contribute to the more rapid washin of inhalational anesthetics in early life [27, 28].

Disease characteristics may also contribute to the variability in the absorption of inhaled anesthetics. Right-to-left shunts affect the washin of inhalational anesthetics to a greater extent than left-to-right shunts. Induction of anesthesia may be slowed by right-to-left shunting of blood in neonates suffering cyanotic congenital cardiac disease or intrapulmonary (right-to-left) conditions. This slowing is greater with the less soluble anesthetics (e.g., nitrous oxide, sevoflurane) than the more soluble ones (e.g., halothane). Left-to-right shunts usually have minimal impact on uptake because cardiac output is increased so that systemic tissue perfusion is maintained at normal levels.

Distribution

Distribution describes the movement from systemic circulation into various body compartments, tissues, and cells. Distribution is influenced by body composition, protein binding, hemodynamics (e.g., regional blood flow) and membrane permeability. Disease processes may also impact the distribution of drugs.

Body Composition

Total body water and extracellular fluid (ECF) [29] decrease throughout gestation, the neonatal period, and childhood (Fig. 3.3), whereas the percent of body weight contributed by fat increases from 3 % in a 1.5-kg preterm neonate to 12 % in a full-term neonate and then doubles by 4–5 months of postnatal age. These changes in the body composition substantively affect the volumes of distribution of drugs. Polar drugs such as depolarizing and non-depolarizing neuromuscular-blocking drugs (NMBDs) distribute rapidly into the ECF, but enter cells more slowly. The initial dose of such drugs is consequently greater in the neonate than in the child or adult. Lipid-soluble drugs may also have a larger volume of distribution in neonates. The volume of distribution at steady state of fentanyl is 5.9 (SD 1.5) L/kg in a neonate compared with 1.6 (SD 0.3) L/kg in an adult [30]. This may explain the reduced respiratory depression after doses as large as 10 μg/kg in full-term neonates. However, high-dose therapy (50 μg/kg) results in a prolonged effect in neonates due to reduced clearance. In the case of propofol,

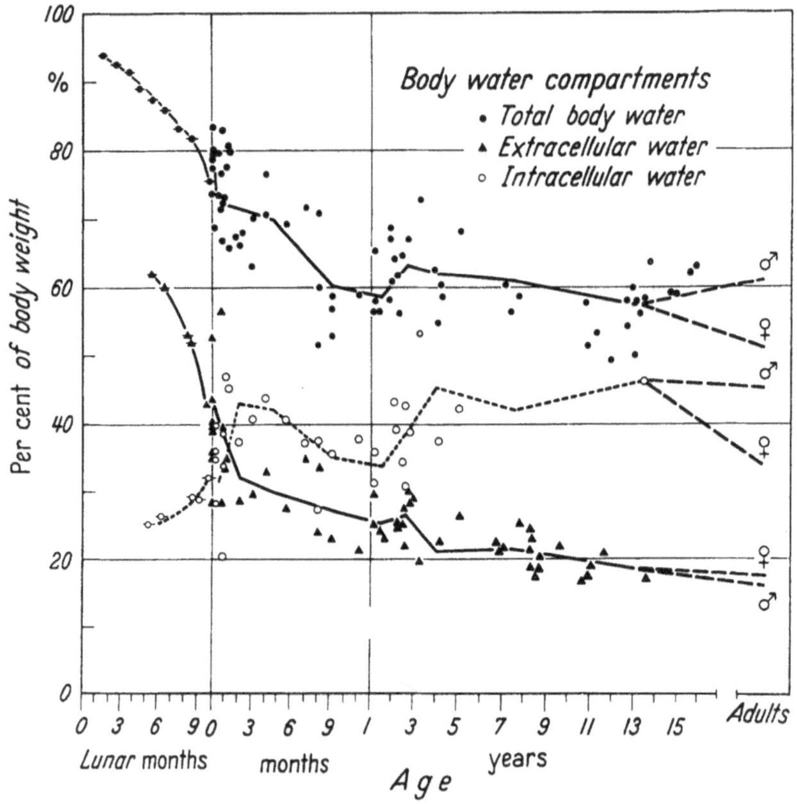

Fig. 3.3 Body water compartment changes during growth (used with permission from Friis-Hansen B. Changes in body water compartments during growth. In: Linneweh F, editor. Die Physiologische Entwicklung des Kindes. Berlin, Germany. Springer-Verlag. 1959)

reduction in the plasma concentration after induction of anesthesia is attributable to redistribution rather than rapid clearance. Neonates have less body fat and muscle content than older children. Hence, less propofol is apportioned to these "deep" compartments, attenuating the redistribution of propofol. If repeat doses of propofol are administered, they may accumulate in the blood and brain and delay recovery.

Plasma Proteins

The plasma alpha 1-acid glycoprotein (AAG) and albumin concentrations in neonates are reduced, albeit with a broad range of scatter (e.g., AAG 0.32–0.92 g/L), but reach adult concentrations by 6 months of postnatal age [31–33]. AAG is an acute phase reactant that increases after surgical stress. This increases the total plasma concentrations for low to intermediate extraction drugs such as bupivacaine that bind to AAG [34].

The concentration of unbound bupivacaine, however, will not change because the clearance of unbound bupivacaine depends only on the intrinsic metabolizing capacity of the liver. Any increase in unbound concentrations, for example, during long-term epidural infusions, is attributable to a reduced clearance rather than a decrease in the AAG concentration [35]. Total bupivacaine concentrations increase in the first 24 h after surgery in neonates who are receiving a continuous epidural infusion of bupivacaine; unbound bupivacaine concentrations, however, have not been studied. This increase in total bupivacaine is attributable in part to an increase of AAG. This increase in total bupivacaine, combined with reports of seizures in infants given epidural bupivacaine infusion, has led to recommendations to stop epidural infusions at 24 h. However, it is the unbound bupivacaine concentration that is responsible for the CNS effects, and this is determined by the clearance of the unbound bupivacaine. Clearance, the pivotal variable in the elimination of unbound bupivacaine, is reduced in neonates. In addition, clearance shows large interindividual variability, which means that unbound bupivacaine concentrations may increase steadily in some individuals with very low clearance. The lack of knowledge regarding the clearance of bupivacaine in each neonate precludes pronouncing the duration of a safe bupivacaine infusion for all [36].

Plasma albumin concentrations are least in preterm neonates but increase steadily, approximating adult values by 5 months of postnatal age. Binding capacity approaches adult values by 1 year of age. In addition, free fatty acids and unconjugated bilirubin compete with acidic drugs (e.g., ibuprofen, ceftriaxone) for albumin binding. The induction dose of thiopental in neonates is less than it is in children. It is possible that this is related to the decreased binding of thiopental to plasma albumin; 13 % of the drug is unbound in neonates compared with 7 % in adults [37].

Regional Blood Flows

The initial phase of distribution reflects the magnitude of regional blood flow. Consequently, the brain, heart, and liver, which receive the largest fraction of cardiac output, are first exposed. Drugs are then redistributed to other relatively well-perfused tissues, such as the skeletal muscle. There is a much slower tertiary distribution to relatively under-perfused tissues of the body that is noted with long-term drug infusions. In addition to perinatal circulatory changes (e.g., ductus venosus, ductus arteriosus), there are maturational differences in relative organ mass and regional blood flow, while a symptomatic patent ductus arteriosus may also result in differences in distribution. Blood flow as a fraction of the cardiac output, to the kidney and brain, increases with age, whereas blood flow to the liver decreases through the neonatal period [38]. Cerebral and hepatic mass as proportions of body weight in the infant are much greater than in the adult [39]. While onset times are generally faster for neonates than adults (a size effect), reduced cardiac output and cerebral perfusion in neonates mean that the expected onset time after an intravenous induction is slower in neonates, although reduced protein binding may counter this observation for some drugs. Offset time is also delayed because redistribution to well-perfused and deep under-perfused tissues is more limited.

Blood-Brain Barrier

The blood-brain barrier (BBB) is a network of tight junctions that restricts paracellular diffusion of compounds between the blood and brain. Confusion over the importance of this barrier in the neonate exists, partly because of early studies on respiratory depression caused by morphine and meperidine [40]. Early investigations found that the respiratory depression after morphine was greater than that after meperidine. This difference was attributed to greater brain concentrations of morphine because of the poorly developed BBB in the neonate [40]. It was postulated that BBB permeability to water-soluble drugs, such as morphine, changes with maturation [40]. However, the neonatal respiratory depression observed after morphine could have been explained by pharmacokinetic age-related changes. For example, the volume of distribution of morphine in term neonates 1–4 days (1.3 L/kg) is reduced compared with that in infants 8–60 days of age (1.8 L/kg) and in adults (2.8 L/kg) [41]. Consequently, we might expect greater initial concentrations of morphine in neonates than in adults, resulting in more pronounced respiratory depression in the former. Respiratory depression, measured by carbon dioxide response curves or by arterial oxygen tension, is similar from 2 to 570 days of age at the same morphine blood concentration [42]. The BBB theory in this particular circumstance lacks strong evidence. It is more likely that the increased neonatal respiratory depression after morphine is due to pharmacokinetic age-related changes.

The BBB may have impact, however, in other ways. Small molecules are thought to access fetal and neonatal brains more readily than in adults [43]. BBB function improves gradually, possibly reaching maturity by full-term age [43]. Kernicterus, for example, is more common in preterm neonates than in full-term neonates. In contrast to drugs bound to plasma proteins, unbound lipophilic drugs passively diffuse across the BBB equilibrating very quickly. This may contribute to bupivacaine's propensity for seizures in neonates. Decreased protein binding, as in the neonate, results in a greater proportion of unbound drug that is available for passive diffusion.

In addition to passive diffusion, there are specific transport systems that mediate active transport. Pathological CNS conditions can cause BBB breakdown and alter these transport systems. Fentanyl is actively transported across the BBB by a saturable ATP-dependent process, whereas ATP-binding cassette proteins such as *P*-glycoprotein actively pump out opioids such as fentanyl and morphine [44]. *P*-Glycoprotein modulation significantly influences opioid brain distribution and onset time, magnitude and duration of analgesic response [45]. Modulation may occur during disease processes, fever, or in the presence of other drugs (e.g., verapamil, magnesium) [44]. Recent evidence identified *P*-glycoprotein in the brain of fetuses as early as 22 weeks' gestation [46]. The prevalence and concentration of *P*-glycoprotein increased with fetal maturation. Genetic polymorphisms that affect *P*-glycoprotein-related genes may explain differences in CNS-active drug sensitivity [47, 48].

Elimination

The main routes by which drugs and their metabolites are eliminated from the body are the hepatobiliary system, the kidneys and the lungs. The liver is the primary organ for clearance of most drugs, although the lungs have a major role for anesthetic vapors. Drug-metabolizing enzymes are generally divided into phase I and phase II reactions. Phase I reactions are non-synthetic reactions like oxidation, reduction and hydrolysis. The most important group of enzymes involved in phase I processes are the cytochrome P450 (CYP) isoenzymes. Phase II reactions convert lipid-soluble drugs to water-soluble compounds, e.g., uridine diphosphate-glucuronosyltransferase (UGT). Metabolism may result in transformation to an active drug (e.g., codeine to morphine by CYP2D6, propacetamol to paracetamol by esterase, morphine to morphine-6-glucuronide by UGT2B7) or into a toxic compound (halothane to trifluoroacetyl chloride by CYP2E1 causing halothane hepatitis).

Hepatic Metabolic Clearance

Constitutional, environmental and genetic factors all contribute to the variability in clearance, but in the young neonate, age is the dominant covariate. Most CYP isoenzymes have small phenotypic activity until birth except for CYP3A7 [49, 50].

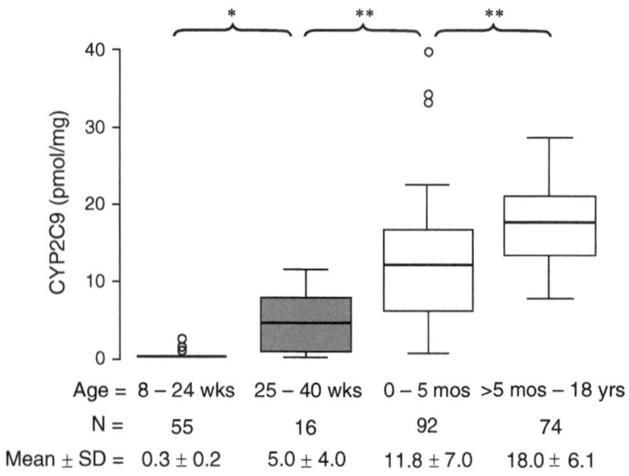

Fig. 3.4 Developmental expression of human hepatic CYP2C9 enzyme (used with permission from Koukouritaki et al. [50])

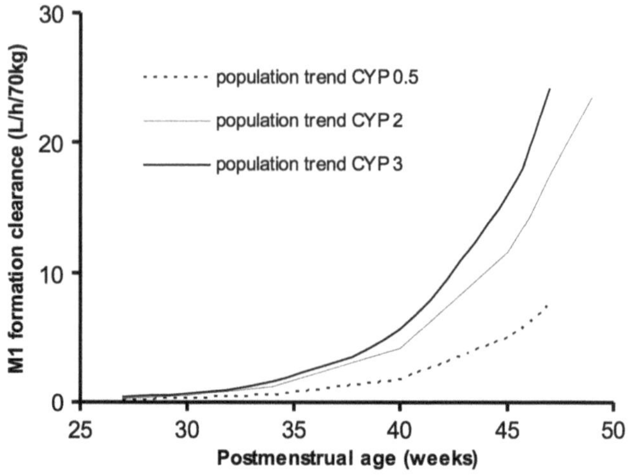

Fig. 3.5 Tramadol M1 metabolite formation clearance (CYP2D6) increases with postmenstrual age. Rate of increase varies with genotype expression. Adopted from Allegaert [14]. Allegaert K, van den Anker JN, de Hoon JN, et al. Covariates of tramadol disposition in the first months of life. Br J Anaesth 2008;100:525–32

CYP3A7 expresses its greatest activity during gestation after which its activity steadily decreases until there is no activity by 2 years [51, 52]. CYP2E1 activity surges after birth [53], CYP2D6 becomes detectable soon thereafter reaching adult levels by 2 weeks of age, and CYP3A4 and CYP2C (Fig. 3.4) are detectable during the first week, whereas CYP1A2 is the last to appear [52, 54]. Neonates depend on the immature CYP3A4 for levobupivacaine or midazolam clearance and on CYP1A2 for ropivacaine clearance, dictating reduced epidural infusion rates in this age group [1, 2, 55, 56].

CYP1A2 is 4–5 % in the neonate reaching 50 % of adult activity levels by 1 year of age [22]. Formation of the M1 metabolite of tramadol, a reflection of CYP2D6 activity [14], appears rapidly at term and reaches 84 % of mature values by 44 weeks' PMA.

Pharmacogenomics (PG) investigates variations of DNA and RNA characteristics related to drug response that incorporates both PK and PD. Large interindividual PK variability depends to a large extent on polymorphisms of the genes that encode for metabolic enzymes [57, 58].

The effect of genetic variability on plasma cholinesterase activity and its effect on the termination of action of succinylcholine is a well-known example [59]. Another example is the CYP2D6 single nuclear polymorphism (SNP), inherited as an autosomal recessive trait that may result in poor analgesia from codeine because the active metabolite morphine is not formed [58, 60]. Both PMA and CYP2D6 activity score explained the interindividual variability in tramadol metabolism (Fig. 3.5) [51, 60]. The interplay between maturation of tramadol clearance, M1 metabolite formation and maturing GFR on M1 concentration (and subsequent analgesia) is shown in Fig. 3.6 [48]. This observation illustrates the potential relevance of polymorphisms in neonatal pharmacology.

Some phase II isoenyzmes are mature in full-term neonates at birth (sulfate conjugation), whereas others are not (acetylation, glycination, glucuronidation) [52, 61]. Glucuronidation is important in the metabolic clearance of drugs (paracetamol, morphine, propofol) frequently administered by anesthesiologists. In the neonate, glucuronidation accounts for only 25 % of the phase II conjugation of acetaminophen, whereas in adults it accounts for ~75 % [22]. Allometric body-size scaling complemented by maturation models [8, 62] has been used to unravel the effects of maturation of the pharmacology of morphine [63–65] and paracetamol [66, 67]. Both drugs are cleared by specific isoforms (UGT1A6 and UGT2B7) [52]. In both instances, clearance is immature in the preterm 24-week PMA neonate and matures to reach adult rates by the end of the first year of life (Fig. 3.7). Dexmedetomidine is also cleared predominantly by the UGT system (UGT1A4 and UGT2B10) and has a similar maturation profile [68].

Glucuronidation is the major metabolic pathway for propofol. This pathway is immature in neonates, although multiple CYP isoenzymes (CYP2B6, CYP2C9, CYP2A6) also contribute to its metabolism and cause a more rapid maturation profile than expected from glucuronidation alone [69] (Fig. 3.7). Urine collections after intravenous bolus of propofol in neonates (PNA 11 days, PMA 38 weeks) support this contention. Urinary metabolites included both propofol glucuronide and 1- and 4-quinol glucuronide in a ratio of 1:2. Hydroxylation to quinol metabolites was active in these neonates [70], contributing to the rapid increase in clearance at this age that is faster than that reported for glucuronide conjugation alone (e.g., paracetamol, morphine).

Disease characteristics also contribute to the variability in UGT-related clearance. Maturation of morphine clearance occurs more quickly in infants undergoing noncardiac surgery compared with those after cardiac surgery [71]. Neonates

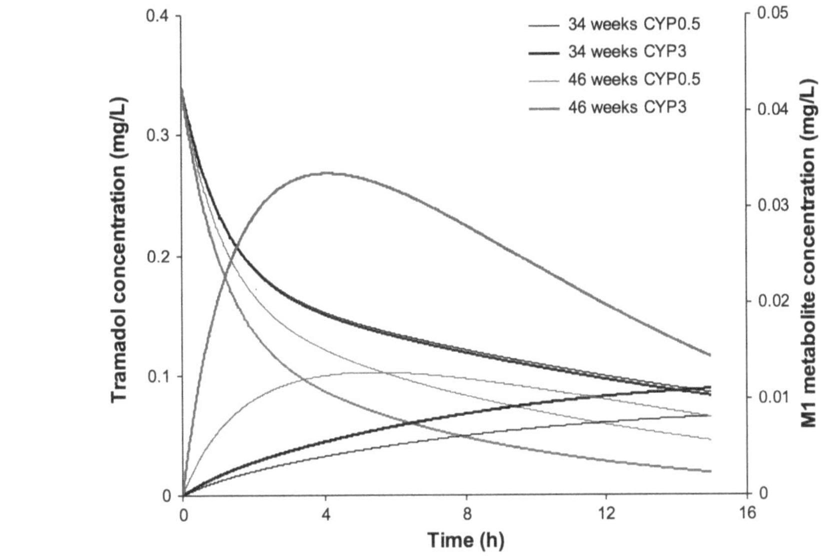

Fig. 3.6 Time-concentration profiles for tramadol and the M1 metabolite in neonates. CYP2D6 activity has been assigned a score of 0–3. Clearance of the parent drug is reduced in the 34-week PMA neonate compared with the 46-week PMA neonate and CYP activity has little impact on profiles. At 46 weeks both total clearance and CYP2D6 activity have increased, resulting in distinct profiles. The M1 metabolite is cleared by renal function, and the rapid maturation of glomerular filtration rate around 40 weeks' PMA has impact on the M1 metabolite profile, resulting in a peak concentration and subsequent decrease (adapted from Allegaert et al. [14])

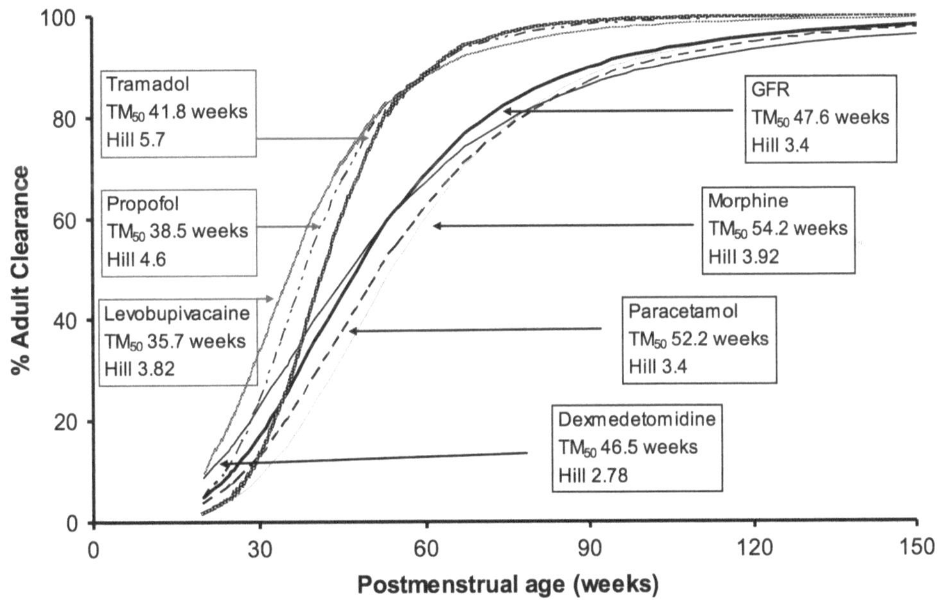

Fig. 3.7 Clearance maturation, expressed as a percentage of mature clearance, of drugs where glucuronide conjugation (paracetamol, morphine, dexmedetomidine) plays a major role. These profiles are closely aligned with glomerular filtration rate (GFR). In contrast, cytochrome P450 isoenzymes also contribute to propofol metabolism and cause a faster maturation profile than expected from glucuronide conjugation alone. Tramadol clearance maturation (phase I, CYP2D6, CYP3A) is also rapid. Maturation parameter estimates were taken from references [14, 56, 62, 64, 68, 84, 118]

requiring extracorporeal membrane oxygenation [72] or positive pressure ventilation [64] also have reduced clearance. Similarly, the clearance of propofol is reduced after cardiac surgery in children [73].

Extrahepatic Routes of Metabolic Clearance

Many drugs undergo metabolic clearance at extrahepatic sites. Remifentanil and atracurium are degraded by nonspecific esterases in tissues and erythrocytes, and these processes appear mature at birth, even in preterm neonates [74]. Clearance, expressed per kilogram, is increased in younger children [75–79], likely attributable to size because clearance is similar when scaled to a 70-kg person using allometry [75]. Ester local anesthetics are metabolized by plasma butyryl-cholinesterase, which is thought to be reduced in neonates. The in vitro plasma half-life of 2-chloroprocaine in umbilical cord blood is twice that in maternal blood [80], but there are no in vivo studies of the effects of age on its metabolism. Succinylcholine clearance is increased in neonates [81, 82], suggesting butyryl-cholinesterase activity is mature at birth.

Pulmonary Elimination

The factors that determine anesthetic absorption through the lung (alveolar ventilation, FRC, cardiac output, solubility) also contribute to elimination kinetics. We might anticipate more rapid washout in neonates for any given duration of anesthesia because of the greater alveolar ventilation to FRC ratio, greater fraction of cardiac output perfusing vessel-rich tissues, reduced solubility in blood and tissues, and a reduced distribution to fat and muscle. Furthermore, younger age (as in the neonate) will speed the elimination of more soluble anesthetics such as halothane to a greater extent than the less soluble anesthetics, desflurane and sevoflurane. Halothane, and to a far lesser extent isoflurane (1.5 %) and sevoflurane (5 %), undergoes hepatic metabolism. Halothane is reported to undergo as much as 20–25 % metabolism, but at typical anesthetizing concentrations, hepatic halothane removal is extremely small [83].

Renal Elimination

Renal elimination of drugs and their metabolites occurs primarily by two processes: glomerular filtration and tubular secretion. Glomerular filtration rate (GFR) is only 10 % that of mature value at 25 weeks, 35 % at term and 90 % of the adult GFR at 1 year of age [22, 84]. Aminoglycosides are almost exclusively cleared by renal elimination and maintenance dose is predicted by PMA because it predicts the time course of renal maturation [85]. The kidney is also capable of metabolizing drugs; CYP2E1, which metabolizes ether anesthetics, is active in the kidney. The very presence of CYP2E1 in the kidney has been held responsible for the degradation of ether anesthetics and the release of nephrotoxic fluoride [86].

Immaturity of the clearance pathways can be used to our advantage when managing apnea after anesthesia in the preterm neonate. N_7-Methylation of theophylline to produce caffeine is well developed in the neonate, whereas oxidative demethylation (CYP1A2) responsible for caffeine metabolism is deficient. Theophylline is effective for the management of postoperative apnea in the preterm neonate, in part because it is a prodrug of caffeine, which is effective in controlling apnea in this age group and can only be cleared slowly by the immature kidney [87].

Milrinone, an inodilator, is used increasingly in children after congenital cardiac surgery. Renal clearance is the primary route of elimination. A clearance of 9 L/h/70 kg is reported in adults with congestive heart failure, and we might anticipate that clearance in preterm neonates is reduced to 10 % of this rate because renal function is correspondingly immature in this cohort. This has been confirmed in 26-week PMA preterm infants whose milrinone clearance was 0.96 L/h/70 kg [88]. Similarly the clearance of the neuromuscular-blocking drug (NMBD) d-tubocurare can be directly correlated with GFR [89]. Some drugs such as the nonsteroidal anti-inflammatory drugs (NSAIDs) may compromise renal clearance in early life: ibuprofen reduces GFR by 20 % in preterm neonates, independent of gestational age [90, 91].

Neonatal Pharmacodynamic Differences

Children's responses to drugs have much in common with the responses in adults once developmental PK aspects are considered [92]. The perception that drug effects differ in children arises because these drugs have not been adequately studied in pediatric populations who have size- and age-related effects as well as different diseases. Neonates, however, often have altered pharmacodynamics as well.

The minimum alveolar concentration (MAC) is commonly used to express anesthetic vapor potency. The MAC values for most vapors in neonates are less than those in infants (Fig. 3.8) [27]. The MAC of isoflurane in preterm neonates <32 weeks' gestation was 1.28 %(SD 0.17), and in preterm neonates 32–37 weeks' gestation was 1.41 % (SD 0.18) which in turn is less than in full-term neonates [93].

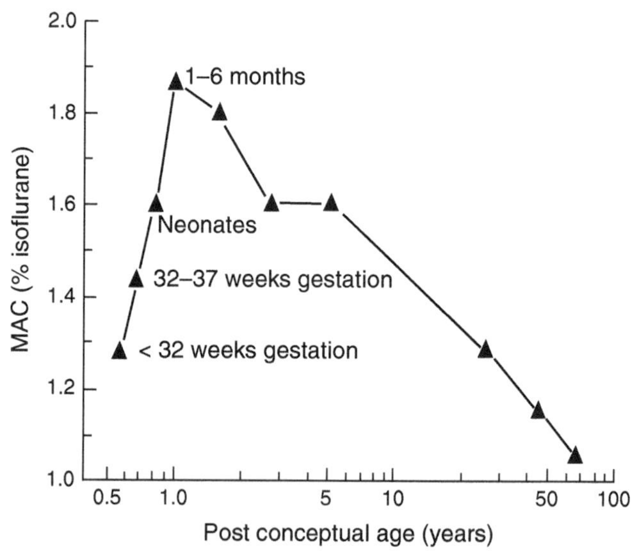

Fig. 3.8 Effect of age on the minimum alveolar concentration (MAC) of isoflurane. MAC increases as age decreases reaching a zenith in infants 1–6 months of age and decreases thereafter as age decreases to 24 weeks' gestation [93]

Similarly, the MAC of halothane in full-term neonates (0.87 %) is less than that in infants (1.20 %), but the decrease in blood pressure and the incidence of hypotension in neonates and infants at approximately 1 MAC of halothane are similar [94].

Changes in regional blood flow may influence the amount of drug that reaches the brain. Inhalational anesthetics are thought to act via gamma-aminobutyric acid ($GABA_A$) receptors, and receptor numbers or developmental shifts in the regulation of chloride transporters in the brain may change with age, altering the response to these anesthetics. Midazolam acts on the same receptors. Data from rodents from immediate neonates to PNA 40 days have shown developmental PD changes for sedation that mimic those observed in human childhood [95]. Such models offer potential to improve our understanding of developmental pharmacology [96].

Neonates demonstrate an increased sensitivity to the effects of neuromuscular-blocking drugs [89]. The reason for this sensitivity is unknown, but the finding is consistent with the observation that there is a threefold reduction in the release of acetylcholine from the infant rat phrenic nerve compared with the adult nerve [97, 98]. Reduced clearance and increased sensitivity prolong the duration of neuromuscular effect.

The duration of regional block with amide local anesthetic agents in infants is reduced compared with older children. Moreover, infants require a larger weight-scaled dose to achieve a similar dermatomal level when local anesthetics are given by subarachnoid block. This may, in part, be due to reduced myelination in infants, greater cerebrospinal fluid volume, increased spacing of nodes of Ranvier and the length of nerve exposed.

There is an age-dependent expression of intestinal motilin receptors and the modulation of antral contractions in neonates. Prokinetic agents may not be useful in very preterm neonates, useful only, in part, in older preterm infants but very useful in full-term infants. Similarly, bronchodilators are ineffective in neonates because of the paucity of bronchial smooth muscle that can cause bronchospasm.

Cardiac calcium stores in the endoplasmic reticulum are reduced in the neonatal heart because of immaturity. Exogenous calcium has a greater impact on contractility in this age group than in older children or adults. Conversely, calcium channel blocking drugs (e.g., verapamil) can cause life-threatening bradycardia and hypotension [99]. Catecholamine release and response to vasoactive drugs vary with age. These pharmacodynamic differences are based in part upon developmental changes in myocardial structure, cardiac innervation and adrenergic receptor function. For example, the immature myocardium has fewer contractile elements and therefore a decreased ability to increase contractility; it also responds poorly to standard techniques of manipulating preload [100]. Dopaminergic receptors are present in the pulmonary vasculature and are believed to be responsible for pulmonary vasoconstriction in preterm neonates. However, systemic vasoconstriction is greater than that observed in the pulmonary circulation, and this differential response contributes to the use of dopamine in neonates with known pulmonary hypertension after cardiac surgery. Neonates have underdeveloped sympathetic innervation and reduced stores of norepinephrine. Signs of cardiovascular α-receptor stimulation may occur at lower doses than β-receptor stimulation because β-receptor maturation lags behind α-receptor maturation during the development of the adrenergic system [101]. The preterm neonate has immature metabolic and elimination pathways leading to increased dopamine concentrations after prolonged infusions [101–104]. These maturational changes in PK and PD may contribute to dopamine's continued popularity in the neonatal nursery while its popularity wanes in the adult population.

Pharmacodynamic Measures

In general, outcome measures are more difficult to assess in neonates than in children or adults. The common effects measured in anesthesia are circulatory and respiratory depression, neuromuscular blockade, depth of anesthesia, and sedation or pain. Circulatory responses may be assessed using heart rate and blood pressure, although more detailed analyses require echocardiogram and electrophysiology of the conduction systems. Similarly, respiratory responses may be assessed in terms of respiratory rate and gas exchange (oximetry and capnometry), but more sophisticated effects require CO_2 response curves and compliance changes. Electromyography response of the adductor pollicis is a consistent effect measure for investigation of neuromuscular blockade in both neonates and adults. Differences are minor, e.g., neonates do not tolerate repetitive stimulations for as long as older children, because the acetylcholine reserves in neonates are limited. In the cases of depth of anesthesia, sedation and pain in neonates, assessing outcome variables becomes more difficult.

A common metric to assess the depth of anesthesia is the electroencephalogram (EEG) or a modification of detected EEG signals (spectral edge frequency, bispectral index, entropy). Physiological studies in adults and children indicate that EEG-derived anesthesia depth monitors provide an imprecise and drug-dependent measure of arousal. They can be used as guides for anesthesia and have improved outcomes in adults. In older children, the physiology, anatomy and clinical observations indicate the performance of the monitors may be similar to that in adults. However, ketamine provides inconsistent estimates of depth of anesthesia with the BIS. In the case of sevoflurane, the BIS in children paradoxically increases at end-tidal concentrations >3 % [105]. In infants the use of these monitors cannot yet be supported in theory or in practice [106, 107]. Both outside and during anesthesia, the EEG in infants is fundamentally different from the EEG in older children; there remains a need for specific neonate-derived algorithms if EEG-derived anesthesia depth monitors are to be used in neonates [108, 109].

The existence of an extensive number of sedation or pain scales does not mean that all assessment-related problems have been solved. Most scores are validated for the acute, procedural setting and perform less reliably for subacute or chronic pain or stress. Scoring systems seldom take into account the limited capacity of the more immature infants to mount a consistent behavioral and physiological response to pain. Validation is based on assessment of intra- and interindividual variability and correlations with neuroendocrine markers of stress or pain. Future research may provide us with objective tools to quantify pain and sedation but will have to take the maturational aspects of the neonate into account.

Induction Agents

Intravenous induction agents exert their anesthetic effects by achieving adequate cerebral concentrations to prevent undesired responses such as movement. Termination of these effects is attributed to redistribution of the drugs away from the brain rather than rapid clearance from the body, an effect that may be delayed in neonates. With less body fat and muscle in neonates, less drug is apportioned to these "deep" compartments. Delayed awakening after intravenous agents occurs in neonates because the concentration of these agents in the brain remains greater than that observed in older children as a consequence of slower redistribution.

Propofol

Mechanism

The hypnotic actions of propofol result from its interaction with the $GABA_A$ receptor [110, 111].

Pharmacodynamics

Integrated PK–PD studies in neonates are lacking, partly due to a lack of consistent effect measures. Consequently, the target concentration for anesthesia in neonates is unknown. The equilibration half-time ($T_{1/2}$keo) for the effect compartment is unknown but is assumed to be smaller [109] than the 3 min described in adults [112, 113]. Reduced numbers of $GABA_A$ receptors in the neonatal brain may contribute to a reduced target concentration to effect a response, but this hypothesis remains untested. A circadian night rhythm effect has been noted in an investigation of infant propofol sedation after major craniofacial surgery [114], but such an effect is unlikely in neonates who do not have established day/night sleep cycles.

Pharmacokinetics

Propofol is metabolized in the liver with an extraction ratio of approximately 0.9. Clearance is limited by the hepatic blood flow and is thus reduced in children in low cardiac output states [73]. Clearance is affected primarily by UGT1A9 (glucuronidation), with contributions from CYP2B6, CYP2C9, and CYP2A6 isoenzymes, resulting in a more rapid maturation profile than expected from glucuronide conjugation alone (Fig. 3.7).

Although propofol is widely used for target-controlled infusion (TCI) anesthesia in children, commonly used TCI data sets [113, 115–117], have only investigated propofol PK in children beyond infancy. In an effort to link neonatal data with those from children [118], Allegaert used allometry and the Hill equation [62] to suggest a maturation half-time of 44 weeks and a Hill coefficient of 4.9 [119]. Clearance at 28 weeks' gestation is only 10 % that of the mature value and by full term reaches 38 %. Clearance in the full-term neonate achieves 90 % of the adult value (1.83 L/min/70 kg) by 30 weeks' PMA. While postmenstrual age (PMA) is the major descriptor of maturation, it is possible that postnatal age (PNA) may also have an additional effect on maturation of propofol clearance above that predicted by PMA [69]. Further longitudinal data that examine individual neonates as they grow are required to clarify this aspect of maturation.

Adverse Effects

Propofol is used for intubation by neonatologists [120, 121] and anesthesiologists [122, 123]. While doses of 2–3 mg/kg are reported [123–125], caution is advocated in early postnatal life where a transient return to fetal circulation is possible ("flip-flop" phenomenon) due to reduced systemic vascular resistance concomitant with increased pulmonary resistance (associated with hypoxemia and acidosis) [126, 127]. Profound low cardiac output state, together with profound oxygen desaturation that was refractory to usual resuscitation measures including most inotropes, has been reported [125, 128, 129]. Additionally, hypotension of 30-min duration has been reported in preterm neonates given propofol 3 mg/kg for procedural sedation in a neonatal intensive care unit [130], although the severity of the hypotension was similar to that reported after volatile anesthetics at 1 MAC [118], Whether these episodes are attributable to hypovolemia or persistent fetal circulation is not clear, although one study was undertaken in preterm infants within a few hours after birth [125]. In other reports where propofol was administered to older preterm infants, hypotension was not detected [121, 131]. We recommend loading these infants with 10–20 mL/kg balanced salt solution before administration of propofol and atropine 0.02 mg/kg IV and preoxygenation if the risk of bradycardia and desaturation during tracheal intubation are possible. Other adverse effects (bradycardia, propofol infusion syndrome, respiratory depression, immune function) are poorly documented in neonates and require further investigation. Neonates can experience pain on injection and the use of lignocaine to ameliorate this effect is suggested.

Thiopental

Mechanism

Thiopental is an analogue of pentobarbitone. The greater lipid solubility of thiopental is achieved by substituting a sulfur atom in place of an oxygen atom on the barbiturate acid ring [132]. Greater penetration of the BBB has been described in neonates compared with older animals, possibly attributable to the greater blood-brain flow in this cohort [133]. The most likely mechanism of action of thiopental is via binding to $GABA_A$ receptors, which increases the duration of GABA-activated chloride opening.

Pharmacodynamics

The ED_{50} of thiopental varies with age: 3.4 mg/kg in neonates, 6.3 mg/kg in infants, 3.9 mg/kg in children aged 1–4 years, 4.5 mg/kg in children 4–7 years, 4.3 mg/kg in children 7–12 years and 4.1 mg/kg in adolescents aged 12–16 years [134, 135]. It remains to be determined whether altered PK or PD responses explain the reduced dose requirements in neonates. The effect site concentration of thiopental for induction of anesthesia in neonates may be less than that in infants because the neonate has relatively immature cerebral cortical function, rudimentary dendritic arborizations and relatively few synapses [136]. However, integrated PK–PD studies with thiopental in neonates have not been performed to support or refute this premise [137]. The plasma concentration (EC_{50}) of thiopental required for induction of anesthesia in adults based on the EEG is 17.9 mcg/mL; comparable data in neonates are lacking [138]. The $T_{1/2}$keo in adults is 0.6 min [138], but there are no estimates in neonates. Children aged 13–68 months given rectal thiopental (44 mg/kg) 45 min prior to surgery were either asleep or adequately sedated with plasma concentrations above 2.8 mcg/mL [139].

Pharmacokinetics

Peak concentrations of thiopental are reached in the brain and other well-perfused organs within one circulation time. Recovery is due to redistribution. Reported pharmacokinetic parameter estimates have been derived from infusions administered for seizure control in neonates suffering hypoxic-ischemic insults. Clearance estimates in neonates ranged from 66 to 320 mL/h/kg with a volume of distribution at steady state (Vss) of 3.6–5.4 L/kg [140–143]. Interindividual variability was considerable [137]. While most clearance estimates are less than those in adults (200 mL/h/kg) [138], interpretation is difficult because the hypoxic-ischemic insult will also affect the clearance. Clearance is through oxidation (CYP2C19) to an inactive metabolite, thiopental carboxylic acid, and neonatal immature hepatic function decreases oxidizing capacity. CYP2C19 microsomal activity is approximately 30 % of mature values in the third trimester and increases dramatically around birth [50]. A recent analysis of thiopental clearance maturation is consistent with the timing of maturation of CYP2C19. Clearance rapidly increases during the neonatal period from 33 mL/h/kg at 24 weeks' PMA to 160 mL/h/kg at term; an adult clearance of 200 mL/h/kg is reported [144]. Neonates (25.7–41.4 weeks' PMA) undergoing surgery on the first day of life yielded an elimination half-life of 8 h (interquartile range (IQR), 2.5–10.8) and a clearance of 92 mL/min/kg (IQR 20 100) [145]. Thiopental has a low hepatic extraction ratio (0.3), exhibiting capacity-limited elimination. In adults, 10–12 % of thiopental is metabolized per hour; comparable data are not available in neonates. Michaelis-Menten kinetics are reported after prolonged infusion in adults. Michaelis-Menten kinetics are also reported in neonates. The Michaelis constant (Km 28.3 mg/L) is similar to that reported for adults (26.7 mg/L). The maximum rate of metabolism (Vmax) increases from 0.44 mg/min/kg at 24 weeks' PMA to 5.26 mg/min/kg at term; an adult Vmax of 7 mg/min/kg is reported [144].

Adverse Effects

These are similar to those described for propofol. Thiopental has little direct effect on vascular smooth muscle tone. Cardiovascular depression is centrally mediated by inhibition of sympathetic nervous activity and direct myocardial depression through effects on trans-sarcolemmal and sarcoplasmic reticulum calcium flux [146]. There is no pain on injection. Because the action of thiopental is terminated by redistribution and metabolism is slow, recovery may be very slow after an infusion of thiopental.

Ketamine

Mechanism of Action

The analgesic properties of ketamine are mediated by multiple mechanisms at central and peripheral sites. The contribution from *N*-methyl-D-aspartate (NMDA) receptor antagonism and interaction with cholinergic, adrenergic, serotonergic and opioid pathways and local anesthetic effects remain to be fully elucidated.

Pharmacodynamics

Ketamine is available as a mixture of two enantiomers; the S(+)-enantiomer has four times the potency of the R(−)-enantiomer. S(+)-ketamine has approximately twice the potency of the racemate. The metabolite norketamine has a potency that is one-third that of its parent. Plasma concentrations associated with hypnosis and amnesia during surgery are 0.8–4 μg/mL; awakening usually occurs at concentrations less than 0.5 μg/mL. Pain thresholds are increased at 0.1 μg/mL [147]. Data from neonates are not available.

Pharmacokinetics

Ketamine is very lipid soluble with rapid distribution. Ketamine undergoes *N*-demethylation to norketamine. Elimination of racemic ketamine is complicated by the R(−)-ketamine enantiomer, which inhibits the elimination of the S(+)-ketamine enantiomer [148]. Clearance in children is similar to adult rates (80 L/h/70 kg, i.e., liver blood flow) within the first 6 months of life, when corrected for size using allometric models [35]. Clearance in the neonate is reduced (26 L/h/70 kg) [149–151], while Vss is increased in neonates (3.46 L/kg at birth, 1.18 L/kg at 4 years, 0.75 L/kg at adulthood [135]). This larger Vss in neonates contributes to the observation that neonates require a fourfold greater dose than 6-year-old children to prevent gross motor movement [152]. There is a high hepatic extraction ratio and the relative bioavailability of oral, nasal, and rectal formulations is 30–50 %.

Adverse Effects

Ketamine can cause psychotic reactions and hallucinations that can cause distress in older children. These effects can be attenuated by benzodiazepines. An antisialagogue may be effective to diminish copious secretions that may occur after parenteral administration. Tolerance in children may occur with repeated use. Hypocapnia may attenuate ketamine-induced increases in intracranial pressure.

Ketamine is infrequently used in neonates, with perhaps the exception of those with right-to-left congenital heart defects. However, even this limited use has come under scrutiny over concerns that NMDA antagonists (e.g., ketamine and $GABA_A$ agonists) cause significant neuronal apoptosis and other cellular dysgenesis during the period of rapid synaptogenesis in newborn animals [153–155]. Neonatal rats that were anesthetized with ketamine but did not undergo any surgical stimulation or inflammatory response sustained widespread neuronal apoptosis and long-term memory deficits.[156, 157]. The severity of these findings appeared to depend on both the dose and duration of exposure and the coadministration of other proapoptotic compounds in these 7-day-old rats. Moreover, these same findings have been reported in other animals including nonhuman primates and in the presence of anesthetics other than ketamine. More recently, interventions have been forthcoming that appear to prevent or attenuate the neurocognitive sequelae from these anesthetics in newborn animals [158–160]. Nonetheless, extrapolating these animal data to the care of human neonates remains contentious [161, 162].

Inhalation Agents

Although inhalational anesthetics have been administered to children for 150 years, the pharmacology of inhalational anesthetics in neonates has only been the subject of investigation for 50 years or less. Research has clarified the pharmacokinetics of inhalational anesthetics in neonates, their MAC values and cardiorespiratory responses to clarify the pharmacology of inhalational anesthetics in this vulnerable age group. These developments have allowed practitioners to provide safe anesthesia while attenuating the incidence and severity of adverse events.

Physicochemical Properties

The chemical structures of the current inhalational agents are based on a polyhalogenated ether skeleton (with one exception): isoflurane and desflurane are methyl ethyl ether anesthetics and sevoflurane is a methyl isopropyl (Table 3.1). The single exception to the ether skeleton is halothane, a polyhalogenated alkane that is infrequently used today. Desflurane differs from its older cousin, isoflurane, only in the substitution of a fluoride atom for a chloride on the alpha carbon of isoflurane, whereas sevoflurane differs by the substitution of a trifluoromethyl group for chloride on the alpha carbon of isoflurane. The minor atomic substitutions and structural differences among these ether anesthetics confer substantial differences in their physicochemical and pharmacological properties that are elucidated in Table 3.1.

Pharmacokinetics

In the 1960s, investigators determined that the washin curves for halothane (Fig. 3.9) and nitrous oxide in neonates were more rapid than in adults [26, 163]. While the rate of increase of alveolar to inspired partial pressures of nitrous oxide in adults is rapid, achieving an FA/FI ratio of 0.8 within 10 min, it is even more rapid in neonates and infants, achieving a ratio of 0.9 within 5 min. The fundamental principle underlying the pharmacokinetics of these anesthetics in neonates is the movement of inhalational anesthetics among organs in the body. Outside of the body, inhalational anesthetics exist in the gas phase where the concentrations or partial pressures are interchangeable (assuming the ideal gas law). However

Table 3.1 Pharmacology of inhaled anesthetics

	Halothane	Enflurane	Isoflurane	Sevoflurane	Desflurane
Pharmacology					
Chemical structure	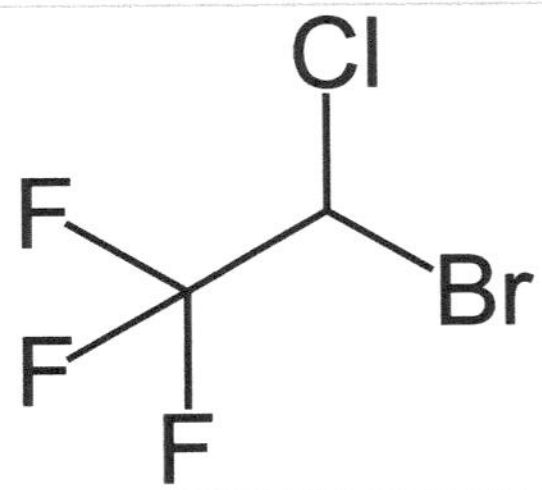	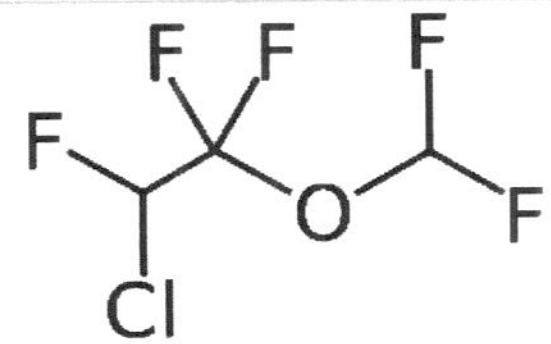	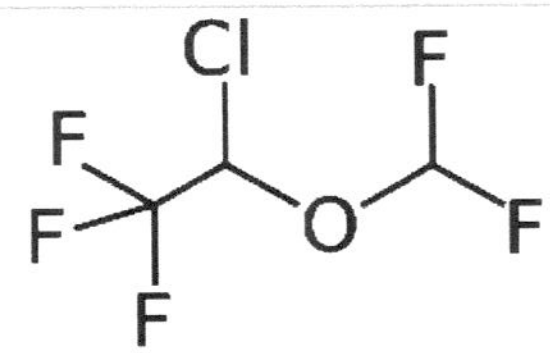	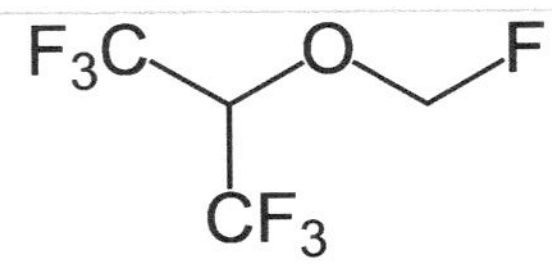	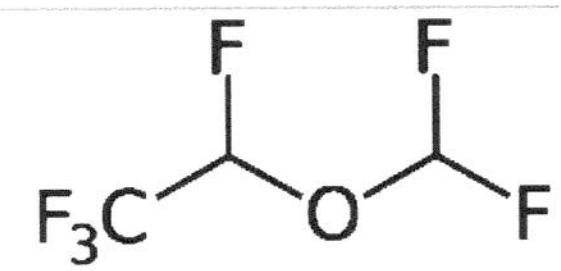
Molecular weight	197.4	184.5	184.5	200.1	168
Boiling point (°C)	50.2	56.5	48.5	58.6	23.5
Vapor pressure (mmHg)	244	172	240	185	664
Saturation concentration (%)	34	24	34	26	93
Odour	Mild, pleasant	Etheric	Etheric	Pleasant	Etheric
Solubility					
$\lambda_{b/g}$ adults	2.4	1.9	1.4	0.66	0.42
$\lambda_{b/g}$ neonates	2.14	1.78	1.19	0.66	–
$\lambda_{brain/b}$ adults	1.9	1.3	1.6	1.7	1.2
$\lambda_{brain/b}$ neonates	1.5	0.9	1.3	–	–
$\lambda_{fat/b}$ adults	51.1	–	45	48	27
MAC					
MAC_{adults}	0.75	1.7	1.2	2.05	7.0
$MAC_{neonates}$	0.87	–	1.60	3.2	9.2

The pharmacology, solubility and MAC of five potent inhalational anesthetics. Note that the boiling point of desflurane is close to room temperature and that the solubility of the anesthetics in blood and fat decreases from left to right across the table, whereas MAC increases from left to right

b/g blood/gas, *brain/b* brain/blood, *fat/b* fat/blood, *MAC* minimum alveolar concentration (percent), λ partition coefficient. Data from

1. Lerman J, Gregory GA, Willis MM, Eger EI 2nd. Age and solubility of volatile anesthetics in blood. Anesthesiology 1984;61:139–43.
2. Malviya S, Lerman J. The blood/gas solubilities of sevoflurane, isoflurane, halothane, and serum constituent concentrations in neonates and adults. Anesthesiology 1990;72:793–6.
3. Yasuda N, Targ AG, Eger EI II. Solubility of I-653, sevoflurane, isoflurane, and halothane in human tissues. Anesth Analg 1989;69:370-3.
4.. Lerman J, Schmitt-Bantel BI, Gregory GA, et al. Effect of age on the solubility of volatile anesthetics in human tissues. Anesthesiology 1986;65:307–11.
5. Data from Steward A, Allott PR, Cowles AL, Mapleson WW. Solubility coefficients for inhaled anesthetics for water, oil and biological media. Br J Anaesth 1973:45;282–93.
6. de Jong RH, Eger EI II. MAC expanded: AD50 and AD95 values of common inhalation anesthetics in man. Anesthesiology 1975:42;384–9.

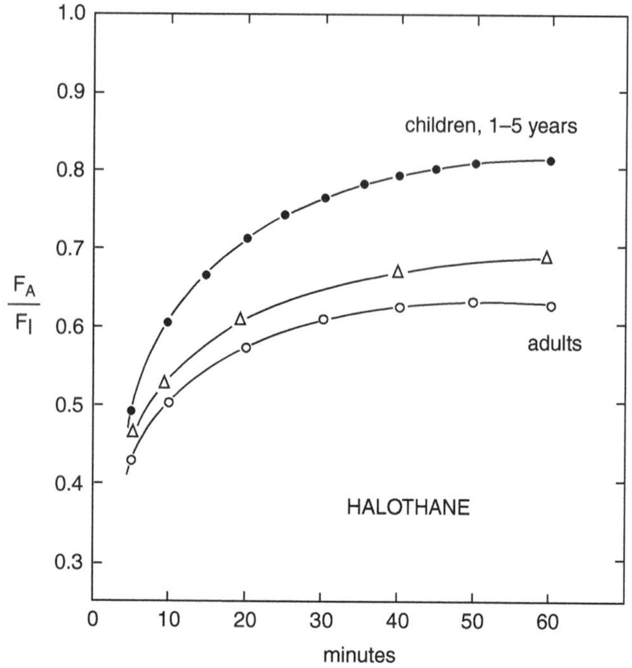

Fig. 3.9 Rate of rise of alveolar to inspired partial pressures of halothane in children and adults (reproduced with permission, Salanitre & Rackow [26])

Table 3.2 Determinants of the rapid washin of inhalational agents in infants

1. Greater alveolar ventilation to functional residual capacity ratio
2. Greater fraction of the cardiac output distributed to the vessel-rich group
3. Reduced tissue/blood solubility
4. Reduced blood/gas solubility

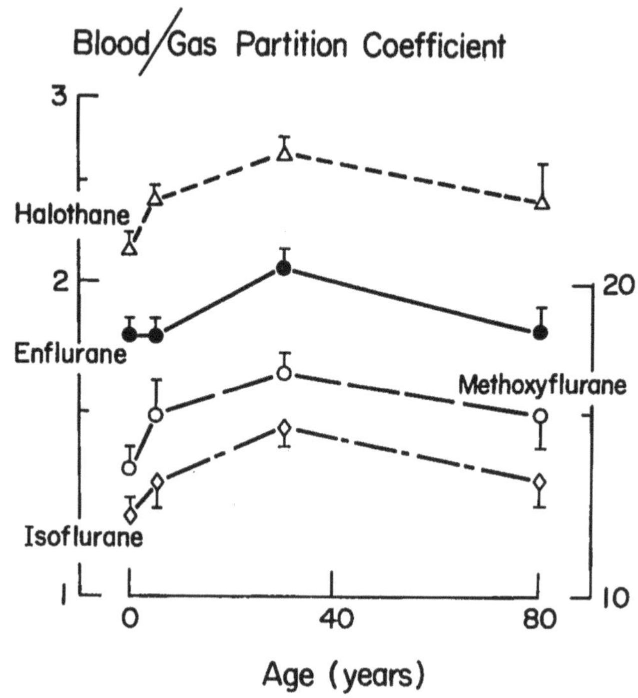

Fig. 3.10 Effect of age on the blood/gas partition coefficient of the four inhalational agents, isoflurane, enflurane, halothane and methoxyflurane. The solubility of all four agents in neonates is 18 % less than in adults (reproduced with permission, Lerman et al. [165])

inside the body, the concentrations of these anesthetics in any liquid or solid tissue exceed the equivalent partial pressure because they are bound to proteins and lipids. In addition, these anesthetics move across membranes (from the functional residual capacity (FRC) to the blood or blood to tissue phases) without impediment, along partial pressure gradients, not concentration gradients. Conceptually, this is identical to our understanding of the movement of other gases such as oxygen and carbon dioxide in the body. Inhalational anesthetics move across membranes seeking to equilibrate partial pressures, even though the concentrations of anesthetics in the tissues differ. As a result, we only refer to inhalational anesthetics in terms of their partial pressures inside the body.

Four factors explain the more rapid washin of inhalational anesthetics in neonates compared with older children and adults (Table 3.2). The first factor is the delivery of anesthetics to the lungs. Alveolar ventilation determines the rate of delivery of anesthetic to the lungs and thus to the FRC [164]. The greater the ratio of the alveolar ventilation to FRC, the more rapidly the anesthetic partial pressure in the FRC increases. In neonates, this ratio is 5:1, threefold greater than in adults, 1.5:1. The remaining three factors explain the rapid washin of anesthetics in neonates by their effects on the uptake of anesthetics from the lungs. Although a greater cardiac output should actually slow the washin of anesthetic into the FRC, in neonates it speeds the washin. The reason for this is that the greater cardiac output in neonates is primarily distributed to the vessel-rich group (VRG) of tissues (brain, heart, kidneys, and gastrointestinal and endocrine organs), which in the neonate comprises a large fraction (18 %) of the body weight compared with 5 % in the child/adult. Because the VRG receives such a large proportion of the cardiac output, the anesthetic partial pressures in the VRG equilibrate very rapidly, leaving much of the blood returning to the heart with partial pressures that are similar to those in the blood that left the heart. Hence, a diminishing quantity of inhalational anesthetic is taken up from the FRC into the pulmonary blood, allowing the partial pressure in the FRC to increase. At the same time, the blood and tissue solubilities of inhalational anesthetics in neonates are less than those in older children and adults (Fig. 3.10, Table 3.1) [28, 165, 169]. This is true for the more soluble inhalational anesthetics with 18 % less solubilities in neonates compared with older children and adults. However, in the cases of the less soluble anesthetics, sevoflurane and desflurane, the solubilities in neonates likely do not differ substantially from those in adults [28]. Hence, blood solubility differences of the less soluble inhalational anesthetics do not contribute substantively to the rapid washin of sevoflurane and desflurane in neonates. Similarly, age-related differences in hemoglobin, serum concentration of α-1-acid glycoprotein and prematurity do not significantly affect the solubility of most inhalational anesthetics in the blood [166, 167]. Accordingly, the uptake of anesthetics by blood and tissues in neonates is relatively small leaving the partial pressure in the FRC to increase unabated.

To understand the washin of inhalational anesthetics, it is useful to consider a model such as a reservoir (a sink) to represent the FRC, with water flowing into the sink analogous to alveolar ventilation bringing the anesthetic gases into the FRC. For simplicity, the outlet from the reservoir is plugged in this model. The rate of rise of the level (e.g., washing of anesthetic) follows an exponential curve, the variables of which are determined by the volume of the reservoir and the flow into the reservoir. The equation that describes such a washin is a simple, first-order exponential equation:

$$C / C_0 = 1 - e^{-kt}, \quad \text{where } k \text{ is } 1/\tau, \tag{3.1}$$

where τ is the time constant defined by Eq. (3.2):

$$\tau(\text{min}) = \frac{\text{volume of functional residual capacity (L)}}{\text{alveolar ventilation (L / min)}}. \tag{3.2}$$

Four time constants are required to achieve 98 % equilibration of anesthetic partial pressures in the reservoir. Hence, with an FRC of 0.5 L and an alveolar ventilation of 1 L/min, τ is 0.5 and the time to reach 98 % equilibration of inspired, and alveolar anesthetic partial pressure is 2 min.

Similarly, the increase in anesthetic partial pressure in tissues is determined by a simple first-order exponential curve dependent on the delivery of anesthetic to the tissues (tissue blood flow) and the capacity of the tissues for anesthetic to reach partial pressure equilibration (the product of the volume of the tissue and the solubility of anesthetic in the tissue). This is expressed by an equation similar to that of Eq. (3.2) as follows:

$$\tau_{\text{brain}} = \frac{\text{volume of the brain (mL)} \times \text{brain / blood solubility}}{\text{brain blood flow (mL / min)}}. \tag{3.3}$$

Understanding the washin of inhalational anesthetic into the brain is key to appreciating the pharmacokinetics of induction of anesthesia with an inhalational anesthetic. Assuming the blood flow to the brain is 50 mL/min/100 g of brain (and the brain density is 1 g/mL) and the brain/blood solubility for a particular inhalational anesthetic in an adult is 2.0, then the time constant is

$$\tau_{\text{brain}} = \frac{100 \text{ mL} \times 2}{50 \text{ mL / min}} = 4 \text{ min}.$$

Thus, the time to reach 98 % equilibration of anesthetic partial pressures is 16 min. If the brain/blood solubility were half, 1.0, as might be in the case of a neonate, then the time to 98 % equilibration would decrease by 50 % to 8 min, resulting in a more rapid onset of anesthesia in the neonate and cardiorespiratory sequelae.

The washin curves for the commonly used inhalational anesthetics have been reported for adults [168]. The alveolar to inspired concentrations for halothane reach 0.35 in the first minute of the start of anesthesia, independent of how aggressive the alveolar ventilation (see Fig. 3.11). In the neonate, the washin of halothane in the first minute is probably closer to 0.5, based on the more rapid washin of halothane in neonates [26]. With a maximum inspired concentration for halothane of 5 % and a MAC in neonates of 0.87 %, the alveolar partial pressure would be 5×0.5/0.87 or

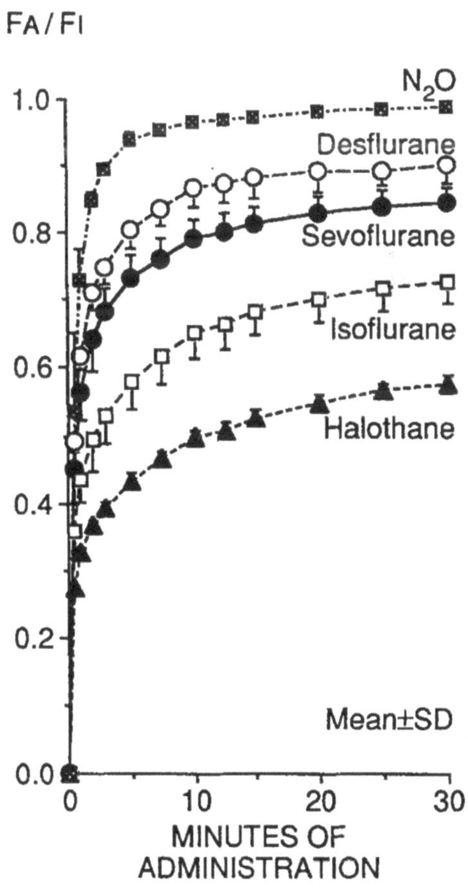

Fig. 3.11 Washin of N_2O, desflurane, sevoflurane, isoflurane and halothane in adults. The order of washin parallels the solubility of these agents in blood (reproduced with permission from Yasuda N, et al. [168])

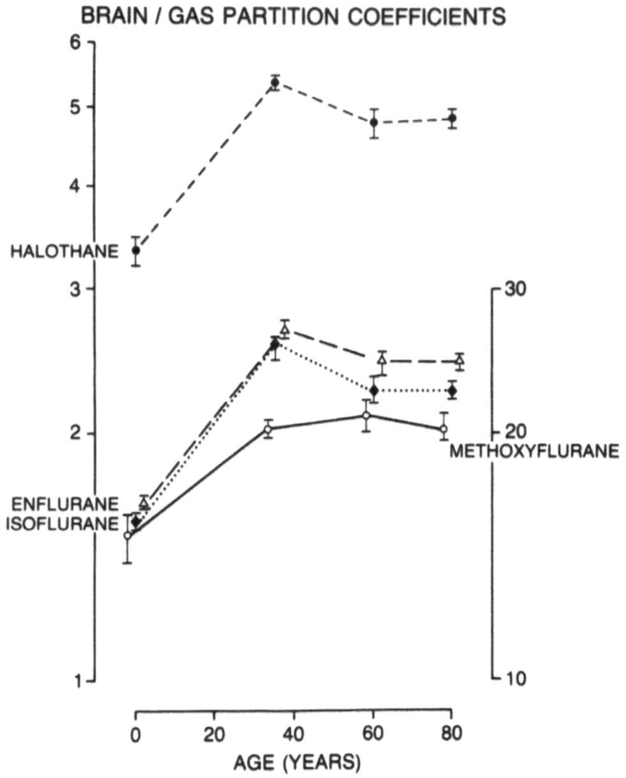

Fig. 3.12 Effect of age on the solubility of isoflurane, enflurane, halothane and methoxyflurane in the human brain. The solubilities of all anesthetics in the neonatal brain are less than those in older adults (reproduced with permission, Lerman J, et al. [169])

2.9 × MAC. If sevoflurane were substituted for halothane, then the washin in the first minute would be ~0.5 for both adults and neonates (as sevoflurane is an insoluble anesthetic). With an inspired concentration of 8 % and a MAC of 3.3 %, the alveolar partial pressure would be 8 × 0.5/3.3 or 1.2 × MAC, which is less than one-half that with halothane. Thus, sevoflurane is less likely to cause hemodynamic depression in the neonate in the early period of anesthesia as would halothane, but obversely, sevoflurane does not achieve as deep a level of anesthesia as halothane in the first minute.

The rate of increase of alveolar to inspired partial pressures of inhalational anesthetics varies inversely with the solubility in blood as follows: nitrous oxide > desflurane > sevoflurane > isoflurane > enflurane > halothane > methoxyflurane (Fig. 3.11) [168]. After a stepwise change in the inspired partial pressure of less soluble anesthetics, the alveolar partial pressure equilibrates very rapidly with the new inspired partial pressure. Since the washout of these anesthetics is equally rapid (see below), the inspired partial pressure can be returned to its initial value rapidly by decreasing the inspired partial pressure. Thus, anesthetic depth can be controlled more rapidly with the less soluble than with the more soluble inhalational anesthetics.

The solubilities of the inhalational anesthetics in the vessel-rich tissues in neonates are approximately one-half that in adults (Fig. 3.12) [169]. These reduced tissue solubilities for halothane, isoflurane, enflurane, and methoxyflurane are attributable to two differences in the composition of tissues in neonates compared with those in adults: (1) greater water content and (2) decreased protein and lipid concentrations. The reduced tissue solubilities decrease the time for partial pressure equilibration of anesthetics in tissues (see time constant for tissues, above). Although the partial pressures of inhalational agents in tissues cannot easily be measured in vivo, they may be estimated by measuring the anesthetic partial pressure in the exhaled or alveolar gases. Thus, the reduced tissue solubilities of inhalational anesthetics speed the washin of anesthetic partial pressures in neonates compared with adults.

The pharmacokinetics of inhalational anesthetics during the first 15–20 min depends primarily on the characteristics of the vessel-rich group, whereas the pharmacokinetics during the subsequent 20–200 min depends on the characteristics of the muscle group [164]. The solubility of inhalational anesthetics in the skeletal muscle varies directly with age in a logarithmic relationship [169]. This effect of age on the solubility of anesthetics in muscle has been attributed to age-dependent increases in protein concentration in the first five decades of life and in fat content in the subsequent three decades of life [169]. Since the muscle mass in the neonate is small, this effect is attenuated.

The net effect of these differences between neonates and adults is to speed the equilibration of anesthetic partial pressures in alveoli and tissues and thereby speed the rate of equilibration of alveolar to inspired anesthetic partial pressures of soluble anesthetics in neonates compared with adults [26, 163]. However, the difference in the rate of washin of less soluble anesthetics between neonates and adults may be less pronounced than that of more soluble anesthetics.

Ventilation

Changes in alveolar ventilation directly affect the washin of inhalational anesthetics: as alveolar ventilation increases, the washin of the anesthetics increases (Fig. 3.13) [164]. Ventilation is the primary determinant of the delivery of anesthetics to the lungs to effect the washin of the anesthetics. The effect of ventilation on the washin is more pronounced with more soluble anesthetics, e.g., halothane, and less pronounced or limited with less soluble anesthetics, sevoflurane and desflurane. The reason for the differential effect of ventilation rests with the dependency of the anesthetic on its speed of delivery to achieve partial pressure equilibration. Those anesthetics that are more soluble in blood (and tissues) are taken up more rapidly by blood (and tissues), thus slowing their washin. Conversely, those that are less soluble in blood are taken up very little by blood, facilitating a more rapid washin.

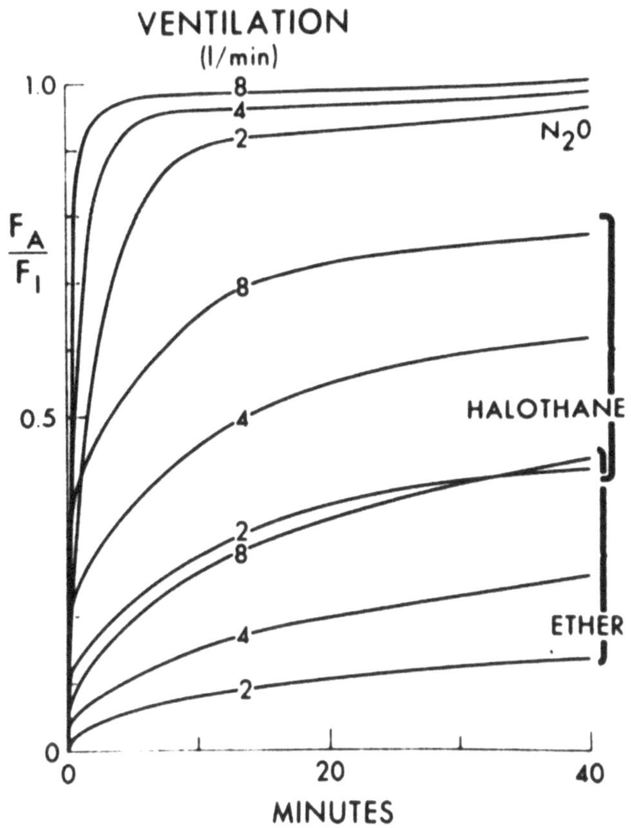

Fig. 3.13 Effect of alveolar ventilation on the washin of soluble (ether), intermediate (halothane), and insoluble (N_2O) anesthetics. Changes in ventilation affect the washin of more soluble than less soluble anesthetics (reproduced with permission, Eger EI 2nd. Anesthetic uptake and action. Baltimore: Williams & Wilkins; 1974) [164]

Cardiac Output

Changes in cardiac output inversely affect the washin of inhalational anesthetics compared with ventilation: the greater the cardiac output through the lungs, the more rapidly anesthetic is removed from the lungs and the slower the washin of anesthetic into the alveoli [164]. In the neonate, the effect of cardiac output is paradoxical as the greater cardiac output actually speeds the washin since most of the cardiac output is directed to the VRG, which comprises 18 % of the cardiac output, that speeds the equilibration of alveolar to inspired anesthetic partial pressure.

Induction

The more rapid washin of insoluble versus soluble anesthetics is generally believed to parallel a more rapid induction of anesthesia with the former, although this notion is probably untrue. Whereas the washin is determined by the pharmacokinetics of the agents, the speed of induction of anesthesia depends upon both pharmacokinetic and pharmacodynamic factors including: (1) the rate of equilibration of anesthetic partial pressures (determined by the four factors in Table 3.2), (2) the maximum inspired concentration, (3) airway irritability and (4) the MAC value. It is the interaction of these four factors that determines the relative speed of induction of anesthesia.

The rate of washin of inhalational anesthetic into the lungs varies inversely with the solubility of inhalational anesthetics in the blood (N_2O > desflurane > sevoflurane > isoflurane > halothane > methoxyflurane) [168]. Only two of these anesthetics are truly devoid of airway irritability when delivered by mask, sevoflurane and halothane. Although less soluble anesthetics washin to the FRC more rapidly than more soluble anesthetics, this more rapid washin is offset by the maximum inspired concentration (overpressure technique) and their greater MAC (Table 3.1). Using Fig. 3.11, we can explain why neonates may appear to be unconscious early in the induction but still respond to painful stimuli as we frequently experience. See below for full discussion.

Control of Anesthetic Depth

Two feedback mechanisms modulate the depth of anesthesia during inhalational anesthesia: respiratory and cardiovascular. During spontaneous ventilation, respiratory depression limits the depth of anesthesia. As the depth of anesthesia increases, alveolar ventilation decreases, the neonate arouses from anesthesia as the anesthetics are redistributed away from the VRG, and spontaneous ventilation increases. This is a *negative feedback* effect [170]. This protective mechanism permits the use of inspired concentrations of inhalational anesthetics severalfold greater than MAC (overpressure technique) while protecting against excessive circulatory depression. However, if ventilation is controlled, this protective mechanism is bypassed. The alveolar to inspired anesthetic partial pressure ratio increases relentlessly as cardiac output decreases. This decrease in cardiac output limits its removal of anesthetic from the lung leading to a further increase in the alveolar partial pressure of anesthetic. This is a *positive feedback* effect [170]. In such a circumstance, this leads to a downward spiral that might profoundly depress the cardiovascular system and lead to death if the cycle is not interrupted. In dogs breathing spontaneously, concentrations of halothane up to 6 % are tolerated without cardiovascular collapse because the negative feedback mechanism of respiratory depression prevents excessive concentrations within the lungs, whereas if ventilation were controlled, concentrations of halothane ≥4 % will profoundly depress the cardiovascular system and lead to death [170]. Large concentrations of inhalational anesthetics (overpressure technique) are commonly administered during inhalational inductions either as stepwise increases in concentration or as a single-breath large concentration. These large concentrations can be tolerated providing spontaneous ventilation is maintained. If, however, the pattern of ventilation changes from spontaneous to controlled, then circulatory collapse may occur.

This holds particular relevance for neonates. When halothane was administered to neonates, hypotension (and bradycardia) occurred; however, when sevoflurane was introduced, a similar response was not observed, despite the more rapid washin of this new insoluble anesthetic. The reason rests more with the deliverable MAC values for each agent rather than the pharmacokinetics. With a maximum deliverable inspired concentration of 5 % halothane and a MAC in neonates of 0.87 %, 5.7 inspired MAC multiples could be delivered. However, with a maximum deliverable inspired concentration of 8 % sevoflurane and a MAC in neonates of 3.3 %, only 2.4 inspired MAC multiples, less than half that deliverable by halothane, can be delivered to the neonate. These calculations demonstrate the greater safety associated with the use of sevoflurane in neonates compared with halothane.

Shunts

Shunts exist in two forms: left to right or right to left. Left-to-right shunts refer to conditions in which blood recirculates through the lungs (usually an intracardiac defect such as a ventricular septal defect). Right-to-left shunts refer to conditions in which venous blood returning to the heart bypasses the lungs (as in an intracardiac (cyanotic heart defect) or intrapulmonary (pneumonia or an endobronchial intubation) defect). The effects of shunts on the rate of equilibration of alveolar to inspired anesthetic partial pressures are poorly understood. In general, left-to-right shunts do not significantly affect the pharmacokinetics of potent inhalational agents, provided cardiac output remains unchanged. In contrast, right-to-left shunts can significantly delay the washin of inhalational anesthetics [171]. The magnitude of the delay with a right-to-left shunt depends on the solubility of the anesthetic: the less soluble the anesthetic (nitrous oxide, desflurane and sevoflurane), the more delayed the washin compared with that of the more soluble anesthetics. These effects are independent of the anatomical level of right-to-left shunts: intracardiac or intrapulmonary (as in the case of an endobronchial intubation).

To understand why right-to-left shunts affect the pharmacokinetics of inhalational anesthetics and less soluble anesthetics in particular, it is useful to consider a simplified model of the lung in which each lung is represented by one alveolus and each lung is perfused by one pulmonary artery (Fig. 3.14) [27]. When the tracheal tube is positioned with its tip at the mid-trachea level (Fig. 3.14a), ventilation is divided equally between both lungs, thereby yielding equal anesthetic partial pressures in both pulmonary veins ($P_V = 1$). However, if the tip of the tube is advanced into the right bronchus (Fig. 3.14b), all of the ventilation is delivered to one lung, that is, the ventilation to that lung is doubled,

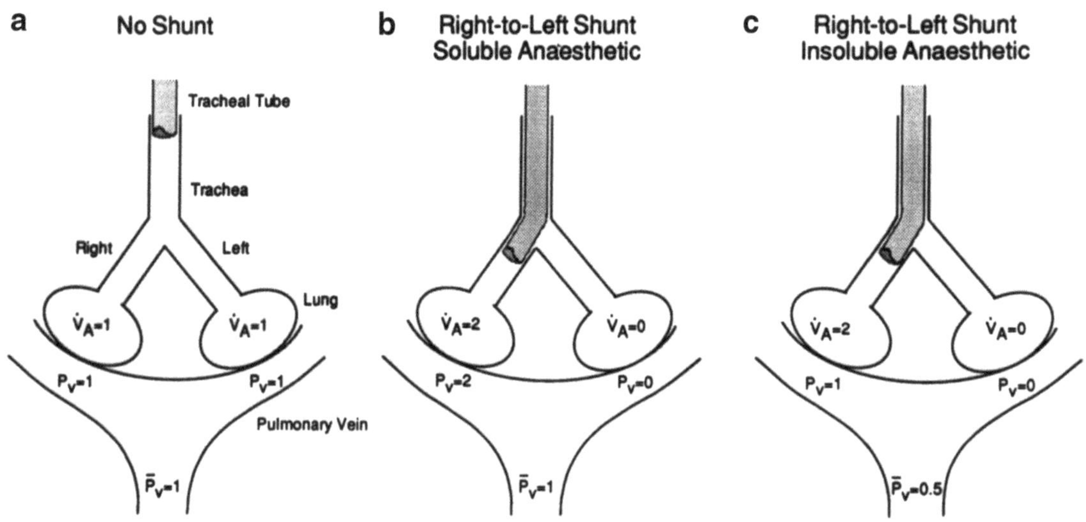

Fig. 3.14 Effect of shunt on the washin of anesthetic partial pressure in blood. (**a**) illustrates the normal washin with no shunt, equal ventilation to both lungs and normocapnia. (**b**) illustrates the effect of a right-to-left shunt (via an endobronchial intubation) on the washin of a soluble anesthetic. Normocapnia is maintained and hypoxic pulmonary vasoconstriction is negligible. The doubled ventilation to the intubated lung offsets the effect of the shunt. The washin is similar to (**a**). However, (**c**) illustrates the dramatic effect of a right-to-left shunt on the washin with a less soluble anesthetic. Since the increased alveolar ventilation to the intubated lung does not substantively affect the washin to the lung, when the blood from the ventilated lung combines with that from the shunted lung, the net effect is a slower washin of anesthetic (with permission, Lerman J. [27])

whereas ventilation to the non-ventilated lung is zero. Under these conditions, the partial pressure of CO_2 remains unchanged. When a soluble anesthetic is administered as in the case of Fig. 3.14b, the partial pressure of anesthetic in the combined pulmonary veins is approximately the same as in the presence of a tracheal intubation. The similar anesthetic partial pressure occurs because the increased ventilation to the ventilated lung compensates to a large extent for the shunt and speeds the increase in alveolar to inspired anesthetic partial pressures. However, when a less soluble anesthetic is administered in the presence of a right-to-left shunt, the effects on the washin of the inhalational agent are quite different. In this case, the increase in ventilation to the ventilated lung minimally increases the washin of the anesthetic (Fig. 3.14c) because changes in ventilation do not substantively affect the washin of insoluble anesthetics (Fig. 3.13). As a consequence, minimal increase in washin to the ventilated lung cannot offset the effects of the shunt. The anesthetic partial pressure in the combined pulmonary vein thus lags behind the partial pressure in the veins when both lungs are ventilated. Induction of anesthesia with a less soluble anesthetic is thereby slower in the presence of a right-to-left shunt than in the absence of a shunt. The less soluble anesthetics, desflurane and sevoflurane, are two such anesthetics whose washin characteristics may be significantly compromised in the presence of a right-to-left shunt.

The washin of halothane was recently evaluated in children with fenestrated Fontan before and after closure of the fenestration [171]. The authors noted that before the fenestration was closed (right-to-left shunt open), the washin of halothane as determined by the increase in arterial to inspired partial pressures was delayed compared with that after the fenestration was closed. Closure of the fenestration increased the pulmonary to systemic blood flow ratio from 0.58 to 0.88. Importantly, they noted that the increase in the end-tidal partial pressure of halothane did not parallel the arterial partial pressure. This observation is consistent with published evidence that the correlation between the end-tidal and arterial partial pressures of a gas (carbon dioxide) in children with cyanotic heart disease is poor [172].

Metabolism

The metabolism of inhalational anesthetics is discussed below under Renal and Hepatic Effects.

Emergence

The washout of inhalational agents follows an exponential decay (the inverse of the washin curve) [168]. The order of the washout of the anesthetics parallels their blood/gas solubilities, that is, the anesthetic that is washed out first, desflurane, is the least soluble in blood [168]. The order of washout in children is expected to be similar to that in adults.

Recovery of motor function in rats parallels the washout of inhalational anesthetics from fastest to slowest: desflurane < sevoflurane < isoflurane < halothane [173]. Notably, the rate of recovery increases in parallel with the duration of anesthesia [173]. In studies in which the recovery from two or more inhalational agents was compared, the end-tidal concentrations of the anesthetics were maintained at approximately 1 MAC until the conclusion of surgery, after which the anesthetics were abruptly discontinued [174–176]. In this paradigm, it is not surprising to find that the rates of recovery paralleled the rates of washout, which in turn paralleled the solubilities of the inhalational agents. In clinical practice however, anesthetic concentrations are gradually tapered as the end of surgery approached. This practice may attenuate the differences in the rates of recovery among inhalational agents reported previously.

In neonates, recovery after inhalational anesthesia is somewhat slower than that predicted solely by the washout curves. In part, this area of investigation has been hampered by a lack of consensus on the essential factors associated with emergence in the neonate [177]. Many anesthesiologists have struggled to explain why neonates recover at a slower rate than expected after a brief anesthetic with only inhalational anesthesia. No clear answers to explain this curiosity have been forthcoming.

Pharmacodynamics

In 1969, the MAC of halothane was noted to increase as age decreased [178]. The MAC of halothane reached its maximum value (1.1 %) in the youngest age group, which included 2 neonates and 4 infants 1–6 months of age. Based on this MAC measurement, one study cautioned against the use of halothane in neonates because it caused more hypotension than it did in older infants [179]. We postulated at the time that neonates were more sensitive to the myocardial depressant effects of halothane than children. Subsequently, when we determined the MAC of halothane in neonates as a group distinct from older infants 1–6 months of age, the MAC in the former group, 0.87 SD 0.1 %, was 15–25 % less than that in the latter, 1.2 % [94]. Furthermore, when 1 MAC of inhalational anesthetics was administered, the systolic blood pressure and heart rate responses in neonates were similar to those in older infants [94, 180, 181]. The MAC values in full-term neonates for the inhalational anesthetics in use today are 1.60 SD 0.01 % for isoflurane [182], 9.0 SD % for desflurane [180] and 3.3 SD 0.2 % for sevoflurane [181]. In addition, there is evidence that the primary cause of the increased sensitivity of neonates to cardiodepression by inhalational anesthetics may also be explained by immaturity of the cardiovascular system [183]. Using echocardiography, the cardiodepressant effects of halothane and isoflurane in concentrations up to 1.5 MAC in neonates were noted to be greater than in older infants [184]. The increased susceptibility of neonates to the depressant effects of inhalational anesthetics has been attributed, in part, to a decrease in myocardial contractile elements, a decrease in calcium sensitivity of myocardial fibers [183] and an incomplete sympathetic innervation of the heart and vascular system. Evidence also indicates that both pressor and depressor baroresponses are depressed in the presence of isoflurane in the preterm and full-term neonate [185]. These data suggest that the magnitude of the cardiovascular depression by inhalational anesthetics at 1 MAC in neonates is similar to that reported in older infants and that at concentrations in excess of 1 MAC, it may be greater than in older infants.

In order to attenuate the cardiodepressant effects of inhalational anesthetics in neonates, heart rate should be maintained and preload optimized. Neonatal myocardium evolves during the first month after birth, improving in compliance [186]. Because neonates depend on a rapid heart rate to maintain cardiac output, cardiovascular depression, particularly in the presence of halothane, can be reversed or offset in part by intravenous atropine (0.02 mg/kg) [184, 187]. To optimize preload, balanced salt solution or albumen, in a volume of 5–20 mL/kg, should be administered before anesthesia is induced [93, 184]. Neonates who have had cardiorespiratory dysfunction in the presurgical period or were managed in the neonatal intensive care unit often present to the operating room relatively dehydrated because of aggressive diuretic therapy and/or third-space fluid losses. After rehydration but in the absence of chronotropic agents, systolic arterial pressure decreases ≈ 20–25 % at 1 MAC halothane, desflurane, and sevoflurane compared with awake values in neonates, with either no changes or minimal decreases in heart rate [94, 180, 181]. Similar responses have been reported with 1 MAC of these anesthetics in infants 1–6 months of age.

Curiously, the MAC values for sevoflurane in neonates and infants 1–6 months of age are similar 3.3 and 3.2 %, respectively [181]. It remains unclear why the relationship between the MAC of sevoflurane and age in childhood differs from that for the other inhalational anesthetics. Whether the conformational structure of sevoflurane, a methyl isopropyl ether, or some other physicochemical characteristic is responsible for this unique relationship between MAC of sevoflurane and age is unclear.

The MAC of isoflurane decreases steadily in neonates as gestational age decreases to 24 weeks (Fig. 3.8) [93]. Not only did this study characterize the relationship between the MAC for isoflurane in preterm neonates and age, but it also confirmed the notion that neonates as young as 24 weeks' gestation respond to noxious stimuli in a predictable manner. Although several explanations have been posited to explain the age-dependent change in MAC in the perinatal period including residual effects of placentally transmitted female hormones, central nervous system substance P and maturation of central nervous system, the cause remains speculative.

Several factors moderate the MAC of inhalational anesthetics in infants and children. The MAC of halothane in children with cerebral palsy and severe mental retardation is approximately 25 % less than that in children without disabilities [188].

Whether these same relationships hold true in neonates has not been established. Acute administration of barbiturates and benzodiazepines decreases MAC [189, 190]; chronic administration of similar medications (such as in the case of children who have been treated with anticonvulsants) does not appear to affect MAC [191]. The effects of specific anticonvulsants such as valproic acid and phenytoin on the MAC of inhalational agents require clarification. Adults who are homozygote for melano-cortin for desflurane require ~20 % more anesthetic (6.2 % vs 5.2 %) than for brunettes [192].

The additivity of MAC fractions of inhalational agents (as well as nitrous oxide) is well established. However, the concept of additivity in children does not hold true for all inhalational agents: the additive contribution for nitrous oxide holds true for the MAC of halothane and isoflurane [193, 194] but not for the MAC of sevoflurane and desflurane [180, 181, 195] children 1–3 years, only 24 %, and that of desflurane only 22 %. Whether the same holds true in neonates is unknown. Additional evidence from the MAC response to tracheal intubation supports this attenuated effect of nitrous oxide on the MAC of sevoflurane in children [196]. This differential effect of nitrous oxide on the MAC values of inhalational agents in children and of its effect on the MAC of sevoflurane and desflurane between children and adults have not been explained.

Nitrous oxide is commonly used to supplement general anesthesia. However, nitrous oxide is infrequently used in neonates, particularly preterm neonates, who require emergency surgery and who are at risk of pulmonary or retinal complications from high oxygen tensions. The avoidance of nitrous oxide in neonates who have bowel obstruction or gas-filled closed spaces is well accepted [197]. However, its avoidance in neonates who are at risk of oxygen toxicity is less clear. It has been recommended that the PaO_2 be limited to a maximum value of 80 mm Hg (that is, an SaO_2 of 93 %) to prevent the effects of oxygen toxicity. This value lies at the shoulder of the steep descending portion of the oxyhemoglobin dissociation curve. If nitrous oxide were used to maintain the arterial oxygen tension below this value, then any minor difficulty with the airway could lead to a rapid hemoglobin oxygen desaturation. This potential problem would be mitigated if nitrogen were used instead of nitrous oxide, since the former is 34 times less soluble in blood than the latter.

In these circumstances nitrous oxide should be avoided and replaced with an air/oxygen mixture.

The MAC responses to stimuli other than skin incision, i.e., tracheal intubation, LMA insertion, extubation and return of wakefulness (MAC awake), have also been determined in children, although their applicability to neonates has not been established [198]. The MAC response to tracheal intubation is 10–50 % greater than the MAC for skin incision for halothane [199, 200], enflurane [201], and sevoflurane [196, 202, 203], whereas the MAC for tracheal extubation is approximately 10–25 % less than the MAC for isoflurane [204], desflurane [205 and sevoflurane [206, 207]. The MAC response to tracheal intubation during sevoflurane anesthesia in children is attenuated in the presence of adjuvants such as clonidine [203]. None of these effects have been validated in neonates.

Central Nervous System

For the past decade, the anesthesia literature has been dominated and preoccupied with the effects of anesthesia on neuroapoptosis in the neonatal brain. Neuroapoptosis is discussed further in Chaps. 4 (Anesthetic techniques for Neonatal Anesthesia) and 15 (Anesthetic Complications in the Neonate) and will not be repeated here.

Although cerebral blood flow (CBF) is autoregulated, there are limits in mean blood pressures beyond which CBF is pressure passive. Evidence suggests that neurological sequelae are increasingly likely when the CBF decreases below 20mL/kg/min. However, there is a dearth of evidence to support this notion in neonates and during general anesthesia [208].

CBF to the cortex is 3–4-fold greater than to white matter, in part, explaining the increasing vulnerability to periventricular leukomalacia in the perinatal period.

All potent inhalational agents depress the central nervous system with dose-dependent decreases in the cerebral vascular resistance and the cerebral metabolic rate for oxygen. The decrease in vascular resistance causes a reciprocal increase in CBF that starts at 0.6 MAC [209]. The extent of the increase in CBF, however, depends on the inhalational agent: halothane > enflurane > isoflurane [209]. The effects of sevoflurane on CBF are similar to those of isoflurane; however, the effects of desflurane differ substantively. Desflurane blunts the cerebral autoregulatory response [210, 211]. The net effect of inhalational agents is an increase in the ratio of the cerebral blood flow to metabolic rate, with desflurane increasing the ratio the greatest.

The effects of inhalational agents on the central nervous system in neonates and children have not been fully elucidated. Preliminary data suggest that cerebral blood flow velocity in children varies directly with the end-tidal carbon dioxide partial pressure during halothane anesthesia [212]. Cerebral blood flow velocity increases as the concentration of halothane increases [213], but does not change significantly in the presence of increasing concentrations of isoflurane.

The EEG activity of desflurane and sevoflurane is similar to that of isoflurane [214, 215]. The electroencephalographic (EEG) activity during halothane anesthesia differs substantially from that during sevoflurane anesthesia [216]. In the case of halothane, the EEG is characterized by slow waves superimposed on fast rhythms (α and β waves), whereas in the case of sevoflurane, the EEG is characterized by mainly sharp slow waves. Furthermore, the shift of power of the EEG from low (1–4 Hz) to medium frequencies (8–30 Hz) is greater for halothane than it is for sevoflurane. The unique EEG tracing in the neonate evolves rapidly in the first few months after birth [217]. During the neonatal period, up to 2 % sevoflurane exerts limited effects on the EEG; however, by 3–5 months of postnatal age, the EEG is responsive to increasing sevoflurane concentrations. The clinical relevance of these EEG differences remains unclear at this time, although the BIS responses, which are derived from the EEG, to sevoflurane differ substantively from those of halothane [105, 218]. Since brain monitors are not used in neonates, this issue is moot.

In children who are anesthetized with sevoflurane, both epileptiform activity in the form of myoclonic movement of the extremities and transient spike and wave complexes on EEG have been reported [219–222].

In two children with histories of epilepsy, diffuse spike and wave complexes were noted on EEG at 5 and 7 % inspired concentrations [220]. In a third child without a history of seizures, a 30-s burst of spike and wave complexes was recorded during sevoflurane anesthesia for spinal surgery but recognized only after the event resolved [222]. None of these three children exhibited clinical evidence of seizure activity. To determine whether these involuntary movements could have as their origin a cortical focus, the EEG was analyzed for evidence of seizure activity in children who had been anesthetized with either halothane or sevoflurane [216]. None of the children displayed either clinical or EEG evidence of seizure activity. The EEG patterns for both halothane and sevoflurane were characteristic even though all of the children had been premedicated with midazolam. The association between myoclonic movement and seizures during sevoflurane anesthesia remains tenuous [223]. A single case of a seizure has been reported in a neonate after sevoflurane anesthesia [224]. However, 3–5 % of children experience at least 1 seizure in childhood, with the greatest incidence occurring in infants <1 year of age [225, 226]. Since epileptiform activity does not portend frank seizures, its clinical relevance during sevoflurane is unknown. Recognizing that idiopathic seizures occur far more frequently than seizures resulting from sevoflurane, the source for such seizures should be sought beyond sevoflurane.

Cardiovascular System

Inhalational agents affect the cardiovascular system either directly (by depressing myocardial contractility or the conduction system or by dilating the peripheral vasculature) or indirectly (by affecting the balance of parasympathetic and sympathetic nervous systems and neurohumoral, renal or reflex responses). The cardiovascular responses to inhalational agents in children are further complicated by maturational changes in the cardiovascular system and its responsiveness to these anesthetics [183, 186]. This is particularly a concern in neonates, although few studies have specifically addressed myocardial contractility in the neonate.

Assessment of cardiovascular variables in infants and children presents a challenge for clinicians. Blood pressure may be measured either invasively (arterial line) or noninvasively. Electrocardiography is routinely used in all age groups to detect arrhythmias. In contrast to blood pressure and electrocardiography, measurement of cardiac output and myocardial contractility is much more difficult to quantify in this age group. Two-dimensional echocardiography and impedance cardiometry have been used to estimate cardiac output and myocardial contractility in infants and children [184, 227–229], although the echocardiographic measurements are subject to variability depending on the preload and afterload. Load-independent derived echocardiographic variables (stress-velocity and stress-shortening indices) have since improved the accuracy of echocardiographic estimates of myocardial function and are used with increasing frequency [230].

In neonates, several factors affect the blood pressure responses to inhalational agents including the particular inhalational anesthetic, the dose, the preload status of the infant, the presence of coexisting diseases and the techniques used to measure the systemic pressure (invasive vs noninvasive) and cardiac function (echocardiography). Most studies demonstrated modest, dose-dependent decreases in blood pressure with all of the inhalational agents. At ~1 MAC, systolic blood pressure decreased ~24 % with halothane, 30 % with sevoflurane and 34 % with desflurane [94, 180, 181]. Systolic pressures may further decrease with concentrations up to 1.5 MAC. Few data exist regarding the hemodynamic responses beyond 1.5 MAC. On balance, all of the inhalational agents (in concentrations up to 1.5 MAC) modestly depress the systemic blood pressure with increasing dose.

The effects of inhalational anesthetics on myocardial contractility and cardiac output in the neonate are incompletely understood. Cardiac output in neonates decreases at 1.0 and 1.5 MAC halothane and isoflurane similarly [184]. Knowing the limited effects of sevoflurane and desflurane on myocardial contractility, one might expect that these anesthetics decrease cardiac output and myocardial contractility at 1 and 1.5 MAC less than halothane [231]. The effects of large concentrations of sevoflurane and desflurane on cardiac function in neonates have been difficult given very large MAC values in this age group. Intravenous atropine and a bolus of balanced salt solution restore, in part, the depressed circulation in neonates [187, 232, 233].

The mechanism by which inhalational agents depress myocardial function remains controversial. Studies in both animal and human myocardial cells suggest that the potent inhalational agents, halothane, isoflurane and sevoflurane, directly depress myocardial contractility by decreasing intracellular Ca^{2+} flux. Inhalational agents decrease the Ca^{2+} flux by their action on the calcium channels themselves, the ion exchange pumps and the sarcoplasmic reticulum [183]. Inhalational agents may also attenuate contractility of ventricular myocytes via voltage-dependent L-type calcium channels (which are responsible for release of large amounts of calcium from the sarcoplasmic reticulum) [183, 186, 234, 235].

That neonates and infants are more sensitive to the depressant actions of inhalational agents than older children is supported by experimental evidence of maturational differences between neonatal and adult rat, rabbit, and feline myocardium [235–238]. Structural differences that may account, in part, for the changes in myocardial sensitivity to inhalational agents with age include a reduction in contractile elements, immature sarcoplasmic reticulum and functional differences in calcium sensitivity of the contractile elements, calcium channels and the sodium–calcium pump in the neonatal myocardium [183, 234–236, 238–241]. The determinants of Ca^{2+} homeostasis in ventricular myocardial cells in the neonate depend on trans-sarcolemma Ca^{2+} flux to a far greater extent than on the sarcoplasmic reticulum [183]. This is based upon a growing body of experimental evidence that includes the finding that the concentration of the Na^+–Ca^{2+} exchange protein in the neonatal myocardium, a protein that regulates trans-sarcolemma flux of Ca^{2+}, exceeds that in adult cells by 2.5-fold and that its concentration decreases with age as the concentration of voltage-dependent L-type calcium channel increases [236]. Furthermore, halothane reversibly inhibits the Na^+–Ca^{2+} exchange protein in immature myocardial cells [236]. The sarcoplasmic reticulum is poorly developed in neonatal myocardial cells, and this finding weighs heavily against the SR being the major source of Ca^{2+} required for myocardial contractility.

The baroreflex response is also depressed in neonates with both halothane [242] and isoflurane [185], albeit to a greater extent with the former than the latter. In view of the greater incidence of hypotension in neonates and infants than older children, an intact baroreflex could offset, in part, the cardiovascular consequences. However, inhalational agents blunt this response, leaving the infant vulnerable to the cardiovascular depressant actions of inhalational agents. Prophylactic anticholinergics and preload augmentation may attenuate the decrease in cardiac output in the presence of inhaled anesthetics.

Inhalational anesthetics vary in their effect on cardiac rhythm. Halothane may slow the heart rate, in some cases leading to junctional rhythms, bradycardia and asystole. These are dose-dependent responses. Three mechanisms have been proposed to explain the genesis of halothane-associated dysrhythmias: a direct effect on the sinoatrial node, a vagal effect, or an imbalance in the parasympathetic/sympathetic tone. It has also been suggested that the etiology of the bradycardia during halothane anesthesia may be a withdrawal of sympathetic tone. Bradycardia is particularly marked in the neonate, presumably because parasympathetic influences predominate over the sparse sympathetic innervation of the myocardium in this age group. Junctional rhythms are also common during halothane anesthesia. Atrial or ventricular ectopic beats are rare except in the presence of hyper- or hypocapnia. In infants anesthetized with halothane, 10 μg/kg atropine increases heart rate ≥50 % and promotes sinus rhythm [243]. This dose of atropine also increases blood pressure in infants ≥6 months of age and children.

Halothane also sensitizes the myocardium to catecholamines, particularly during hypercapnia. It decreases the threshold for ventricular extrasystoles during epinephrine administration by threefold [244–246]. In contrast, isoflurane, desflurane and sevoflurane maintain or increase heart rate during the early induction period of anesthesia [176, 180, 181, 227, 229, 231, 247–250]. When bradycardia occurs in an anesthetized neonate, the primary cause is always hypoxia, even during anesthesia, before other causes such as a direct drug effect are given serious consideration. The ether anesthetics, isoflurane, desflurane and sevoflurane, do not sensitize the myocardium to catecholamines to the same extent as halothane [244, 245, 251]. The mechanism by which the sinus node controls automaticity is incompletely understood but may include K currents, hyperpolarization-activated current and T and L forms of Ca^{2+} currents [183]. Moreover, developmental changes in these channels likely account, in part, for the differential effects of inhalational agents on heart rate with age [239].

Respiratory System

Inhalational agents significantly affect respiration in infants in a dose-dependent fashion via effects on the respiratory center, chest wall muscles, and reflex responses. Halothane depresses respiration by decreasing tidal volume and attenuating the response to carbon dioxide [252–254]. This depression is offset, in part, by an increase in the respiratory rate [253, 254]. These ventilatory responses to halothane are age dependent; minute ventilation in infants decreases to a greater extent than in children [255]. In infants and young children, intercostal muscle activity is inhibited at greater concentrations than the diaphragm [252, 256]. This effect is most pronounced in preterm and full-term neonates and infants and when an endotracheal tube is used in place of an LMA [257]. Isoflurane, enflurane, sevoflurane and desflurane depress the ventilatory drive and tidal volume and attenuate the respiratory responses to carbon dioxide [253, 254, 258–264]. The increase in respiratory frequency that follows respiratory depression may not restore minute ventilation to preanesthetic levels.

Sevoflurane depresses respiration to a similar extent as halothane up to 1.4 MAC, but depresses respiration to a greater extent than halothane at concentrations >1.4 MAC in adults [260]. Sevoflurane does not decrease the tone of the intercostal muscles to the same extent as halothane [256, 260]. The compensatory changes in respiratory rate differ among the anesthetics; respiratory rate increases at ≥1.4 MAC halothane, is unchanged with isoflurane but decreases at ≥1.4 MAC enflurane [253, 254]. When 8 % sevoflurane was compared with 5 % halothane, minute ventilation and tidal volume decreased and respiratory rate increased with both agents to similar extents [265].

Table 3.3 In vivo metabolism of inhalational agents

Inhalational agent	% Metabolized
Methoxyflurane	50 %
Halothane	20 %
Sevoflurane	5 %
Enflurane	2.4 %
Isoflurane	0.2 %
Desflurane	0.02 %

Renal

The potent inhalational agents may affect renal function via four possible mechanisms: cardiovascular, autonomic, neuroendocrine and metabolic. Although the first three mechanisms pose no direct threat to renal function, the fourth mechanism, metabolism, is a serious clinical concern that has resulted in renal dysfunction and death after some inhalational anesthetics.

Inhalational agents are metabolized in vivo to varying extents (Table 3.3). Halothane is the inhalational anesthetic still in use that is most metabolized, but releases very little fluoride in the inorganic form. Most of the fluoride that is liberated from the metabolism of halothane exists in an organic form, trifluoroacetate. This compound has been linked to halothane hepatitis (see below). Metabolism of inhalational agents by the CYP450 2E21 releases inorganic fluoride [266]. Sevoflurane releases the most fluoride, followed by isoflurane and desflurane based on the extent of metabolism (Table 3.3). Even after 131 MAC·h isoflurane, the cumulative inorganic fluoride concentration is small [267]. The metabolism of sevoflurane yields both an inorganic and organic fluoride moiety [268]. The organic form, hexafluoroisopropanol (HFIP), is rapidly conjugated and excreted by the kidneys [268]. It poses no serious threat to renal function in humans; however, inorganic fluoride that is released from these three ether anesthetics has garnered great interest in the relationship between inhalational anesthetics and renal function.

Peak plasma concentrations of inorganic fluoride after exposure to inhalational agents follow an order that is similar to that in Table 3.3: methoxyflurane > sevoflurane > enflurane > isoflurane > halothane ≈ desflurane [269–273]. In the case of methoxyflurane, two metabolites are produced: inorganic fluoride and oxalic acid. Both have been implicated in the pathogenesis of renal dysfunction although clinically, the renal injury was more consistent with the concentration of inorganic fluoride rather than oxalic acid [274, 275]. Subsequent studies demonstrated that >2.5 MAC·h methoxyflurane resulted in subclinical nephrotoxicity provided the plasma concentration of inorganic fluoride exceeded 50 μM and that >5 MAC·h resulted in frank nephrotoxicity if the concentrations exceeded 90 μM [275a]. These clinical concerns led to the voluntary withdrawal of methoxyflurane from clinical practice.

In contrast to the adult experience with methoxyflurane, renal dysfunction was not a feature after this anesthetic in children. The peak plasma concentrations of inorganic fluoride in children anesthetized with methoxyflurane were significantly less than that in adults after an equivalent anesthetic exposure [276]. The reduced plasma concentrations of fluoride in children were attributed to several possible factors including a decreased metabolism of methoxyflurane, a greater uptake of fluoride by bone, an increased excretion of fluoride ions or a reduced renal sensitivity to fluoride in children [276]. Another plausible explanation for the reduced plasma concentrations of inorganic fluoride in children may have been an immature CYP4502E1 isoenzyme system in the kidneys (see below).

That the plasma concentrations of inorganic fluoride in children who were anesthetized with sevoflurane were similar to or greater than those after enflurane raised concerns about possible renal dysfunction after prolonged exposure to sevoflurane [277–279]. Preliminary evidence suggested that inorganic fluoride should not be a serious clinical problem in children since the peak plasma concentrations of inorganic fluoride after sevoflurane anesthesia were similar to those in adults: <20 μM after ≈ 1 MAC•h, which decreased to <10 μM by 4 h after discontinuation of anesthesia [279].

However, peak plasma concentrations of inorganic fluoride paralleled the MAC·h exposure to sevoflurane in both children and adults [279]. Concerns regarding the risk of renal dysfunction after sevoflurane were heightened after reports that the peak plasma concentration of inorganic fluoride in some adults exceeded the purported threshold for nephrotoxicity (90 μM). Despite the large plasma concentrations of inorganic fluoride after sevoflurane anesthesia, there was no evidence of renal dysfunction.

To understand anesthetic-induced nephrotoxicity, it was suggested that the primary isoenzyme responsible for the degradation of enflurane, isoflurane, sevoflurane and methoxyflurane anesthetics was CYP450 2E1 [266, 280–282]; secondary isoenzymes implicated in renal defluorination include CYP450 2A6 and 3A [280]. Subsequently, large quantities of CYP450 2E1 were found not only within the liver (where degradation of ether inhalational agents yielded large plasma concentrations of inorganic fluoride) but also within the kidneys [86]. The affinity of renal CYP450 2E1 for methoxyflurane was found to be fivefold greater than that for sevoflurane [86]. This provided further evidence that the renal dysfunction after ether inhalational agents was likely due to the local production of inorganic fluoride within the renal medulla rather than excessive plasma concentrations of inorganic fluoride. Because CYP450 2E1 has a greater affinity for methoxyflurane than sevoflurane, this explains why renal dysfunction occurred after methoxyflurane and not sevoflurane and was independent of the circulating inorganic fluoride concentrations [86, 283]. Consequently, there is no restriction on the duration of sevoflurane exposure with respect to the risk of fluoride-induced renal dysfunction.

Sevoflurane may also indirectly affect renal function through by-products of its metabolism in the presence of carbon dioxide absorbents, soda lime. These by-products are five in number, but two are potentially nephrotoxic compounds, known as compounds A and B. Compound A is produced in concentrations that may achieve toxicity (at least in rats), whereas B achieves much smaller concentration. Compound A is nephrotoxic in rats, but has not been associated with nephrotoxicity in humans. It is the reason the fresh gas flow has been set to a minimum value of 2 L/min in the presence of sevoflurane in some countries (see below),, although this is a moot point if absorbents devoid of sodium hydroxide and potassium hydroxide (e.g., Amsorb®) are used (see below).

Hepatic

In vivo metabolism of inhalational agents varies with age; increasing within the first two years of life to reach adult values. The developmental changes in metabolism may be attributed to several factors including reduced activity of the hepatic microsomal enzymes, reduced fat stores, and more rapid elimination of inhalational agents in infants and children compared to adults. Halothane, isoflurane, enflurane, sevoflurane and desflurane have all been associated with postoperative liver dysfunction and/or failure [284–288]. Halothane and sevoflurane have also been associated with transient hepatic dysfunction in infants and children, but not in neonates [289–293, 749]. Several case reports of transient postoperative liver failure and one case of fulminant hepatic failure and death have been attributed to "halothane hepatitis" that was confirmed serologically with antibodies to halothane-altered hepatic cell membrane antigens in children [289]. The exact mechanism of the hepatic dysfunction after halothane remains unclear, although some have speculated that it is caused by an immunologic response to a metabolite of halothane. This putative toxic metabolite, a trifluoroacetyl halide compound, is produced during oxidative metabolism of halothane. It is believed that this compound induces an immunologic response in the liver by binding covalently to hepatic microsomal proteins thereby forming an immunologically active hapten. A subsequent exposure to the inhalational agent then incites an immunologic response in the liver [294]. Hepatic enzymes may also be induced by previous administration of drugs such as barbiturates, phenytoin and rifampin. Although some have admonished clinicians of the risks of repeat anesthetics with halothane in children, in view of the millions of uneventful repeat halothane anesthetics in infants and children worldwide, there is insufficient evidence at present to support such an admonition in this population.

Clinical Effects

Induction Techniques

Although the physicochemical characteristics of the ether series of anesthetics would predict that anesthesia could be induced smoothly and more rapidly with these agents than with halothane (Table 3.1) [165, 169], this has not proved to be the case. All of the methyl ethyl ether anesthetics irritate the upper airway in children resulting in a high incidence of breath-holding, coughing, salivation, excitement, laryngospasm and hemoglobin oxygen desaturation [175, 247, 295–300].

Consequently, most clinicians avoid inhalational inductions with these anesthetics.

In contrast to the irritant airway effects of the methyl ethyl ether anesthetics, the methyl isopropyl ether anesthetic, sevoflurane, is well tolerated when administered by mask to infants and children at any concentration [174, 176, 183, 301–311]. The incidences of coughing, breath-holding, laryngospasm, and hemoglobin oxygen desaturation during inhalational inductions with sevoflurane whether by slow incremental increases in concentration or a single breath are similar to those that occur during inductions with halothane. The observation that the airway reflex responses are infrequent after a single-breath induction with 8 % sevoflurane or 5 % halothane casts doubt on the adage that high concentrations of inhalational agents trigger airway reflex responses [306]. In fact, the induction is so smooth with sevoflurane even in neonates that dialling 8 % sevoflurane in one step is routine to achieve rapid induction of anesthesia in the neonate without triggering airway reflexes. By increasing the inspired concentration in one step, the period of excitement or agitation during induction is minimized.

Both intravenous and inhalational agents have been used for induction of anesthesia in neonates with congenital heart disease. Sevoflurane compares favorably with halothane for induction of anesthesia in such patients scheduled for cardiac surgery and may be preferred because it maintains cardiovascular stability to a greater extent than halothane, but similar to isoflurane [312–314].

Central Neuroexcitation

Paroxysmal increases in blood pressure (both systolic and diastolic pressures) and heart rate have been reported in adults after a rapid increase in the inspired concentration of isoflurane or desflurane [315–317]. Neuroexcitatory responses have not been reported in neonates with either of these agents nor have they been reported during sevoflurane or halothane anesthesia at any age [317]. This rapid increase in the inspired concentration of isoflurane or desflurane triggers a massive sympathetic response, mediated by norepinephrine and/or epinephrine, and results in tachycardia and hypertension [318, 319]. Further increases in the inspired concentration of the inciting agent, in an effort to control the tachycardia and hypertension, will not control these responses but will perpetuate or possibly augment the response. In order to restore normal vital signs, the inciting agent must be discontinued and replaced with another inhalational or intravenous agent. Repetitive small increases (1 %) in the inspired concentration of the putative agent produce transient but attenuated catecholamine bursts and cardiovascular responses compared with larger increases in concentration [320, 321]. Fentanyl (2 μg/kg), esmolol and clonidine have all been effective in preventing, attenuating or eliminating these sympathetic responses [322–324]. The site or sites responsible for triggering a neuroexcitatory response are unknown, although the rapidity of the response suggests that the lung is a primary site [325]. Others, however, dispute this notion contending that two sites must be responsible for triggering the sympathetic discharge, the lung and a vessel-rich organ [326]. Of these two sites, the vessel-rich organ, is believed to mediate the greater response [326].

Emergence

Emergence or recovery has been arbitrarily divided into early (extubation, eye opening following commands) and late (drinking, discharge time from recovery or hospital). Although most studies have demonstrated a more rapid early recovery after less soluble anesthetics [230, 301, 327–329], few have demonstrated a more rapid late recovery with these anesthetics than the more soluble anesthetics [174, 176, 330, 331]. Clinicians have been at a loss to explain why neonates/infants with pyloric stenosis recover slowly after a pure inhalational anesthetic. In theory, they should recover rapidly based on the rapid washout of the sevoflurane; however, this has not been our experience. Recovery only appears rapid if desflurane is used without opioids.

The speed of recovery from anesthesia should follow the order of washout of the inhalational agents: desflurane > sevoflurane > isoflurane > halothane > methoxyflurane [168].

Those agents with lower solubility in blood and tissues are eliminated more rapidly than those with greater solubility; the contribution of metabolism to recovery is minor because the relative rate of metabolism is small compared with the duration of exposure to anesthetics. Although some advocate switching inhalational agents from a more soluble to less soluble agent toward the end of surgery for economy and to facilitate a rapid emergence, the only evidence suggests that switching from isoflurane to desflurane 30 min before the end of anesthesia in adults does not speed emergence [332]. However, these results were based on specific set of clinical conditions in adults that may not be applicable to all conditions or to neonates.

The incidence of complications such as airway reflex responses and vomiting during emergence from anesthesia is similar with all inhalational agents [248, 296, 301, 303, 328–331, 333]. In the case of neonates, airway reflex responses are very common, whereas vomiting and emergence delirium after anesthesia are not.

Emergence Delirium

The introduction of the new inhalational agents, desflurane and sevoflurane, has rekindled interest in a clinical entity known as "emergence delirium". Emergence delirium is defined as a dissociated state of consciousness in which a child is inconsolable, irritable, uncompromising and/or uncooperative. The child is often demanding that all monitors and all bandages be removed and that they be dressed in their own clothing. Parents who witness this transient state, which lasts 10–20 min and occurs primarily in preschool age toddlers, usually volunteer that this behavior is unusual and uncustomary for their child. However, emergence delirium is rare and unreported in neonates. The incidence of emergence delirium after isoflurane, sevoflurane, and desflurane appears to be similar, but significantly greater than after halothanef [301, 328, 329, 331, 334–336]. The etiology of emergence delirium is unknown. Although pain was initially thought to be responsible for triggering this disorder, a report of a high incidence of delirium after sevoflurane anesthesia for MRI established that pain was not the primary causative agent of delirium after these newer anesthetics [337]. The diagnosis of delirium after inhalational anesthesia was bolstered by the introduction of the Pediatric Anesthesia Emergence Delirium (PAED) scale [338], although this scale has not been validated in neonates. Several preventative measures and interventions have been proposed for the child with delirium after anesthesia [339].

Neuromuscular Junction

Inhalational agents potentiate the actions of non-depolarizing muscle relaxants [340–342] and decrease neuromuscular transmission [343], the latter however only at large concentrations. The mechanism of the reduced neuromuscular transmission is unknown but may be arise from the depression of the central nervous system. The mechanism of the potentiation of non-depolarizing muscle relaxants by inhalational agents is also unknown but is likely attributable to actions of inhalational agents at the neuromuscular junction rather than pharmacokinetic or central nervous system effects. The potentiation of action of non-depolarizing relaxants follows the order: isoflurane ≈ desflurane ≈ sevoflurane > enflurane > halothane > nitrous oxide/narcotic technique [340, 344]. However, this potentiation may depend on the type of non-depolarizing relaxant studied (longer-acting relaxants are affected to a greater extent than intermediate-acting relaxants) [340, 341, 345] and the concentration of inhalational agent (smaller concentrations may not demonstrate any differences among inhalational agents, whereas greater concentrations may demonstrate differences) [341]. During 0.6 MAC isoflurane, it took 56 min after 0.45 mg/kg and 100 min after 0.6 mg/kg rocuronium to recover the first twitch to 75 % of baseline [346].

Malignant Hyperthermia

All inhalational anesthetics (except xenon) trigger MH reactions in susceptible patients [347–356]. To date, MH has not been reported in a neonate. Nonetheless, neonates with a family history of MH should be managed with standard MH precautions. For the management of MH-susceptible patients, the reader should refer to the MHAUS website (http://www.MHAUS.org) or the local national MH website.

Stability

Inhalational agents may be degraded via one of several pathways in the presence of most CO_2 absorbents to form several potentially toxic by-products. Enflurane, isoflurane and desflurane (but not halothane and sevoflurane) react with desiccated soda lime to produce carbon monoxide. Both halothane and sevoflurane may be degraded when incubated with some CO_2 absorbents, yielding compounds that are potentially organ toxic (see Canizarro reaction below) [357]. Two new absorbents may address these clinical risks: molecular sieves [358] and absorbents lacking sodium and potassium accelerants (e.g., Amsorb™) [359–361]. Amsorb™ absorbs CO_2 without releasing carbon monoxide or compound A [359, 360]. Carbon dioxide absorbents differ in their composition and, therefore, in their affinity to interact with inhaled agents. Soda lime contains 95 % calcium hydroxide, either sodium or potassium hydroxide, and the balance as water. Baralyme contains 80 % calcium hydroxide, 20 % barium hydroxide and the balance as water. Amsorb™ contains 70 % calcium hydroxide, 0.7 % calcium chloride, 0.7 % calcium sulfate, 0.7 % polyvinylpyrrolidone and the balance as water. Amsorb™ and other nonreactive absorbents contain neither sodium nor potassium hydroxide, compounds added to improve CO_2 absorption efficiency [360, 362].

Carbon monoxide may be released into the anesthetic breathing circuit when isoflurane or desflurane is incubated with a desiccated CO_2 absorbent. The absorbent within a CO_2 canister may become desiccated if dry fresh gas flows through the canister at a rate sufficient to remove most of the moisture (i.e., >5 L/min continuously through the absorbent canister for 24 h or greater while it is not in service). If the circuit reservoir bag is detached from the canister while fresh gas is flowing, then gas flows through the canister and exits through two sites: a smaller fraction of the fresh gas exits through the inspiratory limb of the canister and a larger fraction of gas flows retrograde through the canister and exits at the site where the reservoir bag should be attached. If the reservoir bag is attached to the canister, then less gas flows retrograde through the canister and the time to desiccate the absorbent is markedly prolonged. Once the absorbent becomes desiccated, carbon monoxide may be released into the inspiratory limb of the breathing circuit if one of the methyl ethyl ether inhalational agents (desflurane, isoflurane or enflurane) is administered [363–365]. The magnitude of the carbon monoxide production follows the order from greatest to least: desflurane ≥ enflurane > isoflurane >> halothane = sevoflurane. Other factors that determine the magnitude of the carbon monoxide concentration produced include the concentration of the inhalational agent, the dryness of the absorbent, the type of absorbent, and the temperature of the absorbent [363]. Currently, carbon monoxide is not detectable by most freestanding anesthetic agent analysers, pulse oximetry or blood/gas analysers (with the exception of co-oximeters), although it is detectable by mass spectrometry. The key to this problem is prevention: turn off the anesthetic machine at the end of the day, disconnect the fresh gas hose to the absorbent canister, leave the reservoir bag connected to the canister, and avoid contact between the desiccated absorbent and the three ether anesthetics, desflurane, enflurane and isoflurane. Others have suggested that high-flow anesthesia should be avoided whenever a circle circuit is used to prevent inadvertent desiccation of absorbent. If the absorbent is desiccated, then some recommend "rehydrating" the absorbent, although this too is fraught with potential problems (including clumping of the absorbent) [366]. If in fact, the absorbent is suspected of being desiccated, then the authors recommend replacing the absorbent before introducing an inhalational agent. Alternatives to conventional absorbents such as the molecular sieve and Amsorb™ may very well obviate all reactions that occur with current absorbents [359, 360]. When these same ether anesthetics are incubated with desiccated Amsorb™, carbon monoxide is not produced [359, 360]. The incidence of carbon monoxide poisoning during anesthesia remains an extremely rare complication when soda lime is used as the CO_2 absorbent. In contrast, the incidence of carbon monoxide poisoning is zero with Amsorb™.

Sevoflurane is both absorbed and degraded via the Cannizzaro reaction in the presence of absorbent resulting in five degradation products [367, 368]. Although the degradation of sevoflurane by the absorbent was initially posited to delay the washin of sevoflurane, recent evidence suggests that the quantity of sevoflurane degraded is of little clinical significance to the speed of washin of sevoflurane [369]. Of the five degradation products between sevoflurane and soda lime, compounds A and B appear in the greatest concentrations in the inspired limb of the breathing circuit. Compound A, fluoromethyl-2,2-difluoro-1-(trifluoromethyl) vinyl ether (also known as PIFE), is nephrotoxic in rats at concentrations ≥100 ppm and has an LC50 of 1100 ppm. Compound B, a methoxyethyl ether compound that is minimally volatile at room temperature, is present in closed circuits at <5 ppm and poses little risk to animals and humans. The remaining three metabolites, compounds C, D, and E, are present in such low concentrations in the breathing circuit that they do not merit further consideration. In a low-flow closed circuit model with an inspired concentration of 2.5 % sevoflurane, the concentration of compound A peaks at 20–40 ppm after several hours of anesthesia [369–373]. Studies are conflicting regarding the risks of using fresh gas flows <2 lpm with sevoflurane and in patients with pre-existing renal dysfunction [374]. In children, compound A concentrations are ≤16 ppm after 5.6 MAC·h sevoflurane in a closed circuit with 2 L/min fresh gas flow [375]. Factors that are known to increase the production of compound A include an increase in the inspired concentration of sevoflurane, Baralyme > soda lime and an increase in the temperature of the absorbent [367, 368].

Studies in rats indicate that under low-flow conditions, compound A is nephrotoxic [376–378].

In contrast, similar studies in humans have yielded inconsistent results [370–372, 379]. The mechanism behind compound A-induced nephrotoxicity is believed to be β-lyase-dependent metabolism to nephrotoxic fluorinated compounds, although this has been the subject of intense debate [283, 380, 381]. More recent evidence suggests that differences in the evidence of nephrotoxicity from compound A in rats and humans relate to differences in metabolic pathways between species [382, 383].

At the present time, sevoflurane is the only inhalational agent for which some federal authorities have recommended minimum fresh gas flow guidelines when it is administered in an anesthetic circuit with soda lime. The minimum fresh gas flow guideline of 2 L/min for >1 h of anesthesia is mandated in only five countries worldwide. The remaining countries where sevoflurane is used have no restriction on the minimum fresh gas flow that can be used in a closed circuit.

Analgesic Drugs

Acetaminophen (Paracetamol)

Mechanism of Action

Acetaminophen is widely used in the management of pain, but lacks anti-inflammatory effects. Acetaminophen has a central analgesic effect that is mediated through activation of descending serotonergic pathways. Prostaglandin H_2 synthetase (PGHS) is the enzyme responsible for metabolism of arachidonic acid to the unstable prostaglandin H_2. The two major forms of this enzyme are the constitutive PGHS-1 (COX-1) and the inducible PGHS-2 (COX-2). PGHS comprises two sites: a cyclooxygenase (COX) site and a peroxidise (POX) site. The conversion of arachidonic acid to PGG_2, the precursor of the prostaglandins (Fig. 3.15), depends on a tyrosine-385 radical at the COX site. Formation of a ferryl protoporphyrin IX radical cation from the reducing agent Fe^{3+} at the POX site is essential for the conversion of tyrosine 385 to its radical form. Acetaminophen acts as a reducing cosubstrate on the POX site and reduces the availability of the ferryl protoporphyrin IX radical cation (Fig. 3.16). This effect can be reduced by the presence of hydroperoxide-generating lipoxygenase enzymes within the cell (peroxide tone) or by swamping the POX site with substrate such as PGG_2. Peroxide tone and swamping explain acetaminophen's lack of peripheral analgesic effect, platelet effect and anti-inflammatory effects. Alternatively, acetaminophen effects may be mediated by an active metabolite (p-aminophenol). P-Aminophenol is conjugated with arachidonic acid by fatty acid amide hydrolase to form AM404. AM404 exerts its effect through cannabinoid receptors [384].

Analgesic Pharmacodynamics

Acetaminophen is believed to be an effective antipyretic at serum concentrations of 10–20 mg/L, and these concentrations have been extrapolated to those that provide analgesia. However, the often-cited source for the antipyretic serum concentrations of 10–20 mg/L makes reference to an unpublished source without further elaboration [385]. The calculated ED_{50} for rectal acetaminophen to avoid any supplemental opioids after day-stay surgery is 35 mg/kg [386]. Time delays of approximately one hour between peak concentration and peak effect have been reported [387, 750].

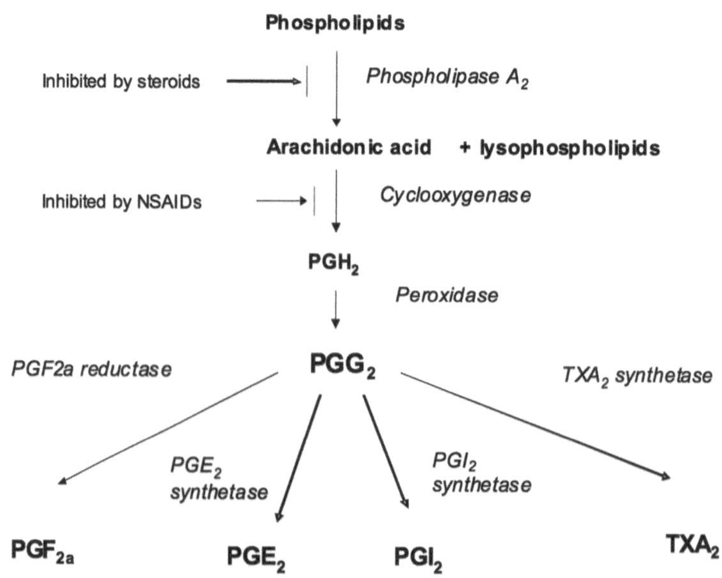

Fig. 3.15 Phospholipid metabolism to the prostaglandins

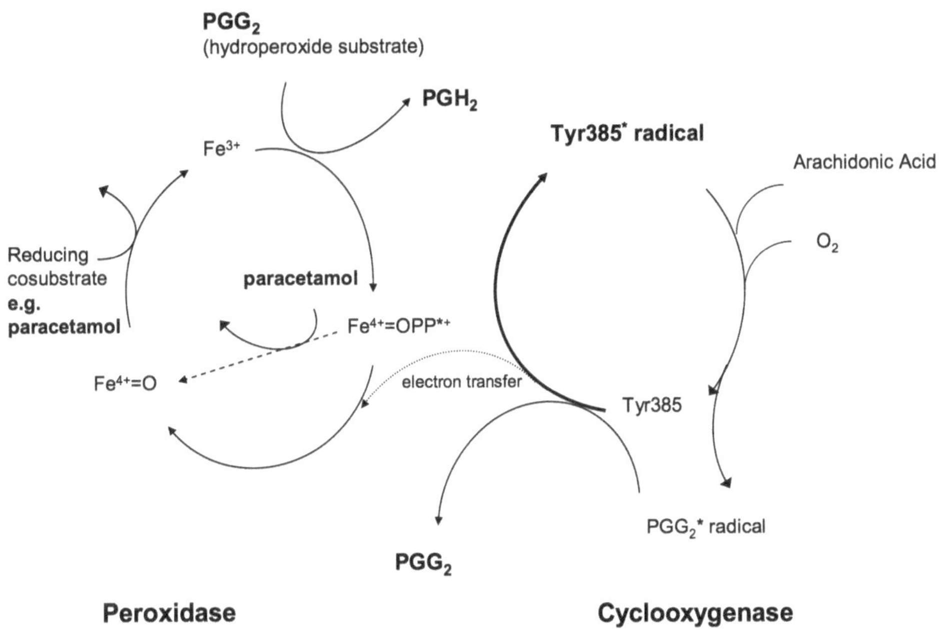

Fig. 3.16 Prostaglandin H_2 synthetase (PGHS) is the enzyme responsible for metabolism of arachidonic acid to the unstable prostaglandin H_2. Formation of tyrosine-385 radical (Tyr385*) at the COX site is dependent on the reduction of a ferryl protoporphyrin IX radical cation ($Fe^{4+}=OPP^{*+}$) at the POX site. Paracetamol is a reducing cosubstrate that partially reduces $Fe^{4+}=OPP^{*+}$, decreasing the amount available for regeneration of Tyr385*. Figure adopted. Aronoff DM, Oates JA, Boutaud O. New insights into the mechanism of action of acetaminophen: Its clinical pharmacologic characteristics reflect its inhibition of the two prostaglandin H2 synthetases. Clin Pharmacol Ther 2006;79:9–19

Pain fluctuations, pain type and placebo effects complicate interpretation of the clinical studies. Population parameter estimates of a maximum effect of oral acetaminophen are 5.17 (the greatest possible pain relief (VAS 0–10) would equate to an Emax of 10) and an EC_{50} of 9.98 mg/L [388]. The equilibration half-time ($T_{1/2}$keo) of the analgesic effect compartment was 53 min with a target effect compartment concentration of 10 mg/L associated with a pain reduction of 2.6/10 [387, 750]. Recent evidence using IV paracetamol generated somewhat different estimates of population parameters with a maximum effect of 4.15 pain units and an EC_{50} of 2.07 mg/L. However, the equilibration half-time ($T_{1/2}$keo) of the analgesic effect compartment was almost double that for oral acetaminophen, 1.58 h [389].

There are few data examining acetaminophen analgesia in neonates. The existing data suggest poor analgesic effect after oral and rectal formulations, after painful procedures [390, 391], after circumcision [392], and during heel prick [393]. This is in contrast to the documented analgesic effect in infants and children [386, 388, 394]. It is unclear why the analgesic effect of acetaminophen in neonates is so poor, but it may be attributable to inadequate serum concentrations, type of pain stimulus or assessment tools for the discrimination of pain. Intravenous paracetamol has been successfully used for neonatal analgesia in the perioperative period [395, 396].

Pharmacokinetics

The relative bioavailability of rectal to oral acetaminophen formulations (rectal/oral) is approximately 0.5 in children, but the relative bioavailability is greater in neonates and approaches unity [23]. There are two intravenous paracetamol formulations available and care must be taken with choice of formulation [397]. One is an acetaminophen formulation, whereas the other, propacetamol (*N-acetylpara-aminophenoldiethyl* aminoacetic ester), is a water-soluble prodrug of acetaminophen that can be administered intravenously over 15 min. It is rapidly hydroxylated into acetaminophen (1 g propacetamol = 0.5 g acetaminophen) [67].

Acetaminophen has a pKa of 9.5, and in the alkaline medium of the duodenum, acetaminophen is non-ionized. Consequently, the absorption half-time of the non-ionized form from the duodenum is rapid in children ($T_{1/2}$abs 4.5 min) who were given acetaminophen as an elixir [397]. The absorption half-time in infants under the age of 3 months was delayed, ($T_{1/2}$abs 16.6 min) consistent with delayed gastric emptying in young infants [20, 21]. Rectal absorption is slow and erratic with large variability. For example, absorption parameters for the triglyceride base were $T_{1/2}$abs 1.34 h (CV 90 %) with a lag time before absorption began of 8 min (31 %). The absorption half-life for rectal formulations was prolonged in infants less than 3 months (1.51 times greater) compared with those in older children [66].

Sulfate metabolism is the dominant route of elimination in neonates, while glucuronide conjugation (UGT1A6) is dominant in adults [22]. Glucuronide/sulfate ratios range from 0.12 in preterm neonates of 28–32 weeks' PCA, 0.28 in those at 32–36 weeks' PCA [399] and 0.34 in full-term neonates <2 days old [400]. A total body clearance of 0.74 L/h/70 kg at 28 weeks' PMA and 4.9 (CV 38 %) L/h/70 kg in full-term neonates after enteral acetaminophen has been reported using an allometric ¾ power model [66]. Clearance increases over the first year of life and reaches 80 % of that in older children by 6 months of postnatal age [23, 62]. Similar clearance estimates are reported in neonates after intravenous formulations of acetaminophen with weight accounting for almost 60 % of the variability in clearance with age (Fig. 3.7) [401–403, 751]. The relative bioavailability of the oral formulation is 0.9. The volume of distribution for acetaminophen is 49–70 L/70 kg. The volume of distribution decreases exponentially with a maturation half-life of 11.5 weeks from 109.7 L/70 kg at 28 weeks postconception to 72.9 L/70 kg by 60 weeks [23] reflective of fetal body composition, and water distribution changes over the first few months of life.

Adverse Effects

The toxic metabolite of acetaminophen, *N*-acetyl-*p*-*benzoquinone* imine (NAPQI), is formed by the cytochrome P450s CYP2E1, 1A2, and 3A4. This metabolite binds to intracellular hepatic macromolecules to produce cell necrosis and damage. Infants less than 90 days' PNA have decreased expression of CYP2E1 activity in vitro compared with older infants, children, and adults [53, 404]. CYP3A4 appears during the first week after birth [404], whereas CYP1A2 appears later [54, 404]. Neonates can produce hepatotoxic metabolites (e.g., NAPQI), but the reduced activity of cytochrome P-450 in neonates may explain the rare occurrence of acetaminophen-induced hepatotoxicity in neonates.

Two European centers have published intravenous dosing guidelines for acetaminophen in neonates [397, 405] and the drug is widely used by anesthetists in the UK. Preliminary data [402, 406, 407] from neonates suggest that current dosing regimens are safe. It must be stressed, however, that these are preliminary data only. The combined subject numbers were only 239 neonates. These numbers are too few to exclude the possibility of future hepatotoxicity; caution and continued monitoring of neonates given acetaminophen are vital. The two studies had daily doses that varied by a factor of two. Both authors report satisfactory analgesia, and so it is probably safer to recommend the smaller rather than the larger dosing regimen. Clearance variability and the lack of a suitable marker of reduced clearance in the first few days after birth also support a recommendation of the smaller dose [403]. Several reports have noted accidental 10-fold overdoses of acetaminophen to young infants that fortunately resolved without sequelae [408, 409, 748]. Extreme care must be taken when administering this medication to neonates.

Nonsteroidal Anti-Inflammatory Drugs

Mechanism of Action

The nonsteroidal anti-inflammatory drugs (NSAIDs) are a heterogeneous group of compounds that share common antipyretic, analgesic and anti-inflammatory effects. NSAIDs act by reducing prostaglandin biosynthesis through inhibition of cyclooxygenase (COX) site of the PGHS enzyme. The prostanoids produced by the COX-1 isoenzyme protect the gastric mucosa, regulate renal blood flow, and induce platelet aggregation. NSAID-induced gastrointestinal toxicity, for example, is likely mediated through blockade of COX-1 activity, whereas the anti-inflammatory effects of NSAIDs are likely mediated primarily through inhibition of the inducible isoform, COX-2.

Pharmacodynamics

The NSAIDs are commonly used in children for antipyresis and analgesia. The anti-inflammatory properties of the NSAIDs have, in addition, been used in such diverse disorders as juvenile idiopathic arthritis (JIA), renal and biliary colic, dysmenorrhea, Kawasaki disease, and cystic fibrosis. The NSAIDs indomethacin and ibuprofen are also used to treat delayed closure of patent ductus arteriosus (PDA) in preterm infants.

There are no linked PK–PD studies of NSAID analgesia or fever in neonates or infants. Investigation of a concentration-response relationship for PDA closure shows that a target serum concentration of 3.5 mg/L is associated with 90 % PDA closure. Dosing increases with PMA to achieve this target because clearance increases with age [410].

NSAID-associated analgesia has been compared to analgesia from other analgesics or analgesic modalities, e.g., caudal blockade, acetaminophen or morphine in children. These data confirm that NSAIDs in children are effective analgesic drugs, improving the quality of analgesia, but they do not quantify the effect. It is not possible to develop an understanding of the dose-effect relationship from these data, nor is it possible to determine if equipotent doses are being compared. The onset of analgesia may correlate with CSF concentrations. CSF penetration after ketorolac, diclofenac, ibuprofen, and indomethacin is rapid in children with peak concentrations reached approximately 30 min after IV administration of routine doses [411–414].

Pharmacokinetics

NSAIDs are rapidly absorbed in the gastrointestinal tract after oral administration in children. The relative bioavailability of oral preparations approaches unity. The rate and extent of absorption after rectal administration of NSAIDs such as ibuprofen, diclofenac, flurbiprofen, indomethacin and nimesulide are less than after the oral routes.

The apparent volume of distribution is small in adults (<0.2 L/kg) but larger in children. The volume of distribution in preterm neonates (22–31 weeks of gestational age) given IV ibuprofen was 0.62 (S.D. 0.04) L/kg [415]. The ibuprofen central volume decreased dramatically after closure of the PDA in preterm neonates (0.244 vs 0.171 L/kg) [416]. The NSAIDs, as a group, are weakly acidic, lipophilic and highly protein bound. The bound fraction is larger in preterm neonates and children, but less than in adults. The impact of altered protein binding is probably minimal with routine dosing because NSAIDs cleared by the liver have a low hepatic extraction ratio [417].

NSAIDs undergo extensive phase I and phase II enzyme biotransformation in the liver, with subsequent excretion into urine or bile. Renal elimination is not an important elimination pathway for the commonly used NSAIDs. Pharmacokinetic parameter estimate variability is large, in part, attributable to covariate effects of age, size, and pharmacogenomics. Ibuprofen, for example, is metabolized by the CYP2C9 and CYP2C8 subfamily. Considerable variation exists in the expression of CYP2C activities among individuals, and functional polymorphism of the gene coding for CYP2C9 has been described [418]. CYP2C9 activity is low immediately after birth (21 % of adult), subsequently increasing progressively to reach a peak activity within 3 months, when expressed as mg/kg/h [52, 419]. Clearance (L/h/kg) is generally greater in children than it is in adults, as we might expect when the linear per kilogram model is used. Ibuprofen clearance increases from 2.06 mL/h/kg at 22–31 weeks' PCA [415] and 9.49 mL/h/kg at 28 weeks' PCA [416] to 140 mL/kg/min at 5 years [420]. Similar data exist for indomethacin [421–423].

Many NSAIDs exhibit stereoselectivity [424]. Ibuprofen stereoselectivity is reported in preterm neonates (<28-week gestation). R- and S-ibuprofen half-lives were about 10 h and 25.5 h, respectively. The mean clearance of R-ibuprofen (12.7 mL/h) was about 2.5-fold greater than for S-ibuprofen (5.0 mL/h) [425].

During pregnancy, there is relatively little transfer of NSAIDs from maternal to fetal blood. Very small quantities of NSAIDs are secreted into breast milk. Similarly, infant exposure to ketorolac via breast milk is estimated to be only 0.4 % of maternal exposure [426].

Drug Interactions

NSAIDs undergo drug interactions through altered clearance and competition for active renal tubular secretion with other organic acids. A large fractional protein binding has been proposed to explain drug interactions between NSAIDs and oral anticoagulant agents, oral hypoglycemics, sulphonamides, bilirubin and other protein-bound drugs. An influential paper by Aggeler et al. [427] showed that warfarin administered with phenylbutazone increased both the plasma warfarin concentrations and the prothrombin time in normal volunteers. Phenylbutazone displaces warfarin from its albumin binding sites in vitro, but this observation should not be extrapolated to explain changes in prothrombin time. The observed effect is due to changes in competition for similar drug metabolic clearance pathways and not from changes in protein binding [417].

Adverse Effects

NSAIDs have the potential to cause gastrointestinal irritation, blood clotting disorders, renal impairment, neutrophil dysfunction and bronchoconstriction; effects are attributed to COX-1/COX-2 ratios, although this concept may be an oversimplification.

Ibuprofen reduces the GFR by 20 % in preterm neonates, affecting aminoglycoside clearance, an effect that appears to be independent of gestational age [90]. No significant difference in the change in cerebral blood volume, change in cerebral blood flow or tissue oxygenation index was found between administration of ibuprofen and placebo in neonates [428].

The risk of acute GI bleeding in children given short-term ibuprofen was estimated to be 7.2/100,000 (CI 2–18/100,000) [429, 430], a prevalence not different from children given acetaminophen. The incidence of clinically significant gastropathy in children given NSAIDs for JIA is comparable to that in adults given long-term NSAIDs [431, 432], but the prevalence of gastroduodenal injury may be very much greater depending on the assessment criteria (e.g., abdominal pain, anemia, endoscopy) applied. Data for neonates are not available.

The commonly used NSAIDs have reversible antiplatelet effects, which are attributable to the inhibition of thromboxane synthesis. Bleeding time is usually slightly increased, but remains within normal limits in children with normal coagulation systems. Neonates given prophylactic ibuprofen to induce PDA closure did not have an increased frequency of intraventricular hemorrhage [433].

Opioid Analgesic Drugs

Morphine

Morphine is the most commonly used opioid in neonates and infants. Morphine's main analgesic effect is by supraspinal μ_1-receptor activation. The μ_2-receptor in the spinal cord plays an important analgesic role when the drug is administered by the intrathecal or epidural route [434]. Morphine is soluble in water, but lipid solubility is poor compared with other opioids. Morphine's low oil/water partition coefficient of 1.4 and its pKa of 8 (10–20 % unionized drug at physiologic pH) contribute to delayed onset of peak action with slow CNS penetration.

Pharmacodynamics

Target analgesic plasma concentrations are believed to be 10–20 ng/mL after major surgery in neonates and infants [71, 435]. The concentration required for sedation during mechanical ventilation may be greater (125 ng/mL) [436]. The large pharmacokinetic and pharmacodynamic variability requires that morphine is often titrated to effect using small incremental doses (0.02 mg/kg) in neonates and infants suffering postoperative pain [437]. The effect compartment equilibration half-time ($T_{1/2}$keo) for morphine is ~17 min in adults [438] and is estimated to be 8 min in the full-term neonate [439]. The role of morphine for nursing procedures in the neonatal unit remains controversial. Morphine did not reduce pain responses during endotracheal suctioning, despite plasma concentrations up to 400 ng/mL [64]. Intermittent intravenous acetaminophen reduces the morphine requirements in neonates after major surgery [396].

The principle metabolites of morphine, morphine-3-glucuronide (M3G) and morphine-6-glucuronide (M6G), have pharmacologic activity. Contributions to both the desired effect (analgesia) and the undesired effects (nausea, respiratory depression) of M6G are the subject of clinical controversy [440]. It has been suggested that M3G antagonizes morphine and contributes to the development of tolerance [441].

Opioid analgesics including morphine are widely used to control painful responses in neonates. However, evidence from animals suggests that their use may cause long-term adverse sequelae. In humans, the neonatal use of morphine exerted no long-term effects measured in children 8–9 years of age in terms of intelligence, behavior and visual motor function [442].

Pharmacokinetics

Morphine is primarily metabolized by the hepatic enzyme UGT2B7 into M3G and M6G. Sulphation and renal clearance are minor pathways in adults but are more dominant in neonates. Clearance is perfusion limited with a high hepatic extraction ratio. Oral bioavailability is ~35 % due to this first pass effect. The metabolites are cleared by the kidney and, in part, by biliary excretion. Impaired renal function leads to M3G and M6G accumulation.

Morphine clearance matures with PMA reaching adult values at 6–12 months [64]. Clearance increases from 3.2 L/h/70 kg at 24 weeks' PMA to 9.3 L/h/70 kg at 32 weeks' PMA and 19 L/h/70 kg at term (Fig. 3.7). The volume of distribution is increased in preterm ventilated neonates (190 L/70 kg) compared with full-term neonates whose lungs were not ventilated (122 L/70 kg) [64]. The volume of distribution in term neonates increased from 83 L/70 kg at birth to a mature value of 136 L/70 kg within 3 months. Metabolite (M3G, M6G) clearance increases with age similar to that described for GFR maturation in infants [63] (Fig. 3.17).

Although an infusion of 5–10 mcg/kg/h will achieve a target concentration of 10 ng/mL in a typical term neonate, clearance is affected by PMA and pathology [65, 443]. Recent evidence indicates that morphine infusions of 4-5 mcg/kg/h provides effective analgesia with minimal risk of

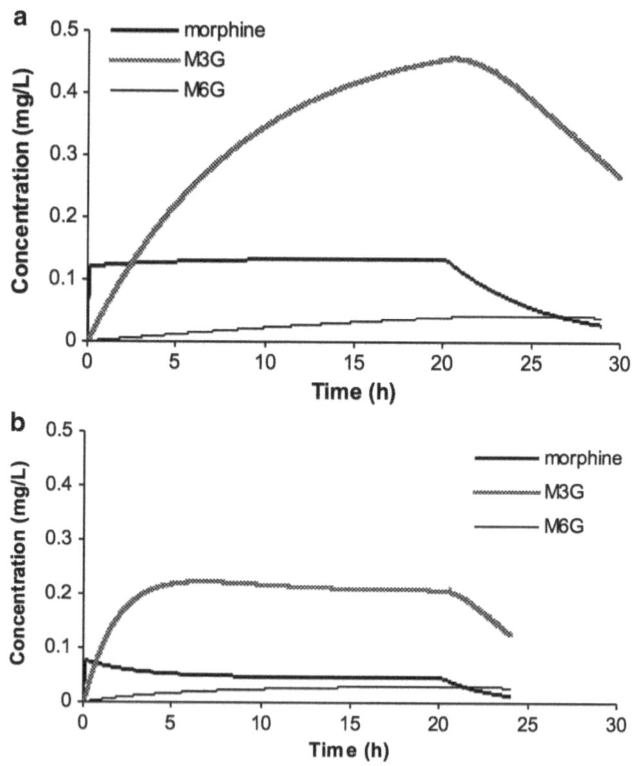

Fig. 3.17 Morphine administered as a bolus 0.07 mg/kg with subsequent infusion 0.03 mg/kg/h in a neonate (**a**) and a 1-year-old child (**b**). The concentrations of parent drug and metabolites are different in the two individuals because of the complex interplays between formation and elimination clearances. (Data from Bouwmeester NJ, Anderson BJ, Tibboel D, Holford NH. Developmental pharmacokinetics of morphine and its metabolites in neonates, infants and young children. Br J Anaesth. 2004;92:208–17) [63]

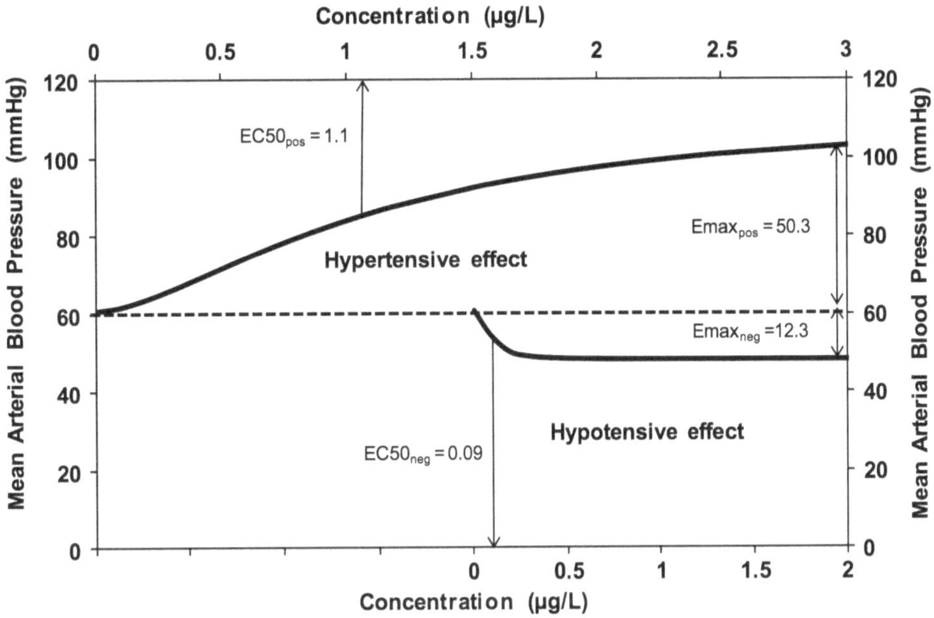

Fig. 3.18 Composite Emax model, showing hyper- and hypotensive effect of dexmedetomidine on mean arterial blood pressure. From Potts [623]

overdose in neonates <10 days PNA whereas morphine infusions of 11–23 mcg/kg/h provide reasonable analgesia in older neonates and infants [444]. Morphine pharmacokinetic parameters show large interindividual variability contributing to the range of morphine serum concentrations observed during constant infusions. Protein binding of morphine is small in preterm neonates and has minimal impact on the disposition changes with age. The M6G/morphine ratio also changes with age (Fig. 3.18) because of desynchrony between the maturation of metabolite formation and elimination pathways, but the clinical effect of these ratio changes is unclear.

Although morphine is usually administered intravenously to neonates, other routes have been used. A large variability in the analgesic effect of morphine has been observed after rectal administration; this is a major disadvantage of this route. Although this route is commonly used [445], delayed absorption with multiple doses causing respiratory arrest has been reported [446]. Morphine (25–50 mcg/kg) can also be given via the caudal route to neonates [447, 448]. While systemic absorption is slow, morphine spreads within the CSF to the brainstem where it may cause respiratory depression lasting from 6 h to >18 h [449].

Adverse Effects

Respiratory depression may occur at concentrations of 20 ng/mL [42] in infants and children, but concentration-response relationships in neonates, particularly preterm neonates prone to physiological apnea, are unknown. Hypotension, bradycardia and flushing reflect morphine's histamine-releasing characteristics. These are more pronounced with rapid intravenous bolus administration [450, 451]. The incidence of vomiting in postoperative children is related to the morphine dose. Morphine doses in excess of 0.1 mg/kg are associated with a >50 % incidence of vomiting in infants and children [398, 452, 453].

It is difficult to quantify this adverse effect in awake healthy neonates who commonly regurgitate after feeding.

Withdrawal symptoms may be observed in neonates after cessation of a continuous morphine infusion for >2 weeks and after infusion periods <2 weeks if the morphine infusion rate is >40 μg/kg/h. Strategies to prevent withdrawal from morphine include the use of neuraxial analgesia, nurse-controlled sedation management protocols, ketamine or naloxone mixed with morphine infusion and alternate agents (e.g., methadone) with lower potential for tolerance [454, 455].

Fentanyl

Fentanyl offers greater hemodynamic stability than morphine, a rapid onset ($T_{1/2}$keo = 6.6 min in adults) a short duration of effect. Its relative increased lipid solubility and small molecular conformation enables efficient penetration of the BBB and redistribution.

Pharmacodynamics

Fentanyl is a potent μ-receptor agonist with a potency 70–125 times greater than that of morphine. A plasma concentration of 15–30 ng/mL is required to provide total intravenous anesthesia (TIVA) in adults, whereas the EC_{50}, based on EEG evidence is 10 ng/mL [456, 457]. Fentanyl has been shown to effectively prevent preterm neonates from surgical stress responses and to improve postoperative outcome [458]. Single doses of fentanyl (3 mcg/kg) can reduce the physiologic and behavioral measures of pain and stress associated with mechanical ventilation in preterm infants [459]. Fentanyl has similar respiratory depression in infants and adults when plasma concentrations are similar [460].

Pharmacokinetics

Fentanyl is metabolized by oxidative *N*-dealkylation (CYP3A4) into nor-fentanyl and hydroxylized. All metabolites are inactive and a small amount of fentanyl is eliminated via the kidneys unchanged. Fentanyl clearance is 70–80 % of adult values in term neonates and, when standardized to a 70-kg person, reaches adult values (approx. 50 L/h/70 kg) within the first 2 weeks of life [35]. Clearance matures with gestational age: 7 ml/min/kg at 25 weeks' PMA, 10 ml/min/kg at 30 weeks' PMA and 12 ml/min/kg at 35 weeks' PMA [461]. Fentanyl's volume of distribution at steady state (Vss) is ~5.9 L/kg in term neonates and decreases with age to 4.5 L/kg during infancy, 3.1 L/kg during childhood and 1.6 L/kg in adults [30]. This increased Vss results in a smaller blood concentration after bolus administration in neonates and infants. Administration of fentanyl 3 mcg/kg in infants intraoperatively neither depressed respiration nor caused hypoxemia in a placebo-controlled trial [462, 463].

Fentanyl clearance may be impaired with decreased hepatic blood flow, e.g., from increased intra-abdominal pressure in neonatal omphalocele repair [464]. Infants with cyanotic heart disease had reduced Vss and greater plasma concentrations of fentanyl with infusion therapy [465]. These greater plasma concentrations resulted from a reduced clearance (34 L/h/70 kg) that was attributed to hemodynamic disturbance and consequent reduced hepatic blood flow [466].

Fentanyl is widely distributed with a short duration of effect as a result of redistribution to deep, lipid-rich compartments. Fentanyl redistributes slowly from lipid-rich tissues after discontinuation of therapy, resulting in prolonged periods of sedation and respiratory depression. Although CYP3A4 is subject to single nuclear polymorphisms with slow and rapid metabolizers, redistribution rather than clearance is responsible for offset of the drug effect after single-dose therapy. The context-sensitive half-time (CSHT) after a 1 h infusion of fentanyl is ~20 min, which increases to 270 min after an 8-h infusion in adults [467]. While the CSHT is reduced in children [468], there are no data in neonates. Alternative administration routes (e.g., transdermal and transmucosal) have not been studied in neonates [469]. Epidural fentanyl is widely combined with an amide local anesthetic for provision of postoperative analgesia, although there is limited evidence to support such a combination in young children when a therapeutic concentration of local anesthetic is administered [470]. Spread beyond the level of administration is dose dependent, but limited and respiratory depression is uncommon [471, 472].

Adverse Effects

Neonatal tolerance to synthetic opioids develops more rapidly (3–5 days) than it does with morphine (2 weeks) and diamorphine (>2 weeks) [473]. Fentanyl also has a propensity for muscular rigidity and laryngospasm with doses as little as 2 mcg/kg IV in neonates [474, 475]. Other drugs metabolized by CYP3A4 (e.g., cyclosporin, erythromycin) may compete for clearance and increase fentanyl plasma concentrations.

Respiratory depression (hours) may outlast fentanyl's analgesic effect (35–45 min) due to the prolonged CSHT and/or recirculation of fentanyl bound to the stomach's acid medium (up to 20 % of an IV dose) or delayed release from peripheral compartments.

Remifentanil

Remifentanil resembles fentanyl, sufentanil, and alfentanil in chemical structure. It is a selective μ-receptor agonist with a greater potency than alfentanil. Its brief elimination half-life of 3–6 min [77, 476] means it is usually given as an infusion [477, 478]. Intravenous remifentanil doses of 0.25 μg/kg/min appear to be safe and effective in neonates [479, 480].

Pharmacodynamics

A target plasma concentration of 2–3 mcg/L is adequate for laryngoscopy and 6–8 mcg/L for laparotomy, and 10–12 mcg/L might be sought to ablate the stress response associated with cardiac surgery [481]. Analgesic concentrations are 0.2–0.4 mcg/L. The $T_{1/2}$keo is 1.16 min in adults [76], but the neonatal $T_{1/2}$keo has not been reported. Analgesic alternatives should be available for when the short-duration analgesic effect from remifentanil has dissipated. Reports of a rapid development of μ-receptor tolerance with remifentanil use are conflicting. Activity at δ-opioid receptors may contribute [482].

Pharmacokinetics

Remifentanil is metabolized by nonspecific esterases in tissues and erythrocytes to carbonic acid [483, 484]; these esterases appear to be mature even in preterm neonates [74]. Carbonic acid is excreted through the kidneys. Metabolism is independent of liver and renal functions. Clearance in patients with butyryl-cholinesterase deficiency is unaffected.

Remifentanil clearance can be described in all age groups by simple application of an allometric model [485]. This standardized clearance of 2,790 mL/min/70 kg is similar to that reported by others in children [77, 486] and adults [76, 483]. The smaller the child, the greater the clearance when expressed as mL/min/kg. Clearances decrease with age, with rates of 90 mL/kg/min in infants <2 years of age, 60 mL/kg/min in children 2–12 years of age and 40 mL/kg/min in adults [75, 485, 486]. The steady state volume of distribution was greatest in infants <2 months of age (452 mL/kg) and decreased to 308 mL/kg in children 2 months to 2 years and to 240 mL/kg in children >2 years [77]. Elimination half-life appears to be constant, ~3 to 6 min independent of the age of the patient and duration of the infusion [77, 476]. Intravenous remifentanil doses of 0.25 μg/kg/min appear to be safe and effective in neonates [479, 480], but PK–PD data in this age group remain limited.

Although covariate effects such as cardiac surgery appear to have a muted effect on PK, as is seen with propofol, cardiopulmonary bypass (CPB) does have an impact. Remifentanil dosage adjustments are required during and after CPB due to marked changes in its volume of distribution [487]. Other PK changes during CPB are consistent with adult data in which a decreased metabolism occurred with a reduced temperature [488] and with reports of greater clearance after CPB (increased metabolism) compared with during CPB [486].

Adverse Effects

Respiratory depression is concentration dependent [489, 490]. Muscle rigidity remains a concern with bolus doses above 3 mcg/kg used for intubation in neonates [491]. The initial loading dose of remifentanil may cause hypotension and [492] bradycardia prompting some to target the plasma rather than effect site concentration when initiating infusion. This hypotensive response has been quantified in children undergoing cranioplasty surgery. A steady state remifentanil concentration of 14 mcg/L would typically achieve a 30 % decrease in MAP. This concentration is twice that required for laparotomy but is easily achieved with a bolus injection. The $T_{1/2}$keo of 0.86 min for this hemodynamic effect [493] is less than remifentanil-induced spectral edge changes described in adults ($T_{1/2}$keo = 1.34 min) [76, 494]. Neonatal data are very limited.

Because the inhibitory neurotransmitter, glycine, is included in the formulation of remifentanil, it should not be used for spinal or epidural applications [495].

Alfentanil

Alfentanil is a synthetic opioid that is chemically related to fentanyl. It has a rapid onset ($T_{1/2}$keo =0.9 min in adults), a brief duration of action and one-fourth the potency of fentanyl. Alfentanil has reduced lipid solubility and causes less histamine release than fentanyl [496]. The analgesic dose of alfentanil for endotracheal intubation and suctioning in preterm neonates is 10–20 μg/kg [497–499]. A target plasma concentration of 400 ng/mL is used in anesthesia. Metabolism is through oxidative *N*-dealkylation by CYP3A4 and *O*-dealkylation and then conjugation to end products that are excreted via the kidney [500]. The plasma protein binding of alfentanil increases from 65 % in preterm neonates to 79 % in term infants and then to ~90 % in adults [501, 502]. The volume of distribution (Vss) in children (0.163 L/kg) is one-third that in adults (0.457 L/kg) [503]. Clearance in neonates (20–60 mL/min/70 kg) is one-tenth that in adults (250–500 mL/min/70 kg [698]). In preterm neonates, the half-life is as long as 6–9 h [504, 505]. Alfentanil cannot be used without neuromuscular-blocking drugs in neonates because of the frequency of rigidity [497, 506].

Sufentanil

Sufentanil is 5–10 times more potent than fentanyl, with a $T_{1/2}$keo of 6.2 min in adults [507]. A concentration of 5–10 ng/mL is required for TIVA and 0.2–0.4 ng/mL for analgesia. Pharmacodynamic differences are suggested in neonates. The plasma concentration of sufentanil at the time of additional anesthetic supplementation to suppress hemodynamic responses to surgical stimulation was 2.51 ng/mL in neonates, significantly greater than the concentrations of 1.58, 1.53, and 1.56 ng/mL observed in infants, children and adolescents, respectively [508].

Elimination of sufentanil has been suggested by *O*-demethylation and *N*-dealkylation in animal studies. Like fentanyl and alfentanil, the P-450 CYP3A4 enzyme is responsible for the *N*-dealkylation [509]. Clearance in neonates undergoing cardiovascular surgery (6.7 ± 6.1 mL/kg/min) is reduced compared with values of 18.1 ± 2.7, 16.9 ± 3.2 and 13.1 ± 3.6 mL/kg/min in infants, children and adolescents, respectively [508]. Clearance rates in infants (27.5 ± 9.3 mL/kg/min) were greater than those in children (18.1 ± 10.7 mL/kg/min) in another study of children undergoing cardiovascular surgery [510]. Maturation of clearance is rapid [511], and clearance maturation standardized to a 70-kg person using allometry is similar to that of other drugs that depend on CYP3A4 for metabolism (e.g., levobupivacaine, fentanyl, alfentanil) (Fig. 3.7) [512]. The volume of distribution at steady state (Vss) was 4.15 ± 1.0 L/kg in neonates, greater than the values of 2.73 ± 0.5 and 2.75 ± 0.5 L/kg observed in children and adolescents, respectively [508, 513]. Clearance in healthy children (2–8 years) was greater (30.5 ± 8.8 mL/kg/min) than those undergoing cardiac surgery [513]. Decreased hepatic blood flow reduces clearance [513].

The free fraction of sufentanil decreases with increasing age (neonates 19 %, infants 11 %, children and adults 8 %) and is strongly correlated with the alpha 1-acid glycoprotein plasma concentration [501]. The reduced concentration of alpha 1-acid glycoprotein in neonates and infants [514] increases the free fraction of sufentanil in these age groups. Although sufentanil, fentanyl, alfentanil, and remifentanil have >70 % protein binding and have high hepatic (or nonhepatic for remifentanil) extraction ratios, protein binding changes are probably clinically unimportant [515] because the dose is titrated to effect, and variability in the clearance has a much greater impact.

Epidural sufentanil (0.7–0.75 mcg/kg) has been effective in children lasting >3 h [516–518] although pruritus can be bothersome [516]. Nasal sufentanil may have a role for sedation in children although data in neonates are lacking [519–521].

Codeine

Codeine, or methylmorphine, is a morphine-like opioid with 1/10 the potency of morphine. It is mainly metabolized by glucuronidation, but minor pathways are *N*-demethylation to norcodeine and *O*-demethylation to morphine. Approximately 10 % of codeine is metabolized to morphine. As the affinity of codeine for opioid receptors is very low, the analgesic effect of codeine is mainly due to its metabolite, morphine [522]. Codeine is effectively a prodrug analgesic. The continued use of this minor opium alkaloid for pediatric analgesia remains baffling [523] and is subject to debate because it is a prodrug [524]. The CYP2D6 enzyme catalyses the metabolism of codeine to morphine. A genetic polymorphism of this enzyme causes distinct phenotypes responsible for the presence of ultrarapid extensive, extensive and slow codeine metabolizers [525–527, 753]. Between 7 % and 10 % of the European population are believed to be slow metabolizers of codeine [526, 528, 529], but this percentage varies with race [526, 528]. In poor metabolizers, codeine confers little or no analgesia, although adverse effects persist [529]. In ultrarapid metabolizers on the other hand, a large incidences of adverse effects might be expected including apnea and death, because of large plasma morphine concentrations [754]. A consensus guideline has been drafted on whether genetic testing for CYP2D6 polymorphisms should be undertaken before patients are prescribed codeine and if they are tested, subsequent managements based on the genetic results [530].

Codeine can be administered by intramuscular, oral and rectal routes. Intravenous codeine is not recommended because of hypotensive effects [531]. Blood concentrations after rectal codeine are less than those after intramuscular codeine because of incomplete, slower, more variable absorption [532]. Codeine is often used in combination with acetaminophen or NSAIDs. The addition of codeine to acetaminophen has been shown to improve postoperative pain relief in infants [533]. The analgesic effect of the combination of acetaminophen (10–15 mg/kg) and codeine (1–1.5 mg/kg) was comparable to that of ibuprofen (5–10 mg/kg) in children after tonsillectomy [534]. Codeine has been used in infants and neonates after major surgery as an adjunct to acetaminophen or NSAIDs (optimal oral codeine dosage of 1–1.5 mg/kg every 4–6 h, oral acetaminophen of 20 mg/kg every 6 h in infants older than 3 months) [535]. It is anticipated that analgesic alternatives should be available for when the short-duration analgesic effect from remifentanil has dissipated, preterm neonates would gain little analgesic benefit from codeine because the conversion rate to morphine is limited. Maturation of CYP2D6 should follow that of M1 production from tramadol (Fig. 3.5), a metabolite also produced by CYP2D6. There is rapid maturation of this enzyme after 40 weeks' PMA, suggesting that post-term neonates could benefit, although there are no studies investigating this drug in neonates.

The pharmacokinetics of codeine is poorly described in children despite several decades of use. A volume of distribution (V) of 3.6 L/kg and a clearance (CL) of 0.85 L/h have been described in adults, but there are few data detailing the developmental changes in pediatric pharmacokinetics. The neonatal half-life in neonates (4.5 h) is greater than that in the infant (2.6 h) as a result of immature clearance [536]. Administration (especially of codeine preparations with an antihistamine and a decongestant) in the neonate may cause intoxication [537]. A neonate has died from morphine poisoning when his mother used codeine while breastfeeding. The mother, an ultrarapid metabolizer (UM), produced much more morphine when taking codeine than most people do [538, 539]. Further evidence suggests that the combination of an UM of CYP2D6 and decreased expression of the *P*-glycoprotein gene, ABCB1, which codes for transport of codeine (and other compounds) out of the central nervous system, predicted 87 % of the infant and maternal central nervous system depression to codeine [530]. When guidelines were followed to improve the safety of codeine during breastfeeding, genotyping did not predict neonatal sedation. Rather, neonatal sedation (2.1 %) occurred only when mother's codeine consumption exceeded the recommended guidelines [540].

The adverse effects of codeine are broadly similar to those of other opioids. Adverse effects at low doses appear to be directly related to morphine plasma concentrations but are caused by codeine at greater doses [541]. There is a broad belief that codeine causes fewer adverse effects, such as sedation and respiratory depression, compared with other opioids, but there is little evidence for this notion. The analgesic effect of codeine is dependent on its conversion to morphine. Consequently other medications competing for the CYP2D6 enzyme (e.g., quinidine) may decrease the analgesic effect of codeine.

Meperidine (Pethidine)

Meperidine is a weak opioid, primarily μ-receptor, agonist that has a potency of 1/10 that of morphine. The analgesic effects are detectable within 5 min of intravenous administration and peak effect is reached within 10 min in adults [542, 543]. Meperidine is metabolized by *N*-demethylation to meperidinic acid and normeperidine. Meperidine clearance in infants and children is approximately 8–10 mL/min/kg [506, 544]. Elimination in neonates is greatly reduced, and elimination half-time in neonates, who have received pethidine by placental transfer, may be 2–7 times greater than that in adults [545]. The Vss in infants, 7.2 (3.3–11) L/kg [544], is greater than that in children 2–8 years of 2.8 SD 0.6 L/kg [544].

Meperidine was initially synthesized as an anticholinergic agent but was soon discovered to have analgesic properties. Although meperidine's anticholinergic effects were demonstrated in vitro, the anticholinergic effects on the biliary and renal tracts have not been demonstrated in vivo. Studies have clearly demonstrated that meperidine is no more effective for treating biliary or renal tract spasm than comparative μ opioids [546]. Because morphine results in better analgesia with fewer adverse effects, there are no particular advantages of meperidine as an analgesic [547]. Accumulation of the metabolite normeperidine results in seizures and dysphoria [548], although metabolism of meperidine to normeperidine is reduced 7-fold in neonates compared with adults [545].

Intramuscular administration of meperidine was frequently used in pediatric patients in the past, but this route of administration is used uncommonly today because it is painful and may lead to sterile abscesses. Meperidine was used for a number of years as a component of various "lytic cocktails" that provided sedation. It was administered either rectally or orally. The safety of these admixtures, especially in neonates, is dubious and used now infrequently [549]. Meperidine's local anesthetic properties have been found useful for epidural techniques [550].

Methadone

Methadone is a synthetic opioid with an analgesic potency similar to that of morphine but with a more rapid distribution and a slower elimination. Methadone is used as a maintenance drug in opioid-addicted adults to prevent withdrawal. Methadone might have beneficial effects because it is a long-acting synthetic opioid with a very high bioavailability (80 %) by the enteral route. It also has NMDA receptor antagonistic activity. Agonism of this receptor is associated with opioid tolerance and hyperalgesia. Methadone is a racemate and clinical effect is due to the R-methadone isomer. Methadone is 2.5–20 times more analgesic than morphine [551].

Although only limited data on the efficacy and safety of methadone are available, methadone is widely used for the treatment of opioid withdrawal in neonates and children [454, 552, 553]. Intravenous methadone has been shown to be an effective analgesic for postoperative pain relief [554], and oral administration has been recommended as the first-line opioid for severe and persistent pain in children [555]. It seems also to be a safe enteral alternative for intravenous opioids in palliative pediatric oncological patients [556]. Although a predominant role for methadone in the management of prolonged pain in neonates has been suggested, its use needs to be evaluated in a clinical research setting [455].

Methadone has high lipid solubility [557] with a large volume of distribution of 6–7 L/kg in children and adults [558–560]. Clearance in children 1–18 years was 5.4 SD 3.2 mL/min/kg [560]. There are few PK data available for infants under 1 year of age. The few neonatal data on methadone pharmacokinetics show an increased elimination half-life with enormous interindividual variability (3.8–62 h) [455]. This increased elimination half-life can be attributed to increased distribution volume in neonates; clearance in neonates is similar to adults due to active CYP3A7 [755]. A physiological-based PK model using CYP3A activity maturation has been proposed to estimate methadone time-concentration profiles from neonates to adults [561], although validation in neonates is pending.

The increased lipid solubility and greater duration of effect give this drug a potential role in a single-shot epidural.

Sedatives

Benzodiazepines

These drugs produce anxiolysis, amnesia, and hypnosis. They are commonly used as adjuncts to both local and general anesthesia. Midazolam is the most common benzodiazepine used perioperatively. It is water soluble in an acid pH carrier, but becomes lipid soluble at physiological pH. This facilitates rapid BBB entry. Midazolam is highly bound to serum albumin (>96 %). It is a medium extraction drug with changes in plasma protein concentrations having limited effect on its clearance. However, a reduced albumin concentration will increase the unbound fraction after bolus intravenous administration.

Mechanism of Action

Benzodiazepines bind to $GABA_A$ receptors, increasing chloride entry into cells. This renders these receptors resistant to excitation because they are hyperpolarized.

Pharmacodynamics

PK–PD relationships have been described for intravenous midazolam in adults. When an EEG signal is used as an effect measure, the EC_{50} is 35–77 ng/mL, with a $T_{1/2}$keo of 0.9–1.6 min described [562–564]. While the $T_{1/2}$keo is increased in the elderly and in low cardiac output states, estimates in neonates are lacking. PK–PD relationships are more difficult to describe after oral midazolam because the active metabolite, 1-hydroxy metabolite (1-OHMDZ), has approximately half the activity of the parent drug [565].

Sedation in children is more difficult to quantify. No PK–PD relationship was established in children 2 days to 17 years who were given a midazolam infusion in intensive care. Midazolam dosing could, however, be effectively titrated to the desired level of sedation, assessed by the COMFORT scale [566]. Consistent with this finding, desirable sedation in children after cardiac surgery was achieved at mean serum concentrations between 100 and 500 ng/mL [567–569].

Pharmacokinetics

Midazolam is metabolized mainly by hepatic hydroxylation (CYP3A4) [49]. These hydroxymetabolites are glucuronidated and excreted in the urine. CYP3A7 is the dominant CYP3A enzyme in utero; it is expressed in the fetal liver and appears to have activity from as early as 50–60 days after conception. CYP3A4 expression increases dramatically after the first week of life in term neonates. Hepatic CYP3A4 activity begins to dramatically increase at about 1 week of age, reaching 30–40 % of adult expression by 1 month [512]. Midazolam clearance does not parallel CYP3A4 activity because the former also depends on the size of the liver, its blood flow and environmental factors. Midazolam has a hepatic extraction ratio in the intermediate range of 0.3–0.7. Metabolic clearance depends on both liver perfusion and enzyme activity.

Clearance is reduced in neonates (0.8–2.2 mL/min/kg) [570–575], but increases exponentially after 39 weeks' PMA [573, 576]. Central volume of distribution is related to weight (V1 0.591 SD 0.065 L/kg), whereas peripheral volume of distribution remains constant (V2 0.42 SD 0.11 L) in 187 neonates 0.7–5.2 kg [573]. It has been suggested that midazolam self-induces its own clearance [567]. The latter observation from infants after cardiac surgery likely results from the improved hepatic function after the insult of cardiopulmonary bypass. Neonates who require extracorporeal membrane oxygenation (ECMO) have an increase in Vss during ECMO therapy (0.8 L/kg to 4.1 L/kg) caused by sequestration of midazolam by the circuitry, although clearance (1.4 SD 0.15 mL/min/kg) was unchanged [577].

Clearance may be reduced in the presence of pathology. A reduced clearance of midazolam has been reported after circulatory arrest for cardiac surgery [578]. Covariates such as renal failure, hepatic failure [569] and concomitant administration of CYP3A inhibitors [579] are important predictors of altered midazolam and metabolite pharmacokinetics in pediatric intensive care patients [580]. The clearance of midazolam was reduced by 30 % in neonates receiving sympathomimetic amines, probably as a consequence of the underlying compromised hemodynamics [573].

Adverse Effects

Metabolites can accumulate in the presence of renal failure, causing increased sedation. Respiratory depression, and hypotension after midazolam are well recognized. Cessation of long-term sedation with midazolam can cause withdrawal symptoms often manifest as irritability, agitation, tremors and sleeplessness.

Alpha-2 Agonists

Clonidine

Clonidine is an alpha-2 adrenoreceptor agonist that produces sedation, anxiolysis, analgesia and hypotension. It is commonly used in the caudal and epidural space where it prolongs the duration of analgesia approximately 3 h [581–586].

Pharmacodynamics

A plasma clonidine concentration in the range of 0.3–0.8 mcg/L confers satisfactory preoperative sedation in children 1–11 years with substantively greater concentrations, 4-6 mcg/L, required for sedation in the pediatric ICU [587, 756]. The plasma concentration that provides analgesia in adults is 1.5–2 mcg/L [588–590]. Clonidine-mediated analgesia, sedation and anxiolysis are dose dependent in adults [591–593].

When administered intravenously at clinically relevant doses, alpha-2 agonists have a biphasic effect on blood pressure and cause a dose-dependent decrease in heart rate. This biphasic effect results from two different sites of alpha-2 adrenoreceptor stimulation – an initial direct action on peripheral vascular resistance and a delayed central sympatholysis [594, 595]. The net effect of these responses was a 26.3 % reduction in mean arterial blood pressure after intravenous doses of 2.5 mcg/kg in children 1–10 years [596].

Pharmacokinetics

Approximately 50 % of clonidine is eliminated unchanged by the kidney and there is considerable interindividual variability [593, 597, 598]. It remains unclear which drug-metabolizing enzymes are responsible for nonrenal clearance. The exact fraction of clonidine that undergoes hepatic biotransformation is unclear, but has been reported to be between 40 % and 60 % after intravenous administration [593, 597–599]. The major metabolite of clonidine is p-hydroxyclonidine, formed by hydroxylation of the phenol ring, which is present at <10 % of the concentration in the urine [597]. CYP2D6 is involved in this process. There are limited neonatal pharmacokinetics data and none in preterm infants. A pooled pediatric analysis reported the clearance of clonidine at birth to be 3.8 L/h/70 kg (0.12 L/h/kg), a rate that matured with a half-time of 25.7 weeks to reach 82 % adult rate by 1 year postnatal age. The central volume of distribution (V1) was 62.5 (71.1 %) L/70 kg, intercompartment clearance (Q) 157 (77.3 %) L/h/70 kg and peripheral volume of distribution (V2) 119 (22.9 %) L/70 kg. The volumes of distribution, but not clearance, increased after cardiac surgery (V1 123 %, V2 126 %). There was a lag time of 2.3 (CV 73.2 %) min before absorption began in the rectum after administration of a rectal solution [600]. The absorption half-life from the epidural space was slower than that from the rectum (0.98 CV 24.5 % h vs 0.26 CV 32.3 % h). The relative bioavailability of epidural and rectal clonidine was unity ($F = 1$) compared with intravenous administration [601]. In a study of 36 neonates (0.5–26 days' PNA) who were given oral clonidine for neonatal abstinence syndrome, the estimated apparent clearance was 0.16 L/h/kg [602], which is consistent with intravenous clearance estimates given probable reduced oral bioavailability; oral bioavailability is 0.55 in children [603].

Dexmedetomidine

Dexmedetomidine has a seven times greater specificity for the alpha-2 adrenoreceptor than clonidine. Dexmedetomidine is a unique alpha-2 adrenoreceptor agonist that, unlike traditional sedative agents, is reported to produce its sedative effect, at least in part, through an endogenous sleep-promoting pathway that does not produce clinically significant respiratory depression [604–608]. Use of dexmedetomidine in neonatal intensive care and sedation practice is increasing [609–611]. Dexmedetomidine use in neonates and children has even expanded to include prevention of emergence delirium, postoperative pain and burn management, invasive and noninvasive procedural sedation, and the management of opioid withdrawal [604–606, 612–620].

Pharmacodynamics

A plasma concentration in excess of 0.6 $\mu g.L^{-1}$ is estimated to produce satisfactory sedation in adult ICU patients [621], and similar target concentrations are estimated in children, but there is a lack of neonatal experience [622]. Dexmedetomidine administered as a single bolus dose in infants after cardiac surgery produces a biphasic effect of mean arterial blood pressure (Fig. 3.18). The peripheral vasopressor effect was directly related to plasma concentration with an $Emax_{pos}$ of 50.3 (CV 44.50 %) mmHg, an EC_{50pos} of 1.1 (48.27 %) $\mu\ L^{-1}$ and a $Hill_{pos}$ coefficient of 1.65. The delayed central sympatholytic response was described with an $Emax_{neg}$ of -12.30 (CV 37.01 %) mmHg, an EC_{50neg} of 0.10 (104.40 %) $\mu\ L^{-1}$ and a $Hill_{neg}$ coefficient of 2.35. The equilibration half-time ($T_{1/2}$keo) was 9.66 (165.23 %) min [623]. These results have been reproduced in children presenting for sedation during radiological procedures. There was a 5 % incidence of hypertension in these patients; the incidence was greatest in those under 1 year of age and those who required an additional bolus dose to maintain sedation [624].

Upper airway changes associated with increasing doses of dexmedetomidine (1–3 mcg/kg) in children with and without obstructive sleep apnea (OSA) are small in magnitude and do not appear to be associated with clinical signs of airway obstruction [625, 626]. Even though these changes are small, all precautions to manage airway obstruction should be taken when dexmedetomidine is used for sedation [625]. Upper airway changes during dexmedetomidine (2 mcg/kg/h) compared with propofol sedation yielded similar airway support requirements [627]. A study in neonates has not yet been performed.

Pharmacokinetics

Population parameter estimates for a two-compartment model were clearance (CL) of 42.1 (CV 30.9 %) L/h/70 kg, central volume of distribution (V1) of 56.3 (61.3 %) L/70 kg, intercompartment clearance (Q) of 78.3 (37.0 %) L/70 kg and peripheral volume of distribution (V2) of 69.0 (47.0 %) L/70 kg. Clearance increases from 18.2 L/h/70 kg at birth in a full-term neonate to reach 84.5 % of the mature value by 1-year postnatal age. Children given a dexmedetomidine infusion after cardiac surgery had reduced clearance (83.0 %) compared with a population given a bolus dose [622, 628]. Similar parameter estimates with reduced clearance in children receiving dexmedetomidine infusion after cardiac surgery have been described by others.

Adverse Effects

Intravenous use of dexmedetomidine for CT scanning has been associated with modest fluctuations in heart rate and blood pressure that required no pharmacologic interventions or reporting as adverse events [629]. Similar results were noted for MRI scanning, although many required adjunct medications to complete the studies [630, 631]. While the use of high-dose dexmedetomidine (≥2 mcg/kg/h) was associated with decreases in heart rate and blood pressure outside the established "awake" normal values for children, the deviations were generally within 20 % of normal, although some infants developed profound bradycardias and hypotension. No adverse sequelae were reported [632]. Less favorable results have been noted in the electrophysiology laboratory. Heart rate decreased while arterial blood pressure increased significantly after 1 mcg/kg IV over 10 min followed by a 10-min continuous infusion of 0.7 mcg/kg/h. Sinus node function was significantly affected and atrioventricular nodal function was also depressed [633].

Alternately, dexmedetomidine has been used to terminate supraventricular tachycardia and compared with adenosine [634]. Dexmedetomidine appears to be as effective and possibly more effective than adenosine for this indication, although a prospective study is warranted before dexmedetomidine can be advocated for the electrophysiology laboratory. Dexmedetomidine has also been studied in the cardiac catheterization laboratory in children with and without pulmonary hypertension [635]. A loading dose of dexmedetomidine caused a decrease in heart rate and an increase in mean arterial pressure and systemic vascular resistance. Furthermore, neither cardiac index nor pulmonary vascular resistance changed significantly in those with and without pulmonary hypertension.

Local Anesthetic Agents

Mechanism of Action

Local anesthetics are grouped as either amino amides (lignocaine, bupivacaine) or amino esters (prilocaine, tetracaine), although their mechanisms of action are the same. They act principally by inactivating the fast sodium channels that initiate neural action potentials. Inactivation occurs on the cytosolic aspect of the membrane. Drug must first traverse this phospholipid bilayer membrane before having an effect. Effect from individual agents depends on the molecular size, lipid solubility, unbound drug availability, and degree of ionization at physiological pH. Neonates have reduced concentrations of AAG and this increases the unbound concentration [636, 637] compared with adults. A decrease in pH will also increase the unbound concentration in plasma. Neonates with their greater metabolic rate and reduced bicarbonate stores may be more prone to acidosis during convulsions caused by local anesthetic toxicity increasing susceptibility to subsequent cardiac toxicity. A decrease in intracellular pH also causes ion trapping of the active moiety of the local anesthetic molecule leading to further exacerbation of toxicity [638].

Cardiac sodium channels are more sensitive and stereospecific than nerve channels. Consequently, the R(+) enantiomer of bupivacaine has greater toxicity than the S(−) enantiomer (levobupivacaine) in cardiac myocytes [639]. Local anesthetics also affect potassium and calcium ion channels. Nodal conduction in the heart depends on calcium channel activity and influence at this site can cause dysrhythmias. Neonates have a relative immaturity of the sarcoplasmic reticular regulation of cytosolic calcium, and force development and relaxation in the immature heart depend more on the trans-sarcolemma calcium flux than in the adult.

Unmyelinated fibers are more sensitive to local anesthetic effects than myelinated fibers and myelination is incomplete at birth. Local anesthetics need to block 2–3 adjacent nodes of Ranvier to block conduction in myelinated fibers. Thinly myelinated fibers have shorter distances between nodes than thickly myelinated fibers. Consequently, neonates and infants need only small concentrations of local anesthetic to achieve a similar blockade as that observed in adults [640].

Pharmacodynamics

Local anesthetics are antiepileptics at reduced concentrations, acting either on GABA-glutamate regulation or by blocking sodium channels in a manner similar to phenytoin. At serum concentrations less than 5–7 μg/mL, lidocaine possesses anticonvulsant properties in infants [641–643]. At concentrations greater than 7–10 μg/mL, lidocaine causes convulsions, while at serum concentrations greater than 15–20 μg/mL, lidocaine induces global depression with coma and cardiovascular collapse. The effect of local anesthetics on sodium channel preparations is difficult to quantify because they depend on the type of channel investigated, biochemical and electrophysiological conditions or stereospecificity [643]. Sodium channels expressed in nerve fibers have an EC_{50} ranging from ~100 μM to 800 μM for lidocaine and to 150 μM for bupivacaine [645–647]. Successful neuronal blockade in vivo requires concentrations 200 times greater because penetration of the perineural area is poor. Vascular removal and degree of ionization result in only a small amount of drug reaching the sodium channel. Hydrophobic drugs (e.g., bupivacaine) cross into neural tissue more readily than those that are more hydrophilic (e.g., prilocaine).

Pharmacokinetics

The major hepatic clearance pathway for lignocaine to its active metabolites monoethylglycinexylidide and glycinexylidide is CYP1A2. Lignocaine is a high-extraction drug that displays perfusion-limited clearance. Clearance is equivalent to hepatic blood flow and a reduction in hepatic blood flow reduces clearance. Lignocaine total body clearance in neonates, expressed per kilogram, is similar to that reported in adults (0.55 vs. 0.61 L/h/kg). While hepatic blood flow is increased in neonates [38, 49], CYP1A2 activity is not detectable until well after birth. CYP3A4, which has a minor role in lignocaine clearance in adults, is also immature in neonates. CYP3A7 is expressed in the fetal liver and may contribute to clearance. Neonates excrete a greater fraction of the dose unchanged in urine and the urinary metabolites, which account for more than 70 % of the dose in adults and account for less than 30 % of the dose in neonates [84, 648].

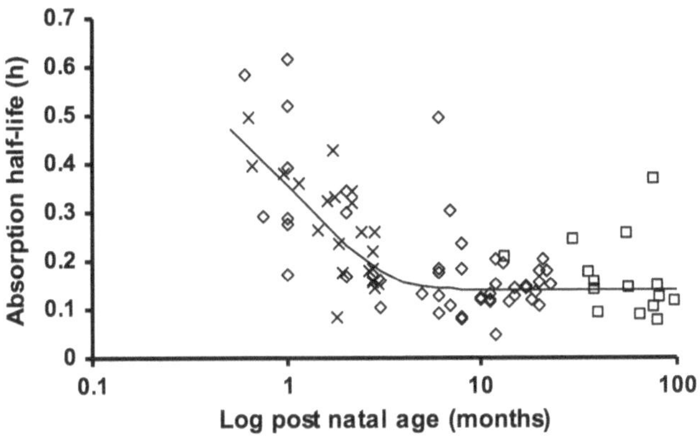

Fig. 3.19 Individual predicted levobupivacaine absorption half-time (Tabs), standardized to a 70-kg person, is plotted against postnatal age. The *solid line* represents the nonlinear relation between Tabs and postnatal age. From Chalkiadis [654]

Renal function is also immature in neonates, and consequently we might anticipate reduced clearance of lignocaine in neonates. Allometric scaling reveals a standardized clearance that is one-third that of adults. CYP3A4 assumes a greater role in the clearance of bupivacaine and levobupivacaine. Bupivacaine is predominantly metabolized into pipecoloxylidide by CYP3A4. Maturation patterns are similar for bupivacaine and levobupivacaine. Levobupivacaine clearance is 5.8 L/h/70 kg at 1-month PNA and increases with a maturation half-time of 2.3 months to reach 80 % of the mature value of 22.1 L/h/70 kg by 6-month postnatal age (Fig. 3.19). Ropivacaine is mainly metabolized into 3′- and 4′-OH-ropivacaine by the CYP1A2 and, to a minor extent, to pipecoloxylidide by CYP3A4. An unbound clearance of 120 L/h/70 kg at 30-day postnatal age is 33 % that of the mature estimate for ropivacaine [55, 649]. Bupivacaine and ropivacaine have extraction ratios of 35 % in adults and are considered capacity limited for clearance. Failure to appreciate reduced clearance in neonates has resulted in convulsions during continuous epidural infusion [650, 651]. Safe continuous epidural bupivacaine infusion rates of 0.2–0.25 mg/kg/h (maximum 72 h) in neonates and 0.4–0.5 mg/kg/h in children were empirically derived [1]. These empirically derived rates in neonates and children result in steady state concentrations of about 1 mg/L and mirror age-related clearance changes. The volume of distribution of lignocaine in neonates is twice that of adults (2.75 vs 1.1 L/kg) [648] and is also increased for ropivacaine in neonates [652], but no age-related volume changes are reported for bupivacaine or its enantiomer, levobupivacaine [56, 649, 653–655].

In contrast to the amino amide local anesthetics, esters are rapidly metabolized by plasma cholinesterases. The clearance in adults, 2.37 L/min, far exceeds the hepatic blood flow, supporting its extensive extrahepatic metabolism [655]. Some patients have reduced cholinesterase blood concentrations with consequent reduced clearance. There are a great number of plasma cholinesterase genotypes leading to wide variations in plasma cholinesterase activity [656].

Disposition may be altered by anatomical differences between infant and child. In neonates and young infants, an epidural catheter can be threaded easily from the caudal space to the thoracic region. Anatomical studies have shown that in neonates and young infants, the epidural fat is spongy and gelatinous in appearance with distinct spaces between individual fat globules [657]. With increasing age, fat becomes more tightly packed and fibrous. Local anesthetics bind to epidural fat. The absorption half-life (Tabs) (Fig. 3.20) and the time to peak concentration (Tmax) are increased in this neonatal age group [56]. Reduced clearance and slow absorption both contribute to the observed increase in Tmax in neonates. The prolonged absorption half-time would be consistent with increased epidural fat rather than reduced epidural fat, and the increased Tabs may have more to do with the surface area available for absorption in the epidural space. Observations in neonatal lambs with surgically created left-to-right shunts revealed both reduced clearance and volume of distribution of lignocaine [658]. These data are yet to be confirmed in humans.

Adverse Effects

The major adverse effects are related to cardiovascular and central nervous systems. Cardiac toxicity is more commonly reported in children than neurotoxicity, although this may be attributable to masking of neurotoxic symptoms and signs during anesthesia. The use of benzodiazepines may suppress seizure activity, while inhalational drugs may exacerbate cardiovascular signs.

Plasma concentrations of lignocaine from 10 mcg/mL and bupivacaine of 3–5 mcg/mL in adults may be expected to produce adverse effects. However, adverse events range in severity and correlate poorly with the total concentrations. The rate of increase of plasma concentration, protein binding, ionization, arterial oxygen tension and maturity of the blood-brain barrier also influences the risk of toxicity. Neonates, with their reduced protein binding resulting in greater unbound concentrations, immature BBB, metabolic acidosis during seizure activity, propensity to desaturate rapidly and immature cardiac physiology, are at greater risk of adverse effects [659].

Levobupivacaine and ropivacaine are less cardiotoxic than bupivacaine. A mean plasma concentration of levobupivacaine in healthy adults of 2.38 mg/L is less cardiodepressive than a bupivacaine concentration of 1.87 mg/L [660], but there are no recommendations regarding the "safe" serum concentration of levobupivacaine in children.

Prilocaine mixed with lignocaine is a common component of a topical local anesthetic cream, EMLA® (eutectic mixture of local anesthetics). Neonates have a tendency to form methemoglobin because they have reduced methemoglobin reductase activity, and fetal hemoglobin is more readily oxidized compared with adult hemoglobin. This, combined with increased percutaneous absorption, resulted in reluctance to use repeat lidocaine-prilocaine cream in neonates [25], although single-dose application is safe [661].

Neuromuscular-Blocking Drugs

Neonatal Physiology

The neuromuscular junction is immature and structurally different in neonates, the skeletal muscle properties change in infancy, the proportion of muscle in relation to body weight is reduced, the extracellular fluid that neuromuscular-blocking drugs (NMBDs) distribute to is increased, the metabolic clearance pathways are often immature, and the relationship between parasympathetic and sympathetic tone unbalanced in early life. It is not surprising that NMBDs behave quite differently in neonates both in their desired effects and adverse effects.

Fetal neonatal postjunctional acetylcholine receptors differ from adult receptors [662, 663]. Adult receptors possess five subunits—two α and one β, δ and ε subunits. Preterm neonates (<31-week PMA) have a γ-subunit instead of an ε-subunit in their neuromuscular receptor [664]. Fetal receptors have a greater opening time than adult receptors, allowing more sodium to enter the cell with a consequent larger depolarizing potential. The resulting increased sensitivity to acetylcholine is at odds with the observed increased sensitivity to NMBDs, but may compensate for reduced acetylcholine stores in the terminal nerve endings [665].

Neuromuscular transmission is immature in neonates and infants until the age of 2 months [666, 667].

Neonates deplete acetylcholine vesicle reserves more quickly than do infants >2 months old and in children [666] in response to tetanic nerve stimulation. Data from phrenic nerve-hemidiaphragm preparations from rats aged 11–28 days suggests this is due to a low quantal content of acetylcholine in neonatal end plate potentials [98]. Neonates display an increased sensitivity to NMBDs. An alternative proposal to explain this increased sensitivity is based on NMBD synergism observations [668, 669]. Neonates display poor synergism, and this has been explained on the basis that NMBDs occupy only one of the two α-subunit receptor sites in neonates as opposed to two in children and adults [669]. If this is true, then neonates may use NMBDs more efficiently than children. Skeletal muscle fibers can be grouped into two broad types: type I fibers are rich in oxidative enzymes and type II fibers that are rich in glycolytic enzymes [670]. Preterm infants tolerate respiratory loads poorly. The diaphragm in the preterm neonate contains only 10 % of the slowly contracting type I fibers. This proportion increases to 25 % at term and to 55 % by 2 years of age [671]. A similar maturation pattern has been observed for the intercostal muscles [671]. Type I fibers tend to be more sensitive to NMBDs than type II fibers, and consequently the diaphragmatic function in neonates may be better preserved and recover earlier than peripheral muscles [672–675]. Total body water and extracellular fluid (ECF) [29] are greatest in preterm neonates and decrease throughout gestation and postnatal life, whereas fat as a percentage of body weight is 3 % in a 1.5-kg preterm neonate, 12 % in a term neonate and 25 % by 4–5 months of postnatal age. Muscle contributes only 10 % of body weight in neonates, and 33 % by the end of childhood. These body component changes affect the volumes of distribution of drugs. Polar drugs such as depolarizing and non-depolarizing neuromuscular-blocking drugs (NMBDs) distribute rapidly into the ECF but enter cells more slowly. Consequently, a larger initial dose of such drugs is required in infants compared with children or adults. Increasing the muscle bulk contributes new acetylcholine receptors. This greater number of receptors requires a greater amount of drug to block activation of receptor ion channels.

Pharmacodynamics

Age-related variability in the dose required to achieve a predetermined level of neuromuscular blockade has been reported for non-depolarizing NMBDs during balanced thiopental-N_2O-fentanyl anesthesia. The ED_{95} of vecuronium was 47 SD 11 mcg/kg in neonates and infants, 81 SD 12 mcg/kg in children between 3 and 10 years of age and 55 SD 12 mcg/kg in patients aged 13 years or older.

Similar profiles have been reported for other NMBDs (Fig. 3.20) [675–680]. In addition, duration of neuromuscular blockade is greater in neonates than it is in children [681].

The reduced dose requirement in neonates is attributable to immaturity of the neuromuscular junction. The increased volume of distribution from an expanded ECF in neonates means a similar initial dose is given to neonates and teenagers. The reason for the larger dose requirement in children compared with adults is unclear but it may be the result of increased muscle bulk.

Investigation of concentration-response relationships is more revealing. The plasma concentration required in neonates to achieve the same level of neuromuscular block as in children or adults is 20–50 % less [89, 682–685], consistent with immaturity of the neuromuscular junction. Plasma concentration requirements are reduced by volatile anesthetic

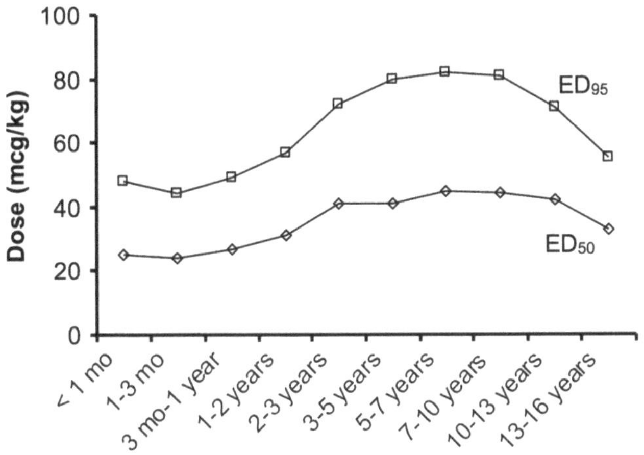

Fig. 3.20 Dose changes with age for vecuronium during balanced anesthesia. ED_{50} is the dose that achieves 50 % of the maximum response, while ED_{95} is the dose that achieves 95 % of the maximum response. Data from Meretoja et al. [676]

agents [345, 686, 687]. The onset time for NMBDs in neonates is faster than it is in older children than adults. Onset time (time to maximal effect) after vecuronium of 70 mcg/kg was most rapid for infants (1.5 SD 0.6 min) compared with that for children (2.4 SD 1.4 min) and adults (2.9 SD 0.2 min) [681].

These observations are similar to those reported for other intermediate- and long-acting NMBDs [672]. Rocuronium is currently the most popular NMBD in children, but studies in neonates are limited. In a study of 0.45 or 0.6 mg/kg rocuronium IV during isoflurane anesthesia in neonates and infants, the onset of neuromuscular blockade in neonates was exceedingly rapid onset (~15–30 s) compared with older infants (60 s), although recovery to a TOF of 70 % was slower in neonates, 62 min with 0.45 mg/kg and 95 min with 0.6 mg/kg compared with older infants by almost 50 % [346]. In late preterm infants, 0.5 mg/kg rocuronium was administered to facilitate tracheal intubation during fentanyl analgesia. Although paralysis was determined visually, by the absence of respiration and movement, the time to onset of neuromuscular weakness was ~55 s. Recovery from neuromuscular blockade was determined by the return of respiration and/or movement. Recovery averaged only 10 min after 0.5 mg/kg rocuronium but ranged from 2 to 60 min [688]. In a study of rocuronium of 0.3 mg/kg IV in neonates, infants, and children anesthetized with halothane, the onset of neuromuscular blockade was less, the frequency of a TOF >70 % greater and the duration of blockade greater in neonates and infants <6 months of age compared with older infants 6–24 months of age and children >2 years of age [689]. The current data indicates the dose of rocuronium in neonates must be carefully scaled back (to 0.3–0.45 mg/kg) to account for its protracted duration of action. The more rapid onset of these drugs in neonates has been attributed to a greater cardiac output seen with the per kilogram model [672].

Cardiac output is used as a surrogate measure for muscle perfusion. Onset time is a function of size. An onset time standardized to a 70-kg person using an allometric ¼ power model is around 3 min. In children with low cardiac output or decreased muscle perfusion, onset times are prolonged. The onset time of neuromuscular paralysis is proportional to $T_{1/2}$keo. An increase in the $T_{1/2}$keo of d-tubocurare with increasing inspired halothane concentration has been demonstrated [690]. The reason for the delayed action of tubocurarine may be that halothane is both a negative inotrope [691] and decreases muscle blood flow [692].

Succinylcholine remains the NMBD with the more rapid onset. The onset time of a paralyzing dose (1.0 mg/kg) of succinylcholine 1 mg/kg is 35–55 s in children and adolescents. The onset time after 3 mg/kg in neonates is faster (30–40 s) [693]. Onset time is dependent on both age and dose; the younger the child and the greater the dose, the shorter the onset time. The onset times of equipotent doses of succinylcholine (0.9 min) and mivacurium (1.4 min) in infants (2–12 months) and children (1–12 years) are very similar [694]. Consequently an argument can be made for the use of larger dose of an intermediate-duration NMBD rather than succinylcholine for rapid sequence intubation. However, use of increased dose of such drugs in the neonate will also prolong neuromuscular blockade. There is also potential for increased adverse effects (e.g., pain on injection, tachycardia). Phase II blockade may also develop with high or repeat succinylcholine dosing [695]. Succinylcholine may be given as an intramuscular injection for intubation in children [696]. There are few data available from neonates, but infant studies suggest that a dose of up to 5 mg/kg may be required to achieve satisfactory intubating conditions [697]. Onset to maximum blockade is slow (4 SD 6 min), and mean full recovery of T1 occurred in 15.6 SD 0.9 min after injection [697]. The slow onset time limits the usefulness of this technique. Intralingual or submental routes have also been used in children but there are no neonatal data.

Pharmacokinetics

The dose of NMBDs at different ages depends on a complex interweaving of pharmacodynamic and pharmacokinetic factors. Fisher et al. [89] unravelled some of these aspects for d-tubocurarine in children (Table 3.4). The volume of distribution mirrors ECF changes and can be predicted using either an allometric ¾ power model or the surface area model, both of which approximate ECF changes with weight. This occurs because ECF is a major contributor to the volume of distribution at steady state (Vss). These volume

Table 3.4 Age-related pharmacokinetics (SD) of d-tubocurarine

	Weight (kg)	CL (mL/min/kg)	CL surface area (mL/min/m²)	CL allometric 3/4 (mL/min/70 kg)
(A) Total body clearance				
Neonate (1 day to 2 months)	3.5	3.7 (2.1)	56 (32)	122 (70)
Infant (2 months to 1 year)	7	3.3 (0.4)	59 (7)	130 (15)
Child (1–12 years)	22	4 (1.1)	110 (30)	210 (58)
Adult (12–30 years)	60	3 (0.8)	115 (31)	202 (54)

(B) Volume of distribution at steady state	Weight (kg)	Vdss (L/kg)	Vdss surface area (L/m²)	Vdss allometric (power 1) (L/70 kg)	Vdss allometric (power ¾) (L/70 kg)
Neonate	3.5	0.74 (0.33)	11 (5)	52 (23)	25 (11)
Infant	7	0.52 (0.22)	9 (4)	36 (15)	21 (9)
Child	22	0.41 (0.12)	11 (3)	29 (8)	22 (6)
Adult	60	0.3 (0.1)	12 (4)	21 (7)	20 (7)

(C) Half-times	Chronological time (min)			Physiological time (min)		
	$T_{1/2}\alpha$	$T_{1/2}\beta$	$T_{1/2}$keo	$T_{1/2}\alpha$	$T_{1/2}\beta$	$T_{1/2}$keo
Neonate	4.1 (2.2)	174 (60)	6.3 (3.5)	8.7 (4.7)	368 (127)	13.3 (7.4)
Infant	7.0 (4)	130 (54)	7.5 (3.5)	12.9 (7.4)	240 (100)	13.9 (6.5)
Child	6.7 (2.4)	90 (23)	7.9 (2.7)	8.9 (3.2)	120 (31)	10.6 (3.6)
Adult	7.9 (4.1)	89 (18)	6.8 (1.9)	8.2 (4.3)	93 (19)	7.1 (2.0)

Data taken from Fisher DM et al. *Anesthesiology* 1982; 57: 203–8 [89]

changes are true for both depolarizing (succinylcholine) [698–700] and non-depolarizing NMBDs [701].

The clearance of d-tubocurarine, standardized to an allometric or surface area model, is reduced in neonates and infants compared with older children and adults [89]. These age-related clearance changes follow age-related maturation of glomerular filtration in the kidney [84], which is the elimination route of d-tubocurarine. Total plasma clearance of other non-depolarizing muscle relaxants cleared by renal (alcuronium) and/or hepatic pathways (pancuronium, pipecuronium, rocuronium and vecuronium) is all reduced in neonates [682, 684, 702–704]. In contrast, the clearances of atracurium and cisatracurium are neither renal nor hepatic dependent but rather depend on Hofmann elimination, ester hydrolysis and other unspecified pathways [705]. Clearance of these drugs is increased in neonates when expressed as per kilogram [706–708]. When clearance is standardized using allometric ¾ power scaling, the clearances for atracurium and cisatracurium are similar throughout all age groups. The clearance of succinylcholine, expressed as per kilogram, also decreases as age increases [81, 82]. Succinylcholine is hydrolyzed by butyryl-cholinesterase. These observations are consistent with that observed for the clearance of remifentanil [485], which is also cleared by plasma esterases. These clearance pathways are mature at birth. Conversion of d-tubocurarine half-times from chronological time to physiologic time is revealing. $T_{1/2}\alpha$ increases with age in chronological time, but in physiologic time it is the same at all ages, as we would expect from a distribution phase standardized by allometry. $T_{1/2}\beta$ decreases with age in physiologic time, consistent with reduced clearance related to volume in the very young. The $T_{1/2}$keo is large in neonates and infants, reduced in children and further reduced in adults. The cause of this change with age is uncertain but may be related to increased muscle bulk and concomitant increased muscle perfusion in older children and adults.

Antagonism of Neuromuscular Blockade

Although edrophonium may establish a faster onset of effect, final recovery is invariably greater with neostigmine, which is why the latter is recommended for routine pediatric practice [709, 710]. The distribution volumes of neostigmine are similar in infants (2–10 months), children (1–6 years), and adults (Vss of 0.5 L/kg), whereas the elimination half-life is less in the pediatric patients [711]. Clearance decreases as age increases (13.6, 11.1, 9.6 mL/min/kg in infants, children and adults 29–48 years) [711] as we might expect from allometric scaling. The dose of neostigmine required to reverse d-tubocurare blockade was 30–40 % less for infants and children than for adults (expressed as per kilogram) with a duration of effect of neostigmine similar in both pediatric and adult patients. Other studies have confirmed that a train-of-four (TOF) ratio recovers to 0.7 in less than ten minutes when a 90 % neuromuscular blockade from pancuronium is antagonized with neostigmine 30–40 μg/kg in infants, children or adults [710, 712–714]. Neonates recover more rapidly to full strength after neostigmine antagonism than older children [710, 715].

For example, antagonizing an atracurium-induced 90 % neuromuscular block in infants and children by neostigmine 50 μg/kg was fastest in the youngest age group [709]. The time to a TOF ratio of 0.7 was 4 min in neonates and infants, 6 min in 2–10-year-old children and 8 min in adolescents. These observations are consistent with allometric models for size [35].

Sugammadex is a new drug that reverses the NMB effects of rocuronium and, to a lesser extent, vecuronium. It has a cylinder-like cyclodextrin structure that irreversibly encapsulates rocuronium into its cavity. An early sugammadex study in children suggests that sugammadex of 2 mg/kg reverses a rocuronium-induced moderate neuromuscular blockade in infants, children and adolescents [716].

The average time to recover a TOF ratio of 0.9 at the time of appearance of the second twitch response was 1.2, 1.1, and 1.2 min in children, adolescents, and adults, respectively. Sugammadex is cleared through the renal system and the elimination kinetics are known to be prolonged in renal failure.

Although GFR is immature in neonates, this is unlikely to be of consequence here. Sugammadex has been used in patients with end-stage renal failure [717–719] with similar reversal characteristics as those with normal renal function.

Adverse Effects

Succinylcholine is the most pilloried NMBD despite its importance for rapid sequence intubation [720–722]. Its molecular structure resembles that of two acetylcholine molecules joined by an ester linkage. Consequently, stimulation of cholinergic autonomic receptors can be associated with cardiac arrhythmias, increased salivation and bronchial secretions. Muscle fasciculation is also associated with mild hyperkalemia (0.2 mmol/L), increased intragastric and intraocular pressure, masseter spasm, and skeletal muscle pains. Severe hyperkalemia may occur in patients with burns, paraplegia, trauma or disuse atrophy. This may be associated with rhabdomyolysis and myoglobinemia in those patients suffering certain neuromuscular disorders (e.g., Duchenne's muscular dystrophy). These disorders are not always diagnosable in neonates. Congenital myotonic dystrophy, for example, may present with mild respiratory dysfunction or feeding difficulty in the neonate. The response to succinylcholine in these neonates, however, remains dramatic with sustained muscle contraction [723]. Succinylcholine is a trigger agent for malignant hyperthermia. Succinylcholine has a prolonged effect in children with butyryl-cholinesterase deficiency. This is an inherited disease due to the presence of one or more abnormal genes (atypical, fluoride-resistant, and silent genes) [656]. On the other hand, one genetic variant, the Cynthiana or Nietlich variant, represents an ultrarapid degradation of succinylcholine [724].

The non-depolarizing NMBDs all have different adverse effects that are often used to therapeutic advantage. d-Tubocurarine may produce hypotension and bronchospasm after large doses and a rapid administration. Pancuronium confers sympathomimetic effects as a result of blocking the reuptake of noradrenaline; the resultant tachycardia may augment cardiac output during induction for cardiac surgery in neonates. Doses in excess of the ED_{95} of rocuronium have also proven popular for cardiac surgery to capitalize on its vagolytic activity that increases heart rate. Unfortunately, rocuronium also causes local pain when injected rapidly and may trigger anaphylaxis. Atracurium can liberate histamine precipitating bronchospasm and hypotension. These effects are attenuated with the isomer cisatracurium.

Anticholinergic Drugs

These drugs block acetylcholine at the postganglionic cholinergic (parasympathetic) endings. They also block the direct vasodilator effect of acetylcholine on blood vessels (antimuscarinic) and in the CNS. They cause mydriasis and tachycardias, increase intraocular pressure, inhibit sweating, reduce salivation, decrease lower esophageal sphincter tone and have similar effects on tone in the digestive and urinary tracts. Atropine, scopolamine, and glycopyrrolate are the three commonly used anticholinergic drugs in anesthesia. Differences in clinical effects are not very prominent in healthy patients [725].

While these drugs are commonly administered with the anticholinesterases to reverse residual neuromuscular blockade, their routine use in neonatal anesthesia is declining [726]. The benefits of reduced secretions or prevention of bradycardia during otolaryngological surgery, eye surgery and endoscopic procedures in children less than one year of age justify their use by some [727], but this continues to be debated [728]. Bradycardia and desaturation continue to complicate neonatal intubation [729]. Anticholinergics were used in the past to reduce salivation associated with ketamine, but the use of ketamine is also declining in neonates, while neuroapoptotic effects are investigated.

Atropine

Atropine is metabolized in the liver by *N*-demethylation followed by conjugation with glucuronic acid [730]; both processes are immature in the neonate. Approximately 50 % of the drug is eliminated by the kidneys unchanged. An old technique to diagnose atropine poisoning was to put a drop of the victim's urine into the eye of a cat and observe for mydriasis.

It is anticipated that the clearance of atropine is reduced in neonates because of immature renal and hepatic functions, although confirmatory data remain elusive. Children <2 years of age demonstrate an increased volume of distribution as steady state (3.2 SD 1.5 vs. 1.3 SD 0.5 L/kg) compared with those older than 2 years [731]. Clearance was similar in those aged less than 2 years (6.8 SD 5.3 mL/min/kg) and those older than 2 years (6.5 SD 1.6 mL/min/kg). The elimination half-life in healthy adults is 3 SD 0.9 h, whereas that in term neonates is 4 times greater [454]. No data have been forthcoming in preterm neonates [731, 732]. Pharmacodynamic responses to atropine in neonates have been limited. Infants <6 months of age required a larger dose of atropine to increase the heart rate compared with older children during halothane anesthesia [243]. Indeed, a small dose, 5 mcg/kg, did not change the heart rate. In addition, a wide range of doses of atropine (5–40 mcg/kg) had no substantive effect on the systolic blood pressure. However, current pediatric literature cautions against doses of atropine less than 0.1 mg independent of the child's weight [733], although some have voiced their criticism of this dosing [733]. If one adhered to this minimum dose recommendation, one would have to give a 1-kg infant 100 mcg/kg for anticholinergic prophylaxis, a dose that constitutes a massive anticholinergic overdose. The rationale for this dosing must be evidence based. Historically, this recommendation appears to be founded in an early study in children and adults who received atropine, of whom only 5 subjects were between 6 weeks and 2.9 years of age [735]. They found that repeated doses of atropine of 1.8 μg/kg IV did not increase the heart rate in the younger age group as much as the older children and adults, leading them to caution against small doses of atropine in young children. However, no bradycardias occurred. Recently, the electrophysiological responses to atropine of 5 mcg/kg IV during sevoflurane anesthesia were reported in 60 infants <15 kg; no bradycardia or life-threatening arrhythmias were detected as expected [736]. These data provide compelling evidence that there is no minimum dose of atropine; 5 mcg/kg IV does not cause bradycardia or other arrhythmias in infants.

Maximum heart rate change and minimum saliva flow occurred within 7–8 min after intravenous drug administration in adults, but data in neonates are lacking [737].

Scopolamine

Scopolamine is a tertiary amine with greater CNS effects than atropine, causing sedation and amnesia. Its moderate antiemetic activity [738] is of limited use in neonates. The drug, combined with morphine, was a popular intramuscular premedication in the past, but is unsuitable for use in neonates. Routine intramuscular premedication has lost favor and intramuscular morphine-scopolamine causes hypercarbia and oxygen desaturation [739]. Scopolamine is less effective for blocking the cardiac vagal response and has a greater drying effect compared with atropine, although these differences in clinical effects are not very prominent in healthy patients [725]. A direct correlation between serum concentrations of scopolamine and changes in EEG signals in adults is reported, but there are no neonatal data [740].

Scopolamine has a distribution volume of 1.4 L/kg [741] in adults. Glucuronide conjugation, sulfate conjugation and hydrolysis by the CYP3A family are involved in its clearance [740]. Both glucuronidation and the CYP3A enzyme systems are immature at birth and clearance is likely reduced. The pharmacokinetics of scopolamine is poorly understood [741].

Glycopyrrolate

Glycopyrrolate is quaternary ammonium compound with poor CNS penetration. It has pronounced antisialagogue activity [742], but there were no differences in heart rate, demeanor or facial flushing after intramuscular injection of atropine or glycopyrrolate in 80 infants under 1 year of age [743].

Glycopyrrolate remains popular for antagonizing the parasympathomimetic effects of neostigmine and is as effective as atropine for preventing the oculocardiac reflex [744].

Absorption from the gastrointestinal tract tract is poor (10–25 %) [745]. Clearance in children less than 1 year of age ($n=8$) was 1.01 L/kg/h (range 0.32–1.85 L/kg/h) and Vss of 1.83 L/kg (range 0.70–3.87 L/kg), but there are no neonatal data. The renal system accounts for 85 % of elimination [746] and clearance is anticipated to be reduced in neonates because renal function is immature [84].

Adverse Effects

Poisoning signs and symptoms in adults can be described as "hot as a hare, blind as a bat, dry as a bone, red as a beet and mad as a hen" [747]. These relate to the peripheral effects of dry mouth, blurred vision, and hot, dry skin; central effects contribute hyperpyrexia, restlessness, anxiety, excitement, hallucinations, delirium and mania. Cerebral depression and death can occur in severe poisoning. The mydriatic effect on the eye when solanaceous plant (e.g., *Atropa belladonna*) extract is used topically has been employed by women to lure male suitors even though it causes the female to be somewhat uncertain of her beau's features.

The vagal response is greater in neonates than adults. The resulting tachycardia may be beneficial during anesthesia in neonates with their rate-dependent cardiac output. Propofol in combination with remifentanil can cause profound bradycardia during induction, as may repeat dosing of succinylcholine, laryngeal instrumentation, and surgical manipulation of the eye, testes, and hollow viscera. Prophylactic use of atropine may preclude bradycardia under these circumstances [748]. Hypoxemia, however, is the commonest cause of bradycardia and this must be managed with oxygen, not atropine.

References

1. Berde C. Convulsions associated with pediatric regional anesthesia. Anesth Analg. 1992;75:164–6.
2. Arnold JH, Truog RD, Scavone JM, Fenton T. Changes in the pharmacodynamic response to fentanyl in neonates during continuous infusion. J Pediatr. 1991;119:639–43.
3. Sheiner LB. The population approach to pharmacokinetic data analysis: rationale and standard data analysis methods. Drug Metab Rev. 1984;15:153–71.
4. Sheiner LB, Stanski DR, Vozeh S, Miller RD, Ham J. Simultaneous modeling of pharmacokinetics and pharmacodynamics: application to D-tubocurarine. Clin Pharmacol Ther. 1979;25:358–71.
5. Tod M, Jullien V, Pons G. Facilitation of drug evaluation in children by population methods and modelling. Clin Pharmacokinet. 2008;47:231–43.
6. West GB, Brown JH. The origin of allometric scaling laws in biology from genomes to ecosystems: towards a quantitative unifying theory of biological structure and organization. J Exp Biol. 2005;208:1575–92.
7. West GB, Brown JH, Enquist BJ. A general model for the origin of allometric scaling laws in biology. Science. 1997;276:122–6.
8. Anderson BJ, Holford NH. Mechanism-based concepts of size and maturity in pharmacokinetics. Annu Rev Pharmacol Toxicol. 2008;48:303–32.
9. Johnson TN. The problems in scaling adult drug doses to children. Arch Dis Child. 2008;93:207–11.
10. Edginton AN, Schmitt W, Voith B, Willmann S. A mechanistic approach for the scaling of clearance in children. Clin Pharmacokinet. 2006;45:683–704.
11. Peeters MY, Allegaert K, van Oud-Alblas HJB, et al. Prediction of propofol clearance in children from an allometric model developed in rats, children and adults versus a 0.75 fixed-exponent allometric model. Clin Pharmacokinet. 2010;49:269–75.
12. Hill AV. The possible effects of the aggregation of the molecules of haemoglobin on its dissociation curves. J Physiol. 1910;14:iv–vii.
13. Richards FJ. A flexible growth function for empirical use. J Exp Bot. 1959;10:290–301.
14. Allegaert K, Anderson BJ, Verbesselt R, et al. Tramadol disposition in the very young: an attempt to assess in vivo cytochrome P-450 2D6 activity. Br J Anaesth. 2005;95:231–9.
15. Conney AH, Davison C, Gastel R, Burns JJ. Adaptive increases in drug-metabolizing enzymes induced by phenobarbital and other drugs. J Pharmacol Exp Ther. 1960;130:1–8.
16. Perucca E. Clinically relevant drug interactions with antiepileptic drugs. Br J Clin Pharmacol. 2006;61:246–55.
17. Strolin Benedetti M, Ruty B, Baltes E. Induction of endogenous pathways by antiepileptics and clinical implications. Fundam Clin Pharmacol. 2005;19:511–29.
18. Corcos L, Lagadic-Gossmann D. Gene induction by Phenobarbital: an update on an old question that receives key novel answers. Pharmacol Toxicol. 2001;89:113–22.
19. Eker HE, Yalcin Cok O, Aribogan A, Arslan G. Children on phenobarbital monotherapy requires more sedatives during MRI. Paediatr Anaesth. 2011;21(10):998–1002.
20. Grand RJ, Watkins JB, Torti FM. Development of the human intestinal tract: a review. Gastroenterology. 1976;70:790–810.
21. Liang J, Co E, Zhang M, Pineda J, Chen JD. Development of gastric slow waves in preterm infants measured by electrogastrography. Am J Physiol. 1998;274:G503–8.
22. Funk RS, Brown JT, Abdel-Rahman SM. Pediatric pharmacokinetics: human development and drug disposition. Pedaiatr Clin N Am. 2012;59:1001–16.
23. Anderson BJ, van Lingen RA, Hansen TG, Lin YC, Holford NH. Acetaminophen developmental pharmacokinetics in premature neonates and infants: a pooled population analysis. Anesthesiology. 2002;96:1336–45.
24. van Hoogdalem E, de Boer AG, Breimer DD. Pharmacokinetics of rectal drug administration, Part I. General considerations and clinical applications of centrally acting drugs. Clin Pharmacokinet. 1991;21:11–26.
25. Taddio A, Stevens B, Craig K, et al. Efficacy and safety of lidocaine-prilocaine cream for pain during circumcision. N Engl J Med. 1997;336:1197–201.
26. Salanitre E, Rackow H. The pulmonary exchange of nitrous oxide and halothane in infants and children. Anesthesiology. 1969;30:388–94.
27. Lerman J. Pharmacology of inhalational anaesthetics in infants and children. Paediatr Anaesth. 1992;2:191–203.
28. Malviya S, Lerman J. The blood/gas solubilities of sevoflurane, isoflurane, halothane, and serum constituent concentrations in neonates and adults. Anesthesiology. 1990;72:793–6.
29. Friis-Hansen B. Body water compartments in children: changes during growth and related changes in body composition. Pediatrics. 1961;28:169–81.
30. Johnson KL, Erickson JP, Holley FO, et al. Fentanyl pharmacokinetics in the paediatric population. Anesthesiology. 1984;61:A441.
31. Luz G, Innerhofer P, Bachmann B, Frischhut B, Menardi G, Benzer A. Bupivacaine plasma concentrations during continuous epidural anesthesia in infants and children. Anesth Analg. 1996;82:231–4.
32. Luz G, Wieser C, Innerhofer P, Frischhut B, Ulmer H, Benzer A. Free and total bupivacaine plasma concentrations after continuous epidural anaesthesia in infants and children. Paediatr Anaesth. 1998;8:473–8.
33. Huang Z, Ung T. Effect of alpha-1-acid glycoprotein binding on pharmacokinetics and pharmacodynamics. Curr Drug Metab. 2013;14:226–38.
34. Erichsen CJ, Sjovall J, Kehlet H, Hedlund C, Arvidsson T. Pharmacokinetics and analgesic effect of ropivacaine during continuous epidural infusion for postoperative pain relief. Anesthesiology. 1996;84:834–42.
35. Anderson BJ, McKee AD, Holford NH. Size, myths and the clinical pharmacokinetics of analgesia in paediatric patients. Clin Pharmacokinet. 1997;33:313–27.
36. Bosenberg AT, Thomas J, Cronje L, et al. Pharmacokinetics and efficacy of ropivacaine for continuous epidural infusion in neonates and infants. Paediatr Anaesth. 2005;15:739–49.
37. Russo H, Bressolle F. Pharmacodynamics and pharmacokinetics of thiopental. Clin Pharmacokinet. 1998;35:95–134.
38. Bjorkman S. Prediction of drug disposition in infants and children by means of physiologically based pharmacokinetic (PBPK) modelling: theophylline and midazolam as model drugs. Br J Clin Pharmacol. 2005;59:691–704.
39. Johnson TN, Tucker GT, Tanner MS, Rostami-Hodjegan A. Changes in liver volume from birth to adulthood: a meta-analysis. Liver Transpl. 2005;11:1481–93.

40. Way WL, Costley EC, Way EL. Respiratory sensitivity of the newborn infant to meperidine and morphine. Clin Pharmacol Ther. 1965;6:454–61.
41. Pokela ML, Olkkola KT, Seppala T, Koivisto M. Age-related morphine kinetics in infants. Dev Pharmacol Ther. 1993;20:26–34.
42. Lynn AM, Nespeca MK, Opheim KE, Slattery JT. Respiratory effects of intravenous morphine infusions in neonates, infants, and children after cardiac surgery. Anesth Analg. 1993;77:695–701.
43. Engelhardt B. Development of the blood-brain barrier. Cell Tissue Res. 2003;314:119–29.
44. Henthorn TK, Liu Y, Mahapatro M, Ng KY. Active transport of fentanyl by the blood-brain barrier. J Pharmacol Exp Ther. 1999;289:1084–9.
45. Hamabe W, Maeda T, Kiguchi N, Yamamoto C, Tokuyama S, Kishioka S. Negative relationship between morphine analgesia and P-glycoprotein expression levels in the brain. J Pharmacol Sci. 2007;105:353–60.
46. Daood MJ, Tsai C, Addab-Barmada M, Watchko JF. ABC transporter (P-gp/ABCB1, MRPl/ABCC1, BCRP/ABCG2) expression in the developing human CNS. Neuropediatrics. 2008;39:211.
47. Choudhuri S, Klaassen CD. Structure, function, expression, genomic organization, and single nucleotide polymorphisms of human ABCB1 (MDR1), ABCC (MRP), and ABCG2 (BCRP) efflux transporters. Int J Toxicol. 2006;25:231–59.
48. Hajj A, Khabbaz L, Laplanche JL, Peoc'h K. Pharmacogenetics of opiates in clinical practice: the visible tip of the iceberg. Pharmacogenomics. 2013;14:575–85.
49. Hines RN, McCarver DG. The ontogeny of human drug-metabolizing enzymes: phase I oxidative enzymes. J Pharmacol Exp Ther. 2002;300:355–60.
50. Koukouritaki SB, Manro JR, Marsh SA, et al. Developmental expression of human hepatic CYP2C9 and CYP2C19. J Pharmacol Exp Ther. 2004;308:965–74. Epub 2003 Nov 21.
51. Allegaert K, van de Velde M, van den Anker J. Neonatal clinical pharmacology. Pediatr Anesth. 2014;24(1):30–8. doi:10.1111/pan.12176.
52. Cuzzolin L. Drug metabolizing enzymes in the perinatal and neonatal period: differences in the expression and activity. Curr Drug Metab. 2013;14:167–73.
53. Johnsrud EK, Koukouritaki SB, Divakaran K, Brunengraber LL, Hines RN, McCarver DG. Human hepatic CYP2E1 expression during development. J Pharmacol Exp Ther. 2003;307:402–7.
54. Kearns GL, Abdel-Rahman SM, Alander SW, Blowey DL, Leeder JS, Kauffman RE. Developmental pharmacology–drug disposition, action, and therapy in infants and children. N Engl J Med. 2003;349:1157–67.
55. Anderson BJ, Hansen TG. Getting the best from pediatric pharmacokinetic data. Paediatr Anaesth. 2004;14:713–15.
56. Chalkiadis GA, Anderson BJ. Age and size are the major covariates for prediction of levobupivacaine clearance in children. Paediatr Anaesth. 2006;16:275–82.
57. de Wildt SN, Kearns GL, Leeder JS, van den Anker JN. Cytochrome P450 3A: ontogeny and drug disposition. Clin Pharmacokinet. 1999;37:485–505.
58. Ma JD, Lee KC, Kuo GM. Clinical application of pharmacogenomics. J Pharm Pract. 2012;25:417–27.
59. Davis L, Britten JJ, Morgan M. Cholinesterase: its significance in anaesthetic practice. Anaesthesia. 1997;52:244–60.
60. Neville KA, Becker ML, Goldman JL, Kearns GL. Developmental pharmacogenomics. Pediatr Anesth. 2011;21:255–65.
61. McCarver DG, Hines RN. The ontogeny of human drug-metabolizing enzymes: phase II conjugation enzymes and regulatory mechanisms. J Pharmacol Exp Ther. 2002;300:361–6.
62. Anderson BJ, Holford NH. Mechanistic basis of using body size and maturation to predict clearance in humans. Drug Metab Pharmacokinet. 2009;24:25–36.
63. Bouwmeester NJ, Anderson BJ, Tibboel D, Holford NH. Developmental pharmacokinetics of morphine and its metabolites in neonates, infants and young children. Br J Anaesth. 2004;92:208–17.
64. Anand KJ, Anderson BJ, Holford NH, et al. Morphine pharmacokinetics and pharmacodynamics in preterm and term neonates: secondary results from the NEOPAIN trial. Br J Anaesth. 2008;101:680–9.
65. Holford NHG, Ma SC, Anderson BJ. Prediction of morphine dose in humans. Pediatr Anesth. 2012;22:209–22.
66. Anderson BJ, Woollard GA, Holford NH. A model for size and age changes in the pharmacokinetics of paracetamol in neonates, infants and children. Br J Clin Pharmacol. 2000;50:125–34.
67. Anderson BJ, Pons G, Autret-Leca E, Allegaert K, Boccard E. Pediatric intravenous paracetamol (propacetamol) pharmacokinetics: a population analysis. Pediatr Anesth. 2005;15:282–92.
68. Potts AL, Warman GR, Anderson BJ. Dexmedetomidine disposition in children: a population analysis. Paediatr Anaesth. 2008;18:722–30.
69. Allegaert K, Peeters MY, Verbesselt R, et al. Inter-individual variability in propofol pharmacokinetics in preterm and term neonates. Br J Anaesth. 2007;99:864–70.
70. Allegaert K, Vancraeynest J, Rayyan M, et al. Urinary propofol metabolites in early life after single intravenous bolus. Br J Anaesth. 2008;101(6):827–31.
71. Lynn A, Nespeca MK, Bratton SL, Strauss SG, Shen DD. Clearance of morphine in postoperative infants during intravenous infusion: the influence of age and surgery. Anesth Analg. 1998;86:958–63.
72. Peters JW, Anderson BJ, Simons SH, Uges DR, Tibboel D. Morphine pharmacokinetics during venoarterial extracorporeal membrane oxygenation in neonates. Intensive Care Med. 2005;31:257–63.
73. Rigby-Jones AE, Nolan JA, Priston MJ, Wright PM, Sneyd JR, Wolf AR. Pharmacokinetics of propofol infusions in critically ill neonates, infants, and children in an intensive care unit. Anesthesiology. 2002;97:1393–400.
74. Welzing L, Ebenfeld S, Dlugay V, Wiesen MH, Roth B, Mueller C. Remifentanil degradation in umbilical cord blood of preterm infants. Anesthesiology. 2011;114:570–7.
75. Rigby-Jones AE, Priston MJ, Thorne GC, Tooley MA, Sneyd JR, Wolf AR. Population pharmacokinetics of remifentanil in critically ill post cardiac neonates, infants and children. Br J Anaesth. 2005;95:578P–9.
76. Minto CF, Schnider TW, Egan TD, et al. Influence of age and gender on the pharmacokinetics and pharmacodynamics of remifentanil. I. Model development. Anesthesiology. 1997;86:10–23.
77. Ross AK, Davis PJ, Dear Gd GL, et al. Pharmacokinetics of remifentanil in anesthetized pediatric patients undergoing elective surgery or diagnostic procedures. Anesth Analg. 2001;93:1393–401.
78. Kan RE, Hughes SC, Rosen MA, Kessin C, Preston PG, Lobo EP. Intravenous remifentanil: placental transfer, maternal and neonatal effects. Anesthesiology. 1998;88:1467–74.
79. Egan TD. Pharmacokinetics and pharmacodynamics of remifentanil: an update in the year 2000. Curr Opin Anaesthesiol. 2000;13:449–55.
80. Zsigmond EK, Downs JR. Plasma cholinesterase activity in newborns and infants. Can Anaesth Soc J. 1971;18:278–85.
81. Cook DR, Wingard LB, Taylor FH. Pharmacokinetics of succinylcholine in infants, children, and adults. Clin Pharmacol Ther. 1976;20:493–8.
82. Goudsouzian NG, Liu LM. The neuromuscular response of infants to a continuous infusion of succinylcholine. Anesthesiology. 1984;60:97–101.
83. Sawyer DC, Eger 2nd EI, Bahlman SH, Cullen BF, Impelman D. Concentration dependence of hepatic halothane metabolism. Anesthesiology. 1971;34:230–5.

84. Rhodin MM, Anderson BJ, Peters AM, et al. Human renal function maturation: a quantitative description using weight and postmenstrual age. Pediatr Nephrol. 2009;24:67–76.
85. Langhendries JP, Battisti O, Bertrand JM, et al. Adaptation in neonatology of the once-daily concept of aminoglycoside administration: evaluation of a dosing chart for amikacin in an intensive care unit. Biol Neonate. 1998;74:351–62.
86. Kharasch ED, Hankins DC, Thummel KE. Human kidney methoxyflurane and sevoflurane metabolism. Intrarenal fluoride production as a possible mechanism of methoxyflurane nephrotoxicity. Anesthesiology. 1995;82:689–99.
87. McNamara DG, Nixon GM, Anderson BJ. Methylxanthines for the treatment of apnea associated with bronchiolitis and anesthesia. Paediatr Anaesth. 2004;14:541–50.
88. Paradisis M, Jiang X, McLachlan AJ, Evans N, Kluckow M, Osborn D. Population pharmacokinetics and dosing regimen design of milrinone in preterm infants. Arch Dis Child Fetal Neonatal Ed. 2007;92:F204–9.
89. Fisher DM, O'Keeffe C, Stanski DR, Cronnelly R, Miller RD, Gregory GA. Pharmacokinetics and pharmacodynamics of d-tubocurarine in infants, children, and adults. Anesthesiology. 1982;57:203–8.
90. Allegaert K, Cossey V, Debeer A, et al. The impact of ibuprofen on renal clearance in preterm infants is independent of the gestational age. Pediatr Nephrol. 2005;20:740–3. Epub 2005 Mar 23.
91. Allegaert K, Cossey V, Langhendries JP, et al. Effects of co-administration of ibuprofen-lysine on the pharmacokinetics of amikacin in preterm infants during the first days of life. Biol Neonate. 2004;86:207–11.
92. Stephenson T. How children's responses to drugs differ from adults. Br J Clin Pharmacol. 2005;59:670–3.
93. LeDez KM, Lerman J. The minimum alveolar concentration (MAC) of isoflurane in preterm neonates. Anesthesiology. 1987;67:301–7.
94. Lerman J, Robinson S, Willis MM, Gregory GA. Anesthetic requirements for halothane in young children 0-1 month and 1-6 months of age. Anesthesiology. 1983;59:421–4.
95. Koch SC, Fitzgerald M, Hathway GJ. Midazolam potentiates nociceptive behavior, sensitizes cutaneous reflexes, and is devoid of sedative action in neonatal rats. Anesthesiology. 2008;108:122–9.
96. Tobin JR. Paradoxical effects of midazolam in the very young. Anesthesiology. 2008;108:6–7.
97. Meakin G, Morton RH, Wareham AC. Age-dependent variation in response to tubocurarine in the isolated rat diaphragm. Br J Anaesth. 1992;68:161–3.
98. Wareham AC, Morton RH, Meakin GH. Low quantal content of the endplate potential reduces safety factor for neuromuscular transmission in the diaphragm of the newborn rat. Br J Anaesth. 1994;72:205–9.
99. Radford D. Side effects of verapamil in infants. Arch Dis Child. 1983;58:465–6.
100. Steinberg C, Notterman DA. Pharmacokinetics of cardiovascular drugs in children. Inotropes and vasopressors. Clin Pharmacokinet. 1994;27:345–67.
101. Seri I, Tulassay T, Kiszel J, Machay T, Csomor S. Cardiovascular response to dopamine in hypotensive preterm neonates with severe hyaline membrane disease. Eur J Pediatr. 1984;142:3–9.
102. Cuevas L, Yeh TF, John EG, Cuevas D, Plides RS. The effect of low-dose dopamine infusion on cardiopulmonary and renal status in premature newborns with respiratory distress syndrome. Am J Dis Child. 1991;145:799–803.
103. Seri I, Tulassay T, Kiszel J, et al. Effect of low-dose dopamine infusion on prolactin and thyrotropin secretion in preterm infants with hyaline membrane disease. Biol Neonate. 1985;47:317–22.
104. Seri I. Dopamine and natriuresis. Mechanism of action and developmental aspects. Am J Hypertens. 1990;3:82S–6.
105. Kim HS, Oh AY, Kim CS, Kim SD, Seo KS, Kim JH. Correlation of bispectral index with end-tidal sevoflurane concentration and age in infants and children. Br J Anaesth. 2005;95:362–6.
106. Davidson AJ. Measuring anesthesia in children using the EEG. Pediatr Anesth. 2006;16:374–87.
107. Davidson AJ, Huang GH, Rebmann CS, Ellery C. Performance of entropy and Bispectral Index as measures of anaesthesia effect in children of different ages. Br J Anaesth. 2005;95:674–9.
108. Davidson AJ, Sale SM, Wong C, et al. The electroencephalograph during anesthesia and emergence in infants and children. Paediatr Anaesth. 2008;18:60–70.
109. Jeleazcov C, Schmidt J, Schmitz B, Becke K, Albrecht S. EEG variables as measures of arousal during propofol anaesthesia for general surgery in children: rational selection and age dependence. Br J Anaesth. 2007;99:845–54.
110. Solt K, Forman SA. Correlating the clinical actions and molecular mechanisms of general anesthetics. Curr Opin Anaesthesiol. 2007;20:300–6.
111. Grasshoff C, Drexler B, Rudolph U, Antkowiak B. Anaesthetic drugs: linking molecular actions to clinical effects. Curr Pharm Des. 2006;12:3665–79.
112. Billard V, Gambus PL, Chamoun N, Stanski DR, Shafer SL. A comparison of spectral edge, delta power, and bispectral index as EEG measures of alfentanil, propofol, and midazolam drug effect. Clin Pharmacol Ther. 1997;61:45–58.
113. Marsh B, White M, Morton N, Kenny GN. Pharmacokinetic model driven infusion of propofol in children. Br J Anaesth. 1991;67:41–8.
114. Peeters MY, Prins SA, Knibbe CA, et al. Propofol pharmacokinetics and pharmacodynamics for depth of sedation in nonventilated infants after major craniofacial surgery. Anesthesiology. 2006;104:466–74.
115. Kataria BK, Ved SA, Nicodemus HF, et al. The pharmacokinetics of propofol in children using three different data analysis approaches (see comments). Anesthesiology. 1994;80:104–22.
116. Gepts E, Camu F, Cockshott ID, Douglas EJ. Disposition of propofol administered as constant rate intravenous infusions in humans. Anesth Analg. 1987;66:1256–63.
117. Absalom A, Amutike D, Lal A, White M, Kenny GN. Accuracy of the 'Paedfusor' in children undergoing cardiac surgery or catheterization. Br J Anaesth. 2003;91:507–13.
118. Allegaert K, de Hoon J, Verbesselt R, Naulaers G, Murat I. Maturational pharmacokinetics of single intravenous bolus of propofol. Paediatr Anaesth. 2007;17:1028–34.
119. Anderson BJ. Pediatric models for adult target-controlled infusion pumps. Paediatr Anaesth. 2009;20(3):223–32.
120. Ghanta S, Abdel-Latif ME, Lui K, Ravindranathan H, Awad J, Oei J. Propofol compared with the morphine, atropine, and suxamethonium regimen as induction agents for neonatal endotracheal intubation: a randomized, controlled trial. Pediatrics. 2007;119:e1248–55.
121. Papoff P, Mancuso M, Caresta E, Moretti C. Effectiveness and safety of propofol in newborn infants. Pediatrics. 2008;121:448. author reply -9.
122. Veyckemans F. Propofol for intubation of the newborn? Pediatr Anesth. 2001;11:630–1.
123. Westrin P. The induction dose of propofol in infants 1-6 months of age and in children 10-16 years of age. Anesthesiology. 1991;74:455–8.
124. Allegaert K. Is propofol the perfect hypnotic agent for procedural sedation in neonates? Curr Clin Pharmacol. 2009;4:84–6.
125. Welzing L, Kribs A, Eifinger F, Huenseler C, Oberthuer A, Roth B. Propofol as an induction agent for endotracheal intubation can cause significant arterial hypotension in preterm neonates. Pediatr Anesth. 2010;20:605–11.

126. Clarke WR. The transitional circulation: physiology and anesthetic implications. J Clin Anesth. 1990;2:192–211.
127. Williams GD, Jones TK, Hanson KA, Morray JP. The hemodynamic effects of propofol in children with congenital heart disease. Anesth Analg. 1999;89:1411–16.
128. Veyckemans F. Propofol for intubation of the newborn? Pediatr Anesth. 2001;11:629–32.
129. Lerman J, Heard C, Steward DJ. Neonatal tracheal intubation: an imbroglio unresolved. Pediatr Anesth. 2010;20:585–90.
130. Vanderhaegen J, Naulaers G, Van Huffel S, Vanhole C, Allegaert K. Cerebral and systemic hemodynamic effects of intravenous bolus administration of propofol in neonates. Neonatology. 2009;98:57–63.
131. Nauta M, Onland W, De Jaegere A. Propofol as an induction agent for endotracheal intubation can cause significant arterial hypotension in preterm infants. Pediatr Anesth. 2011;21:711–12.
132. Domek NS, Barlow CF, Roth LJ. An ontogenetic study of phenobarbital-C-14 in cat brain. J Pharmacol Exp Ther. 1960; 130:285–93.
133. Mirkin BL. Perinatal pharmacology: placental transfer, fetal localization, and neonatal disposition of drugs. Anesthesiology. 1975;43:156–70.
134. Westrin P, Jonmarker C, Werner O. Thiopental requirements for induction of anesthesia in neonates and in infants one to six months of age. Anesthesiology. 1989;71:344–6.
135. Jonmarker C, Westrin P, Larsson S, Werner O. Thiopental requirements for induction of anesthesia in children. Anesthesiology. 1987;67:104–7.
136. Glantz LA, Gilmore JH, Hamer RM, Lieberman JA, Jarskog LF. Synaptophysin and postsynaptic density protein 95 in the human prefrontal cortex from mid-gestation into early adulthood. Neuroscience. 2007;149:582–91.
137. Norman E, Malmqvist U, Westrin P, Fellman V. Thiopental pharmacokinetics in newborn infants: a case report of overdose. Acta Paediatr. 2009;98:1680–2.
138. Stanski DR, Maitre PO. Population pharmacokinetics and pharmacodynamics of thiopental: the effect of age revisited [see comments]. Anesthesiology. 1990;72:412–22.
139. Lindsay WA, Shepherd J. Plasma levels of thiopentone after premedication with rectal suppositories in young children. Br J Anaesth. 1969;41:977–84.
140. Bonati M, Marraro G, Celardo A, et al. Thiopental efficacy in phenobarbital-resistant neonatal seizures. Dev Pharmacol Ther. 1990;15:16–20.
141. Garg DC, Goldberg RN, Woo-Ming RB, Weidler DJ. Pharmacokinetics of thiopental in the asphyxiated neonate. Dev Pharmacol Ther. 1988;11:213–18.
142. Demarquez JL, Galperine R, Billeaud C, Brachet-Liermain A. High-dose thiopental pharmacokinetics in brain-injured children and neonates. Dev Pharmacol Ther. 1987;10:292–300.
143. Gaspari F, Marraro G, Penna GF, Valsecchi R, Bonati M. Elimination kinetics of thiopentone in mothers and their newborn infants. Eur J Clin Pharmacol. 1985;28:321–5.
144. Larsson P, Anderson BJ, Norman E, Westrin P, Fellman V. Thiopentone elimination in newborn infants: exploring Michaelis-Menten kinetics. Acta Anaesthesiol Scand. 2011; 55:444–51.
145. Norman E, Westrin P, Fellman V. Placental transfer and pharmacokinetics of thiopentone in newborn infants. Arch Dis Child. 2010;95:F277–82.
146. Komai H, Rusy BF. Effect of thiopental on Ca2+ release from sarcoplasmic reticulum in intact myocardium. Anesthesiology. 1994;81:946–52.
147. Grant IS, Nimmo WS, McNicol LR, Clements JA. Ketamine disposition in children and adults. Br J Anaesth. 1983;55:1107–11.
148. Ihmsen H, Geisslinger G, Schuttler J. Stereoselective pharmacokinetics of ketamine: R(-)-ketamine inhibits the elimination of S(+)-ketamine. Clin Pharmacol Ther. 2001;70:431–8.
149. Cook RD, Davis PJ. Pediatric anesthesia pharmacology. In: Lake CL, editor. Pediatric cardiac anesthesia. 2nd ed. East Norwalk: Appleton & Lange; 1993. p. 134.
150. Hartvig P, Larsson E, Joachimsson PO. Postoperative analgesia and sedation following pediatric cardiac surgery using a constant infusion of ketamine. J Cardiothorac Vasc Anesth. 1993;7:148–53.
151. Chang T, Glazko AJ. Biotransformation and disposition of ketamine. Int Anesthesiol Clin. 1974;12:157–77.
152. Lockhart CH, Nelson WL. The relationship of ketamine requirement to age in pediatric patients. Anesthesiology. 1974;40:507–8.
153. Scallet AC, Schmued LC, Slikker Jr W, et al. Developmental neurotoxicity of ketamine: morphometric confirmation, exposure parameters, and multiple fluorescent labeling of apoptotic neurons. Toxicol Sci. 2004;81:364–70.
154. Paule MG, Li M, Allen RR, et al. Ketamine anesthesia during the first week of life can cause long-lasting cognitive deficits in rhesus monkeys. Neurotoxicol Teratol. 2011;33:220–30.
155. Brambrink AM, Evers AS, Avidan MS, et al. Ketamine-induced neuroapoptosis in the fetal and neonatal rhesus macaque brain. Anesthesiology. 2012;116:372–84.
156. Fredriksson A, Archer T, Alm H, Gordh T, Eriksson P. Neurofunctional deficits and potentiated apoptosis by neonatal NMDA antagonist administration. Behav Brain Res. 2004;153:367–76.
157. Wang C, Sadovova N, Fu X, et al. The role of the N-methyl-D-aspartate receptor in ketamine-induced apoptosis in rat forebrain culture. Neuroscience. 2005;132:967–77.
158. Shih J, May LDV, Gonzalez HE, et al. Delayed environmental enrichment reverses sevoflurane-induced memory impairment in rats. Anesthesiology. 2012;116:586–602.
159. Turner CP, Gutierrez S, Liu C, et al. Strategies to defeat ketamine-induced neonatal brain injury. Neuroscience. 2012;210:384–92.
160. Oz S, Ivashko-Pachima Y, Gozes I. The ADNP derived peptide, NAP modulates the tubulin pool: implication for neurotrophic and neuroprotective activities. PLoS One. 2012;7(12):e51458.
161. Soriano SG, Anand KJ, Rovnaghi CR, Hickey PR. Of mice and men: should we extrapolate rodent experimental data to the care of human neonates? Anesthesiology. 2005;102:866–8.
162. Anand KJ, Hall RW, Desai N, et al. Effects of morphine analgesia in ventilated preterm neonates: primary outcomes from the NEOPAIN randomised trial. Lancet. 2004;363:1673–82.
163. Steward DJ, Creighton RE. The uptake and excretion of nitrous oxide in the newborn. Can Anaesth Soc J. 1978;25:215–17.
164. Eger II EI. Anesthetic uptake and action. Baltimore: Williams & Wilkins; 1974.
165. Lerman J, Willis MM, Gregory GA, Eger II EI. Age and the solubility of volatile anesthetics in blood. Anesthesiology. 1984;61:139–43.
166. Lerman J, Gregory GA, Eger II EI. Hematocrit and the solubility of volatile anesthetics in blood. Anesth Analg. 1984;63:911–14.
167. Sinclair L, Strong HA, Lerman J. Effects of AAGP, local anesthetics and pH on the partition coefficients of halothane, enflurane and sevoflurane in blood and buffered saline (abstract). Can J Anaesth. 1988;35:S99.
168. Yasuda N, Lockhart SH, Eger II EI, Weiskopf RB, Liu J, Laster M, Taheri S, Peterson NA. Comparison kinetics of sevoflurane and isoflurane in humans. Anesth Analg. 1991;72:316–24.
169. Lerman J, Schmitt-Bantel BI, Willis MM, Gregory GA, Eger II EI. Effect of age on the solubility of volatile anesthetics in human tissues. Anesthesiology. 1986;65:63–7.

170. Gibbons RT, Steffey EP, Eger II EI. The effect of spontaneous versus controlled ventilation on the rate of rise of alveolar halothane concentration in dogs. Anesth Analg. 1977;56:32–4.
171. Huntington JH, Malviya S, Voepel-Lewis T, Lloyd TR, Massey KD. The effect of a right-to-left intracardiac shunt on the rate of rise of arterial and end-tidal halothane in children. Anesth Analg. 1999;88:759–62.
172. Burrows FA. Physiologic dead space, venous admixture, and the arterial to end-tidal carbon dioxide difference in infants and children undergoing cardiac surgery. Anesthesiology. 1989;70:219–25.
173. Eger II EI, Johnson BH. Rates of awakening from anesthesia with I-653, halothane, isoflurane and sevoflurane: a test of the effect of anesthetic concentration and duration in rats. Anesth Analg. 1987;66:977–82.
174. Naito Y, Tamai S, Shingu K, Fujimori R, Mori K. Comparison between sevoflurane and halothane for paediatric ambulatory anaesthesia. Br J Anaesth. 1991;67:387–9.
175. Davis PJ, Cohen IT, McGowan FX, Latta K. Recovery characteristics of desflurane versus halothane for maintenance of anesthesia in pediatric ambulatory patients. Anesthesiology. 1994;84:298–302.
176. Sarner JB, Levine M, Davis PJ, Lerman J, Cook RD, Motoyama EK. Clinical characteristics of sevoflurane in children: a comparison with halothane. Anesthesiology. 1995;82:38–46.
177. Bould MD, Sury MR. Defining awakening from anesthesia in neonates: a consensus study. Pediatr Anesth. 2011;21:259–63.
178. Gregory GA, Eger II EI, Munson ES. The relationship between age and halothane requirement in man. Anesthesiology. 1969;30: 488–91.
179. Diaz JH, Lockhart CH. Is halothane really safe in infancy? Anesthesiology. 1979;51:S313.
180. Taylor RH, Lerman J. Minimum alveolar concentration (MAC) of desflurane and hemodynamic responses in neonates, infants and children. Anesthesiology. 1991;75:975–9.
181. Lerman J, Kleinman S, Yentis SW, Sikich N. Pharmacology of sevoflurane in infants and children. Anesthesiology. 1994;80:814–24.
182. Cameron CB, Robinson S, Gregory GA. The minimum anesthetic concentration of isoflurane in children. Anesth Analg. 1984; 63:418–20.
183. Baum VC, Palmisano BW. The immature heart and anesthesia. Anesthesiology. 1997;87:1529–48.
184. Murray DJ, Forbes RB, Mahoney LT. Comparative hemodynamic depression of halothane versus isoflurane in neonates and infants: an echocardiographic study. Anesth Analg. 1992;74:329–37.
185. Murat I, Lapeyre G, Saint-Maurice C. Isoflurane attenuates baroreflex control of heart rate in human neonates. Anesthesiology. 1989;70:395–400.
186. Wolf AR, Humphry AT. LImitations and vulnerabilities of the neonatal cardiovascular system: considerations for anesthetic management. Pediatr Anesth. 2014;24:5–9.
187. Barash PG, Glanz S, Katz JD, Taunt K, Talner NS. Ventricular function in children during halothane anaesthetic: an echocardiographic evaluation. Anesthesiology. 1978;49:79–85.
188. Frei FJ, Haemmerle MH, Brunner R, Kern C. Minimum alveolar concentration for halothane in children with cerebral palsy and severe mental retardation. Anaesthesia. 1997;52:1056–60.
189. Tsunoda Y, Hattori Y, Takatsuka E, et al. Effects of hydroxyzine, diazepam and pentazocine on halothane minimum alveolar anesthetic concentration. Anesth Analg. 1973;52:390–4.
190. Perisho JA, Beuchel DR, Miller RD. The effect of diazepam (Valium®) on minimum alveolar anaesthetic requirement (MAC) in man. Can Anaesth Soc J. 1971;18:536–40.
191. Viegas O, Stoelting RK. Halothane MAC in dogs unchanged by phenobarbital. Anesth Analg. 1976;55:677–9.
192. Liem EB, Lin CM, Suleman MI, et al. Anesthetic requirement is increased in redheads. Anesthesiology. 2004;101:279–83.
193. Murray DJ, Mehta MP, Forbes RB, Dull DL. Additive contribution of nitrous oxide to halothane MAC in infants and children. Anesth Analg. 1990;71:120–4.
194. Murray DJ, Mehta MP, Forbes RB. The additive contribution of nitrous oxide to isoflurane MAC in infants and children. Anesthesiology. 1991;75:186–90.
195. Fisher DM, Zwass MS. MAC of desflurane in 60 % nitrous oxide in infants and children. Anesthesiology. 1992;76:354–6.
196. Swan HD, Crawford MW, Pua HL, Stephens D, Lerman J. Additive contribution of nitrous oxide to sevoflurane MAC for tracheal intubation in children. Anesthesiology. 1999;91:667–71.
197. Mellor DJ, Lerman J. Anesthesia for neonatal emergencies. Semin Perinatol. 1998;22:363–79.
198. Anderson BJ, Lerman J, Coté CJ, editors. Pharmacokinetics and pharmacology of drugs used in children. A practice of anesthesia for infants and children. 5th ed. Philadelphia, PA: Elsevier; 2013. Chap 6.
199. Yakaitis RW, Blitt CD, Angiulo JP. End-tidal halothane concentration for endotracheal intubation. Anesthesiology. 1977;47:386–8.
200. Watcha MF, Forestner JE, Connor MT, Dunn CM, Gunter JB, et al. Minimum alveolar concentration of halothane for tracheal intubation in children. Anesthesiology. 1988;69:412–16.
201. Yakaitis RW, Blitt CD, Angiulo JP. End-tidal enflurane concentration for endotracheal intubation. Anesthesiology. 1979;50:59–61.
202. Taguchi M, Watanabe S, Asakura N, Inomata S. End-tidal sevoflurane concentrations for laryngeal mask airway insertion and for tracheal intubation in children. Anesthesiology. 1994;81:628–31.
203. Nishina K, Mikawa K, Shiga M, Maekawa N, Obara H. Oral clonidine premedication reduces minimum alveolar concentration of sevoflurane for tracheal intubation in children. Anesthesiology. 1997;87:1324–7.
204. Neelakanta G, Miller J. Minimum alveolar concentration of isoflurane for tracheal extubation in deeply anesthetized children. Anesthesiology. 1994;80:811–13.
205. Cranfield KAW, Bromley LM. Minimum alveolar concentration of desflurane for tracheal extubation in deeply anaesthetized, unpremedicated children. Br J Anaesth. 1997;78:370–1.
206. Higuchi H, Ura T, Taoda M, Tanaka K, Satoh T. Minimum alveolar concentration of sevoflurane for tracheal extubation in children. Acta Anaesth Scand. 1997;41:911–13.
207. Inomata S, Suwa T, Toyooka H, Suto Y. End-tidal sevoflurane concentration for tracheal extubation and skin incision in children. Anesth Analg. 1998;87:1263–7.
208. Vutskits L. Cerebral blood flow in the neonate. Pediatr Anesth. 2014;24:22–9.
209. Eger II EI. Isoflurane: a review. Anesthesiology. 1981;55:559–76.
210. Bedforth NM, Girling KJ, Skinner HJ, et al. Effects of desflurane on cerebral autoregulation. Br J Anaesth. 2001;87:193–7.
211. Holmstrom A, Rosen I, Akeson J. Desflurane results in higher cerebral blood flow than sevoflurane or isoflurane at hypocapnia in pigs. Acta Anaesthesiol Scand. 2004;48:400–4.
212. Leon J, Bissonnette B. Cerebrovascular response to carbon dioxide in children anaesthetized with halothane and isoflurane. Can J Anaesth. 1991;38:817–24.
213. Paut O, Lazzell VA, Bissonnette B. The effect of low concentrations of halothane on the cerebrovascular circulation in young children. Anesthesia. 2000;55:528–31.
214. Scheller MS, Tateishi A, Drummond JC, Zornow MH. The effects of sevoflurane on cerebral blood flow, cerebral metabolic rate for oxygen, intracranial pressure, and the electroencephalogram are similar to those of isoflurane in the rabbit. Anesthesiology. 1988;68:548–51.
215. Rampil IJ, Weiskopf RB, Brown J, Eger II EI, Johnson B, Holmes MA, Donegan JH. I-653 and isoflurane produce similar dose-related changes in the electroencephalogram of pigs. Anesthesiology. 1988;69:298–302.

216. Constant I, Dubois MC, Piat V, Moutard ML, McCue M, Murat I. Changes in electroencephalographic and autonomic cardiovascular activity during induction of anesthesia with sevoflurane compared with halothane or in children. Anesthesiology. 1999;91:1604–15.
217. Hayashi K, Shigemi K, Sawa T. Neonatal electroencephalography shows low sensitivity to anesthesia. Neurosci Lett. 2012;517:87–91.
218. Edwards JJ, Soto RG, Bedford RF. Bispectral Index™ values are higher during halothane vs. sevoflurane anesthesia in children, but not in infants. Acta Anaesthesiol Scand. 2005;49:1084–7.
219. Adachi M, Ikemoto Y, Kubo K, Takuma C. Seizure-like movements during induction of anesthesia with sevoflurane. Br J Anaesth. 1992;68:214–15.
220. Komatsu H, Taie S, Endo S, et al. Electrical seizures during sevoflurane anesthesia in two pediatric patients with epilepsy. Anesthesiology. 1994;81:1535–7.
221. Zacharias M. Convulsive movements with sevoflurane in children. Anaesth Intensive Care. 1997;25:727.
222. Woodforth IJ, Hicks RG, Crawford MR, Stephen JP, et al. Electroencephalographic evidence of seizure activity under deep sevoflurane anesthesia in a nonepileptic patient. Anesthesiology. 1997;87:1579–82.
223. Voss LJ, Sleigh JW, Barnard JPM, et al. The howling cortex: seizures and general anesthetic drugs. Anesth Analg. 2008;107:1689–703.
224. Hsieh SW, Lan KM, Luk HN, et al. Postoperative seizures after sevoflurane anesthesia in a neonate. Acta Anaesthesiol Scand. 2004;48:662.
225. Hauser WA, Annegers JF, Kurland LT. Incidence of epilepsy and unprovoked seizures in Rochester, Minnesota: 1935–1984. Epilepsia. 1993;34:453–8.
226. Friedman MJ, Sharieff GQ. Seizures in children. Pediatr Clin N Am. 2006;53:257–77.
227. Wolf WJ, Neal MB, Peterson MD. The hemodynamic and cardiovascular effects of isoflurane and halothane anesthesia in children. Anesthesiology. 1986;64:328–33.
228. Murray D, Vandewalker G, Matherne P, Mahoney LT. Pulsed doppler and two-dimensional echocardiography: comparison of halothane and isoflurane on cardiac function in infants and small children. Anesthesiology. 1987;67:211–17.
229. Kawana S, Wachi J, Nakayama M, et al. Comparison of haemodynamic changes induced by sevoflurane and halothane in paediatric patients. Can J Anaesth. 1995;42:603–7.
230. Holzman RS, Vandervelde VE, Kaus SJ, et al. Sevoflurane depresses myocardial contractility less than halothane during induction of anesthesia in children. Anesthesiology. 1996;85:1260–7.
231. Wodey E, Pladys P, Copin C, et al. Comparative hemodynamic depression of sevoflurane versus halothane in infants. Anesthesiology. 1997;87:795–800.
232. Friesen RH, Lichtor JL. Cardiovascular depression during halothane anesthesia in infants: a study of three induction techniques. Anesth Analg. 1982;61:42–5.
233. Sagarminaga J, Wynands JE. Atropine and the electrical activity of the heart during induction of anaesthesia in children. Can Anaesth Soc J. 1963;10:328–41.
234. Schmidt U, Schwinger RH, Bohm S, et al. Evidence for an interaction of halothane with the L-type Ca2+ channel in human myocardium. Anesthesiology. 1993;79:332–9.
235. Baum VC, Wetzel GT. Sodium-calcium exchange in neonatal myocardium: reversible inhibition by halothane. Anesth Analg. 1994;78:1105–9.
236. Kanaya N, Kawana S, Tsuchida H, Miyamoto A, Ohshika H, Namiki A. Comparative myocardial depression of sevoflurane, isoflurane, and halothane in cultured neonatal rat ventricular myocytes. Anesth Analg. 1998;87:1041–7.
237. Rao CC, Boyer MS, Krishna G, Paradise RR. Increased sensitivity of the isometric contraction of the neonatal isolated rat atria to halothane, isoflurane, and enflurane. Anesthesiology. 1986; 64:13–8.
238. Krane EJ, Su JY. Comparison of the effects of halothane on newborn and adult rabbit myocardium. Anesth Analg. 1987;66:1240–4.
239. Palmisano BW, Mehner RW, Stowe DF, Bosnjak ZJ, Kampine JP. Direct myocardial effects of halothane and isoflurane: comparison between adult and infant rabbits. Anesthesiology. 1994;81:718–29.
240. Murat I, Hoerter J, Ventura-Clapier R. Developmental changes in effects of halothane and isoflurane on contractile properties of rabbit cardiac skinned fibers. Anesthesiology. 1990;73:137–45.
241. Murat I, Ventura-Clapier R, Vassort G. Halothane, enflurane, and isoflurane decrease calcium sensitivity and maximal force in detergent treated rat cardiac fibers. Anesthesiology. 1988;69:892–9.
242. Gregory GA. The baroresponses of preterm infants during halothane anesthesia. Can Anaesth Soc J. 1982;29:105–7.
243. Palmisano BW, Setlock MA, Brown MP, Siker D, Tripuraneni R. Dose-response for atropine and heart rate in infants and children anesthetized with halothane and nitrous oxide. Anesthesiology. 1991;75:238–42.
244. Hayashi Y, Sumikawa K, Tashiro C, Yamatodani A, Yoshiya I. Arrhythmogenic threshold of epinephrine during sevoflurane, enflurane, and isoflurane anesthesia in dogs. Anesthesiology. 1988;69:145–7.
245. Johnston RR, Eger II EI, Wilson C. A comparative interaction of epinephrine with enflurane, isoflurane, and halothane in man. Anesth Analg. 1976;55:709–12.
246. Karl HW, Swedlow MD, Lee KW, Downes JJ. Epinephrine-halothane interactions in children. Anesthesiology. 1983;58:142–5.
247. Taylor RH, Lerman J. Induction and recovery characteristics for desflurane in children. Can J Anaesth. 1992;39:6–13.
248. Piat V, Dubois M-C, Johanet S, Murat I. Induction and recovery characteristics and hemodynamic responses to sevoflurane and halothane in children. Anesth Analg. 1994;79:840–4.
249. Kern C, Erb T, Frei F. Haemodynamic response to sevoflurane compared with halothane during inhalational induction in children. Paediatr Anaesth. 1997;7:439–44.
250. Friesen RH, Lichtor JL. Cardiovascular effects of inhalation induction with isoflurane in infants. Anesth Analg. 1983;62:411–14.
251. Weiskopf RB, Eger II EI, Holmes MA, et al. Epinephrine-induced premature ventricular contractions and changes in arterial blood pressure and heart rate during I-653, Isoflurane, and halothane anesthesia in swine. Anesthesiology. 1989;70:293–8.
252. Lindahl SGE, Yates AP, Hatch DJ. Respiratory depression at different end-tidal halothane concentrations. Anaesthesia. 1987;42:1267–75.
253. Murat I, Chaussain J, Hamza J, Saint-Maurice CL. The respiratory effects of isoflurane, enflurane and halothane in spontaneously breathing children. Anaesthesia. 1987;42:711–18.
254. Wren WS, Allen P, Synnott A, O'Keeffe D, O'Griofa P. Effects of halothane, isoflurane and enflurane on ventilation in children. Br J Anaesth. 1987;59:399–409.
255. Brown KA, Reich O, Bates JHT. Ventilatory depression by halothane in infants and children. Can J Anaesth. 1995;42:588–96.
256. Brown KA, Aun C, Stocks J, Jackson E, Mackersie A, Hatch D. A comparison of the respiratory effects of sevoflurane and halothane in infants and young children. Anesthesiology. 1998;89:86–92.
257. Reignier J, Ben Ameur M, Ecoffey C. Spontaneous ventilation with halothane in children. Anesthesiology. 1995;83:674–8.
258. Doi M, Ikeda K. Respiratory effects of sevoflurane. Anesth Analg. 1987;66:241–4.

259. Murat I, Saint-Maurice JP, Beydon L, Macgee K. Respiratory effects of nitrous oxide during isoflurane anaesthesia in children. Br J Anaesth. 1986;58:1122–9.
260. Doi M, Ikeda K. Postanesthetic respiratory depression in humans: a comparison of sevoflurane, isoflurane and halothane. J Anesth. 1987;1:137–42.
261. Yamakage M, Tamiya K, Horikawa D, et al. Effects of halothane and sevoflurane on the paediatric respiratory pattern. Paediatr Anaesth. 1994;4:53–6.
262. Mori N, Suzuki M. Sevoflurane in paediatric anaesthesia: effects on respiration and circulation during induction and recovery. Paediatr Anaesth. 1996;6:95–102.
263. Komatsu H, Chujo K, Morita J, et al. Spontaneous breathing with the use of a laryngeal mask airway in children: comparison of sevoflurane and isoflurane. Paediatr Anaesth. 1997;7:111–15.
264. Behforouz N, Dubousset AM, Jamali S, Ecoffey C. Respiratory effects of desflurane anesthesia on spontaneous ventilation in infants and children. Anesth Analg. 1998;87:1052–5.
265. Walpole R, Olday J, Haetzman M, et al. A comparison of the respiratory effects of high concentrations of halothane and sevoflurane. Pediatr Anesth. 2001;11:157–60.
266. Kharasch ED, Thummel KE. Identification of cytochrome P450 2E1 as the predominant enzyme catalyzing human liver microsomal defluorination of sevoflurane, isoflurane, and methoxyflurane. Anesthesiology. 1993;79:795–807.
267. Arnold JH, Truog RD, Rice SA. Prolonged administration of isoflurane to pediatric patients during mechanical ventilation. Anesth Analg. 1993;76:520–6.
268. Kharasch ED, Karol MD, Lanni C, Sawchuk R. Clinical sevoflurane metabolism and disposition I. Sevoflurane and metabolite pharmacokinetics. Anesthesiology. 1995;82:1369–78.
269. Mazze RI, Calverley RK, Smith T. Inorganic fluoride nephrotoxicity: prolonged enflurane and halothane anesthesia in volunteers. Anesthesiology. 1977;46:265–71.
270. Higuchi H, Sumikura H, Sumita S, et al. Renal function in patients with high serum fluoride concentrations after prolonged sevoflurane anesthesia. Anesthesiology. 1995;83:449–58.
271. Frink EJ, Malan TP, Isner J, et al. Renal concentrating function with prolonged sevoflurane or enflurane anesthesia in volunteers. Anesthesiology. 1994;80:1019–25.
272. Munday IT, Stoddart PA, Jones RM, Lytle J, Cross MR. Serum fluoride concentration and urine osmolality after enflurane and sevoflurane anesthesia in male volunteers. Anesth Analg. 1995;81:353–9.
273. Jones RM, Koblin DD, Cashman JN, et al. Biotransformation and hepato-renal function in volunteers after exposure to desflurane (I-653). Br J Anaesth. 1990;64:482–7.
274. Cousins MH, Mazze RI, Kosek JC, et al. The etiology of methoxyflurane nephrotoxicity. J Pharm Exp Ther. 1974;190:530–41.
275. Cousins MJ, Mazze RI. Methoxyflurane nephrotoxicity: a study of dose response in man. JAMA. 1973;225:1611–16.
276. Stoelting RK, Peterson C. Methoxyflurane anesthesia in pediatric patients: evaluation of anesthetic metabolism and renal function. Anesthesiology. 1975;42:26–9.
277. Oikkonen M, Meretoja O. Serum fluoride in children anaesthetized with enflurane. Eur J Anaesth. 1989;6:401–7.
278. Hinkle AJ. Serum inorganic fluoride levels after enflurane in children. Anesth Analg. 1989;68:396–9.
279. Levine MF, Sarner J, Lerman J, Davis P, Sikich N, Maloney K, Motoyama E, Cook DR. Plasma inorganic fluoride concentrations after sevoflurane anesthesia in children. Anesthesiology. 1996;84:348–53.
280. Kharasch ED, Armstrong AS, Gunn K, Artru A, Cox K, Karol MD. Clinical sevoflurane metabolism and disposition: II. The role of cytochrome P450 2E1 in fluoride and hexafluoroisopropanol formation. Anesthesiology. 1995;82:1379–88.
281. Kharasch ED, Thummel KE, Mautz D, Bosse S. Clinical enflurane metabolism by cytochrome P450-2E1. Clin Pharm Ther. 1994;55:434–40.
282. Kharasch ED, Hankins DC, Cox K. Clinical isoflurane metabolism by CYP450 2E1. Anesthesiology. 1999;90:766–71.
283. Gentz BA, Malan Jr TP. Renal toxicity with sevoflurane: a storm in a teacup? Drugs. 2001;61:2155–62.
284. Carey RMT, Van Dyke RA. Halothane hepatitis: a critical review. Anesth Analg. 1972;51:135–60.
285. Lewis JH, Zimmerman HJ, Ishak KG, Mullick FG. Enflurane hepatotoxicity: a clinicopathological study of 24 cases. Ann Intern Med. 1983;98:984–92.
286. Carrigan TW, Straughen WJ. A report of hepatic necrosis and death following isoflurane anesthesia. Anesthesiology. 1987;67:581–3.
287. Martin JL, Pleverk DJ, Flannery KD, Charlton M, et al. Hepatotoxicity after desflurane anesthesia. Anesthesiology. 1995;83:1125–9.
288. Turillazzi E, D'Errico S, Neri M, et al. A fatal case of fulminant hepatic necrosis following sevoflurane anesthesia. Toxicol Pathol. 2007;35:840–5.
289. Kenna JG, Neuberger J, Mieli-Vergani G, Mowat AP, Williams R. Halothane hepatitis in children. Br Med J. 1989;294:1209–11.
290. Ogawa M, Doi K, Mitsufuji T, Satoh K, Takatori T. Drug induced hepatitis following sevoflurane anesthesia in a child. Masui. 1991;40:1542–5.
291. Watanabe K, Hatakenaka S, Ikemune K, Chigyo Y, Kubozono T, Arai T. A case of suspected liver dysfunction induced by sevoflurane anesthesia. Masui. 1993;42:902–5.
292. Taivainen T, Tiainen P, Meretoja OA, Raiha L, Rosenberg PH. Comparison of the effects of sevoflurane and halothane on the quality of anaesthesia and serum glutathione transferase alpha and fluoride in paediatric patients. Br J Anaesth. 1994;73:590–5.
293. Jang Y, Kim I. Severe hepatotoxicity after sevoflurane anesthesia in a child with mild renal dysfunction. Pediatr Anesth. 2005;15:1140–4.
294. Wark H, Earl J, Chau DD, Overton J. Halothane metabolism in children. Br J Anaesth. 1990;64:474–81.
295. Fisher DM, Robinson S, Brett CM, Perin G, Gregory GA. Comparison of enflurane, halothane, and isoflurane for diagnostic and therapeutic procedures in children with malignancies. Anesthesiology. 1985;63:647–50.
296. Wren WS, McShane AJ, McMarthy JG, Lamont BJ, Casey WF, Hannon VM. Isoflurane in paediatric anaesthesia: induction and recovery from anaesthesia. Anaesthesia. 1985;40:315–23.
297. Phillips AJ, Brimacombe JR, Simpson DL. Anaesthetic induction with isoflurane or halothane: oxygen saturation during induction with isoflurane or halothane in unpremedicated children. Anaesthesia. 1988;43:927–9.
298. Crean PM, Laird CRD, Keilty SR, Black GW. The influence of atropine premedication on the induction of anesthesia with isoflurane in children. Paediatr Anaesth. 1991;1:37–9.
299. Lindgren L, Randell T, Saarnivaara L. Comparison of inhalation induction with isoflurane and halothane in children. Eur J Anaesth. 1991;8:33–7.
300. Zwass MS, Fisher DM, Welborn LG, et al. Induction and maintenance characteristics of anesthesia with desflurane and nitrous oxide in infants and children. Anesthesiology. 1992;76:373–8.
301. Lerman J, Davis PJ, Welborn LG, et al. Induction, recovery, and safety characteristics of sevoflurane in children undergoing ambulatory surgery: a comparison with halothane. Anesthesiology. 1996;84:1332–40.
302. Black A, Sury RJ, Hemington L, Howard R, Mackersie A, Hatch DJ. A comparison of the induction characteristics of sevoflurane and halothane in children. Anaesthesia. 1996;51:539–42.

303. Sigston PE, Jenkins AMC, Jackson EA, Sury MRJ, Mackersie AM, Hatch DJ. Rapid inhalation induction in children: 8 % sevoflurane compared with 5 % halothane. Br J Anaesth. 1997;78:362–5.
304. Ariffin SA, Whyte JA, Malins AF, Cooper GM. Comparison of induction and recovery between sevoflurane and halothane supplementation of anaesthesia in children undergoing outpatient dental extractions. Br J Anaesth. 1997;78:157–9.
305. Baum VC, Yemen TA, Baum LD. Immediate 8 % sevoflurane induction in children, a comparison with incremental sevoflurane and incremental halothane. Anesth Analg. 1997;85:313–16.
306. Agnor RC, Sikich N, Lerman J. Single breath vital capacity rapid inhalation induction in children: 8 % sevoflurane versus 5 % halothane. Anesthesiology. 1998;89:379–84.
307. Morimoto Y, Mayhew JF, Knox SL, Zornow MH. Rapid induction of anesthesia with high concentration of halothane or sevoflurane in children. J Clin Anesth. 2000;12:184–8.
308. Ho KY, Chua WL, Lim SS, Ng AS. A comparison between single- and double-breath vital capacity inhalation induction with 8 % sevoflurane in children. Pediatr Anesth. 2004;14:457–61.
309. Fernandez M, Lejus C, Rivault O, et al. Single-breath vital capacity rapid inhalation induction with sevoflurane: feasibility in children. Pediatr Anesth. 2005;15:307–13.
310. Lejus C, Bazin V, Fernandez M, et al. Inhalation induction using sevoflurane in children the single-breath vital capacity technique compared to the tidal volume technique. Anaesthesia. 2006; 61:535–40.
311. Lee SY, Cheng SL, Ng SB, Lim SL. Single-breath vital capacity high concentration sevoflurane induction in children: with or without nitrous oxide? Br J Anaesth. 2013;110:81–6.
312. Russell IA, Miller Hance WC, Gregory G, et al. The safety and efficacy of sevoflurane anesthesia in infants and children with congenital heart disease. Anesth Analg. 2001;92:1152–8.
313. Dalal PG, Corner A, Chin C, et al. Comparison of the cardiovascular effects of isoflurane and sevoflurane as measured by magnetic resonance imaging in children with congenital heart disease. J Clin Anesth. 2008;20:40–4.
314. Rivenes SM, Lewin MB, Stayer SA, et al. Cardiovascular effects of sevoflurane, isoflurane, halothane, and fentanyl-midazolam in children with congenital heart disease: an echocardiographic study of myocardial contractility and hemodynamics. Anesthesiology. 2001;94:223–9.
315. Ebert TJ, Muzi M. Sympathetic hyperactivity during desflurane anesthesia in healthy volunteers: a comparison with isoflurane. Anesthesiology. 1993;79:444–53.
316. Ishikawa T, Nishino T, Hiraga K. Immediate responses of arterial blood pressure and heart rate to sudden inhalation of high concentrations of isoflurane in normotensive and hypertensive patients. Anesth Analg. 1993;77:1022–5.
317. Ebert TJ, Muzi M, Lopatka CW. Neurocirculatory responses to sevoflurane in humans: a comparison to desflurane. Anesthesiology. 1995;83:88–95.
318. Yli-Hankala A, Randell T, Seppala T, et al. Increases in hemodynamic variables and catecholamine levels after rapid increase in isoflurane concentration. Anesthesiology. 1993;78:266–71.
319. Weiskopf RB, Moore MA, Eger II EI, et al. Rapid increase in desflurane concentration is associated with greater transient cardiovascular stimulation than with rapid increase in isoflurane concentration in humans. Anesthesiology. 1994;80:1035–45.
320. Weiskopf RB, Eger II EI, Noorani M, Daniel M. Repetitive rapid increases in desflurane concentration blunt transient cardiovascular stimulation in humans. Anesthesiology. 1994;81:843–9.
321. Moore MA, Weiskopf RB, Eger II EI, et al. Rapid 1 % increases of end-tidal desflurane concentration to greater than 5 % transiently increases heart rate and blood pressure in humans. Anesthesiology. 1994;81:94–8.
322. Tanaka S, Tsuchida H, Namba H, Namiki A. Clonidine and lidocaine inhibition of isoflurane-induced tachycardia in humans. Anesthesiology. 1994;81:1341–9.
323. Weiskopf RB, Eger II EI, Noorani M. Fentanyl, esmolol and clonidine blunt the transient cardiovascular stimulation induced by desflurane in humans. Anesthesiology. 1994;81:1350–5.
324. Devcic A, Muzi M, Ebert TJ. The effects of clonidine on desflurane-mediated sympathoexcitation in humans. Anesth Analg. 1995;80:773–9.
325. Muzi M, Ebert TJ, Hope WG, Robinson BJ, Bell LB. Site(s) medicating sympathetic activation with desflurane. Anesthesiology. 1996;85:737–47.
326. Weiskopf RB, Eger II EI, Daniel M, Noorani M. Cardiovascular stimulation induced by rapid increases in desflurane concentration in humans results from activation of tracheopulmonary and systemic receptors. Anesthesiology. 1995;83:1173–8.
327. O'Brien K, Robinson DN, Morton N. Induction and emergence in infants less than 60 weeks post-conceptual age: comparison of thiopental, halothane, sevoflurane and desflurane. Br J Anaesth. 1998;80:456–9.
328. Welborn LG, Hannallah RS, Norden JM, et al. Comparison of emergence and recovery characteristics of sevoflurane, desflurane, and halothane in pediatric ambulatory patients. Anesth Analg. 1996;83:917–20.
329. Valley RD, Ramza JT, Calhoun P, et al. Tracheal extubation of deeply anesthetized pediatric patients: a comparison of isoflurane and sevoflurane. Anesth Analg. 1999;88:742–5.
330. Meretoja OA, Taivainen T, Raiha L, et al. Sevoflurane-nitrous oxide or halothane-nitrous oxide for paediatric bronchoscopy and gastroscopy. Br J Anaesth. 1996;76:767–71.
331. Sury MRJ, Black A, Hemington L, et al. A comparison of the recovery characteristics of sevoflurane and halothane in children. Anaesthesia. 1996;51:543–6.
332. Neumann MA, Weiskopf RB, Gong DH, Eger II EI, Ionescu P. Changing from isoflurane to desflurane toward the end of anesthesia does not accelerate recovery in humans. Anesthesiology. 1998;88:914–21.
333. Davis PJ, Greenberg JA, Gendelman M, Fertal K. Recovery characteristics of sevoflurane and halothane in preschool-aged children undergoing bilateral myringotomy and pressure equalization tube insertion. Anesth Analg. 1999;88:34–8.
334. Aono J, Ueda W, Mamiya K, Takimoto E, Manabe M. Greater incidence of delirium during recovery from sevoflurane anesthesia in preschool boys. Anesthesiology. 1997;87:1298–300.
335. Kuratani N, Oi Y. Greater incidence of emergence agitation in children after sevoflurane anesthesia as compared with halothane. A meta-analysis of randomized controlled trials. Anesthesiology. 2008;109:225–32.
336. Sethi S, Ghai B, Ram J, Wig J. Postoperative emergence delirium in pediatric patients undergoing cataract surgery – a comparison of desflurane and sevoflurane. Pediatr Anesth. 2013;23:1131–7.
337. Cravero J, Surgenor S, Whalen K. Emergence agitation in paediatric patients after sevoflurane anaesthesia and no surgery: a comparison with halothane. Pediatr Anesth. 2000;10:419–24.
338. Sikich N, Lerman J. Development and psychometric evaluation of the pediatric anesthesia emergence delirium scale. Anesthesiology. 2004;100:1138–45.
339. Dahmani S, Stany I, Brasher C, et al. Pharmacological prevention of sevoflurane- and desflurane-related emergence agitation in children: a meta-analysis of published studies. Br J Anaesth. 2010;104:216–23.
340. Ali HH, Savarese JJ. Monitoring of neuromuscular function. Anesthesiology. 1976;45:216–49.

341. Rupp SM, Miller RD, Gencarelli PJ. Vecuronium-induced neuromuscular blockade during enflurane, isoflurane, and halothane anesthesia in humans. Anesthesiology. 1984;60:102–5.
342. Chapple DJ, Clark JS, Hughes R. Interaction between atracurium and drugs used in anaesthesia. Br J Anaesth. 1983;55:17S–22.
343. Caldwell JE, Laster MJ, Magorian T, et al. The neuromuscular effects of desflurane, alone and combined with pancuronium or succinylcholine in humans. Anesthesiology. 1991;74:412–18.
344. Kobayashi O, Ohta Y, Kosaka F. Interaction of sevoflurane, isoflurane, enflurane and halothane with non-depolarizing muscle relaxants and their prejunctional effects at the neuromuscular junction. Acta Med Okayama. 1990;44:209–15.
345. Brandom BW, Cook DR, Woelfel SK, Rudd GD, Fehr B, Lineberry CG. Atracurium infusion requirements in children during halothane, isoflurane, and narcotic anesthesia. Anesth Analg. 1985;64:471–6.
346. Rapp HJ, Altenmueller CA, Waschke C. Neuromuscular recovery following rocuronium bromide single dose in infants. Pediatr Anesth. 2004;14:329–35.
347. Lerman J, Relton JES. Anaesthesia for malignant hyperthermia susceptible patients. In: Britt BA, editor. Malignant hyperthermia. Boston: Martinus Nijhoff Publishing; 1987. p. 369–92.
348. Britt BA, Kalow W. Malignant hyperthermia: a statistical review. Can Anaesth Soc J. 1970;17:293–315.
349. Pan TH, Wollack AR, DeMarco JA. Malignant hyperthermia associated with enflurane anesthesia: a case report. Anesth Analg. 1975;54:47–9.
350. Relton JES, Creighton RE, Johnston AE, Pelton DA, Conn AW. Hyperpyrexia in association with general anaesthesia in children. Can Anaesth Soc J. 1966;13:419–24.
351. Joseph MM, Shah K, Viljoen JF. Malignant hyperthermia associated with isoflurane anesthesia. Anesth Analg. 1982;61:711–12.
352. Otsuka H, Komura Y, Mayumi T, et al. Malignant hyperthermia during sevoflurane anesthesia in a child with central core disease. Anesthesiology. 1991;75:699–701.
353. Ochiai R, Toyoda Y, Nishio I, et al. Possible association of malignant hyperthermia with sevoflurane anesthesia. Anesth Analg. 1992;74:616–18.
354. Wedel DJ, Gammel SA, Milde JH, Iaizzo PA. Delayed onset of malignant hyperthermia induced by isoflurane and desflurane compared with halothane in susceptible swine. Anesthesiology. 1993;78:1138–44.
355. Ducart A, Adnet P, Renaud B, Riou B, Krivosic-Horber R. Malignant hyperthermia during sevoflurane administration. Anesth Analg. 1995;80:609–11.
356. Michalek-Sauberer A, Fricker R, Gradwohl I, Gilly H. A case of suspected malignant hyperthermia during desflurane administration. Anesth Analg. 1997;85:461–2.
357. Yamakage M, Takahashi K, Takahashi M, et al. Performance of four carbon dioxide absorbents in experimental and clinical settings. Anaesthesia. 2009;64:287–92.
358. Fee JPH, Murray JM, Luney SR. Molecular sieves: an alternative method of carbon dioxide removal which does not generate compound A during simulated low-flow sevoflurane anaesthesia. Anaesthesia. 1995;50:841–5.
359. Renfrew CW, Murray JM, Fee JPH. A new approach to carbon dioxide absorbents. Acta Scand Anaesth. 1998;41 Suppl 12:58–60.
360. Murray JM, Renfrew CW, Bedi A, et al. Amsorb: a new carbon dioxide absorbent for use in anesthetic breathing systems. Anesthesiology. 1999;91:1342–8.
361. Keijzer C, Perez RSGM, de Lange JJ. Compound A and carbon monoxide production from sevoflurane and seven different types of carbon dioxide absorbent in a patient model. Acta Anaesthesiol Scand. 2007;51:31–7.
362. Versichelen LFM, Bouche MPLA, Rolly G, et al. Only carbon dioxide absorbents free of both NaOH and KOH do not generate compound A during in vitro close-system sevoflurane. Evaluation of five absorbents. Anesthesiology. 2001;95:750–5.
363. Fang ZX, Eger II EI, Laster MJ, et al. Carbon monoxide production from degradation of desflurane, enflurane, isoflurane, halothane and sevoflurane by soda lime and Baralyme. Anesth Analg. 1995;80:1187–93.
364. Moon RE. Carbon monoxide gas may be linked to CO2 absorbent. Anesth Patient Saf Found Newslett. 1991;6:8.
365. Frink EJ, Nogami WM, Morgan SE, Salmon RC. High carboxyhemoglobin concentrations occur in swine during desflurane anesthesia in the presence of partially dried carbon dioxide absorbents. Anesthesiology. 1997;87:308–16.
366. Baxter PJ, Kharasch ED. Rehydration of desiccated baralyme prevents carbon monoxide formation from desflurane in an anesthesia machine. Anesthesiology. 1997;86:1061–5.
367. Hanaki C, Fujui K, Morio M, Tashima T. Decomposition of sevoflurane by sodalime. Hiroshima J Med Sci. 1987;36:61–7.
368. Morio M, Fujii K, Satoh N, et al. Reaction of sevoflurane and its degradation products with soda lime. Toxicity of the byproducts. Anesthesiology. 1992;77:1155–64.
369. Liu J, Laster MJ, Eger II EI, Taheri S. Absorption and degradation of sevoflurane and isoflurane in a conventional anesthetic circuit. Anesth Analg. 1991;72:785–9.
370. Ebert TJ, Frink Jr EJ, Kharasch ED. Absence of biochemical evidence for renal and hepatic dysfunction after 8 hours of 1.25 minimum alveolar concentration of sevoflurane anesthesia in volunteers. Anesthesiology. 1998;88:601–10.
371. Ebert TJ, Messana LD, Uhrich TD, Staacke TS. Absence of renal and hepatic toxicity after four hours of 1.25 minimum alveolar anesthetic concentration sevoflurane anesthesia in volunteers. Anesth Analg. 1998;86:662–7.
372. Kharasch ED, Frink Jr EJ, Zager R, et al. Assessment of low-flow sevoflurane and isoflurane effects on renal function using sensitive markers of tubular toxicity. Anesthesiology. 1997;86:1238–53.
373. Eger II EI, Gong D, Koblin DD, et al. Dose-related biochemical markers of renal injury after sevoflurane versus desflurane anesthesia in volunteers. Anesth Analg. 1997;85:1154–63.
374. Hideyuki H, Yushi A, Hiroki W, et al. The effects of low-flow sevoflurane and isoflurane anesthesia on renal function in patients with stable moderate renal insufficiency. Anesth Analg. 2001;92:650–5.
375. Frink EJ, Green Jr WB, Brown EA, et al. Compound A concentrations during sevoflurane anesthesia in children. Anesthesiology. 1996;84:566–71.
376. Gonsowski CT, Laster MJ, Eger II EI, et al. Toxicity of compound A in rats: effect of increasing duration of administration. Anesthesiology. 1994;80:566–73.
377. Gonsowski CT, Laster MJ, Eger II EI, et al. Toxicity of compound A in rats: effect of a 3-hour administration. Anesthesiology. 1994;80:556–65.
378. Keller KA, Callan C, Prokocimer P, et al. Inhalation toxicity study of a haloalkene degradant of sevoflurane, compound A (PIFE), in sprague-dawley rats. Anesthesiology. 1995(1220–32).
379. Eger II EI, Koblin DD, Bowland T, et al. Nephrotoxicity of sevoflurane versus desflurane anesthesia in volunteers. Anesth Analg. 1997;85:160–8.
380. Iyer RA, Frink EJ, Ebert TJ, Anders MW. Cysteine conjugate β-lyase-dependent metabolism of compound A (2-[fluoromethoxy]-1,1,3,3,3-pentafluoro-1-propene) in human subjects anesthetized with sevoflurane and in rats given compound A. Anesthesiology. 1998;88:611–18.
381. Martin JL, Laster MJ, Kandel L, et al. Metabolism of compound A by renal cysteine-s-conjugate β-lyase is not the mechanism of compound A-induced renal injury in the rat. Anesth Analg. 1996;82:770–4.

382. Kharasch ED, Schroeder JL, Sheffels P, et al. Influence of sevoflurane on the metabolism and renal effects of compound A in rats. Anesthesiology. 2005;103:1183–8.
383. Kharasch ED, Schroeder JL, Bammler T, et al. Gene expression profiling of nephrotoxicity from the sevoflurane degradation product fluoromethyl-2,2-difluoro-1-(trifluoromethyl)vinyl ether ("compound A") in rats. Toxicol Sci. 2006;90:419–31.
384. Anderson BJ. Paracetamol (Acetaminophen): mechanisms of action. Paediatr Anaesth. 2008;18:915–21.
385. Peterson RG, Rumack BH. Pharmacokinetics of acetaminophen in children. Pediatrics. 1978;62:877.
386. Korpela R, Korvenoja P, Meretoja OA. Morphine-sparing effect of acetaminophen in pediatric day-case surgery. Anesthesiology. 1999;91:442–7.
387. Anderson BJ, Gibb IA. Paracetamol (acetaminophen) pharmacodynamics; interpreting the plasma concentration. Arch Dis Child. 2007;93:241–7, 149.
388. Anderson BJ, Woollard GA, Holford NH. Acetaminophen analgesia in children: placebo effect and pain resolution after tonsillectomy. Eur J Clin Pharmacol. 2001;57:559–69.
389. Allegaert K, Naulaers G, Vanhaesebrouch S, Anderson BJ. The paracetamol concentration-effect relation in neonates. Pediatr Anesth. 2013;23:45–50.
390. Lingen van RA, Deinum HT, Quak CM, Okken A, Tibboel D. Multiple-dose pharmacokinetics of rectally administered acetaminophen in term infants. Clin Pharmacol Ther. 1999;66:509–15, 152.
391. van Lingen RA, Quak CM, Deinum HT, et al. Effects of rectally administered paracetamol on infants delivered by vacuum extraction. Eur J Obstet Gynecol Reprod Biol. 2001;94:73–8.
392. Howard CR, Howard FM, Weitzman ML. Acetaminophen analgesia in neonatal circumcision: the effect on pain. Pediatrics. 1994;93:641–6.
393. Shah V, Taddio A, Ohlsson A. Randomised controlled trial of paracetamol for heel prick pain in neonates. Arch Dis Child Fetal Neonatal Ed. 1998;79:F209–11.
394. Rod B, Monrigal JP, Lepoittevin L, Granry JC, Cavellat M. Treatment of postoperative pain in children in the recovery room. Use of morphine and propacetamol by the intravenous route. Cah Anesthesiol. 1989;37:525–30.
395. Agrawal S, Fitzsimons JJ, Horn V, Petros A. Intravenous paracetamol for postoperative analgesia in a 4-day-old term neonate. Paediatr Anaesth. 2007;17:70–1.
396. Ceelie I, de Wildt SN, van Dijk M, et al. Effect of intravenous paracetamol on postoperative morphine requirements in neonates and infants undergoing major noncardiac surgery: a randomized controlled trial. JAMA. 2013;309:149–54.
397. Allegaert K, Murat I, Anderson BJ. Not all intravenous paracetamol formulations are created equal. Paediatr Anaesth. 2007;17:811–12.
398. Anderson BJ, Pearce S, McGann JE, Newson AJ, Holford NH. Investigations using logistic regression models on the effect of the LMA on morphine induced vomiting after tonsillectomy. Paediatr Anaesth. 2000;10:633–8.
399. van Lingen RA, Deinum JT, Quak JM, et al. Pharmacokinetics and metabolism of rectally administered paracetamol in preterm neonates. Arch Dis Child Fetal Neonatal Ed. 1999;80:F59–63.
400. Miller RP, Roberts RJ, Fischer LJ. Acetaminophen elimination kinetics in neonates, children, and adults. Clin Pharmacol Ther. 1976;19:284–94.
401. Allegaert K, Anderson BJ, Naulaers G, et al. Intravenous paracetamol (propacetamol) pharmacokinetics in term and preterm neonates. Eur J Clin Pharmacol. 2004;8:8.
402. Palmer GM, Atkins M, Anderson BJ, et al. I.V. acetaminophen pharmacokinetics in neonates after multiple doses. Br J Anaesth. 2008;101:523–30.
403. Anderson BJ, Allegaert K. Intravenous neonatal paracetamol dosing: the magic of 10 days. Paediatr Anaesth. 2009;19:289–95.
404. Hines RN. Ontogeny of human hepatic cytochromes P450. J Biochem Mol Toxicol. 2007;21:169–75.
405. Bartocci M, Lundeberg S. Intravenous paracetamol: the 'Stockholm protocol' for postoperative analgesia of term and preterm neonates. Paediatr Anaesth. 2007;17:1120–1.
406. Wilson-Smith EM, Morton NS. Survey of i.v. paracetamol (acetaminophen) use in neonates and infants under 1 year of age by UK anesthetists. Paediatr Anaesth. 2009;19:329–37.
407. Allegaert K, Rayyan M, De Rijdt T, Van Beek F, Naulaers G. Hepatic tolerance of repeated intravenous paracetamol administration in neonates. Paediatr Anaesth. 2008;18:388–92.
408. Beringer RM, Thompson JP, Parry S, Stoddart PA. Intravenous paracetamol overdose: two case reports and a change to national treatment guidelines. Arch Dis Child. 2011;96:307–8.
409. Nevin DG, Shung J. Intravenous paracetamol overdose in a preterm infant during anesthesia. Pediatr Anesth. 2009;20:105–7.
410. Shaffer CL, Gal P, Ransom JL, et al. Effect of age and birth weight on indomethacin pharmacodynamics in neonates treated for patent ductus arteriosus. Crit Care Med. 2002;30:343–8.
411. Mannila A, Kumpulainen E, Lehtonen M, et al. Plasma and cerebrospinal fluid concentrations of indomethacin in children after intravenous administration. J Clin Pharmacol. 2007;47:94–100.
412. Kokki H, Kumpulainen E, Laisalmi M, Savolainen J, Rautio J, Lehtonen M. Diclofenac readily penetrates the cerebrospinal fluid in children. Br J Clin Pharmacol. 2008;65:879–84.
413. Kumpulainen E, Kokki H, Laisalmi M, et al. How readily does ketorolac penetrate cerebrospinal fluid in children? J Clin Pharmacol. 2008;48:495–501.
414. Kokki H, Kumpulainen E, Lehtonen M, et al. Cerebrospinal fluid distribution of ibuprofen after intravenous administration in children. Pediatrics. 2007;120:e1002–8.
415. Aranda JV, Varvarigou A, Beharry K, et al. Pharmacokinetics and protein binding of intravenous ibuprofen in the premature newborn infant. Acta Paediatr. 1997;86:289–93.
416. Van Overmeire B, Touw D, Schepens PJ, Kearns GL, van den Anker JN. Ibuprofen pharmacokinetics in preterm infants with patent ductus arteriosus. Clin Pharmacol Ther. 2001;70:336–43.
417. Benet LZ, Hoener BA. Changes in plasma protein binding have little clinical relevance. Clin Pharmacol Ther. 2002;71:115–21.
418. Hamman MA, Thompson GA, Hall SD. Regioselective and stereoselective metabolism of ibuprofen by human cytochrome P450 2C. Biochem Pharmacol. 1997;54:33–41.
419. Tanaka E. Clinically important pharmacokinetic drug-drug interactions: role of cytochrome P450 enzymes. J Clin Pharm Ther. 1998;23:403–16.
420. Scott CS, Retsch-Bogart GZ, Kustra RP, Graham KM, Glasscock BJ, Smith PC. The pharmacokinetics of ibuprofen suspension, chewable tablets, and tablets in children with cystic fibrosis. J Pediatr. 1999;134:58–63.
421. Wiest DB, Pinson JB, Gal PS, et al. Population pharmacokinetics of intravenous indomethacin in neonates with symptomatic patent ductus arteriosus. Clin Pharmacol Ther. 1991;49:550–7.
422. Smyth JM, Collier PS, Darwish M, et al. Intravenous indometacin in preterm infants with symptomatic patent ductus arteriosus. A population pharmacokinetic study. Br J Clin Pharmacol. 2004;58:249–58.
423. Olkkola KT, Maunuksela EL, Korpela R. Pharmacokinetics of postoperative intravenous indomethacin in children. Pharmacol Toxicol. 1989;65:157–60.
424. Lynn AM, Bradford H, Kantor ED, et al. Postoperative ketorolac tromethamine use in infants aged 6-18 months: the effect on morphine usage, safety assessment, and stereo-specific pharmacokinetics. Anesth Analg. 2007;104:1040–51. tables of contents.

425. Gregoire N, Gualano V, Geneteau A, et al. Population pharmacokinetics of ibuprofen enantiomers in very premature neonates. J Clin Pharmacol. 2004;44:1114–24.
426. Brocks DR, Jamali F. Clinical pharmacokinetics of ketorolac tromethamine. Clin Pharmacokinet. 1992;23:415–27.
427. Aggeler PM, O'Reilly RA, Leong L, Kowitz PE. Potentiation of anticoagulant effect of warfarin by phenylbutazone. N Engl J Med. 1967;276:496–501.
428. Naulaers G, Delanghe G, Allegaert K, et al. Ibuprofen and cerebral oxygenation and circulation. Arch Dis Child Fetal Neonatal Ed. 2005;90:F75–6.
429. Lesko SM, Mitchell AA. An assessment of the safety of pediatric ibuprofen. A practitioner-based randomized clinical trial. JAMA. 1995;273:929–33.
430. Lesko SM, Mitchell AA. The safety of acetaminophen and ibuprofen among children younger than two years old. Pediatrics. 1999;104:e39.
431. Keenan GF, Giannini EH, Athreya BH. Clinically significant gastropathy associated with nonsteroidal antiinflammatory drug use in children with juvenile rheumatoid arthritis. J Rheumatol. 1995;22:1149–51.
432. Dowd JE, Cimaz R, Fink CW. Nonsteroidal antiinflammatory drug-induced gastroduodenal injury in children. Arthritis Rheum. 1995;38:1225–31.
433. Ment LR, Vohr BR, Makuch RW, et al. Prevention of intraventricular hemorrhage by indomethacin in male preterm infants. J Pediatr. 2004;145:832–4.
434. Paul D, Bodnar RJ, Gistrak MA, Pasternak GW. Different mu receptor subtypes mediate spinal and supraspinal analgesia in mice. Eur J Pharmacol. 1989;168:307–14.
435. Bouwmeester NJ, Anand KJ, van Dijk M, Hop WC, Boomsma F, Tibboel D. Hormonal and metabolic stress responses after major surgery in children aged 0-3 years: a double-blind, randomized trial comparing the effects of continuous versus intermittent morphine. Br J Anaesth. 2001;87:390–9.
436. Chay PC, Duffy BJ, Walker JS. Pharmacokinetic-pharmacodynamic relationships of morphine in neonates. Clin Pharmacol Ther. 1992;51:334–42.
437. Anderson BJ, Persson M, Anderson M. Rationalising intravenous morphine prescriptions in children. Acute Pain. 1999;2:59–67.
438. Inturrisi CE, Colburn WA. Application of pharmacokinetic-pharmacodynamic modeling to analgesia. In: Foley KM, Inturrisi CE, editors. Advances in pain research and therapy opioid analgesics in the management of clinical pain. New York: Raven Press; 1986. p. 441–52.
439. van Lingen RA, Simons SH, Anderson BJ, Tibboel D. The effects of analgesia in the vulnerable infant during the perinatal period. Clin Perinatol. 2002;29:511–34.
440. Wittwer E, Kern SE. Role of morphine's metabolites in analgesia: concepts and controversies. AAPS J. 2006;8:E348–52.
441. Gong QL, Hedner J, Bjorkman R, Hedner T. Morphine-3-glucuronide may functionally antagonize morphine-6-glucuronide induced antinociception and ventilatory depression in the rat. Pain. 1992;48:249–55.
442. de Graaf J, van Lingen RA, Valkenburg AJ, et al. Does neonatal morphine use affect neuropsychological outcomes at 8 to 9 years of age? Pain. 2013;154:449–58.
443. Taylor J, Liley A, Anderson BJ. The relationship between age and morphine infusion rate in children. Paediatr Anaesth. 2013;23:40–4.
444. Krekels EHJ, Tibboel D, de Wildt SN, et al. Evidence-based morphine dosing for postoperative neonates and infants. Clin Pharmacokinet. 2014;53:553–63.
445. Lundeberg S, Beck O, Olsson GL, Boreus LO. Rectal administration of morphine in children. Pharmacokinetic evaluation after a single-dose. Acta Anaesthesiol Scand. 1996;40:445–51.
446. Gourlay GK, Boas RA. Fatal outcome with use of rectal morphine for postoperative pain control in an infant. BMJ. 1992; 304:766–7.
447. Mayhew JF, Brodsky RC, Blakey D, Petersen W. Low-dose caudal morphine for postoperative analgesia in infants and children: a report of 500 cases. J Clin Anesth. 1995;7:640–2.
448. Haberkern CM, Lynn AM, Geiduschek JM, et al. Epidural and intravenous bolus morphine for postoperative analgesia in infants. Can J Anaesth. 1996;43:1203–10.
449. Nichols DJ, Yaster M, Lynn AM, et al. Disposition and respiratory effects of intrathecal morphine in children. Anesthesiology. 1993;79:733–8.
450. Kart T, Christrup LL, Rasmussen M. Recommended use of morphine in neonates, infants and children based on a literature review: Part 2–Clinical use. Paediatr Anaesth. 1997;7:93–101.
451. Kart T, Christrup LL, Rasmussen M. Recommended use of morphine in neonates, infants and children based on a literature review: Part 1–Pharmacokinetics. Paediatr Anaesth. 1997;7:5–11.
452. Anderson BJ, Ralph CJ, Stewart AW, Barber C, Holford NH. The dose-effect relationship for morphine and vomiting after day-stay tonsillectomy in children. Anaesth Intensive Care. 2000;28:155–60.
453. Weinstein MS, Nicolson SC, Schreiner MS. A single dose of morphine sulfate increases the incidence of vomiting after outpatient inguinal surgery in children. Anesthesiology. 1994;81:572–7.
454. Suresh S, Anand KJS. Opioid tolerance in neonates: a state of the art review. Paediatr Anaesth. 2001;11:511–21.
455. Chana SK, Anand KJ. Can we use methadone for analgesia in neonates? Arch Dis Child Fetal Neonatal Ed. 2001;85:F79–81.
456. Scott JC, Stanski DR. Decreased fentanyl and alfentanil dose requirements with age. A simultaneous pharmacokinetic and pharmacodynamic evaluation. J Pharmacol Exp Ther. 1987;240:159–66.
457. Wynands JE, Townsend GE, Wong P, Whalley DG, Srikant CB, Patel YC. Blood pressure response and plasma fentanyl concentrations during high- and very high-dose fentanyl anesthesia for coronary artery surgery. Anesth Analg. 1983;62:661–5.
458. Anand KJ, Sippell WG, Aynsley-Green A. Randomised trial of fentanyl anaesthesia in preterm babies undergoing surgery: effects on the stress response. Lancet. 1987;1:62–6.
459. Guinsburg R, Kopelman BI, Anand KJ, de Almeida MF, Peres Cde A, Miyoshi MH. Physiological, hormonal, and behavioral responses to a single fentanyl dose in intubated and ventilated preterm neonates. J Pediatr. 1998;132:954–9.
460. Hertzka RE, Gauntlett IS, Fisher DM, Spellman MJ. Fentanyl-induced ventilatory depression: effects of age. Anesthesiology. 1989;70:213–18.
461. Saarenmaa E, Neuvonen PJ, Fellman V. Gestational age and birth weight effects on plasma clearance of fentanyl in newborn infants. J Pediatr. 2000;136:767–70.
462. Barrier G, Attia J, Mayer MN, Amiel-Tison C, Shnider SM. Measurement of post-operative pain and narcotic administration in infants using a new clinical scoring system. Intensive Care Med. 1989;15:S37–9.
463. Billmire DA, Neale HW, Gregory RO. Use of i.v. fentanyl in the outpatient treatment of pediatric facial trauma. J Trauma. 1985;25:1079–80.
464. Koehntop DE, Rodman JH, Brundage DM, et al. Pharmacokinetics of fentanyl in neonates. Anesth Analg. 1986;65:227–32.
465. Koren G, Goresky G, Crean P, Klein J, MacLeod SM. Pediatric fentanyl dosing based on pharmacokinetics during cardiac surgery. Anesth Analg. 1984;63:577–82.
466. Koren G, Goresky G, Crean P, Klein J, MacLeod SM. Unexpected alterations in fentanyl pharmacokinetics in children undergoing cardiac surgery: age related or disease related? Dev Pharmacol Ther. 1986;9:183–91.

467. Hughes MA, Glass PS, Jacobs JR. Context-sensitive half-time in multicompartment pharmacokinetic models for intravenous anesthetic drugs. Anesthesiology. 1992;76:334–41.
468. Ginsberg B, Howell S, Glass PS, et al. Pharmacokinetic model-driven infusion of fentanyl in children. Anesthesiology. 1996;85:1268–75.
469. Zernikow B, Michel E, Anderson BJ. Transdermal fentanyl in childhood and adolescence: a comprehensive literature review. J Pain. 2007;8:187–207.
470. Lerman J, Nolan J, Eyres R, et al. Efficacy, safety, and pharmacokinetics of levobupivacaine with and without fentanyl after continuous epidural infusion in children: a multicenter trial. Anesthesiology. 2003;99:1166–74.
471. Goodarzi M. Comparison of epidural morphine, hydromorphone and fentanyl for postoperative pain control in children undergoing orthopaedic surgery. Paediatr Anaesth. 1999;9:419–22.
472. Ganesh A, Adzick NS, Foster T, Cucchiaro G. Efficacy of addition of fentanyl to epidural bupivacaine on postoperative analgesia after thoracotomy for lung resection in infants. Anesthesiology. 2008;109:890–4.
473. Franck LS, Vilardi J, Durand D, Powers R. Opioid withdrawal in neonates after continuous infusions of morphine or fentanyl during extracorporeal membrane oxygenation. Am J Crit Care. 1998;7:364–9.
474. Muller P, Vogtmann C. Three cases with different presentation of fentanyl-induced muscle rigidity–a rare problem in intensive care of neonates. Am J Perinatol. 2000;17:23–6.
475. Fahnenstich H, Steffan J, Kau N, Bartmann P. Fentanyl-induced chest wall rigidity and laryngospasm in preterm and term infants. Crit Care Med. 2000;28:836–9.
476. Reich A, Beland B, van Aken H. Intravenous narcotics and analgesic agents. In: Bissonnette B, Dalens BJ, editors. Pediatric anesthesia. New York: McGraw-Hill; 2002. p. 259–77.
477. Patel SS, Spencer CM. Remifentanil. Drugs. 1996;52:417–27.
478. Duthie DJ. Remifentanil and tramadol. Br J Anaesth. 1998;81:51–7.
479. Davis PJ, Galinkin J, McGowan FX, et al. A randomized multicenter study of remifentanil compared with halothane in neonates and infants undergoing pyloromyotomy. I. Emergence and recovery profiles. Anesth Analg. 2001;93:1380–6.
480. Chiaretti A, Pietrini D, Piastra M, et al. Safety and efficacy of remifentanil in craniosynostosis repair in children less than 1 year old. Pediatr Neurosurg. 2000;33:83–8.
481. Mani V, Morton NS. Overview of total intravenous anesthesia in children. Paediatr Anaesth. 2010;20(3):211–22.
482. Zhao M, Joo DT. Enhancement of spinal N-methyl-D-aspartate receptor function by remifentanil action at delta-opioid receptors as a mechanism for acute opioid-induced hyperalgesia or tolerance. Anesthesiology. 2008;109:308–17.
483. Egan TD. Remifentanil pharmacokinetics and pharmacodynamics. A preliminary appraisal. Clin Pharmacokinet. 1995;29:80–94.
484. Dershwitz M, Hoke JF, Rosow CE, et al. Pharmacokinetics and pharmacodynamics of remifentanil in volunteer subjects with severe liver disease. Anesthesiology. 1996;84:812–20.
485. Rigby-Jones AE, Priston MJ, Sneyd JR, et al. Remifentanil-midazolam sedation for paediatric patients receiving mechanical ventilation after cardiac surgery. Br J Anaesth. 2007;99:252–61.
486. Davis PJ, Wilson AS, Siewers RD, Pigula FA, Landsman IS. The effects of cardiopulmonary bypass on remifentanil kinetics in children undergoing atrial septal defect repair. Anesth Analg. 1999;89:904–8.
487. Sam WJ, Hammer GB, Drover DR. Population pharmacokinetics of remifentanil in infants and children undergoing cardiac surgery. BMC Anesthesiol. 2009;9:5.
488. Michelsen LG, Holford NH, Lu W, Hoke JF, Hug CC, Bailey JM. The pharmacokinetics of remifentanil in patients undergoing coronary artery bypass grafting with cardiopulmonary bypass. Anesth Analg. 2001;93:1100–5.
489. Barker N, Lim J, Amari E, Malherbe S, Ansermino JM. Relationship between age and spontaneous ventilation during intravenous anesthesia in children. Paediatr Anaesth. 2007;17:948–55.
490. Litman RS. Conscious sedation with remifentanil during painful medical procedures. J Pain Symptom Manage. 2000;19:468–71.
491. Choong K, AlFaleh K, Doucette J, et al. Remifentanil for endotracheal intubation in neonates: a randomised controlled trial. Arch Dis Child Fetal Neonatal Ed. 2010;95:F80–4.
492. Penido MG, Garra R, Sammartino M, Silva YP. Remifentanil in neonatal intensive care and anaesthesia practice. Acta Paediatr. 2010;99:1454–63.
493. Standing JF, Hammer GB, Sam WJ, Drover DR. Pharmacokinetic-pharmacodynamic modeling of the hypotensive effect of remifentanil in infants undergoing cranioplasty. Paediatr Anaesth. 2010;20:7–18.
494. Anderson BJ, Holford NH. Leaving no stone unturned, or extracting blood from stone? Paediatr Anaesth. 2010;20:1–6.
495. Thompson JP, Rowbotham DJ. Remifentanil–an opioid for the 21st century. Br J Anaesth. 1996;76:341–3.
496. Olkkola KT, Hamunen K. Pharmacokinetics and pharmacodynamics of analgesic drugs. In: Anand KJ, Stevens B, McGrath P, editors. Pain in neonates. 2nd ed. Amsterdam: Elsevier; 2000. p. 135–58. Revised and enlarged edition.
497. Saarenmaa E, Huttunen P, Leppaluoto J, Fellman V. Alfentanil as procedural pain relief in newborn infants. Arch Dis Child Fetal Neonatal Ed. 1996;75:F103–7.
498. Pokela ML. Effect of opioid-induced analgesia on beta-endorphin, cortisol and glucose responses in neonates with cardiorespiratory problems. Biol Neonate. 1993;64:360–7.
499. Pokela ML, Koivisto M. Physiological changes, plasma beta-endorphin and cortisol responses to tracheal intubation in neonates. Acta Paediatr. 1994;83:151–6.
500. Davis PJ, Cook DR. Clinical pharmacokinetics of the newer intravenous anaesthetic agents. Clin Pharmacokinet. 1986;11:18–35.
501. Meuldermans W, Woestenborghs R, Noorduin H, Camu F, van Steenberge A, Heykants J. Protein binding of the analgesics alfentanil and sufentanil in maternal and neonatal plasma. Eur J Clin Pharmacol. 1986;30:217–19.
502. Wilson AS, Stiller RL, Davis PJ, et al. Fentanyl and alfentanil plasma protein binding in preterm and term neonates. Anesth Analg. 1997;84:315–18.
503. Meistelman C, Saint-Maurice C, Lepaul M, Levron JC, Loose JP, Mac GK. A comparison of alfentanil pharmacokinetics in children and adults. Anesthesiology. 1987;66:13–6.
504. Marlow N, Weindling AM, Van Peer A, Heykants J. Alfentanil pharmacokinetics in preterm infants. Arch Dis Child. 1990;65:349–51.
505. Killian A, Davis PJ, Stiller RL, Cicco R, Cook DR, Guthrie RD. Influence of gestational age on pharmacokinetics of alfentanil in neonates. Dev Pharmacol Ther. 1990;15:82–5.
506. Pokela ML, Olkkola KT, Koivisto M, Ryhanen P. Pharmacokinetics and pharmacodynamics of intravenous meperidine in neonates and infants. Clin Pharmacol Ther. 1992;52:342–9.
507. Hilberman M, Hyer D. Potency of sufentanil. Anesthesiology. 1986;64:665–8.
508. Greeley WJ, de Bruijn NP, Davis DP. Sufentanil pharmacokinetics in pediatric cardiovascular patients. Anesth Analg. 1987;66:1067–72.
509. Tateishi T, Krivoruk Y, Ueng YF, Wood AJ, Guengerich FP, Wood M. Identification of human liver cytochrome P-450 3A4 as the enzyme responsible for fentanyl and sufentanil N-dealkylation. Anesth Analg. 1996;82:167–72.
510. Davis PJ, Cook DR, Stiller RL, Davin-Robinson KA. Pharmacodynamics and pharmacokinetics of high-dose

sufentanil in infants and children undergoing cardiac surgery. Anesth Analg. 1987;66:203–8.
511. Greeley WJ, de Bruijn NP. Changes in sufentanil pharmacokinetics within the neonatal period. Anesth Analg. 1988;67:86–90.
512. Lacroix D, Sonnier M, Moncion A, Cheron G, Cresteil T. Expression of CYP3A in the human liver–evidence that the shift between CYP3A7 and CYP3A4 occurs immediately after birth. Eur J Biochem. 1997;247:625–34.
513. Guay J, Gaudreault P, Tang A, Goulet B, Varin F. Pharmacokinetics of sufentanil in normal children. Can J Anaesth. 1992;39:14–20.
514. Lerman J, Strong A, LeDez KM, et al. Effects of age on the serum concentration of a1-acid glycoprotein and the binding of lidocaine in pediatric patients. Clin Pharm Ther. 1989;46:219–25.
515. Benet LZ, Hoener B-a. Changes in plasma protein binding have little clinical consequence. Clin Pharm Ther. 2002;71:115–21.
516. Cho JE, Kim JY, Kim JE, Chun DH, Jun NH, Kil HK. Epidural sufentanil provides better analgesia from 24 h after surgery compared with epidural fentanyl in children. Acta Anaesthesiol Scand. 2008;52:1360–3.
517. Bichel T, Rouge JC, Schlegel S, Spahr-Schopfer I, Kalangos A. Epidural sufentanil during paediatric cardiac surgery: effects on metabolic response and postoperative outcome. Paediatr Anaesth. 2000;10:609–17.
518. Benlabed M, Ecoffey C, Levron JC, Flaisler B, Gross JB. Analgesia and ventilatory response to CO2 following epidural sufentanil in children. Anesthesiology. 1987;67:948–51.
519. Helmers JH, Noorduin H, Van Peer A, Van Leeuwen L, Zuurmond WW. Comparison of intravenous and intranasal sufentanil absorption and sedation. Can J Anaesth. 1989;36:494–7.
520. Henderson JM, Brodsky DA, Fisher DM, Brett CM, Hertzka RE. Pre-induction of anesthesia in pediatric patients with nasally administered sufentanil. Anesthesiology. 1988;68:671–5.
521. Roelofse JA, Shipton EA, de la Harpe CJ, Blignaut RJ. Intranasal sufentanil/midazolam versus ketamine/midazolam for analgesia/sedation in the pediatric population prior to undergoing multiple dental extractions under general anesthesia: a prospective, double-blind, randomized comparison. Anesth Prog. 2004;51:114–21.
522. Williams DG, Hatch DJ, Howard RF. Codeine phosphate in paediatric medicine. Br J Anaesth. 2001;86:413–21.
523. Cartabuke RS, Tobias JD, Taghon T, Rice J. Current practices regarding codeine administration among paediatricians and pediatric subspecialists. Clin Pediatr. 2014;53(1):26–30.
524. Tremlett M, Anderson BJ, Wolf A. Pro-con debate: is codeine a drug that still has a useful role in pediatric practice? Paediatr Anaesth. 2010;20:183–94.
525. Chen ZR, Somogyi AA, Bochner F. Polymorphic O-demethylation of codeine. Lancet. 1988;2:914–15.
526. Sindrup SH, Brosen K. The pharmacogenetics of codeine hypoalgesia. Pharmacogenetics. 1995;5:335–46.
527. Koren G, Madadi P. Pharmacogenetic insights into codeine analgesia: implication to codeine use. Pharmacogenomics. 2008;9:1267–84.
528. Williams DG, Patel A, Howard RF. Pharmacogenetics of codeine metabolism in an urban population of children and its implications for analgesic reliability. Br J Anaesth. 2002; 89:839–45.
529. Eckhardt K, Li S, Ammon S, Schanzle G, Mikus G, Eichelbaum M. Same incidence of adverse drug events after codeine administration irrespective of the genetically determined differences in morphine formation. Pain. 1998;76:27–33.
530. Madadi P, Amstutz U, Rieder M, et al. Clinical practice guideline: CYP2D6 genotyping for safe and efficacious codeine therapy. J Popul Ther Clin Pharmacol. 2013;20:e369–96.
531. Parke TJ, Nandi PR, Bird KJ, Jewkes DA. Profound hypotension following intravenous codeine phosphate. Three case reports and some recommendations. Anaesthesia. 1992;47:852–4.
532. McEwan A, Sigston PE, Andrews KA, et al. A comparison of rectal and intramuscular codeine phosphate in children following neurosurgery. Paediatr Anaesth. 2000;10:189–93.
533. Tobias JD, Lowe S, Hersey S, Rasmussen GE, Werkhaven J. Analgesia after bilateral myringotomy and placement of pressure equalization tubes in children: acetaminophen versus acetaminophen with codeine. Anesth Analg. 1995;81:496–500.
534. St Charles CS, Matt BH, Hamilton MM, Katz BP. A comparison of ibuprofen versus acetaminophen with codeine in the young tonsillectomy patient. Otolaryngol Head Neck Surg. 1997;117:76–82.
535. Cunliffe M. Codeine phosphate in children: time for re-evaluation? Br J Anaesth. 2001;86:329–31.
536. Quiding H, Olsson GL, Boreus LO, Bondesson U. Infants and young children metabolise codeine to morphine. A study after single and repeated rectal administration. Br J Clin Pharmacol. 1992;33:45–9.
537. Magnani B, Evans R. Codeine intoxication in the neonate. Pediatrics. 1999;104:e75.
538. Ciszkowski C, Madadi P, Phillips MS, Lauwers AE, Koren G. Codeine, ultrarapid-metabolism genotype, and postoperative death. N Engl J Med. 2009;361:827–8.
539. Madadi P, Shirazi F, Walter FG, Koren G. Establishing causality of CNS depression in breastfed infants following maternal codeine use. Paediatr Drugs. 2008;10:399–404.
540. Kelly LE, Chaudhry SA, Rieder MJ, et al. A clinical tool for reducing central nervous system depression among neonates exposed to codeine through breast milk. PLoS One. 2013;8:e70073.
541. Poulsen L, Brosen K, Arendt-Nielsen L, Gram LF, Elbaek K, Sindrup SH. Codeine and morphine in extensive and poor metabolizers of sparteine: pharmacokinetics, analgesic effect and side effects. Eur J Clin Pharmacol. 1996;51:289–95.
542. Koren G, Maurice L. Pediatric uses of opioids. Pediatr Clin N Am. 1989;36:1141–56.
543. Jaffe JH, Martine WR. Opioid analgesics and antagonists. In: Goodman Gilman A, Rall TW, Nies AS, Taylor P, editors. The pharmacological basis of therapeutics. New York: Pergamon Press; 1990. p. 485–531.
544. Hamunen K, Maunuksela EL, Seppala T, Olkkola KT. Pharmacokinetics of i.v. and rectal pethidine in children undergoing ophthalmic surgery. Br J Anaesth. 1993;71:823–6.
545. Caldwell J, Wakile LA, Notarianni LJ, et al. Maternal and neonatal disposition of pethidine in childbirth–a study using quantitative gas chromatography-mass spectrometry. Life Sci. 1978;22: 589–96.
546. Latta KS, Ginsberg B, Barkin RL. Meperidine: a critical review. Am J Ther. 2002;9:53–68.
547. Vetter TR. Pediatric patient-controlled analgesia with morphine versus meperidine. J Pain Symptom Manage. 1992;7:204–8.
548. Berde CB, Sethna NF. Analgesics for the treatment of pain in children. N Engl J Med. 2002;347:1094–103.
549. Cote CJ, Karl HW, Notterman DA, Weinberg JA, McCloskey C. Adverse sedation events in pediatrics: analysis of medications used for sedation. Pediatrics. 2000;106:633–44.
550. Ngan Kee WD. Intrathecal pethidine: pharmacology and clinical applications. Anaesth Intensive Care. 1998;26:137–46.
551. Sabatowski R, Kasper SM, Radbruch L. Patient-controlled analgesia with intravenous L-methadone in a child with cancer pain refractory to high-dose morphine. J Pain Symptom Manage. 2002;23:3–5.
552. Suresh S, Anand KJ. Opioid tolerance in neonates: mechanisms, diagnosis, assessment, and management. Semin Perinatol. 1998;22:425–33.
553. Tobias JD. Tolerance, withdrawal, and physical dependency after long-term sedation and analgesia of children in the pediatric intensive care unit. Crit Care Med. 2000;28:2122–32.

554. Berde CB, Beyer JE, Bournaki MC, Levin CR, Sethna NF. Comparison of morphine and methadone for prevention of postoperative pain in 3- to 7-year-old children. J Pediatr. 1991;119:136–41.
555. Shir Y, Shenkman Z, Shavelson V, Davidson EM, Rosen G. Oral methadone for the treatment of severe pain in hospitalized children: a report of five cases. Clin J Pain. 1998;14:350–3.
556. Davies D, DeVlaming D, Haines C. Methadone analgesia for children with advanced cancer. Pediatr Blood Cancer. 2008;51:393–7.
557. Berkowitz BA. The relationship of pharmacokinetics to pharmacological activity: morphine, methadone and naloxone. Clin Pharmacokinet. 1976;1:219–30.
558. Kaufmann JJ, Koski WS, Benson DN, Semo NM. Narcotic and narcotic antagonist pKa's and partition coefficients and their significance in clinical practice. Drug Alcohol Depend. 1975;1:103–14.
559. Gourlay GK, Wilson PR, Glynn CJ. Pharmacodynamics and pharmacokinetics of methadone during the perioperative period. Anesthesiology. 1982;57:458–67.
560. Berde CB, Sethna HF, Holzman RS, Reidy P, Gondek EJ. Pharmacokinetics of methadone in children and adolescents in the perioperative period. Anesthesiology. 1987;67:A519.
561. Yang F, Tong X, McCarver DG, Hines RN, Beard DA. Population-based analysis of methadone distribution and metabolism using an age-dependent physiologically based pharmacokinetic model. J Pharmacokinet Pharmacodyn. 2006;33:485–518.
562. Mandema JW, Tuk B, van Steveninck AL, Breimer DD, Cohen AF, Danhof M. Pharmacokinetic-pharmacodynamic modeling of the central nervous system effects of midazolam and its main metabolite alpha-hydroxymidazolam in healthy volunteers. Clin Pharmacol Ther. 1992;51:715–28.
563. Greenblatt DJ, Ehrenberg BL, Gunderman J, et al. Pharmacokinetic and electroencephalographic study of intravenous diazepam, midazolam, and placebo. Clin Pharmacol Ther. 1989;45:356–65.
564. Buhrer M, Maitre PO, Crevoisier C, Stanski DR. Electroencephalographic effects of benzodiazepines. II. Pharmacodynamic modeling of the electroencephalographic effects of midazolam and diazepam. Clin Pharmacol Ther. 1990;48:555–67.
565. Johnson TN, Rostami-Hodjegan A, Goddard JM, Tanner MS, Tucker GT. Contribution of midazolam and its 1-hydroxy metabolite to preoperative sedation in children: a pharmacokinetic-pharmacodynamic analysis. Br J Anaesth. 2002;89:428–37.
566. de Wildt SN, de Hoog M, Vinks AA, Joosten KF, van Dijk M, van den Anker JN. Pharmacodynamics of midazolam in pediatric intensive care patients. Ther Drug Monit. 2005;27:98–102.
567. Hartwig S, Roth B, Theisohn M. Clinical experience with continuous intravenous sedation using midazolam and fentanyl in the paediatric intensive care unit. Eur J Pediatr. 1991;150:784–8.
568. Lloyd-Thomas AR, Booker PD. Infusion of midazolam in paediatric patients after cardiac surgery. Br J Anaesth. 1986;58:1109–15.
569. Booker PD, Beechey A, Lloyd-Thomas AR. Sedation of children requiring artificial ventilation using an infusion of midazolam. Br J Anaesth. 1986;58:1104–8.
570. Lee TC, Charles BG, Harte GJ, Gray PH, Steer PA, Flenady VJ. Population pharmacokinetic modeling in very premature infants receiving midazolam during mechanical ventilation: midazolam neonatal pharmacokinetics. Anesthesiology. 1999;90:451–7.
571. Harte GJ, Gray PH, Lee TC, Steer PA, Charles BG. Haemodynamic responses and population pharmacokinetics of midazolam following administration to ventilated, preterm neonates. J Paediatr Child Health. 1997;33:335–8.
572. de Wildt SN, Kearns GL, Hop WC, Murry DJ, Abdel-Rahman SM, van den Anker JN. Pharmacokinetics and metabolism of intravenous midazolam in preterm infants. Clin Pharmacol Ther. 2001;70:525–31.
573. Burtin P, Jacqz-Aigrain E, Girard P, et al. Population pharmacokinetics of midazolam in neonates. Clin Pharmacol Ther. 1994;56:615–25.
574. Jacqz-Aigrain E, Daoud P, Burtin P, Maherzi S, Beaufils F. Pharmacokinetics of midazolam during continuous infusion in critically ill neonates. Eur J Clin Pharmacol. 1992;42:329–32.
575. Jacqz-Aigrain E, Wood C, Robieux I. Pharmacokinetics of midazolam in critically ill neonates. Eur J Clin Pharmacol. 1990;39:191–2.
576. Anderson BJ, Larsson P. A maturation model for midazolam clearance. Paediatr Anaesth. 2011;21:302–8.
577. Mulla H, McCormack P, Lawson G, Firmin RK, Upton DR. Pharmacokinetics of midazolam in neonates undergoing extracorporeal membrane oxygenation. Anesthesiology. 2003;99:275–82.
578. Mathews HM, Carson IW, Lyons SM, et al. A pharmacokinetic study of midazolam in paediatric patients undergoing cardiac surgery. Br J Anaesth. 1988;61:302–7.
579. Hiller A, Olkkola KT, Isohanni P, Saarnivaara L. Unconsciousness associated with midazolam and erythromycin. Br J Anaesth. 1990;65:826–8.
580. de Wildt SN, de Hoog M, Vinks AA, van der Giesen E, van den Anker JN. Population pharmacokinetics and metabolism of midazolam in pediatric intensive care patients. Crit Care Med. 2003;31:1952–8.
581. Nishina K, Mikawa K. Clonidine in paediatric anaesthesia. Curr Opin Anaesthesiol. 2002;15:309–16.
582. Bergendahl H, Lonnqvist PA, Eksborg S. Clonidine in paediatric anaesthesia: review of the literature and comparison with benzodiazepines for premedication. Acta Anaesthesiol Scand. 2006;50:135–43.
583. Ansermino M, Basu R, Vandebeek C, Montgomery C. Nonopioid additives to local anaesthetics for caudal blockade in children: a systematic review. Paediatr Anaesth. 2003;13:561–73.
584. Manickam A, Vakamudi M, Parameswari A, Chetan C. Efficacy of clonidine as an adjuvant to ropivacaine for caudal analgesia in children undergoing subumbilical surgery. J Anaesthesiol Clin Pharm. 2012;28:185–9.
585. Engelman E, Marsala C. Bayesian enhanced meta-analysis of post-operative analgesic efficacy of additives for caudal analgesia in children. Acta Anaesth Scand. 2012;56:817–32.
586. Schnabel A, Poepping DM, Pogatzki-Zahn EM, Zahn PK. Efficacy and safety of clonidine as additive for caudal regional anesthesia: a quantitative systematic review of randomized controlled trials. Paediatr Anaesth. 2011;21:1219–30.
587. Sumiya K, Homma M, Watanabe M, et al. Sedation and plasma concentration of clonidine hydrochloride for pre-anesthetic medication in pediatric surgery. Biol Pharm Bull. 2003;26:421–3.
588. Hall JE, Uhrich TD, Ebert TJ. Sedative, analgesic and cognitive effects of clonidine infusions in humans. Br J Anaesth. 2001;86:5–11.
589. Marinangeli F, Ciccozzi A, Donatelli F, et al. Clonidine for treatment of postoperative pain: a dose-finding study. Eur J Pain. 2002;6:35–42.
590. Bernard JM, Hommeril JL, Passuti N, Pinaud M. Postoperative analgesia by intravenous clonidine. Anesthesiology. 1991;75:577–82.
591. Dollery CT, Davies DS, Draffan GH, et al. Clinical pharmacology and pharmacokinetics of clonidine. Clin Pharmacol Ther. 1976;19:11–7.
592. Milne B. Alpha-2 agonists and anaesthesia. Can J Anaesth. 1991;38:809–13.

593. Davies DS, Wing AM, Reid JL, Neill DM, Tippett P, Dollery CT. Pharmacokinetics and concentration-effect relationships of intervenous and oral clonidine. Clin Pharmacol Ther. 1977; 21:593–601.
594. Kamibayashi T, Maze M. Clinical uses of alpha2 -adrenergic agonists. Anesthesiology. 2000;93:1345–9.
595. Talke P. Pharmacodynamics of alpha2-adrenoceptor agonists. Best Pract Res Clin Anaesthesiol. 2000;14:271–83.
596. Lonnqvist PA, Bergendahl H. Pharmacokinetics and haemodynamic response after an intravenous bolus injection of clonidine in children. Paediatr Anaesth. 1993;3:359–64.
597. Lowenthal DT, Matzek KM, MacGregor TR. Clinical pharmacokinetics of clonidine. Clin Pharmacokinet. 1988;14:287–310.
598. Arndts D, Doevendans J, Kirsten R, Heintz B. New aspects of the pharmacokinetics and pharmacodynamics of clonidine in man. Eur J Clin Pharmacol. 1983;24:21–30.
599. Arndts D. New aspects of the clinical pharmacology of clonidine. Chest. 1983;83:397–400.
600. Lonnqvist PA, Bergendahl HT, Eksborg S. Pharmacokinetics of clonidine after rectal administration in children. Anesthesiology. 1994;81:1097–101.
601. Potts AL, Larsson P, Eksborg S, Warman G, Lonnqvist P-A, Anderson BJ. Clonidine disposition in children; a population analysis. Pediatr Anesth. 2007;17:924–33.
602. Xie HG, Cao YJ, Gauda EB, Agthe AG, Hendrix CW, Lee H. Clonidine clearance matures rapidly during the early postnatal period: a population pharmacokinetic analysis in newborns with neonatal abstinence syndrome. J Clin Pharmacol. 2011;51(4):502–11.
603. Larsson P, Nordlinder A, Bergendahl HT, et al. Oral bioavailability of clonidine in children. Pediatr Anesth. 2011;21:335–40.
604. Ibacache ME, Munoz HR, Brandes V, Morales AL. Single-dose dexmedetomidine reduces agitation after sevoflurane anesthesia in children. Anesth Analg. 2004;98:60–3.
605. Tobias JD. Dexmedetomidine to treat opioid withdrawal in infants following prolonged sedation in the pediatric ICU. J Opioid Manag. 2006;2:201–5.
606. Tobias JD. Dexmedetomidine: applications in pediatric critical care and pediatric anesthesiology. Pediatr Crit Care Med. 2007;8:115–31.
607. Mason KP, O'Mahony E, Zurakowski D, Libenson MH. Effects of dexmedetomidine sedation on the EEG in children. Paediatr Anaesth. 2009;19:1175–83.
608. Mason KP, Lerman J. Dexmedetomidine in children: current knowledge and future applications. Anesth Analg. 2011;113: 1129–42.
609. O'Mara K, Gal P, Ransom JL, et al. Successful use of dexmedetomidine for sedation in a 24-week gestational age neonate. Ann Pharmacother. 2009;43:1707–13.
610. Chrysostomou C, Schulman SR, Castellanos MH, et al. A Phase II/III, multicentre, safety, efficacy, and pharmacokinetic study of dexmedetomidine in preterm and term neonates. J Pediatr. 2013;Pii:S0022-3476(13)01230-4. Epub ahead of print.
611. O'Mara K, Gal P, Wimmer J, et al. Dexmedetomidine versus standard therapy with fentanyl for sedation in mechanically ventilated premature neonates. J Pediatr Pharmacol Ther. 2012;17:252–62.
612. Tobias JD. Controlled hypotension in children: a critical review of available agents. Paediatr Drugs. 2002;4:439–53.
613. Nichols DP, Berkenbosch JW, Tobias JD. Rescue sedation with dexmedetomidine for diagnostic imaging: a preliminary report. Paediatr Anaesth. 2005;15:199–203.
614. Hammer GB, Philip BM, Schroeder AR, Rosen FS, Koltai PJ. Prolonged infusion of dexmedetomidine for sedation following tracheal resection. Paediatr Anaesth. 2005;15:616–20.
615. Walker J, Maccallum M, Fischer C, Kopcha R, Saylors R, McCall J. Sedation using dexmedetomidine in pediatric burn patients. J Burn Care Res. 2006;27:206–10.
616. Koroglu A, Teksan H, Sagir O, Yucel A, Toprak HI, Ersoy OM. A comparison of the sedative, hemodynamic, and respiratory effects of dexmedetomidine and propofol in children undergoing magnetic resonance imaging. Anesth Analg. 2006;103:63–7.
617. Fagin A, Palmieri T, Greenhalgh D, Sen S. A comparison of dexmedetomidine and midazolam for sedation in severe pediatric burn injury. J Burn Care Res. 2012;33:759–63.
618. Schnabel A, Reichi SU, Poepping DM, et al. Efficacy and safety of intraoperative dexmedetomidine for acute postoperative pain in children: a meta-analysis of randomized controlled trials. Pediatr Anesth. 2013;23:170–9.
619. Olutoye OA, Glover CD, Diefenderfer JW, et al. The effect of intraoperative dexmedetomidine on postoperative analgesia and sedation in pediatric patients undergoing tonsillectomy and adenoidectomy. Anesth Analg. 2010;111:490–5.
620. Chen JY, Lia JE, Liu TJ, et al. Comparison of the effects of dexmedetomidine, ketamine, and placebo on emergence agitation after strabismus surgery in children. Can J Anesth. 2013;60: 385–92.
621. Hsu YW, Cortinez LI, Robertson KM, et al. Dexmedetomidine pharmacodynamics: part I: crossover comparison of the respiratory effects of dexmedetomidine and remifentanil in healthy volunteers. Anesthesiology. 2004;101:1066–76.
622. Potts AL, Anderson BJ, Warman GR, Lerman J, Diaz SM, Vilo S. Dexmedetomidine pharmacokinetics in pediatric intensive care–a pooled analysis. Paediatr Anaesth. 2009;19:1119–29.
623. Potts AL, Anderson BJ, Holford NH, Vu TC, Warman GR. Dexmedetomidine hemodynamics in children after cardiac surgery. Paediatr Anaesth. 2010;20:425–33.
624. Mason KP, Zurakowski D, Zgleszewski S, Prescilla R, Fontaine PJ, Dinardo JA. Incidence and predictors of hypertension during high-dose dexmedetomidine sedation for pediatric MRI. Paediatr Anaesth. 2010;20(6):516–23.
625. Mahmoud M, Radhakrishman R, Gunter J, et al. Effect of increasing depth of dexmedetomidine anesthesia on upper airway morphology in children. Paediatr Anaesth. 2010;20:506–15.
626. Mahmoud M, Jung D, Salisbury S, et al. Effect of increasing depth of dexmedetomidine and propofol anesthesia on upper airway morphology in children and adolescents with obstructive sleep apnea. J Clin Anesth. 2013;25(7):529–41. pii:S0952-8180(13)00203-1. Epub ahead of print.
627. Mahmoud M, Gunter J, Donnelly LF, Wang Y, Nick TG, Sadhasivam S. A comparison of dexmedetomidine with propofol for magnetic resonance imaging sleep studies in children. Anesth Analg. 2009;109:745–53.
628. Su F, Nicolson SC, Gastonguay MR, et al. Population pharmacokinetics of dexmedetomidine in infants after open heart surgery. Anesth Analg. 2010;110:1383–92.
629. Mason KP, Zgleszewski SE, Prescilla R, Fontaine PJ, Zurakowski D. Hemodynamic effects of dexmedetomidine sedation for CT imaging studies. Paediatr Anaesth. 2008;18:393–402.
630. Siddappa R, Riggins J, Kariyanna S, et al. High-dose dexmedetomidine sedation for pediatric MRI. Pediatr Anesth. 2011;21:153–8.
631. Heard C, Burrows F, Johnson K, et al. A comparison of dexmedetomidine-midazolam with propofol for maintenance of anesthesia in children undergoing magnetic resonance imaging. Anesth Analg. 2008;107:1832–9.
632. Mason KP, Zurakowski D, Zgleszewski SE, et al. High dose dexmedetomidine as the sole sedative for pediatric MRI. Paediatr Anaesth. 2008;18:403–11.

633. Hammer GB, Drover DR, Cao H, et al. The effects of dexmedetomidine on cardiac electrophysiology in children. Anesth Analg. 2008;106:79–83. table of contents.
634. Chrysostomou C, Morell VO, Wearden P, et al. Dexmedetomidine: therapeutic use for the termination of reentrant supraventricular tachycardia. Congenit Heart Dis. 2013;8:48–56.
635. Friesen RH, Nichols CS, Twite MD, et al. The hemodynamic response to dexmedetomidine loading dose in children with and without pulmonary hypertension. Anesth Analg. 2013;117: 953–9.
636. Coyle DE, Denson DD, Thompson GA, Myers JA, Arthur GR, Bridenbaugh PO. The influence of lactic acid on the serum protein binding of bupivacaine: species differences. Anesthesiology. 1984;61:127–33.
637. Lerman J, Strong HA, LeDez KM, Swartz J, Rieder MJ, Burrows FA. Effects of age on the serum concentration of alpha 1-acid glycoprotein and the binding of lidocaine in pediatric patients. Clin Pharmacol Ther. 1989;46:219–25.
638. Eyres RL. Local anaesthetic agents in infancy. Paediatr Anaesth. 1995;5:213–18.
639. Valenzuela C, Snyders DJ, Bennett PB, Tamargo J, Hondeghem LM. Stereoselective block of cardiac sodium channels by bupivacaine in guinea pig ventricular myocytes. Circulation. 1995;92:3014–24.
640. Hoerter JA, Vassort G. Participation of the sarcolemma in the control of relaxation of the mammalian heart during perinatal development. Adv Myocardiol. 1982;3:373–80.
641. Hellstrom-Westas L, Svenningsen NW, Westgren U, Rosen I, Lagerstrom PO. Lidocaine for treatment of severe seizures in newborn infants. II. Blood concentrations of lidocaine and metabolites during intravenous infusion. Acta Paediatr. 1992;81:35–9.
642. Hellstrom-Westas L, Westgren U, Rosen I, Svenningsen NW. Lidocaine for treatment of severe seizures in newborn infants. I. Clinical effects and cerebral electrical activity monitoring. Acta Paediatr Scand. 1988;77:79–84.
643. Hattori H, Yamano T, Hayashi K, et al. Effectiveness of lidocaine infusion for status epilepticus in childhood: a retrospective multi-institutional study in Japan. Brain Dev. 2008;30:504–12.
644. Vladimirov M, Nau C, Mok WM, Strichartz G. Potency of bupivacaine stereoisomers tested in vitro and in vivo: biochemical, electrophysiological, and neurobehavioral studies. Anesthesiology. 2000;93:744–55.
645. Wang GK, Wang SY. Altered stereoselectivity of cocaine and bupivacaine isomers in normal and batrachotoxin-modified Na+channels. J Gen Physiol. 1992;100:1003–20.
646. Sheets MF, Hanck DA. Outward stabilization of the S4 segments in domains III and IV enhances lidocaine block of sodium channels. J Physiol. 2007;582:317–34.
647. Chevrier P, Vijayaragavan K, Chahine M. Differential modulation of Nav1.7 and Nav1.8 peripheral nerve sodium channels by the local anesthetic lidocaine. Br J Pharmacol. 2004;142:576–84.
648. Mihaly GW, Moore RG, Thomas J, Triggs EJ, Thomas D, Shanks CA. The pharmacokinetics and metabolism of the anilide local anaesthetics in neonates. I. Lignocaine. Eur J Clin Pharmacol. 1978;13:143–52.
649. Rapp HJ, Molnar V, Austin S, et al. Ropivacaine in neonates and infants: a population pharmacokinetic evaluation following single caudal block. Paediatr Anaesth. 2004;14:724–32.
650. Agarwal R, Gutlove DP, Lockhart CH. Seizures occurring in pediatric patients receiving continuous infusion of bupivacaine. Anesth Analg. 1992;75:284–6.
651. McCloskey JJ, Haun SE, Deshpande JK. Bupivacaine toxicity secondary to continuous caudal epidural infusion in children. Anesth Analg. 1992;75:287–90.
652. Aarons L, Sadler B, Pitsiu M, et al. Population pharmacokinetic analysis of ropivacaine and its metabolite 2', 6'-pipecoloxylidide from pooled data in neonates, infants, and children. Br J Anaesth. 2011;107:409–24.
653. Tucker GT, Mather LE. Clinical pharmacokinetics of local anaesthetics. Clin Pharmacokinet. 1979;4:241–78.
654. Chalkiadis GA, Anderson BJ, Tay M, et al. Pharmacokinetics of levobupivacaine after caudal epidural administration in infants less than 3 months of age. Br J Anaesth. 2005;95:524–9.
655. Tucker GT. Pharmacokinetics of local anaesthetics. Br J Anaesth. 1986;58:717–31.
656. Galley HF, Mahdy A, Lowes DA. Pharmacogenetics and anesthesiologists. Pharmacogenomics. 2005;6:849–56.
657. Bosenberg AT, Bland BA, Schulte Steinberg O, Downing JW. Thoracic epidural anesthesia via caudal route in infants. Anesthesiology. 1988;69:265–9.
658. Bokesch PM, Castaneda AR, Ziemer G, Wilson JM. The influence of a right-to-left cardiac shunt on lidocaine pharmacokinetics. Anesthesiology. 1987;67:739–44.
659. Mirkin BL. Developmental pharmacology. Annu Rev Pharmacol. 1970;10:255–72.
660. Bardsley H, Gristwood R, Baker H, Watson N, Nimmo W. A comparison of the cardiovascular effects of levobupivacaine and rac-bupivacaine following intravenous administration to healthy volunteers. Br J Clin Pharmacol. 1998;46:245–9.
661. Brisman M, Ljung BM, Otterbom I, Larsson LE, Andreasson SE. Methaemoglobin formation after the use of EMLA cream in term neonates. Acta Paediatr. 1998;87:1191–4.
662. Mishina M, Takai T, Imoto K, et al. Molecular distinction between fetal and adult forms of muscle acetylcholine receptor. Nature. 1986;321:406–11.
663. Jaramillo F, Schuetze SM. Kinetic differences between embryonic- and adult-type acetylcholine receptors in rat myotubes. J Physiol. 1988;396:267–96.
664. Hesselmans LF, Jennekens FG, Van den Oord CJ, Veldman H, Vincent A. Development of innervation of skeletal muscle fibers in man: relation to acetylcholine receptors. Anat Rec. 1993;236:553–62.
665. Jaramillo F, Vicini S, Schuetze SM. Embryonic acetylcholine receptors guarantee spontaneous contractions in rat developing muscle. Nature. 1988;335:66–8.
666. Goudsouzian NG. Maturation of neuromuscular transmission in the infant. Br J Anaesth. 1980;52:205–14.
667. Goudsouzian NG, Standaert FG. The infant and the myoneural junction. Anesth Analg. 1986;65:1208–17.
668. Meretoja OA, Brandom BW, Taivainen T, Jalkanen L. Synergism between atracurium and vecuronium in children. Br J Anaesth. 1993;71:440–2.
669. Meretoja OA, Taivainen T, Jalkanen L, Wirtavuori K. Synergism between atracurium and vecuronium in infants and children during nitrous oxide-oxygen-alfentanil anaesthesia. Br J Anaesth. 1994;73:605–7.
670. Day NS, Blake GJ, Standaert FG, Dretchen KL. Characterization of the train-of-four response in fast and slow muscles: effect of d-tubocurarine, pancuronium, and vecuronium. Anesthesiology. 1983;58:414–17.
671. Keens TG, Bryan AC, Levison H, Ianuzzo CD. Developmental pattern of muscle fiber types in human ventilatory muscles. J Appl Physiol. 1978;44:909–13.
672. Meretoja OA. Neuromuscular blocking agents in paediatric patients: influence of age on the response. Anaesth Intensive Care. 1990;18:440–8.
673. Donati F, Antzaka C, Bevan DR. Potency of pancuronium at the diaphragm and the adductor pollicis muscle in humans. Anesthesiology. 1986;65:1–5.
674. Laycock JR, Baxter MK, Bevan JC, Sangwan S, Donati F, Bevan DR. The potency of pancuronium at the adductor pollicis

and diaphragm in infants and children. Anesthesiology. 1988;68:908–11.
675. Laycock JR, Donati F, Smith CE, Bevan DR. Potency of atracurium and vecuronium at the diaphragm and the adductor pollicis muscle. Br J Anaesth. 1988;61:286–91.
676. Meretoja OA, Wirtavuori K, Neuvonen PJ. Age-dependence of the dose-response curve of vecuronium in pediatric patients during balanced anesthesia. Anesth Analg. 1988;67:21–6.
677. Meakin G, Shaw EA, Baker RD, Morris P. Comparison of atracurium-induced neuromuscular blockade in neonates, infants and children. Br J Anaesth. 1988;60:171–5.
678. Basta SJ, Ali HH, Savarese JJ, et al. Clinical pharmacology of atracurium besylate (BW 33A): a new non-depolarizing muscle relaxant. Anesth Analg. 1982;61:723–9.
679. Woelfel SK, Brandom BW, McGowan Jr FX, Cook DR. Clinical pharmacology of mivacurium in pediatric patients less than off years old during nitrous oxide-halothane anesthesia. Anesth Analg. 1993;77:713–20.
680. Goudsouzian NG, Denman W, Schwartz A, Shorten G, Foster V, Samara B. Pharmacodynamic and hemodynamic effects of mivacurium in infants anesthetized with halothane and nitrous oxide. Anesthesiology. 1993;79:919–25.
681. Fisher DM, Miller RD. Neuromuscular effects of vecuronium (ORG NC45) in infants and children during N2O, halothane anesthesia. Anesthesiology. 1983;58:519–23.
682. Fisher DM, Castagnoli K, Miller RD. Vecuronium kinetics and dynamics in anesthetized infants and children. Clin Pharmacol Ther. 1985;37:402–6.
683. Fisher DM, Canfell PC, Spellman MJ, Miller RD. Pharmacokinetics and pharmacodynamics of atracurium in infants and children. Anesthesiology. 1990;73:33–7.
684. Wierda JM, Meretoja OA, Taivainen T, Proost JH. Pharmacokinetics and pharmacokinetic-dynamic modelling of rocuronium in infants and children. Br J Anaesth. 1997;78:690–5.
685. Kalli I, Meretoja OA. Infusion of atracurium in neonates, infants and children. A study of dose requirements. Br J Anaesth. 1988;60:651–4.
686. Alifimoff JK, Goudsouzian NG. Continuous infusion of mivacurium in children. Brit J Anaesth 1989; 63:520–4.
687. Woelfel SK, Dong ML, Brandom BW, Sarner JB, Cook DR. Vecuronium infusion requirements in children during halothane-narcotic-nitrous oxide, isoflurane-narcotic-nitrous oxide, and narcotic-nitrous oxide anesthesia. Anesth Analg. 1991;73:33–8.
688. Feltman DM, Weiss MG, Nicoski P, et al. rocuronium for nonemergent intubation of term and preterm infants. J Perinatol. 2011;31:38–43.
689. Driessen JJ, Robertson EN, Van Egmond J, et al. The time-course of action and recovery of rocuronium 0.3 mg/kg^{-1} in infants and children during halothane anaesthesia measured with acceleromyography. Pediatr Anesth. 2000;10:493–7.
690. Stanski DR, Ham J, Miller RD, Sheiner LB. Pharmacokinetics and pharmacodynamics of d-tubocurarine during nitrous oxide-narcotic and halothane anesthesia in man. Anesthesiology. 1979;51:235–41.
691. Prys-Roberts C, Lloyd JW, Fisher A, et al. Deliberate profound hypotension induced with halothane: studies of haemodynamics and pulmonary gas exchange. Br J Anaesth. 1974;46:105.
692. Pauca AL, Hopkins AM. Acute effects of halothane, nitrous oxide and thiopentone on upper limb blood flow. Br J Anaesth. 1972;43:326–33.
693. Meakin G, Walker RW, Dearlove OR. Myotonic and neuromuscular blocking effects of increased doses of suxamethonium in infants and children. Br J Anaesth. 1990;65:816–18.
694. Cook DR, Gronert BJ, Woelfel SK. Comparison of the neuromuscular effects of mivacurium and suxamethonium in infants and children. Acta Anaesthesiol Scand Suppl. 1995;106:35–40.
695. DeCook TH, Goudsouzian NG. Tachyphylaxis and phase II block development during infusion of succinylcholine in children. Anesth Analg. 1980;59:639–43.
696. Gronert BJ, Brandom BW. Neuromuscular blocking drugs in infants and children. Pediatr Clin N Am. 1994;41:73–91.
697. Sutherland GA, Bevan JC, Bevan DR. Neuromuscular blockade in infants following intramuscular succinylcholine in two or five per cent concentration. Can Anaesth Soc J. 1983;30:342–6.
698. Anderson BJ, Meakin GH. Scaling for size: some implications for paediatric anaesthesia dosing. Paediatr Anaesth. 2002; 12:205–19.
699. Cook DR, Fisher CG. Neuromuscular blocking effects of succinylcholine in infants and children. Anesthesiology. 1975;42: 662–5.
700. Meakin G, McKiernan EP, Morris P, Baker RD. Dose-response curves for suxamethonium in neonates, infants and children. Br J Anaesth. 1989;62:655–8.
701. Cook DR. Muscle relaxants in infants and children. Anesth Analg. 1981;60:335–43.
702. Matteo RS, Lieberman IG, Salanitre E, McDaniel DD, Diaz J. Distribution, elimination, and action of d-tubocurarine in neonates, infants, children, and adults. Anesth Analg. 1984;63:799–804.
703. Tassonyi E, Pittet JF, Schopfer CN, et al. Pharmacokinetics of pipecuronium in infants, children and adults. Eur J Drug Metab Pharmacokinet. 1995;20:203–8.
704. Meretoja OA, Erkola O. Pipecuronium revisited: dose-response and maintenance requirement in infants, children, and adults. J Clin Anesth. 1997;9:125–9.
705. Fisher DM, Canfell PC, Fahey MR, et al. Elimination of atracurium in humans: contribution of Hofmann elimination and ester hydrolysis versus organ-based elimination. Anesthesiology. 1986;65:6–12.
706. Brandom BW, Stiller RL, Cook DR, Woelfel SK, Chakravorti S, Lai A. Pharmacokinetics of atracurium in anaesthetized infants and children. Br J Anaesth. 1986;58:1210–13.
707. Imbeault K, Withington DE, Varin F. Pharmacokinetics and pharmacodynamics of a 0.1 mg/kg dose of cisatracurium besylate in children during N2O/O2/propofol anesthesia. Anesth Analg. 2006;102:738–43.
708. Reich DL, Hollinger I, Harrington DJ, Seiden HS, Chakravorti S, Cook DR. Comparison of cisatracurium and vecuronium by infusion in neonates and small infants after congenital heart surgery. Anesthesiol. 2004;101:1122–7.
709. Kirkegaard-Nielsen H, Meretoja OA, Wirtavuori K. Reversal of atracurium-induced neuromuscular block in paediatric patients. Acta Anaesthesiol Scand. 1995;39:906–11.
710. Meakin G, Sweet PT, Bevan JC, Bevan DR. Neostigmine and edrophonium as antagonists of pancuronium in infants and children. Anesthesiology. 1983;59:316–21.
711. Fisher DM, Cronnelly R, Miller RD, Sharma M. The neuromuscular pharmacology of neostigmine in infants and children. Anesthesiology. 1983;59:220–5.
712. Meretoja OA, Taivainen T, Wirtavuori K. Cisatracurium during halothane and balanced anaesthesia in children. Paediatr Anaesth. 1996;6:373–8.
713. Meistelman C, Debaene B, d'Hollander A, Donati F, Saint-Maurice C. Importance of the level of paralysis recovery for a rapid antagonism of vecuronium with neostigmine in children during halothane anesthesia. Anesthesiology. 1988;69:97–9.
714. Debaene B, Meistelman C, d'Hollander A. Recovery from vecuronium neuromuscular blockade following neostigmine administration in infants, children, and adults during halothane anesthesia. Anesthesiology. 1989;71:840–4.
715. Bevan JC, Purday JP, Reimer EJ, Bevan DR. Reversal of doxacurium and pancuronium neuromuscular blockade with neostigmine in children. Can J Anaesth. 1994;41:1074–80.

716. Plaud B, Meretoja O, Hofmockel R, et al. Reversal of rocuronium-induced neuromuscular blockade with sugammadex in pediatric and adult surgical patients. Anesthesiology. 2009;110:284–94.
717. Robertson EN, Driessen JJ, Vogt M, De Boer H, Scheffer GJ. Pharmacodynamics of rocuronium 0.3 mg kg(-1) in adult patients with and without renal failure. Eur J Anaesthesiol. 2005;22:929–32.
718. Staals LM, Snoeck MM, Driessen JJ, Flockton EA, Heeringa M, Hunter JM. Multicentre, parallel-group, comparative trial evaluating the efficacy and safety of sugammadex in patients with end-stage renal failure or normal renal function. Br J Anaesth. 2008;101:492–7.
719. Staals LM, Snoeck MM, Driessen JJ, et al. Reduced clearance of rocuronium and sugammadex in patients with severe to end-stage renal failure: a pharmacokinetic study. Br J Anaesth. 2010;104:31–9.
720. Morell RC, Berman JM, Royster RI, Petrozza PH, Kelly JS, Colonna DM. Revised label regarding use of succinylcholine in children and adolescents. Anesthesiology. 1994;80:242–5.
721. Badgwell JM, Hall SC, Lockhart C. Revised label regarding use of succinylcholine in children and adolescents. Anesthesiology. 1994;80:243–5.
722. Goudsouzian NG. Recent changes in the package insert for succinylcholine chloride: should this drug be contraindicated for routine use in children and adolescents? (Summary of the discussions of the anesthetic and life support drug advisory meeting of the Food and Drug Administration, FDA building, Rockville, MD, June 9, 1994). Anesth Analg. 1995;80:207–8.
723. Anderson BJ, Brown TC. Anaesthesia for a child with congenital myotonic dystrophy. Anaesth Intensive Care. 1989;17:351–4.
724. Lockridge O. Genetic variants of human serum cholinesterase influence metabolism of the muscle relaxant succinylcholine. Pharmacol Ther. 1990;47:35–60.
725. Ali-Melkkila T, Kanto J, Iisalo E. Pharmacokinetics and related pharmacodynamics of anticholinergic drugs. Acta Anaesthesiol Scand. 1993;37:633–42.
726. Johr M. Is it time to question the routine use of anticholinergic agents in paediatric anaesthesia? Paediatr Anaesth. 1999;9:99–101.
727. Rautakorpi P, Manner T, Kanto J. A survey of current usage of anticholinergic drugs in paediatric anaesthesia in Finland. Acta Anaesthesiol Scand. 1999;43:1057–9.
728. Shaw CA, Kelleher AA, Gill CP, Murdoch LJ, Stables RH, Black AE. Comparison of the incidence of complications at induction and emergence in infants receiving oral atropine vs no premedication. Br J Anaesth. 2000;84:174–8.
729. Venkatesh V, Ponnusamy V, Anandaraj J, et al. Endotracheal intubation in a neonatal population remains associated with a high risk of adverse events. Eur J Pediatr. 2011;170:223–7.
730. Hinderling PH, Gundert-Remy U, Schmidlin O. Integrated pharmacokinetics and pharmacodynamics of atropine in healthy humans. I: Pharmacokinetics. J Pharm Sci. 1985;74:703–10.
731. Virtanen R, Kanto J, Iisalo E, Iisalo EU, Salo M, Sjovall S. Pharmacokinetic studies on atropine with special reference to age. Acta Anaesthesiol Scand. 1982;26:297–300.
732. Pihlajamaki K, Kanto J, Aaltonen L, Iisalo E, Jaakkola P. Pharmacokinetics of atropine in children. Int J Clin Pharmacol Ther Toxicol. 1986;24:236–9.
733. Kleinman ME, Chameides L, Schexnayder SM, et al. Pediatric advanced life support: 2010 American Heart Association guidelines for cardiopulmonary resuscitation and emergency cardiovascular care. Pediatrics. 2010;126:e1361–99.
734. Barrington KJ. The myth of a minimum dose for atropine. Pediatrics. 2011;127:783–4.
735. Dauchot P, Gravenstein JS. Effects of atropine on the electrocardiogram in different age groups. Clin Pharm Ther. 1971;12:274–80.
736. Eisa L, Passi Y, Lerman J, et al. Do small doses of atropine cause bradycardia in young children? ASA. 2013. Abstract:A3074.
737. Hinderling PH, Gundert-Remy U, Schmidlin O, Heinzel G. Integrated pharmacokinetics and pharmacodynamics of atropine in healthy humans. II: Pharmacodynamics. J Pharm Sci. 1985;74:711–17.
738. Kranke P, Morin AM, Roewer N, Wulf H, Eberhart LH. The efficacy and safety of transdermal scopolamine for the prevention of postoperative nausea and vomiting: a quantitative systematic review. Anesth Analg. 2002;95:133–43. table of contents.
739. Alswang M, Friesen RH, Bangert P. Effect of preanesthetic medication on carbon dioxide tension in children with congenital heart disease. J Cardiothorac Vasc Anesth. 1994;8:415–19.
740. Renner UD, Oertel R, Kirch W. Pharmacokinetics and pharmacodynamics in clinical use of scopolamine. Ther Drug Monit. 2005;27:655–65.
741. Kanto J, Klotz U. Pharmacokinetic implications for the clinical use of atropine, scopolamine and glycopyrrolate. Acta Anaesthesiol Scand. 1988;32:69–78.
742. Warran P, Radford P, Manford ML. Glycopyrrolate in children. Br J Anaesth. 1981;53:1273–6.
743. Cozanitis DA, Jones CJ, Erkola O. Anticholinergic premedication in infants: a comparison of atropine and glycopyrrolate on heart rate, demeanor, and facial flushing. Pediatr Pharmacol. 1984;4:7–10.
744. Meyers EF, Tomeldan SA. Glycopyrrolate compared with atropine in prevention of the oculocardiac reflex during eye-muscle surgery. Anesthesiology. 1979;51:350–2.
745. Rautakorpi P, Manner T, Ali-Melkkila T, Kaila T, Olkkola K, Kanto J. Pharmacokinetics and oral bioavailability of glycopyrrolate in children. Pharmacol Toxicol. 1998;83:132–4.
746. Rautakorpi P, Ali-Melkkila T, Kaila T, et al. Pharmacokinetics of glycopyrrolate in children. J Clin Anesth. 1994;6:217–20.
747. Cohen LH, Thale T, Tissenbaum MJ. Acetylcholine treatment of schizophrenia. Arch Neurol Psychiatr. 1944;51:171–5.
748. Blanc VF. Atropine and succinylcholine: beliefs and controversies in paediatric anaesthesia. Can J Anaesth. 1995;42:1–7.
749. De la Pintiere A, Beuchée A, Bétrémieux PE. Intravenous propacetamol overdose in a term newborn. Arch Dis Child Fetal Neonatal Ed. 2003;88:F351–2.
750. Khalil S, Glorimar M. Sevoflurane-induced hepatotoxicity? Pediatr Anesth. 2006;16:806.
751. Murat I, Baujard C, Foussat C, et al. Tolerance and analgesic efficacy of a new i.v. paracetamol solution in children after inguinal hernia repair. Paediatr Anaesth. 2005;15:663–70.
752. Allegaert K, Palmer GM, Anderson BJ. The pharmacokinetics of intravenous paracetamol in neonates: size matters most. Arch Dis Child. 2011;96:575–80.
753. Crews KR, Gaedigk A, Dunnenberger HM, et al. Clinical pharmacogenetics implementation consortium (CPIC) guidelines for codeine therapy in the context of cytochrome P450 2D6 (CYP2D6) genotype. Clin Pharm Ther 2012;91:321–6.
754. Kelly LE, Rieder M, van den Anker J, et al. More codeine fatalities after tonsillectomy in North American children. Pediatrics: 2012;129(5);1343–7.
755. Ward RM, Drover DR, Hammer GB, Stemland CJ, Kern S, Tristani-Firouzi M, Lugo RA, Satterfield K, Anderson BJ. The pharmacokinetics of methadone and its metabolites in neonates, Infants and children. Pediatr Anesth 2014: 591–601.
756. Hunseler C, Balling G, Rohlig C, et al. Continuous infusion of clonidine in ventilated newborns and infants: a randomized controlled trial. Pediatr Crit Care Med 2014; 15:511–22.

Selection of Anesthesia Techniques for the Neonate

4

Nada Sabourdin, Nicolas Louvet, and Isabelle Constant

General Principles

What Are the Aims of Anesthesia in the Neonate?

To adopt the optimal anesthetic strategy for neonates, we first must establish the goals of anesthesia. For neonates, the goals of anesthesia are the same as they are for adults: to abolish consciousness, prevent the storage of unpleasant memories, avoid nociceptive responses to stress (pain), and provide immobility to enable the surgeon to work under the best possible conditions. Regarding consciousness, formation of memories, and recall in the neonate, the physiological specifics require more detailed discussion, which follows below. In the cases of nociception and immobility, the evidence has established unequivocally that the anatomical and physiological pathways of nociception and movement are present and functional even before birth, although they may not have exactly the same central modulation. Thus, analgesia and immobility are concepts that can be easily applied to neonates with some pharmacokinetic and pharmacodynamic nuances.

Consciousness is a concept that physicists, philosophers, psychologists, doctors, theologians, neurophysiologists, or anatomists have tried to explain for centuries without success. Even though the concept of consciousness itself remains imprecise, indirect evidence of consciousness has been detected in the first months of life [1]. Evidence ranges from behavioral observations [2] to electrophysiological data [3] to functional imaging. If there is a dearth of evidence that consciousness exists in the early neonatal, it may be due to our inability to observe and measure it rather than to its lack of existence. For example, 30 years ago, fetal consciousness was an inconceivable concept, but today it is a hotly debated subject. Despite the lack of evidence confirming the presence of consciousness and awareness in the neonate, the conservative approach is to assume that they are conscious and aware until we have proof to the contrary.

The concept of memory as it relates to the neonate raises several questions. First, are the physiological pathways of memory developed and mature in the neonate? The creation of a memory involves complex cerebral networks, but three structures, in particular, play important roles in this process: the thalamus, the hippocampus, and the amygdala. The interaction of these three structures can be presented as follows: all the sensory ascending stimuli are integrated at a subcortical level by the thalamus, which acts as the control tower, and then relayed to specific areas within the brain. Some of these areas are cortical, like the olfactory or visual cortex, and lead to a conscious perception. Other areas are subcortical and lead to unconscious perceptions or reactions. The cortical data are then associated and encoded in their general context by the hippocampus, to form memory, which includes information such as "what," "where," "when," etc. The limbic system, which manages emotions, and especially the amygdala, is responsible for emotional modulation and amplification. Events occurring in a strong emotional context are much more profoundly remembered than neutral events. In humans, anatomical studies have demonstrated that the amygdala is mature in neonates, whereas the hippocampus reaches maturity by the end of the first decade. The perceptions of neonates are thus strongly influenced by the emotional context in which they occur. It might imply that the memories of neonates are "mainly emotional," perceptive. This differential maturation process of cerebral structures could shift the balance from "understanding" towards "feeling" as the principal determinant of the formation of a memory.

N. Sabourdin • N. Louvet
Department of Anesthesiology, Armand Trousseau Hospital, 26 Avenue du Dr Arnold Netter, 75571 Paris Cedex 12, France

I. Constant (✉)
Department of Anesthesiology, Armand Trousseau Hospital, 26 Avenue du Dr Arnold Netter, 75571 Paris Cedex 12, France

Service d'Anesthésie-Réanimation chirurgicale, Hôpital d'enfants Armand Trousseau, 26 Avenue du Dr Arnold Netter, 75571 Paris Cedex 12, France
e-mail: isabelle.constant@trs.aphp.fr

J. Lerman (ed.), *Neonatal Anesthesia*, DOI 10.1007/978-1-4419-6041-2_4,

If some of the physiological pathways of memory are present in the neonate, do we have evidence that they are functional? There is abundant evidence that some forms of memory exist in the neonatal, and even antenatal, periods. Neonates develop haptic, iconic, and echoic memories that mature with age [4–6]. Neonatal olfactory preferences [7–9], auditory recognition of voices [10, 11], and music [12, 13], for example, may have their provenances in prenatal experiences.

Memory is classically differentiated into explicit and implicit memory, based on the kind of recall processes involved. Explicit memory is characterized by conscious and voluntary recalling of a reportable memory. Implicit memory applies to subconscious recalling, potentially responsible for changes in behavior or emotional disturbances. Implicit memory is also involved in animal conditioning. Even if these two entities are separated semantically, memory is only one process and can be compared to an iceberg in which the visible (above sea level) part represents explicit memory and the non-visible (submerged) part represents implicit memory. In neonates, the distinction between explicit and implicit memory may not be applicable. Indeed, "reportability" of explicit memory is difficult to evidence before language acquisition. Animal studies have demonstrated that young animals are more sensitive to fear conditioning than are old animals. In humans, long-lasting implicit memories have been reported. Repeated experience during the first year of life can influence the performance of children 2 years later [14]. More recently, several recalls have been evidenced by demonstrating different behavioral patterns, related to the presence or absence of analgesia during painful stimuli in the neonatal period [15]. These data suggest that neonates and infants have a very active implicit memory, which is a basis for their behavioral adaptation to environment.

Finally, it seems necessary to avoid conscious and unconscious perception, integration, and memorization of stressful experiences commonly encountered in the perioperative context, such as fear, cold, hunger, noise, lights, handling, uncomfortable position, unfamiliar voices, faces or smells, and also pain. This will not only limit the temporary unpleasantness of hospitalization but might also preclude long-term behavioral or emotional disturbances that a neonatal surgery might experience. In other words, in neonates as in adults, we should provide adequate levels of anesthesia to suppress consciousness, ensure analgesia, and prevent memorization.

Which Agents Should We Use to Achieve These Goals?

Hypnotics abolish consciousness, and analgesics decrease afferent nociception, but no specific drug targets memory. Two indirect actions may limit the formation of memories. *Hypnotics* prevent the cortical integration involved in explicit memory by depressing cortical activity. Relatively small doses of hypnotics can achieve this by decreasing the integration of the ascending peripheral input. Although their main target is cortical, these drugs also act at a subcortical level, if their dose is sufficient [15]. The same concept may hold true for increasing doses of general anesthetics such as propofol in which function MRI demonstrated an interruption between the putamen and other subcortical regions of the brain with progressive decreases in level of consciousness [16, 17]. Hypnotics first inhibit explicit memory and consciousness as the dose increases, then they inhibit movement at surgical incision (MAC), and finally, they inhibit the hemodynamic responses to incision (MAC BAR). These effects result from their actions at different levels within the nervous system: respectively the cortex, the spinal cord, and the brainstem. Hypnotics also limit emotional modulation, by a direct action on the amygdala. In addition, we can diminish the peripheral input that reaches the thalamus, by administering opioids. They act preferentially at the medullar and subcortical level, blocking the transmission of ascending nociceptive information and blunting autonomic responses. As the dose of opioids increases, they will also cause sedation.

Finally, amnesia occurs from a balance between the inhibitory effect of anesthetics and subcortical modulation of encoding and storage by unconscious emotional stimuli. The concept of balanced-anesthesia is now well established in neonates as in other subjects. The advantage of this technique is that it associates different drugs with different targets for a desired combined effect. This association can potentiate the effects of each product, facilitating reduced effective concentrations, thereby limiting deleterious side effects of the drugs used.

Are Anesthetics Toxic to Newborn Brains?

The beginning of the twenty-first century witnessed new concerns about the potential neurotoxicity of anesthetic drugs on the developing brain of young infants.

The sentinel evidence of this neurotoxicity had its provenance in pregnant female rats that received halothane during pregnancy and subsequently gave birth to newborn rats with altered synaptogenesis and neurobehavioral challenges [18]. Subsequently, widespread neuronal degeneration (neuroapoptosis) was reported in newborn rat pups that received prolonged ketamine anesthesia [19]. This provided the first evidence that both the structure and function of the central nervous system in neonatal rodents may be adversely affected by anesthetics [20]. In newborn rodents, neuroapoptosis proved to be most severe on the 7th postnatal day. All newborn animals studied from rodents to nonhuman primates

Table 4.1 Effects of drugs on neurocognitive function in newborn animals

Proapoptotic
• Isoflurane, sevoflurane, desflurane, N_2O
• Ketamine, propofol, thiopental, midazolam, diazepam, $MgSO_4$, dexamethasone, CO_2
Antiapoptotic
• Lithium, melatonin, clonidine
• Preconditioning (with ketamine), NAP, TRP601
• Vitamin D_3
• Environmental enrichment
Non-apoptotic
• Dexmedetomidine, opioids, ± xenon, local anesthetics
Unknown
• Muscle relaxants

Terms
N_2O is nitrous oxide
$MgSO_4$ is magnesium sulfate
CO_2 is carbon dioxide
NAP (davunetide) is the abbreviation for a short peptide fragment (NAPVSIPQ) derived from the activity-dependent neuroprotective protein
TRP601 is the abbreviated term for the irreversible caspase inhibitor, pentapeptide quinolin-2-carbonyl-VD(OMe)VAD(OMe)-CH_2-O(2,6 F_2)Ph
J. Lerman 2013

demonstrated similar neuroapoptotic responses to anesthesia. Newborn animals that were anesthetized with a host of different anesthetics (proapoptotic) (Table 4.1) for periods quite uncharacteristic for neonatal surgery in humans (e.g., 4–6 or more hours) developed neuroanatomical and neuropathological changes. However, some anesthetics did not cause apoptosis (N_2O, Midazolam) when they were administered alone, but they did cause neuroapoptosis when they were combined [20–23]. Other drugs prevented apoptosis (antiapoptotic), whereas others yet were non-apoptotic or unknown (Table 4.1). Additionally, neuroapoptosis in newborn animals was shown to depend on both the dose of the proapoptotic drugs, the greater the dose, the more severe the apoptosis, and the duration of exposure, more than 3 h of high-dose ketamine or 1 or more hours of 2 % isoflurane was needed to induce neuroapoptosis [24–26]. In fact, even though most anesthetics cause harm to susceptible newborns animals, others cause no harm and some actually may be protective. In most studies, the neuropathology was characterized by a decrease in neuronal density, oligodendrocyte degeneration, suppression of neurogenesis, and synaptic remodeling as well as short- and long-term behavior and cognitive dysfunction [22, 27–32] (Table 4.2). Several recent reviews summarized the animal studies, neuropathological data, and clinical evidence [33–38].

Numerous investigators have questioned the appropriateness of the model used to address this question. In most experiments, fewer than two-thirds of the animals survive until the conclusion of the study, begging the question how could such a model hold relevance to human anesthesia at all. Second, most experiments did not monitor cardiorespiratory variables throughout to ensure that they did not the harm the animals. Third, the MAC of the inhalational anesthetics is not constant over time in these animals. Finally, the care provided to these newborns after the anesthetics may not have been optimal [39].

Despite the obvious concern regarding the potential harm apoptosis may cause in humans if similarly affected, great strides have also been made in identifying strategies to block and prevent neuroapoptosis in newborn rodents. Several drugs have been identified as having antiapoptotic properties (Table 4.1). Preconditioning (with ketamine) and vitamin D3 have both been effective individually in attenuating apoptosis [40]. Additional neuroprotective strategies using NAP and TRP601, the former a derivative of the activity-dependent neuroprotective protein [41] and the latter an irreversible caspase inhibitor [42], both substantively decrease the severity of the apoptosis in newborn animal models [41, 42]. In addition, environmental enrichment, which attenuated brain injury during recovery in adult rodents, effected similar salutary effects in newborn rodents exposed to anesthesia [39, 43, 44].

The mechanisms of the neurotoxicity induced by anesthetic agents in the immature animal brain remain incompletely understood. We know that most anesthetics act by activating $GABA_A$ receptors and/or inhibiting NMDA receptors (exceptions include clonidine/dexmedetomidine and opioids). These neurotransmitters play a vital role in the normal development and maturation of the brain, particularly but not exclusively, during the vulnerable period of rapid synaptogenesis. During rapid brain growth, neurons that are superfluous and no longer required become quiescent, which triggers caspase 3 activation. This activates apoptosis and the superfluous cells involute and disappear. This remodeling

Table 4.2 Functional deficits associated with specific anesthetic agents identified in animal studies

Anesthetics	Learning	Spatial memory	Social memory	Spontaneous motor activity	Attention	Behavior
Isoflurane	x	x		x	x	x
Sevoflurane	x		x			
Nitrous oxide	x	x		x	x	x
Propofol	x	x		x		
Ketamine	x	x		x	x	x
Midazolam (as part of a cocktailn)	x	x		x	x	x
Barbiturates	x	x				

Data Courtesy of Dr. Lena Sun
Presented at the Postgraduate Assembly, New York State Society of Anesthesiologists Annual meeting, December 2011

process enables the brain to remove superfluous neurons and expand other parts of the brain. Anesthetics that modify GABA- and NMDA-mediated neurotransmission might disrupt this process by depressing the neurons and "putting the neurons to sleep," triggering apoptosis even though the neurons were not scripted for removal. This "abnormal neuronal inhibition" could trigger apoptotic cell death in vulnerable neurons, or alter the normal synaptogenesis [27], causing a decrease in neuronal density and synaptic remodeling. The *balance* between NMDA- and GABA-mediated neuronal activity could also affect dendritic spine development and neuronal connectivity [45]. However, these theories should be regarded with caution, since the activity of $GABA_A$ receptor, for example, one of the main inhibitory systems in the mature brain, displays excitatory properties in the immature cortical neuron [46].

What is the relevance of neuroapoptosis in terms of future neurological development? Apoptosis is a normal process during brain development in mammalian species. In humans, 50–70 % of the neuronal cells will have undergone "physiological" apoptosis by the end of the cerebral maturation [47, 48]. If this process is arrested, cerebral malformations and premature death occur in a mouse model [49]. It remains to be determined if the apoptosis observed after anesthesia targets neurons that would have spontaneously died in the natural course of development or if it destroys neurons that were destined to be part of the final cerebral network. However, we do not even know if such a fixed predestination of neurons exists or if the central nervous system is able to compensate for one neuronal death by "sparing" another cell.

Many have criticized the notion of extrapolating neuronal and neurocognitive sequelae in animal studies to human neonates. These issues have been addressed in several reviews or editorials [50–54].

The corresponding period of neuronal susceptibility in humans, if one indeed exists, is unclear. It was believed, on a weight basis approach, that the brain growth spurt period in humans started in the third trimester of gestation and lasted until the third year of life [55–57]. A cell count approach points to the interval between 28 and 33 weeks of gestation as the period of maximal neurogenesis [46]. Recently, modern "neuroinformatic" methods set the peak window of vulnerability to 17–22 weeks of gestation, until the early postnatal period [58]. In this area, we still lack strong evidence defining a potential "danger" period of susceptibility to anesthetic neurotoxicity in humans.

Other questions relate to the dose and duration of anesthetic drugs used in the animal studies. Animals require comparatively greater doses of intravenous drugs than humans, on a weight basis, or with an allometric approach, to achieve the same pharmacodynamic goals [59, 60]. As a result, most of the animal studies are performed with doses that exceed the therapeutic range in humans, but that are relevant for the considered animal models [24, 61]. Anesthetic side effects, for example, at therapeutic concentrations, may be more marked in rodents than in humans, including hemodynamic and metabolic disturbances, and may confound the neurological sequelae [52, 59]. The MAC of inhalational anesthetics is believed to remain fairly constant across species. In a comparative study of isoflurane, sevoflurane, and desflurane, apoptosis was equally severe after all three anesthetics after 6 h [62]. In contrast, neuroapoptosis in newborn rats that were exposed to 1 h of isoflurane was similar to controls and significantly less than that in rats exposed to 6 h of isoflurane, although one study demonstrated neuroapoptosis after 1 h of 2 % isoflurane [25, 26]. However, recent evidence suggests that the MAC of sevoflurane in newborn rats decreases with tail-clamping over time, raising questions regarding the equivalent MAC values in neonatal animals [39]. Many studies in newborn animals have been performed with strict control of hemodynamic, respiratory, and metabolic variables and, despite the controls, still yielded substantive neuroapoptosis. Moreover, histopathologic findings describe apoptotic and not ischemic or excitotoxic mechanisms involved in neuronal cell death observed after exposure to anesthetic drugs.

Finally, all animal studies of neuroapoptosis after anesthetic drugs have been undertaken without surgical or painful stimulation, since pain and/or inflammation by themselves induce neuroapoptosis. In a surgical setting, anesthetics attenuate the potential damage of nociceptive stimulation. Two studies addressed the effects of anesthetics on neuronal function/integrity during an inflammatory insult. These studies yielded conflicting results leaving this concern unresolved [63–65].

A crucial question that is currently being investigated is the relevance of all these in vitro and animal findings in the human neonate. Does anesthesia in the young infant transiently or permanently alter his neurologic development, cognitive performance, or behavioral characteristics? Several case-controlled or cohort studies have sought evidence to answer this question. Although several studies have pointed to an association between children who received multiple general anesthetics before 3 years of age and learning disabilities, these studies have been difficult to interpret due to the presence of multiple confounding variables [66–72]. One notable study of identical twins indicated that intellectual indices did not differ between twins who were discordant for receiving anesthesia at a young age. In sum, the current clinical evidence does not establish an association between general anesthesia in young children and cognitive dysfunction. Prospective studies are required to clarify this issue [73, 74]. Nonetheless, some have taken the enormous leap of faith by assuming that the current clinical evidence heralds similar outcomes in humans and have recommended delaying elective surgery in neonates until they are older [75, 76]. However, few surgeries in neonates are totally elective. Locoregional may be preferred to general anesthesia and the use of drugs that do not trigger apoptosis, preferred to those that do, where possible. In addition, an enriched postoperative environment and strategic interventions (see above) may attenuate the risk of neurocognitive pathology. A measured response is far more appropriate than delaying all surgeries in neonates, in which parents and guardians review the risk-benefit ratio of proceeding versus delaying surgery and anesthesia, with the responsible physicians and surgeons.

A second issue that has raised concerns regarding the safe use of inhalational anesthetics in children has been epileptiform EEG activity. The immature neonatal cortex is relatively more vulnerable and sensitive to anesthetics than the mature cerebral cortex. The baseline EEG pattern of a neonate is characterized by slow oscillations, reflecting immature brain functioning. The complexity of the EEG increases with age, from neonates to adults. Evidence suggests that infants require less sevoflurane to reach a given target of cortical inhibition (BIS 50) than do older children [77]. Similarly, Rigouzzo et al. reported that subtotal cortical inhibition (defined by the occurrence of burst suppression patterns on the EEG) was observed with lower concentrations in infants than in older children. Taken together these studies suggest that infants are more sensitive to cortical inhibition produced by sevoflurane.

In terms of surgical incision, greater end-tidal concentrations of sevoflurane are required to inhibit movement as evidenced by the greater MAC values for 0–6 months compared with older children. These data suggest that in the neonate, subcortical structures, at least at the level of the spinal cord, are less sensitive to sevoflurane-induced inhibition.

The balance between cortical and subcortical processes in the neonate appears to differ from that in older children or adults. If we seek to inhibit the subcortical structures to prevent movement and negative subconscious memory formation with potential behavioral consequences, we require larger end-tidal concentrations of sevoflurane in neonates. However, if the cortex is more sensitive to sevoflurane, then these larger concentrations may introduce a risk of neuronal toxicity. So the questions are what is our goal and what level of theoretical risk can we accept?

Fortunately, opioids provide subcortical inhibition and decreased sympathetic activity, allowing reduced doses of hypnotics while reducing concerns regarding toxicity.

If all of the preceding were true, then the challenge for the anesthesiologist is to find a compromise between subcortical inhibition and potential toxicity of general anesthetics in neonates. Opioids may provide the solution with a balanced anesthetic, although judicious choice of the correct opioid and the correct dose is required to preclude delayed recovery and delayed tracheal extubation.

Optimal Risk-Benefit Ratio

To optimize the risk-benefit ratio of anesthesia in the neonate (if neurotoxicity proves to hold true in humans), the clinical approach to provide anesthesia for surgery and procedures will be to use anesthetics that are not neurotoxic, to administer adjuvant agents that prevent apoptosis (see above), and/or use regional anesthesia.

Techniques of Anesthesia

Spinal Anesthesia

Spinal anesthesia for the neonate was initially developed in the eighties for its potential benefit to preclude postoperative apnea in the premature and ex-premature infant [78, 79]. In 1998, a landmark study demonstrated a significantly small incidence of postoperative apnea in premature infants who underwent inguinal hernia repair under spinal anesthesia compared with those under general anesthesia with thiopental and halothane [80]. For the premature and ex-premature infant, the risk of apnea decreases steadily between birth and

60 weeks post-conceptional age (PCA), when it is <1 %. At 45 weeks PCA, this risk is approximately of 5 % [81, 82]. Anemia (hematocrit <30 %) [83, 84], hypothermia [85], and other comorbidities such as impaired neurologic or respiratory function increase the risk of postoperative apnea [80–82, 86–89]. It has become an increasingly common practice to consider spinal anesthesia as the preferred technique for brief surgical procedures in the inguinal and lower abdominal areas in ex-premature neonates. This practice has remained unchanged over the past two decades despite the introduction of newer, less soluble inhalational anesthetics.

One study indicated that sevoflurane might induce more cardiorespiratory complications in ex-premature neonates with a preexisting impaired respiratory function than spinal anesthesia, although spinal anesthesia was associated with a substantial failure rate [90]. In a Cochrane review on "regional (spinal, epidural, caudal) versus general anesthesia in preterm infants undergoing inguinal herniorrhaphy in early infancy" [91], the authors concluded that there is "no reliable evidence concerning the effect of spinal as compared to general anesthesia on the incidence of post-operative apnea, bradycardia, or oxygen desaturation in ex-preterm infants undergoing herniorrhaphy" based on 3 published studies that included 108 infants. However, the results were confounded by the concomitant administration of sedatives, mostly ketamine or benzodiazepine, to several infants in the spinal anesthesia arms of the studies. The authors hypothesized that if those who had received sedatives were excluded, spinal anesthesia would have likely been beneficial in terms of postoperative respiratory events.

Because of the significant risk of postoperative apnea, ex-premature infants aged less than 60 weeks PCA require 12 h of apnea-free respiratory monitoring after surgery, irrespective of the anesthetic provided. It has not yet been clearly established whether spinal anesthesia or anesthesia with sevoflurane alone or with local block can abbreviate the period of postoperative monitoring. Some have proposed that certain infants greater than 46 weeks PCA without anemia or comorbidities may be discharged earlier, if they prove to be at a reduced risk for postoperative apnea [92]. This recommendation requires prospective evaluation.

In addition to the possible benefit of avoiding general anesthesia in the neonate, spinal anesthesia has several additional advantages in the preoperative period. It allows a comfortable and safe anesthetic for the infant, who continues to breathe spontaneously; and as opposed to older children, spinal anesthesia does not induce clinically significant autonomic disturbances in the neonate. In particular, arterial blood pressure remains stable [93, 94]. Therefore, cardiorespiratory homeostasis in the neonate is usually maintained during spinal anesthesia. In addition, infants who have received spinal anesthesia are often very calm and peaceful during surgery. Some actually fall asleep during the surgery. Interestingly, the BIS has been recorded in unpremedicated ex-preterm infants undergoing surgery with spinal anesthesia. The BIS decreased during the first 25 min after the spinal, to reach a nadir of 60, that remained unchanged for the next 20 min, but finally returned to 100 during the final 20 min [95]. To explain this response, the authors posited a decrease in the ascending sensory input to the brain, permitting sleep.

Complications with spinal anesthesia are rare, even in large series [89, 96–98]. Recent evidence suggests that complications after neuraxial analgesia in neonates may be as small as 0.29 % [99]. The theoretical risk of septic or aseptic meningitis is very small and has only been reported in two children. In both instances, the role of dural puncture remained uncertain [100, 101]. A high blockade incurring the need for ventilatory assistance (0.67 % in one series) or intubation (0.33 %) [98] is unlikely, if the correct dose is administered, and the infant remains strictly horizontal. Neuraxial hematoma has not been reported in a child, although it has been described in an infant undergoing diagnostic lumbar puncture, who had undiagnosed hemophilia A [102]. The usefulness of testing for coagulation indices in children undergoing lumbar punctures under spinal anesthesia remains contentious. The results are often abnormal, particularly in the premature (<45 weeks PCA), without a clinically significant hemorrhagic tendency [103].

Based on clinical observations of transient or persistent neurological symptoms after spinal anesthesia in adults [104], a direct cytotoxicity of local anesthetics has been suspected and investigated. This neurotoxicity was first characterized in animal studies [105] and then in in vitro human neuronal cells models [106]. The mechanisms are still unclear and probably multiple. However, all local anesthetics, and particularly bupivacaine and lidocaine, have triggered dose-dependent neuronal cell dysfunction, death, or apoptosis, at in vitro concentrations similar to or less than clinical concentrations observed in the CSF after standard spinal anesthesia. Recent evidence suggested that spinal anesthesia does not trigger apoptosis in newborn rodents that received spinal anesthesia on postnatal day 7, 14, and 21 [25]. However, the period of rapid synaptogenesis may peak earlier in the dorsal horn of the spinal cord, e.g., on day 3, not day 7, as in the cortex and basal ganglia [99]. Accordingly, it remains possible that despite the current evidence to the contrary, the spinal cord might be vulnerable to apoptosis in the neonatal period.

The main concern regarding spinal anesthesia in the neonate is its failure rate. The reported failure rate of spinal anesthesia is between 3 % and 20 %, depending on the experience of the anesthesiologist with spinal blocks [89, 90, 98, 107–109].

Regarding the anesthetic potency of spinal anesthesia, in addition to interindividual variability, the duration of analgesia and motor block varies according to the type and dosage of the local anesthetic chosen, but usually lasts a minimum of 60 min [89], which sets the limit of the duration of any surgical procedure performed under spinal anesthesia.

In conclusion, spinal anesthesia displays numerous advantages over general anesthesia and is associated with few complications. Although particularly useful in the ex-preterm infant of less than 60 weeks' PCA, it may be considered in the neonate undergoing any sub-mesocolic surgery of less than 60 min in duration. Recent concerns about potential local anesthetic neurotoxicity have been articulated in the literature. However, the evidence arises primarily from animal and experimental studies, and their clinical relevance to humans has yet to be established. When the location and duration of surgery make it appropriate, spinal anesthesia may be the optimal option for the neonate.

General Anesthesia

According to the clinical context, and in particular, the probability of full stomach, a rapid sequence induction (RSI) may be preferred.

RSI for General Anesthesia

An RSI is currently performed for every child who has a full stomach, in order to minimize the risk of regurgitation of gastric contents and pulmonary aspiration. To minimize this risk, a proper delay should be observed before induction of anesthesia in the case of non-urgent procedures. The lack of a sufficient fasting period is one of the most common circumstances leading to an RSI.

Current fasting rules were developed based on the best estimate times for gastric emptying of the food product in question. These rules are age independent, although some studies (gastric emptying of infant formula) have only been undertaken in select age groups. Clear fluids may be ingested up to 2 h before anesthesia/surgery in neonates and all older children [110–113]. A Cochrane review on pediatric fasting concluded that ad libitum clear fluid intake until 2 h before surgery improved the child's well-being and did not increase the risk of regurgitation [114]. Breast milk may be ingested up to 4 h before anesthesia, and artificial milk (e.g., cow's milk) may be ingested up to 6 h before anesthesia [112, 113, 115]. If it is necessary to start surgery before the stomach is considered empty, an RSI should be performed.

Alternately, some conditions associated with functional or mechanical ileus in the neonatal period require an RSI independent of the fasting interval. The most frequent pathologies are those of the digestive tract: atresia, obstruction, volvulus or perforation, necrotizing enterocolitis, omphalocele, gastroschisis, and congenital diaphragmatic hernia. Pyloric stenosis, which occurs at the end of the first month of postnatal life, is classically considered a condition with "full stomach," although several institutions routinely perform inhalational inductions of anesthesia in these infants without substantial consequences. In the first months of life, children with hiatal hernia, untreated or persistent esophageal reflux, may also be at risk for regurgitation and considered candidates for an RSI.

Awake Versus Anesthetized Tracheal Intubation

After more than 20 years of debate, routine awake intubation in the neonate has been supplanted by premedication and anesthesia [116]. Today, there remain few reasons to perform tracheal intubation without any premedication in elective intubations [117], although many continue to recommend awake intubations during resuscitation, deteriorating critically ill neonates (and those in respiratory failure) and in those with difficult airways [118]. Recent surveys in France and in the UK [119] revealed that 80 and 90 %, respectively, of elective intubations in neonates were performed with general anesthesia. Several publications reviewed the advantages and disadvantages of premedication (e.g., sedation or general anesthesia) before intubation [120, 121]. Their conclusions consistently suggest that awake intubation in the neonate should be avoided. The physiological consequences [122] of such a procedure include:

1. Intense pain. The short- and long-term negative consequences of pain in the neonatal period are now well recognized and documented.
2. An increase in arterial blood pressure.
3. An increase in the intracranial pressure, often measured as the anterior fontanel pressure, and modifications in cerebral blood flow velocity [123, 124]. There is no evidence that awake intubation is associated with intracerebral or intracranial hemorrhage.
4. A decrease in heart rate due to the vagal reaction to intense pain. Tachycardia has also been observed.
5. A decrease in blood oxygen saturation.

In the past, some clinicians feared the hemodynamic consequences of anesthetic drugs in the neonate. Bradycardia and hypotension were observed during halothane anesthesia in the neonate, although current drugs used in appropriate doses provide hemodynamic stability. In a study in which tracheal intubation was performed in 33 neonates either awake or during sevoflurane anesthesia, adverse events occurred less frequently in the anesthetized group. In particular, they noted the incidence of bradycardia decreased from 44.4 to 8.3 % in the anesthetized group, although the duration of laryngoscopy and intubation was 16 s with sevoflurane and 61 s awake [125]. Inability to perform awake intubations in ~10 s points to a serious failure in mastering the skills of awake tracheal intubation in neonates and raises serious concerns about the veracity of any of these studies [126].

Some also feared the loss of spontaneous ventilation would expose the neonates to the risk of severe hemoglobin desaturations. If the anesthesiologist is skilled to manage the airway in the neonate, mask ventilation will maintain normal oxygenation and ventilation. In fact, fewer desaturations occur when the child is anesthetized before tracheal intubation rather than awake during the procedure [125]. This may be attributed to effective preoxygenation with 100 % O_2 in the absence of a child who is struggling, gasping, and crying, particularly during prolonged attempted laryngoscopies.

Premedication provides better conditions for intubation, particularly in the hands of less experienced laryngoscopists. With premedication, the neonate does not move or resist, laryngoscopy is easier to perform [125], and the vocal cords are abducted. In addition, premedication decreases the time to intubation, the number of attempts before a successful intubation, and intubation-related airway injuries [127–129].

Preoxygenation

Preoxygenation is an essential component of an RSI. The aim of preoxygenation is to provide maximal oxygen reserves to allow the greatest duration of apnea without desaturation, in order to avoid hypoxemia before the trachea is intubated. This topic has been poorly assessed in children, especially neonates. However, some of the few pediatric studies include a subgroup of infants less than 1 year of age. We can only extrapolate their results to the first month of life to appreciate the implications.

The younger the age of the child, the less the time interval between removing the facemask and the onset of hemoglobin desaturation. In healthy infants whose lungs were ventilated manually, saturation decreased from 100 to 95 % in approximately 90 s after the onset of apnea and then from 95 to 90 % rapidly (<10 s) [130, 131]. In older children (2–7 years old), 2 min of preoxygenation almost doubled the duration of apnea without incurring hypoxia [132] and that extending the duration of preoxygenation beyond 2 min did not improve the results. When this schema was tested in infants, 1 year and 3 months of age, 2 min of preoxygenation resulted in desaturation to <95 % in 110 s. Desaturation <90 % occurred only 8 s later [133].

Using an end-tidal oxygen fraction of 0.9 as the target end-point for preoxygenation, infants 0–6 months of age required 36 ± 11.4 s or ~60 s [134] for preoxygenation. These results suggested that a brief duration of preoxygenation may be effective in infants, provided the facemask is held tightly against the face during the preoxygenation period.

Cricoid Pressure

Cricoid pressure has been traditionally applied to all patients undergoing RSI to prevent the regurgitation and aspiration of gastric fluids. However, several incidents have been reported [135] in which cricoid pressure caused a clinical problem: excessive pressure [136], incorrect location, and inappropriate timing of the procedure. To be effective, but not traumatic, cricoid pressure must be applied precisely. The usual recommendation is to apply a force of 30–44 N to the cricoid ring with loss of consciousness [137], irrespective of the age of the child. However, a recent bronchoscopic study determined that only 5 N force is required to compress the lumen of the cricoid ring by 50 % in infants [138].

Several others have questioned the effectiveness of cricoid pressure [139]. In adults, an MRI investigation determined that the esophageal lumen was not obliterated by cricoid pressure, but rather it moved laterally from the spinal axis in more than 90 % of patients [140]. In contrast, another MRI study indicated that cricoid pressure obliterated the hypopharyngeal lumen, irrespective of the position and diameter of the esophagus [141]. There appears to be no technique to ensure that in any patient, cricoid pressure reliably obliterates the esophageal lumen.

Even if cricoid pressure were correctly applied, there is no evidence that RSI prevents gastric fluid aspiration. Aspiration is a very rare event with approximately 24 instances of aspiration in 63,180 pediatric general anesthetics, all of whom had cricoid pressure applied during the induction [142]. Moreover, cricoid pressure can impair view of the glottis during laryngoscopy [143–145]. This is particularly important in infants and neonates in whom the adult hand applying the cricoid pressure can limit the mouth opening. In addition, a relatively small force applied to the neck might cause subglottic obstruction in young children [138]. If tracheal intubation is impeded for any of the above reasons, cricoid pressure must be released in order to permit rapid tracheal intubation, which remains the top priority of an RSI. To conclude, cricoid pressure is no longer considered a mandatory ingredient in an RSI, provided the reasons are clearly articulated [139, 146].

Gastric Emptying

Passing an oro- or nasogastric tube before an RSI is neither required nor effective in completely emptying the stomach. However, a gastric tube may be useful in the presence of preoperative ileus or digestive tract obstruction. Since neonates are exclusively fed liquids, a gastric tube may significantly reduce the volume of the gastric fluid contents, although pulmonary aspiration may still occur. If a gastric tube is in place, it is not necessary to remove it before induction [147], and it does not impair the effectiveness of cricoid pressure [143]. The anesthesiologist may however prefer if the gastric tube is removed to ensure clear visualization of the larynx.

Mask Ventilation

Although mask ventilation with oxygen is not usually recommended during an RSI in order to avoid gastric insufflation and regurgitation, it must be performed if severe hemoglobin desaturation occurs before the trachea is intubated. Neonates should never be allowed to become hypoxic out of concern that mask ventilation might theoretically cause pulmonary aspiration. The incidence of pulmonary aspiration during and after an RSI in infants and children is rare, whereas the incidence of hypoxemia and their harmful consequences is quite frequent. Some advocate mask ventilation to provide safer intubating conditions during RSI in neonates by limiting the peak airway pressures to <10 cmH_2O to avoid desaturations without inflating the stomach [148, 149]. This is particularly relevant in the neonate: without preoxygenation, severe desaturation occurs within 10 s of apnea in the healthy neonate. This is often too brief an interval to complete induction of anesthesia, neuromuscular blockade, and tracheal intubation.

Anesthetic Agents for RSI

The optimal combination of anesthetics to achieve a rapid, secure, and successful intubation in the neonate has not been determined. The RSI classically associates a hypnotic and a neuromuscular blocking agent, administered intravenously in rapid sequence in predetermined doses, with a rapid injection and effect. The objective is to minimize the period between the loss of upper airway protective reflexes and tracheal intubation, when the risk of pulmonary aspiration into the unprotected airway is greatest. Most of the drugs used in adults for RSI are considered equally safe and effective in children, even in neonates.

Regarding intravenous hypnotics, *thiopental* (3–5 mg/kg) or propofol (3–5 mg/kg) can be used for a rapid induction, although for propofol, there is a dearth of studies in very young children. The ED_{50} for thiopental in neonates (to tolerate a facemask for 30 s) is 3.4 ± 0.2 mg/kg [150]. The ED_{50} for propofol in neonates has not been determined.

In neonates, *thiopental* allows a quick and smooth induction of anesthesia and preserves hemodynamic stability [151]. In the first month of life, the dose of thiopental is 45 % less than it is in older infants 1–6 months of age, probably attributable to the reduced protein binding, more permeable blood-brain barrier, and increased brain sensitivity to thiopental [150]. However, the elimination half-life of thiopental in neonates exceeds 14 h, 2.5-fold greater than midazolam [152]. When administered with succinylcholine, thiopental increases the success rate and shortens the time interval to tracheal intubation [128]. *Propofol* has a time of onset similar to that of thiopental, but a much briefer duration of action, which is an advantage in the context of RSI. Propofol is also more effective than thiopental in limiting the hypertensive response to laryngoscopy in children 1–6 months and to reduce the delay before extubation [153]. Propofol confers two additional advantages: it attenuates airway reactivity and decreases the muscular tension of the jaw muscles. When associated with succinylcholine in healthy children 0–3 months undergoing pyloromyotomy, propofol caused only moderate decease in blood pressure [154]. Propofol may enhance right-to-left shunting in the immediate neonatal period (via a patent foramen ovale, ductus arteriosus), because it reduces systemic vascular resistance more than pulmonary resistance. This may explain the three reports of profound hypotension and prolonged hypoxemia in neonates [155]. When used in preterm neonates (30 weeks gestational age, <8 h postnatal age) in a dose of 1 mg/kg IV bolus, propofol decreased the mean arterial blood pressure by 33 %, from 38 (29–42) mmHg to 24 (22–40) mmHg [156]. This decrease in systemic blood pressure is similar to that associated with one MAC inhalational anesthetics in neonates [157, 158]. Administration of 10–20 ml/kg boluses of balanced salt solution before administration of propofol (and inhalational anesthetics) may attenuate these hemodynamic effects. Pain during IV injection of propofol is common in neonates, leading to a brisk withdrawal of the limb. This may lead to accidental disconnection or loss of the line, at a critical stage of induction. Several strategies have been shown to be effective to attenuate the pain during injection including administration of nitrous oxide by mask and a mini-Bier block with lidocaine [159–161]. In the absence of effective preventative treatment, the anesthesiologist should secure the limb gently while propofol is injected and until the neonate is deeply anesthetized.

In the context of neonatal RSI, the use of *ketamine* for induction of anesthesia has not been embraced because of its potential to increase systemic blood pressure and cerebral blood flow in premature infants. In the case of neonates who are hemodynamically unstable, intravenous fentanyl has been the preferred agent.

Succinylcholine (2 mg/kg) is the muscle relaxant of choice for RSI because of its rapid onset and brief duration of action [162]. The younger the child, the briefer the duration of the paralysis after succinylcholine [163]. All muscle relaxants, especially succinylcholine [128, 164], greatly improve the conditions for tracheal intubation [165]. However, life-threatening side effects have caused many to fear the use of succinylcholine in young children [121]. Bradycardia may occur after a single dose of IV succinylcholine in infants, but is easily prevented by pretreatment with 0.02 mg/kg IV atropine. More ominously, acute hyperkalemia and rhabdomyolysis may occur after succinylcholine when it is administered to a neonate with an undiagnosed myopathy, such as Werdnig–Hoffman disease or muscular dystrophy. Although these diseases are rare, if electrocardiographic evidence of hyperkalemia occurs after succinylcholine, IV calcium chloride (10 mg/kg), not dantrolene, should be administered intravenously. Malignant hyperthermia (MH) is an exceedingly uncommon disease in neonates, but there may be a family history of MH that will require avoiding succinylcholine and inhalational anesthetics (except nitrous oxide and xenon).

Rocuronium has emerged as the intermediate muscle relaxant of choice in infants and children when succinylcholine is contraindicated or eschewed. Although doses as large as 0.9 mg/kg IV provide excellent conditions for tracheal intubation in less than 1 min, the children in that study were greater than 1 year of age [166]. In contrast to succinylcholine, the duration of action of rocuronium is greater with increasing doses and younger age patients. The optimal dose of rocuronium for RSI in neonates has not been determined. Published studies indicate fairly rapid onset times with 0.45 and 0.6 mg/kg IV rocuronium, although these doses were studied in the presence of inhalational anesthetics [167]. The downside to using such large doses of rocuronium in neonates is the time to recover: 62 and 95 min, respectively [121, 167]. If the surgery is expected to be brief, as in a pyloric stenosis, then the use of large doses of rocuronium will markedly delay emergence and extubation. The prolonged duration of action of rocuronium, then, must be taken into consideration when choosing both the neuromuscular blocking agent and its dose.

With the increasing use of propofol in neonates and during RSI, anticholinergics may continue to play a substantive role. Propofol enhances parasympathetic activity, which can explain the bradycardia often observed after induction of anesthesia. In adults, the decrease in heart rate after propofol in patients who were also receiving a continuous infusion of remifentanil was abolished by pretreatment with 0.5 mg IV atropine [168]. Since cardiac output depends to a large extent on heart rate in neonates, a bradycardia will compromise the cardiac output and decrease tissue oxygenation. In addition, neonates are prone to developing hypoxemia during prolonged apneas such as during RSI. For both of these reasons, intravenous atropine is justified in this population and should be integrated in the standard RSI of infants when using propofol.

Induction of General Anesthesia for Elective Surgery

In the past, anesthetists feared the hemodynamic and respiratory consequences of anesthetic agents in children. Halothane in particular caused profound hypotension, bradycardia, arrhythmias, and apnea. Hypnotics, opioids, and muscle relaxants could produce severe hypotension, tachycardia, bradycardia, dysrhythmia, chest rigidity, or respiratory depression. These could lead to fatal hemodynamic or respiratory failure. To lessen the risk of such adverse events in neonates, practitioners administered the smallest possible doses of these drugs and the most limited number of different drugs. In addition, many older drugs had prolonged durations of action diverse dose-dependent side effects that led to a polypharmacy approach to minimize these effects.

With the introduction of receptor-specific and better-tolerated anesthetics, induction of general anesthesia for elective surgery even in neonate is infrequently met with the past concerns. As cardiopulmonary morbidity has substantively decreased, latent fears have emerged about potential deleterious effects of anesthetics on neurologic development. Currently, these latter fears should not deter the clinician from administering an appropriate anesthetic to a neonate to ensure their safe conduct through the surgery.

Intravenous Induction

Intravenous anesthesia is a common induction technique in neonates globally, since most neonatal surgery occurs in the peripartum period, is associated with a full stomach, and requires an RSI. These neonates arrive in the operating room from the NICU with an IV (or PICC line) in place. Thiopental or propofol is commonly used for induction of anesthesia in a similar dose and with the same limitations as in RSI.

Tracheal intubation can be performed effectively after IV propofol alone, but not so after thiopental or other IV agents [169]. This property of propofol may be attributed to its ability to profoundly depress the laryngeal reflexes and relax the oropharyngeal muscles [170]. When compared with a combination of morphine, atropine, and succinylcholine, propofol 2.5 mg/kg led to a more rapid, successful intubation, less desaturation episodes, and a more rapid recovery time in 63 premature neonates undergoing non-urgent procedures [171]. However, it should be noted that most anesthesiologists would use a larger dose of propofol if it were the only induction agent, the times to intubation were 120 versus 260 s for propofol versus the three drug regimen, times that far exceed those acceptable to anesthesiologists, and all neonates were intubated nasally. Finally, the intubations were performed by registrars, not attending faculty, again raising doubts about the external validity of the data. Similar criticisms hold true for much of the evidence emerging from the neonatology literature [126]. When inducing anesthesia with propofol, the clinician should gently hold the limb where the IV is located, in order to prevent brisk withdrawal movements that might result in loss of the line before all the drugs are injected. The IV site should also be visible at least until all the drugs have been infused. Accidental disconnections can lead to underdosage and airway or hemodynamic reactivity during laryngoscopy. The injection may be done slowly, titrating the optimal dose of hypnotic drugs to the clinical state of the neonate. Pain during injection of propofol is an issue in neonates, even if local anesthetics are added to the propofol. However, it may be attenuated by the prior injection of an opioid (see Anesthetics for RSI, above).

Inhalational Induction

An inhalational induction is a suitable technique to induce anesthesia in the neonate undergoing elective surgery. In this age group, induction is rapid, smooth, technically easy to perform, and pain free. One of its main advantages is that it does not require that IV access be established while the infant is awake, a procedure that can be particularly difficult, prolonged, painful, and stressful for the struggling infant as well as for the anesthesiologist. Sevoflurane is the inhalational agent of choice for induction of anesthesia in infants. Because of its excellent cardiovascular profile, large concentrations of sevoflurane can be administered without causing excessive circulatory depression, unlike halothane. However, theoretical concerns have been raised regarding its potential to trigger epileptiform EEG activity [172]. The probability of epileptiform EEG activity increases in the presence of large concentrations of sevoflurane [173, 174] and hyperventilation and decreases in the presence of midazolam, opioids, and nitrous oxide [173]. Rare instances of tonic–clonic activity have been reported during and after sevoflurane anesthesia (fewer than 20 in the literature), but in only one case in a neonate [175]. In fact, with the exception of a report in one adult, EEG evidence of seizures during sevoflurane anesthesia has not been proven [176]. Severe EEG epileptiform signs during sevoflurane usually occur during deep anesthesia and precede the appearance of burst suppression. Currently, the long-term morbidity of such epileptiform EEG patterns is unknown, although we do know that epileptiform EEG patterns only weakly portend seizures. Given the large number of inhalational inductions performed with sevoflurane in neonates, infants, and children globally and the dearth of reports of seizures and seizure-like activity, the risk and consequences associated with epileptiform EEG activity are probably very minor.

Tracheal intubation can be performed with sevoflurane alone in most infants and children [177]. The main factor associated with the success is to provide sufficient time from the beginning of the inhalational induction until an adequate depth of anesthesia have been achieved, one that is often associated with the loss of spontaneous ventilation [178]. Both positive end-expiratory pressure (10 cmH_2O) and assisted ventilation speed the rapid onset of a deep level of anesthesia [179]. Alternately, the time to tracheal intubation may be abbreviated by supplementing the inhalational induction with IV drugs such as propofol, opioids, and muscle relaxants [180]. These strategies have been studied in children and likely may be extended to neonates, although evidence in neonates remains lacking. In neonates, the time to induce anesthesia is rapid; however, with a MAC of 3.2 % sevoflurane, the maximum MAC multiple that can be achieved within the first minute or two of anesthesia is only 1.2 (unlike halothane which can achieve a MAC multiple of 2.5 within the same time) (see Pharmacology chapter). Hence, to speed the induction of deep anesthesia, an IV dose of 2–3 mg/kg propofol may be administered [180].

The analgesic properties and adverse events of all opioids are dose dependent. But each opioid differs in its potency, onset of action, and duration of action.

Fentanyl (1–5 μg/kg) is one of the most frequently used analgesics for tracheal intubation in the NICU [119, 181]. This synthetic opioid has an analgesic potency 50–100 times that of morphine. It is quite lipid soluble and highly bound to plasma proteins. Its onset of clinical activity is approximately 1 min, with a duration of effect after a single IV dose of 30–45 min. Fentanyl's large hepatic extraction ratio implies that its termination of the action depends on both liver blood flow and CYP450 3A4/7 activity [182]. However, when hepatic blood flow is attenuated, as in several neonatal abdominal pathologies with increased intra-abdominal pressure, the elimination rate may be dramatically reduced (approaching zero), with a correspondingly greater half-life [183, 184].

Fentanyl should be injected slowly IV since it is associated with thoracic rigidity when injected rapidly. It provides excellent conditions for rapid intubation and with few hemodynamic adverse events when it is combined with atropine and a neuromuscular blockade [121, 165, 185]. Whether administered in bolus doses or as a continuous infusion, fentanyl maintains excellent hemodynamic stability [186].

Sufentanil is a synthetic opioid that is ten times more potent than fentanyl. It is highly lipid soluble and strongly bound to alpha-1-acid glycoprotein. In the neonate, the elimination half-life of sufentanil is increased. This is attributable to an increased volume of distribution and diminished clearance [187, 188]. It has an excellent hemodynamic tolerance, even at large doses [189]. Sufentanil can attenuate the cardiovascular response to intubation. Studies performed on a neonatal population are lacking, but some data on children 2–9 years of age, 0.3 μg/kg sufentanil combined with 2.5 mg/kg of propofol, and vecuronium, effectively blunted the cardiovascular responses to tracheal intubation [190]. The ED_{50} for sufentanil for excellent intubating conditions decreased as the expired fraction of sevoflurane increased in children [191]. For example, at 3 % of sevoflurane, the ED_{50} was 0.32 μg/kg sufentanil. However, considering the significant pharmacokinetic changes that occur during the first month of life, the extrapolation of these results to neonates should be viewed cautiously.

Although fentanyl and sufentanil remain the most frequent opioids administered to neonates before laryngoscopy and tracheal intubation, even shorter-acting opioids such as alfentanil and remifentanil have been evaluated.

Alfentanil is a synthetic opioid, derived from fentanyl. It is 5–10 times less potent than fentanyl and has a shorter onset and duration of action, mainly because of its reduced volume of distribution. Alfentanil is strongly bound to albumin but also to the plasma alpha-1 acid glycoprotein, a molecule present at reduced concentrations in the plasma of neonates compared with older children or adults [192]. Thus, like sufentanil, its free fraction is increased. The metabolism of alfentanil is mainly via hepatic enzymes, using metabolic pathways that are still immature at birth. In neonates, the elimination half-life is tenfold greater than in infants and children [193], attributable primarily to its decreased clearance [194]. This limits the interest of alfentanil in neonates. In adults, a bolus of alfentanil reduces the hemodynamic response to tracheal intubation, but causes bradycardia at doses in excess of 30 μg/kg [195, 196]. In children aged 3–10 years, the optimal bolus dose for intubation after 1 min exposure to 5 % sevoflurane, in 50 % of the population, was 11.5 μg/kg, without major adverse effects [197]. In children, when combined with propofol, a bolus of 15 μg/kg of alfentanil facilitated a comfortable tracheal intubation and blunted the subsequent hemodynamic response [198, 199]. In neonates, a bolus of 9–15 μg/kg of alfentanil facilitates tracheal intubation and decreases the stress response to that procedure. However, alfentanil may induce a greater incidence of muscle rigidity than other opioids [200].

Remifentanil is the most recent synthetic opioid to become commercially available. In contrast to other opioids, remifentanil is metabolized by nonspecific plasma and tissue esterases, with activities at birth similar to those in adults. Thus, the elimination of remifentanil is rapid and independent of hepatic and renal functions. Its elimination half-life is very brief irrespective of the dose; its context-sensitive half-life is also independent of the age of the child, dose, and duration of infusion, approximately 3–5 min. Side effects associated with bolus doses of opioids may be problematic with IV remifentanil: bradycardia, chest wall rigidity, respiratory depression, nausea and vomiting, and hyperalgesia [121, 201, 202]. Remifentanil is 26- to 65-fold more potent than fentanyl, primarily binding to μ opioid receptors and secondarily to κ and σ receptors. There is no defined dosing in neonates. IV doses range from 1 to 5 μg/kg for boluses and from 0.025 to 5 μg/kg/min for infusions, depending on the concurrent medications [202]. In neonates, a single bolus of 3 μg/kg IV remifentanil for non-urgent intubation yielded less favorable intubating conditions than a combination of fentanyl and succinylcholine [203]. In children 3–10 years of age, the optimal bolus dose of IV remifentanil for successful tracheal intubation during 5 % sevoflurane was 0.56 μg/kg [204]. Remifentanil boluses have also been evaluated as adjuvants to propofol during intravenous induction of anesthesia in infants and children [205]. Although neonates have not been studied as a group separate from infants, the ED_{50} and ED_{95} for remifentanil after propofol 5 mg/kg in neonates and infants <3 months of age to provide excellent intubating conditions were 3.1 and 5.0 mg/kg [206]. A continuous infusion of remifentanil has also been recommended to complement sevoflurane during induction of anesthesia. Here too, studies in neonates are lacking. In children 3–10 years old, the ED_{50} sevoflurane during 0.2 μg/kg/min of remifentanil was 1.81 % [207]. The principle of providing opioid analgesia before intubation seems reasonable, but neither the opioid nor the dose and timing is known to optimize the risk-benefit ratio in the neonate. Nonetheless, it is important to administer sufficient doses of hypnotics, like sevoflurane, to attenuate the nociceptive response to laryngoscopy at a cortical and even subcortical level, even in the absence of analgesics. Thus far, the effects of large concentrations of hypnotics or the combination of hypnotics and opioids during induction of anesthesia in neonates are unknown.

Muscle Relaxants for Tracheal Intubation

All muscle relaxants improve the conditions for tracheal intubation in neonates. However, in most instances in children, relaxants are unnecessary to achieve a quick and stress-free intubation. Many authors advocate relaxant-free techniques for tracheal intubation in children, with appropriate doses of hypnotics and opioids [208]. These drugs inhibit consciousness, blunt the hemodynamic response to nociceptive stimuli, and, in sufficient amount, prevent movement (see below). Given the risks associated with the use of neuromuscular blocking agents, including anaphylaxis and difficulty to antagonize in young infants, clinicians should carefully weigh their risk-benefit ratio in neonates.

Succinylcholine should be used only for rapid sequence inductions and in emergencies (e.g., laryngospasm), because of its potential side effects. For the remainder of circumstances, a non-depolarizing agent can be used.

Infants are more sensitive to non-depolarizing neuromuscular blocking agents (ND-NMB agents) than are older children: fewer than 50 % of the receptors have to be occupied to achieve intubating conditions in young infants compared with 90 % of the receptors in adults [209]. Hence, neonates require smaller doses of succinylcholine to achieve a targeted effect, and the duration of paralysis will be greater than in children [210]. Increasing the amount of injected NMB agent will speed the time to peak effect, but prolong the duration of action of the NMB agent [211].

The advantage of rocuronium is its rapid onset of action: 0.6 mg/kg induced good intubation conditions in 60 s in children anesthetized with propofol [212]. In contrast, rocuronium has a prolonged and unpredictable duration of action in neonates [167]. For a full discussion of the dosing of rocuronium in neonates, see above.

Mivacurium and atracurium have a brief duration of action, but greater time to profound neuromuscular block (2–3 min) than other muscle relaxants. Mivacurium 200 μg/kg IV provides good intubating conditions after 90 s in children [213]. Several studies showed that fentanyl decreased the number of attempts and the incidence of desaturation during tracheal intubation in premature and full-term neonates [185, 214]. Muscle relaxation occurred by 94 s with a time to return of spontaneous movements of ~15 min. Intubating conditions were scored as excellent. However, this protocol did not include any hypnotic drug, and no study compared mivacurium-fentanyl to a hypnotic-fentanyl combination in neonates.

Mivacurium is degraded spontaneously by pseudocholinesterase, leaving no active metabolites. On the other hand, atracurium is degraded spontaneously by Hoffman degradation, a process that depends only on pH and temperature [215]. In patients with a deficiency in plasma pseudocholinesterase (estimated frequency 1/2,000), mivacurium may cause prolonged neuromuscular blockade. In neonates, the activity of these esterases is less than in older patients, approximately 50 % of the adult normal rate. The maturation profile is still unclear: there may be a rapid increase in the pseudocholinesterase in the first month of life and then a slower increase towards adult values [216]. In a neonatal case report of prolonged neuromuscular blockade after an injection of 0.2 mg/kg of mivacurium, plasma levels of cholinesterases were not instructive, and the diagnosis could only be confirmed by molecular investigation [217].

Cisatracurium is one of the ten stereoisomers that comprise the muscle relaxant, atracurium [215]. Cisatracurium induces less histamine release than atracurium. A dose of 0.15 mg/kg provides excellent intubation conditions after 120 s in infants anesthetized with nitrous oxide-thiopental-fentanyl anesthesia [215]. In the same study, the onset time was more rapid and the recovery time greater in younger patients.

Nitrous Oxide

In children, N_2O speeds induction of anesthesia with sevoflurane, imparting no foul odor and limited respiratory and hemodynamic adverse effects [218]. However, nitrous oxide may not be ideal for anesthesia in the neonate for the several reasons. First, since many surgeries in neonates are emergencies that involve bowel obstruction or a risk of bowel distention, N_2O is often relatively contraindicated. Second, loss of the neonatal airway during induction of anesthesia with N_2O speeds the rate of desaturation as the ratio of oxygen consumption to lung oxygen reserve would be very large. Third, N_2O has been shown to stimulate opioid and adrenergic centers that activate descending inhibitory neurons (DINS) in adults. These DINS transmit from supraspinal centers in the brain to the posterior horn of the spinal cord. When activated, DINS provide potent antinociception. In the neonate, the DINS are poorly developed and immature [219], thus limiting the analgesic effects of N_2O [220]. Fourth, N_2O potentiates the neurotoxicity of other anesthetic agents on the developing brain in neonatal animals [20], although there is no evidence that N_2O is neurotoxic in humans. Fifth, when administered concomitantly with propofol or sevoflurane, N_2O decreases the regional oxygen extraction fraction and creates a possible imbalance in the cerebral metabolic rate [221]. Finally, nitrous oxide impairs the metabolism of vitamin B12, folate, and methionine synthetase that may lead to myelosuppression and megaloblastic anemia [222], although this usually requires a prolonged exposure.

In conclusion, the combination of propofol, opiates, or muscle relaxants to an inhalational induction provides better conditions for tracheal intubation and permits the use of smaller concentrations of sevoflurane, although the optimal doses of these compounds have not yet been determined in neonates.

Tracheal Intubation: Oral or Nasal Route?

The decision to intubate the trachea in the neonate orally or nasally is often an institutional or clinician's preference, based on local practice and experience.

Oral tracheal intubation is quicker [223] and easier to perform than nasal intubation, thereby reducing the period of apnea and the time interval during which the airway is unprotected. A Cochrane review of nasal versus oral tracheal intubation for the mechanical ventilation of neonates in the neonatal intensive care unit yielded only two studies, thus precluding any definitive recommendations. However, they did note from one of the studies, that hemodynamic responses were similar when hypnosis and analgesia were provided, that failed intubation occurred more frequently after nasal compared with oral intubations, and that atelectasis occurred more frequently after nasal intubation [224].

Mobility of nasotracheal tubes during head movement may be less than that of orotracheal tubes, an effect that may reduce the rate of accidental extubation or endobronchial intubation. However, a Cochrane review (above) noted that the incidence of complications, including accidental extubation, was similar with nasal and oral intubations. Published studies in neonates and preterm infants (560–2,000 g) with orotracheal tubes demonstrated that 55° flexion of the neck yielded less movement of the tip of the tube than 55° extension of the neck (3.1 versus 7.4 mm) [225–227]. In 15 neonates and infants, ages 14 days to 15 months, extension of the neck resulted in 6.5 mm of cephalad displacement of the tip of the orotracheal tube, almost twice the 3.5 mm of the tip of displacement of the nasotracheal tube [228]. Given the short length of the trachea in neonates (4–4.5 cm), extension of the neck in a neonate with an orotracheal tube could lead to an unexpected extubation.

In conclusion, there is no solid argument to recommend one route of tracheal intubation in neonates. Nasotracheal intubation tends to be more difficult and take more time, thereby increasing the risk of desaturation, although it is more secure and less likely to become extubated. In contrast, orotracheal intubation is easier, faster, but may facilitate more accidental extubations. Carefully taped tracheal tubes will minimize excessive tube displacement, although nasotracheal tubes are associated with less displacement. The final decision will depend on both the clinician's experience, the size of the infant, the context of surgery, and the postoperative destination of the infant.

Maintenance of Anesthesia

Hypnosis

Short-acting inhalational anesthetics are appropriate hypnotics for maintenance of anesthesia in neonates. Sevoflurane offers several advantages over intravenous anesthetics in that it is suited for an inhalational induction, is minimally metabolized, has rapid pharmacokinetics, and is safe in infants with cardiorespiratory disease. However, sevoflurane does potentiate NMBD [210]. Alternately, desflurane is unsuited for inhalational induction and increases airway resistance [229] but has more favorable pharmacokinetics primarily due to its limited solubility in blood and tissues, resulting in more rapid recovery and return to spontaneous respiration compared with the older more soluble anesthetics, is metabolized to a lesser extent than sevoflurane, and confers no end-organ toxicity [230].

Maintenance of anesthesia via the intravenous route in neonates is also fraught with pitfalls for several reasons [231]. First, the IV lines are particularly fragile in neonates. Subcutaneous infiltration or accidental disconnection may occur most dangerously during maintenance of anesthesia. This is particularly problematic with IVs cited in the antecubital fossa. Moreover, once the drapes cover the neonate, and surgery begins, the IV site is often concealed from the anesthesiologist's sight and control. There are no monitoring devices that can alert the anesthesiologist to an occluded or disconnected intravenous catheter. As a result, the patient might awaken, move, or display pain-related hemodynamic disturbances while still anesthetized. Second, the effect-site concentration of propofol during anesthesia cannot be measured, unlike the breath-by-breath data provided by the gas analyzer for inhalational anesthetics. There is considerable interindividual variability in the pharmacokinetic–pharmacodynamic profile of propofol in the first weeks of life [232]. Because we lack a reliable device to monitor the depth of anesthesia in infants, patients may be under- or overdosed with propofol. For inhaled anesthetics, there is a more constant relationship at all ages between the expired fraction of drugs and clinical stages of depth of anesthesia (e.g., MAC). And last, no devices allowing target-controlled infusion are available for young children, which make the continuous infusion of propofol more susceptible to human errors when calculating and programming the infusion rates. In the future, if TCI devices and adequate monitors are developed, TIVA may prove to be safer and easier to perform in neonates.

Propofol infusion syndrome (PRIS) is a rare but potentially fatal complication that was first described in the 1990s in PICU in children sedated for prolonged (>48 h) periods with large infusions rates (>5 mg/kg/h) of propofol. PRIS is characterized by refractory bradycardia, lipemic plasma, metabolic acidosis, and rhabdomyolysis that deteriorate to renal and hepatic failure and asystole. However, an increasing number of episodes of suspected PRIS have been reported after propofol infusions that were brief in duration, during general anesthesia for surgical procedures, and in children as well as in adults [233–235]. Young age, a large infusion dose of propofol (>5 mg/kg/h) and prolonged duration (>48 h), critical illness, high fat/low carbohydrate intake, inborn error in mitochondrial fatty acid oxidation, and concomitant catecholamine infusion or steroids have been identified as risk factors for developing PRIS [235]. A suspected case of PRIS with metabolic anomalies and bradycardia has been described in a preterm infant (24 weeks gestation), who underwent a propofol anesthetic at 33 weeks PCA. The infant received 80 and 60 mg/kg/h of propofol for 2 h [236]. Unexplained bradycardia or lactic acidosis during propofol anesthesia should lead the clinician to suspect PRIS. In such a case, the propofol infusion should be stopped and replaced with another anesthetic. In addition, to standard cardiovascular support, it is essential to administer glucose in order to prevent lipolysis in the process of energy production, especially in young infants whose glycogen stores are very small. If adjuvant agents such as opioids are administered concurrently with the propofol infusion, smaller doses of propofol may be required to sedate the patient and, in so doing, obviate the development of PRIS. Treatment of PRIS has included hemodialysis to remove the lipids from circulation. However, no definitive treatment has been uniformly successful in reversing PRIS. Prevention is the most important strategy. Limiting the dose and duration of the propofol infusion, supplementing the sedation/anesthesia with opioids or other anesthetics and glucose infusions (to avoid starvation), and hemodialysis/extracorporeal membrane oxygenator and glucagon may be salutary for cases of possible PRIS [235].

Analgesia

Thirty years ago, neonates underwent surgery with little to no analgesia. In the 1980s, several investigators both measured and acknowledged the capability of the human neonate to perceive pain and a number demonstrated the importance of treating the pain. Indeed, further research uncovered that the neonate is actually more sensitive to painful stimuli than are older subjects [237, 238]. First, several seminal studies documented the short-term consequences of pain (and the stress response) in the neonate in terms of changes in hemodynamics, metabolism, agitation, and recovery [239, 240]. Second, subsequent studies determined that painful experiences such as neonatal circumcision caused long-term behavioral changes [241]. Some of these early painful experiences resulted in persistent alterations in pain sensitivity [242, 243].

How could a child or adult "remember" a painful neonatal experience? Pain sensitivity and behavioral changes depend on "implicit memory." Pain-induced *neurotoxicity* and *neuroplasticity* can account for some of the symptoms. Unrelieved neonatal pain causes apoptosis in cortical and subcortical areas, associated with abnormal neurocognitive development in rats [63]. Interestingly, the development of memory was also impaired in this model. Changes caused by early painful experiences can also be observed in the peripheral nervous system: neonatal skin wounds caused a prolonged increase in the innervation of the wound site in rats [243]. In a study using functional MRI, pain-specific cortical and subcortical hyperactivation was demonstrated in children 11–16 years of age, who were born preterm, and who had undergone painful procedures as neonates [244]. Finally, a painful stimulus may activate the amygdala even during general anesthesia, thereby increasing the probability of recall, even if subconscious.

Once the negative consequences of untreated pain were strongly established, clinicians increased their prescriptions of perioperative analgesics for neonates. In the past two or more decades, the attitudes of anesthesiologists and other physicians changed radically shifting from "no analgesia" to "as much analgesia as possible" in neonates. The dose of analgesics was limited by the absence of pain or the presence of side effects, most notably respiratory depression in the neonate.

Published studies in the early 2000s raised new questions about the benefits of routine use of analgesics in neonates. The first doubts arose from the NEOPAIN trial in which preemptive morphine infusions administered to premature neonates neither reduced the incidence of severe neurological adverse events nor reduced the mortality compared with placebo. Moreover, intermittent morphine boluses were associated with a greater incidence of these complications [245]. However, these findings should not deter us from delivering adequate analgesia to neonates, as recommended by international guidelines.

In terms of the pharmacokinetic profiles of opioids in neonates, large interindividual variability precludes a relationship between the opioid concentrations and the effect site. Compared with adults, protein binding of opioids is diminished, free fractions are increased, the blood-brain barrier is more permeable, distribution volumes are increased, clearances are decreased, and elimination half-lives are greater in neonates than in older children [246]. Protein binding and hepatic metabolism undergo dramatic changes and maturation throughout the neonatal and infant periods. Alpha-1-acid glycoprotein is the main binding protein for fentanyl, sufentanil, and alfentanil [247]. Neonates and young infants have less AAG concentrations, a phenomenon that may in part explain the greater free fraction and larger volumes of distribution of these opioids [248].

At birth, most metabolic pathways are immature, especially those involving hepatic enzymes. The CYP450 3A4, which is a major hepatic enzyme of the metabolism of fentanyl and sufentanil [249], is nonfunctional at birth (replacing the fetal CYP3A7 isozyme), but matures during the first weeks of life [250, 251]. Moreover, many of the P450 cytochromes are subject to genetic polymorphisms that can modulate their activity [252]. The maturation processes, combined with the genetic variability, result in important interindividual differences in the responses to opioid during the neonatal period.

In neonates, *fentanyl* and *sufentanil* are the most frequently used opioids during general anesthesia. They both provide relative hemodynamic stability [253]. In the very young patient, their pharmacokinetic and pharmacodynamic characteristics make their administration sometimes difficult to adjust.

When used in a single-dose before tracheal intubation, both IV fentanyl (1–5 μg/kg) and sufentanil (0.2–0.3 μg/kg) have a rapid onset of action and a short duration of action. In contrast, the pharmacokinetics of sufentanil make it a more appropriate opioid for maintenance of anesthesia: if used in repeated injections or continuous infusion, fentanyl will accumulate in peripheral tissues (fat, muscle), and thus its context-sensitive half-life will increase [254]. This effect is even more pronounced in neonates, because of the immaturity of metabolic pathways.

Alfentanil's rapid onset and short duration of action are of interest when it is used as a single dose for brief surgical procedures. In the neonate, pyloric stenosis is a good indication for this opioid. Theoretically, alfentanil can be delivered as a continuous infusion, but in this case, its short duration of action is no longer an advantage over fentanyl or sufentanil. It accumulates in a large peripheral compartment, and, like fentanyl, its context-sensitive half-life increases [254]. Moreover, it is metabolized by the same cytochromes as fentanyl and sufentanil and, thus, is susceptible to the same interindividual variability through genetic and developmental variability.

Remifentanil is an ultrashort-acting opioid that is rapidly metabolized by tissues esterases (that reach maturity at birth) to inactive metabolites. Remifentanil achieves its maximum end-organ effect rapidly after the infusion begins. Not surprisingly, these characteristics lead to a context-sensitive half-life that is constant, independent of its duration of infusion, even in neonates and infants [255]. However, evidence suggests that the rate of recovery after remifentanil in neonates less than 1 week old may be greater than it is in infants 7 days to 3 months of age [256]. Pharmacodynamically, remifentanil may induce bradycardia, an effect classically attributed to the parasympathomimetic properties of remifentanil, a direct negative chronotropic effect [257]. The decrease in heart rate attributable to remifentanil after 5 μg/kg was infused over 1 min, peaks at 3 and 5 min after the infusion, but was less impressive in infants ≤2 months than in older children, although only 8 infants ≤2 months were included [258].

Regarding the routine use of remifentanil for maintenance of anesthesia, several issues persist. Pharmacokinetic models integrated in electronic devices for neonates have not been developed. Further, chest wall rigidity and postoperative hyperalgesia remain concerns after IV boluses of the opioid.

In conclusion, the choice of the optimal analgesic for general anesthesia in the neonate depends on the type and duration of surgical procedure as well as the mode of postoperative management expected, i.e., rapid extubation or persistent ventilation.

Although the neurotoxicity of NMDA antagonists and $GABA_A$ agonists in animal models are a cause for concern, until further data are available in humans, we do not recommend a change in practice. We strongly recommend the use of potent opioids such as fentanyl or sufentanil, although the use of remifentanil is increasing. Growing interest about the properties of remifentanil and abundance of clinical trials in neonates might soon allow its safe use in this age group. Until reliable and valid pain/analgesia monitors are developed, it remains difficult to distinguish between "not enough" and "too much" analgesia.

Muscle Relaxants

In the past, when pain and recall were neglected concepts in the newborn, muscle relaxants were commonplace in pediatric anesthetists. But with the advances in modern anesthesia, the occasional episodes of anaphylaxis associated with the use of NMBDs, and the release of safer opioids and hypnotics, NMBDs have become less popular [259–261]. Moreover, fears of residual neuromuscular block and incomplete antagonism with anticholinesterases have led many practitioners to restrict the use of NMBDs to facilitating tracheal intubation. However, non-depolarizing NMBDs may also improve surgical conditions during maintenance of anesthesia, although the indications are actually quite few. If NMBDs are required during critical periods of surgery, bolus doses are preferred over infusions. If NMBDs are administered, neuromuscular monitoring should be used. Alternately, bolus doses of propofol have proven to be very effective to "relax" the abdomen when it appears to be tight, or the bowels will not return easily to the abdomen as the surgery concludes. Although untested, this approach to relax the abdomen with propofol is exceedingly effective and does not appear to prolong emergence. If NMBDs are used, it cannot be emphasized enough that neonates require smaller doses, and even these smaller doses have prolonged effects and have less predictable duration of action.

The release of sugammadex may change the reluctance on the part of anesthesiologists towards using rocuronium and vecuronium in neonates and infants [209]. This drug irreversibly binds these two NMBDs and completely removes them from clinical activity. Sugammadex is associated with relatively few side effects. Neither pharmacodynamic nor pharmacokinetic data on the use of sugammadex in neonates are available.

Conclusion

There are many controversies in neonatal anesthesia, and in this chapter, we sought to explore several of these. In so doing, we have outlined both the advantages and disadvantages of each approach, what is known and unknown about the evidence, and where future studies are most needed.

References

1. Davidson AJ. The aims of anesthesia in infants: the relevance of philosophy, psychology and a little evidence. Paediatr Anaesth. 2007;17(2):102–8.
2. Lewis M. The emergence of consciousness and its role in human development. Ann N Y Acad Sci. 2003;1001:104–33.
3. Tononi G, et al. Investigating neural correlates of conscious perception by frequency-tagged neuromagnetic responses. Proc Natl Acad Sci USA. 1998;95(6):3198–203.
4. Sann C, Streti A. Inter-manual transfer of object texture and shape in human neonates. Neuropsychologia. 2008;46:698–703.
5. Marcus L, Lejeune F, Berne-Audéoud F, et al. Tactile sensory capacity of the preterm infant: manual perception of shape from 28 gestational weeks. Pediatrics. 2012;130:e88–94.
6. Cecchini M, Baroni E, Di Vito C, et al. Newborn preference for a new face vs. a previously seen communicative or motionless face. Infant Behav Dev. 2011;34:424–33.
7. Marlier L, Schaal B, Soussignan R. Bottle-fed neonates prefer an odor experienced in utero to an odor experienced postnatally in the feeding context. Dev Psychobiol. 1998;33(2):133–45.
8. Marlier L, Schaal B, Soussignan R. Neonatal responsiveness to the odor of amniotic and lacteal fluids: a test of perinatal chemosensory continuity. Child Dev. 1998;69(3):611–23.
9. Delaunay-El Allam M, Soussignan R, Patris B, et al. Long-lasting memory for an odor acquired at the mother's breast. Dev Sci. 2010;13(6):849–63.
10. Kisilevsky BS, et al. Fetal sensitivity to properties of maternal speech and language. Infant Behav Dev. 2009;32(1):59–71.
11. Partanen E, Kujala T, Naatanen R, et al. Learning-induced neural plasticity of speech processing before birth. Proc Natl Acad Sci USA. 2013;110(37):15145–50.
12. James DK, Spencer CJ, Stepsis BW. Fetal learning: a prospective randomized controlled study. Ultrasound Obstet Gynecol. 2002;20(5):431–8.
13. Granier-Deferre C, Bassereau S, Ribeiro A, et al. A melodic contour repeatedly experienced by human near-term fetuses elicits a profound cardiac reaction one month after birth. PLoS One. 2011;6(2):e17304.
14. Myers NA, Perris EE, Speaker CJ. Fifty months of memory: a longitudinal study in early childhood. Memory. 1994;2(4):383–415.
15. Antognini JF, et al. Preserved reticular neuronal activity during selective delivery of supra-clinical isoflurane concentrations to brain in goats and its association with spontaneous movement. Neurosci Lett. 2004;361(1–3):94–7.

16. Gili T, Saxena N, Diukova A, et al. The thalamus and brainstem act as key hubs in alterations of human brain network connectivity induced by mild propofol sedation. J Neurosci. 2013;33(9):4024–31.
17. Mhuircheartaigh RN, Rosenom-Lanng D, Wise R, et al. Cortical and subcortical connectivity changes during decreasing levels of consciousness in humans: a functional magnetic resonance imaging study using propofol. J Neurosci. 2010;30(27):9095–102.
18. Uemura E, Levin ED, Bowman RE. Effects of halothane on synaptogenesis and learning behavior in rats. Exp Neurol. 1985;89(3):520–9.
19. Ikonomidou C, et al. Blockade of NMDA receptors and apoptotic neurodegeneration in the developing brain. Science. 1999;283(5398):70–4.
20. Jevtovic-Todorovic V, et al. Early exposure to common anesthetic agents causes widespread neurodegeneration in the developing rat brain and persistent learning deficits. J Neurosci. 2003;23(3):876–82.
21. Fredriksson A, et al. Neonatal exposure to a combination of N-methyl-D-aspartate and gamma-aminobutyric acid type A receptor anesthetic agents potentiates apoptotic neurodegeneration and persistent behavioral deficits. Anesthesiology. 2007;107(3):427–36.
22. Young C, et al. Potential of ketamine and midazolam, individually or in combination, to induce apoptotic neurodegeneration in the infant mouse brain. Br J Pharmacol. 2005;146(2):189–97.
23. Ma D, et al. Xenon mitigates isoflurane-induced neuronal apoptosis in the developing rodent brain. Anesthesiology. 2007;106(4):746–53.
24. Jr Slikker W, Zou X, Hotchkiss CE, et al. Ketamine-induced neuronal cell death in the perinatal rhesus monkey. Toxicol Sci. 2007;98:145–58.
25. Yahalom B, Athiraman U, Soriano SG, et al. Spinal anesthesia in infant rats: development of a model and assessment of neurologic outcomes. Anesthesiology. 2011;114:1325–35.
26. Johnson SA, Young C, Olney JW. Isoflurane-induced neuroapoptosis in the developing brain of nonhypoglycemic mice. J Neurosurg Anesthesiol. 2008;20:21–8.
27. Briner A, et al. Volatile anesthetics rapidly increase dendritic spine density in the rat medial prefrontal cortex during synaptogenesis. Anesthesiology. 2010;112(3):546–56.
28. Fredriksson A, et al. Neurofunctional deficits and potentiated apoptosis by neonatal NMDA antagonist administration. Behav Brain Res. 2004;153(2):367–76.
29. Paule MG, et al. Ketamine anesthesia during the first week of life can cause long-lasting cognitive deficits in rhesus monkeys. Neurotoxicol Teratol. 2011;33(2):220–30.
30. Yu D, Jiang Y, Gao J, et al. Repeated exposure to propofol potentiates neuroapoptosis and long-term behavioural deficits in neonatal rats. Neurosci Lett. 2013;534:41–6.
31. Ramage TM, Chang FL, Shih J, et al. Distinct long-term neurocognitive outcomes after equipotent sevoflurane or isoflurane anaesthesia in immature rats. Br J Anaesth. 2013;110:i39–46.
32. Briner A, Nikonenko I, De Roo M, et al. Developmental stage-dependent persistent impact of propofol anesthesia on dendritic spines in the rat medial prefrontal cortex. Anesthesiology. 2011;115(2):282–93.
33. Loepke AW, Soriano SG. An assessment of the effects of general anesthetics on developing brain structure and neurocognitive function. Anesth Analg. 2008;106(6):1681–707.
34. Istaphanous GK, Loepke AW. General anesthetics and the developing brain. Curr Opin Anaesthesiol. 2009;22(3):368–73.
35. Istaphanous GK, Ward CG, Loepke AW. The impact of the perioperative period on neurocognitive development, with a focus on pharmacological concerns. Best Pract Res Clin Anaesthesiol. 2010;24(3):433–49.
36. Davidson A, Flick RP. Neurodevelopmental implications of the use of sedation and analgesia in neonates. Clin Perinatol. 2013;40:559–73.
37. Sanders RD, Hassell J, Davidson AJ, et al. Impact of anaesthetics and surgery on neurodevelopment: an update. Br J Anaesth. 2013;110(S1):i53–72.
38. Reddy SV. Effect of general anesthetics on the developing brain. J Anaesthesiol Clin Pharmacol. 2012;28:6–10.
39. Shih J, May LDV, Gonzalez HE, et al. Delayed environmental enrichment reverses sevoflurane-induced memory impairment in rats. Anesthesiology. 2012;116:586–602.
40. Turner CP, Gutierrez S, Liu C, et al. Strategies to defeat ketamine-induced neonatal brain injury. Neuroscience. 2012;210:384–92.
41. Gozes I. Microtubules (tau) as an emerging therapeutic target: NAP (Davunetide). Curr Pharm Des. 2011;17:3413–7.
42. Chauvier D, Renolleau S, Holifanjanianina S, et al. Targeting neonatal ischemic brain injury with a pentapeptide-based irreversible caspase inhibitor. Cell Death Dis. 2011;2:e203. doi:10.1038/cddis.2011.87.
43. Itoh T, Imano M, Nishida S, et al. Exercise inhibits neuronal apoptosis and improves cerebral function following rat traumatic brain injury. J Neural Transm. 2011;118:1263–72.
44. Sim YJ, Kim H, Kim JY, et al. Long-term treadmill exercise overcomes ischemia-induced apoptotic neuronal cell death in gerbils. Physiol Behav. 2005;84:733–8.
45. De Roo M, et al. Anesthetics rapidly promote synaptogenesis during a critical period of brain development. PLoS One. 2009;4(9):e7043.
46. Ben-Ari Y, et al. GABA: a pioneer transmitter that excites immature neurons and generates primitive oscillations. Physiol Rev. 2007;87(4):1215–84.
47. Rabinowicz T, et al. Human cortex development: estimates of neuronal numbers indicate major loss late during gestation. J Neuropathol Exp Neurol. 1996;55(3):320–8.
48. Oppenheim RW. Cell death during development of the nervous system. Annu Rev Neurosci. 1991;14:453–501.
49. Kuida K, et al. Decreased apoptosis in the brain and premature lethality in CPP32-deficient mice. Nature. 1996;384(6607):368–72.
50. Olney JW, et al. Anesthesia-induced developmental neuroapoptosis. Does it happen in humans? Anesthesiology. 2004;101(2):273–5.
51. Anand KJ. Anesthetic neurotoxicity in newborns: should we change clinical practice? Anesthesiology. 2007;107(1):2–4.
52. Jevtovic-Todorovic V, Olney JW. PRO: anesthesia-induced developmental neuroapoptosis: status of the evidence. Anesth Analg. 2008;106(6):1659–63.
53. Loepke AW, Jr McGowan FX, Soriano SG. CON: the toxic effects of anesthetics in the developing brain: the clinical perspective. Anesth Analg. 2008;106(6):1664–9.
54. Perouansky M, Jr Hemmings HC. Neurotoxicity of general anesthetics: cause for concern? Anesthesiology. 2009;111(6):1365–71.
55. Dobbing J, Sands J. Comparative aspects of the brain growth spurt. Early Hum Dev. 1979;3(1):79–83.
56. Dekaban AS. Changes in brain weights during the span of human life: relation of brain weights to body heights and body weights. Ann Neurol. 1978;4(4):345–56.
57. Jr Slikker W, Paule MG, Wright LKM, et al. Systems biology approaches for toxicology. J Appl Toxicol. 2007;27:201–17.
58. Clancy B, et al. Extrapolating brain development from experimental species to humans. Neurotoxicology. 2007;28(5):931–7.
59. Loepke AW, et al. The physiologic effects of isoflurane anesthesia in neonatal mice. Anesth Analg. 2006;102(1):75–80.
60. Green CJ, et al. Ketamine alone and combined with diazepam or xylazine in laboratory animals: a 10 year experience. Lab Anim. 1981;15(2):163–70.

61. Cattano D, Young C, Straiko MMW, et al. Subanesthetic doses of propofol induce neuroapoptosis in the infant mouse brain. Anesth Analg. 2008;106:1712–4.
62. Istaphanous GK, et al. Anesthesiology 2011:114;578.
63. Anand KJS, et al. Ketamine reduces the cell death following inflammatory pain in newborn rat brain. Pediatr Res. 2007;62(3): 283–90.
64. Liu JR, Liu Q, Li J, et al. Noxious stimulation attenuates ketamine-induced neuroapoptosis in the developing rat brain. Anesthesiology. 2012;117:64–71.
65. Shu Y, Zhou Z, Wan Y, et al. Nociceptive stimuli enhance anesthetic-induced neuroapoptosis in the rat developing brain. Neurobiol Dis. 2012;45:743–50.
66. Wilder RT, Flick RP, Sprung J, et al. Early exposure to anesthesia and learning disabilities in a population-based birth cohort. Anesthesiology. 2009;110:796–804.
67. DiMaggio C, et al. A retrospective cohort study of the association of anesthesia and hernia repair surgery with behavioral and developmental disorders in young children. J Neurosurg Anesthesiol. 2009;21(4):286–91.
68. DiMaggio C, Sun LS, Li G. Early childhood exposure to anesthesia and risk of developmental and behavioral disorders in a sibling birth cohort. Anesth Analg. 2011;113:1143–51.
69. Ing C, Dimaggio C, Whitehouse A, et al. Long-term differences in language and cognitive function after childhood exposure to anesthesia. Pediatrics. 2012;130:e476–85.
70. Flick RP, Katusic SK, Colligan RC, et al. Cognitive and behavioral outcomes after early exposure to anesthesia and surgery. Pediatrics. 2011;128:e1053–61.
71. Sprung J, Flick RP, Katusic SK, et al. Attention-deficit/hyperactivity disorder after early exposure to procedures requiring general anesthesia. Mayo Clin Proc. 2012;87:120–9.
72. Block RI, Thomas JJ, Bayman EO, Choi JY, Kimble KK, Todd MM. Are anesthesia and surgery during infancy associated with altered academic performance during childhood? Anesthesiology. 2012;117:494–503.
73. Davidson AJ, McCann ME, Morton NS, Myles PS. Anesthesia and outcome after neonatal surgery: the role for randomized trials. Anesthesiology. 2008;109:941–4.
74. Sun LS, Li G, DiMaggio CJ, et al. Feasibility and pilot study of the Pediatric Anesthesia Neuro Development Assessment (PANDA) project. J Neurosurg Anesthesiol. 2012;24:382–8.
75. Kinsler V, Bulstrode N. The role of surgery in the management of congenital melanocytic naevi in children: a perspective from Great Ormond Street Hospital. J Plast Reconstr Aesthet Surg. 2009;62(5):595–601.
76. Rappaport B, Mellon D, Simone A, et al. Defining safe use of anesthesia in children. N Engl J Med. 2011;364:1387–90.
77. Davidson AJ, et al. Performance of entropy and Bispectral Index as measures of anaesthesia effect in children of different ages. Br J Anaesth. 2005;95(5):674–9.
78. Abajian JC, et al. Spinal anesthesia for surgery in the high-risk infant. Anesth Analg. 1984;63(3):359–62.
79. Kurth CD, et al. Postoperative apnea in preterm infants. Anesthesiology. 1987;66(4):483–8.
80. Allen GS, et al. Postoperative respiratory complications in ex-premature infants after inguinal herniorrhaphy. J Pediatr Surg. 1998;33(7):1095–8.
81. Cote CJ, et al. Postoperative apnea in former preterm infants after inguinal herniorrhaphy. A combined analysis. Anesthesiology. 1995;82(4):809–22.
82. Malviya S, Swartz J, Lerman J. Are all preterm infants younger than 60 weeks postconceptual age at risk for postanesthetic apnea? Anesthesiology. 1993;78(6):1076–81.
83. Welborn LG, et al. Anemia and postoperative apnea in former preterm infants. Anesthesiology. 1991;74(6):1003–6.
84. Zagol K, Lake DE, Vergales B, et al. Anemia, apnea of prematurity, and blood transfusions. J Pediatr. 2012;161:417–21.
85. Henderson-Smart DJ, Steer PA. Caffeine versus theophylline for apnea in preterm infants. Cochrane Database Syst Rev (1):CD000273.
86. Welborn LG, et al. Postoperative apnea in former preterm infants: prospective comparison of spinal and general anesthesia. Anesthesiology. 1990;72(5):838–42.
87. Murphy JJ, Swanson T, Ansermino M, Milner R. The frequency of apneas in premature infants after inguinal hernia repair: do they need overnight monitoring in the intensive care unit? J Pediatr Surg. 2008;43:865–8.
88. Shenkman Z, Erez I, Freud E, et al. Risk factors for spinal anesthesia in preterm infants undergoing inguinal hernia repair. J Pediatr (Rio J). 2012;88:222–6.
89. Frawley G, Ingelmo P. Spinal anaesthesia in the neonate. Best Pract Res Clin Anaesthesiol. 2010;24:337–51.
90. William JM, et al. Post-operative recovery after inguinal herniotomy in ex-premature infants: comparison between sevoflurane and spinal anaesthesia. Br J Anaesth. 2001;86(3):366–71.
91. Craven PD, et al. Regional (spinal, epidural, caudal) versus general anaesthesia in preterm infants undergoing inguinal herniorrhaphy in early infancy. Cochrane Database Syst Rev. 2003;3, CD003669.
92. Walther-Larsen S, Rasmussen LS. The former preterm infant and risk of post-operative apnoea: recommendations for management. Acta Anaesthesiol Scand. 2006;50(7):888–93.
93. Dohi S, Naito H, Takahashi T. Age-related changes in blood pressure and duration of motor block in spinal anesthesia. Anesthesiology. 1979;50(4):319–23.
94. Oberlander TF, et al. Infants tolerate spinal anesthesia with minimal overall autonomic changes: analysis of heart rate variability in former premature infants undergoing hernia repair. Anesth Analg. 1995;80(1):20–7.
95. Hermanns H, et al. Sedation during spinal anaesthesia in infants. Br J Anaesth. 2006;97(3):380–4.
96. Lacroix F. Epidemiology and morbidity of regional anaesthesia in children. Curr Opin Anaesthesiol. 2008;21(3):345–9.
97. Giaufre E, Dalens B, Gombert A. Epidemiology and morbidity of regional anesthesia in children: a one-year prospective survey of the French-Language Society of Pediatric Anesthesiologists. Anesth Analg. 1996;83(5):904–12.
98. Williams RK, et al. The safety and efficacy of spinal anesthesia for surgery in infants: the Vermont Infant Spinal Registry. Anesth Analg. 2006;102(1):67–71.
99. Walker SM, Yaksh TL. Neuraxial analgesia in neonates and infants: a review of clinical and preclinical strategies for the development of safety and efficacy data. Anesth Analg. 2012;115: 638–62.
100. Easley RB, et al. Aseptic meningitis after spinal anesthesia in an infant. Anesthesiology. 1999;91(1):305–7.
101. Luz G, et al. Spinal anaesthesia and meningitis in former preterm infants: cause-effect? Paediatr Anaesth. 1999;9(3):262–4.
102. Faillace WJ, Warrier I, Canady AI. Paraplegia after lumbar puncture. In an infant with previously undiagnosed hemophilia A. Treatment and peri-operative considerations. Clin Pediatr (Phila). 1989;28(3):136–8.
103. De Saint Blanquat L, et al. Preoperative coagulation tests in former preterm infants undergoing spinal anaesthesia. Paediatr Anaesth. 2002;12(4):304–7.
104. Pollock JE. Transient neurologic symptoms: etiology, risk factors, and management. Reg Anesth Pain Med. 2002;27(6):581–6.
105. Selander D. Neurotoxicity of local anesthetics: animal data. Reg Anesth. 1993;18(6 Suppl):461–8.
106. Perez-Castro R, et al. Cytotoxicity of local anesthetics in human neuronal cells. Anesth Analg. 2009;108(3):997–1007.

107. Shenkman Z, et al. Spinal anesthesia in 62 premature, former-premature or young infants–technical aspects and pitfalls. Can J Anaesth. 2002;49(3):262–9.
108. Frumiento C, Abajian JC, Vane DW. Spinal anesthesia for preterm infants undergoing inguinal hernia repair. Arch Surg. 2000;135(4):445–51.
109. Polaner DM, Drescher J. Pediatric regional anesthesia: what is the current safety record? Paediatr Anaesth. 2011;21:737–42.
110. Cook-Sather SD, Litman RS. Modern fasting guidelines in children. Best Pract Res Clin Anaesthesiol. 2006;20(3):471–81.
111. Soreide E, et al. Pre-operative fasting guidelines: an update. Acta Anaesthesiol Scand. 2005;49(8):1041–7.
112. Apfelbaum JL, Caplan RA, Connis RT, et al. American Society of Anesthesiologsts committee on Standard and practice parameters. Practice guidelines for preoperative fasting and the use of pharmacologic agents to reduce the risk of pulmonary aspiration: application to healthy patients undergoing elective procedures. Anesthesiology. 2011;114:495–511.
113. Smith I, Kranke P, Murat I, et al. Perioperative fasting in adults and children: guidelines from the European Society of Anaesthesiology. Eur J Anaesthesiol. 2011;28:556–9.
114. Brady MC, et al. Preoperative fasting for preventing perioperative complications in children. Cochrane Database Syst Rev. 2009;4, CD005285.
115. Cavell B. Gastric emptying in infants fed human bilk or infant formula. Acta Paediatr Scand. 1981;70:639–41.
116. Kelleher J, Mallya P, Wyllie J. Premedication before intubation in UK neonatal units: a decade of change? Arch Dis Child Fetal Neonatal Ed. 2009;94:F332–5.
117. Carbajal R, Eble B, Anand KJ. Premedication for tracheal intubation in neonates: confusion or controversy? Semin Perinatol. 2007;31(5):309–17.
118. Kumar P, Denson SE, Mancuso TJ, Committee on Fetus and Newborn, Section on Anesthesiology and Pain Medicine. Clinical report-premedication for nonemergency endotracheal intubation in the neonate. Pediatrics. 2010;125:608–15.
119. Chaudhary R, et al. Use of premedication for intubation in tertiary neonatal units in the United Kingdom. Paediatr Anaesth. 2009;19(7):653–8.
120. Duncan HP, Zurick NJ, Wolf AR. Should we reconsider awake neonatal intubation? A review of the evidence and treatment strategies. Paediatr Anaesth. 2001;11(2):135–45.
121. Barrington KJ. Premedication for endotracheal intubation in the newborn infant. Paediatr Child Health. 2011;16:159–64.
122. Marshall TA, et al. Physiologic changes associated with endotracheal intubation in preterm infants. Crit Care Med. 1984;12(6):501–3.
123. Stow PJ, McLeod ME, Burrows FA, et al. Anterior fontanelle pressure responses to tracheal intubation in the awake and anaesthetized infant. Br J Anaesth. 1986;60:167–70.
124. Millar C, Bissonnette B. Awake intubation increases intracranial pressure without affecting cerebral blood flow velocity in infants. Can J Anaesth. 1994;41:281–7.
125. Hassid S, et al. Randomized controlled trial of sevoflurane for intubation in neonates. Paediatr Anaesth. 2007;17(11):1053–8.
126. Lerman J, Heard C, Steward DJ. Neonatal tracheal intubation: an imbroglio unresolved. Paediatr Anaesth. 2010;20:585–90.
127. Oei J, et al. Facilitation of neonatal nasotracheal intubation with premedication: a randomized controlled trial. J Paediatr Child Health. 2002;38(2):146–50.
128. Cook-Sather SD, et al. A comparison of awake versus paralyzed tracheal intubation for infants with pyloric stenosis. Anesth Analg. 1998;86(5):945–51.
129. Bhutada A, et al. Randomised controlled trial of thiopental for intubation in neonates. Arch Dis Child Fetal Neonatal Ed. 2000;82(1):F34–7.
130. Kinouchi K, et al. Duration of apnea in anesthetized infants and children required for desaturation of hemoglobin to 95 %. The influence of upper respiratory infection. Anesthesiology. 1992;77(6):1105–7.
131. Patel R, et al. Age and the onset of desaturation in apnoeic children. Can J Anaesth. 1994;41(9):771–4.
132. Xue F, et al. Children's development effecting blood oxygen desaturation following apnea. Chin Med J (Engl). 1995;108(6):434–7.
133. Xue FS, et al. Study of the safe threshold of apneic period in children during anesthesia induction. J Clin Anesth. 1996;8(7):568–74.
134. Jr Morrison JE, et al. Preoxygenation before laryngoscopy in children: how long is enough? Paediatr Anaesth. 1998;8(4):293–8.
135. Ho AM, et al. Airway difficulties caused by improperly applied cricoid pressure. J Emerg Med. 2001;20(1):29–31.
136. Francis S, Russell WC, Thompson JP. Complete airway obstruction in a ventilated patient after oesophageal dilatation. Br J Anaesth. 2002;89(3):517–9.
137. Landsman I. Cricoid pressure: indications and complications. Paediatr Anaesth. 2004;14(1):43–7.
138. Walker RW, Ravi R, Haylett K. Effect of cricoid force on airway calibre in children: a bronchoscopic assessment. Br J Anaesth. 2010;104(1):71–4.
139. Lerman J. On cricoid pressure: "may the force be with you". Anesth Analg. 2009;109(5):1363–6.
140. Smith KJ, et al. Cricoid pressure displaces the esophagus: an observational study using magnetic resonance imaging. Anesthesiology. 2003;99(1):60–4.
141. Rice MJ, et al. Cricoid pressure results in compression of the post-cricoid hypopharynx: the esophageal position is irrelevant. Anesth Analg. 2009;109(5):1546–52.
142. Warner MA, et al. Perioperative pulmonary aspiration in infants and children. Anesthesiology. 1999;90(1):66–71.
143. Brimacombe JR, Berry AM. Cricoid pressure. Can J Anaesth. 1997;44(4):414–25.
144. Benumof JL. Difficult laryngoscopy: obtaining the best view. Can J Anaesth. 1994;41(5 Pt 1):361–5.
145. Oh J, Lim T, Chee Y, et al. Videographic analysis of glottic view with increasing cricoid pressure force. Ann Emerg Med. 2013;61:407–13.
146. Ovassapian A, Salem MR. Sellick's maneuver: to do or not do. Anesth Analg. 2009;109(5):1360–2.
147. Vanner RG, Asai T. Safe use of cricoid pressure. Anaesthesia. 1999;54(1):1–3.
148. Weiss M, Gerber A. Rapid sequence induction in children—it's not a matter of time! Or is it? Paediatr Anaesth. 2008;18(10):980.
149. Bordes M, Cros AM. Inhalation induction with sevoflurane in paediatrics: what is new? Ann Fr Anesth Reanim. 2006; 25(4):413–6.
150. Westrin P, Jonmarker C, Werner O. Thiopental requirements for induction of anesthesia in neonates and infants one to six months of age. Anesthesiology. 1989;71:344–6.
151. Tibballs J, Malbezin S. Cardiovascular responses to induction of anaesthesia with thiopentone and suxamethonium in infants and children. Anaesth Intensive Care. 1988;16(3):278–84.
152. Bach V, et al. A randomized comparison between midazolam and thiopental for elective cesarean section anesthesia: III. Placental transfer and elimination in neonates. Anesth Analg. 1989;68(3):238–42.
153. Schrum SF, et al. Comparison of propofol and thiopental for rapid anesthesia induction in infants. Anesth Analg. 1994;78(3):482–5.
154. Dubois MC, et al. Anesthesia in the management of pyloric stenosis. Evaluation of the combination of propofol-halogenated anesthetics. Ann Fr Anesth Reanim. 1993;12(6):566–70.
155. Veyckemans F. Propofol for intubation of the newborn? Paediatr Anaesth. 2001;11(5):630–1.

156. Welzing L, et al. Propofol as an induction agent for endotracheal intubation can cause significant arterial hypotension in preterm neonates. Paediatr Anaesth. 2010;20(7):605–11.
157. Lerman J, et al. The pharmacology of sevoflurane in infants and children. Anesthesiology. 1994;80(4):814–24.
158. Taylor RH, Lerman J. Minimum alveolar concentration of desflurane and hemodynamic responses in neonates, infants, and children. Anesthesiology. 1991;75:975–9.
159. Picard P, Tramer MR. Prevention of pain on injection with propofol: a quantitative systematic review. Anesth Analg. 2000;90:963–9.
160. Jalota L, Kalira V, George E, et al. Prevention of pain on injection of propofol: systematic review and meta-analysis. BMJ. 2011;342:d1110.
161. Beh T, Splinter W, Kim J. In children, nitrous oxide decreases pain on injection of propofol mixed with lidocaine. Can J Anaesth. 2002;49:1061–3.
162. Rawicz M, Brandom BW, Wolf A. The place of suxamethonium in pediatric anesthesia. Paediatr Anaesth. 2009;19(6):561–70.
163. Meakin G, Walker RW, Dearlove OR. Myotonic and neuromuscular blocking effects of increased doses of suxamethonium in infants and children. Br J Anaesth. 1990;65(6):816–8.
164. Khammash H, et al. Surfactant therapy in full-term neonates with severe respiratory failure. Pediatrics. 1993;92(1):135–9.
165. Lemyre B, Cheng R, Gaboury I. Atropine, fentanyl and succinylcholine for non-urgent intubations in newborns. Arch Dis Child Fetal Neonatal Ed. 2009;94(6):F439–42.
166. Cheng CA, Aun CS, Gin T. Comparison of rocuronium and suxamethonium for rapid tracheal intubation in children. Paediatr Anaesth. 2002;12(2):140–5.
167. Rapp HJ, Altenmueller CA, Waschke C. Neuromuscular recovery following rocuronium bromide single dose in infants. Pediatr Anaesth. 2004;14:329–35.
168. Maruyama K, et al. Can intravenous atropine prevent bradycardia and hypotension during induction of total intravenous anesthesia with propofol and remifentanil? J Anesth. 2010;24(2):293–6.
169. Taha S, Siddik-Sayyid S, Alameddine M, et al. Propofol is superior to thiopental for intubation without muscle relaxants. Can J Anaesth. 2005;52:249–53.
170. Barker P, Langton JA, Wilson IG, Smith G. Movements of the vocal cords on induction of anaesthesia with thiopentone or propofol. Br J Anaesth. 1992;69:23–5.
171. Ghanta S, et al. Propofol compared with the morphine, atropine, and suxamethonium regimen as induction agents for neonatal endotracheal intubation: a randomized, controlled trial. Pediatrics. 2007;119(6):e1248–55.
172. Constant I, Seeman R, Murat I. Sevoflurane and epileptiform EEG changes. Paediatr Anaesth. 2005;15:266–74.
173. Vakkuri A, et al. Sevoflurane mask induction of anaesthesia is associated with epileptiform EEG in children. Acta Anaesthesiol Scand. 2001;45(7):805–11.
174. Yli-Hankala A, et al. Epileptiform electroencephalogram during mask induction of anesthesia with sevoflurane. Anesthesiology. 1999;91(6):1596–603.
175. Hsieh SW, Lan KM, Luk HN, Jawan B. Postoperative seizures after sevoflurane anesthesia in a neonate. Acta Anaesthesiol Scand. 2004;48:662.
176. Pilge S, Jordan D, Kochs EF, Schnieder G. Sevoflurane-induced epileptiform electroencephalographic activity and generalized tonic-clonic seizures in a volunteer study. Anesthesiology. 2013;119:447.
177. Wappler F, et al. Inhalational induction of anaesthesia with 8 % sevoflurane in children: conditions for endotracheal intubation and side-effects. Eur J Anaesthesiol. 2003;20(7):548–54.
178. Politis GD, et al. Factors associated with successful tracheal intubation of children with sevoflurane and no muscle relaxant. Anesth Analg. 2002;95(3):615–20. table of contents.
179. Meier S, et al. The effect of chin lift, jaw thrust, and continuous positive airway pressure on the size of the glottic opening and on stridor score in anesthetized, spontaneously breathing children. Anesth Analg. 2002;94(3):494–9. table of contents.
180. Lerman J, et al. Propofol for tracheal intubation in children anesthetized with sevoflurane: a dose-response study. Paediatr Anaesth. 2009;19(3):218–24.
181. Lago P, et al. Pain management in the neonatal intensive care unit: a national survey in Italy. Paediatr Anaesth. 2005;15(11):925–31.
182. Saarenmaa E, Neuvonen PJ, Fellman V. Gestational age and birth weight effects on plasma clearance of fentanyl in newborn infants. Pediatrics. 2000;136:767–70.
183. Collins C, et al. Fentanyl pharmacokinetics and hemodynamic effects in preterm infants during ligation of patent ductus arteriosus. Anesth Analg. 1985;64(11):1078–80.
184. Koehntop DE, et al. Pharmacokinetics of fentanyl in neonates. Anesth Analg. 1986;65(3):227–32.
185. Dempsey EM, et al. Facilitation of neonatal endotracheal intubation with mivacurium and fentanyl in the neonatal intensive care unit. Arch Dis Child Fetal Neonatal Ed. 2006;91(4):F279–82.
186. Hamon I, et al. Effects of fentanyl administration on general and cerebral haemodynamics in sick newborn infants. Acta Paediatr. 1996;85(3):361–5.
187. Davis PJ, et al. Pharmacodynamics and pharmacokinetics of high-dose sufentanil in infants and children undergoing cardiac surgery. Anesth Analg. 1987;66(3):203–8.
188. Greeley WJ, de Bruijn NP. Changes in sufentanil pharmacokinetics within the neonatal period. Anesth Analg. 1988; 67(1):86–90.
189. Moore RA, et al. Hemodynamic and anesthetic effects of sufentanil as the sole anesthetic for pediatric cardiovascular surgery. Anesthesiology. 1985;62(6):725–31.
190. Xue FS, et al. Different small-dose sufentanil blunting cardiovascular responses to laryngoscopy and intubation in children: a randomized, double-blind comparison. Br J Anaesth. 2008;100(5):717–23.
191. Soulard A, et al. Optimal dose of sufentanil in children for intubation after sevoflurane induction without neuromuscular block. Br J Anaesth. 2009;102(5):680–5.
192. Lerman J, Strong JA, LeDez KM, et al. Effects of age on the serum concentration of α_1-acid glycoprotein and the binding of lidocaine in pediatric patients. Clin Pharm Ther. 1989;46:219–22.
193. Marlow N, et al. Alfentanil pharmacokinetics in preterm infants. Arch Dis Child. 1990;65(4):349–51.
194. Davis PJ, et al. Pharmacokinetics of alfentanil in newborn premature infants and older children. Dev Pharmacol Ther. 1989; 13(1):21–7.
195. Pathak D, et al. Effects of alfentanil and lidocaine on the hemodynamic responses to laryngoscopy and tracheal intubation. J Clin Anesth. 1990;2(2):81–5.
196. Martineau RJ, et al. Alfentanil controls the haemodynamic response during rapid-sequence induction of anaesthesia. Can J Anaesth. 1990;37(7):755–61.
197. Kwak HJ, et al. Optimal bolus dose of alfentanil for successful tracheal intubation during sevoflurane induction with and without nitrous oxide in children. Br J Anaesth. 2010;104(5):628–32.
198. McConaghy P, Bunting HE. Assessment of intubating conditions in children after induction with propofol and varying doses of alfentanil. Br J Anaesth. 1994;73(5):596–9.
199. Steyn MP, et al. Tracheal intubation without neuromuscular block in children. Br J Anaesth. 1994;72(4):403–6.
200. Pokela ML, et al. Alfentanil-induced rigidity in newborn infants. Anesth Analg. 1992;75(2):252–7.
201. Allegaert K, Thewissen L, van den Anker JN. Remifentanil in neonates: a promising compound in search of its indications? Pediatr Neonatol. 2012;53:387–8.

202. Penido MG, Garra R, Sammartino M, et al. Remifentanil in neonatal intensive care and anaesthesia practice. Acta Paediatr. 2010;99:1454–63.
203. Choong K, et al. Remifentanil for endotracheal intubation in neonates: a randomised controlled trial. Arch Dis Child Fetal Neonatal Ed. 2010;95(2):F80–4.
204. Min SK, et al. The optimal dose of remifentanil for intubation during sevoflurane induction without neuromuscular blockade in children. Anaesthesia. 2007;62(5):446–50.
205. Crawford MW, Hayes J, Tan JM. Dose-response of remifentanil for tracheal intubation in infants. Anesth Analg. 2005;100(6):1599–604.
206. Hume-Smith H, et al. The effect of age on the dose of remifentanil for tracheal intubation in infants and children. Paediatr Anaesth. 2010;20(1):19–27.
207. He L, et al. Effects of different doses of remifentanil on the end-tidal concentration of sevoflurane required for tracheal intubation in children. Anaesthesia. 2009;64(8):850–5.
208. Morton NS. Tracheal intubation without neuromuscular blocking drugs in children. Paediatr Anaesth. 2009;19(3):199–201.
209. Meretoja OA. Neuromuscular block and current treatment strategies for its reversal in children. Paediatr Anaesth. 2010;20(7):591–604.
210. Brandom BW, Fine GF. Neuromuscular blocking drugs in pediatric anesthesia. Anesthesiol Clin North America. 2002;20(1):45–58.
211. Eikermann M, et al. Optimal rocuronium dose for intubation during inhalation induction with sevoflurane in children. Br J Anaesth. 2002;89(2):277–81.
212. Fuchs-Buder T, Tassonyi E. Intubating conditions and time course of rocuronium-induced neuromuscular block in children. Br J Anaesth. 1996;77(3):335–8.
213. McCluskey A, Meakin G. Dose-response and minimum time to satisfactory intubation conditions after mivacurium in children. Anaesthesia. 1996;51(5):438–41.
214. Roberts KD, et al. Premedication for nonemergent neonatal intubations: a randomized, controlled trial comparing atropine and fentanyl to atropine, fentanyl, and mivacurium. Pediatrics. 2006;118(4):1583–91.
215. Meakin GH. Role of muscle relaxants in pediatric anesthesia. Curr Opin Anaesthesiol. 2007;20(3):227–31.
216. Whittaker M. Plasma cholinesterase variants and the anaesthetist. Anaesthesia. 1980;35(2):174–97.
217. Doucet O, et al. Prolonged neuromuscular blockade with mivacurium in a newborn. Ann Fr Anesth Reanim. 1998;17(7):725–7.
218. Dubois MC, et al. Comparison of three techniques for induction of anaesthesia with sevoflurane in children. Paediatr Anaesth. 1999;9(1):19–23.
219. Fitzgerald M. The development of nociceptive circuits. Nat Rev Neurosci. 2005;6(7):507–20.
220. Fujinaga M, et al. Nitrous oxide lacks the antinociceptive effect on the tail flick test in newborn rats. Anesth Analg. 2000;91(1):6–10.
221. Kaisti KK, et al. Effects of sevoflurane, propofol, and adjunct nitrous oxide on regional cerebral blood flow, oxygen consumption, and blood volume in humans. Anesthesiology. 2003;99(3):603–13.
222. Weimann J. Toxicity of nitrous oxide. Best Pract Res Clin Anaesthesiol. 2003;17(1):47–61.
223. Xue FS, et al. The circulatory responses to tracheal intubation in children: a comparison of the oral and nasal routes. Anaesthesia. 2007;62(3):220–6.
224. Spence K, Barr P. Nasal versus oral intubation for mechanical ventilation of newborn infants. Cochrane Database Syst Rev 1999 (2): Art No. CD000948. (updated 2009).
225. Kuhns LR, Poznanski AK. Endotrachel tube position in the infant. J Pediatr. 1971;78:991–6.
226. Todres ID, deBros F, Kramer SS, et al. Endotracheal tube displacement in the newborn infant. J Pediatr. 1976;89:126–7.
227. Rost JR, Frush DP, Auten RL. Effect of neck position on endotracheal tube location in low birth weight infants. Pediatr Pulmonol. 1999;27:199–202.
228. Olufolabi AJ, Charlton GA, Spargo PM. Effect of head posture on tracheal tube position in children. Anaesthesia. 2004;59(11):1069–72.
229. von Ungern-Sternberg BS, et al. Desflurane but not sevoflurane impairs airway and respiratory tissue mechanics in children with susceptible airways. Anesthesiology. 2008;108(2):216–24.
230. Sale SM, et al. Prospective comparison of sevoflurane and desflurane in formerly premature infants undergoing inguinal herniotomy. Br J Anaesth. 2006;96(6):774–8.
231. Lerman J, Johr M. Inhalational anesthesia vs total intravenous anesthesia (TIVA) for pediatric anesthesia. Paediatr Anaesth. 2009;19(5):521–34.
232. Hannallah RS, et al. Propofol: effective dose and induction characteristics in unpremedicated children. Anesthesiology. 1991;74(2):217–9.
233. Fudickar A, Bein B. Propofol infusion syndrome: update of clinical manifestation and pathophysiology. Minerva Anestesiol. 2009;75(5):339–44.
234. Laquay N, et al. [Propofol infusion syndrome]. Ann Fr Anesth Reanim. 2010;29(5):377–86.
235. Diedrich DA, Brown DR. Analytic reviews: propofol infusion syndrome in the ICU. J Intensive Care Med. 2011;26:59–72.
236. Sammartino M, et al. Propofol overdose in a preterm baby: may propofol infusion syndrome arise in two hours? Paediatr Anaesth. 2010;20:973–4.
237. Anand KJ. Consensus statement for the prevention and management of pain in the newborn. Arch Pediatr Adolesc Med. 2001;155(2):173–80.
238. Anand KJ. Clinical importance of pain and stress in preterm neonates. Biol Neonate. 1998;73(1):1–9.
239. Anand KJ, Hickey PR. Pain and its effects in the human neonate and fetus. N Engl J Med. 1987;317(21):1321–9.
240. Anand KJ, Sippell WG, Aynsley-Green A. Pain, anaesthesia, and babies. Lancet. 1987;2(8569):1210.
241. Taddio A, et al. Effect of neonatal circumcision on pain responses during vaccination in boys. Lancet. 1995;345(8945):291–2.
242. Peters JW, et al. Does neonatal surgery lead to increased pain sensitivity in later childhood? Pain. 2005;114(3):444–54.
243. Reynolds ML, Fitzgerald M. Long-term sensory hyperinnervation following neonatal skin wounds. J Comp Neurol. 1995; 358(4):487–98.
244. Hohmeister J, et al. Cerebral processing of pain in school-aged children with neonatal nociceptive input: an exploratory fMRI study. Pain. 2010;150(2):257–67.
245. Anand KJ, et al. Effects of morphine analgesia in ventilated preterm neonates: primary outcomes from the NEOPAIN randomised trial. Lancet. 2004;363(9422):1673–82.
246. Jablonka DH, Davis PJ. Opioids in pediatric anesthesia. Anesthesiol Clin North America. 2005;23(4):621–34. viii.
247. Meuldermans WE, Hurkmans RM, Heykants JJ. Plasma protein binding and distribution of fentanyl, sufentanil, alfentanil and lofentanil in blood. Arch Int Pharmacodyn Ther. 1982;257(1):4–19.
248. Meistelman C, et al. Effects of age on plasma protein binding of sufentanil. Anesthesiology. 1990;72(3):470–3.
249. Tateishi T, et al. Identification of human liver cytochrome P-450 3A4 as the enzyme responsible for fentanyl and sufentanil N-dealkylation. Anesth Analg. 1996;82(1):167–72.
250. Lacroix D, et al. Expression of CYP3A in the human liver-evidence that the shift between CYP3A7 and CYP3A4 occurs immediately after birth. Eur J Biochem. 1997;247(2):625–34.
251. Kearns GL, et al. Developmental pharmacology–drug disposition, action, and therapy in infants and children. N Engl J Med. 2003;349(12):1157–67.

252. Zhou SF, Liu JP, Chowbay B. Polymorphism of human cytochrome P450 enzymes and its clinical impact. Drug Metab Rev. 2009;41(2):89–295.
253. Glenski JA, et al. Comparison of the hemodynamic and echocardiographic effects of sufentanil, fentanyl, isoflurane, and halothane for pediatric cardiovascular surgery. J Cardiothorac Anesth. 1988;2(2):147–55.
254. Egan TD, et al. The pharmacokinetics of the new short-acting opioid remifentanil (GI87084B) in healthy adult male volunteers. Anesthesiology. 1993;79(5):881–92.
255. Davis PJ, Cladis FP. The use of ultra-short-acting opioids in paediatric anaesthesia: the role of remifentanil. Clin Pharmacokinet. 2005;44(8):787–96.
256. Wee LH, et al. Remifentanil infusion for major abdominal surgery in small infants. Paediatr Anaesth. 1999;9(5):415–8.
257. Tirel O, et al. Effect of remifentanil with and without atropine on heart rate variability and RR interval in children. Anaesthesia. 2005;60(10):982–9.
258. Ross AK, et al. Pharmacokinetics of remifentanil in anesthetized pediatric patients undergoing elective surgery or diagnostic procedures. Anesth Analog. 2001;93(6):1393–401. table of contents.
259. Sadleir PHM, Clarke RC, Bunning DL, et al. Anaphylaxis to neuromuscular blocking drugs: incidence and cross-reactivity in Western Australia from 2002 to 2011. Br J Anaesth. 2013; 110:981–7.
260. Nel L, Eren E. Peri-operative anaphylaxis. Br J Clin Pharmacol. 2011;71:647–58.
261. Mertes PM, Alla F, Tréchot P, et al. Anaphylaxis during anesthesia in France: an 8-year national survey. J Allergy Clin Immunol. 2011;128:366–73.
262. Weber F. Evidence for the need for anaesthesia in the neonate. Best Pract Res Clin Anaesthesiol. 2010;24:475–84.
263. Hermann C, et al. Long-term alteration of pain sensitivity in school-aged children with early pain experiences. Pain. 2006;125(3): 278–85.

Neonatal Airway Management

5

Paul A. Stricker, John E. Fiadjoe, and Ronald S. Litman

Expertise in neonatal airway management requires an understanding of early human anatomical development as well as a set of clinical skills to provide safe mask ventilation and tracheal intubation in this extremely small-sized population of patients. Since neonatal airway experiences are not a daily occurrence in most anesthesiology training programs, this skill set is acquired only after repeated patient encounters over a prolonged period of time that may span years or decades. In this chapter, we review the foundations upon which management of the neonatal airway is based. The reader should note that these foundations are largely based on our collective experience, which is complemented by case reports and case series that reflect the experience of others as there is a dearth of prospective studies on airway management in the neonate. The chapter is divided into three sections: (1) anatomy and physiology of the neonatal upper airway, (2) techniques for standard neonatal airway management, and (3) techniques for managing the anatomically abnormal neonatal airway.

Neonatal Upper Airway Anatomy

Management of the neonatal airway is primarily governed by the unique anatomical features of the upper airway at this early age. The occipital portion of the neonatal skull is relatively larger than that of older infants and children (neurocranium-to-face size ratio is 8:1 in neonates, 6:1 in 2-year-olds, and 4:1 in 5-year-olds [1, 2]). This anatomical feature provides a natural state of cervical flexion that facilitates direct laryngoscopy in the supine child [3] but may predispose to upper airway obstruction during spontaneous respiration and mask ventilation [4]. Many neonatal and pediatric textbooks have emphasized the importance of obligate nasal breathing in neonates, as a means to facilitate and coordinate the suck-swallow-breathing mechanism. Although neonates born with congenital choanal atresia occasionally develop life-threatening upper airway obstruction [5], healthy neonates are able to coordinate both mouth and nasal breathing [6].

A major anatomical consideration in the management of the neonatal airway stems from the relatively cephalad position of the larynx (i.e., close proximity of the uvula and epiglottis) that facilitates the swallowing-breathing mechanism in neonates. The larynx descends from the C2–C3 level to C4–C5 level by 3 years of age, increasing the distance between the larynx and other facial structures such as the mandible [7]. The tip of the epiglottis also descends throughout childhood from C2 to C3 [8]. This more cephalad position of the larynx in neonates enables a direct view of the glottic aperture with a straight rather than curved laryngoscope blade.

The high compliance of the neonatal chest wall (due to incomplete ossification of the ribs and weak intercostal muscles) prevents the passive outward recoil that contributes to maintenance of functional residual capacity (FRC) in older children. In contrast, neonates preserve FRC volumes using their laryngeal adductor muscles as expiratory "valves" to restrict exhalation and maintain positive end-expiratory pressure in a process referred to as "laryngeal braking" [9–11].

Neonatal Upper Airway Reflexes

Neonatal upper airway reflexes protect against inhalation of foreign substances into the lower respiratory tract. Although these reflexes have been studied in both the awake and sedated states, much less is known about their effects at deeper levels of anesthetic-induced unconsciousness.

In children beyond early infancy, mechanisms that protect against the ingestion of foreign materials into the lower

P.A. Stricker, MD • J.E. Fiadjoe, MD
University of Pennsylvania School of Medicine,
The Children's Hospital of Pennsylvania, Philadelphia, PA USA

R.S. Litman, DO (✉)
Department of Anesthesiology and Critical Care,
University of Pennsylvania School of Medicine,
34th St & Civic Center Blvd., Philadelphia, PA 19104, USA
e-mail: litmanr@email.chop.edu

J. Lerman (ed.), *Neonatal Anesthesia*, DOI 10.1007/978-1-4419-6041-2_5,

respiratory tract include swallowing and coughing [12]. Neonates and young infants, however, primarily manifest this protection as central apnea (with bradycardia), upper airway obstruction [13], laryngospasm, and arousal [14]. These laryngeal chemoreflexes mature rapidly during early development [15]. In addition, these adaptive responses are more prominent in direct relationship to a younger gestational age [13, 16–21] and may play a role in the etiology of sudden infant death syndrome (SIDS) [22]. The apneic reflex (with bradycardia) may be prolonged in the presence of sedative or anesthetic agents [23–25], hypoxemia [26, 27], anemia [28], and RSV infection [29, 30]. The administration of central stimulants such as theophylline may abbreviate this reflex [24].

Neonatal Airway Management

Routine airway management for neonates presents challenges that are not confronted in older children. Neonates usually require emergency surgeries; thus the issues that pertain to the urgent nature of the surgery add to the difficulties and risks. In this section, we consider the unique aspects of neonatal airway management that are encountered during the preanesthetic assessment and preparation and routine airway management techniques.

Preanesthetic Assessment

Preanesthetic assessment of the neonate includes a thorough review of previous airway management episodes. If tracheal intubation has been performed previously, the involved providers should be queried and the medical records reviewed to clarify any difficulties that were encountered. For all neonates, the underlying diagnoses and conditions should be reviewed with specific attention to the upper and lower airways, since the airway management may have to be tailored accordingly. Some conditions that lack direct airway involvement may indirectly impact on the airway. For example, the neonate with a giant omphalocele may rapidly desaturate during induction of anesthesia due to pulmonary hypoplasia and a reduced FRC. Similarly, neonates with congenital diaphragmatic hernia require special attention to limit the peak inspiratory pressures during induction of anesthesia to prevent intestinal insufflation during mask ventilation and a pneumothorax after tracheal intubation.

Physical examination of the airway should focus on the presence of anatomical abnormalities that may hinder face mask ventilation or direct laryngoscopy. Physical findings such as micrognathia should alert the anesthesiologist to prepare appropriate techniques for a difficult airway. Diagnosing micrognathia in neonates may be tricky; careful examination of the facial profile with the neonate in the neutral position may reveal a mandible that is recessed in relation to the maxilla.

Preoperative Preparation

All equipment that may be required to manage the airway should be prepared before the infant arrives in the operating room or before anesthesia is induced for procedures in the neonatal intensive care unit. Induction agents and emergency medications (as appropriate) should be prepared in unit doses to reduce drug errors should an urgent intraoperative situation ensue. The functionality of the selected laryngoscope handle and blade together with backup equipment should be verified before induction of anesthesia. A styleted tracheal tube for the anticipated tube size as well as one that is one-half size smaller and larger should be available, as well as appropriately sized oral airways for managing upper airway obstruction. Because of its important role as a ventilation rescue device, a laryngeal mask should also be immediately available. If difficulty with face mask ventilation or tracheal intubation is anticipated, additional equipment (vide infra) and personnel should be available.

Induction of Anesthesia

Face Mask Ventilation

The neonate should be positioned supine to facilitate mask ventilation and direct laryngoscopy. The selected mask size and fit should be checked before induction of anesthesia. A properly sized mask covers the nose and mouth without overlying the eyes or extending beyond the chin. Face masks designed to minimize dead space may be advantageous in the neonatal population. The Rendall-Baker face mask has been mostly replaced by the cuffed (cushioned), low-profile face mask, which seals against air leaks around the mouth and nose. After loss of consciousness, upper airway obstruction is relieved primarily by chin lift, which is easily accomplished by placing the body of the left-hand middle finger across the bony portion of the chin, and extending the neck (Fig. 5.1). However, in anesthetized neonates, this maneuver closes the mouth, which may obstruct the upper airway, a problem often incompletely relieved by simply extending the neck. Furthermore, digital pressure is often inadvertently applied to the submental triangle, which may further obstruct the upper airway. An essential maneuver to establish a patent airway in neonates and young infants is temporomandibular joint subluxation, which is accomplished by placing the operator's fifth digit(s) in the retromandibular notch, at the apex of the ascending ramus of the mandible, immediately below the external auditory canal and behind the pinna. The condyles are pulled in an upward direction, toward the frontal hairline (i.e., a full "jaw thrust") [31]. This maneuver anteriorly translocates the jaw as well as rotates the temporomandibular joint, thereby opening the mouth and pulling the tongue off the posterior pharyngeal wall. The face mask is

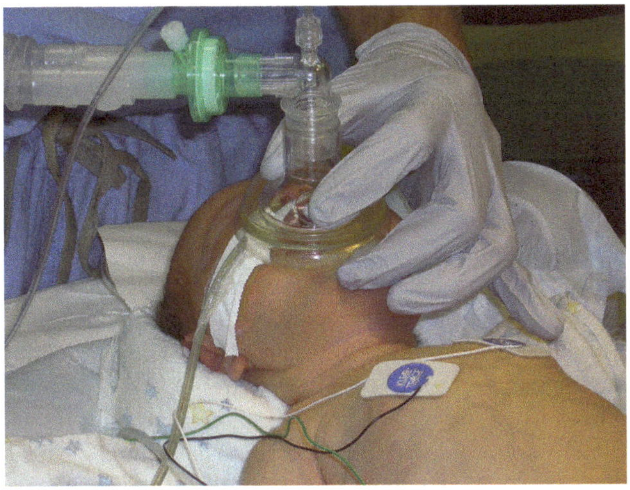

Fig. 5.1 When mask ventilating a small infant, the middle finger rests on the mandible to provide chin lift without compression of soft tissues in the submental triangle

held on the face using the operator's thumbs. A far less effective "jaw-thrust maneuver" that is widely taught involves applying digital pressure to the angle of the mandible. In this maneuver, the mandible is translocated anteriorly, but the temporomandibular joint does not rotate. This partially relieves the airway obstruction. Given the lack of familiarity with the proper application of the full "jaw thrust," many prefer yet another maneuver, to insert an oral airway device. This latter technique is not uniformly effective as too large an oral airway may push the epiglottis into the glottic opening and too small an airway may push the tongue into the glottic opening. Furthermore, in the neonate with a difficult airway, the oral airway may be more difficult to seat properly. Hence, it is crucial to understand how to optimize the upper airway in the neonate by manipulating the temporomandibular joint rather than relying on oral airways.

In most neonates, effective face mask ventilation can be accomplished at peak inspiratory pressures of <15 cm H_2O and rates of 20–40 breaths per minute. Maintaining positive end-expiratory pressure during ventilation (5–10 cm H_2O) promotes alveolar patency and improves gas exchange. Occasionally, an alveolar recruitment maneuver is required (see below).

Laryngeal Mask Airways and Supraglottic Devices

Although tracheal intubation remains the standard of care for intraoperative airway management in emergency surgery, some practitioners prefer a supraglottic device for elective surgery in neonates [32]. Initial studies and clinical experience with the Classic Laryngeal Mask Airways (LMAs) in neonates demonstrated a greater failure rate during insertion and decreased efficacy with the size 1 LMA compared with larger size airways in older children [33]. This was attributed to a cuff design flaw that failed to account for the unique anatomy of the neonatal airway. However, clinical experience suggests that placing an LMA is no more difficult in this age group than older children, although these small LMAs may be dislodged easily. Therefore, the capnogram must be observed continuously.

LMAs may offer advantages over tracheal intubation during airway resuscitation outside of the operating room because the LMA is simple to insert, requires technical skills that are easily acquired, and is associated with a high success rate, even in the hands of inexperienced operators [34]. Recent studies have demonstrated that the failure rates for tracheal intubation by resident pediatricians in the delivery room is substantial [35–38]. In one study, 87 % of residents reported their level of confidence with tracheal intubation as good or excellent after the completion of residency training, despite their failure to satisfy objective standards for technical competence [38]. Limited evidence to date suggests that the LMA is effective in neonatal resuscitation in infants >34 weeks and possibly comparable to tracheal intubation, although the LMA has not been compared with bag-mask ventilation [39, 40]. It remains to be established whether the LMA or other supraglottic airway should be used for primary airway management in neonatal resuscitation [41]. However, its use has been recommended as a secondary tool in near-term and term neonates who have failed resuscitation with bag-mask ventilation or tracheal intubation [42].

The ProSeal LMA is a laryngeal mask airway with a wider laryngeal bowl and a channel for gastric drain tube insertion. This device is now available in a size 1 and has been studied in neonates and infants weighing 2–5 kg [43, 44]. The initial results suggest that in addition to the 100 % success rate inserting the ProSeal LMA [43, 44], the quality of the initial airway, the effectiveness of the seal, and the maximum tidal volume were significantly better than with the cLMA [43, 44].

Laryngeal tube suction II (LTS II; VBM Medizintechnik, Sulz, Germany) is another supraglottic airway device available in a size suitable for use in neonates. It is inserted blindly in a manner similar to the LMA. The LTS II has an esophageal and a pharyngeal cuff that are interconnected as well as a channel for placement of a gastric drain tube. Ventilation is delivered through multiple holes in the tube that are positioned between these two cuffs. While a case series describing the utility of this device in 10 neonates and infants has been published [32], larger prospective trials evaluating its safety or efficacy in neonates have not yet been conducted.

The LMA can also be utilized as a valuable adjunct for tracheal tube placement in neonates with difficult airways. This is reviewed in the following sections of the chapter.

Laryngoscopy and Orotracheal Intubation

Indications for tracheal intubation are traditionally determined by the surgical procedure, duration of the surgery, risk of aspiration of gastric contents, and pulmonary function. In anesthetized neonates, airway maintenance with a face mask is less desirable because of the high dead space-to-tidal volume ratio and concerns for the development of atelectasis. As a general rule, tracheal intubation is indicated for open cavity procedures of the abdomen or chest, intracranial procedures, and in cases where control of arterial PCO_2 is required. It is also indicated when the anesthesiologist has limited access to the airway during surgeries such as those involving the head and neck and when positions other than supine are required. Tracheal intubation and mechanical ventilation are also useful in neonates to avoid atelectasis that could develop during prolonged anesthesia with spontaneous ventilation.

The "sniffing position" is classically described as the optimal head position to facilitate direct laryngoscopy and tracheal intubation. In adults, a number of recent publications suggested that the sniffing position offers no advantage over simple head extension [45, 46]. In children, there is better alignment of pharyngeal structures with simple neck extension as compared with the "sniffing position." [47] Because of the relatively large occiput, the neonate may naturally be in the sniffing position without active head flexion. The large occiput of the neonate, when placed on a pillow, flexes the head and, in some extreme cases, may contribute to airway obstruction. Comparative trials to determine the optimal position for laryngoscopy and intubation in neonates have not been performed.

Direct laryngoscopy is the most common method of achieving tracheal intubation in neonates. Traditionally, the Miller blade has been favored in this age group because of anatomical considerations including a relatively cephalad larynx and to facilitate alignment of the oral and laryngeal axes [3], although there is no evidence that the straight blade provides either an improved view or easier tracheal intubation than the curved blade in neonates [48–50]. The Miller blade offers greater control and displacement of the base of the tongue, particularly for difficult intubations. The smaller size and reduced profile of the Miller blade (alternatively, the Wisconsin or Wis-Hipple size 0 blade) may also give the operator more room to pass the tracheal tube through the mouth and pharynx into the trachea rather than down the visual path under the blade. When laryngoscopy is performed with a straight blade, the blade is usually inserted into the mouth in the midline after sweeping the tongue to the left. However, when faced with a difficult intubation, this blade is preferably introduced at the right commissure of the lips, not in the midline, an approach known as the paraglossal approach [51, 52]. The blade follows the right alveolar groove until the tip reaches the epiglottis, at which point the epiglottis is lifted exposing the glottis. This approach yields a superior access to the glottis over the midline approach as the angle of the blade and the distance to the larynx are both reduced compared with the same variables that are associated with inserting the blade into the mouth in the midline.

Traditionally, the Miller is advanced to lift the epiglottis to expose the larynx. Some however use this blade in a manner analogous to the curved blade by advancing it into the vallecula to lift the tongue. If the glottis exposure is suboptimal after advancing the laryngoscope and positioning it, the laryngoscopist can externally manipulate the larynx to bring the glottis into view. A small amount of external, posterior pressure with or without lateral displacement often significantly improves laryngeal exposure and facilitates intubation. This practice should be a reflex maneuver for the pediatric anesthesiologist to improve the view of the glottis. In neonates, laryngeal manipulation can be performed using the operator's fifth digit of the left hand (Fig. 5.2).

In select circumstances outside of the obstetric delivery room, tracheal intubation may be performed in unmedicated neonates who might not tolerate the cardiovascular depressant effects of anesthetic or sedative drugs or whose airways are compromised or potentially difficult to secure. However, infants and neonates experience pain, and performing laryngoscopy without sedative premedication or general anesthesia has untoward cardiovascular (and behavioral) effects and should be avoided whenever possible [53–55]. Furthermore, the administration of anesthetic, sedative, and neuromuscular-

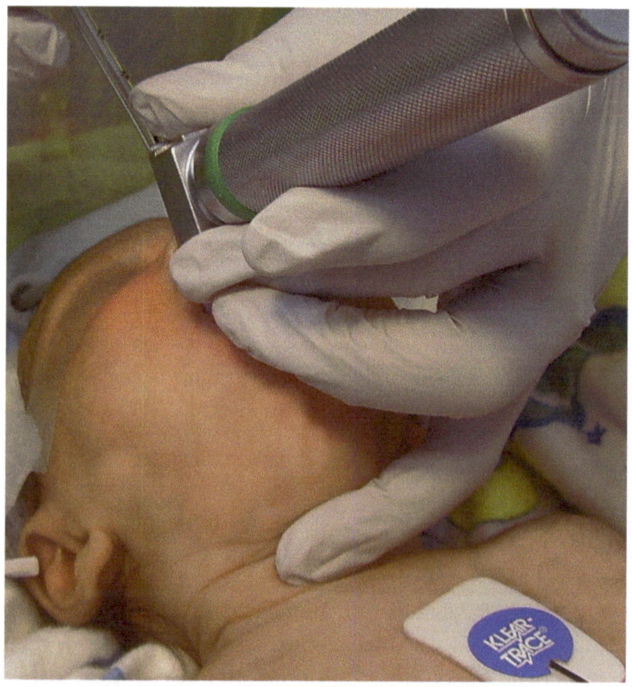

Fig. 5.2 Orotracheal intubation in the neonate is facilitated by using the fifth finger of the left hand, which provides posterior or lateral external displacement of the larynx

blocking drugs improves conditions for intubation and decreases the likelihood of trauma to the airway [56–59]. A consensus statement published by The International Evidence-Based Group for Neonatal Pain states "tracheal intubation without the use of analgesia or sedation should be performed only for urgent resuscitations in the delivery room or for life-threatening situations associated with the unavailability of intravenous access" [54]. In selected cases, such as when face mask ventilation or tracheal intubation is expected to be difficult, intubation may be performed after sedative premedication rather than general anesthesia. Various medication regimens have been evaluated for nonemergency tracheal intubation in the neonatal ICU [60–63], although most studies are seriously flawed precluding the determination of a preferred regimen [64].

Tracheal intubation in an unsedated critically ill neonate may be a lifesaving maneuver. Although it has been eschewed by many, if the need arises, it is important to know how to perform an "awake" intubation. This is not a technique that should be first attempted in a lifesaving situation. When planning an awake intubation, the operator should ensure that the stomach is empty (e.g., suction is readily available), and atropine 0.02 mg/kg IV and oxygen have been administered. In advance of the intubation, a styleted tracheal tube of the appropriate size (in a hockey stick configuration), laryngoscope handle and appropriate size blade, and suction should be available. An experienced assistant holds the infant's arms fully extended against the side of the head to prevent the head and upper torso from wiggling and the shoulders from lifting off the table during laryngoscopy. Once laryngoscopy begins, tracheal intubation should be completed within 10–12 s. The laryngoscope blade should be inserted into the mouth at the right commissure aiming the tip of the blade toward the midline in one fluid motion. The laryngoscope should be held in one hand and the tracheal tube in the other. As soon as the neonate gags as the blade is inserted, the epiglottis should be lifted and the tube passed between the vocal cords. When carbon dioxide is detected, 2–3 mg/kg IV propofol or other anesthetics may then be administered to attenuate any cardiovascular responses to laryngoscopy. The tracheal tube should then be taped and secured at an appropriate depth.

Nasotracheal Intubation

Nasotracheal intubation is more challenging to perform than orotracheal intubation, especially in neonates. Although no studies have specifically reported the sequelae after nasotracheal intubation in neonates, complications in older children include epistaxis, retropharyngeal perforation, sinusitis, bacteremia, and turbinate avulsion [65–70]. Nonetheless, this approach is preferred for neonates undergoing cardiac surgery, posterior fossa neurosurgery, and for prolonged intubation in the intensive care in many institutions. A topical vasoconstrictor such as 0.025 % oxymetazoline may be applied before intubation to prevent bleeding from the nasal mucosa. The dose of the vasoconstrictor should be carefully calculated as severe hypertension and reflex bradycardia progressing to cardiac arrest have been reported after inadvertent overdoses of phenylephrine [71–74] and oxymetazoline [75, 76]. Hence, these agents should be used judiciously in neonates. An alternative technique to minimize nasal bleeding is to telescope the tracheal tube into the flange end of a red rubber catheter and draw the lubricated catheter containing the tube through the nose [77].

Tracheal Tube Size Selection

A variety of methods exist for determining the expected uncuffed tracheal tube diameter in children, including formulas based on age and height. However, in neonates, the diameter of the tracheal tube is determined empirically, based on the neonate's weight. For neonates <1.5 kg, we use a size 2.5 mm ID uncuffed tube, for those between 1.6 and 3.5 kg, we use a size 3.0 mm ID uncuffed tube, and for those weighing >3.5 kg, a 3.5 mm ID uncuffed tube. In the latter part of the first year after birth, for infants weighing 5 kg or more, we use a 4.0 mm ID tube. The appropriate tube size for each neonate may need to be adjusted based on preexisting medical conditions (e.g., subglottic stenosis, Down syndrome) (Fig. 5.3a–c) and whether the tube is cuffed or uncuffed.

Uncuffed Versus Cuffed Tracheal Tubes

Uncuffed tracheal tubes have traditionally been used in neonates out of the concern that a cuffed tube may cause subglottic injury. However, modern cuffed tracheal tubes with high-volume, low-pressure cuffs have not been associated with an increased incidence of subglottic airway injury or an increased incidence of post-extubation stridor during general anesthesia in children and may reduce operating room pollution and anesthetic gas waste compared with uncuffed tubes [78, 79, 80]. No long-term studies with cuffed tubes have been published in neonates. However, one study in the pediatric intensive care unit reported no cases of post-extubation stridor or significant long-term sequelae when cuffed tracheal tubes were in place for up to 6 days, although only 21 infants were allocated cuffed tubes [81]. In a recent study with the Microcuff® tube in young children, 326 infants were studied with a 2.8 % incidence of stridor [79]. The number of neonates in the latter study was not reported as a distinct group. Recently, post-extubation stridor was reported in three neonates after the use of Microcuff® tubes, although the tubes that were used were NOT recommended for their ages [82]. *Readers should be cognizant of two additional issues regarding the Microcuff® tubes: 1. the 3.0 (not 3.5) mm ID Microcuff® tube is recommended for full-term neonates >3 kg up to 8 months of age, and 2. if the cuff of the Microcuff® tube is inflated, it is prudent to monitor the cuff pressure throughout the anesthetic to preclude excess cuff pressures, although the critical pressure that interrupts mucosal blood flow in the neonate is unknown.*

When a cuffed tube is used, the cuff inflation volume should be adjusted to achieve the desired leak pressure. The Microcuff® tracheal tube seals the airway at pressures that are less than traditional cuffed tubes. Accordingly, the time interval until the cuff pressure requires adjustment with the Microcuff® tube exceeds that with traditional polyvinylchloride tracheal tube [83]. Irrespective of the brand of tracheal tube used and whether nitrous oxide is used or not, it is prudent to either monitor the cuff pressure intermittently or deflate and reinflate the cuff periodically to preclude excessive cuff pressures and possible mucosal ischemia.

Cuffed tracheal tubes offer a number of theoretical and practical advantages over uncuffed tubes. Theoretical advantages include a better seal of the trachea from macroaspiration than uncuffed tubes (Fig. 5.3e), although the incidence of aspiration pneumonia with an uncuffed tube is exceedingly small and aspiration is known to occur even with cuffed tubes. In addition, they enable the use of small fresh gas flows (and associated economic advantages) and decrease operating room pollution, although fresh gas flows in North America are minimal with uncuffed tubes [80, 84]. Third, cuffed tracheal tubes reduce the number of laryngoscopies to achieve a proper size tube as well as reducing the associated morbidity from multiple tube changes, although the morbidity from reintubation is exceedingly small in experienced hands. Subglottic damage after intubation has been attributed, for the most part, to intubation with oversized tubes, prolonged intubation, the use of cuffed tubes, and head movement [104]. There are, nonetheless, at least two practical advantages of cuffed tubes. The first is to facilitate ventilation of lungs with reduced lung compliance such as in chronic lung disease. The second is for surgical procedures close to the airway, where these tubes limit the escape of oxygen-enriched gases thereby decreasing the risk of fires.

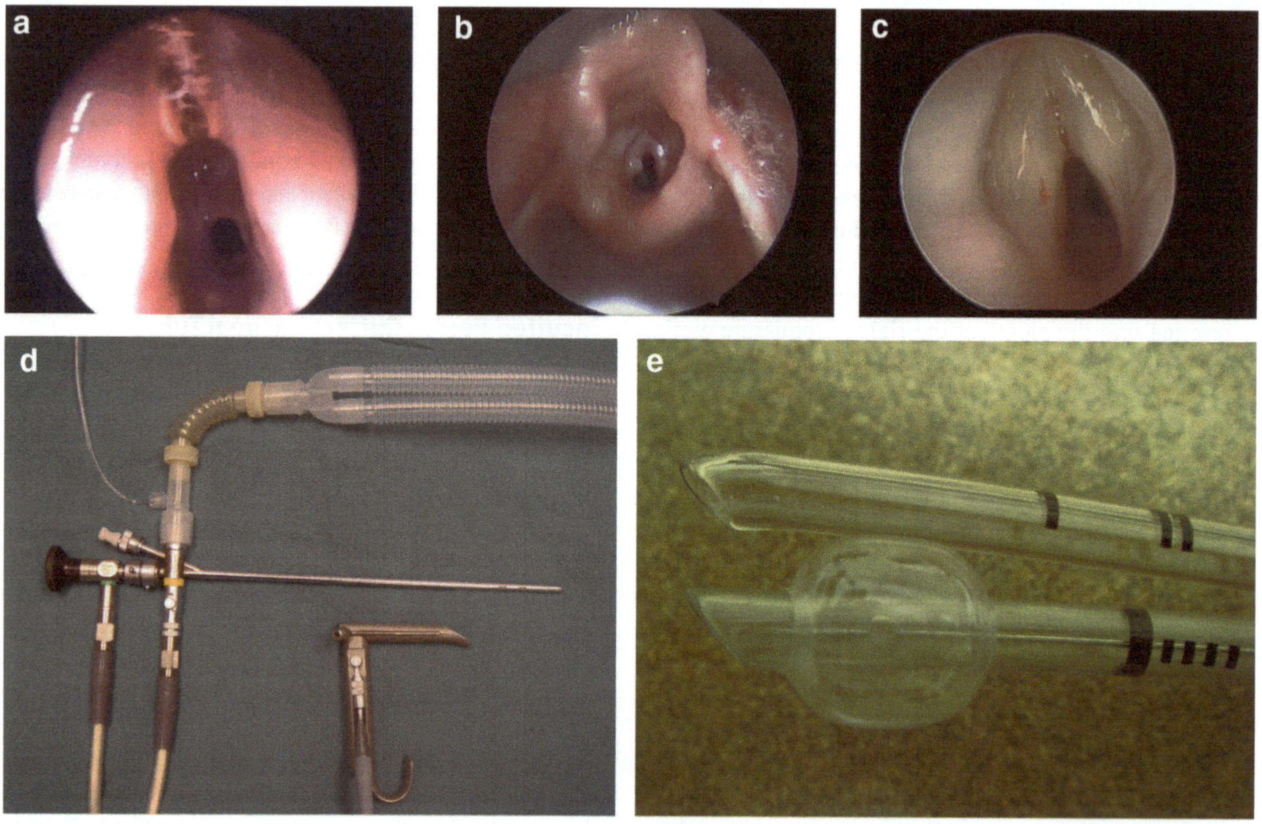

Fig. 5.3 (**a**) Bronchoscopic view of a subglottic web. (**b**) Bronchoscopic view of subglottic cysts. Courtesy of Dr. M. Benoit, Department of Otolaryngology, Strong Hospital, University of Rochester, NY. (**c**) Bronchoscopic view of subglottic stenosis after prolonged intubation. Courtesy of Dr. M. Benoit, Department of Otolaryngology, Strong Hospital, University of Rochester, NY. (**d**) A rigid bronchoscope with telescope and light source. Anesthesia breathing circuit with a flexible connector attached to the ventilation port of the bronchoscope. In the *lower right* of the photo, an anterior commissure laryngoscope is shown. (**e**) An uncuffed and an inflated Microcuff® cuffed tracheal tube for comparison. Note the absence of the Murphy eye in the Microcuff® tube. The heavy *black line* on the Microcuff® tube corresponds with the vocal cord position in the neonate

Uncuffed tubes remain advantageous when a maximal internal airway diameter is a priority, as in spontaneous respiration. Because the resistance to turbulent airflow is inversely proportional to the fifth power of the radius of the tube, the work of breathing spontaneously may become impaired by selecting a cuffed tracheal tube with a radius that is smaller than the equivalent uncuffed tube. In addition, suctioning and pulmonary toilet are more difficult in tubes of smaller internal diameters. The magnitude of the differences in diameter is magnified in smaller size tubes that are used in preterm and very low birth weight infants.

Assessing Tube Size for Intubation

It is important to estimate the diameter of the tracheal tube that will fit the neonate's airway in preparation of tracheal intubation. A tube whose outer diameter is too large will be too snug in the cricoid ring and will exert excessive pressure on the subglottic or tracheal mucosa, resulting in mucosal ischemia. In the short term, this can lead to edema of the loose pseudostratified columnar epithelium that lines the subglottic region and to stridor from an edematous narrowed airway after extubation. In the long term, it may contribute to the development of scarring and subglottic stenosis.

The diameter of the uncuffed tracheal tube that is most appropriate for a neonate may be assessed using either the "air leak test" or by manually assessing the resistance to its passage through the subglottis. For the "air leak test," the tip of the tube is positioned mid-trachea and the adjustable pressure-limiting (APL) valve is closed. While the pressure within the breathing circuit increases, a stethoscope is positioned over the suprasternal notch. The pressure at which a leak is first auscultated is noted. Indirect evidence indicates that the leak pressure should be limited to 15–20 cm H_2O to minimize the risk of mucosal edema and tissue damage in adults [86]. Comparable evidence in neonates has not been forthcoming. When performing the "air leak test," it is important to avoid a slow and prolonged leak test as this might compromise the circulation, similar to that observed during a prolonged Valsalva maneuver.

A second sizing approach is to choose the tube that passes through the glottis and subglottis without substantial manual resistance. If resistance is detected as the tube passes through the subglottic region, then a half-size smaller tube should be inserted. If the tube passes easily through the subglottis, it is important to auscultate for excessive gas leak to ensure that the tube is not too small for the larynx, otherwise it is replaced with a tube a half-size larger.

It is noteworthy that the recommended diameter for Microcuff® tracheal tubes is 3.0 mm ID for neonates >3 kg and up to 8 months. The diameter is 3.5 mm ID for infants >8 months of age. These sizes are one-half size smaller than those recommended for uncuffed tubes in neonates and infants of the corresponding ages. We recommend the readers follow the manufacturer's guidelines for the appropriate tube size.

Positioning the Tracheal Tube Tip

Ideally, the tip of the tracheal tube should be mid-tracheal level. A variety of formulae have been developed to predict the optimal positional length of the tracheal tube within the trachea. In neonates, a commonly used rule of thumb is the "123–789 rule," where a 1 kg baby should have the tube taped at approximately 7 cm at the maxillary alveolar ridge, a 2 kg baby should have the tube taped at 8 cm, and a 3 kg baby should have the tube taped at 9 cm for a mid-tracheal position. When the cuff passes just beyond the vocal cords or in the case of an uncuffed tube, the tip passes 1–2 cm beyond the vocal cords; the centimeter marking on the tube at the level of the gums (or incisors) should be noted. Some operators advance the uncuffed tube until the breath sounds become unilateral, i.e., a right endobronchial intubation producing no breath sounds over the left chest. The centimeter depth at which breath sounds become unilateral is identified as the level of the carina. The tube is then withdrawn until it rests approximately midway between the carina and the vocal cords. Knowing the centimeter marking with this depth of insertion as well as the depth of the carina gives the anesthesiologist an idea of how much tracheal tube displacement can safely occur before an endobronchial intubation or tracheal extubation occurs. The distance between the glottis and the carina in full-term neonates is approximately 4–5 cm [87, 88]. Therefore, once the distance to the carina is found, the tracheal tube is pulled back approximately 2 cm to achieve a position that is mid-tracheal. A shortened tracheal length (i.e., a more cephalad bifurcation) is associated with certain medical conditions such as trisomy 21 [89] and myelomeningocele [90, 91]. These neonates are therefore at greater risk of accidental right main bronchial intubation, even when the tube is believed to be mid-tracheal. One should always be wary of a tracheal takeoff of the right upper lobe bronchus if a mild hemoglobin oxygen desaturation persists or air entry is diminished in the right upper chest. Confirmation of a mid-tracheal tube position can be determined by palpating the tube tip or the cuff in the suprasternal notch and by chest radiograph [92].

Investigators have determined that the markings on the Microcuff® tube just proximal to the cuff more reliably ensure a properly positioned tube tip and cuff in the trachea than the cm markings at the lips (Fig. 5.3e) [93]. Since the Microcuff® tube has no Murphy eye and does have a cuff, it is prudent to respect this recommendation and use the tube markings near the tip when positioning the tracheal tube rather than the distance at the lips.

Rapid Sequence Intubation in Neonates

The traditional rapid sequence induction (RSI) without ventilation is not usually feasible in neonates because of their relatively greater oxygen consumption, reduced FRC, and increased closing volumes compared with older children, all of which result in rapid desaturation and hypoxemia during the apneic period. Furthermore, it is difficult to preoxygenate the neonate because they cry and move, preventing the application of a tight face mask, and breathe shallowly. These factors lead most pediatric anesthesiologists to perform a "modified" RSI induction in neonates [94]. With this technique, the lungs are gently ventilated manually after loss of consciousness via a face mask using low airway pressures (<10–15 cm H_2O), which prevent a significant decrease in oxyhemoglobin saturation.

Controversy exists regarding the effectiveness of cricoid pressure to prevent regurgitation in patients after induction of anesthesia [95]. Although a full discussion of this subject is beyond the scope of this chapter, what is known is that the force required to occlude the lumen of the esophagus in neonates has not been established, that a force as little as 5 N may deform the airway in the infant [96], and that the esophagus is often displaced laterally, an effect that is far more prevalent in younger children [97]. In adults, the application of up to 50 newtons cricoid pressure reduced the visibility of the glottis by 50 % [98]. Furthermore, at 30 newtons cricoid pressure, the duration of fiber-optic intubation was prolonged compared with no cricoid pressure [99]. Although comparable data in neonates and children are not available, it is reasonable to expect the effect of cricoid pressure on visibility of the glottis opening to be limited even further. In the absence of evidence that cricoid pressure prevents regurgitation, we do not recommend the routine application of cricoid pressure in neonates. Nonetheless, supplementary maneuvers to minimize aspiration of gastric contents include emptying the stomach with a red rubber catheter before induction of anesthesia, as well as rapidly administering the induction agents and rapidly securing the airway with a tracheal tube. In the event that cricoid pressure is applied, it should be maintained until complete neuromuscular blockade is established. In support of this practice, appropriately applied cricoid pressure has been shown to be effective in preventing gastric inflation during gentle bag-mask ventilation in anesthetized infants and children [100]. If the initial attempt at tracheal intubation fails while cricoid pressure continues to be applied, gentle face mask ventilation should be performed. If ventilation is difficult while cricoid pressure is applied, despite the use of adjunctive devices such as an oral or nasopharyngeal airway or an LMA, cricoid pressure should be lessened or released [101, 102]. The evidence that cricoid pressure prevents pulmonary regurgitation in this clinical setting remains unproven [85].

Table 5.1 Difficult airway in neonates

Difficult mask ventilation
Maxillary hypoplasia
Crouzon's syndrome
Apert's syndrome (acrocephalosyndactyly type I)
Pfeiffer's syndrome
Choanal atresia
Marshall–Smith syndrome
Rubinstein–Taybi syndrome
Possible difficult laryngoscopy/intubation
(a) *Micrognathia*
Pierre Robin sequence
Stickler syndrome
Smith–Lemli–Opitz syndrome
Treacher Collins syndrome
Goldenhar's syndrome; hemifacial microsomia
First arch syndrome; midfacial cleft
(b) *Possible micrognathia and other soft tissue facial anomalies*
Arthrogryposis trisomy 8
Trisomy 9
Trisomy 13 (Patau syndrome)
Trisomy 18 (Edwards syndrome)
CHARGE association
Cornelia de Lange syndrome
Velocardiofacial syndrome (Shprintzen syndrome)
Freeman–Sheldon syndrome (whistling face syndrome)
(c) *Macroglossia*
Beckwith-Wiedemann syndrome
Congenital hypothyroidism
Down syndrome
Cystic hygroma
Congenital lingual tumor/intraoral tumor
Mucopolysaccharidoses (Hurler, Hunter, Morquio, and Maroteaux–Lamy syndromes)[a]
Lipoid proteinosis trisomy 4p
Weaver syndrome
(d) *Intraoral/tracheal pathology*
Microstomia
Congenital temporomandibular joint dysfunction
Laryngeal/vallecular cyst, laryngeal web
Laryngotracheal cleft
Laryngeal/tracheal hemangiomas
Tracheal and subglottic stenosis
Other defects that may complicate the airway
Cervical spine immobility
Arthrogryposis
Emery–Dreifuss muscular dystrophy
Fibrodysplasia ossificans progressiva syndrome

[a]Data from Frawley G, Fuenzalida D, Donath S, Yaplito-Lee J, Peters H. A retrospective audit of anesthetic techniques and complications in children with mucopolysaccharidoses. Pediatr Anesth 2012: 22; 737–744

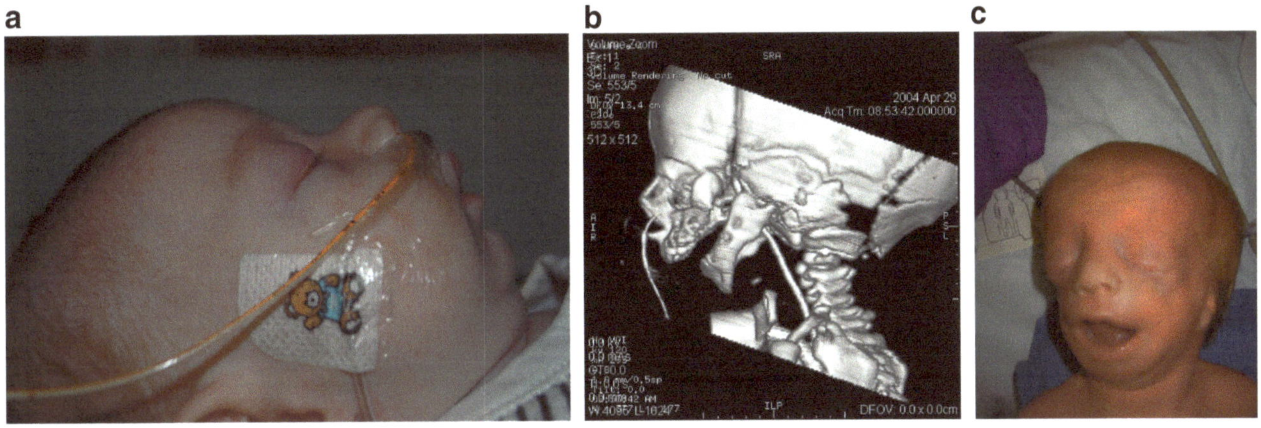

Fig. 5.4 (**a**) Lateral profile of a 3-week-old male with Pierre Robin sequence. Note the retrognathic chin, which will impair laryngoscopy and tracheal intubation. (**b**) A three dimensional CT reconstruction of a neonate with Pierre Robin sequence. Note the hypoplastic mandibular body length and severely obtuse gonial angle (see text). Courtesy of Dr. J. Girotto, Department of Plastic Surgery, Strong Hospital, University of Rochester, NY. (**c**) Neonate with Treacher Collins syndrome. Note the small mandible, deformed ears, and teardrop eyelids, which are characteristic facial features of this syndrome

Management of the Difficult Airway

The neonatal airway represents the extremes of the differences between pediatric and adult airways. Epidemiologically, difficult airways occur more frequently in infants <1 year of age (with neonates comprising the second most common age group), Mallampati 3 or 4, ASA physical status III and IV, cardiac and craniofacial surgeries, and a low BMI [103]. Consequently, anesthesiologists find airway management in this population to be the most challenging. The spectrum of congenital and acquired [104, 105], airway disorders ranges from difficult mask ventilation to difficult tracheal intubation due to a panoply of different causes (Table 5.1).

The difficult airway in the neonate presents several unique challenges, as well as sharing many challenges that parallel those of the older child. The dimensions of the face, mandible, and neck present challenges for maintaining a patent airway with the face mask. Superimposed on the difficulties of the normal neonatal airway, the flat face, maxillary hypoplasia, and small mouth of the neonate with Crouzon's disease and Apert's syndrome often lead to an obstructed airway. In many instances, an oropharyngeal airway or laryngeal mask airway will relieve the obstruction. However, direct laryngoscopy and orotracheal intubation is usually uncomplicated. As infants with these syndromes mature, mask anesthesia remains a challenge, whereas direct laryngoscopy remains uncomplicated. Neonates with Pierre Robin sequence (Fig. 5.4a) [106], Treacher Collins syndrome (Fig. 5.4c), and Goldenhar's syndrome may also present challenging but not insurmountable airways. Mask anesthesia may be difficult as the mandibular deformities render temporomandibular joint subluxation difficult (Fig. 5.4b) [107]. Pierre Robin sequence is characterized by a triad of micrognathia, glossoptosis, and respiratory distress in the first 24–48 h after birth. Direct laryngoscopy may be particularly challenging in neonates with Pierre Robin sequence in part as a result of a short mandibular body length (Fig. 5.4b) [107]. However, the airway becomes easier to manage with age such that by 2 years of age, the mandible is often aligned with the maxilla [108]. In contrast, laryngoscopy in neonates with Treacher Collins syndrome is easier at birth and becomes progressively more difficult with increasing age [108, 109]. This may be directly attributable to a shortened ascending ramus of the mandible [107]. In both Pierre Robin sequence and Treacher Collins syndrome, the gonial angle (or the angle between the ascending ramus and body of the mandible) is significantly more obtuse than in unaffected neonates, which may contribute to difficult laryngoscopy exposure. Neonates with Goldenhar's syndrome may be split in airway management: 50 % have airways that are not difficult to manage, and 50 % are exceedingly difficult to manage. Interestingly, the difficulty presented by the airway in this last syndrome does not change with age.

Neonates with subglottic webs (Fig. 5.3a), hemangiomas, cysts (Fig. 5.3b), tumors, and laryngomalacia as well as those with subglottic stenosis from prior tracheal intubation (Fig. 5.3c) may present a challenge to those using a face mask as well as a laryngoscope blade [110, 111]. The degree of airway obstruction and the dynamic changes that may occur with induction of anesthesia are often unknown in neonates with these defects.

Before embarking on an anesthetic for a child with a difficult airway, it is essential that a proper operating room and airway equipment setup is in place as well as expert assistance present before induction of anesthesia [112]. In elective cases, severely dysmorphic neonates and those with only a single means of accessing their airways (e.g., severe temporomandibular joint dysfunction that limits mouth opening and eliminates the ability to rescue ventilation with an LMA) should be evaluated by an otolaryngologist before induction of general anesthesia. This allows the otolaryngologist to assess the airway for alternate approaches to tracheal intubation (such as rigid bronchoscopy or surgical tracheostomy) (Fig. 5.2d) in the event that noninvasive attempts at tracheal intubation also fail. The availability of an otolaryngologist does not necessarily guarantee an expeditious airway rescue since the anatomical reasons that may lead to a failed intubation may also create difficulties for a tracheostomy [113].

The approach to the anticipated difficult neonatal airway is similar to that in older children. Although general anesthesia is the preferred approach to securing the airway in these infants, topical administration of local anesthesia supplemented with sedation and awake tracheal intubation should also be considered as alternative approaches. During induction of general anesthesia, spontaneous ventilation is preferred as it ensures ventilation is maintained and inhalational anesthesia can be reversed should the operators fail to secure the airway. However, spontaneous ventilation may be difficult to maintain in some neonates (particularly in the preterm neonate and those with hypoplastic mandibles) because of the small dimensions of their upper airways, sensitivity to inhalational agents, and chest wall instability in addition to the defect at the root of the difficult airway. The decision to administer a muscle relaxant depends on the risk/benefit ratio of paralysis including difficulty ventilating the lungs and realizing a "cannot-intubate-cannot-ventilate" scenario may develop, although the latter is rare in neonates [114–116]. Induction of anesthesia must be carried out carefully, avoiding upper airway obstruction, which in most neonates, results in the rapid onset of arterial hemoglobin desaturation.

Topical anesthesia applied to the airway combined with sedation has been used to blunt cardiorespiratory responses during laryngoscopy. However, a recent review (in older children) suggested that not only does topical local anesthesia not reduce the incidence of perioperative airway reflexes, but that it actually may paradoxically increase the incidence of laryngospasm, although this was only an observational study [117]. Alternately, sedation may be provided by midazolam and fentanyl, propofol, dexmedetomidine, or ketamine administered intravenously [57, 63, 118–122]. These approaches have all been used to secure the airway, although the responses were generally optimally controlled when a muscle relaxant was coadministered. Lastly, an awake intubation may be necessary in order to secure the difficult airway, particularly in the absence of otolaryngology support or alternatives. The approach described earlier in this chapter to performing an awake orotracheal intubation should be followed closely in order to reliably and rapidly secure the airway in the neonate. Once the airway is secured and carbon dioxide is identified in the airway, then a bolus of intravenous propofol should be administered immediately to induce general anesthesia.

We remain firmly committed to perfecting our skills with the laryngoscope and direct laryngoscopy. The discussion above provides a detailed description of how to properly use the Miller blade in neonates with a difficult airway. Nonetheless, in some circumstances, the airway cannot be secured by direct laryngoscopy and alternative airway devices are required. The following describes those airway devices.

Adjuncts such as an oropharyngeal airway or LMA may be useful, particularly in the child with a dysmorphic face, in whom the jaw thrust [31] only partially preserves the patent upper airway. The LMA has served as an effective bridge to tracheostomy in several difficult airway reports in neonates [108, 114, 123]. The appropriate size LMA should always be readily available in the event it is needed urgently. Before instrumenting the airway however, intravenous access should be established to facilitate the administration of resuscitative medications.

Several different video and optical technologies are available to manage difficult neonatal airways [108]. Much of the evidence for the effectiveness of these devices is based on investigations in adults and older children. As a result, the information presented here is a synthesis of published reports and the clinical experience of the authors using these devices in neonates.

The Storz Video (Karl Storz GmbH, Tuttlingen, Germany, Fig. 5.5) and the GlideScope (Verathon, Bothell, Washington, Fig. 5.6) are two video laryngoscopes that may be used to facilitate tracheal intubation in neonates [124, 127]. The Storz video laryngoscope consists of a size 0 and 1 straight

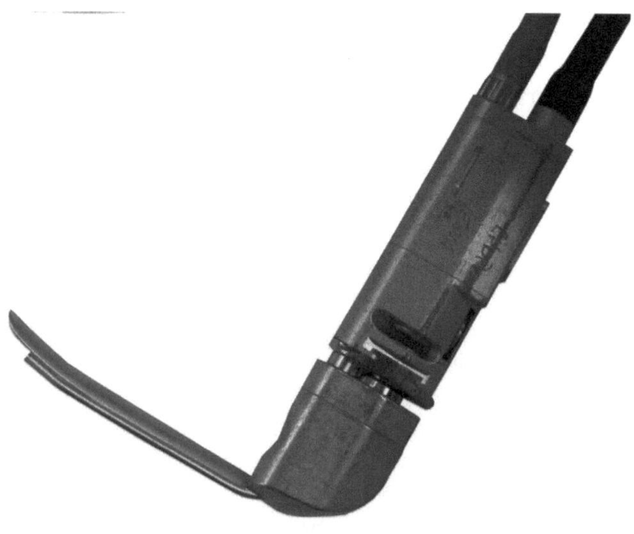

Fig. 5.5 Neonatal-sized Storz video laryngoscope

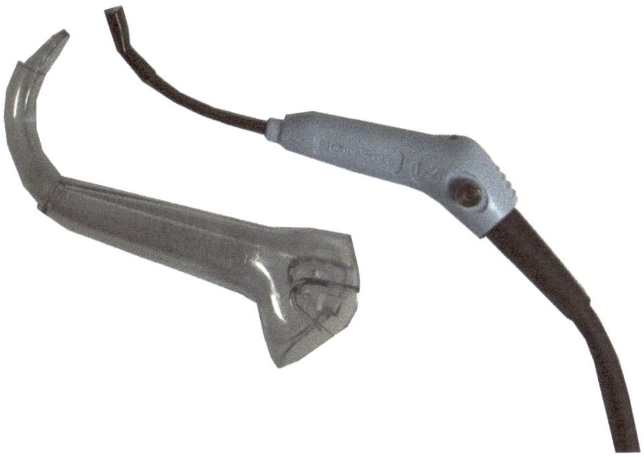

Fig. 5.6 Neonatal-sized GlideScope

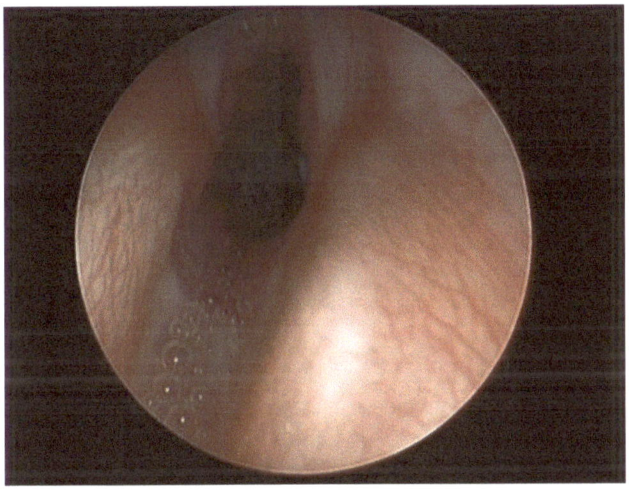

Fig. 5.7 Laryngeal cleft

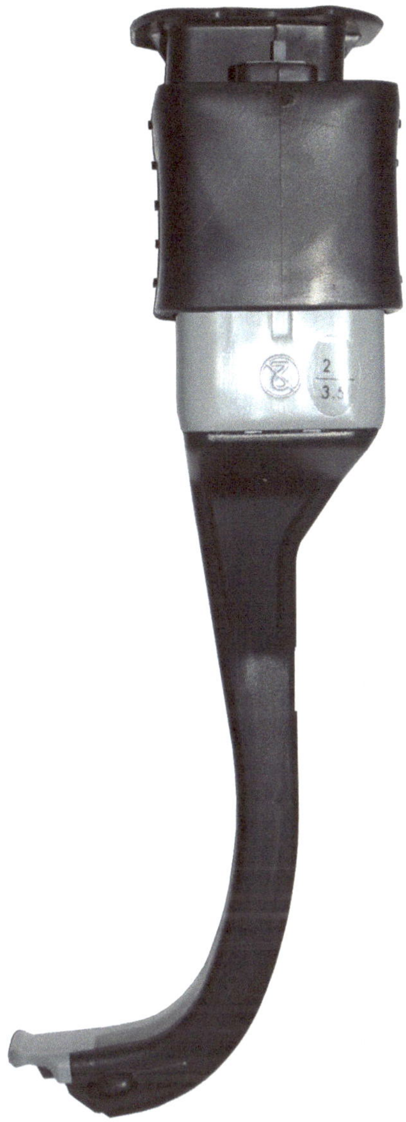

Fig. 5.8 Neonatal-sized Airtraq optical laryngoscope

blade, which incorporates a 2.8 mm image and light bundle within a stainless steel tube. This video laryngoscope has been used successfully in the delivery room, to facilitate tracheal intubation in neonates as small as 500 g [125]. The detailed view from the camera allows visual inspection of the airway in those suspected of having vocal cord dysfunction, laryngeal clefts (Fig. 5.7), and gastroesophageal reflux.

Despite the large number of publications on the GlideScope video laryngoscope in adults and older children, there are few publications documenting its use in infants and neonates [126]. The redesigned GlideScope Cobalt is a MAC-style plastic blade that fits onto a video baton. It is available in all pediatric sizes and almost always provides a clear, crisp view of the glottic opening, except in the most anatomically deformed neonates. However, there is a learning curve to navigating the tracheal tube through the oropharynx and into the glottic opening, while focusing on the video screen. Once this maneuver has been mastered, the device provides a reliably high success rate in most neonates with craniofacial anomalies as long as mouth opening is sufficient to accept the blade. The tracheal tube should be visualized throughout its advancement so as to avoid injury to the airway in neonates with limited oropharyngeal space.

The Airtraq optical laryngoscope (Prodol, Vizcaya, Spain) is a single-use curved laryngoscope that uses mirrors and prisms to transmit the image from the tip of the device to a viewfinder (Fig. 5.8) [127]. It has a conduit for the tracheal tube along its side that directs the tracheal tube toward the glottic opening as it is advanced. The Airtraq has been used successfully in managing the difficult airway in the neonate, although there are no controlled systematic evaluations in this population [127–132]. Despite the built-in channel, one publication described two cases (one neonate and one infant) in which a full glottic view was obtained, and yet difficulty was encountered directing the tube into the trachea.

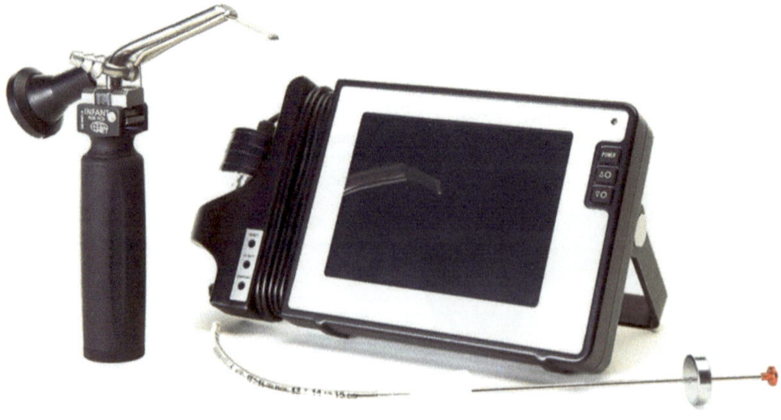

Fig. 5.9 Neonatal-sized Truview EVO2 (courtesy of Dan White, Truphatek, Inc.)

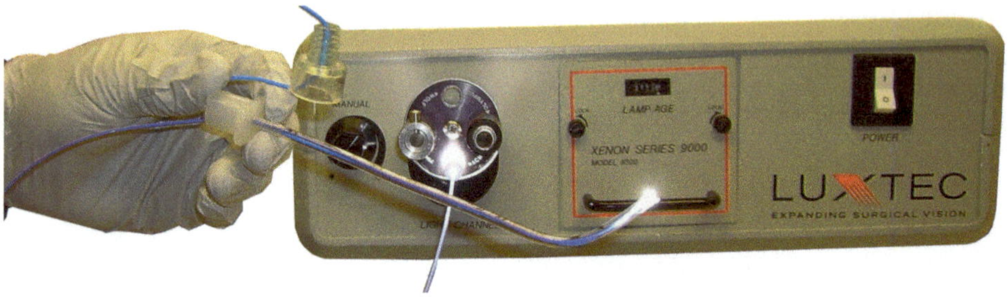

Fig. 5.10 A single fiber-optic light bundle is attached to a rheostat-controlled light source and placed inside a styleted endotracheal tube to form a "homegrown" lighted stylet

The authors attributed the failures to the bulk of the device that limited its maneuverability [133]. Others have had success utilizing a gum elastic bougie to facilitate placement of the tracheal tube when the standard approach failed [134].

The Truview EVO2 (Truphatek, Netanya, Israel) incorporates a prismatic lens in an angulated rigid blade (Fig. 5.9) [127]. It has a side port for oxygen insufflation during intubation. When the Truview was compared with the Miller blade in neonates, the former provided improved Cormack-Lehane views and a clinically insignificant increase in the time to tracheal intubation [135]. Caution should be exercised when insufflating oxygen at excessive flows (i.e., Bonfils recommends <3 l per minute of oxygen flow) through these intubation devices as subcutaneous emphysema has been reported [136].

When using any of the video-assisted intubation devices described above (with the exception of the Airtraq), the selected tracheal tube should be prepared with a lightly lubricated stylet before laryngoscopy. Although the stylet is not absolutely necessary in all cases, an anterior curve matching the blade angle of the selected device facilitates tube placement. Laryngoscopy is performed by introducing the blade in the midline or to the right of the tongue, and airway structures are progressively visualized until the blade tip is placed either in the vallecula or under the epiglottis. Vallecular placement with engagement of the glossoepiglottic ligament will elevate the epiglottis exposing the glottic opening in most infants. On occasion, the epiglottis obstructs the camera view because of its length in neonates and infants. In this case, the epiglottis should be gently lifted with the blade to expose the glottic inlet. After a satisfactory view has been obtained, the tracheal tube is passed along the shaft of the blade (unlike the lateral insertion typical with standard direct laryngoscopy). This insertion technique guarantees that the tracheal tube will come into the view of the video camera as it is advanced and reduces the risk of soft tissue injury.

The lighted stylet remains a viable option for intubating the neonate with a difficult airway [137, 138]. A stylet for neonatal use can easily be fashioned from readily available equipment in the operating room. A single fiber-optic light bundle (20 g Fiberoptic Endoilluminator, Cat No. MVS1011, Storz, St. Louis, MO, USA) can be inserted into the chosen tracheal tube alongside a rigid stylet, and the fiber-optic bundle is then connected to a rheostat-controlled fiber-optic light source (Fig. 5.10) [138]. Transillumination of light in the neck is used to guide the placement of the tracheal tube; however, because of the relative lack of subcutaneous fat in neonatal patients, changes in light intensity with esophageal

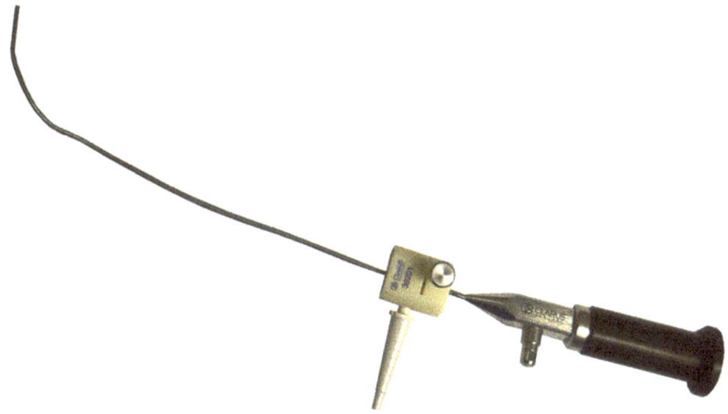

Fig. 5.11 Neonatal-sized Shikani Optical Stylet

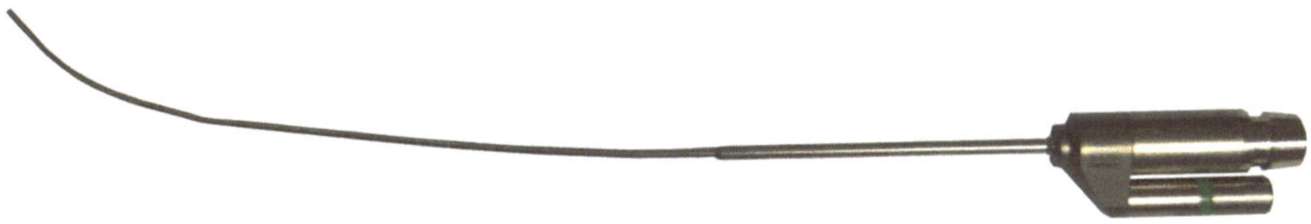

Fig. 5.12 Neonatal-sized Bonfils fiber-optic laryngoscope

placement may not be readily appreciated. Thus, lighted stylet intubation in the neonate requires an element of feel and observing continuous illumination of the transilluminated light. A brief disappearance and reappearance of the transilluminated light suggests esophageal placement, and the visualization of a cone of light in the caudad direction suggests correct glottic positioning.

Optical stylets combine the rigidity of the lighted stylet with fiber optics to allow direct visualization during intubation. The Shikani Optical Stylet (SOS; Fig. 5.11) and the Bonfils fiber-optic laryngoscope (Fig. 5.12) represent two designs with neonatal application. The SOS is malleable whereas the Bonfils is rigid with a fixed curve of 40°. Both are limited by the presence of secretions but have been successfully utilized in neonates. Optical stylets can be combined with the anterior commissure laryngoscope or a standard laryngoscope to facilitate intubation; the laryngoscope displaces soft tissue and provides an unobstructed path for the stylet to be maneuvered [139]. Some authors have reported less success with the Bonfils when compared with standard laryngoscopy [140], while others question its utility in children [141, 142]. The Bonfils has been used successfully with a 2.5 mm tracheal tube in a small-for-gestational-age neonate in whom direct laryngoscopy failed [143].

The flexible fiber-optic bronchoscope remains the gold standard for managing the neonate with a difficult airway. A working channel has been incorporated into neonatal size bronchoscopes with variable effectiveness in removing secretions [144]. If difficulty is encountered with the oral and nasal approaches, fiber-optic intubation through the nose or an LMA should be considered. This technique has been used successfully for tracheal intubation in this age group. A correctly positioned LMA simplifies intubation with the flexible fiber-optic bronchoscope and allows continuous ventilation via a swivel adapter [145–151]. With the increasing use of cuffed tubes in children, practitioners should be aware that most neonatal LMAs will not allow the passage of cuffed tracheal tubes without some modifications to the pilot balloon cuff. [152] The exception to this observation is the air-Q intubating LMA (Mercury Medical, Clearwater, FL) which readily accepts the pilot balloon of the cuffed tube [153, 154]. In neonates with severe upper airway obstruction, the LMA can be placed in the awake infant and followed by induction of general anesthesia and fiber-optic intubation [155–158]. Placement of a modified nasal airway provides an alternative option for oxygenation during intubation in a neonate. In small infants with the potential for life-threatening upper airway obstruction during administration of general anesthesia (e.g., large cystic hygroma), moderate sedation may be considered using small, incremental doses of ketamine and midazolam after the application of topical anesthesia [159].

In neonates, multiple attempts at tracheal intubation can rapidly result in upper airway edema that is sufficiently significant to compromise ventilation. An otolaryngologist should be consulted for evaluation for a tracheostomy if the intubation of the airway is essential. In the unlikely event of life-threatening airway obstruction unrelieved by an LMA, needle cricothyroidotomy is the recommended invasive technique for nonsurgically trained providers to establish life-sustaining oxygenation. However, the neonatal cricothyroid membrane is described as slit-like with overlap of the cricoid and thyroid cartilages [160]. The neonatal cricothyroid membrane is too small for surgical cricothyroidotomy to be performed measuring 2.61 mm in length and 3.03 mm in width in neonatal cadavers, dimensions that are too small for a neonatal tracheal tube [161]. Attempts to pass a tracheal or tracheostomy tube could result in laryngeal fracture or severe airway injury. The lack of a laryngeal prominence in the neonate combined with a more cephalad glottic position makes localizing the membrane in the neonate more difficult than in the adult. After identification of the cricothyroid membrane, a 16- to 18-gauge needle/catheter with a saline-filled 3 ml syringe attached should be inserted in a caudad direction through the membrane. Aspiration of air confirms entry into the tracheal air column; the catheter is left in place and the needle is removed. Before ventilation is attempted, it is crucial to verify that the tip of the needle and catheter are within the air column of the trachea rather than extratracheal, e.g., in subcutaneous tissue or cerebrospinal fluid, lest potential fatal sequelae occur. A number of techniques to deliver oxygen and connect to the in situ catheter (including using a stopcock, 3 cc syringe barrel, and a 15 mm adapter) have been described, using pressures of 25–35 psi obtained from a high-pressure oxygen source [160]. Commercial devices (e.g., Enk oxygen flow modulator set, Cook Critical Care, Bloomington, Indiana) are available for regulating oxygen insufflation.

The difficult neonatal airway represents one of the most challenging clinical scenarios for the pediatric anesthesiologist. If the difficult airway is anticipated, then appropriate planning may take place. However, in those rare instances in which the difficult airway is unanticipated, it may be prudent to ensure appropriate management by referring to a difficult pediatric airway algorithm [112, 162]. Consistent success requires adequate preparation, maintenance of skill with indirect visualization devices, and assembling the appropriate personnel when assistance is required.

Airway Management and Ex Utero Intrapartum Treatment

Rare conditions may occasionally result in compromised and potentially life-threatening neonatal airway immediately after birth. These conditions include (but are not limited to) congenital cystic hygroma of the neck, congenital high airway obstruction syndrome (CHAOS) caused by obstruction at the level of the larynx or trachea, and cervical teratoma (see Fig. 5.13) or other tumor of the face, mouth, and neck. Antenatal diagnosis permits scheduling the time of delivery to ensure that an ex utero intrapartum treatment (EXIT) technique is prepared to manage the neonates airway [163–165]. The EXIT procedure is performed on the partially delivered fetus while it continues to receive oxygen through an intact uteroplacental circulation. EXIT procedures include direct laryngoscopy/bronchoscopy and tracheal intubation, tracheostomy, or tumor resection. Figures 5.14a, b show a neonate and MRI scan of that neonate who presented antenatally with

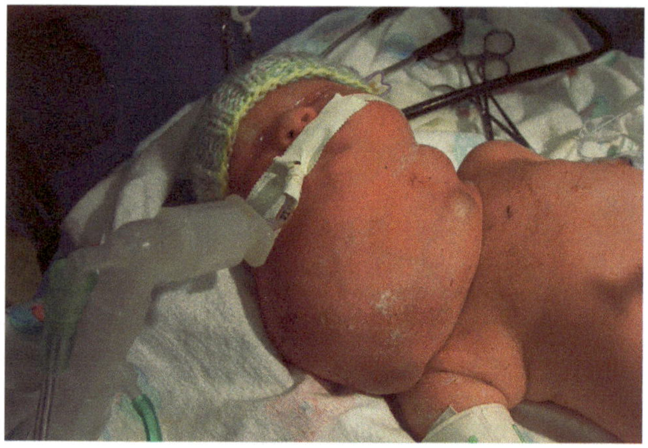

Fig. 5.13 Cervical teratoma

a

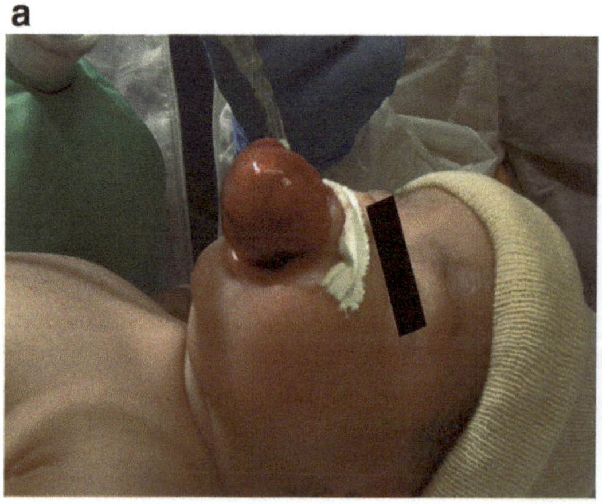

b

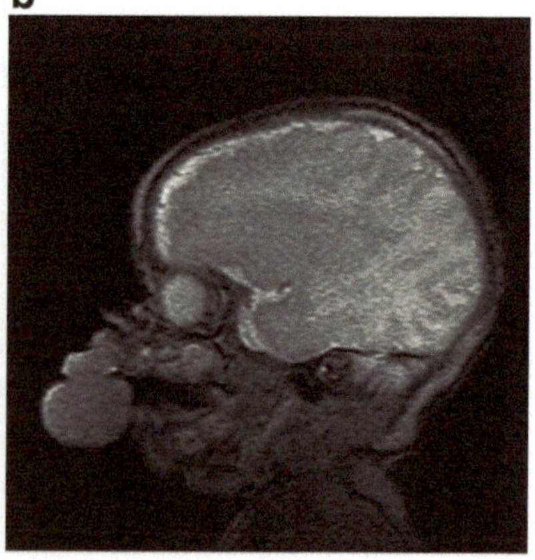

Fig. 5.14 (**a**) Neonate with a hamartoma of the hard palate. (**b**) CT scan of the neonate in Fig. 5.11a demonstrating a clear and patent nasopharyngeal airway

a hamartoma of the hard palate. An EXIT procedure was undertaken, although orotracheal intubation was successful performed by anesthesia upon delivery. The benign tumor was subsequently resected. In some centers, such as ours, airway management is performed entirely by the surgical team. Once the neonate's airway is secured using a tracheal tube or surgical airway (depending on the size and location of the obstructing lesion), the placental cord may be severed.

Fetal anesthetic management consists of transplacental transfer of volatile anesthetics (via the mother who receives general endotracheal anesthesia) and an intramuscular injection of atropine, fentanyl, and vecuronium into the fetus, once it is exposed via a uterine incision. Muscle relaxation is critical to prevent the fetus from taking a breath, which would cause a switch from fetal to transitional circulatory pattern.

EXIT procedures may also be performed for resection of congenital pulmonary masses and cannulation for extracorporeal membrane oxygenator (ECMO) support for select congenital cardiac conditions. One of the original indications for the EXIT procedure was to remove a tracheal plug that was placed during mid-gestation in an attempt to promote pulmonary development in fetuses with congenital diaphragmatic hernia [166].

References

1. Dorst JP. Changes of the skull during childhood. In: Newton TH, Potts DG, editors. Radiology of the skull and brain. St Louis: Mosby; 1971.
2. Sullivan PG. Skull, jaw, and teeth growth patterns. In: Falkner FTJM, editor. Human growth: a comprehensive treatise. New York: Plenum Press; 1971.
3. Westhorpe RN. The position of the larynx in children and its relationship to the ease of intubation. Anaesth Intensive Care. 1987;15:384–8.
4. Praud JP, Reix P. Upper airways and neonatal respiration. Respir Physiol Neurobiol. 2005;149:131–41.
5. Cozzi F, Steiner M, Rosati D, Madonna L, Colarossi G. Clinical manifestations of choanal atresia in infancy. J Pediatr Surg. 1988;23:203–6.
6. Miller MJ, Martin RJ, Carlo WA, Fouke JM, Strohl KP, Fanaroff AA. Oral breathing in newborn infants. J Pediatr. 1985; 107:465–9.
7. Sasaki CT, Levine PA, Laitman JT, Crelin Jr ES. Postnatal descent of the epiglottis in man. A preliminary report. Arch Otolaryngol. 1977;103:169–71.
8. Schwartz DS, Keller MS. Maturational descent of the epiglottis. Arch Otolaryngol Head Neck Surg. 1997;123:627–8.
9. Radvanyi-Bouvet MF, Monset-Couchard M, Morel-Kahn F, Vicente G, Dreyfus-Brisac C. Expiratory patterns during sleep in normal full-term and premature neonates. Biol Neonate. 1982;41:74–84.
10. Mortola JP, Milic-Emili J, Noworaj A, Smith B, Fox G, Weeks S. Muscle pressure and flow during expiration in infants. Am Rev Respir Dis. 1984;129:49–53.
11. Vandam LD. The functional anatomy of the lung. Anesthesiology. 1952;13:130–41.
12. Page M, Jeffery HE. Airway protection in sleeping infants in response to pharyngeal fluid stimulation in the supine position. Pediatr Res. 1998;44:691–8.
13. Pickens DL, Schefft GL, Thach BT. Pharyngeal fluid clearance and aspiration preventive mechanisms in sleeping infants. J Appl Physiol. 1989;66:1164–71.
14. Thach BT. Some aspects of clinical relevance in the maturation of respiratory control in infants. J Appl Physiol. 2008;104:1828–34.
15. Thach BT. Maturation and transformation of reflexes that protect the airway from liquid aspiration from fetal to adult life. Am J Med. 2001;111(Suppl 8A):69S–77S.
16. Perkett EA, Vaughan RL. Evidence for a laryngeal chemoreflex in some human preterm infants. Acta Paediatr Scand. 1982;71:969–72.
17. Pickens DL, Schefft G, Thach BT. Prolonged apnea associated with upper airway protective reflexes in apnea of prematurity. Am Rev Respir Dis. 1988;137:113–8.
18. Davies AM, Koenig JS, Thach BT. Upper airway chemoreflex responses to saline and water in preterm infants. J Appl Physiol. 1988;64:1412–20.
19. Davies AM, Koenig JS, Thach BT. Characteristics of upper airway chemoreflex prolonged apnea in human infants. Am Rev Respir Dis. 1989;139:668–73.
20. Pickens DL, Schefft GL, Storch GA, Thach BT. Characterization of prolonged apneic episodes associated with respiratory syncytial virus infection. Pediatr Pulmonol. 1989;6:195–201.
21. Wennergren G, Hertzberg T, Milerad J, Bjure J, Lagercrantz H. Hypoxia reinforces laryngeal reflex bradycardia in infants. Acta Paediatr Scand. 1989;78:11–7.
22. Wetmore RF. Effects of acid on the larynx of the maturing rabbit and their possible significance to the sudden infant death syndrome. Laryngoscope. 1993;103:1242–54.
23. Donnelly DF, Haddad GG. Effect of graded anesthesia on laryngeal-induced central apnea. Respir Physiol. 1986;66:235–45.
24. Lee JC, Stoll BJ, Downing SE. Properties of the laryngeal chemoreflex in neonatal piglets. Am J Physiol. 1977;233:R30–6.
25. Kurth CD, Hutchison AA, Caton DC, Davenport PW. Maturational and anesthetic effects on apneic thresholds in lambs. J Appl Physiol. 1989;67:643–7.
26. Lanier B, Richardson MA, Cummings C. Effect of hypoxia on laryngeal reflex apnea–implications for sudden infant death. Otolaryngol Head Neck Surg. 1983;91:597–604.
27. Sladek M, Grogaard JB, Parker RA, Sundell HW. Prolonged hypoxemia enhances and acute hypoxemia attenuates laryngeal reflex apnea in young lambs. Pediatr Res. 1993;34:813–20.
28. Fagenholz SA, Lee JC, Downing SE. Association of anemia with reduced central respiratory drive in the piglet. Yale J Biol Med. 1979;52:263–70.
29. Lindgren C, Jing L, Graham B, Grogaard J, Sundell H. Respiratory syncytial virus infection reinforces reflex apnea in young lambs. Pediatr Res. 1992;31:381–5.
30. Lindgren C, Grogaard J. Reflex apnoea response and inflammatory mediators in infants with respiratory tract infection. Acta Paediatr. 1996;85:798–803.
31. Larson Jr PC. Laryngospasm-the best treatment. Anesthesiology. 1998;89:1293–4.
32. Scheller B, Schalk R, Byhahn C, Peter N, L'Allemand N, Kessler P, Meininger D. Laryngeal tube suction II for difficult airway management in neonates and small infants. Resuscitation. 2009;80:805–10.
33. Mizushima A, Wardall GJ, Simpson DL. The laryngeal mask airway in infants. Anaesthesia. 1992;47:849–51.
34. Brimacombe J. The advantages of the LMA over the tracheal tube or facemask: a meta-analysis. Can J Anaesth. 1995;42:1017–23.

35. O'Donnell CP, Kamlin CO, Davis PG, Morley CJ. Endotracheal intubation attempts during neonatal resuscitation: success rates, duration, and adverse effects. Pediatrics. 2006;117: e16–21.
36. Bismilla Z, Finan E, McNamara PJ, LeBlanc V, Jefferies A, Whyte H. Failure of pediatric and neonatal trainees to meet Canadian Neonatal Resuscitation Program standards for neonatal intubation. J Perinatol. 2010;30:182–7.
37. Leone TA, Rich W, Finer NN. Neonatal intubation: success of pediatric trainees. J Pediatr. 2005;146:638–41.
38. Falck AJ, Escobedo MB, Baillargeon JG, Villard LG, Gunkel JH. Proficiency of pediatric residents in performing neonatal endotracheal intubation. Pediatrics. 2003;112:1242–7.
39. Grein AJ, Weiner GM. Laryngeal mask airway versus bag-mask ventilation or endotracheal intubation for neonatal resuscitation. Cochrane Database Syst Rev. 2009; 1: CD003314.pub2
40. Zhu XY, Lin BC, Zhang QS, et al. A prospective evaluation of the efficacy of the laryngeal mask airway during neonatal resuscitation. Resuscitation. 2011;82:1405–9.
41. Schmolzer GM, Agarwal M, Kamlin CO, Davis PG. Supraglottic airway devices during neonatal resuscitation: an historical perspective, systematic review and meta-analysis of available clinical trials. Resuscitation. 2013;84(6):722–30.
42. Zanardo V, Weiner G, Micaglio M, Doglioni N, Buzzacchero R, Trevisanuto D. Delivery room resuscitation of near-term infants: role of the laryngeal mask airway. Resuscitation. 2010; 81:327–30.
43. Micaglio M, Bonato R, De Nardin M, Parotto M, Trevisanuto D, Zanardo V, Doglioni N, Ori C. Prospective, randomized comparison of ProSeal and Classic laryngeal mask airways in anaesthetized neonates and infants. Br J Anaesth. 2009;103:263–7.
44. Lopez-Gil M, Mantilla I, Blanco T, et al. The size 1 ProSeal™ laryngeal mask airway in infants: a randomized, noncrossover study with the Classic™ laryngeal mask airway. Pediatr Anesth. 2012;22:365–70.
45. Adnet F, Baillard C, Borron SW, Denantes C, Lefebvre L, Galinski M, Martinez C, Cupa M, Lapostolle F. Randomized study comparing the "sniffing position" with simple head extension for laryngoscopic view in elective surgery patients. Anesthesiology. 2001; 95:836–41.
46. Adnet F, Borron SW, Dumas JL, Lapostolle F, Cupa M, Lapandry C. Study of the "sniffing position" by magnetic resonance imaging. Anesthesiology. 2001;94:83–6.
47. Vialet R, Nau A, Chaumoitre K, Martin C. Effects of head posture on the oral, pharyngeal and laryngeal axis alignment in infants and young children by magnetic resonance imaging. Paediatr Anaesth. 2008;18:525–31.
48. Greenland KB, Eley V, Edwards MJ, Allen P, Irwin MG. The origins of the sniffing position and the Three Axes Alignment Theory for direct laryngoscopy. Anaesth Intensive Care. 2008;36 Suppl 1:23–7.
49. Doherty JS, Froom SR, Gildersleve CD. Pediatric laryngoscopes and intubation aids old and new. Paediatr Anaesth. 2009;19 Suppl 1:30–7.
50. Robertshaw FL. A new laryngoscope for infants and children. Lancet. 1962;2:1034.
51. Henderson JJ. The use of paraglossal straight blade laryngoscopy in difficult tracheal intubation. Anaesthesia. 1997;52: 552–60.
52. Achen B, Terblanche OC, Finucane BT. View of the larynx obtained using the Miller blade and paraglossal approach, compared to that with the Macintosh blade. Anaesth Intensive Care. 2008;36:717–21.
53. Anand KJ, Maze M. Fetuses, fentanyl, and the stress response: signals from the beginnings of pain? Anesthesiology. 2001; 95:823–5.
54. Anand KJ. Consensus statement for the prevention and management of pain in the newborn. Arch Pediatr Adolesc Med. 2001;155:173–80.
55. Anand KJS, Phil D, Hickey PR. Pain and its effects in the human neonate and fetus. N Engl J Med. 1987;317:1321–48.
56. Kumar P, Denson SE, Mancuso TJ. Premedication for nonemergency endotracheal intubation in the neonate. Pediatrics. 2010;125:608–15.
57. Roberts KD, Leone TA, Edwards WH, Rich WD, Finer NN. Premedication for nonemergent neonatal intubations: a randomized, controlled trial comparing atropine and fentanyl to atropine, fentanyl, and mivacurium. Pediatrics. 2006;118:1583–91.
58. Lemyre B, Cheng R, Gaboury I. Atropine, fentanyl and succinylcholine for non-urgent intubations in newborns. Arch Dis Child Fetal Neonatal Ed. 2009;94:F439–42.
59. Carbajal R, Eble B, Anand KJ. Premedication for tracheal intubation in neonates: confusion or controversy? Semin Perinatol. 2007;31:309–17.
60. Ghanta S, Abdel-Latif ME, Lui K, Ravindranathan H, Awad J, Oei J. Propofol compared with the morphine, atropine, and suxamethonium regimen as induction agents for neonatal endotracheal intubation: a randomized, controlled trial. Pediatrics. 2007;119:e1248–55.
61. Lemyre B, Doucette J, Kalyn A, Gray S, Marrin ML. Morphine for elective endotracheal intubation in neonates: a randomized trial [ISRCTN43546373]. BMC Pediatr. 2004;4:20.
62. Bhutada A, Sahni R, Rastogi S, Wung JT. Randomised controlled trial of thiopental for intubation in neonates. Arch Dis Child Fetal Neonatal Ed. 2000;82:F34–7.
63. Dempsey EM, Al Hazzani F, Faucher D, Barrington KJ. Facilitation of neonatal endotracheal intubation with mivacurium and fentanyl in the neonatal intensive care unit. Arch Dis Child Fetal Neonatal Ed. 2006;91:F279–82.
64. Lerman J, Heard C, Steward DJ. Neonatal tracheal intubation: an imbroglio unresolved. Pediatr Anesth. 2010;20:585–90.
65. Tintinalli JE, Claffey J. Complications of nasotracheal intubation. Ann Emerg Med. 1981;10:142–4.
66. Krebs MJ, Sakai T. Retropharyngeal dissection during nasotracheal intubation: a rare complication and its management. J Clin Anesth. 2008;20:218–21.
67. Hansen M, Poulsen MR, Bendixen DK, Hartmann-Andersen F. Incidence of sinusitis in patients with nasotracheal intubation. Br J Anaesth. 1988;61:231–2.
68. Oncag O, Cokmez B, Aydemir S, Balcioglu T. Investigation of bacteremia following nasotracheal intubation. Paediatr Anaesth. 2005;15:194–8.
69. Wilkinson JA, Mathis RD, Dire DJ. Turbinate destruction–a rare complication of nasotracheal intubation. J Emerg Med. 1986; 4:209–12.
70. Williams AR, Burt N, Warren T. Accidental middle turbinectomy: a complication of nasal intubation. Anesthesiology. 1999;90: 1782–4.
71. Baldwin FJ, Morley AP. Intraoperative pulmonary oedema in a child following systemic absorption of phenylephrine drops. Br J Anaesth. 2002;88:440–2.
72. Greher M, Hartmann T, Winkler M, Zimpfer M, Crabnor CM. Hypertension and pulmonary edema associated with subconjunctival phenylephrine in a 2-month-old child during cataract extraction. Anesthesiology. 1998;88:1394–6.
73. Groudine SB, Hollinger I, Jones J, DeBouno BA. New York State guidelines on the topical use of phenylephrine in the operating room. The Phenylephrine Advisory Committee. Anesthesiology. 2000;92:859–64.
74. Riegle EV, Gunter JB, Lusk RP, Muntz HR, Weiss KL. Comparison of vasoconstrictors for functional endoscopic sinus surgery in children. Laryngoscope. 1992;102:820–3.

75. Thrush DN. Cardiac arrest after oxymetazoline nasal spray. J Clin Anesth. 1995;7:512–4.
76. Sprung J, Alhaddad ST. Use of anticholinergics to treat bradycardia caused by alpha1-adrenergic agonist overdose is not safe. J Clin Anesth. 1996;8:426–7.
77. Watt S, Pickhardt D, Lerman J, Armstrong J, Creighton PR, Feldman L. Telescoping tracheal tubes into catheters minimizes epistaxis during nasotracheal intubation in children. Anesthesiology. 2007;106:238–42.
78. Murat I. Cuffed tubes in children: a 3-year experience in a single institution. Pediatr Anaesth. 2001;11:748–9.
79. Weiss M, Dullenkopf A, Fischer JE, Gerber AC. Group EPEIS: Prospective randomized controlled multi-centre trial of cuffed or uncuffed endotracheal tubes in small children. Br J Anaesth. 2009;103:867–73.
80. Eschertzhuber S, Salgo B, Schmitz A, Roth W, Frotzler A, Keller CH, Gerber AC, Weiss M: Cuffed endotracheal tubes in children reduce sevoflurane and medical gas consumption and related costs. Acta Anaesthesiol Scand. 2010;54:855–8.
81. Deakers TW, Reynolds G, Stretton M, Newth CJ. Cuffed endotracheal tubes in pediatric intensive care. J Pediatr. 1994;125:57–62.
82. Sathyamoorthy M, Lerman J, Lakshminrusimha S. Inspiratory stridor after tracheal intubation with a Microcuff tracheal tube in three young infants. Anesthesiology. 2013;118:748–50.
83. Dullenkopf A, Gerber A, Weiss M. The Microcuff tube allows a longer time interval until unsafe cuff pressures are reached in children. Can J Anaesth. 2004;51:997–1001.
84. Khine HH, Corddry DH, Kettrick RG, Martin TM, McCloskey JJ, Rose JB, Theroux MC, Zagnoev M. Comparison of cuffed and uncuffed endotracheal tubes in young children during general anesthesia. Anesthesiology. 1997;86:627–31.
85. El Orbany M, Connolly LA. Rapid sequence induction and intubation: current controversy. Anesth Analg. 2010;110:1318–25.
86. Seegobin RD, Van Hasselt GL. Endotracheal cuff pressure and tracheal mucosal blood flows: endoscopic study of four large volume cuffs. BMJ. 1984;288:965–8.
87. Butz Jr RO. Length and cross-section growth patterns in the human trachea. Pediatrics. 1968;42:336–41.
88. Griscom NT, Wohl ME. Dimensions of the growing trachea related to age and gender. AJR. 1986;146:233–7.
89. Hansen DD, Haberkern CM, Jonas RA, Davis PJ, McGowan FX. Case conference. Case 1-1991. J Cardiothorac Vasc Anesth. 1991;5:81–5.
90. Wells TR, Jacobs RA, Senac MO, Landing BH. Incidence of short trachea in patients with myelomeningocele. Pediatr Neurol. 1990;6:109–11.
91. Wells AL, Wells TR, Landing BH, Cruz B, Galvis DA. Short trachea, a hazard in tracheal intubation of neonates and infants: syndromal associations. Anesthesiology. 1989;71:367–73.
92. Bednarek FJ, Kuhns LR. Endotracheal tube placement in infants determined by suprasternal palpation: a new technique. Pediatrics. 1975;56:224–9.
93. Weiss M, Gerber AC, Dullenkopf A. Appropriate placement of intubation depth marks in a new cuffed paediatric tracheal tube. Br J Anaesth. 2005;94:80–7.
94. Weiss M, Gerber AC. Rapid sequence induction in children – it's not a matter of time! Paediatr Anaesth. 2008;18:97–9.
95. Lerman J. On cricoid pressure: "may the force be with you". Anesth Analg. 2009;109:1363–6.
96. Walker RW, Ravi R, Haylett K. Effect of cricoid force on airway calibre in children: a bronchoscopic assessment. Br J Anaesth. 2010;104:71–4.
97. Dotson K, Kiger J, Carpenter C, Lewis M, Hill J, Raney L, Losek JD. Alignment of cricoid cartilage and esophagus and its potential influence on the effectiveness of Sellick maneuver in children. Pediatr Emerg Care. 2010;26:722–5.
98. Oh J, Lim T, Chee Y, et al. Videographic analysis of glottic view with increasing cricoid pressure force. Ann Emerg Med. 2012;61(4):407–13.
99. Arenkiel B, Smitt M, Olsen KS. The duration of fibre-optic intubation is increased by cricoid pressure. A randomised double-blind study. Acta Anaesthesiol Scan. 2013;57:358–63.
100. Moynihan RJ, Brock-Utne JG, Archer JH, Feld LH, Kreitzman TR. Effect of cricoid pressure on preventing gastric insufflation in infants and children. Anesthesiology. 1993;78:652–6.
101. Landsman I. Cricoid pressure: indications and complications. Pediatr Anaesth. 2004;14:43–7.
102. Mac GP, Ball DR. The effect of cricoid pressure on the cricoid cartilage and vocal cords: an endoscopic study in anaesthetised patients. Anaesthesia. 2000;55:263–8.
103. Heinrich S, Birkholz T, Ihmsen H, et al. Incidence and predictors of difficult laryngoscopy in 11,219 pediatric anesthesia procedures. Pediatr Anesth. 2012;22:729–36.
104. Holzki J, Laschat ML, Puder C. Iatrogenic damage to the pediatric airway, mechanisms and scar development. Pediatr Anesth. 2009;19 Suppl 1:131–46.
105. Wei JL, Bond J. Management and prevention of endotracheal intubation injury in neonates. Curr Opin Otolaryngol Head Neck Surg. 2011;19:474–7.
106. Marston AP, Lander TA, Tibesar RJ, Sidman JD. Airway management for intubation in newborns with Pierre Robin Sequence. Laryngoscope. 2012;122:1401–4.
107. Chung MT, Levi B, Hyun JS, et al. Pierre Robin sequence and Treacher Collins hypoplastic mandible comparison using three-dimensional morphometric analysis. J Craniofacial Surg. 2012;23:1959–63.
108. Sims C, von Ungern-Sternberg BS. The normal and the challenging pediatric airway. Pediatr Anesth. 2012;22:521–6.
109. Hosking J, Zoanetti D, Carlyle A, Anderson P, Costi D. Anesthesia for Treacher Collins syndrome: a review of airway management in 240 pediatric cases. Pediatr Anesth. 2012;22:752–8.
110. Laya BF, Lee EY. Congenital causes of upper airway obstruction pediatric patients: updated imaging techniques and review of imaging findings. Semin Roentgenol. 2012;47:147–58.
111. Wright CT, Goudy SL. Congenital laryngomalacia: symptom duration and need for surgical intervention. Ann Otol Rhinol Laryngol. 2012;131:57–60.
112. Weiss M, Engelhardt T. Proposal for the management of the unexpected difficult pediatric airway. Pediatr Anesth. 2010;20:454–64.
113. Chen YL, Wu KH. Airway management of patients with craniofacial abnormalities: 10-year experience at a teaching hospital in Taiwan. J Chin Med Assoc. 2009;72:468–70.
114. Wrightson F, Soma M, Smith JH. Anesthetic experience of 100 pediatric tracheostomies. Paediatr Anaesth. 2009;19:659–66.
115. Spencer C, Kapila A. Difficult neonatal airway. Paediatr Anaesth. 2010;20:283–4.
116. Brooks P, Ree R, Rosen D, Ansermino M. Canadian pediatric anesthesiologists prefer inhalational anesthesia to manage difficult airways. Can J Anaesth. 2005;52:285–90.
117. Hamilton ND, Hegarty M, Calder A, et al. Does topical lidocaine before tracheal intubation attenuate airway responses in children? An observational audit. Pediatr Anesth. 2012;22:345–50.
118. Chaudhary R, Chonat S, Gowda H, et al. Use of premedications for intubation in tertiary neonatal units in the United Kingdom. Pediatr Anesth. 2009;19:653–8.
119. Kelleher J, Mallya P, Wyllie J. Premedication before intubation in UK neonatal units: a decade of change? Arch Dis Child Fetal Neonatal Ed. 2009;94:F332–5.
120. Kumar P, Denson SE, Mancuso TJ, Committee on Fetus and Newborn, Section on Anesthesiology and Pain Medicine. Clinical

report-premedication for nonemergency endotracheal intubation in the neonate. Pediatrics. 2010;125:608–15.

121. Durrmeyer X, Vutskits L, Anand KJS, Rimensberger PC. Use of analgesic and sedative drugs in the NICU: integrating clinical trials and laboratory data. Pediatr Res. 2010;67:117–27.
122. Shiota M, Oda Y, Taniguchi M, et al. Dexmedetomidine infusion for sedation in the intensive care setting in an infant with airway compromise due to congenital mediastinal neuroblastoma. Pediatr Anesth. 2010;22:581–610.
123. Draskovic B, Uram-Benka A, Kljajic V. Laryngeal mask airway as the only choice for primary airway control in newborn with tracheal stenosis. Med Pregl. 2010;63:275–9.
124. Hackell RS, Held LD, Stricker PA, Fiadjoe JE. Management of the difficult infant airway with the Storz Video Laryngoscope: a case series. Anesth Analg. 2009;109:763–6.
125. Vanderhal AL, Berci G, Simmons CJ, Hagiike M. A videolaryngoscopy technique for the intubation of the newborn: preliminary report. Pediatrics. 2009;124:339–46.
126. Fiadjoe JE, Gurnaney H, Dalesio N, et al. A prospective randomized equivalence trial of the Glidescope Cobalt® video laryngoscope to traditional direct laryngoscopy in neonates and infants. Anesthesiology. 2012;16:622–8.
127. Holm-Knudsen R. The difficult pediatric airway – a review of new devices for indirect laryngoscopy in children younger than two years of age. Pediatr Anesth. 2011;2:98–103.
128. Hirabayashi Y, Shimada N, Nagashima S. Tracheal intubation using pediatric Airtraq optical laryngoscope in a patient with Treacher Collins syndrome. Pediatr Anaesth. 2009;19:915–6.
129. Pean D, Desdoits A, Asehnoune K, Lejus C. Airtraq laryngoscope for intubation in Treacher Collins syndrome. Paediatr Anaesth. 2009;19:698–9.
130. Vlatten A, Soder C. Airtraq optical laryngoscope intubation in a 5-month-old infant with a difficult airway because of Robin Sequence. Paediatr Anaesth. 2009;19:699–700.
131. Xue FS, He N, Liu JH, Liao X, Xu XZ, Zhang YM. More maneuvers to facilitate endotracheal intubation using the Airtraq laryngoscope in children with difficult airways. Paediatr Anaesth. 2009;19:916–8.
132. Hirabayashi Y, Shimada N. Airtraq optical laryngoscope: initial clinical experience in 20 children. J Anesth. 2010;24:148–9.
133. Holm-Knudsen RJ, White J. The Airtraq may not be the solution for infants with difficult airways. Pediatr Anaesth. 2010;20:374–5.
134. Lafrikh A, Didier A, Bordes M, Semjen F, Nouette-Gaulain K. Two consecutive intubations using neonatal Airtraq in an infant with difficult airway. Ann Fr Anesth Reanim. 2010;29: 245–6.
135. Singh R, Singh P, Vajifdar H. A comparison of Truview infant EVO2 laryngoscope with the Miller blade in neonates and infants. Pediatr Anaesth. 2009;19:338–42.
136. Sorbello M, Paratore A, Morello G, Merli G, Belluoccio AA, Petrini F. Bonfils fiberscope: better preoxygenate rather than oxygenate! Anesth Analg. 2009;108:386.
137. Krucylak CP, Schreiner MS. Orotracheal intubation of an infant with hemifacial microsomia using a modified lighted stylet. Anesthesiology. 1992;77:826–7.
138. Cook-Sather SD, Schreiner MS. A simple homemade lighted stylet for neonates and infants: a description and case report of its use in an infant with the Pierre Robin anomalad. Paediatr Anaesth. 1997;7:233–5.
139. Handler SD, Keon TP. Difficult laryngoscopy/intubation: the child with mandibular hypoplasia. Ann Otol Rhinol Laryngol. 1983; 92:401–4.
140. Vlatten A, Aucoin S, Litz S, Macmanus B, Soder C. A comparison of bonfils fiberscope-assisted laryngoscopy and standard direct laryngoscopy in simulated difficult pediatric intubation: a manikin study. Pediatr Anaesth. 2010;20:559–65.
141. Baker P, Mahadevan M. The Bonfils fiberscope is not suitable for neonatal intubation. Paediatr Anaesth. 2009;19:418.
142. Houston G, Bourke P, Wilson G, Engelhardt T. Bonfils intubating fibrescope in normal paediatric airways. Br J Anaesth. 2010;105:546–7.
143. Caruselli M, Zannini R, Giretti R, Rocchi G, Camilletti G, Bechi P, Ventrella F, Pallotto R, Pagni R. Difficult intubation in a small for gestational age newborn by bonfils fiberscope. Paediatr Anaesth. 2008;18:990–1.
144. Biban P, Rugolotto S, Zoppi G. Fiberoptic endotracheal intubation through an ultra-thin bronchoscope with suction channel in a newborn with difficult airway. Anesth Analg. 2000;90:1007.
145. Lesmes C, Siplovich L, Katz Y. Fiberoptic bronchoscopy in children using the laryngeal mask airway. Pediatr Surg Int. 2000;16:179–81.
146. Weiss M, Gerber AC, Schmitz A. Continuous ventilation technique for laryngeal mask airway (LMA) removal after fiberoptic intubation in children. Paediatr Anaesth. 2004;14:936–40.
147. Somri M, Gaitini L, Yanovski B, Tome R, Resnikov I, Karsh K, Shaoul R. Flexible upper videoendoscopy through a modified endoscopy mask in infants and young children. Am J Otolaryngol. 2009;49:191–5.
148. Asai T. Increasing the margin of safety during intubation through the laryngeal mask (a reply to Drs Jagannathan and Sohn). Paediatr Anaesth. 2008;18:983–4.
149. Jagannathan N, Sohn LE. Increasing the margin of safety during tracheal intubation through the laryngeal mask airway in neonates and infants. Paediatr Anaesth. 2008;18:898–9.
150. Hinton AE, O'Connell JM, van Besouw JP, Wyatt ME. Neonatal and paediatric fibre-optic laryngoscopy and bronchoscopy using the laryngeal mask airway. J Laryngol Otol. 1997;111:349–53.
151. Baker PA, Aftimos S, Anderson BJ. Airway management during an EXIT procedure for a fetus with dysgnathia complex. Paediatr Anaesth. 2004;14:781–6.
152. Weiss M, Goldmann K. Caution when using cuffed tracheal tubes for fibreoptic intubation through paediatric-sized laryngeal mask airways. Acta Anaesthesiol Scand. 2004;48:523.
153. Kovatsis PG, Fiadjoe JE, Stricker PA. Simple, reliable replacement of pilot balloons for a variety of clinical situations. Paediatr Anaesth. 2010;20:490–4.
154. Fiadjoe JE, Stricker PA, Kovatsis P, Isserman RS, Harris B, McCloskey JJ. Initial experience with the air-Q as a conduit for fiberoptic tracheal intubation in infants. Pediatr Anaesth. 2010;20:205–6.
155. Cain JM, Mason LJ, Martin RD. Airway management in two of newborns with Pierre Robin Sequence: the use of disposable vs multiple use LMA for fiberoptic intubation. Paediatr Anaesth. 2006;16:1274–6.
156. Asai T, Nagata A, Shingu K. Awake tracheal intubation through the laryngeal mask in neonates with upper airway obstruction. Paediatr Anaesth. 2008;18:77–80.
157. Johnson CM, Sims C. Awake fibreoptic intubation via a laryngeal mask in an infant with Goldenhar's syndrome. Anaesth Intensive Care. 1994;22:194–7.
158. Stricker PA, Budac S, Fiadjoe JE, Rehman MA. Awake laryngeal mask insertion followed by induction of anesthesia in infants with the Pierre Robin sequence. Acta Anaesthesiol Scand. 2008;52:1307–8.
159. Bryan Y, Chwals W, Ovassapian A. Sedation and fiberoptic intubation of a neonate with a cystic hygroma. Acta Anaesthesiol Scand. 2005;49:122–3.
160. Mace SE, Khan N. Needle cricothyrotomy. Emerg Med Clin North Am. 2008; 26: 1085–101, xi
161. Navsa N, Tossel G, Boon JM. Dimensions of the neonatal cricothyroid membrane – how feasible is a surgical cricothyroidotomy? Paediatr Anaesth. 2005;15:402–6.

162. Litman RS, Fiadjoe JE, Strikcer PA, Coté CJ. The pediatric airway. In: Cote CJ, Lerman J, Anderson B, editors. A practice of anesthesia for infants and children. Philadelphia, PA: Elsevier; 2013. Figure 12-23.
163. Skarsgard ED, Chitkara U, Krane EJ, Riley ET, Halamek LP, Dedo HH. The OOPS procedure (operation on placental support): in utero airway management of the fetus with prenatally diagnosed tracheal obstruction. J Pediatr Surg. 1996;31:826–8.
164. Bouchard S, Johnson MP, Flake AW, Howell LJ, Myers LB, Adzick NS, Crombleholme TM. The EXIT procedure: experience and outcome in 31 cases. J Pediatr Surg. 2002;37:418–26.
165. Moldenhauer JS. Ex utero intrapartum therapy. Semin Pediatr Surg. 2013;22:44–9.
166. Skarsgard ED, Meuli M, VanderWall KJ, Bealer JF, Adzick NS, Harrison MR. Fetal endoscopic tracheal occlusion ('Fetendo-PLUG') for congenital diaphragmatic hernia. J Pediatr Surg. 1996;31:1335–8.

Monitoring the Neonate: Basic Science

6

Mario Patino, C. Dean Kurth, and John McAuliffe

The role of the anesthesiologist is to modify consciousness, pain perception, and memory as well as to protect organ function during surgical procedures and critical illness. In order to fulfill this role, we gather information from bedside patient monitors and use this information to make clinical decisions. Monitoring the neonate poses special challenges because of the rapid physiological changes in the first few days of life, poorly defined measures of consciousness, and the physical limitations of small size relative to the size of the monitoring devices. The circumstances that bring a neonate for a surgical procedure involve life- or major organ system-threatening conditions. As a consequence, protection of organ function becomes a major focus.

Data from monitors should not be confused with information from the monitors. In the absence of a context, data can be a meaningless set of numbers; the raw data must be interpreted to produce information. Modern devices acquire streams of data from which useful information is extracted by applying processing algorithms. Nearly all algorithms are based on a set of assumptions in order to achieve computational tractability. The validity of these assumptions under the conditions that the data is gathered determines the usefulness of the information. The clinician evaluating the information should be aware of the capabilities and limitations of the monitoring technologies so that correct interpretations are made, as the information is processed in the context of the illness or surgical procedure to formulate a "diagnosis" and to plan an appropriate treatment in order to achieve the best possible outcome for the patient.

M. Patino, MD • C.D. Kurth, MD (✉)
Department of Anesthesia, Cincinnati Children's Hospital Medical Center, University of Cincinnati College of Medicine, 3333 Burnet Ave, Cincinnati, OH 45229, USA
e-mail: dean.kurth@cchmc.org

J. McAuliffe, MD
Department of Anesthesiology, Division of Neurobiology, Cincinnati Children's Hospital Medical Center, University of Cincinnati College of Medicine, 3333 Burnet Ave, Cincinnati, OH 45229, USA

This chapter focuses on monitoring three major organ systems: the respiratory system, the cardiovascular system, and the nervous system. The array of monitoring technologies is vast; consequently, we will limit the discussion to bedside noninvasive technologies applied in the ICU and the operating room. These noninvasive devices can be classified according to the signals analyzed: optical, electrical, mechanical, acoustic, and chemical. Table 6.1 lists these devices and the systems that can be monitored using them.

Before starting any surgical procedure, it is necessary to determine which organ systems are at risk of injury, the degree of risk, the manifestation of injury, and the impact of injury on the outcome of the operative procedure. This process guides the selection of specific systems to be monitored and the type of monitor to be used. Monitoring is a cognitive exercise in integrating and interpreting information from multiple sources to assign a value of "normal" or "abnormal" to the present functional state and to predict outcome.

The Respiratory System

Neonates have less ability to compensate for impairment in respiratory function than adults. Consequently, continuous monitoring of the respiratory system in neonates during surgery and anesthesia is particularly critical. The main devices to monitor the respiratory system include pulse oximetry, oxygen and carbon dioxide gas analyzers, as well as ventilatory pressure, volume, and rate (apnea) monitors.

Pulse Oximetry: The use of pulse oximetry to measure arterial oxygen saturation in anesthesiology is standard of care. Pulse oximetry relies on the Beer–Lambert law, which relates the concentration of a chromophore to light absorption, optical path length, and extinction coefficient. In pulse oximetry, the chromophores of interest are oxy and deoxyhemoglobin. Because there are two chromophores, two wavelengths in which the extinction coefficient of oxy and deoxyhemoglobin differ are required to determine

J. Lerman (ed.), *Neonatal Anesthesia*, DOI 10.1007/978-1-4419-6041-2_6,

Table 6.1 Organ systems and available noninvasive monitors

Organ system	Optical signals	Electrical signals	Mechanical signals	Acoustic signals	Chemical signals
Central nervous system	NIRS	aEEG EMG ABR SSEP			
Respiratory	Gas analysis	Impedance plethysmography	Peak pressure Tidal volume Minute ventilation	Acoustic flow sensors	$EtCO_2$ FiO_2
Cardiovascular	Pulse oximetry Hb concentration Plethysmography index	ECG Impedance plethysmography	NIBP	Echocardiography	

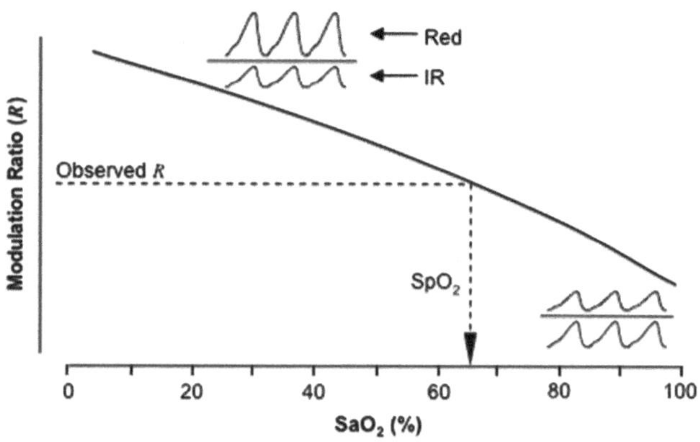

Fig. 6.1 Pulse oximeter SpO_2 is calculated from the empirical relationship between arterial oxygen saturation and R, the absorbance ratio at red and infrared light

oxygen saturation. These are 660 and 940 nm. Neonatal hemoglobin and adult hemoglobin have identical absorption spectrum, and thus pulse oximetry is equally accurate in neonates as in adults. The pulse oximeter calculates oxygen saturation as the ratio of absorbance of the pulsatile optical signal and the non-pulsatile optical signal at two wavelengths, represented by

$$R = (AC_{660} / DC_{660}) / (AC_{940} / DC_{940})$$

where AC is the pulsatile signal and DC is the non-pulsatile signal. The pulse oximeter converts R to oxygen saturation through an empirically derived curve (Fig. 6.1). Of note, the relationship between R and arterial saturation is curvilinear but closely approximates a straight line over a 20 % range in arterial saturation. The calibration curve is constructed by having healthy adults breathe hypoxic gas mixtures and comparing R to CO-oximeter-measured arterial saturation [1]. This calibration curve originates from arterial saturation of 80–100 %; values less than 80 % are extrapolated from the curve and are less accurate because of the curvilinearity (Fig. 6.1). However, it is possible to construct a calibration curve over a different range than 80–100 %; for example, the Masimo "Blue Sensor" is calibrated for the 60–80 % range for use in congenital heart disease.

It is important to distinguish fractional oximetry from functional oximetry. Fractional oximetry calculates the fraction of oxyhemoglobin in relation to the four different species of hemoglobin:

$$\text{Fractional}\,SaO_2 = O_2Hb / (O_2Hb + Hb + MetHb + COHb)$$

Fractional SaO_2 is calculated by pulse CO-oximetry (Masimo Corporation) using at least four different wavelengths. On the other hand, functional oximetry is the saturation determined by traditional pulse oximeters that use only two wavelengths:

$$\text{Functional}\,SpO_2 = O_2Hb / (O_2Hb + Hb)$$

Pulse oximetry suffers from several limitations. Under conditions of hypothermia, vasoconstriction, hypotension, and motion, pulse oximeters are less accurate and less reliable. Advances in signal processing over the years have improved the accuracy and reliability under these conditions, as does placing the sensor on structures closer to the central circulation (e.g., ear lobe, alar nose, and tongue). Polycythemia and anemia do not affect the accuracy of pulse oximetry. During significant hypoxemia, pulse oximeter measurements exceed the actual saturation, although during acute desaturations, the oximeters usually underestimate the actual saturation. During methemoglobinemia, the SpO_2 becomes 85 % regardless of the actual arterial saturation because of the absorbance spectra of methemoglobin relative to hemoglobin. During carbon monoxide exposure, SpO_2 overestimates arterial saturation because oxy- and carboxyhemoglobin absorb red light similarly.

In neonates, pulse oximetry is particularly useful to the monitor preductal and postductal arterial saturation, especially in those predisposed to persistent fetal circulation. A decrease in the postductal SpO_2 compared with preductal SpO_2 of more than 10 % indicates significant pulmonary hypertension and shifts toward fetal circulation. If a right-to-left shunt occurs at the foramen ovale, such a difference would not occur. The preductal and postductal SpO_2 during a PDA closure may serve as a guide to avoid erroneous ligation of other great vessels since the PDA can be larger than the aorta and the left pulmonary artery. In some circumstances, maintenance of the transitional circulation is essential to maintain pulmonary and/or systemic blood flow, such as single ventricle lesions, pulmonary atresia, or transposition of great arteries. Monitoring SpO_2 estimates the ratio between the pulmonary flow and systemic flow (Qp/Qs) and can serve to gauge the balance of pulmonary blood to systemic blood flow.

Monitoring SpO_2 can also track changes in the arterial oxygenation from the fetus to the neonate during the first minutes after birth. During fetal life, normal SpO_2 is approximately 72 %. During the initial hours after birth, there is a rapid and progressive increase in SpO_2 to the mid-90s [2]. Pulse oximetry has also been evaluated as a screening tool for congenital heart disease in the newborn nursery. If SpO_2 does not reach the mid-90s by day two of life, it suggests cyanotic congenital heart disease. Studies have shown pulse oximetry has a specificity of 99 % and a sensitivity of 72 %, superior to a clinical evaluation, to diagnose cyanotic congenital heart disease [3,4]. Oxygen toxicity in preterm infants contributes to development of retinopathy of prematurity, and pulse oximetry is used to maintain SpO_2 between 90 and 94 % to limit this risk. Saturations <90 % reduce the risk of retinopathy of prematurity even further but increase the mortality rate and thus are not recommended [5]. Excessive oxygen administration may also be deleterious during resuscitation [6,7]. During neonatal resuscitation, the American Heart Association recommends monitoring the preductal SpO_2 to titrate the oxygen administration [8].

Inspired and Expired Gas Analysis: Measurement of oxygen, carbon dioxide, and anesthetics remains fundamental to anesthesia practice. Initially these concentrations were measured by mass spectrometry but were replaced by infrared spectrophotometry, as CO_2, N_2O, and inhaled anesthetics have different absorption spectra at 7–13 μm. As with NIRS and pulse oximetry, the concentration of the gases is calculated using the Beer–Lambert law. Oxygen concentration cannot be measured by this technique because it does not absorb infrared light; rather, it is measured by electrochemical or paramagnetic methods.

Expired CO_2 concentration or end-tidal CO_2 ($EtCO_2$) can be plotted against time to show the changes of CO_2 concentration during inspiration and expiration. The continuous measurement of $EtCO_2$ is standard of care in anesthesia practice. Two monitoring systems exist to measure $EtCO_2$: sidestream and mainstream capnography.

Sidestream capnography uses thin tubing connected to the breathing circuit to continuously aspirate gas that flows to a spectrophotometry cell. The flow sampling rates are between 50 and 500 ml/min. In neonates, the high-flow sampling should not be used because it will entrain inspiratory gas leading to an underestimation of the $EtCO_2$ or dramatically decreasing alveolar ventilation if the fresh gas flow is small. Other limitations include water vapor condensation obstructing the tubing, leaks or disconnections at the cell analyzer, and several-second delay from actual to monitored changes in the $EtCO_2$.

Mainstream capnography incorporates the infrared analyzer at the breathing circuit without need for sampling tubing. This results in a more rapid gas analysis. Mainstream capnography offers an advantage in neonates because it eliminates the risks of excessive gas sampling and errors from sampling dead space. However, its disadvantages include the weight of the analyzer kinking the tracheal tube, need for frequent calibration, and water vapor condensation leading to errors and unreliable measurements.

The capnograph provides important clinical information during neonatal anesthesia (Fig. 6.2). The waveform is divided into an inspiratory phase and 3 expiratory phases. The first expiratory phase results from gas in the large airways (anatomical dead space). The second expiratory phase

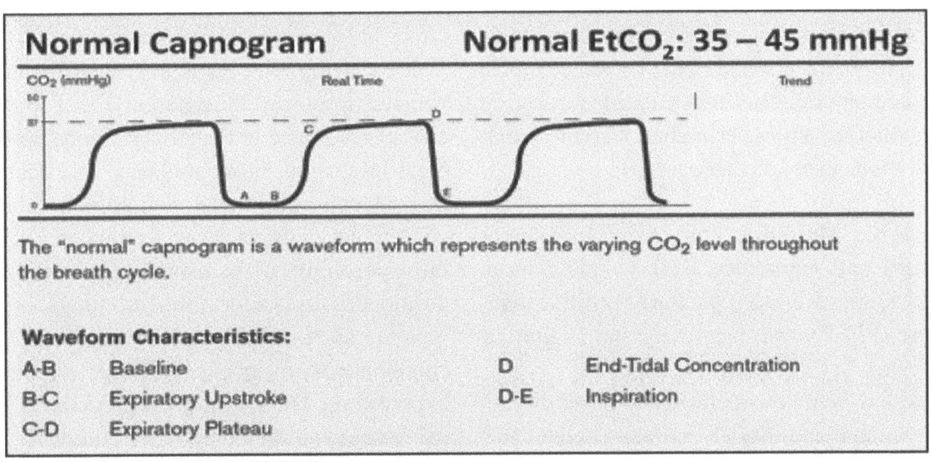

Fig. 6.2 A typical capnogram illustrating the change in carbon dioxide tension during the respiratory cycle

results from the mixed sampling of large airways and alveolar gas (transitional phase). The third expiratory phase results from alveolar gas (plateau phase). During inspiration the $EtCO_2$ rapidly drops to zero. Because of normal physiologic alveolar dead space, a gradient of 1–5 mm Hg normally exists between the $PaCO_2$ and $EtCO_2$. This gradient significantly increases under conditions that increase dead space or decrease cardiac output, which in neonates include right-to-left pulmonary shunt associated with congenital heart disease, meconium aspiration, respiratory distress syndrome, and shock. Also phase III of expiration can change from plateau to an upward slope during conditions of increase alveolar dead space. The $PaCO_2$–$EtCO_2$ gradient should be monitored to gauge pulmonary function. For example, during bronchospasm, the slope of phase III increases from areas of airway obstruction that contain greater CO_2 partial pressures and takes more time to be exhaled.

Apnea Monitors: These monitors are classified based on detection of chest movement (transthoracic impedance), ventilation (capnography), oxygenation (pulse oximetry), or airflow (acoustic). Of the monitors, transthoracic impedance and pulse oximetry are the most popular. Typically, transthoracic impedance is incorporated into ECG monitoring. A small current is transmitted from one ECG pad to another one, and changes in the impedance to this current due to the chest expansion or contraction allow measurement of a respiratory rate. Since transthoracic impedance detects chest movement but not airflow, it misses obstructive apnea, which provides an erroneous respiratory rate. Pulse oximetry is a poor technology to detect apnea because oxygenation changes take time to decrease after the absence of ventilation, especially in neonates who are breathing supplemental oxygen. Capnography as an apnea monitor suffers from unreliability as nasal secretions may obstruct gas sampling to give spurious alarms of apnea. Monitoring the airflow with acoustic sensors located on the neck or chest offers theoretical advantages over transthoracic impedance, capnography, and pulse oximetry. Acoustic apnea monitors sense vibratory sounds produced by turbulent flow in the large airways and converts a sound signal into an electrical signal from which respiratory rate is calculated. Acoustical respiratory rate monitoring has better accuracy and less bias than capnography or impedance technologies [9].

Pulmonary Mechanic Monitors: Pulmonary mechanics includes inspiratory and expiratory tidal volumes, peak inspiratory pressure, mean airway pressure, positive end-expiratory pressure (PEEP), and inspiratory and expiratory cycle time.

Inspiratory tidal gas volume is defined by the setting on the ventilator. Traditional anesthesia ventilators deliver this predetermined volume which can differ substantially from the actual tidal volume, especially in neonates, because of the compliance of the breathing circuit in relation to pulmonary and chest wall compliance and the fresh gas flows. As a result of its unpredictability, mechanical ventilation in neonates historically used a pressure control mode, which is independent of the breathing circuit compliance and of the fresh gas flows [10,11]. However, during pressure mode ventilation, the actual tidal volume varies according to the total compliance and the airway resistance. Thus, tidal volume may suffer if total compliance decreases or airway resistance increases. Examples of such situations include acute pulmonary edema, insertion of chest or abdominal sponges or retractors, or tracheal tube obstruction.

Advances in the anesthesia ventilators have made the delivery of predetermined tidal volumes during volume control ventilation more predictable. These anesthesia machines monitor compliance in the breathing circuit and compensate for it by adjusting the delivered tidal volume, for example, if fresh gas flows or compliance changes. A common circumstance that changes compliance in the breathing circuit is contraction or expansion of the tubing of the breathing circuit. The anesthesia machine tests for compliance as part of the machine check to compensate appropriately for the different circuit compliance. Thus, the compliance test must be done again if the circuit is changed, contracted, or extended. When the tidal volume of contemporary anesthesia ventilators was set to volume control mode in a model of different lung compliances, they found that volume control ventilation could be used in neonatal anesthesia with state-of-the-art ventilators [12]. However, despite these compensatory mechanisms, modern ventilators are unable to compensate for large circuit leaks regardless of the ventilation control mode, volume, or pressure mode. The use of cuffed tracheal tubes eliminates the main source of circuit leaks in neonates.

During a normal breath, the expired tidal volume is less than the inspired tidal volume because of the greater oxygen uptake at the alveolar–capillary membrane compared with the carbon dioxide output from the capillaries into the alveoli. Measurement of expired tidal volume occurs close to the expiratory valve, which tends to overestimate the actual volume.

Monitoring peak inspiratory pressure and tidal volume in neonates provides information about lung compliance and airway resistance to detect conditions such as an endobronchial intubation, bronchospasm, and tracheal tube obstruction. Monitoring these variables also helps to prevent volutrauma or barotrauma during the ventilator support in the operating room, especially in those neonates with pulmonary disease or immature lungs, in whom small tidal volumes and inspiratory pressures decrease the risk of bronchopulmonary dysplasia, a strategy referred to as permissive hypercapnia. During surgical procedures in which substantial changes in the compliance can occur, the peak inspiratory pressure should be modified accordingly to avoid pressure or volume trauma to the lung parenchyma.

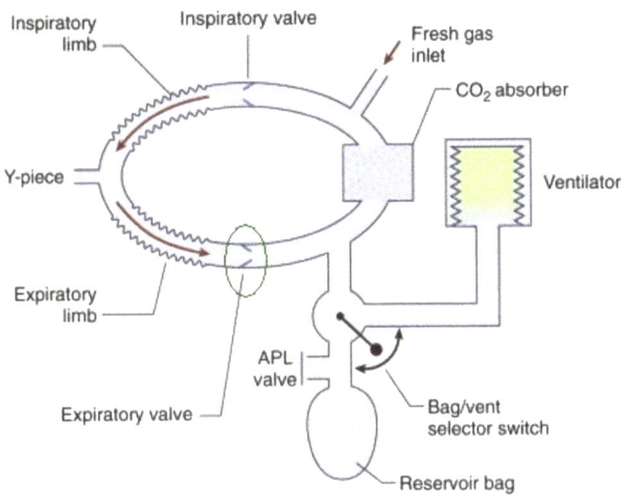

Fig. 6.3 The anesthesia breathing circuit and ventilator and reservoir bag for an anesthesia workstation

The anesthesia circuit incorporates pneumatic or electronic devices to measure airway pressure (Fig. 6.3). The sensor location varies with the anesthesia workstations, ideally closer to the tracheal tube (Y-piece) to increase its reliability. However, this location increases the dead space, along with risks of disconnections or tracheal kinking. Most frequently, the location is close to the expiratory or inspiratory valves. The device incorporates a diaphragm connected to the breathing circuit which changes in diameter according to the airway pressure, activating a pressure relief valve once the selected peak pressure has been reached. It also detects a leak in the system if a minimal threshold pressure is not reached.

The Cardiovascular System

The cardiovascular system delivers substrate to tissue, transports hormones and other message compounds from one organ to another, and removes waste products from the organs. The most easily measured substrate is oxygen, and the most easily measured waste product is carbon dioxide. Quantitative assessment of oxygen delivery requires measurement of cardiac output, oxygen saturation, and hemoglobin concentration. The small size of low- and very-low-birth-weight infants makes use of invasive monitors difficult or impossible and is complicated by the presence of variable shunts which can change over time, making estimates of left ventricular output misleading.

Echocardiography: Acoustic-based technologies have improved dramatically over the last decade. Echocardiography uses both one- and two-dimensional analysis to generate images and superimpose flow information on the image. Color Doppler translates information about flow direction and velocity into a color map and is useful to assess shunts. Doppler measurements are most accurate when the direction of sound wave propagation is directly in line with the direction of blood flow; that is, the insonation angle is zero. The ratio of the observed velocity to the actual velocity is the cosine of the angle of insonation.

The velocity of blood exiting either the left or right ventricle is time dependent. The integral of the velocity–time curve (VTI) can be used to estimate stroke volume if the cross-sectional area is known. Ventricular output is then the product of

$$\text{Output} = \text{HR} \times \text{Area} \times \text{VTI}$$

The cross-sectional area is best measured at right angles to the direction of flow, which necessitates a second window for area measurement. The presence of ductal shunts reduces the usefulness of LV output as a measure of systemic flow. RV output equals venous return in the absence of atrial level shunting or anomalous pulmonary venous return, and as a consequence RV output is a better measure of systemic flow than LV output [13]. Measurement of cross-sectional area of the pulmonary outflow tract requires a significant level of skill and is usually done at the level of the insertion of the pulmonary valve leaflets.

Low-birth-weight infants and infants with significant respiratory compromise are especially prone to low systemic blood flow in the first 24 h of life. The peak velocity in the main pulmonary artery can be measured and is a useful screening tool. Peak PA velocities of greater than 0.45 m/s are unlikely to be associated with low systemic flow states, while peak velocities less than 0.35 m/s have a significant correlation with low systemic flow states [14].

Direct measures of cardiac function in the neonate, especially the preterm neonate, are complicated by the fact that the anterior wall of the LV moves much less than the lateral and posterior walls. Fractional shortening measured using LV anteroposterior diameter will be inaccurate as a consequence. For this reason a short axis view of the LV is used to derive the heart rate-corrected velocity of circumferential fiber shortening (VCF_C). The relationship between VCF_C and LV wall stress has been proposed as a load-independent metric of cardiac performance. The calculation of wall stress requires measuring end-systolic blood pressure, end-systolic posterior LV wall thickness, and end-diastolic LV diameter; two of these parameters must be echo derived. If VCF_C is plotted against LV wall stress, there can be considerable overlap between infants with normal systemic blood flow (SBF) and those with low SBF. However, infants with myocardial dysfunction will have a greater falloff in VCF_C with increases in LV wall stress than infants without myocardial dysfunction [15]. Values greater than 1.0 cirs/s at any wall stress value were almost exclusively associated with the normal SBF group [15]. Thus the absolute value of VCF_C may be a useful screen for poor function, but when measured at two different wall stress values, the slope may be a better measure of function.

Echocardiography displays some limitations, most notable, the presence of an experienced echocardiographer in the neonatal ICU and/or operating room. Consequently there is a need for alternatives that are less dependent on highly trained personnel. One such device is the ultrasound cardiac output monitor (USCOM), a device that measures cardiac output from either right or left ventricle in the neonate. The device (USCOM) has been tested against echocardiographic measures in both term infants with no shunts and a small group of preterm infants. In the term infants both RV and LV outputs were measured using USCOM and echo, while only USCOM-derived output was measured in the preterm infants. In term infants, the USCOM-derived RV output was significantly greater than the echo-derived RV output, while there was better agreement between techniques for LV output [16]. The authors concluded that echo-based measures and USCOM measures were not interchangeable. As in the term infants, the USCOM-measured RV output was significantly greater than the LV output in a group of preterm infants suggesting the device systematically overestimates RV output [17]. In a subsequent publication, Meyer et al. suggested that the USCOM device undergo further controlled clinical trials before its wide application in the neonatal ICU [18].

Oscillometry: Several oscillometry-based noninvasive blood pressure (NIBP) devices exist. Each employs the same principles but utilizes a proprietary algorithm to extract systolic, mean, and diastolic blood pressure from a signal generated by pressure fluctuations in the cuff. The amplitude of the fluctuations varies with cuff pressure. If the amplitude of the fluctuation in cuff pressure is plotted as a function of cuff pressure, the result is an oscillogram. Each oscillogram will have a unique shape and set of inflection points. The algorithms are designed to derive systolic, mean, and diastolic pressure from the data stream contained in the oscillogram.

The oscillometric pulse amplitude results from small pressure changes in the cuff due to the expansion and contraction of blood vessels within the limb encircled by the cuff as blood is ejected into the arterial tree. The diastolic pressure is related to a falloff in the rate of decrease in pulse amplitude once the peak has been achieved, and the systolic pressure is related to the steepest rate of rise of pulse amplitude after a minimum value has been crossed.

Automated noninvasive blood pressure (NIPB) greatly simplified monitoring the neonate in the operating room. There is controversy around the accuracy of NIBP especially in very-low-birth-weight infants at the low end of the blood pressure [19–22], the population most susceptible to periventricular leukomalacia, low cerebral blood flow, and inadequate peripheral perfusion. Studies have shown a systematic overestimation of mean pressure by 3–8 mmHg depending on the device used to measure NIBP [23]. The critical question is "what is the lowest tolerable pressure before target organ failure results," a question not easily answered in the neonate. In one study of extremely low-birth-weight infants, mean arterial pressures below 23 mmHg were clearly associated with cerebral dysfunction [24]. The lower limit of blood pressures generally increases with both gestational and postnatal age; however, the lower limit of cerebral blood flow remains to be established [25].

Pulse CO-oximetry: Advanced pulse oximetry technologies can noninvasively detect hypovolemia, hypoperfusion, and anemia, which are common situations in neonatal surgery. These conditions are difficult to monitor in neonates because insertion of arterial catheters and sampling blood remains challenging in this population.

Advances in optical technologies, especially light emitting diodes (LED), permitted the development of pulse CO-oximetry. Conventional pulse oximetry founded in the 1980s uses two LED at 660 nm and 940 nm, respectively, which were the only commercially available LED at that time. Fortunately, the absorption spectrum of oxy- and deoxyhemoglobin was well differentiated at those wavelengths which permitted the measurement of SpO_2. However, carboxyhemoglobin and methemoglobin were not differentiated, and thus conventional pulse oximetry was unable to determine them or total hemoglobin concentration. In the near red and infrared region, many LED are now commercially available to permit multiwavelength pulse oximetry to measure all hemoglobin species as well as total hemoglobin concentration (SpHb), of which Masimo Corporation has been the leader. In addition, intravascular volume and perfusion status can be monitored through the plethysmograph variability index (PVI) and perfusion index (PI), which analyzes the optical signals in a different way than for hemoglobin concentration and oxygen saturation.

PI and PVI evaluate the interrelation between the cardiovascular and respiratory system to detect hemodynamic changes indicative of circulating blood volume and peripheral perfusion, analogous to respiratory variation in the pulse pressure with ventilation during invasive monitoring of the arterial waveform (Fig. 6.4a). This pulse pressure variation depends on the mode of ventilation because the effects on the venous return, right ventricle afterload, left ventricle end-diastolic pressure, and left ventricle afterload vary during spontaneous inspiration or positive pressure ventilation. This dynamic respiratory variation in arterial pulse pressure and systolic blood pressure is regarded as a sensitive indicator of circulating blood volume and as accurate as central venous pressure and pulmonary artery occlusion pressure.

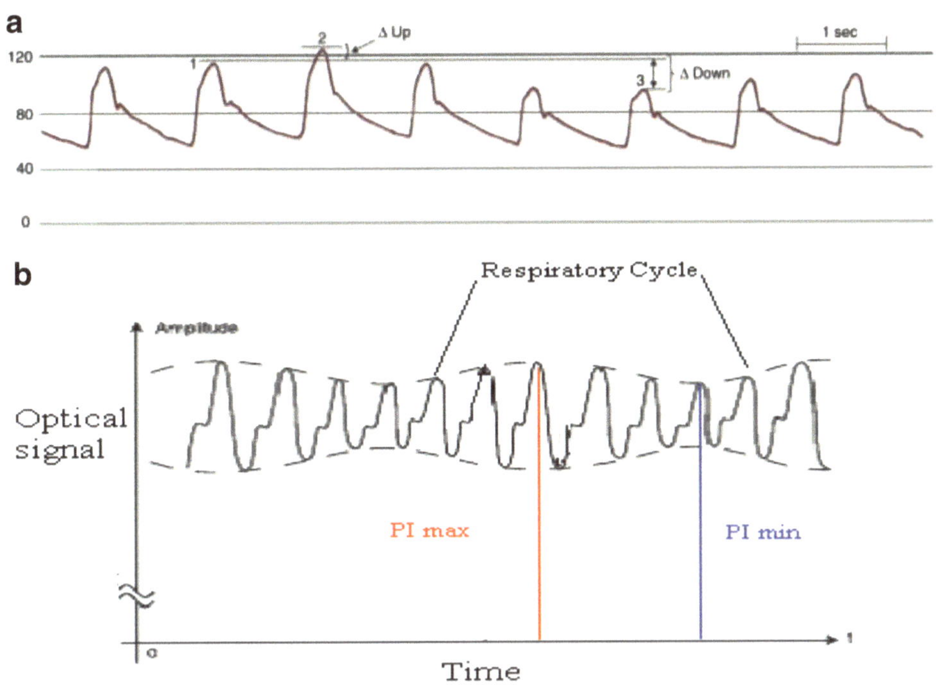

Fig. 6.4 (**a**) Recording from a catheter in the radial artery of a mechanically ventilated adult. During positive pressure ventilation in inspiration, pulmonary flow into the left ventricle increases with a commitment increase in the left ventricular preload and decrease in the left ventricular afterload which in turn increases stroke volume and systolic blood pressure (Δ Up 2). The opposite occurs during expiration (Δ Down 3). Usually this respiratory fluctuation in the systolic blood pressure remains less than 10 mmHg, although it increases with hypovolemia, even though arterial pressure and heart rate remain normal. (**b**) Schematic illustration of PI and PVI. PI is the ratio of the pulsatile optical signal absorbance versus the non-pulsatile optical signal absorbance expressed as a percentage. PVI uses the optical signal variations associated with the respiratory cycle. Note similarity to (**a**)

Pulse index (PI) and the pleth variability index (PVI) are the optical signal components that correlate with the systolic amplitude and the systolic amplitude variation with ventilation, respectively, on the arterial waveform (Fig. 6.4b). The PI is the amplitude difference between the pulsatile and non-pulsatile optical signals and is given as a percentage of the non-pulsatile optical signal which remains constant represented by

$$PI = AC / DC \times 100\%$$

where AC is the amplitude of the alternating pulsatile signal and DC is the amplitude of the direct, non-pulsatile signal. PI directly correlates with the strength of the pulsatile optical signal which correlates with the strength of the manual pulse (Fig. 6.4b). The PI ranges from 0.02 to 20 %, although values above 1 % generally represent normal physiologic conditions. PVI is measured from changes in the PI during a respiratory cycle. PVI is calculated by the difference between the maximum and minimum PI divided by the maximum PI during a respiratory cycle, as shown by

$$PVI = PI\max \quad PI\min / PI\max$$

PVI is given in a percentage (0–100 %), in which higher PVI corresponds to higher pulse oximeter amplitude waveform difference during the respiratory cycle, which correlates with severity of hypovolemia. If hypotension is present, PVI above 12–14 % indicate hypovolemia in which intravenous fluid bolus will improve arterial pressure.

Studies in adults evaluated the clinical utility of PVI. Forget et al. [26] evaluated PVI during general anesthesia for major abdominal surgery, in which fluid management was guided by PVI in one group and not in the other group. The group that received fluid management guided by PVI had decreased blood lactate and received less intravenous crystalloid and total fluids. Canneson et al. [27] showed a good correlation between PVI and respiratory variation of pulse pressure from the invasive arterial waveform. Desebbe et al. [28] found that PVI predicted the hemodynamic changes of positive end-expiratory pressure in mechanically ventilated adults. The use of PVI in spontaneous ventilation is less clear. Keller et al. [29] showed that PVI can detect hemodynamic changes during spontaneous ventilation with passive leg raising. However, PVI did not predict response to fluid bolus for hypotension in spontaneously breathing adults.

Studies in neonates suggest that PI has clinical utility. PI immediately after birth predicted the development of chorioamnionitis, a condition associated with significant morbidity and mortality. PI had a 93.7 % positive predictive value and 100 % negative predictive value in identifying subclinical chorioamnionitis; early detection of chorioamnionitis enabled early treatment which decreased disease severity and admission to a neonatal critical care unit [30]. Similarly, PI has been evaluated to predict the severity of illness for other conditions in neonates [31]. There was an excellent correlation between the PI and the Score for Neonatal Acute Physiology with a 91.2 % positive predictive value and 96.8 % negative predictive value.

Pulse CO-oximetry detects changes in the hemoglobin concentration during surgery earlier than conventional blood draw-based laboratory measurements, decreases the number of blood samples drawn, and guides blood transfusion decisions [32]. Like conventional pulse oximetry, erroneous measurements occur during severe hyperbilirubinemia and the presence of intravascular dyes such as methylene blue. The accuracy of SpHb in healthy adult volunteers undergoing hemodilution showed a bias between SpHb and blood drawn tHb that was less than 2 g/dl for 97 % of all measurements [33]. More recently, the accuracy of SpHb in adults undergoing spine surgery showed the bias between SpHb and tHb was <2 g/dl in 77 % of patients [34]. In pediatrics, the bias and precision of SpHb compared with laboratory blood measurements were 0.9 g/dl and 1.5 g/dl, respectively [35]. An initial in vivo correction after the first measurement improved the accuracy, as SpHb trend was more accurate than absolute measurement of hemoglobin concentration. Advances in the development of sensor size will soon bring this technology for use during neonatal surgery.

The Nervous System

The neonate poses special challenges to neurological monitoring because the immaturity of the nervous system limits the extent of functional information gained by monitoring. However, the future development of the nervous system depends on protecting it during critical illness and detecting and correcting situations that may compromise its well-being. Monitoring the nervous system requires a multimodal approach including electrical activity, oxygenation, and blood flow.

EEG and Amplitude-Integrated EEG (aEEG): The use of EEG in the neonatal intensive care unit has a long history. Due to the small size of the infant's head, the standard montages used in adults were simplified to include recordings from 9 electrodes instead of 21. The neonatal EEG varies considerably with gestational and postnatal age. A developmental glossary of EEG in premature and full-term infant was recently published [36] and the changes were summarized [37] (Fig. 6.5). Given its complexity, interpretation of the neonatal EEG requires an experienced technician and a neurologist, which effectively limit monitoring to only a few hours a day. Amplitude-based EEG was developed in the late 1960s as an alternative tool that provided continuous EEG monitoring that could be used at the bedside by a trained nurse and a non-neurologist clinician.

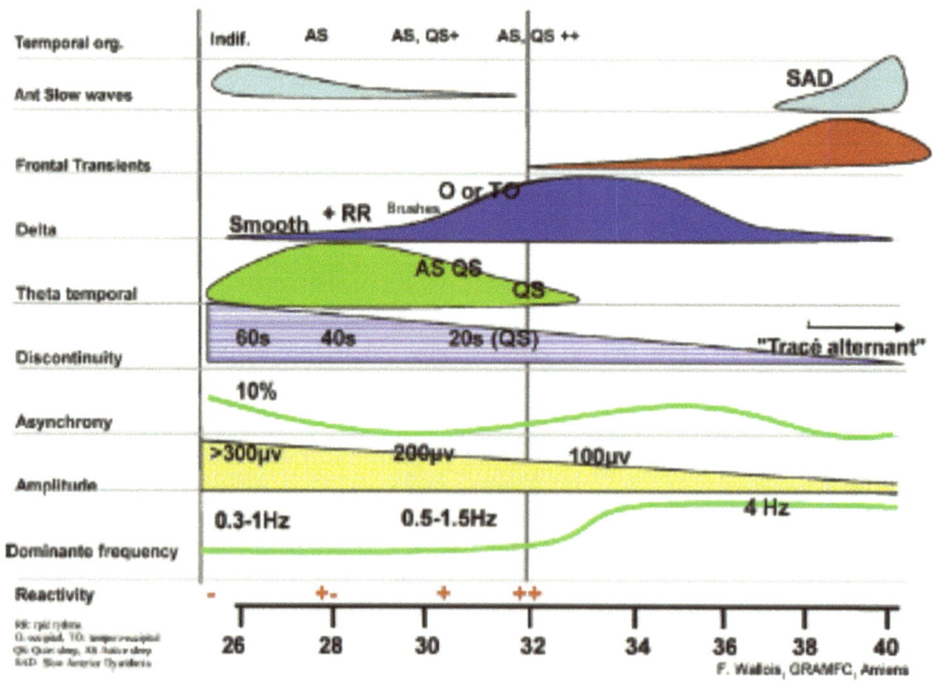

Fig. 6.5 Characteristic changes in EEG during the first few months of life from premature to term infant

The cerebral function monitor, a device using amplitude-based EEG, was originally developed and studied as a tool to predict outcome following cardiac arrest in adults [38,39]. Since the publication of a reference atlas of an EEG in infants in 2003 [40], aEEG has gained popularity in both Europe and North America, as it was found to provide continuous cerebral activity information with minimal interference with care.

The aEEG relies on signals from either a single pair ($P_3 \rightarrow P_4$) of electrodes or two pairs ($C_3 \rightarrow P_3$, $C_4 \rightarrow P_4$). The central–parietal areas are preferred for monitoring the neonate as these areas are at risk for hypoperfusion from vascular watershed phenomenon. Frontal locations are not recommended for two-channel monitoring as this area is electrophysiologically underdeveloped, and seizure activity may not propagate to the frontal region [41].

The aEEG device is portable and designed for ease of use [41,42]. The signal from the electrodes is amplified, filtered (2–15 Hz band pass), rectified, and presented as a peak-to-peak voltage. By filtering out signal frequencies in excess of 15 Hz, interference from muscle activity and electrical devices is eliminated. Filtering out frequencies less than 2 Hz removes low-frequency delta waves. Many algorithms give greater weight to alpha than theta or delta waves although the predominant frequencies present in the premature neonatal EEG are in the delta and theta range. Alpha and beta emerge after 34 weeks of gestation. The aEEG is displayed at slow speeds to reveal trends. Raw EEG can be displayed on screen so that rapid changes such as seizure activity can be seen (Fig. 6.6) [41].

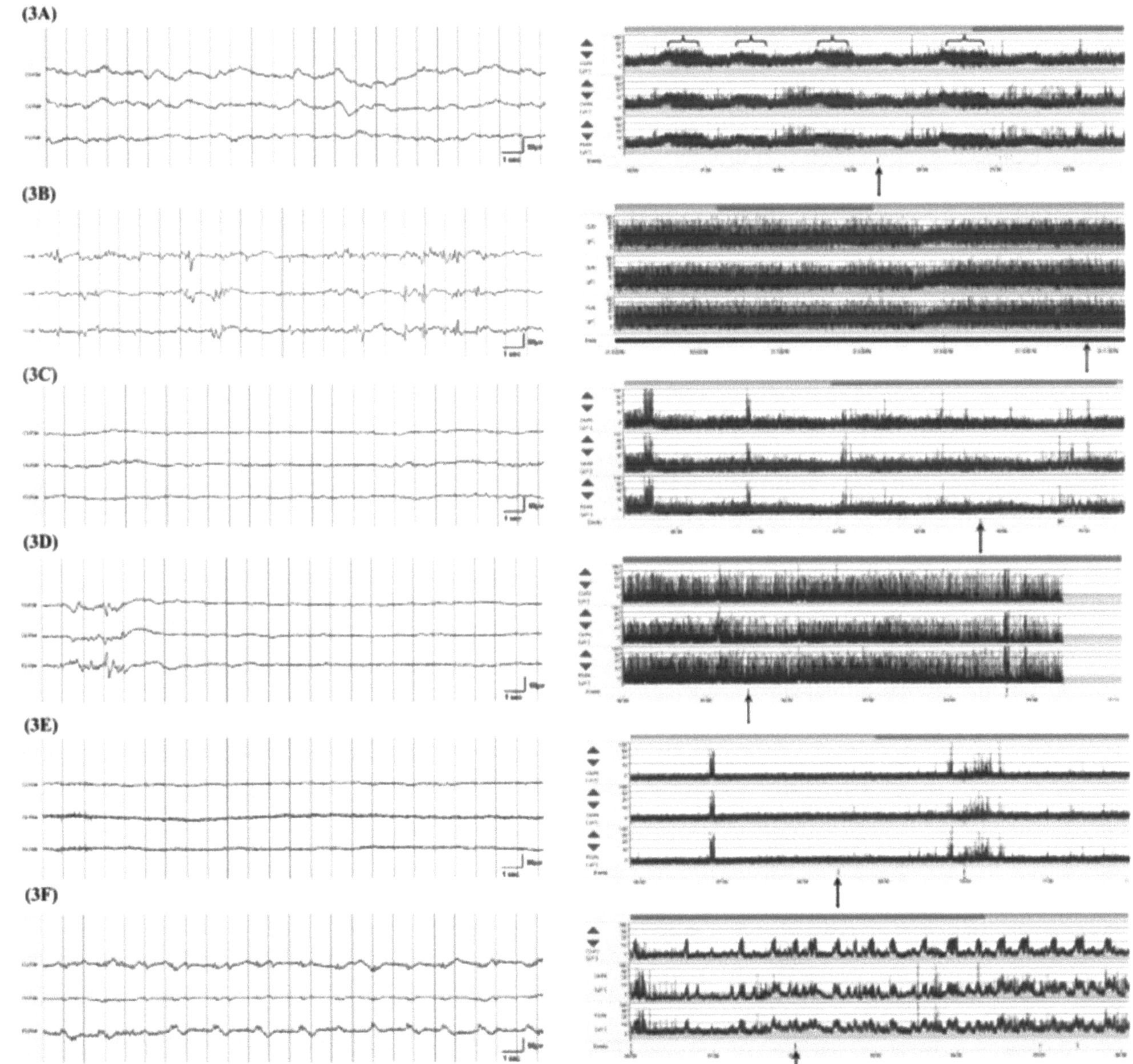

Fig. 6.6 Amplitude EEG patterns during various conditions: a normal aEEG trace (**a**) and a series of abnormal traces including discontinuous activity (**b**), low amplitude (**c**), burst suppression (**d**), flat trace with ECG artifact (**e**), and seizures (**f**)

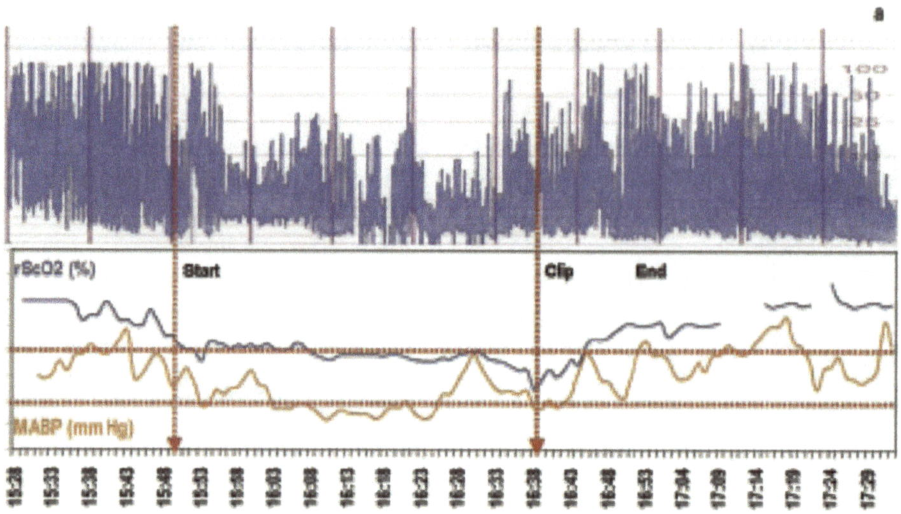

Fig. 6.7 Amplitude EEG, near-infrared spectroscopy, and arterial pressure recordings during neonatal patent ductus ligation

The aEEG displays an upper and lower voltage band. A normal aEEG has a lower voltage greater than 5 μV and an upper value greater than 10 μV [43]. An aEEG trace with a lower band <5 μV and the upper >10 μV is moderately abnormal; the combination of lower band <5 μV and upper band <10 μV is defined as suppressed [43]. An abnormal or suppressed aEEG, when present many hours after birth asphyxia, is very predictive (>70 %) for death or neurological disability [43–45].

Changes in aEEG voltages occur with decreased cerebral perfusion or decreased cerebral metabolism. For example, aEEG amplitude decrements lasting 10–20 minutes were noted in infants given surfactant who experienced a decrease in mean blood pressure and increased pulmonary shunting [46,47]. Decreased aEEG voltages were also noted in a subgroup of infants undergoing ductus ligation under anesthesia who manifested decreases in mean blood pressure and decreases in the NIRS-measured S_cO_2 (see Fig. 6.7) [48].

Amplitude-integrated EEG patterns are related to cerebral perfusion from the first day of life, in both very premature infants and term infants with congenital heart disease [49,50]. The relationship between aEEG and blood pressure is less clear as abnormal aEEG patterns may not manifest in some infants until mean arterial pressure is less than 23 mmHg [24]. aEEG is not adversely affected by mild hypothermia [52]. Collectively, the data suggest that aEEG may be a useful monitor of the adequacy of cerebral perfusion under conditions present in the operating room. However, aEEG output must be scrutinized for artifact by examining the raw EEG as electrical interference and ECG artifact can contaminate the traces [52]. If measures are taken to minimize interference from electrical noise, the aEEG can be a valuable monitor in the operating room.

Neonatal hypoxia–ischemia induces significant changes in the coupling between cerebral perfusion, metabolism, and electrical activity [53]. The aEEG pattern (normal, moderately abnormal, suppressed) correlates with changes in cerebral blood flow and metabolism. Abnormal aEEG is also associated with reduced oxygen consumption in the presence of high cerebral oxygen saturations (e.g., low fractional oxygen extraction) in afterbirth asphyxia [45]. Thorngren-Jerneck et al. showed that abnormal aEEG patterns after neonatal H-I were associated with decreased glucose utilization as measured by positron emission tomography, while normal aEEG patterns were associated with normal glucose utilization [54]. Cooling is frequently instituted as a means of reducing the likelihood of long-term injury in infants who experience hypoxia–ischemia. Abnormal aEEG patterns do not portend a poor neurological outcome in the presence of cooling unless these patterns persist for more than 36 h [55].

Near-Infrared Spectroscopy: Near-infrared spectroscopy (NIRS) is an optical technology based on the relative transparency of biological tissues to near-infrared light (700–900 nm) where oxygen binding chromophores, hemoglobin, and cytochrome oxidase have distinct absorption spectra. Although it is theoretically possible for NIRS to determine the oxygenation of blood and the cell through hemoglobin and cytochrome oxidase, measurement of cytochrome oxidase distinct from hemoglobin has proven difficult in most circumstances. Thus, application of NIRS in the clinical setting has focused on monitoring hemoglobin oxygenation.

NIRS-determined hemoglobin saturation differs from that of pulse oximetry in several respects. First, NIRS interrogates hemoglobin mainly in small vessels (arterioles, capillaries, and venules) to provide a mixed vascular oxygen saturation of the gas-exchanging circulation, whereas pulse oximetry assesses hemoglobin in the arterial circulation. Thus, NIRS cerebral saturation (ScO_2) in normal conditions is 60–80 % because of the dominance of venous blood in the tissue circulation. During cardiac arrest, ScO_2 decreases as brain tissue consumes oxygen, while arterial saturation remains constant or not measurable during the pulseless state. Second, NIRS views the large, total signal of photons passing through the tissue to derive ScO_2, whereas pulse oximetry selects the tiny portion of photons passing through the arteries as a pulse-gated signal to calculate SpO_2. Consequently, pulse oximetry fails during poor perfusion when the pulse signal is extremely weak, whereas NIRS does not suffer from this limitation. Finally, NIRS ScO_2 reflects the balance between oxygen delivery (blood flow, hemoglobin concentration, and arterial saturation) and metabolism (oxygen consumption) and function of the tissue, whereas SpO_2 reflects a component of oxygen delivery and function of the lungs. Thus, a decrease in ScO_2may originate from decreased cerebral blood flow, decreased arterial saturation, decreased blood hemoglobin concentration, or increased cerebral oxygen metabolism, although usually it originates from decreased cerebral blood flow or arterial saturation. As such, combining pulse oximetry with NIRS enables the bedside diagnosis of a pulmonary or cerebral blood flow problem and the institution of appropriate therapy.

It is also possible to measure cerebral blood flow using NIRS and the Fick equation in which oxyhemoglobin or indocyanine green is employed as the tracer. Oxyhemoglobin can become a tracer if the inspired oxygen concentration is increased by an amount sufficient to increase arterial saturation by at least 5 % over 6 s [56,57]. Figure 6.8 illustrates NIRS measurement of oxyhemoglobin, deoxyhemoglobin, and total hemoglobin as oxygen concentration is abruptly increased, from which cerebral blood flow is calculated. Similarly, NIRS can measure cerebral blood flow by rapidly injecting intravenously indocyanine green, an FDA-approved compound strongly absorbing at 800 nm, as the tracer instead of oxyhemoglobin.

Recent advances in theoretical physics and optical technologies improved the capability of NIRS to measure ScO_2. Before 2008, NIRS devices that measured absolute ScO_2were only research oriented and not commercially viable, and the commercially available NIRS devices could only measure trends in ScO_2 not absolute ScO_2values. Currently, Somanetics, CASMED, and Nonin manufacture FDA-approved NIRS devices for neonates that can determine the absolute ScO_2. Evidence suggests these sensors correlate closely although the absolute ScO_2 may differ by as much as 10–15 %, which may complicate the interpretation of clinical studies [58].

What are the critical ScO_2 values that diagnose cerebral hypoxia–ischemia and predict brain damage? In neonatal pigs, cerebral function begins to deteriorate when the ScO_2 decreases to <45 %, noted by slowing of EEG and accumulation of tissue lactate. As ScO_2 decreases to less than 35 %, cerebral energy failure occurs, expressed by loss of tissue ATP and isoelectric EEG [59]. Given normal values for the ScO_2 of 60–80 %, a buffer zone of approximately 15 % exists during which ScO_2 may decrease before brain function begins to change [60,61]. The risk of brain damage is known to depend on the severity and duration of the hypoxic–ischemic insult. For insults producing isoelectric EEG and loss of ATP, less than thirty minutes of hypoxia–ischemia will inflict brain damage. Consequently, insults that decrease the ScO_2 to <35 % require intervention within 30 min to reverse the insult. For insults that cause a ScO_2 between 35 and 45 %, the brain will not exhibit evidence of damage for the first two hours of hypoxia–ischemia, but thereafter, the risk of brain damage increases 15 % for each hour of hypoxia–ischemia [62]. Studies in neonates in the intensive care unit after congenital heart surgery suggest that the risk of brain injury increases after three hours at ScO_2<45 % [63,64]. Thus, interventions are warranted for ScO_2values 35–45 % within 2–3 h of onset.

The most common application of NIRS to neonatal anesthesia has been in congenital heart surgery, and in many centers, it has become standard of care to monitor brain and somatic oxygen saturation. After balloon septostomy for transposition of the great arteries, NIRS showed significant improvement in ScO_2 compared with the group that did not undergo septostomy by 24 h [65]. In critically ill neonates before and after surgery, NIRS is applied on the head and flank or abdomen to determine ScO_2, SkO_2 (kidney), SlO_2 (liver), or SgO_2 (gut) to guide ICU treatments or timing of surgery. Treatments to increase ScO_2 depend on the type of cardiac malformation. For hypoplastic left heart syndrome and other similar physiologies, the following will increase ScO_2: decrease in cerebral oxygen metabolism; administration of inotropes, blood transfusion, or fluid bolus to increase arterial pressure and cardiac output; hypoventilation or ventilation with carbon dioxide to increase arterial PCO_2, cerebral blood flow, and cardiac output; and ventilation with hypoxic gas to decrease pulmonary blood flow and increase cardiac output [66–68]. Administration of oxygen can increase or decrease ScO_2, depending on the malformation and physiology. For example, with hypoplastic left heart syndrome, increasing the FiO_2 increases the SaO_2 to potentially increase ScO_2, whereas increasing the FiO_2 decreases the cardiac output and cerebral blood flow to decrease the ScO_2.

NIRS has also been employed during surgery to guide anesthesia and surgical management. Before and after cardiopulmonary bypass, the anesthesiologist uses NIRS to

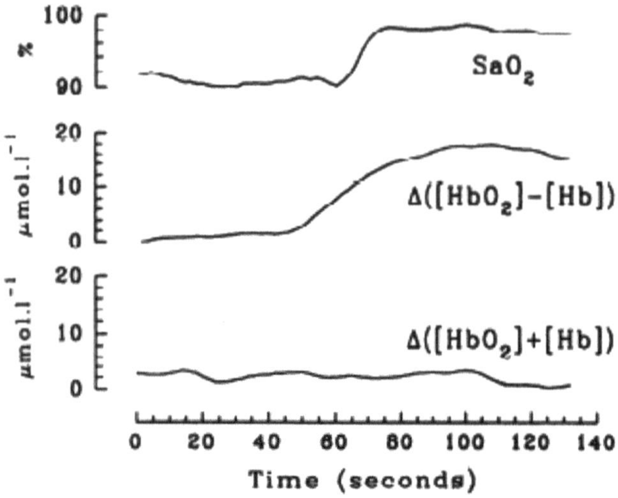

Fig. 6.8 Near-infrared spectroscopy to calculate cerebral blood flow. Inspired oxygen concentration is abruptly increased to raise arterial saturation by 5 %, which induces an increase in tissue oxyhemoglobin concentration detected by NIRS. Application of the Fick equation using oxyhemoglobin as the tracer enables the calculation of cerebral blood flow

diagnose brain and somatic hypoperfusion and ischemia and guide therapies to restore tissue oxygenation, similar to that in the ICU [61,67]. During surgery, NIRS displays characteristic changes that can be used to monitor the brain during cardiopulmonary bypass (CPB) [68,69]. With the institution of CPB, NIRS may be used to verify proper cannula placement as ScO_2 should not decrease [70]. During CPB cooling, ScO_2 should increase to >90 % to reflect brain hypothermia. During hypothermic selective cerebral perfusion or low-flow CPB, ScO_2 should not decrease substantially [71. During reperfusion after deep hypothermic circulatory arrest or selective cerebral perfusion, ScO_2 should increase >80 % to indicate cerebral recirculation. If NIRS does not achieve these values during these situations, the anesthetic and surgical team should search for a reason.

NIRS has also been used as a guide during neonatal resuscitation [72] and in the neonatal ICU to guide resuscitation during circulatory failure, ventilator management during respiratory distress syndrome [73], and extracorporeal membrane oxygenation for respiratory insufficiency from diaphragmatic hernia [52].

Transcranial Doppler: When sound waves are reflected from a moving object, the reflected wave is shifted in frequency from the incident wave; the frequency shift depends on the velocity of the object. If the object is moving toward the sound source, the frequency shift is higher; if the object is moving away from the source, the shift is lower. The frequency shift is also called the Doppler shift after Christian Doppler who described this phenomenon in 1842. Three types of Doppler systems are in use: pulsed wave, continuous wave, and color Doppler. Pulsed wave Doppler allows the user to measure particle velocity up to a limit within a specified region of interest. Continuous wave Doppler has no velocity limit but lacks spatial resolution; the measured velocity is the maximum velocity over the entire beam path. Color Doppler translates information about flow direction and velocity into a color map. Doppler measurements are most accurate when the ultrasound beam is directly in line with the moving particles. The measured velocity falls off as the cosine of the angle between the beam and the vector describing the moving particle path.

Both continuous wave and color Doppler instruments have been used to measure cerebral blood flow velocity in the middle cerebral artery. The continuous wave devices suffer from lack of spatial specificity that can be achieved with pulsed color Doppler techniques. The quality of the measurement can be further improved by obtaining grayscale images so that the insonation angle can be determined exactly. Ultrasound measures of middle cerebral artery blood flow are useful for detection of severe cerebral hypoperfusion in infants at risk for hypotension or large ductal shunts, as retrograde or poor diastolic flow is seen in the large arteries near the circle of Willis in these cases [74]. Normative data for cerebral blood flow velocity in "healthy" preterm neonates has been published [75]. In non-hypotensive neonates, both systolic and diastolic cerebral blood flow velocity increases as a function of postnatal and post-conceptual age [75].

Conversion of velocity to flow requires knowledge of arterial cross-sectional area. This measurement is not easily made and is subject to inaccuracies. However, radiographic data suggests that vessel diameter is relatively constant over short periods of time so that changes in velocity are likely to represent real changes in flow. Practical limitations of space and access to desirable insonation points make application of this modality for estimating cerebral blood flow difficult in the OR environment. There are numerous reports examining the value of Doppler-measured cerebral blood flow before, during, and after cardiopulmonary bypass in neonates [76]. In the setting of selective cerebral perfusion, low-flow cardiopulmonary bypass, and deep hypothermic arrest, transcranial Doppler has been used to detect cerebral hypoperfusion and can guide pump flow rate and surgical and anesthetic therapies intended to prevent cerebral ischemia [76].

Neurophysiological Monitors: During certain surgical procedures, it is desirable to monitor the spinal cord and peripheral nerve function. This is done by measuring the conduction of sensory information from the peripheral nerves to the sensory cortex and assessing the conduction of motor information from the cortex to the skeletal musculature and the functional state of motor axons from nerve roots to muscle. The monitoring modalities are somatosensory evoked potentials (SSEPs), transcranial motor evoked

Table 6.2 SSEP latencies as a function of gestation and age

Gestation/age	Myelination status of pathways	"N12" latency (ms)	"N 20" latency (ms)
32 weeks	ML–PM TCP–UM		68–72
40 weeks	ML–PM TCP–UM/PM		33–38
6 months	ML–PM TCP–PM	6	18
12 months	ML–FM TCP–PM	6	15.5
3 years	ML–FM TCP–FM	6	15
Adult	ML–FM TCP–FM	13	20–21

ML medial lemniscus
TCP thalamocortical projections
UM unmyelinated
PM partially myelinated
FM fully myelinated

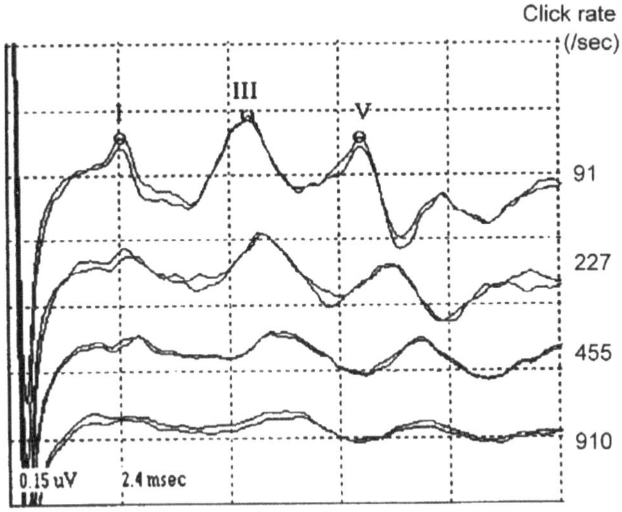

Fig. 6.9 Auditory evoked potential in a premature neonate. ABR from 8-week-old to 32-week-gestation infant at various click rates

potentials (TcMEPs), and electromyography (EMG). These three modalities are used routinely during surgical procedures such as spinal fusion, complex tethered cord releases, and cerebellopontine angle tumor resections. In our experience, one or more of these modalities may prove useful in selected neonatal procedures.

It is possible to record somatosensory evoked potentials (SSEPs) after median nerve [77] and posterior tibial nerve stimulation [78] in preterm and term infants in the awake or lightly sedated state. Neonatal and infant median nerve SSEPs have different morphology and peak latencies compared with adult median nerve SSEPs (Table 6.2). The difference is the result of degree of myelination and other structural differences between the neonatal and the adult peripheral and central nervous systems [79]. In the neonatal ICU setting, both median nerve and posterior tibial nerve SSEPs have prognostic significance for future neurocognitive outcomes in preterm neonates after asphyxia [80,81]. The cortical SSEP signal is easily obliterated by anesthesia and/or deep sedation in the neonate. However, subcortical recording from Erb's point and the posterior neck is more resistant to anesthetic effects and is of interest when the brachial plexus is at risk of injury. Signals from these structures have been recorded and normative data for the expected latencies published [82]. In our experience, a propofol–remifentanil-based technique produces the least suppression of neurophysiologic signals.

The auditory system of the neonate can be monitored using auditory brainstem responses (ABRs) otherwise called brainstem auditory evoked responses. ABRs are similar to SSEPs in that a nerve (the cochlear nerve) and far-field potentials are recorded. ABRs are obtained by presenting a series of clicks in one ear and a masking noise in the opposite ear and recording potentials using electrodes placed at each mastoid and one at the vertex of the head. In order to generate an ABR, the recording must be time locked to the stimulus, filtered, amplified many times, and signal averaged as ABRs have very low amplitude (0.1–0.3 μV), which would be easily overwhelmed by the much higher amplitude EEG signal without special processing.

The ABR from a conscious patient is composed of waves that make up the short, middle, and long latency components of the response. The short-latency responses, called waves I–V, are of interest because they are not easily degraded by sedation and anesthesia. The putative anatomic origin of waves I, III, and V [83] as well as the latency of each wave for different ages [84]. The structures responsible for the generation of ABR waves I–V are supplied by branches of the basilar–vertebral system; consequently, the ABR is very sensitive to brainstem ischemia or hypoperfusion [83].

Recognizable and reproducible ipsilateral ABRs can be detected in preterm infants beginning at about 30–32 weeks' gestation (Fig. 6.9). Reproducing waveforms can be detected on the contralateral side by 34 weeks' gestation. The appearance of wave V on the contralateral side is important, as identification of ABR waves (peaks) is typically done by identifying wave V first and working backwards to identify the other waves. In children and adults wave V is frequently most clearly seen on the contralateral side as auditory pathways cross the midline at the level of the inferior olivary complex. The neural activation triggered by the clicks used in ABR acquisition travels both ipsilateral and crossed pathways. Recently the optimal click rate to assess neurodevelopmental outcomes with the ABR in premature infants 34 weeks postmenstrual age was determined to be 29.9/s [85].

The amplitude of the component waves increases with gestational age, and the latencies to waves I, III, and V decrease with gestational age [86]. Analyzing the ABR in premature

Table 6.3 ABR: change in wave I, II, and V latency with age and wave generators

Gestation/age	Wave I latency (ms)	Wave III latency (ms)	Wave V latency (ms)
32 weeks	1.6±0.23	4.37±0.27	6.75±0.44
40 weeks	1.6±0.23	4.30±0.25	6.63±0.39
6 months	1.6±0.23	4.06±0.19	6.17±0.27
12 months	1.6±0.23	3.91±0.17	5.91±0.21
3 years	1.6±0.23	3.78±0.16	5.66±0.19
Adult	1.6±0.23	3.78±0.15	5.66±0.17
Generators	Distal cochlear nerve	Olivary complex	Contralateral inferior colliculus

infants is particularly challenging, although the characteristics of the developing ABR in infants as young as 26 weeks' gestation have been reported recently [87]. The greatest change in latencies and amplitudes comes after birth. Latencies reach adult values by about 2–3 years of age (Table 6.3), and ABR wave amplitudes reach their maximum at 4 years of age and decline slightly to adult values thereafter [84]. ABR wave amplitude is also sensitive to the rate at which the click stimuli are presented [83]. Infants will maintain ABR wave amplitude at higher stimulus rates than adults [86].

ABRs are frequently used to monitor the eighth cranial nerve (CN VIII) and brainstem during neurosurgical procedures involving the cerebellopontine angle and posterior fossa tumor resections. Traction on CN VIII and changes in blood flow to CN VIII or the cochlear nucleus will affect waves I and II significantly but may also result in loss or amplitude reduction of all other waves as well. Ischemia in the area of the lateral lemniscus or inferior colliculus will affect wave V. A decrease in amplitude of 50 % or more or change in latency of wave V by more than 1 msec may be a sign of brainstem hypoperfusion or incipient ischemia. The ABR is also sensitive to temperature and latency increases of about 7 % for each 1 °C temperature drop; at 26 °C the latencies are double those at 37 °C [88]. ABR amplitude may initially increase as temperature fall, but hypothermia can obliterate the ABR at 20 °C [38,88,89].

Special equipment and trained personnel are required for intraoperative interpretation of ABRs. The acquisition time for a single ABR can be on the order of 3–4 min in order to achieve a reasonable signal-to-noise ratio. However, when available, this modality can provide useful information about the adequacy of brainstem perfusion and auditory pathway function (to the level of the inferior colliculus). All latency changes must be interpreted in the context of estimated brain temperature. Volatile agents, without nitrous oxide, can be used when acquiring ABRs as they are very resistant to anesthesia [90].

Motor evoked potentials are generated by electrically stimulating the motor cortex, either transcranially or directly, and recording compound muscle action potentials (CMAPs) from various muscle groups. The generation of CMAPs is dependent on multiple motor neurons innervating a muscle firing in or nearly in synchrony. In order to achieve firing threshold, individual spinal motor neurons must receive a synchronized descending volley of impulses via the corticospinal tract (CST). The conduction velocity of the axons making up the CST of the neonate are much slower and have a large variance compared to the adult CST, resulting in temporal dispersion of descending signals [91,92]. In addition, direct corticospinal to motor neuron synaptic connections are rare in the neonate and increase with age [93]. Under the influence of anesthesia, the motor neurons in a neonate never simultaneously achieve firing threshold in sufficient numbers to record a CMAP following transcranial stimulation. Special stimulation protocols have been devised to partially overcome some of these limitations enabling motor evoked potentials to be recorded in infants as young as 2 months post term [94,95]. For reasons cited above, the MEPs of very young infants are exquisitely sensitive to anesthesia; thus we employ a propofol–remifentanil-based technique whenever we wish to obtain MEPS for surgical procedures around the spinal cord [90].

Another useful modality for monitoring the integrity of the nervous system is electromyography (EMG). EMG monitors spontaneous muscle activity or stimulated activity. In spontaneous EMG, mechanical or thermal irritation of motor nerves can result in release of neurotransmitter at the myoneural junction to yield a muscle action potential. The number of muscle action potentials recorded is a function of the rate of change of the mechanical or thermal stimulus [96]. Rapid warming from electrocautery use, sudden traction, or mechanical trauma can cause a volley of neural discharges that manifests as a burst or train of EMG activity. Conversely, slowly applied mechanical traction does not always result in spontaneous EMG activity, thus stimulated EMG can be used to test nerves at risk of injury.

In stimulated EMG, the surgeon applies an electrical current and looks for a response from one or more muscle groups innervated by a given nerve root. The recording of a CMAP at a low-threshold current indicates the structure is a nerve. Motor nerve roots can be stimulated to produce a muscle action potentials at very low current levels (<1 mA); the threshold for mixed nerves may be higher (up to 4 mA). During dissection around nerves fibers or roots, stimulation thresholds can provide guidance as to the distance between the nerves and the site of dissection or inform the surgeon that functional neural tissue is present. EMG is unaffected by choice of anesthetic agents as long as neuromuscular blocking agents are not used. The surgeon may opt to use spontaneous and stimulated EMG recording in an attempt to preserve nerve roots during certain surgical procedures.

In the neonate, EMG monitoring is used during the resection of tumors and other malformations that involve the spine including tethered cord and lipomeningomyelocele, when preservation of neurologic function is expected.

References

1. Mannheimer PD. The light-tissue interaction of pulse oximetry. Anesth Analg. 2007;105:S10–17.
2. Brouillette RT, Waxman DH. Evaluation of the newborn's blood gas status. National academy of clinical biochemistry. Clin Chem. 1997;43:215–21.
3. Valmari P. Should pulse oximetry be used to screen for congenital heart disease? Arch Dis Child Fetal Neonatal Ed. 2007;92:F219–24.
4. Arlettaz R, Bauschatz AS, Monkhoff M, Essers B, Bauersfeld U. The contribution of pulse oximetry to the early detection of congenital heart disease in newborns. Eur J Pediatr. 2006;165:94–8.
5. The BOOST II United Kingdom, Australia, and New Zealand Collaborative Groups. Oxygen saturation and outcomes in preterm infants. NEJM. 2013;368:2094–104.
6. Rabi Y, Rabi D, Yee W. Room air resuscitation of the depressed newborn: a systematic review and meta-analysis. Resuscitation. 2007;72:353–63.
7. Saugstad OD, Sejersted Y, Solberg R, Wollen EJ, Bjoras M. Oxygenation of the newborn: a molecular approach. Neonatology. 2012;101:1315–25.
8. Kattwinkel J, Perlman JM, Aziz K, et al. Neonatal resuscitation: 2010 American heart association guidelines for cardiopulmonary resuscitation and emergency cardiovascular care. Pediatrics. 2010;126:e1400–13.
9. Ramsay MAE, Usman M, Lagow E, et al. The accuracy, precision and reliability of measuring ventilatory rate and detecting ventilatory pause by rainbow acoustic monitoring and capnometry. Anesth Analg. 2013;117:69–75.
10. Tobin MJ, Stevenson GW, Horn BJ, Chen EH, Hall SC, Cote CJ. A comparison of three modes of ventilation with the use of an adult circle system in an infant lung model. Anesth Analg. 1998;87:766–71.
11. Stayer SA, Bent ST, Skjonsby BS, Frolov A, Andropoulos DB. Pressure control ventilation: three anesthesia ventilators compared using an infant lung model. Anesth Analg. 2000;91: 1145–50.
12. Bachiller PR, McDonough JM, Feldman JM. Do new anesthesia ventilators deliver small tidal volumes accurately during volume-controlled ventilation? Anesth Analg. 2008;106:1392–400.
13. Evans N. Functional echocardiography in the neonatal intensive care unit. In: Kleinman C, Seri I, Polin R, editors. Hemodynamics and cardiology neonatology: questions and controversies. Philadelphia, PA: Saunders Elsevier; 2008.
14. Evans N. Which inotrope for which baby? Arch Dis Child Fetal Neonatal Ed. 2006;91(3):F213–20.
15. Osborn DA, Evans N, et al. Left ventricular contractility in extremely premature infants in the first day and response to inotropes. Pediatr Res. 2007;61(3):335–40.
16. Patel N, Dodsworth M, et al. Cardiac output measurement in newborn infants using the ultrasonic cardiac output monitor: an assessment of agreement with conventional echocardiography, repeatability and new user experience. Arch Dis Child Fetal Neonatal Ed. 2011;96(3):F206–11.
17. Meyer S, Todd D, et al. Assessment of portable continuous wave Doppler ultrasound (ultrasonic cardiac output monitor) for cardiac output measurements in neonates. J Paediatr Child Health. 2009;45(7–8):464–8.
18. Meyer S, Todd D, et al. Non-invasive cardiac output monitoring in neonates. Arch Dis Child Fetal Neonatal Ed. 2010;95(6):F464.
19. Dannevig I, Dale HC, et al. Blood pressure in the neonate: three non-invasive oscillometric pressure monitors compared with invasively measured blood pressure. Acta Paediatr. 2005;94(2):191–6.
20. Weindling AM, Bentham J. Blood pressure in the neonate. Acta Paediatr. 2005;94(2):138–40.
21. Meyer S, Sander J, et al. Agreement of invasive versus non-invasive blood pressure in preterm neonates is not dependent on birth weight or gestational age. J Paediatr Child Health. 2010;46(5):249–54.
22. Konig K, Casalaz DM, Burke EJ, Watkins A. Accuracy of non-invasive blood pressure monitoring in very preterm infants. Intens Care Med. 2012;38:670.
23. O'Shea J, Dempsey EM. A comparison of blood pressure measurements in newborns. Am J Perinatol. 2009;26(2):113–16.
24. Victor S, Marson AG, et al. Relationship between blood pressure, cerebral electrical activity, cerebral fractional oxygen extraction, and peripheral blood flow in very low birth weight newborn infants. Pediatr Res. 2006;59(2):314–19.
25. Greisen G. Autoregulation of vital and nonvital organ blood flow in the preterm and term neonate. In: Kleinman C, Seri I, Polin R, editors. Hemodynamics and cardiology neonatology: questions and controversies. Philadelphia, PA: Saunders Elsevier; 2008.
26. Forget P, Lois F, et al. Goal-directed fluid management based on the pulse oximeter-derived pleth variability index reduces lactate levels and improves fluid management. Anesth Analg. 2010;111(4):910–14.
27. Cannesson M, Delannoy B, et al. Does the Pleth variability index indicate the respiratory-induced variation in the plethysmogram and arterial pressure waveforms? Anesth Analg. 2008; 106(4):1189–94.
28. Desebbe O, Boucau C, et al. The ability of pleth variability index to predict the hemodynamic effects of positive end-expiratory pressure in mechanically ventilated patients under general anesthesia. Anesth Analg. 2010;110(3):792–8.
29. Keller G, Cassar E, et al. Ability of pleth variability index to detect hemodynamic changes induced by passive leg raising in spontaneously breathing volunteers. Crit Care. 2008;12(2):R37.
30. De Felice C, Del Vecchio A, et al. Early postnatal changes in the perfusion index in term newborns with subclinical chorioamnionitis. Arch Dis Child Fetal Neonatal Ed. 2005;90(5):F411–14.
31. De Felice C, Latini G, et al. The pulse oximeter perfusion index as a predictor for high illness severity in neonates. Eur J Pediatr. 2002;161(10):561–2.
32. Jung et al 2013
33. Macknet MR, Allard M, et al. The accuracy of noninvasive and continuous total hemoglobin measurement by pulse CO-Oximetry in human subjects undergoing hemodilution. Anesth Analg. 2010;111(6):1424–6.
34. Miller RD, Ward TAB, et al. A comparison of three methods of hemoglobin monitoring in patients undergoing spine surgery. Anesth Analg. 2011;112(4):858–63.
35. Jou F, Wesseler JB, et al. Absolute and trend accuracy of continuous and noninvasive hemoglobin in pediatric surgery patients. Presented at annual society for pediatric anesthesia meeting; 2011.
36. Andre M, Lamblin MD, et al. Electroencephalography in premature and full term infants. Developmental features and glossary. Neurophysiol Clin. 2010;40(2):59–124.
37. Wallois F. Synopsis of maturation of specific features in EEG of premature neonates. Neurophysiol Clin. 2010;40(2):125–6.
38. Maynard D, Prior PF, et al. A continuous monitoring device for cerebral activity. Electroencephalogr Clin Neurophysiol. 1969; 27(7):672–3.

39. Maynard D, Prior PF, et al. Device for continuous monitoring of cerebral activity in resuscitated patients. Br Med. 1969;J4(5682):545–6.
40. Hellstrom-Westas L, de Vries LS, et al. An atlas of amplitude-integrated EEGs in the newborn. London: Parthenon Publishing; 2003.
41. El-Dib M, Chang T, et al. Amplitude-integrated electroencephalography in neonates. Pediatr Neurol. 2009;41(5):315–26.
42. Hellstrom-Westas L, Rosen I, et al. Amplitude-integrated electroencephalogram and cerebral injury. Pediatrics. 2003;112(4):1001–2. author reply 1001-1002.
43. al Naqeeb N, Edwards AD, et al. Assessment of neonatal encephalopathy by amplitude-integrated electroencephalography. Pediatrics. 1999;103(6 Pt 1):1263–71.
44. Shalak LF, Laptook AR, et al. Amplitude-integrated electroencephalography coupled with an early neurologic examination enhances prediction of term infants at risk for persistent encephalopathy. Pediatrics. 2003;111(2):351–7.
45. Toet MC, Lemmers PM, et al. Cerebral oxygenation and electrical activity after birth asphyxia: their relation to outcome. Pediatrics. 2006;117(2):333–9.
46. Hellstrom-Westas L, Bell AH, et al. Cerebroelectrical depression following surfactant treatment in preterm neonates. Pediatrics. 1992;89(4 Pt 1):643–7.
47. Skov L, Hellstrom-Westas L, et al. Acute changes in cerebral oxygenation and cerebral blood volume in preterm infants during surfactant treatment. Neuropediatrics. 1992;23(3):126–30.
48. Lemmers PM, Molenschot MC, et al. Is cerebral oxygen supply compromised in preterm infants undergoing surgical closure for patent ductus arteriosus? Arch Dis Child Fetal Neonatal Ed. 2010;95(6):F429–34.
49. West CR, Groves AM, et al. Early low cardiac output is associated with compromised electroencephalographic activity in very preterm infants. Pediatr Res. 2006;59(4 Pt 1):610–15.
50. ter Horst HJ, Mud M, et al. Amplitude integrated electroencephalographic activity in infants with congenital heart disease before surgery. Early Hum Dev. 2010;86(12):759–64.
51. Horan M, Azzopardi D, et al. Lack of influence of mild hypothermia on amplitude integrated-electroencephalography in neonates receiving extracorporeal membrane oxygenation. Early Hum Dev. 2007;83(2):69–75.
52. Toet MC, Lemmers PM. Brain monitoring in neonates. Early Hum Dev. 2009;85(2):77–84.
53. Ioroi T, Peeters-Scholte C, et al. Changes in cerebral haemodynamics, regional oxygen saturation and amplitude-integrated continuous EEG during hypoxia-ischaemia and reperfusion in newborn piglets. Exp Brain Res. 2002;144(2):172–7.
54. Thorngren-Jerneck K, Hellstrom-Westas L, et al. Cerebral glucose metabolism and early EEG/aEEG in term newborn infants with hypoxic-ischemic encephalopathy. Pediatr Res. 2003;54(6):854–60.
55. Hallberg B, Grossmann K, et al. The prognostic value of early aEEG in asphyxiated infants undergoing systemic hypothermia treatment. Acta Paediatr. 2010;99(4):531–6.
56. Edwards AD, Wyatt JS, et al. Cotside measurement of cerebral blood flow in ill newborn infants by near infrared spectroscopy. Lancet. 1988;2(8614):770–1.
57. Yoxall CW, Weindling AM. Measurement of cerebral oxygen consumption in the human neonate using near infrared spectroscopy: cerebral oxygen consumption increases with advancing gestational age. Pediatr Res. 1998;44(3):283–90.
58. Dix LM, van Bel F, Baerts W, Lemmers PM. Comparing near infrared spectroscopy devices and their sensors for monitoring regional cerebral oxygen saturation in the neonates. Pediatr Res. 2013. doi: 10.1038/pr (Epub ahead of print).
59. Kurth CD, Levy WJ, McCann J. Near infrared spectroscopy cerebral oxygen saturation thresholds for cerebral hypoxia ischemia in piglets. J Cereb Blood Flow Metab. 2002;22:335–41.
60. Bernal NP, Hoffman GM, Ghanayem NS, Arca MJ. Cerebral and somatic near infrared spectroscopy in normal newborns. J Pediatr Surg. 2010;45(6):1306–10.
61. Kurth CD, Steven JL, Montenegro LM, Gaynor JW, Spray TL, Nicolson SC. Cerebral oxygen saturation before congenital heart surgery. Ann Thorac Surg. 2001;72:187–92.
62. Kurth CD, McCann J, Wu J, Miles LL, Loepke AW. Cerebral oxygen saturation-time thresholds for cerebral hypoxia-ischemia injury in piglets. Anesth Analg. 2009;108(4):1268–77.
63. Dent CL, Spaeth JP, Jones BV, Schwartz SM, Glauser TA, Hallinan B, Pearl JM, Khoury PR, Brain KCD, MRI. Abnormalities following the Norwood procedure using regional cerebral perfusion. J Thorac Cardiovasc Surg. 2005;130:1523–30.
64. Kussman BD, Wypij D, Laussen PC, Soul JS, Bellinger DC, DiNardo JA, Robertson R, Pigula FA, Jonas RA, Newburger JW. Relationship of intraoperative cerebral oxygen saturation to neurodevelopmental outcome and brain magnetic resonance imaging at 1 year of age in infants undergoing biventricular repair. Circulation. 2010;122(3):245–54.
65. van der Laan ME, Verhagen EA, Bos AF, et al. Effect of balloon atrial septostomy on cerebral oxygenation in neonates with transposition of the great arteries. Pediatr Res. 2013;73:627.
66. Ramamoorthy C, Tabbutt S, Kurth CD, Steven JM, Montenegro LM, Durning S, Wernovsky G, Gaynor WJ, Spray TL, Nicolson SC. Effects of inspired hypoxic and hypercapnic gas mixture cerebral oxygen saturation in neonates with univentricular heart defects. Anesthesiology. 2002;96:283–8.
67. Hoffman GM, Stuth EA, Jaquiss RD, Vanderwal PL, Staudt SR, Troshynski TJ, Ghanayem NS, Tweddell JS. Changes in cerebral and somatic oxygenation during stage 1 palliation of hypoplastic left heart syndrome using continuous regional cerebral perfusion. J Thorac Cardiovasc Surg. 2004; 127(1):223–33.
68. Kurth CD, Steven JM, Nicolson SC, Jacobs ML. Cerebral oxygenation during cardiopulmonary bypass in children. J Thorac Cardiovasc Surg. 1997;113:71–9.
69. Kurth CD, Steven JM, Nicolson SC. Cerebral oxygenation during pediatric cardiac surgery using deep hypothermic circulatory arrest. Anesthesiology. 1995;82:74–82.
70. Gottlieb EA, Fraser Jr CD, Andropoulos DB, Diaz LK. Bilateral monitoring of cerebral oxygen saturation results in recognition of aortic cannula malposition during pediatric congenital heart surgery. Paediatr Anaesth. 2006;16(7):787–9.
71. Andropoulos DB, Stayer SA, McKenzie ED, Fraser Jr CD. Regional low-flow perfusion provides comparable blood flow and oxygenation to both cerebral hemispheres during neonatal aortic arch reconstruction. J Thorac Cardiovasc Surg. 2003;126(6):1712–17.
72. Fuchs H, Lindner W, Buschko A, et al. Brain oxygenation monitoring I during neonatal resuscitation of very low birth weight infants. J Perinatol. 2012;32:356–62.
73. Milan A, Freato F, Vanzo V, et al. Influence of ventilation mode on neonatal cerebral blood flow and volume. Early Hum Dev. 2009;85:415–19.
74. Deeg KH, Rupprecht T. Pulsed Doppler sonographic measurement of normal values for the flow velocities in the intracranial arteries of healthy newborns. Pediatr Radiol. 1989;19(2):71–8.
75. Romagnoli C, Giannantonio C, et al. Neonatal color Doppler US study: normal values of cerebral blood flow velocities in preterm infants in the first month of life. Ultrasound Med Biol. 2006;32(3): 321–31.

76. Polito A, Ricci Z, et al. Cerebral blood flow during cardiopulmonary bypass in pediatric cardiac surgery: the role of transcranial Doppler–a systematic review of the literature. Cardiovasc Ultrasound. 2006;4:47.
77. Smit BJ, de Visser BWO, et al. Somatosensory evoked potentials in very preterm infants. Clin Neurophysiol. 2000;111(5):901–8.
78. Pike AA, Marlow N, et al. Posterior tibial somatosensory evoked potentials in very preterm infants. Early Hum Dev. 1997;47(1):71–84.
79. Gilmore R. Somatosensory evoked potentials in pediatrics – normal. In: Holmes G, Moshe S, Jones H, editors. Clinical neurophysiology of infancy, childhood, and adolescence. Philadelphia, PA: Butterworth Heinemann Elsevier; 2006.
80. Harbord MG, Weston PF. Somatosensory evoked potentials predict neurologic outcome in full-term neonates with asphyxia. J Paediatr Child Health. 1995;31(2):148–51.
81. Pike AA, Marlow N. The role of cortical evoked responses in predicting neuromotor outcome in very preterm infants. Early Hum Dev. 2000;57(2):123–35.
82. Boor R, Goebel B. Maturation of near-field and far-field somatosensory evoked potentials after median nerve stimulation in children under 4 years of age. Clin Neurophysiol. 2000;111(6):1070–81.
83. Møller A. Intraoperative neurophysiological monitoring. Totowa, NJ: Humana Press; 2006.
84. Salamy A. Maturation of the auditory brainstem response from birth through early childhood. J Clin Neurophysiol. 1984;1(3):293–329.
85. Amin SB, Orlando M. Optimum click rate for neurodevelopmental evaluation using auditory brainstem response in premature infants. Am J Perinatol. 2012;29:587–92.
86. Yin R, Wilkinson AR, et al. No close correlation between brainstem auditory function and peripheral auditory threshold in preterm infants at term age. Clin Neurophysiol. 2008;119(4):791–5.
87. Coenraad S, Toll MS, Hoeve HL, Goedegebure A. Auditory brainstem response morphology and analysis in very preterm neonatal intensive care unit infants. Laryngoscope. 2011;121:2245–9.
88. Markand ON, Lee BI, et al. Effects of hypothermia on brainstem auditory evoked potentials in humans. Ann Neurol. 1987;22(4):507–13.
89. Hett DA, Smith DC, et al. Effect of temperature and cardiopulmonary bypass on the auditory evoked response. Br J Anaesth. 1995;75(3):293–6.
90. Francis L, Mohamed M, Patino M, McAuliffe J. Intraoperative neuromonitoring in pediatric surgery. Int Anesthesiol Clin. 2012;50:130–43.
91. Olivier E, Edgley SA, et al. An electrophysiological study of the postnatal development of the corticospinal system in the macaque monkey. J Neurosci. 1997;17(1):267–76.
92. Szelenyi A, de Camargo AB, et al. Neurophysiological evaluation of the corticospinal tract by D-wave recordings in young children. Childs Nerv Syst. 2003;19(1):30–4.
93. Armand J, Olivier E, et al. Postnatal development of corticospinal projections from motor cortex to the cervical enlargement in the macaque monkey. J Neurosci. 1997;17(1):251–66.
94. Journee HL, Polak HE, et al. Conditioning stimulation techniques for enhancement of transcranially elicited evoked motor responses. Neurophysiol Clin. 2007;37(6):423–30.
95. Fulkerson DH, Satyan KB, Wilder LM, et al. Intraoperative monitoring of motor evoked potentials in very young children. J Neurosurg Pediatr. 2011;7:331–7.
96. Julian FJ, Goldman DE. The effects of mechanical stimulation on some electrical properties of axons. J Gen Physiol. 1962;46:297–313.

Further Readings

Tweddell JS, Ghanayem NS, Mussatto KA, et al. Mixed venous oxygen saturation monitoring after stage 1 palliation for hypoplastic left heart syndrome. Ann Thorac Surg. 2007;84:1301–10. discussion 10-1.

Munir S, Guilcher A, et al. Peripheral augmentation index defines the relationship between central and peripheral pulse pressure. Hypertension. 2008;51(1):112–18.

O'Rourke MF, Pauca AL. Augmentation of the aortic and central arterial pressure waveform. Blood Press Monit. 2004;9(4):179–85.

Weindling M, Paize F. Peripheral haemodynamics in newborns: best practice guidelines. Early Hum Dev. 2010;86(3):159–65.

Yoxall CW, Weindling AM, et al. Measurement of cerebral venous oxyhemoglobin saturation in children by near-infrared spectroscopy and partial jugular venous occlusion. Pediatr Res. 1995;38(3):319–23.

Monitoring the Neonate: Practical Considerations

7

David J. Steward

Comprehensive, accurate, timely, and absolutely reliable monitoring is an essential objective for the safe and successful management of the surgical neonate. The achievement of this objective is complicated by two main factors:

1. The small size of the patient increases the difficulty in the application of all types of instrumentation, especially that of vascular access. In addition, the small patient is frequently completely covered during surgery and out of sight or easy reach by the anesthesiologist. Thus, visual observation of the neonate is impossible, leaving the anesthesiologist totally dependent upon the applied monitors. All monitoring lines, probes, or catheters must be functioning perfectly before surgery commences and be protected against any possible compromise intraoperatively such as from pressure from a surgeon's arm. Sampling respiratory gases or blood is also complicated by the small blood volumes that may be sampled from the neonate.
2. The extremely dynamic physiology of the neonate may result in very rapid changes in important parameters. Monitoring systems must be capable of responding instantly to these changes and alerting the anesthesiologist promptly.

This chapter describes and discusses methods for perioperative monitoring of the cardiorespiratory, neurological, and metabolic state of the neonate. The monitors described vary from the simple and noninvasive to the complex and invasive. The selection of the extent of monitoring required for any individual patient will depend upon the severity of the surgical illness and the proposed surgery.

D.J. Steward, MBBS, FRCPC (✉)
Department of Anaesthesia, University of British Columbia, 217 – 2176 Health Sciences Mall, Vancouver, BC, Canada, V6T 1Z3
e-mail: davidjsteward@comcast.net

Cardiorespiratory Monitoring

Historically, the basic monitor for the cardiorespiratory systems has been the stethoscope, either chest wall or esophageal. This is less frequently used today since the introduction of arterial oxygen saturation and end-tidal CO_2 ($EtCO_2$) monitoring but may still be very useful to detect specific conditions and should be applied whenever feasible. A stethoscope is particularly useful as an immediate warning in cases when surgical manipulations may suddenly kink major airways, as in operation for tracheoesophageal fistula. A precordial stethoscope applied to the left chest may also provide early evidence of tracheal tube that migrates endobronchially while positioning the infant. It may also be useful to monitor heart sounds during surgery and might provide other information, e.g., a clue to successful or unsuccessful closure of a persistent ductus arteriosus during thoracoscopic surgery [1]. It is also quite indispensible should other monitors fail. The esophageal stethoscope is a relatively benign instrument, although minor esophageal injuries and complications have been reported [2]. It may cause airway obstruction in infants with vascular ring, even with an endotracheal tube in place. The use of an esophageal stethoscope might result in the esophagus being confused with the trachea during neck operations, and its use should always be communicated to the surgeon [3]. Esophageal stethoscopes often include thermistors to monitor temperature; positioning the stethoscope where the heart sounds are loudest ensures a retrocardiac position of the bulb and central temperature monitoring.

Arterial Hemoglobin Oxygen Saturation Monitoring

Pulse oximetry was introduced in the 1980s and rapidly became an indispensible aid to the management of the neonate in the perioperative period. The pulse oximeter

J. Lerman (ed.), *Neonatal Anesthesia*, DOI 10.1007/978-1-4419-6041-2_7,

probe consists of two light emitting diodes (LEDs) producing respectively red and infrared light with a semiconductor as a detector. The cyclical changes in the absorption of these two wavelengths during arterial pulsations are recorded, and their ratio is derived using an internal algorithm. Optimally the LEDs and the detector should be placed exactly opposite each other with 5–10 mm of intervening tissue. Low readings may occur if the components of the probe are not exactly aligned [4]. In the neonate, the probe is commonly placed across the palm of the hand or foot but also may be applied to the ear lobe, cheek, or tongue [5]. Pulse oximeters vary in their performance but most claim an accuracy of ±2–4 % or less with saturations above 80 %. At low saturations, pulse oximeters are much less accurate. Hence during profound desaturations, they cannot be relied upon. It is also important to realize that the top portion of the oxyhemoglobin desaturation curve is flat; hence at high saturations relatively large changes in arterial pO_2 occur with only minor changes in saturation. Thus, there has been continuing difficulty in defining a "safe" target saturation for the preterm infant in order to avoid the consequences of hyperoxia [6–8]. Different models of pulse oximeter vary in their response time to physiological changes in the patient [9]. In general, those more recent models with "signal extraction technology (SET)" have faster response times.

The pulse oximeter is extremely useful in neonates because desaturation occurs most frequently in this age group [10], but the oximeter is subject to interference from several factors. Motion artifact is usually not a problem during anesthesia but may be significant during the induction and recovery phases. When this may be a problem, the use of models with SET technology (e.g., Masimo) is preferred [9]. A strong external light source may affect the oximeter's performance. The probe should be covered to exclude extraneous light and protected by a rigid frame to prevent pressure on the sensor. In low perfusion states the signals may not be adequate for interpretation, and no result will be displayed; again later model machines with SET may perform better under these conditions. The performance of the pulse oximeter is not affected by changes in the hematocrit, anemia, or bilirubinemia. However in bronze baby syndrome which may occur after phototherapy, SpO_2 readings become unreliable [11]. Dark skin pigmentation also may cause falsely low readings especially at lower levels of saturation (<80 %) [5]. False high readings may occur in the presence of carboxyhemoglobin. Significant levels of methemoglobin bias the reading toward 85 % [5].

In neonatal anesthesia practice it is often advantageous to place two separate pulse oximeter probes on the patient. In some cases it may be desired to monitor both pre-ductal (R arm or head) and post-ductal saturation, and in others the second probe may act simply as a back-up reference [12].

Complications have been reported from the application of oximeter sensors. When applying sensors circumferentially to the finger, caution must be exercised to avoid too tight an application, which might cause injury [13]. When a reusable clip-type sensor is used on the ear, care should be taken to ensure that the clip does not exert excessive pressure [14].

Blood Pressure Monitoring

The basic noninvasive equipment to measure blood pressure is the blood pressure cuff. It is suggested that the width of the cuff used should be 0.44–0.55 × the midpoint circumference of the limb utilized; thus the optimal width in the full-term neonate is approximately 1 in. [15]. In the operating room, the most accurate determination of the systolic pressure can be obtained by placing a Doppler flow probe on an artery distal to the cuff [15]. Measurements taken with an automated oscillometric devices tend to overestimate systolic and mean blood pressures, especially when the neonate is hypotensive [16]. More recent evidence suggests that the greatest discrepancy in noninvasive blood pressures between upper and lower extremities occurred in the smallest infants (<1,000 g) [17]. These devices should not be relied upon in sick infants or those requiring extensive surgery. In healthy infants, blood pressure measurements taken with a cuff applied to the upper and lower extremities are normally similar.

Direct measurement of blood pressure using an intra-arterial line is often required in all critically ill neonates and those requiring major surgery. Arterial lines may be inserted at various sites, and each has advantages and potential disadvantages.

The umbilical artery is relatively easy to access in the immediate neonatal period and has been widely used in neonatal intensive care units. However, serious thromboembolic complications may follow and involve intra-abdominal organs, the lower limbs, and even the spinal cord [18]. Caution should be exercised in the choice of catheter material and design and the fluids administered. Silicon rubber catheters with an end hole are the preferred type of catheters. Hypertonic and alkaline solutions should be avoided. The use of heparin in the infusate may decrease the incidence of line occlusion but does not reduce the incidence of thromboembolism [19]. When managing an infant with an umbilical artery catheter, the anesthesiologist should exercise caution when withdrawing blood samples or flushing the line. Sampling and reinfusing rates should not exceed 1 ml in 30 s in the preterm infant. Rates in excess of this may significantly and adversely affect cerebral blood flow and oxygenation [20].

Radial artery lines are more commonly used for intraoperative monitoring by anesthesiologists. Various methods have been recommended to improve the success of transcutaneous insertion of a catheter in neonates. Smooth insertion of the catheter into small arteries is more likely to be attained if the bevel of the needle is rotated inferiorly once a flashback of blood is observed. In some cases the use of a fine guidewire may be useful to thread an obstructed catheter into the artery. If the artery cannot be palpated readily, a Doppler flowmeter probe or transillumination of the infant's wrist may facilitate its location [21]. In cases of difficulty, it may be necessary to resort to a cutdown for cannulation of the vessel. Allen's test of the adequacy of collateral flow to the hand is difficult to perform in small infants and is unreliable even in adults; hence it is not routinely performed in many centers. Once a radial artery access has been successfully established, the limb should be immobilized on a splint and a secure continuous flush system attached. Normal saline is preferred to glucose-containing solutions for all monitoring lines [22]. Flushing of radial arterial lines should be limited to small volumes and slow rates of injection as retrograde flow into the cerebral circulation may occur with as little as 0.5 ml flush solution [23]. Blood, which has been withdrawn while taking a laboratory sample, should be re-injected into a venous access site rather than an arterial access.

Serious complications with radial artery lines are relatively rare in neonates although instances of ischemic damage to the hand have been described [23–25]. Any evidence of impaired circulation or skin changes distal to the catheter is an indication for its immediate removal. There is no evidence that a cutdown approach to cannulation is accompanied by increased risk of complications [26].

Femoral artery cannulation may be used as an alternative if radial puncture is impossible, and this may better reflect true arterial pressure than does the radial artery in some instances [27]. The risk of infection at the puncture site is not increased with a femoral artery cannulation, although in small infants, the distal circulation should be carefully monitored as perfusion-related complications may occur [28]. Great care should be taken during insertion of femoral lines to avoid needle injury to the hip joint, septic arthritis, and damage to the head of the femur [29]. It is extremely important that the artery be accessed caudal to the level of the inguinal ligament; insertion above the ligament may cause a retroperitoneal hemorrhage. A Seldinger technique with careful aseptic technique is recommended for insertion of an arterial catheter, e.g., 3 Fr, 5 cm polyurethane catheter. The puncture site should be covered with a transparent sterile occlusive dressing and should be regularly inspected. If there is any evidence of impaired circulation in the limb, the catheter should be removed immediately. Sepsis is more likely to occur with femoral (or radial) arterial catheters that are left in place for more than 5 days [28].

The arterial wave form and the actual pressures obtained from arterial catheters in small infants may be affected to a degree by the compliance of the connecting tubing and by a continuous fluid flush. It is also necessary to consider the volume of fluid that is administered in order to continuously flush the tubing. The use of a pressurized bag with a controlled infusion device (e.g., Intraflo or Squeezeflow system) claims to deliver 3 ml/h of flush solution. However, under some circumstances, it may deliver larger volumes of solution, especially when the rapid flush activator is frequently used or malfunctions [30]. This may lead to fluid overload and possible coagulopathy secondary to excessive heparin administration. A cerebral vascular accident may occur when the arterial line is flushed with crystalloid solution continuously, particularly in the radial artery, resulting in an ischemic bolus of crystalloid in the carotid artery. A preferable method to continuously flush arterial lines is to use a syringe pump [30] set to deliver 1 ml/h.

- COOK MEDICAL INC. P.O. Box 4195 Bloomington, IN 47402-4195 U.S.A.
- ICU medical Inc. 951 Calle Amanecer - San Clemente, Ca 92673

Alternative sites to monitor arterial pressure invasively have been suggested. The axillary artery is an attractive alternative as it has a very good collateral circulation and it can be easily palpated. It has successfully been used without serious complication in critically ill neonates [31]. There are also reports of brachial artery cannulation without serious complication [25], although this must be viewed with some caution as this artery has a less well developed collateral circulation.

Central Venous Pressure Monitoring

Central venous catheters (CVCs) may be inserted into the neonate to monitor central pressure and also to permit the infusion of inotropic and hyperosmolar solutions. Transcutaneous insertion of a CVC via the internal jugular vein in the neonate is greatly facilitated by the use of ultrasound [32]. The vein is readily recognized by the ease with which it collapses with slight pressure of the transducer on the neck. Slight pressure over the liver will increase the lumen of the vein and facilitate puncture. It is not usual to place small infants in Trendelenburg position because the tilt adds little to the venous diameter since they are so short. It is common to place a small roll under the shoulders. The left subclavian vein has also been suggested as a route, again preferably with the use of ultrasound to locate the vein accurately [33]. However, the subclavian vein has a smaller diameter in the neonate [34], and its cannulation is associated with a greater incidence of complications, especially pneumothorax. Selecting the correct depth of insertion may be difficult in the small infant. The tip of the catheter should not be inferior to the junction of the superior vena cava with the (R) atrium and this should be confirmed by radiology. If it is further advanced into the (R) atrium, serious complications may result, including arrhythmias, damage to the tricuspid valve, or even cardiac perforation with tamponade. Full aseptic precautions should be observed during central venous cannulation in neonates. When CVCs are to be used to deliver hyperalimentation solutions, extreme care with asepsis is essential as catheter-related sepsis and endocarditis is a common complication.

When it is impossible to access the superior vena cava, a reliable index of central venous pressure may be obtained by monitoring the pressure in the inferior vena cava (IVC) via the femoral vein. Low IVC pressure tends to be only very slightly greater than central venous pressure [35].

Capnography in the Neonate

Capnography provides evidence of ventilation and indirect evidence of cardiac output, pulmonary blood flow, and metabolic state; as such it is an invaluable intraoperative monitor. The shape of the capnogram may be useful to validate readings by observation of an "alveolar plateau" on the tracing. Alterations in this shape may alert the anesthesiologist to developing physiological changes, or technical problems with the circuit and airway. $EtCO_2$ levels also provide an approximation of arterial pCO_2 levels, the accuracy of which is dependent upon many factors. Direct determination of arterial pCO_2 is essential when this level might be crucial. Accuracy in the control of arterial pCO_2 intraoperatively is most desirable as either hypercarbia or hypocarbia may have serious adverse physiological effects.

$EtCO_2$ levels may be measured by either sidestream sampling or mainstream detection methods, both of which have been applied to the neonate [36, 37]. The small tidal volumes and large respiratory rate of the neonate compromise the ability to accurately sample end-tidal gas. Sidestream sampling methods are crucially dependent upon the site of sampling, the sampling rate, and the dead space of sampling tubes. In postsurgical neonates and those in the NICU, microstream sidestream capnography (sampling rate 50 ml/min) and transcutaneous CO_2 correlated reasonably well with the arterial pCO_2 [38, 39]. The increase in apparatus dead space and size of the detector unit adjacent to the tracheal tube are potential problems with mainstream units. Nonetheless, $EtCO_2$ measured using mainstream capnometry in very-low-birth-weight infants correlated reasonably well with the umbilical arterial CO_2 but consistently underestimated the arterial pCO_2 and was more accurate in those with less severe pulmonary disease [40]. A practical consideration at the present time is that most anesthesia machines are equipped with a built-in sidestream monitor.

Gas samples for sidestream monitoring may be collected at the level of the tracheal tube connector or at the tip of the tracheal tube via a fine sampling tube. If collected at the connector, the use of a very low dead space system is desirable [41]. Sidestream sampling using low sampling rates (50 ml/min) from a low dead space (0.5 ml) tracheal tube adaptor in low-birth-weight infants significantly underestimated arterial pCO_2 levels but did detect excessively high and low levels [42]. Samples collected from the tip of the tracheal tube show much better correlation with arterial pCO_2 levels even in the presence of severe lung disease [43]. Double-lumen infant endotracheal tubes with a fine second channel are available for this purpose [43]. A problem with these tubes is that the fine aspirating channel is prone to blockage by secretions.

Mallinckrodt™ Oral/Nasal Tracheal Tube Cuffless Monitoring Lumen Sizes 2.5 up

Mainstream monitored $EtCO_2$ levels are generally less than the arterial pCO_2 especially in infants with significant pulmonary disease [44]. However mainstream $EtCO_2$ may be useful in trending or in warning of significantly abnormal values [44, 45]. The conclusion must be that although $EtCO_2$ is an extremely useful clue to many facets of patient well-being, when you really want to know precisely what is the arterial pCO_2, there is no substitute for an arterial sample!

Body Temperature Monitoring

With a larger surface area to body weight ratio, thin subcutaneous fat layer and the inability to shiver, neonates depend on non-shivering, norepinephrine dependent, thermogenesis from brown fat (in the interscapular and peri-renal areas) for heat production. The maintenance of normothermia and avoidance of cold stress will require careful monitoring. However, there are some important considerations to observe; first there is no uniform "normal" body temperature; different tissues are in different metabolic states and thus will be at different temperatures. Second the core body temperature may be normal, but the infant is maintaining this while in a state of cold stress [46]. If the objective is to maintain the infant in a thermo-neutral state, it is suggested that this may be indicated by a core temperature of 36.7–37.3 °C and a change in core and skin temperatures of less than 0.2–0.3 C°/h [47]. These considerations may influence the choice of temperature monitoring options.

Common sites to monitor the body temperature of the infant are the axilla, rectum, skin, esophagus, and ear.

Measurement of body temperature in the axilla depends upon positioning the probe close to the artery and adducting the arm to close the axillary space; procedures that may not be easy in the neonate. Forces air warmers may directly heat an axillary probe in a neonate. It is also suggested that active non-shivering thermogenesis may influence readings at this site [46].

Rectal temperature is often considered the best index (gold standard) of core temperature, but the readings may be influenced by the depth of insertion, rectal contents and metabolic activity therein, the temperature of an underlying blanket, and the temperature of blood returning from the lower limbs [48]. It is generally recommended that the probe be gently inserted to a depth of 5 cm [49]. The very rare complication of rectal perforation must be considered [50].

Skin temperature is easily measured, and if this is done with a "zero heat flow" method, it may be preferable to continuous rectal temperature monitoring [51]. The "zero heat flow" method requires an insulated probe placed on the skin where it rests on the mattress; this achieves zero heat flow and measures the temperature of deep tissues [52].

When measuring the esophageal temperature, it is important to position the probe in the lower esophagus in relation to the left atrium. This can be achieved by using a combined esophageal stethoscope and temperature sensor, but consider the position of the sensor in relation to the stethoscope. Temperatures in the upper esophagus may be affected by the proximity to the airway.

The ear is not a satisfactory site to monitor temperature in most small infants due to the limitations of the small ear canal. Infrared technology may permit intermittent measurements from the tympanic membrane, and this is sometimes useful postoperatively.

Monitoring Blood Glucose

Perioperative hypoglycemia or excessive hyperglycemia is to be avoided in the neonate. Intermittent tests using a hand-held glucometer are valuable to confirm normal levels and require very little blood. However, the level of significant hypoglycemia or hyperglycemia for the neonate is at the extremes of the range for reasonable accuracy of hand-held units [53]. In addition the results from glucometers (and other point-of-care methods) may be affected by alterations in level of oxygenation, hematocrit, or temperature, by bilirubin and by drugs such as mannitol or dopamine [53, 54]. High hematocrit levels of the neonate may result in low-glucose readings. High arterial pO_2 levels may also result in falsely low-blood glucose readings on models using glucose oxidase technology. A new generation of glucometers specifically designed for the neonate is becoming available, and these are more reliable.

To avoid the obvious disadvantage of intermittent testing, continuous glucose monitoring methods have been developed and have been demonstrated useful to detect unrecognized hypoglycemic episodes [55]. These use a subcutaneous electrode and have been found to function well despite changes in hematocrit and the use of inotropes. However they do require frequent calibration against blood samples. The accuracy of these units declines as hypoglycemic levels are reached, but as this is a continuous monitor, downward trends can be recognized early [55]. Continuous glucose monitoring may be useful during neonatal cardiac procedures and may be vital during the surgery of neonatal insulinoma.

The foregoing would be considered standard monitors to be employed for the neonate during the perioperative period.

References

1. Nezafati MH, Soltani G, Kahrom M. Esophageal stethoscope: an old tool with a new role, detection of residual flow during video-assisted thoracoscopic patent ductus arteriosus closure. J Pediatr Surg. 2010;45(11):2141–5.
2. Friedman M, Toriumi DM. Esophageal stethoscope. Another possible cause of vocal cord paralysis. Arch Otolaryngol Head Neck Surg. 1989;115(1):95–8.
3. Schwartz AJ, Downes JJ. Hazards of a simple monitoring device, the esophageal stethoscope. Anesthesiology. 1977;47(1):64–5.
4. Poets CF, Southall DP. Noninvasive monitoring of oxygenation in infants and children: practical considerations and areas of concern. Pediatrics. 1994;93:737–46.
5. Fouzas S, Priftis KN, Anthracopoulos MB. Pulse oximetry in pediatric practice. Pediatrics. 2011;128:740–52.
6. Castillo A, Sola A, Baquero H, et al. Pulse oxygen saturation levels and arterial oxygen tension values in newborns receiving oxygen therapy in the neonatal intensive care unit: is 85 % to 93 % an acceptable range? Pediatrics. 2008;121(5):882–9.
7. Saugstad OD, Sejersted Y, Solberg R, et al. Oxygenation of the newborn: a molecular approach. Neonatology. 2012;101:315–25.
8. Askie LM. Optimal oxygen saturation in preterm infants: a moving target. Curr Opin Pediatr. 2013;25:188–92.
9. Baquero H, Alvis R, Castillo A, Neira F, Sola A. Avoiding hyperoxia during neonatal resuscitation: time to response of different SpO2 monitors. Acta Pediatr. 2011;100:515–18.
10. de Graaff JC, Bijker JB, Kappen TH, et al. Incidence of intraoperative hypoxemia in children in relation to age. Anesth Analg. 2013;117:169–75.
11. Hussain SA. Pulse oximetry interference in bronze baby syndrome. J Perinatol. 2009;29:828–9.
12. Wouters K. Clinical usefulness of the simultaneous display of pulse oximetry from two probes. Pediatr Anesth. 2008;18:345–6.
13. Wille J, Braams R, Van Haren WH, van der Werken C. Pulse oximeter induced digital injury: frequency rate and possible causative factors. Crit Care Med. 2000;28:3555–7.
14. Urquhart C, Bell G. Ear probe pulse oximeters and neonates. Anaesthesia. 2005;60:294.
15. Sonesson SE, Broberger U. Arterial blood pressure in the very low birthweight neonate. Evaluation of an automatic oscillometric technique. Acta Paediatr Scand. 1987;76:338–41.
16. Emery EF, Greenough A. Non Invasive monitoring in preterm infants receiving intensive care. Eur J Paediatr. 1992;151:136–9.
17. Konig K, Casalaz DM, Burke EJ, Watkins A. Accuracy of non-invasive blood pressure monitoring in very preterm infants. Intens Care Med. 2012;38:670–6.
18. Dannevig I, Dale HC, Liestol K, Lindemann R. Blood pressure in the neonate: three non-invasive oscillometric pressure monitors compared with invasively measured blood pressure. Acta Pediatr Scand. 2005;94:191–6.
19. Ramasethu J. Complications of vascular catheters in the neonatal intensive care unit. Clin Perinatol. 2008;35:199–222.

20. Schulz G, Keller E, Haensse D, Arlettaz R, Bucher HU, Fauchere JC. Slow blood sampling from an umbilical artery catheter prevents a decrease in cerebral oxygenation in the preterm infant. Pediatrics. 2003;111:73–6.
21. Cole FS, Todres ID, Shannon DC. Technique for percutaneous cannulation of the radial artery in the newborn. J Pediatr. 1978;92:105–7.
22. Rais-Bahrami K, Karna P, Dolanski EA. Effect of fluids on life span of peripheral arterial lines. Am J Perinatol. 1990;7:122–4.
23. Butt WW, Gow R, Whyte H, et al. Complications resulting from the use of arterial catheters: retrograde flow and rapid elevation in blood pressure. Pediatrics. 1985;76:250.
24. Cartwright GW, Schreiner RL. Major complication to percutaneous radial artery catheterization in the neonate. Pediatrics. 1980;65:139–41.
25. Schindler E, Kowadl B, Suess H, et al. Catheterization of the radial or brachial artery in neonates and infants. Pediatr Anesth. 2005;15:677–82.
26. Sellden H, Nillson K, Larsson LE, Ekstrom-Jodal B. Radial arterial catheters in children and neonates: a prospective study. Crit Care Med. 1987;15:1106–9.
27. Gallagher JD, Moore RA, McNicholas KW, Jose AB. Comparison of radial and femoral arterial blood pressures in children after cardiopulmonary bypass. J Clin Monit. 1985;1:168–71.
28. Glenski J, Beynen FM, Brady J. A prospective evaluation of femoral artery monitoring in pediatric patients. Anesthesiology. 1987;66:227–9.
29. Asnes RS, Arender GM. Septic arthritis of the hip: a complication of femoral venipuncture. Pediatrics. 1966;38:837–41.
30. Morray J, Todd S. A hazard of continuous flush systems for vascular pressure monitoring in infants. Anesthesiology. 1983;58:187–9.
31. Piotrowski A, Kawczynski P. Cannulation of the axillary artery in critically ill newborn infants. Eur J Pediatr. 1995;154:57–9.
32. Alderson PJ, Burrows FA, Stemp LI, et al. Use of ultrasound to evaluate internal jugular vein anatomy and to facilitate central venous cannulation in paediatric patients. Br J Anaesth. 1993;70:145–8.
33. Haas NA, Haas SA. Central venous catheter techniques in infants and children. Curr Opin Anaesthesiol. 2003;16:291–303.
34. Breschan C, Platzer M, Jost R, Stetner H, Likar R. Size of internal jugular vs subclavian vein in small infants: an observational, anatomical evaluation with ultrasound. Br J Anaesth. 2010;105:179–84.
35. Chait HI, Kuhn MA, Baum VC. Inferior vena caval pressure reliably predicts right atrial pressure in pediatric cardiac surgical patients. Crit Care Med. 1994;22:219–24.
36. McEvedy BA, McLeod ME, Mulera M, et al. End-tidal transcutaneous and arterial CO2 measurements in critically ill neonates: a comparative study. Anesthesiology. 1988;69:112–16.
37. McEvedy BA, McLeod ME, Kirpalani H, et al. End-tidal carbon dioxide measurements in critically ill neonates: a comparison of side-stream and mainstream capnometers. Can J Anaesth. 1990;37:322–6.
38. Tingay DG, Mun KS, Perkins EJ. End tidal carbon dioxide is as reliable as transcutaneous monitoring in ventilated postsurgical neonates. Arch Dis Child Fetal Neonatal Ed. 2013;98:F161–4.
39. Singh BS, Gilbert U, Sing S, Govindaswami B. Sidestream microstream end tidal carbon dioxide measurements and blood gas correlations in neonatal intensive care unit. Pediatr Pulmonol. 2013;48:250–6.
40. Trevisanuto D, Giuliotto S, Cavallin F, et al. End-tidal carbon dioxide monitoring in very low birth weight infants: correlation and agreement with arterial carbon dioxide. Pediatr Pulmonol. 2012;47:367–72.
41. Friederich JA, Brooker RF. A pediatric end tidal carbon dioxide sampling port. Anesth Analg. 1994;79:198.
42. Lopez E, Grabar S, Barbier A, Krauss B, Jarreau PH, Moriette G. Detection of carbon dioxide thresholds using low-flow sidestream capnography in ventilated preterm infants. Intens Care Med. 2009;35:1942–9.
43. Kugelman A, Zelger Aginsky D, Bader D, Shorts I, Riskin A. A novel method of distal end-tidal CO2 capnography in intubated infants: comparison with arterial CO2 and with proximal mainstream end-tidal CO2. Pediatrics. 2008;122:e1219–24.
44. Bhat YR, Abhishek N. Mainstream end-tidal carbon dioxide monitoring in ventilated neonates. Singapore Med J. 2008;49: 199–203.
45. Rozycki HJ, Sysyn GD, Marshall MK, Malooy R, Wiswell TE. Mainstream end-tidal carbon dioxide monitoring in the neonatal intensive care unit. Pediatrics. 1998;101:648–53.
46. Lyon AL, Freer Y. Goals and options in keeping preterm babies warm. Arch Dis Child Fetal Neonatal Ed. 2011;96:F71–4.
47. Sauer PJ, Dane HJ, Visser HK. New standards for neutral thermal environment of healthy very low birth weight infants. Arch Dis Child. 1984;59:18–22.
48. McIntyre J, Hull D. Axillary and rectal temperature measurements in infants. Arch Dis Child. 1992;67:1059.
49. Togawa T. Temperature measurement. Clin Phys Physiol Meas. 1985;6:83–108.
50. Frank JD, Brown S. Thermometers and rectal perforations in the neonate. Arch Dis Child. 1978;53:824–5.
51. Van der Speck RDG, van Lingen RA, Zoeren-Grobben D. Body temperature measurement in VLBW infants by continuous skin measurement is as good or even better alternative than continuous rectal measurement. Acta Paediatr. 2009;98:282–5.
52. Simbrunner G. Temperature measurements and distribution of temperatures throughout the body in neonates. In: Okken A, Koch J, editors. Thermoregulation of sick and low birth weight neonates. Berlin: Springer; 1995.
53. Beardsall K. Measurement of glucose levels in the newborn. Early Hum Dev. 2010;86:263–7.
54. Steven J, Nicholson S. Perioperative management of blood glucose during open heart surgery in infants and children. Pediatr Anesth. 2011;21:630–7.
55. Harris DL, Battin MR, Weston PJ, Harding JE. Continuous glucose monitoring in newborn babies at risk of hypoglycemia. J Pediatr. 2010;157:198–202.

Perioperative Metabolic Care of the Term and Preterm Infant

8

Geoff Frawley, Pablo Ingelmo, and Satyan Lakshminrusimha

Neonatal Body Water Distribution and Metabolism (Fig. 8.1)

The body composition of the fetus changes dramatically during gestation. Total body water, as a proportion of body weight, progressively decreases with advancing gestation (Fig. 8.2). Total body water represents 85 % of body weight in premature infants, 75 % in full-term neonates and 60 % in older children [1]. After birth, excess total body water is mobilized and excreted. Premature infants (Fig. 8.2) mature through several distinct phases before achieving fluid homeostasis. The pre-diuretic phase, which occurs in the first 24–48 postnatal hours, is marked by urine outputs in the range of 0.5–1.5 ml/kg/h. During the subsequent diuretic phase, urine output increases to 3–5 ml/kg/h with a decrease in sodium excretion. As a result, there is 10–15 % weight loss during the first 5–7 postnatal days (with a weight loss of up to 20 % in infants <750 g). The precise mechanisms underlying the contraction of body fluids in the first few postnatal days are not clear but have been attributed, in part, to an atrial natriuretic peptide (ANP) diuresis secondary to increased pulmonary blood flow and stretch of left atrial receptors. Another contributing factor to this diuresis and weight loss during the first postnatal week (largely extracellular fluid loss) is tubular insensitivity to aldosterone [2, 3].

G. Frawley
Department of Anaesthesia and Pain Management, Royal Children's Hospital, Flemington Road, Parkville, VIC 3052, Australia
e-mail: Geoff.frawley@rch.org.au

P. Ingelmo (✉)
Department of Anesthesia, Montreal Children's Hospital, 2300 Tupper Street, C1115, Montreal, QC, Canada, H3H 1P3
e-mail: pabloingelmo@libero.it

S. Lakshminrusimha, MD
Division of Neonatology, Women and Children's Hospital of Buffalo, 219 Bryant Street, Buffalo, NY 14222, USA
e-mail: slakshmi@buffalo.edu

Postnatal Changes in Hypothalamic, Adrenal, and Renal Physiology

Atrial Natriuretic Peptides

The natriuretic peptides are involved in attenuating the renin-angiotensin-aldosterone axis and sympathetic nervous system; suppression of vasopressin release; vasodilatation of the systemic, pulmonary, coronary, and renal circulations; and promotion of natriuresis and diuresis. When compared with older infants and children, neonates in the first few postnatal days have significantly greater circulating levels of natriuretic hormone, perhaps related to the acute increase in ventricular afterload that occurs after birth [3, 4]. Plasma B-type natriuretic peptide (BNP) levels in neonates with respiratory disease, with persistent pulmonary hypertension of the newborn, are significantly greater than in those with normal right ventricular pressure. In children with known congenital heart disease, natriuretic hormone levels vary with the type and severity of the heart defect [5].

Hypothalamic-Pituitary-Adrenal Axis

Remodelling of the adrenal glands after birth occurs via apoptosis of the fetal zone, by remodelling this zone and the development of other zones [6]. At birth, the concentration of free cortisol is only one-third that of maternal levels, with an inverse relationship between cortisol levels and gestational age. The size of the adrenal glands decreases by 25 % during the first 4 postnatal days. In full-term and late preterm neonates, low cord concentrations of ACTH, cortisol and free triiodothyronine are associated with lung fluid retention and transient tachypnea of the newborn (TTN) [7]. Transient insufficiency of the adrenal cortex has been reported in approximately 27 % of ELBW infants and critically ill neonates (defined as an inability to triple the cortisol production rate in response to stress); these infants

J. Lerman (ed.), *Neonatal Anesthesia*, DOI 10.1007/978-1-4419-6041-2_8,

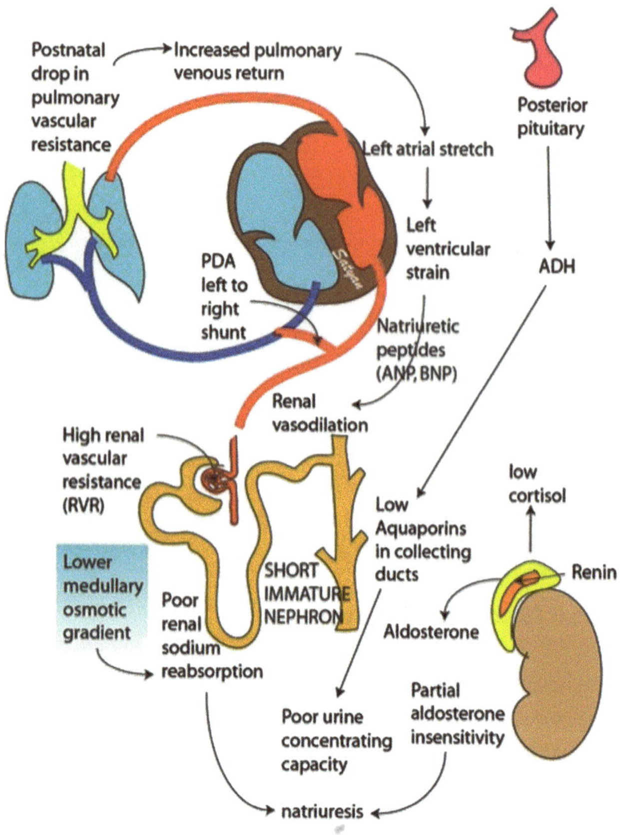

Fig. 8.1 Changes in fluid homeostasis and regulation in neonates (especially preterm neonates) lead to poor concentrating capacity and urinary loss of sodium. Reduction in pulmonary vascular resistance after birth increases pulmonary venous return to the left atrium thereby stretching the atrium. Umbilical cord clamping and removal of the placenta increase systemic vascular resistance and left ventricular strain. Atrial stretch and ventricular strain increase natriuretic peptide levels, which cause renal vasodilation and natriuresis. Although ADH secretion is present, reduced aquaporins in the collecting duct limit the urinary concentrating capacity, particularly in premature infants. Although the renin-angiotensin system is functional with normal/high aldosterone levels, partial aldosterone insensitivity results in a natriuresis. Ductal steal (*left* to *right* shunt across a patent ductus arteriosus—PDA reduces renal perfusion), increased renal vascular resistance, reduced medullary osmotic gradient, short immature nephrons, and reduced cortisol concentrations act in concert to limit the ability of the preterm infant to conserve sodium and water. See text for details

mount a poor response to shock with hypotension that is unresponsive to fluids and inotropes [8–10]. Intravenous pulse doses of hydrocortisone have been shown to be effective in treating inotrope-resistant hypotension in critically ill preterm infants that does not suppress the adrenal gland [9, 11]. However, the vast majority of preterm neonates >30 weeks' gestation demonstrated a positive relationship between their stress response and the urinary cortisol levels [12]. Most neonates with suppressed cortisol levels at birth reach normal plasma cortisol levels within the first 2 weeks after birth [13].

Renin-Angiotensin-Aldosterone

The renin-angiotensin system is very active in the first week of neonatal life resulting in increased vascular tone and increased concentrations of aldosterone [14]. Factors that contribute to increased angiotensinogen and plasma renin activity (PRA) levels include low systemic blood pressure and low renal blood flow, low serum sodium, and a decrease in ECF after birth. The activity of the renin-angiotensin-aldosterone (RAA) system is inversely related to gestational age. The integrity of the renin-angiotensin-aldosterone system at early age contrasts with the inability of the fetal kidney to appropriately control sodium and water reabsorption.

Synthesis of aldosterone in the fetal adrenal gland commences by the 13th gestational week and increases steadily throughout gestation, often exceeding maternal levels at birth. Urinary aldosterone excretion increases significantly in late gestation, between 30 and 41 weeks [2]. In VLBW infants, the adrenal production of aldosterone is reduced compared with that in full-term neonates. This, combined with a partial unresponsiveness of the distal tubule to aldosterone, predisposes these infants to an increased risk of hyponatremia and dehydration. The mechanism of this partial resistance may be explained in part by the reduced expression of renal mineralocorticoid receptors [15]. As aldosterone levels increase with gestational age, distal tubular reabsorption of sodium increases, but even by term, healthy neonates exhibit partial, transient tubular unresponsiveness to aldosterone, resulting in an impaired ability to excrete large or acute sodium loads [2]. In fact at term, plasma levels of aldosterone and renin are increased compared with maternal levels despite the accompanying hyponatremia, hyperkalemia and urinary sodium loss [14]. Aldosterone levels and the distal tubular responses to aldosterone normalize as renal function matures by the end of the first year of life.

Antidiuretic Hormone

Antidiuretic hormone (arginine vasopressin AVP, ADH) increases at birth especially in infants delivered vaginally [16]. ADH secretion is increased in response to stress—during birth, asphyxia or with respiratory distress syndrome (RDS), positive pressure ventilation, pneumothorax, and intracranial hemorrhage. Sensitivity of the volume receptors and osmoreceptors in neonates is similar to the response in adults, but tubular sensitivity to ADH is decreased in preterm infants [17, 18]. The reduced response of the collecting duct's water permeability response to ADH permits the excretion of hypotonic urine in utero and contributes to the neonate's inability to concentrate urine postnatally.

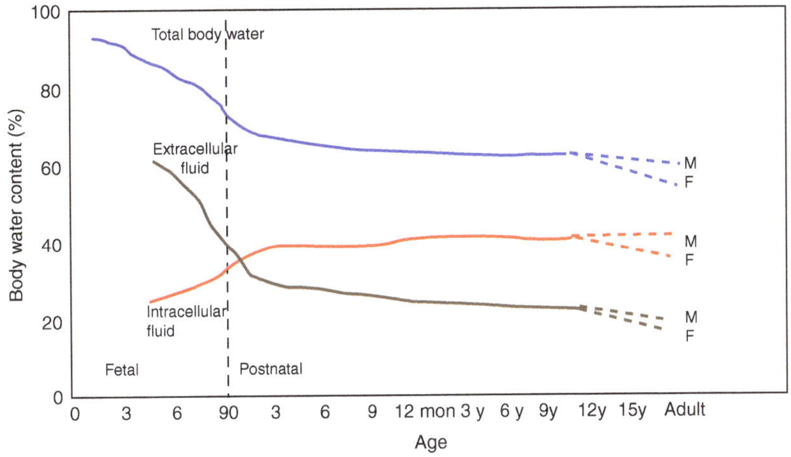

Fig. 8.2 Total body water and intracellular and extracellular water distribution with age

In utero, prostaglandins E2 signal the prostaglandin EP3 receptor to block AQPs [19]. Postnatally, when ADH binds to its receptor on the basolateral membrane of the collecting duct, a series of events culminate in the insertion of aquaporin-2 (AQP2) water channels into the apical membrane of the renal tubule increasing the tubule's water permeability in response to ADH [20]. Aquaporins in the apical membranes of collecting ducts are decreased in premature infants at birth, peak on postnatal day 3 and then decrease to birth concentrations by day 7 [21].

Renal Function: in the neonate is markedly immature compared with that in the older infant, and small for gestational age infants are at increased risk for renal insufficiency [22, 23]. The number of nephrons in the fetus reaches adult numbers by 34–36 weeks' gestation, but the nephrons are shorter and functionally immature [20]. Renal function and the control of fluids and electrolytes are thus impaired in premature infants who are less than 35 weeks postmenstrual age (PMA). Postnatal renal maturation however is more a function of postnatal age than gestational age; thus a preterm infant who is a few weeks old may have more mature renal function than a full-term neonate. After birth, renal blood flow increases in response to increased systemic blood pressure with a resultant increase in glomerular filtration rate. However, the neonatal kidney remains less efficient at excreting an acute sodium or water load than the kidney of an infant or child.

Neonatal Renal Function

Infants tolerate fluid restriction poorly and become dehydrated rapidly as a result of large insensible fluid losses and the inability of the kidneys to concentrate urine. Factors that contribute to this inability to concentrate urine include a decrease in medullary osmotic gradient and a reduced water permeability response of the collecting duct to ADH. The lack of a renal medulla osmotic gradient and the absence of medullary tubules limit the urinary concentrating capacity of the neonatal kidney (600 mOsm/kg in preterm infants and 800 mOsm/kg in full-term neonates) to about half that of the adult value (1,200–1,400 mOsm/kg).

Renal Blood Flow (RBF): RBF at birth is reduced in preterm and full-term infants primarily because the oxygen tension is reduced and the renal vascular resistance (RVR) is increased due to upregulation of the renin-angiotensin system. RBF reaches adult rates by 2 years of age. Angiotensin II is important in utero as it vasoconstricts efferent arterioles, acting as a partial growth factor [19]. RVR is inversely related to gestational age and decreases gradually postnatally, although remaining greater than adults. The presence of a physiologic patent ductus arteriosus with left to right shunting also contributes to low renal blood flow in neonates. During the first twelve hours after birth of full-term neonates, 4–6 % of the cardiac output perfuses the kidney; the perfusion increases to 8–10 % (compared with 25 % in adults) during the first week [19]. A similar pattern of blood flow occurs in preterm infants who are older than 34–35 weeks' gestation with a more gradual decrease in RVR and a slower increase in GFR [24]. A greater proportion of the RBF in infants perfuses the juxtaglomerular nephrons compared with that in adults, in whom the majority of RBF perfuses the cortical area and only 10 % perfuses the medullary area. Because the juxtaglomerular nephrons are more involved in the conservation of rather than excretion of sodium, this explains the limited ability of the infant to excrete a sodium load.

Glomerular Filtration: The glomeruli and nephrons are immature at birth, resulting in a reduced glomerular filtration rate (GFR) and limited concentrating ability. The GFR in the neonate is markedly reduced compared with that in the adult, especially when the infant's smaller size and surface area are taken into account. The reduced GFR in the neonate may be explained by the very low surface area of the glomerular basement membrane [20]. This impairs the neonate's ability to excrete a water load. At 40 weeks postconceptional age, the GFR is 1.5 ml/kg/min (20–40 ml/min/1.73 m^2), increasing to adult levels of 2.0 ml/kg/min (120 ml/min/1.73 m^2) by 2 years of age. The GFR is directly related to gestational age; premature neonates have reduced GFR values that increase slowly compared with those in full-term neonates. In extremely premature infants, the GFR remains reduced until a full complement of nephrons has developed at 35 weeks. The reduced GFR at birth is attributed to low systemic arterial blood pressure, increased renal vascular resistance and reduced ultrafiltration pressure together with a decreased capillary surface area for filtration.

Tubular Function: matures over the first few months postnatally, reaching adult values by 1 year of age. The neonate has a smaller tubular resorptive surface area, fewer solute transporters, decreased Na^+K^+ ATPase activity and altered control of H^+ transport compared with older infants. Most other secretory and absorptive tubular processes, although immature, are relatively well developed by term. Neonates and young infants usually produce urine that is isotonic with plasma, but if required, they can concentrate their urine to achieve an osmolality of 500–700 mOsmol/kg H_2O. Adult values for maximum urine concentrating ability (typically reaching 1,200–1,400 mOsmol/kg H_2O) are achieved by 1 year of age. Glycosuria and aminoaciduria are commonly detected in neonates because of immature active transport pumps in the proximal tubule.

Maintenance Fluid Therapy

Water Requirement

Normal fluid requirements vary markedly in both low birth weight and full-term neonates as well as during infancy (Table 8.1). This variability is caused by differences in caloric expenditures, growth rate, evaporative losses and progress of renal function maturation and proportion of total body water at different ages [26]. Full-term infants require 60 ml/kg/day of fluid on day 1, with increasing incremental requirements that reach 150 ml/kg/day by 1 week postnatally. Premature neonates have larger surface areas relative to their body weights and greater evaporative losses than full-term neonates. As a consequence, premature neonates (≤26 weeks gestational age) require 80 ml/kg/d on day 1 (one-third more than full-term neonates), with increasing incremental requirements that reach 150–180 ml/kg/day by 1 week. In the case of VLBW infants, their surface area-to-weight ratios are approximately three times greater than those in full-term neonates, resulting in greater insensible fluid losses. These losses, combined with the greater urinary excretion of solutes and reduced tubular concentrating ability, further increase the obligatory fluid losses in these infants. Energy expenditure and fluid requirements may also significantly increase during stressful situations such as with surgery (up to 30 % increase), severe sepsis (up to 50 % increase), fever (10 % per degree in excess of 37 °C) and cardiac failure (up to 25 % increase).

Sodium is often not included in the fluids administered to neonates in the first 24–72 h, and the serum sodium can be an accurate marker of the hydration status of the neonate: hyponatremia developing with fluid overload and hypernatremia developing with dehydration.

Careful fluid and electrolyte management is essential for the well-being of the sick surgical neonate. Insufficient administration of fluids can cause hypovolemia, hyperosmolarity, metabolic abnormalities, and renal failure, whereas excess fluid administration can cause generalized edema, congestive heart failure, and pulmonary dysfunction. In the VLBW infant, excess fluid administration may be associated with a patent ductus arteriosus (PDA) because the fluid overload stimulates production of PGE_2, which prevents PDA closure. In the infant with a large PDA, aortic blood is shunted back into the pulmonary artery reducing blood flow down the descending aorta. This reduces intestinal blood

Table 8.1 Average fluid requirements of LBW infants (ml/kg/day) during the first week of life

		Body weight (g)			
Days after birth	Component	750–1,000	1,001–1,250	1,251–1,500	1,501–2,000
1	IWL	65	55	40	30
	Urine	20	20	30	30
	Total	85	75	70	60
2–3	IWL	65	55	40	30
	Urine/stool	40	40	40	45
	Total	105	95	80	75
4–7	IWL	65	55	40	30
	Urine/stool	65	65	65	65
	Total	130	120	105	95

IWL stands for insensible water loss [25]

flow that may result in hypoperfusion, ischemia and necrotizing enterocolitis (NEC). Excess fluid administration may also result in congestive heart failure, intraventricular hemorrhage, NEC and bronchopulmonary dysplasia (BPD).

Sodium and Electrolyte Requirements

Sodium is required for fetal growth, with a normal accretion rate of 1.2 mEq/kg/day between 31 and 38 weeks' gestation. Immediately after birth, both full-term and preterm infants are in negative sodium balance due to the physiologic natriuresis stimulated by ANP changes with birth [3]. The high fractional excretion of Na^+ (FE_{Na^+}) in premature infants can lead to negative Na^+ balance, hyponatremia, neurologic disturbances and poor growth unless sodium is administered at a rate of 3–5 mmol/kg/day. Full-term neonates readily conserve sodium with increased responsiveness of the distal tubule to aldosterone and a rapid increase in Na^+K^+ ATPase activity in the principal cell of the collecting duct after birth. The principal cell is the final determinant of sodium reabsorption and potassium excretion, the latter dependent on potassium channels [20]. Preterm infants demonstrate negative sodium balance for many weeks post delivery because of decreased Na^+K^+ ATPase activity, increased ECF volume and reduced tubular aldosterone sensitivity. Extremely premature infants who become hyponatremic most likely do not have reduced total body sodium, which would permit increasing their sodium intake. These infants require a reduction in total fluid intake. Conversely, the premature infant is unable to rapidly increase sodium excretion in response to an increased concentration of sodium or a large sodium load.

Clinically important disturbances in acid–base status are unusual in full-term neonates, unless protein intake is excessive. Plasma bicarbonate (HCO_3^-) concentrations depend on the renal HCO_3^- threshold, which is reduced in the full-term neonate (19–23 mEq/l) and even less in the premature (18–22 mEq/l) and very low birth weight (<1,300 g) infants (14–18 mEq/l) [19, 20]. The reduced renal HCO_3^- threshold (physiological renal tubular acidosis—RTA) may be caused by the physiologic volume expansion in the premature neonate and the relative immaturity of the tubular transport mechanisms. Sodium bicarbonate or more commonly sodium or potassium acetate supplements of 1–2 mmol/kg/day are generally recommended for very small premature infants. Infants with normal anion gap metabolic acidosis secondary to renal immaturity may have a greater requirement for alkali (acetate) in their parenteral nutrition.

Glucose

The fetal pancreas is able to release insulin in response to the presence of increased glucose and amino acids by the 20th week of gestation, although insulin remains inactive until the onset of corticosteroid action in the second trimester. Insulin then regulates the expression of enzymes related to glycogen and lipid synthesis. As a result, glycogen storage does not begin until the 27th week gestation and increases slowly thereafter until 36 weeks. Hepatic glycogen content then increases quickly until full-term is reached at a rate of 50 mg/g of tissue. This reserve, less than 5 % of the body weight, is rapidly depleted if a source of energy is needed suddenly, explaining why an infant is prone to developing hypoglycemia during the fasting period. The placenta is permeable to triglycerides, free fatty acids, and glycerol, and under the influence of insulin, fatty acid synthesis in the liver and glucose uptake in adipose tissue occur leading to triglyceride synthesis. During the third trimester, fat is stored in adipose tissue, which comprises 16 % of body weight at term, corresponding to an energy reserve of approximately 5,000 kcal.

Endocrine Response at Birth

Birth is associated with an endocrine stress response that is characterized by a massive increase in plasma catecholamine, glucagon and cortisol concentrations. Decreased plasma insulin concentrations as glucagon concentrations increase induce hepatic glycogenolysis, lipolysis, and gluconeogenesis, effects that are also stimulated by increased concentrations of circulating catecholamines at birth. A physiological decrease in blood glucose concentration occurs during the first 2 h after delivery, although the above mechanisms correct this physiologic aberration and initiate homeostasis. Hepatic synthesis through glycogenolysis and gluconeogenesis is the only source of glucose until feeding is established. Estimates of glucose kinetics in full-term neonates suggest that healthy neonates produce glucose at the rate of 5–8 mg kg/min (or 28–45 μmoles kg/min), of which 50–70 % is contributed by gluconeogenesis. Liver glycogen stores are depleted from 50 to 5 mg/g tissue within 12 h of birth, after which energy requirements are supported by oxidative fat metabolism until enteral feeding is established. The rate of lipolysis, as estimated by the rate of appearance of glycerol or fatty acid, corresponds to 6–12 μmoles kg/min.

Hypoglycemia

There is no consensus on the precise definition of hypoglycemia in neonates (although many use a concentration <47 mg/dL as hypoglycemia, rounding to 50 mg/dl) [27], and there are no uniform standards for euglycemia. The physiologically optimal range for plasma glucose concentrations is 70–100 mg/dl (3.9–5.6 mmol/l) with a minimal optimal concentration of glucose, 60 mg/dl (3.3 mmol/l).

Infants who are very immature (ELBW or VLBW) or ill (hypoxia, ischemia, or sepsis) may have greater glucose requirements and are more vulnerable to the consequences of hypoglycemia. Other infants at risk of postnatal hypoglycemia include infants of diabetic mothers, large for gestational age (LGA > 90 ‰) or small for gestational age infants (SGA), infants with Beckwith-Wiedemann syndrome or intrauterine growth retardation (IUGR <10‰), post-asphyxiated infants (APGAR <5 at 5 min) and infants ≤36 weeks' gestation. A glucose infusion rate of 3–4 mg/kg/min should prevent hypoglycemia in full-term infants, whereas an infusion rate of 6–10 mg/kg/min should prevent hypoglycemia in ELBW infants.

In neonates <28 weeks gestational age, hypoglycemia is almost unavoidable in the first few hours after birth if exogenous glucose is not administrated. These infants have limited glycogen stores, decreased availability of amino acids for gluconeogenesis and inadequate lipid stores for the release of fatty acids and fat stores to maintain glucose balance. Ketogenesis is severely limited in preterm infants because they lack fat stores in adipose tissue (fat represents <2 % of total body weight). Depending on its severity, hypoglycemia can produce devastating effects on the central nervous system, especially in neonates [28]. Reduced blood concentrations of glucose invoke a stress response and alter cerebral blood flow and metabolism. During hypoglycemia, brain glucose metabolism decreases by up to 50 % with increased reliance on ketones and lactate as sources for energy. Preterm infants appear less able to counterbalance these developments and to provide alternative fuels for the brain unlike full-term infants. Even moderate hypoglycemia can lead to an adverse neurodevelopmental outcome including an increased risk of motor and developmental delay. Cerebral injury is caused not only by severe prolonged hypoglycemia but also by mild hypoglycemia when it is combined with mild hypoxia or ischemia. MRI detected white matter abnormalities in more than 90 % of full-term neonates with symptomatic hypoglycemia (blood glucose level <45 mg/dL or 2.6 mmol/l) [29, 30].

Hyperglycemia: Hyperglycemia (defined as blood glucose concentration greater than 125 mg/dL or 7 mmol/l or plasma glucose concentration greater than 150 mg/dL or 8.25 mmol/l) is commonly observed during the first week of life in infants born at <30 weeks of gestation. Stress, corticosteroids and methylxanthine therapy and administration of glucose at excessive rates could all cause neonatal hyperglycemia. Glucose infusions are normally maintained at rates between 4 and 7 mg kg/min to ensure basal glucose requirements in neonates. However, hyperglycemia may develop if glucose infusion rates exceed 8 mg/kg/min in infants with birth weights >1 kg and if moderate infusion rates of 4–8 mg/kg/min were administered to VLBW infants with birth weights <1 kg. Hyperglycemia, which usually occurs after an abrupt increase in plasma glucose concentration (e.g., following a bolus of 25 % or 50 % dextrose i.v.), has been associated with a greater risk of intraventricular hemorrhage, although a causal relationship has yet to be proven. In the presence of ischemia or hypoxia, the impaired metabolism of excess glucose causes an accumulation of lactate and a decrease in intracellular pH that subsequently severely compromises cellular function that may result in cell death [28]. However reducing glucose infusions to an extremely low rate to manage hyperglycemia significantly reduces caloric intake, which may have long-term effects on growth and development.

Enteral Nutrition (Trophic Feeding or Minimal Enteral Nutrition)

Feeding is less efficient in some late preterm infants than in full-term neonates because they fatigue quickly and have immature feeding skills prompting oral gavage (tube) feeding until effective oral feeding is achieved [31]. Suck and swallow coordination is often poor in infants born at <34 weeks' gestation. Furthermore, some infants require a longer-than-normal interval between feedings because of delayed gastrointestinal motility and gastric emptying. Furthermore, premature infants <34 weeks' gestation often have intestinal dysmotility that contributes to feeding intolerance with associated anesthetic implications.

Minimal Enteral Nutrition (Trophic Feeding)

Minimal enteral nutrition refers to the practice of early enteral feeding of premature infants. Starting volumes vary from 5 to 25 ml/kg/day with benefits noted at less than 1 ml/kg/day (priming). Minimal trophic feeds (either by bolus or continuous infusion of 10 ml/kg/day) in the first week of life stimulate the gut by increasing the activity of various enzymes, inducing mucosal growth, promoting motility and preventing translocation of bacteria across the gut wall—a significant concern in VLBW infants [32]. Maternal breast milk (colostrum) is preferred; however, positive results have been reported with donor milk and formula feeding. Feeding volumes are kept small, regardless of the size of gastric residuals, with volumes usually less than 20 ml/kg/day. Minimal enteral nutrition is used with caution in any situation associated with gut hypoxia or decreased intestinal blood flow (asphyxia, hypoxemia, hypotension) and/or marked diastolic steal (a patent ductus arteriosus). Continuing feeds during indomethacin treatment is still a controversial issue and clinical practice differs among hospitals.

Normal Enteral Feeds

Maturation of the gastrointestinal tract with increases in the intestinal length and surface area including villus and microvillus growth occur during the last trimester. Human milk is the first choice for preterm and term infants as it provides substantial benefits to premature infants' health including reduced infectious and inflammatory disease and enhanced neurodevelopmental outcome. If unfortified however, human milk may not provide adequate nutrients to meet the demands of premature infants particularly in light of the large variations in the protein and fat content of human milk. Human milk from mothers of preterm infants contains more protein than does the milk from mothers of term infants; initially, it has a protein content of approximately 2.5–3 g/100 mL (colostrum), which decreases to approximately 1.5–2 g/100 mL soon after birth (transitional milk), and finally stabilizes at 0.9–1.4 g/100 mL (mature milk). In general, increased concentration levels of protein persist for the first month of lactation. Thereafter, the protein content of preterm milk decreases and approaches the composition of term human milk. Preterm infants receiving 150 ml/kg per day of fortified human milk receive approximately 3.5 g/kg per day of protein.

Total Parenteral Nutrition

The smaller the infant, the greater the need for parenteral nutrition and the greater the urgency to initiate it. Thus, for infants with birth weights <1,500 g, total parenteral nutrition (TPN) is started at 2–3 days of life when the fluid and sodium status has stabilized. Infants require 90–100 cals/kg of TPN or 110–130 cals/kg of enteral nutrition to optimize growth. When supplementing orogastric feeds, the TPN is increased to 150–160 ml/kg/day as tolerated in order to provide adequate calories for growth. Current practice in many NICUs is to initiate TPN with 3 g/kg of protein soon after birth using "starter" or "vanilla" TPN solutions that are stocked in the NICU. In both human milk and formulae, lipids comprise about 50 % of the total energy and contain the essential fatty acids, linolenic acid and linoleic acid. The primary reason for including parenteral lipids is to provide the essential fatty acids, which are important determinants of membrane lipid composition and central nervous system development. ELBW infants usually receive their dietary fat via parenteral lipid emulsions. There are concerns that lipid infusions in premature neonates may have adverse effects such as impaired oxygenation, increased risk of lung disease, impaired immune function and increased free bilirubin levels. In addition, while there are good reasons for using lipids, a good proportion of these lipids are stored rather than oxidized as fuel.

Fluid Management and Fasting Before Surgery

(a) Elective surgery: Before elective surgery (such as inguinal hernia repair in a growing preterm infant or repair of diaphragmatic hernia), serum electrolytes and fluid status are reviewed and optimized. Preterm infants with BPD are often treated with diuretics to optimize their pulmonary status. Chronic respiratory acidosis with metabolic compensation, hyponatremia, and either hypo- or hyperkalemia is common. Treatment with enteral or parenteral supplements may be necessary before surgery. Neonates should be fasted 2 h after clear fluids, 4 h after human breast milk and 6 h after nonhuman formula [33, 34]. Infants fulfilling these fasting criteria usually have only a minor fluid deficit at the time of surgery, a deficit that is not necessary to correct. When fasting guidelines are not applicable or not followed, some infants may be fasted for several hours before surgery. In this case, preoperative deficits are calculated by multiplying the hourly maintenance fluid requirement by the number of hours of restriction. Murat proposed to replace 50 % of the fasting deficit in the first hour and 25 % in the second and third hours [35]. The amount of fluid given during the first hour should be reduced if neonates are fasting for a shorter period of time or if the neonate is already receiving intravenous fluid before surgery [35].

(b) Emergent surgery: Before emergency surgery, all neonates should be immediately resuscitated with fluids. Abdominal emergencies (volvulus or pneumoperitoneum after NEC) are associated with extravasation of fluid from the vascular space into the lumen. Restoration of intravascular volume using crystalloids (isotonic saline or Ringer lactate), colloids (albumin), or blood products (platelets, packed RBCs, or fresh frozen plasma) is important. Conditions associated with vomiting or aspiration of gastric contents (such as pyloric stenosis, duodenal atresia or stenosis) are associated with abnormalities in serum sodium, potassium, bicarbonate and chloride. Infants with pyloric stenosis present with hypokalemic alkalosis and require resuscitation with fluids that contain adequate amounts of both chloride and potassium before they are scheduled for surgery.

(c) Parenteral nutrition: Continuing TPN with amino acids and lipids before and during surgery is common practice and has the theoretical advantage of providing optimal nutrition during catabolism associated with surgery. Three practical issues regarding the use of parenteral nutrition are the following:

1. Partial parenteral nutrition with feeds: Many infants undergoing semi-elective or elective surgery are receiving partial feeds and partial parenteral nutrition supplementation. The composition of partial parenteral nutrition fluids may include high concentration of

electrolytes (such as sodium, calcium, and potassium) and dextrose to compensate for low mineral content of oral feeds (specifically human milk). When the infant's oral feeds are stopped for preoperative fasting, the partial TPN should not be increased to full volume. Instead, a new TPN solution with optimal glucose and electrolytes at full volume (often 100–150 ml/kg/day) should be initiated. Alternately, the neonate's feeds may be supplemented with a plain crystalloid solution such as dextrose 5 % in water (through a Y connector) to provide a partial TPN solution.

2. Parenteral nutrition is usually administered through a thin percutaneous or peripherally intravascular central catheter (PICC line). These catheters have small internal diameter (usually 1.9-Fr lines) and offer large resistance. They are not suitable for emergency fluid boluses and are at a large risk of rupturing if small syringes (1–3 ml size) are used to inject fluid volumes rapidly because of the great pressures that can build up within the catheter.
3. Y-site compatibility of medications with parenteral nutrition solution: In 2007, Roche laboratories updated their prescribing information for ceftriaxone sodium to include a contraindication for the co-administration with calcium-containing intravenous solutions in neonates due to reported fatal cases of pulmonary and renal precipitates (Rocephin package insert). Readers are referred to a detailed review of compatibilities of medications with lipid- and non-lipid-containing parenteral fluids [36]. Table 8.2 highlights the compatibility of some commonly used medications with 2-in-1 (amino acids + glucose/electrolyte solution) and 3-in-1 (amino acids + lipids + glucose/electrolyte solution) parenteral nutrition solutions.

(d) Steroids: Preterm infants are occasionally treated with courses of corticosteroids such as hydrocortisone or dexamethasone to facilitate extubation, manage lung disease or treat resistant hypotension. Some of these infants may develop adrenocortical insufficiency with a suppressed HPA axis if more than an occasional pulse dose of steroids has been administered. Adrenocortical insufficiency may present with circulatory collapse during the stress associated with surgery. A stress dose of hydrocortisone is required before surgery in these infants to prevent circulatory collapse.

Intraoperative Fluid Requirement

Maintenance

Maintenance fluid requirements are commonly calculated using the formula devised by Holliday and Segar and modified by Oh (Table 8.3) [37]. In 1957, Holliday and Segar described the relationship between physiologic fluid losses and caloric expenditure [37]. They determined that physiologic deficits from urine output and insensible losses of the skin and respiratory tract are equal to approximately 100 ml/100 kcal metabolized per day. For infants 0–10 kg in weight, this is equivalent to 100 ml/kg. Their corresponding rule for hourly water requirement became the well-known rule of 4 + 2 + 1 rule described by Oh (Table 8.3) [38]. Electrolyte requirements were based on the electrolyte composition of human milk and cow's milk. They recommended 2 mEq/100 kcal/day of both potassium and chloride and 3 mEq/100 kcal/day of sodium [37]. The APA consensus guideline on perioperative fluid management in children did not reach agreement on what type and volume of fluid to give a full-term neonate after day 3 of life, but most neonatologists recommend that the maintenance fluid should include 10 % dextrose with Na (3 mmol/kg/day) and K (2 mmol/kg/day) given at a rate of 4 ml/kg/h or 100–120 ml/kg/day [39].

The objective of perioperative fluid therapy is to provide maintenance fluid requirements, maintain normoglycemia, correct fluid deficits and provide the volume of fluid to maintain adequate tissue perfusion. The fluid requirement varies with the type and nature of the fluid deficit (fluid loss or plasma loss) and the effect that these replacement fluids might have on the intravascular volume, coagulation cascade, and microcirculation. Infants at risk of perioperative hypoglycemia, including neonates <48 h old, those receiving TPN, or a preoperative glucose infusion and IUGR or VLBW infants should be given dextrose during surgery. Infants who receive parenteral nutrition preoperatively should continue to receive that same nutrition during surgery (the preferred approach) or a dextrose-containing maintenance fluid. During surgery, the majority of older infants may be given maintenance balanced salt solutions without dextrose, such as 0.9 % sodium chloride or Ringer lactate/Hartmann's solution, provided the blood glucose is monitored during surgery.

The optimal dextrose concentration of maintenance fluid during surgery is controversial. Stress-induced or glucocorticoid-induced hyperglycemia is common during surgery. However, some preterm infants may not be capable of mounting a stress response and in the absence of supplementary glucose infusions, may be at risk for hypoglycemia. Prolonged and severe hypoglycemia is associated with extensive and widespread neuronal injury. Current literature suggests that even transient hypoglycemia may result in neurologic injury in neonates [40]. In older infants, 5 % dextrose solutions should be avoided, but 1–2.5 % dextrose in lactated Ringer or normal saline may be appropriate [41, 42]. Wellborn reported that a 2.5 % dextrose infusion is preferable as 5 % dextrose invariably resulted in moderate to marked hyperglycemia [43–45]. An increased base excess due to lipid mobilization and ketosis has been reported in children who were given dextrose-free Hartmann's solution but did not occur when dextrose (2 % or 5 %) was added to the solution [46].

Table 8.2 Y-site compatibility of medications with parenteral nutrition solution

Medication	2-in-1 TPN	3-in-1 TPN	Comments
Acyclovir	I	I	White precipitate forms immediately
Albumin	C	I	
Alprostadil	C	–	
Amikacin sulphate	C	Conflicting data	
Amphotericin B	I	I	Yellow precipitate formation
Ampicillin	Conflicting but administered in some units		
Atracurium	C	–	
Bumetanide	C	C	
Buprenorphine	C	C	
Caffeine citrate	C	–	
Cefazolin	Incompatible if dextrose concentration is 25 %	C	
Cefotaxime	C	C	
Cefepime	C	–	
Cefoxitin	C	C	
Ceftazidime	C	C	
Ceftriaxone	I	I	
Dexamethasone	C	C	
Diazepam	C	–	
Diphenhydramine	C	C	
Dobutamine	C	C	
Dopamine	C	Conflicting	
Epinephrine	C	–	
Famotidine	C	C	
Fentanyl	C	C	
Furosemide	?		Small amount of precipitate forms in 4 h in select formulations
Heparin	C	I	
Hydrocortisone	C	C	
Insulin	C	C	
Isoproterenol	C	C	
Lorazepam	C	I	
Meperidine	C	C	
Methylprednisolone	C	C	
Metronidazole	C	C	
Midazolam	I	I	White precipitate forms immediately in select formulations
Milrinone	C	–	
Morphine	C	?	
Norepinephrine	C	C	
Ondansetron	C	I	
Oxacillin	C	C	
Penicillin G potassium	C	C	
Pentobarbital	C	I	
Phenobarbital	C	I	
Phenytoin	I	I	
Propofol	C	–	
Ranitidine	C	C	
Sodium bicarbonate	I		Small amount of precipitate forms in 1 h in select formulations
Vancomycin	C	C	
Vecuronium	C	–	

C compatible, *I* incompatible, – data not available, ? data not available, 2-in-1 (amino acids + glucose/electrolyte solution) and 3-in-1 (amino acids + lipids + glucose/electrolyte solution)

Table 8.3 Maintenance fluid requirements

Body weight	Holliday and Segar	Oh
Neonates/young infants 1–10 kg	4 ml/kg/h	4 ml/kg/h
Infants/toddlers 10–20 kg	40 ml/h + 2 ml/kg above 10 kg	20 + (2 × weight in kg) ml/kg/h
Children >20 kg	60 ml/h + 1 ml/kg/h above 20 kg	40 + weight in kg ml/kg/h

Glucose infusion at a rate of 120–300 mg/kg/h (2–5 mg/kg/min) is sufficient to maintain an acceptable blood glucose concentration without risking significant hyperglycemia. When combined with a physiological saline solution, this results in an electrolyte pattern and osmolarity very close to normal physiological extracellular levels [35, 47–49].

Intraoperative Volume Replacement

Intraoperative fluid therapy can be optimally achieved with two different types of fluids administered at different rates: a dextrose-containing solution (preferably TPN) for maintenance fluids at a set rate (usually 100 ml/kg/day or 4 ml/kg/h) and a separate solution to replace liquids (crystalloids such as Ringer lactate or colloids or blood products) (Fig. 8.3).

During surgery, insensible fluid losses (third space losses) vary widely depending on ambient conditions. Premature or low birth weight infants have a greater surface area-to-weight ratio, lose more water by evaporation and consequently require more replacement fluid. Fluid losses from the respiratory tract may be rather significant in small infants and influenced by the degree of humidification of the inspired gases.

Third Space Losses

This refers to the sequestration of fluid to a nonfunctional extracellular space that is beyond osmotic equilibrium with the vascular space [50]. Third space loss is difficult to quantify and may vary from less than 1 ml/kg/h for minor surgical procedures to as great as 15–20 m/kg/h for major abdominal procedures or even up to 50 ml/kg/h during necrotizing enterocolitis surgery in premature infants. Third space loss will be reduced if the procedure were performed laparoscopically.

All losses during surgery should be replaced with an isotonic fluid such as 0.9 % sodium chloride, Ringer lactate/Hartmann's solution, a colloid, or a blood product, depending on the child's hematocrit. Boluses during surgery to correct hypovolemia include colloids, crystalloids (0.9 % saline or

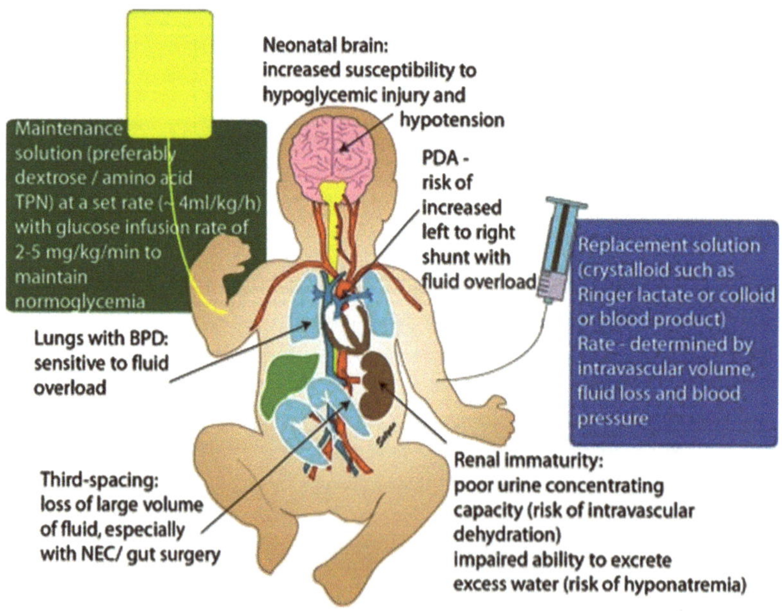

Fig. 8.3 Principles of intraoperative fluid management. Fluid therapy in the operating room consists of two components—maintenance and replacement fluids. The maintenance fluid consists of a dextrose-containing solution (preferably the same preoperative TPN solution) to maintain normoglycemia. The maintenance fluid should be infused at the same rate as preoperatively. The replacement solution should be a balanced salt solution such as Ringer lactate solution or a colloid (albumin) or blood product and is administered to maintain adequate intravascular volume and pressure and to replace any deficit or ongoing losses. Premature infants with bronchopulmonary dysplasia (BPD) and/or a PDA are susceptible to fluid overload. The brain of the neonate is particularly vulnerable to hypoglycemic injury. Cerebral circulation is pressure-passive with limited autoregulation and susceptible to hypotension. Abdominal surgery (especially NEC) is associated with increased "third space" losses into the gut requiring increased replacement fluid therapy. The immature kidney is unable to handle the increased water load, thereby increasing the risk of hyponatremia. See text for details

Ringer lactate/Hartmann's) or blood to maintain the hemoglobin at 10–12 g/dl. Large amounts of normal saline are responsible for hyperchloremic metabolic acidosis, whereas this does not occur after Ringer lactate administration. In stable, critically ill children, a minimum hemoglobin threshold of 7 g/dl for red cell transfusion has been recommended, but no similar consensus has been reached on the minimum hemoglobin threshold for transfusion in infants less than 3 months of age [51–54]. A greater hemoglobin threshold is generally advised to trigger a blood transfusion in full-term and premature neonates, noting that anemic preterm infants are more prone to episodes of postoperative apnea. Neonates with cyanotic congenital heart disease usually require a greater hematocrit in order to maintain systemic oxygenation, and their hemoglobin concentrations should probably be maintained at greater concentrations.

The extent of third space losses during the perioperative period in infants has been challenged in several studies that suggest that the functional fluid space is either unchanged or expanded rather than contracted after surgery [55]. Substantial amounts of fluid accumulate in the interstitial space secondary to factors that include volume overload with crystalloid infusions and iatrogenic deterioration of the vascular barrier [56]. Preterm infants with BPD and/or PDA are sensitive to volume overload resulting in acute respiratory deterioration. It is possible that the practice of liberal isotonic fluid delivery during major pediatric surgery may have adverse implications. We are left to wonder if a smaller amount of crystalloid solution combined with an appropriate colloid might reduce the amount of tissue edema and improve recovery from surgery [57].

Colloids

The choice of colloid for intraoperative fluid management varies from institution to institution. Albumin has been widely favored for the maintenance of colloid osmotic pressure in infants and neonates and continues to be the most frequently used plasma expander in this population [58, 59]. However, the expense of colloids and decreased availability of albumin have led some countries to pursue other options. The Association of Pediatric Anaesthetists of Great Britain and Ireland favors the use of gelatins; the Association of French Speaking Pediatric Anesthetists in France frequently uses hetastarch solutions (HES); however in the USA, albumin remains the first choice [60–62].

Albumin

Albumin has several advantages in neonatal anesthesia. Apart from being the main preserver of the colloid osmotic pressure in plasma (75 %), it also functions as an important binding site for certain metabolites (e.g., bilirubin), free fatty acids and drugs. Of the two available albumin solutions, 5 % albumin solution is osmotically equivalent to an equal volume of plasma, whereas a 25 % solution is osmotically equivalent to five times its plasma volume [63]. In hypotensive premature infants, 4.5 % albumin was demonstrated to be more effective than 20 % albumin. This suggests that the volume of albumin administered is more important than its concentration to maintain or restore cardiovascular stability [64]. Albumin has been associated with a reduction in edema and inspired oxygen concentration requirements in ventilator-dependent hypoalbuminemic preterm infants, compared with infants who received an equal volume of crystalloid maintenance fluid [59]. Side effects from albumin are rare although hemodilution after large volumes of albumin (25 % hemodilution of the blood volume) may lead to a hypocoagulable state through inhibition of platelet aggregation or heparin-like effects on antithrombin III [65].

Nonprotein Colloids: HES

Hydroxyethyl starches (HESs) are a class of synthetic carbohydrate-based colloids that expand the plasma volume with effects lasting 2–6 h. They are prepared in concentrations of 3, 6, and 10 %. New (third)-generation HES fluids are designed with low molecular weight and molar substitution (percent of glucose subunits with hydroxyethyl groups) ratios to minimize side effects, as well as a large ratio of C2:C6 hydroxyethylation to prolong its duration of action [66]. In neonates without cardiac, renal, or hemostatic abnormalities undergoing central line placement, 6 % HES did not increase serum creatinine or bleeding when compared with neonates who received an equal volume of 5 % albumin [67]. However, there was no difference among HES, isotonic saline, and 5 % albumin in the improvement in cardiac output in hypotensive neonates in low cardiac output states [67]. In randomized trials with either normal saline or albumin, HES 130/0.42/6:1 appeared to be safe when used for volume expansion in neonates, infants and children, without serious adverse events [68, 69]. Reported side effects after HES solutions include hypocoagulation, renal toxicity and pruritus, although pruritus is not a concern in neonates. [70]. When 15 ml/kg HES was administered, thromboelastography values after HES 130/0.4 were more impaired than after albumin and gelatin in neonates and infants 3–15 kg [71]. In addition, HES may interfere with the function of von Willebrand factor, factor VIII and platelets, [72] which may present a problem for neonates who require cardiac surgery [73].

Gelatins are polypeptides produced by the degradation of bovine collagen. They have a brief duration of action because of their rapid passage into the interstitial space, rapid glomerular filtration and enzymatic cleavage by proteases.

There are limited data to support the use of gelatin in infants. The Northern Neonatal Nursing Initiative Trial Group was unable to show significant differences in early mortality and morbidity in preterm infants after prophylactic intravenous fresh frozen plasma, gelatin, or glucose [74]. In contrast, a systematic review of randomized controlled trials in adults and children failed to prove that gelatin was safe and effective [75]. Evidence from a septic shock model in animals demonstrated that gelatin and HES maintain plasma volume more effectively than albumin [76]. However, early volume expansion with gelatin in preterm infants was associated with an increased risk of developing NEC compared with neonates who received fresh frozen plasma [77]. The International Guidelines 2000 Conference for Neonatal Resuscitation recommended that emergency volume expansion should be accomplished with either isotonic crystalloid solution or O-negative RBCs [78]. However, the clinical practice guidelines of the Dutch Pediatric Society recommended the use of isotonic saline as safe, effective, and 100 times less expensive than albumin [62].

Postoperative Fluid Maintenance

The APA consensus guideline on perioperative fluid management in children could not reach consensus on the ideal fluid for postoperative maintenance. A survey of postoperative fluids in pediatrics indicated that hypotonic fluids are still commonly prescribed during the perioperative period to children [79–81], although this practice may lead to significant problems. The Royal College of Anaesthetists in conjunction with the Royal College of Pediatrics and Child Health cautioned against the use of 0.18 % saline in 4 % dextrose because of the risk of hyponatremia, especially in infants with conditions associated with increased ADH levels. They recommended that postoperative maintenance fluids should be at least 0.45 % saline, if not 0.9 % saline or Hartmann's solution.

Several reports of morbidity and mortality from severe iatrogenic hyponatremia have drawn the attention of investigators [49]. Hyponatremia (<115 mmol/l) in the perioperative period is primarily the result of extra renal loss of electrolytes in the presence of increased ADH activity and the administration of hypotonic fluids [82, 83]. Hyponatremia produces osmotic movement of free water across cell membranes from the extracellular to the intracellular compartments, the brain being the most seriously affected organ. In early hyponatremia, the brain responds by transporting intracellular sodium to the extracellular environment using the $Na^{+}K^{+}$ ATPase mechanism [84]. Younger children are more susceptible to hyponatremic encephalopathy due to a larger brain-to-skull ratio and greater intracellular concentration of sodium in the brain (about 27 % greater in children than adults) [82]. The inability of the pediatric brain to adapt to excess free water, combined with the large brain-to-skull ratio, explains the relatively rapid onset of cerebral edema in the presence of hyponatremia. The neonatal surgical patient is certainly at risk for increased ADH, as a result of the pain, stress, hypovolemia and/or hemorrhage associated with the perioperative period. Nonosmotic stimuli of ADH secretion include positive pressure ventilation, stress, nausea and vomiting, hypoglycemia, fever, and decreases in intravascular volume [85] as sequelae of illness or surgery [18, 86]. Asphyxiated infants may also have increased circulating arginine vasopressin (which is similar to SIADH), which may predispose these infants to an increased risk of cerebral edema. Immediate management is to restrict fluid intake for 48–72 h, i.e., ≤60 ml/kg/day, or until seizures are no longer a problem. Several studies have suggested that the use of isotonic saline solution, not fluid restriction, decreases the risk of hyponatremia in sick children [86–89].

The updated fluid recommendations by Holliday and Segar for infants and children who remain NPO postoperatively is 2-1-0.5 instead of 4-2-1 as previously recommended for balanced salt solution (in 10 kg increments) in ml/kg/h for infants and children [90]. This regimen, however, was predicated on "turning off" ADH by administering balanced salt solution in sufficient volume [91]. In contrast, the APA consensus guideline failed to issue a fluid maintenance rate for the postoperative period, with some advocating a full maintenance rate as per Holliday and Segar in 1957 [60] and others advocating restricting the children to 60–70 % of full maintenance rates and supplementing that with additional boluses of isotonic fluid as required. Premature neonates may require an additional 30 ml/kg/day because of increased insensible fluid losses and may also require additional sodium supplements (4 mmol/kg/day).

It is a common practice to resume TPN in neonates with a dextrose, electrolyte, amino acid, and lipid solution after surgery at 60–70 % (usually 100 ml/kg/day) of the preoperative rate, with frequent serial monitoring of the serum electrolyte concentrations to preclude hyponatremia. Loss of fluid from the intravascular space due to third space loss is replaced with crystalloid and colloid solutions. Many postoperative infants gain considerable weight due to capillary leak and fluid administration in the perioperative period compromising respiration. Once the preterm infant with BPD is hemodynamically stable, diuresis (sometimes preceded by an infusion of albumin) is necessary to improve respiratory function and facilitate extubation of the trachea. Fluid restriction as described below for postoperative management after cardiac surgery may also have a role in preterm infants with BPD.

Neonatal Endocrine Surgical Stress Response

Adult metabolic studies suggest that critically ill surgical patients have increased resting energy expenditures that are proportional to the severity of the underlying disease process. The stress response in neonates and premature infants however is quantitatively and qualitatively different from that of older individuals. The increases in stress hormones associated with surgery in the neonate exceed those measured in children and adults but under most circumstances return to baseline by 24 h [92]. Neonates <48 h old have a diminished stress response compared with older neonates. One possible explanation for this difference may be the greater secretion of endogenous opioids in the perinatal period blunting the endocrine and metabolic responses [93, 94]. Resting energy expenditures increase only by 20 % in neonates undergoing major surgery but return to normal values within 12 h. It has been suggested that one reason critically ill neonates fuel the metabolic stress response without increasing their resting energy expenditure is that neonates, unlike adults, are still actively growing. Only approximately 65 % of neonatal energy requirements are necessary to meet resting energy expenditure. The remainder is directed primarily to maintain growth and to a lesser extent to regulate temperature and meet the demands of activity. The total energy needs of intravenously fed, full-term, surgical neonates are about 85 kcal kg/day. Sick neonates stop growing, become lethargic and require nursing in a thermoneutral environment. Thus, energy is available to supply the metabolic response to injury without any consistent perturbation in the resting energy expenditure. Other factors such as the use of sedation may further reduce the resting energy expenditure, apportioning more energy for the metabolic response. This suggests that the routine administration of excess calories may not be warranted in critically ill surgical neonates and also supports the hypothesis that neonates redirect energy, normally used for growth, to fuel the stress response [95].

Postoperative Metabolic Needs

Special attention must be directed to providing optimal metabolic care in the postoperative period. Rates of survival for extremely low birth weight (ELBW) (<1,000 g) infants have improved, but delayed-onset growth failure is nearly universal. At the time of birth, only about 18 % of ELBW infants are less than the 10th percentile for weight and length. At 36 weeks corrected gestational age, as the neonates near discharge from the NICU, most ELBW infants are less than the 10th percentile for weight and length. A 26-week gestation 1,000-g birth weight infant begins with body protein stores of approximately 88 g compared with 250 g in a full-term infant. Without protein intake, the infant loses approximately 1.5 % of total body protein per day. After only 3 days without protein intake, body protein stores are reduced by 5 % from birth and are 10 % less than a fetus of comparable age. In contrast, after birth most of the very preterm infants are fed more lipid and glucose and less amino acids and protein than they need. Not surprisingly, therefore, very preterm infants accumulate fat but remain relatively growth restricted at term gestational age compared with those infants who grew normally in utero, and this postnatal growth restriction has long-term adverse growth, development and health consequences.

Special Cases: Cardiac Surgery

Infants presenting for neonatal cardiac surgery require special consideration and represent an exception to the above recommendations. The optimal maintenance fluid infusion rate is often less than has been outlined above in order to manage borderline ventricular function or excessive pulmonary blood flow [96, 97]. Similarly intraoperative fluids must be reduced as fluid overload and renal dysfunction may significantly contribute to morbidity, e.g., after arterial switch surgery in neonates and infants [98, 99]. In addition, the use of intraoperative balanced salt solutions that contain glucose during pediatric cardiac surgery remains controversial because of possible associations with worsened neurological injury compared with results when glucose was not added. The use of glucose-free, balanced salt solutions during pediatric cardiac surgery, however, may result in hypoglycemia during the pre-bypass period. Moderate intraoperative glucose administration (2.5 mg/kg/min) will not cause major hyperglycemia but just may prevent episodes of hypoglycemia. Blood glucose concentrations should always be monitored during neonatal cardiac surgery to preclude swings in the plasma glucose concentrations [100].

Postoperative fluid restriction has also been widely accepted as one of the important strategies to reduce the amount of pulmonary edema and improve respiratory function, prevent intravascular volume overload and reduce multiple-organ dysfunction early after pediatric cardiac surgery, especially in low-weight infants [101]. After cardiopulmonary bypass, there is a tendency for sodium and water retention in association with the systemic inflammatory response to bypass and surgery that increases capillary permeability. Excess postoperative fluids after cardiac surgery correlate significantly and independently with prolonged mechanical ventilation [102]. For bypass cases, fluids are restricted to 50 % of maintenance rates in the immediate postoperative period, whereas in non-bypass cases, it is limited to 60 % of maintenance rates. This fluid regimen should continue until the infant's airway is extubated, after which the fluid rate should increase by 10 % per day [103, 104].

Growth failure and malnutrition are common in neonates with congenital heart disease. The etiology of the growth failure is multifactorial and most likely reflects a hypermetabolic state, inadequate caloric intake, malabsorption and genetic factors [105]. Fluid restriction used for hemodynamic management may also be a contributory factor. Congenital heart disease increases cardiac and respiratory work to a significant effect immediately after cardiac surgery. Adequate enteral nutrition may be difficult to achieve early after cardiac surgery in neonates, but it is essential for growth, wound healing, and the integrity of the immune system. Children with less complex cardiac lesions (e.g., VSD) may need as much as 50 % more calories than healthy infants in order to continue along a normal growth curve. Infants with single-ventricle repairs and aortopulmonary shunts may have relative splanchnic ischemia due to the diastolic runoff from the shunt and be at increased risk for NEC. In most cases, infants who require neonatal surgery have substantive difficulty in gaining weight postoperatively despite these adjustments to the caloric intake. Strategies to optimize the caloric intake and promote weight gain include use of TPN in the early postoperative period, institution of nasogastric feeds and the use of high-calorie enteral feeds [106].

References

1. Hartnoll G, Betremieux P, Modi N. The body water content of extremely preterm infants at birth. Arch Dis Child Fetal Neonatal Ed. 2000;83:F56–9.
2. Martinerie L, Pussard E, Foix-L'Helias L, Petit F, Cosson C, Boileau F, Lombe's M. Physiological partial aldosterone resistance in human newborns. Pediatr Res. 2009;66(3):323–8.
3. Mir T, Laux R, Henning-Hellwage H, Liedke B, Heinze C, von Buelow H, Laer S, Weil J. Plasma concentrations of amino terminal pro atrial natriuretic peptide and amino terminal pro brain natriuretic peptide in healthy neonates: marked rise and rapid increase after birth. Pediatrics. 2003;112(4):896–9.
4. Costello JM, Goodman DM, Green TP. A review of the natriuretic hormone system's diagnostic and therapeutic potential in critically ill children. Pediatr Crit Care Med. 2006;7:308–18.
5. Sanjeev S, Pettersen M, Lua J, Thomas R, Shankaran S, L'Ecuyer T. Role of plasma B-type natriuretic peptide in screening for hemodynamically significant patent Ductus Arteriosus in Preterm Neonates. J Perinatol. 2005;25:709–13.
6. Bolt RJ, van Weissenbruch MM, Popp-Snijders C, Sweep C, Lafeber H, Delemarre-van de Waal HA. Fetal growth and the function of the adrenal cortex in preterm infants. J Clin Endocrinol Metab. 2002;87:1194–9.
7. Atasay B, Ergun H, Okulu E, Mungan Akin I, Arsan S. The association between cord hormones and transient tachypnea of newborn in late preterm and term neonates who were delivered by cesarean section. J Matern Fetal Neonatal Med. 2013; 26(9):877–80.
8. Ng PC. Effect of stress on the hypothalamic-pituitary-adrenal axis in the fetus and newborn. J Pediatr. 2011;158:e41–3.
9. Fernandez EF, Watterberg KL. Relative adrenal insufficiency in the preterm and term infant. J Perinatol. 2009;29:S44–9.
10. Ng PC, Lee CH, Lam CW, et al. Transient adrenocortical insufficiency of prematurity and systemic hypotension. Arch Dis Fetal Neonatal Ed. 2004;89:F119–26.
11. Baker CFW, Barks JDE, Engmann C, et al. Hydrocortisone administration for the treatment of refractory hypotension in critically ill newborns. J Perinatol. 2008;28:412–19.
12. Grofer B, Bodeker RH, Gortner L, Heckmann M. Maturation of adrenal function determined by urinary glucocorticoid steroid excretion rates in preterm infants of more than 30 weeks gestation. Neonataology. 2010;98:200–5.
13. Ng PC. The fetal and neonatal hypothalamic-pituitary-adrenal axis. Arch Dis Child Fetal Neonatal Ed. 2000;82:F250–4.
14. Stephenson T, Broughton Pipkin F, Elias-Jones A. Factors affecting plasma renin and renin substrate in premature infants. Arch Dis Child. 1991;66:1150–4.
15. Martinerie L, Viengchareun S, Delezoide AL, et al. Low renal mineralocorticoid receptor expression at birth contributes to partial aldosterone resistance in neonate. Endocrinology. 2009; 150:4414–24.
16. Ronconi GF, Ronconi M, Presenti P, et al. Influence of the mode of delivery on the plasma levels of ADH in the mother and newborn infant. Pediatr Med Chir. 1985;7:225–8.
17. Burrows FA, Shutak JG, Crone RK. Inappropriate secretion of ADH in a post surgical paediatric population. Crit Care Med. 1983;11:527–31.
18. Rosendahl W, Schulz U, Teufel T, Irtel vB, Gupta D. Surgical stress and neuroendocrine responses in infants and children. J Pediatr Endocrinol. 1995;8:187–94.
19. Ligi I, Boubred F, Grandvuillemin I, et al. The neonatal kidney: implications for drug metabolism and elimination. Curr Drug Metab. 2013;14:174–7.
20. Quigley R. Developmental changes in renal function. Curr Opin Pediatr. 2012;24:184–90.
21. Iacobelli S, Addabbo F, Bonsante F, et al. Aquaporin-2 excretion and renal function during the 1st week of life in preterm newborn infants. Nephron Physiol. 2006;104:121–5.
22. Drukker A, Guignard J-P. Renal aspects of the term and preterm infant: a selective update. Curr Opin Pediatr. 2002;14:175–82.
23. Aly H, Davies J, El-Dib M, Massaro A. Renal function is impaired in small for gestational age premature infants. J Matern Fetal Neonatal. 2013;26(4):388–91.
24. Yared A, Yoskioka T. Autoregulation of glomerular filtration in the young. Semin Nephrol. 1989;9:94–7.
25. Oh W. Fluid and electrolyte therapy in low birth weight infants. Pediatr Rev. 1980;1:313–16.
26. ESPGHAN. Fluid and electrolytes (Na, Cl and K). J Pediatr Gastroenterol Nutr. 2005;41:S33–8.
27. Sweet CB, Grayson S, Polak M. Management strategies for neonatal hypoglycaemia. J Pediatr Pharmacol. 2013;18:199–208.
28. Sieber FE, Traystman RJ. Special issues: glucose and the brain. Crit Care Med. 1992;20:104–14.
29. Inder T. How low can I go? The impact of hypoglycaemia on the immature brain. Pediatrics. 2008;122:440–1.
30. Burns CM, Rutherford MA, Boardman JP, Cowan FM. Pattern of cerebral injury and neurodevelopmental outcomes after symptomatic neonatal hypoglycaemia. Pediatrics. 2008;122:65–74.
31. Hay WW. Strategies for feeding the preterm infant. Neonatology. 2008;94(4):245–54.
32. Reynolds RM, Thureen PJ. Special circumstances: trophic feeds, necrotising enterocolitis and bronchopulmonary dysplasia. Semin Fetal Neonatal Med. 2007;12(1):64–70.
33. Apfelbaum JL, et al. Practice guidelines for preoperative fasting and the use of pharmacologic agents to reduce the risk of pulmonary aspiration: application to healthy patients undergoing elective procedures. An updated report by the American Society of

Anesthesiologists committee on standards and practice parameters. Anesthesiology. 2011;114:495–511.
34. Smith I, et al. Perioperative fasting in adults and children: guidelines from the European society of anaesthesiology. Eur J Anaesthesiol. 2011;28:556–69.
35. Murat I, Dubois M-C. Perioperative fluid therapy in pediatrics. Pediatr Anesth. 2008;18:363–70.
36. Robinson CA, Sawyer JE. Y-site compatibility of medications with parenteral nutrition. J Pediatr Pharmacol Ther. 2009; 14:48–56.
37. Holliday MA, Segar WE. The maintenance need for water in parenteral fluid therapy. Paediatrics. 1957;19:823–32.
38. Oh T. Formulas for calculating fluid maintenance requirements. Anesthesiology. 1980;53:351.
39. APA Consensus Guideline on Perioperative Fluid Management in Children August 2007. http://www.apagbi.org.uk.
40. Dalgic N et al J Pediatr Endocrinol Metab 2002, Kinnala Pediatrics 1999 and Duvanel CB J Pediatrics 1999.
41. Dubois M, Gouyet L, Murat I. Lactated Ringer with 1 % dextrose: an appropriate solution for peri-operative fluid therapy in children. Paediatr Anaesth. 1992;2:99–104.
42. Hongnat J, Murat I, Saint-Maurice C. Evaluation of current paediatric guidelines for fluid therapy using two different dextrose hydrating solutions. Paediatr Anaesth. 1991;1:95–100.
43. Nishina K, Mikawa K, Maekawa N, Asano M, Obara H. Effects of exogenous intravenous glucose on plasma glucose and lipid homeostasis in anesthetized infants. Anesthesiology. 1995; 83:258–63.
44. Berleur MP, Dahan A, Murat I, et al. Perioperative infusions in paediatric patients: rationale for using Ringer-lactate solution with low dextrose concentration. J Clin Pharm Ther. 2003;28:31–40.
45. Geib I, Dubois MC, Gouyet L, et al. Perioperative perfusion in children: evaluation of a new perfusion solution. Ann Fr Anesth Reanim. 1993;12:6–10.
46. Aun CST, Panesar NS. Paediatric glucose homeostasis during anaesthesia. Br J Anaesth. 1990;64:413–18.
47. Berry FA. There is a solution for perioperative fluid management in children. Pediatr Anesth. 2008;18:332–61.
48. Leelanukorum R, Cunliffe M. Intraoperative fluid and glucose management in children. Paediatr Anaesth. 2000;10:353–9.
49. Lonnqvist P. Inappropriate perioperative fluid management in children: time for a solution? Paediatr Anaesth. 2006;17:203–5.
50. Filston HC, Edwards CH, Chitwood R, Larson RM, Marsicano TH, Hill RC. Estimation of postoperative fluid requirements in infants and children. Ann Surg. 1982;196:76–81.
51. Bell EF, Strauss RG, Widness JA, et al. Randomized trial of liberal versus restrictive guidelines for red blood cell transfusion in preterm infants. Pediatrics. 2005;115:1685–91.
52. Kirpalani H, Whyte R. Low versus high haemoglobin concentration threshold for blood transfusion for preventing morbidity and mortality in very low birth weight infants (Review). Cochrane Rev Database Syst Rev 2011;(11):CD000512. Pub2.
53. Morley SL. Red blood cell transfusions in acute paediatrics. Arch Dis Child Educ Pract Ed. 2009;94:65–73.
54. Chen HL, Tseng HI, Lu CC, et al. Effect of blood transfusions on the outcome of very low body weight preterm infants under two different transfusion criteria. Pediatr Neonatol. 2009;50:110–16.
55. Reid DJ. Intracellular and extracellular fluid volume during surgery. Br J Surg. 1968;55:594–6.
56. Chappell D, Jacob M, Hofmann-Kiefer K, et al. A rational approach to perioperative fluid management. Anesthesiology. 2008;109:723–40.
57. Bailey A, McNaull P, Jooste E, Tuchman J. Perioperative crystalloid and colloid fluid management in children: where are we and how did we get there? Anesth Analg. 2010;110:375–90.
58. Robertson NR. Use of albumin in neonatal resuscitation. Eur J Pediatr. 1997;156:428–31.
59. Greenough A. Use and misuse of albumin infusions in neonatal care. Eur J Pediatr. 1998;157:699–702.
60. Schwarz U. Intraoperative fluid therapy in infants and young children. Anaesthetist. 1999;48:41–50.
61. Soderlind M, Salvignol G, Izard P, Lonnqvist PA. Use of albumin, blood transfusion and intraoperative glucose by APA and ADARPEF members: a postal survey. Paediatr Anaesth. 2001; 11:685–9.
62. Boluyt N, Bollen CW, Bos AP, Kok JH, Offringa M. Fluid resuscitation in neonatal and pediatric hypovolemic shock: a Dutch Pediatric Society evidence-based clinical practice guideline. Intensive Care Med. 2006;32:995–1003.
63. De Gaudio AR. Therapeutic use of albumin. Int J Artif Organs. 1995;18:216–24.
64. Emery E, Greenough A, Gamsu H. Randomised controlled trial of colloid infusions in hypotensive preterm infants. Arch Dis Child. 1992;67:1185–90.
65. Tobias MD, Wambold D, Pilla MA, Greer F. Differential effects of serial hemodilution with hydroxyethyl starch, albumin, and 0.9 % saline on whole blood coagulation. J Clin Anesth. 1998;10:366–71.
66. Kozek-Langenecker SA, Jungheinrich C, Sauermann W, Van der Linden P. The effects of hydroxyethyl starch 130/0.4 (6 %) on blood loss and use of blood products in major surgery: a pooled analysis of randomized clinical trials. Anesth Analg. 2008; 107:382–90.
67. Liet JM, Bellouin AS, Boscher C, Lejus C, Roze JC. Plasma volume expansion by medium molecular weight hydroxyethyl starch in neonates: a pilot study. Pediatr Crit Care Med. 2003;4:305–7.
68. Sumpelmann R, Kretz FJ, Luntzer R, et al. Hydroxyethyl starch 130/0.42/6:1 for perioperative volume replacement in 1130 children: results of an European prospective multicentre observational postauthorization safety study (PASS). Paediatr Anesth. 2012;22: 371–8.
69. (Voluven®) or human albumin in children younger than 2 yr undergoing non-cardiac surgery. A prospective, randomized, open label, multicentre trial. Eur J Anaesth 2008;25:437–45
70. Groeneveld AB, Navickis RJ, Wilkes MM. Update on the comparative safety of colloids: a systematic review of clinical studies. Ann Surg. 2011;253:470–83.
71. Haas T, Preinreich A, Oswald E, Pajk W, Berger J, Kuehbacher G, Innerhofer P. Effects of albumin 5 % and artificial colloids on clot formation in small infants. Anaesthesia. 2007;62:1000–7.
72. Rackow EC, Mecher C, Astiz ME, Griffel M, Falk JL, Weil MH. Effects of pentastarch and albumin infusion on cardiorespiratory function and coagulation in patients with severe sepsis and systemic hypoperfusion. Crit Care Med. 1989;17:394–8.
73. Schortgen F, Lacherade JC, Bruneel F, Cattaneo I, Hemery F, Lemaire F, Brochard L. Effects of hydroxyethylstarch and gelatin on renal function in severe sepsis: a multicentre randomised study. Lancet. 2001;357:911–16.
74. Northern Neonatal Nursing Initiative Trial Group. Randomised trial of prophylactic early fresh-frozen plasma or gelatin or glucose in preterm babies: outcome at 2 years. Lancet 1996;348: 229–32
75. Osborn DA, Evans N. Early volume expansion for prevention of morbidity and mortality in very preterm infants. Cochrane Database Syst Rev 2001:CD002055.
76. Marx G, Cobas Meyer M, Schuerholz T, Vangerow B, Gratz KF, Hecker J, Sumpelmann R, Rueckoldt H, Leuwer M. Hydroxyethyl starch and modified fluid gelatin maintain plasma volume in a porcine model of septic shock with capillary leakage. Intensive Care Med. 2002;28:629–35.

77. Thomas-Rueddel DO, Vlasakov V, Reinhart K, et al. Safety of gelatin for volume resuscitation-a systematic review and meta-analysis. Intensive Care Med. 2012;38:1134–42.
78. Niermeyer S, Kattwinkel J, Van Reempts P, et al. International guidelines for neonatal resuscitation: an excerpt from the guidelines 2000 for cardiopulmonary resuscitation and emergency cardiovascular care: international consensus on science. Contributors and reviewers for the neonatal resuscitation guidelines. Pediatrics. 2000;106:E29.
79. Way C, Dhamrait R, Wade A, Walker I. Perioperative fluid therapy in children: a survey of current prescribing practice. Br J Anaesth. 2006;97:371–9.
80. Davies P, Hall T, Ali T, Lakhoo K. Intravenous postoperative fluid prescriptions for children: a survey of practice. BMC Surg. 2008;8:10–4.
81. Snaith R, Peutrell J, Ellis D. An audit of intravenous fluid prescribing and plasma electrolyte monitoring; a comparison with guidelines from the National Patient Safety Agency. Paediatr Anaesth. 2008;18:940–6.
82. Arieff AI, Ayus J, Fraser C. Hyponatremia and death or permanent brain damage in healthy children. BMJ. 1992;304:1218–22.
83. Cunliffe M, Potter F. Four and a fifth and all that. Br J Anaesth. 2006;97:274–7.
84. Moritz ML, Ayus JC. Prevention of hospital-acquired hyponatremia: a case for using isotonic saline. Pediatrics. 2003;111:227–30.
85. Gueli SL, Lerman J. Controversies in pediatric anesthesia: sevoflurane and fluid management. Curr Opin Anaesthesiol. 2013; 26:310–17.
86. Neville KA, Sandeman DJ, Rubinstein A, Henry GM, McGlynn M, Walker JL. Prevention of hyponatremia during maintenance intravenous fluid administration: a prospective randomized study of fluid type versus fluid rate. Pediatrics. 2010;156:313–19.
87. Hoorn EJ, Geary D, Robb M, Halperin ML, Bohn D. Acute hyponatremia related to intravenous fluid administration in hospitalized children: an observational study. Pediatrics. 2004;113: 1279–84.
88. Au AK, Ray PE, McBryde KD, Newman KD, Weinstein SL, Bell MJ. Incidence of postoperative hyponatremia and complications in critically-ill children treated with hypotonic and normotonic solutions. J Pediatr. 2008;152:33–8.
89. Alvarez Montanana P, Modesto I, Alapont V, Perez Ocon A, Ortega Lopez P, Lopez Prats JL, Toledo Parreno JD. The use of isotonic fluid as maintenance therapy prevents iatrogenic hyponatremia in pediatrics: a randomized, controlled open study. Pediatr Crit Care Med. 2008;9:589–97.
90. Holliday MA, Friedman AL, Segar WE, et al. Acute hospital-induced hyponatremia in children: a physiologic approach. J Pediatr. 2004;145:584–7.
91. Holliday MA. Isotonic saline expands extracellular fluid and is inappropriate for maintenance therapy. Pediatrics. 2005;115:193.
92. Anand KJS. Neonatal responses to anaesthesia and surgery. Clin Perinatol. 1990;17:207–14.
93. Schaffer L, Muller-Vincenzi D, Burkhardt T, Rauh M, Ehlert U, Beinder E. Blunted stress response in small for gestational age neonates. Pediatr Res. 2009;65:231–5.
94. McHoney M, Eaton S, Pierro A. Metabolic response to surgery in infants and children. Eur J Pediatr Surg. 2009;19(5):275–85.
95. Jaksic T, Shew S, Keshen T, Dzakovie A, Jahoor F. Do critically ill surgical neonates have increased energy expenditure? J Pediatr Surg. 2001;36(1):63–7.
96. O'Brien F, Walker IA. Fluid homeostasis in the neonate. Pediatr Anesth. 2014;24:49–59.
97. Wolf AR, Humphry AT. Limitations and vulnerabilities of the neonatal cardiovascular system: considerations for anesthetic management. Pediatr Anesth. 2014;24:5–9.
98. Wernovsky G, Wypij D, Jonas R, et al. Postoperative course and hemodynamic profile after the arterial switch operation in neonates and infants. Circulation. 1995;92:2226–35.
99. De Buyst J, Rakza T, Pennaforte T, Johansson AB, Storme L. Hemodynamic effects of fluid restriction in preterm infants with significant patent ductus arteriosus. J Pediatr. 2012;161(3): 404–8.
100. Agus MS, Steil GM, Wypij D, Costello JM, Laussen PC, Langer M, Alexander JL, Scoppettuolo LA, Pigula FA, Charpie JR, Ohye RG, Gaies MG. SPECS Study Investigators: Tight glycemic control versus standard care after pediatric cardiac surgery. N Engl J Med. 2012;367(13):1208–19.
101. Shi S, Zhao ZY, Liu XW, Shu Q, Tan L, Lin R, Shi Z, Fang X. Perioperative risk factors for prolonged mechanical ventilation following cardiac surgery in neonates and young infants. Chest. 2008;134:768–74.
102. Newth CJL, Venkataraman S, Willson DF, Meert KL, Harrison R, Dean JM, Pollack M, Zimmerman J, Anand KJS, Carcillo JA, Nicholson CE. Weaning and extubation readiness in pediatric patients. Pediatr Crit Care Med. 2009;10:1–11.
103. Hazle MA, Gajarski RJ, Yu S, Donohue J, Blatt NB. Fluid Overload in Infants Following Congenital Heart Surgery. Pediatr Crit Care Med. 2013;14(1):44–4.
104. Nicholson GT, Clabby ML, Mahle WT. Is there a benefit to postoperative fluid restriction following infant surgery? Congenit Heart Dis. 2014 Jan 21.
105. Okoromah CAN, Ekure EN, Lesi FEA, Okunowo WO, Tijani BO, Okeiyi JC. Prevalence, profile and predictors of malnutrition in children with congenital heart defects: a case–control observational study. Arch Dis Child. 2011;96:354–360.
106. Schwalbe-Terilli C, Hartman D, Nagle M, Gallagher P, Ittenbach R, Burnham N, Gaynor J, Ravishankar C. Enteral feeding and caloric intake in neonates after cardiac surgery. Am J Crit Care. 2009;18(1):52–7.

9 Neonatal Ventilation

Walid Habre

Adequately ventilating the lungs is crucial in neonates since both hypo- and hyperventilation may confer respiratory and systemic consequences, in addition to contributing to the increased morbidity and mortality in pediatric anesthesia [1, 2]. Recently, enormous efforts have been expended to improve ventilation strategies in neonates using a "protective" and "open-lung" strategy in order to maintain optimal functional residual capacity (FRC) and to prevent ventilation-induced lung injury and bronchopulmonary dysplasia. An increased awareness of the potential harm of hyperventilating the lungs of neonates with large tidal volumes (Vt) that can lead to alveolar overdistension due to excessive shear forces and the liberation of proinflammatory cytokines, which constitute the main features of the so-called ventilation-induced lung injury, have caused a reappraisal of such a practice [3, 4]. Moreover, the resultant hypocapnia from hyperventilation may induce cerebral vasoconstriction and promote the development of cystic periventricular leukomalacia [5]. On the other hand, suboptimal Vt may result in inefficient gas exchange, hypercapnia, and hypoxemia and an increased risk of intraventricular hemorrhage (IVH) [6]. To address these problems, several interesting ventilation modes are now available that can optimize tidal volume and meet the ventilation requirements of the neonate. Despite the introduction of several new ventilation strategies, no single ventilation strategy has proven to be superior over the others in terms of neonatal pulmonary and neurologic outcomes. For every ventilation strategy, real-time pulmonary monitoring should be used in order to compensate for sudden changes in the compliance and resistance of the respiratory system. This chapter reviews the specificities of the respiratory characteristics of neonatal pulmonary function, describes the different ventilation modes available for neonates, and highlights the importance of using a protective and open-lung ventilation strategy.

W. Habre (✉)
Paediatric Anaesthesia Unit, Geneva Children's Hospital, Geneva, Switzerland
e-mail: walid.habre@hcuge.ch

Neonatal Respiratory System

Three specific physiological characteristics distinguish the pulmonary system in the neonate. First, the chest wall, which is comprised of the respiratory muscles and skeletal structures, is very compliant because the ribs are cartilaginous. The horizontal ribs are responsible for the cylinder shape of the infant's thorax, which contrasts with the elliptical-shaped thorax and bucket-handled orientation of the ribs in older children. Moreover, the effectiveness of the intercostal muscles is limited, supporting the chest wall and minimizing its distortion rather than contributing to the increases in tidal volume as occurs in childhood. Thus, the principal muscle responsible for ventilation in the neonate is the diaphragm. However, the diaphragm in the neonate is disadvantaged as it has a smaller muscle mass, has a reduced content of high-endurance (fast twitch 1) muscle fibers, and inserts more horizontally into the chest wall in infants than in older children [7]. This mechanical disadvantage of the chest wall and diaphragm is exaggerated during respiratory distress when oxygen demand is increased. In this case, contraction of the diaphragm causes the lower rib cage to cave inward, thereby reducing the lung volume and offsetting the effect of the diaphragmatic contraction. Together, these chest wall weaknesses limit the neonate's ability to generate an adequate alveolar ventilation since most of the force generated is lost on chest wall deformation and fades quickly due to muscle fatigue [8].

The second important pulmonary feature that distinguishes the neonate is the so-called stiff lung. This results from the increased static elastic recoil pressure. The elastic recoil of the lung depends on the amount of elastic fibers within the lung and the surface tension generated at the air–liquid interface within the alveoli [9]. Surfactant reduces the surface tension within alveoli while maintaining patent terminal

J. Lerman (ed.), *Neonatal Anesthesia*, DOI 10.1007/978-1-4419-6041-2_9,

airways, independent of the alveolar diameter [10]. Moreover, the increased elastin/collagen ratio in neonates increases the forces that tend to collapse alveoli. These forces are counterbalanced in part by the outward opposing forces that prevent the lungs from collapsing. However, because the chest wall is very compliant, the net effect of these two opposing forces reduces the resting lung volume at end expiration. This corresponds to the functional residual capacity (FRC) and represents the resting volume of the respiratory system. Consequently, both the full-term neonate and the preterm infant have a relatively small FRC, even in the presence of efficient surfactant. However, when the amount of surfactant is reduced or respiratory distress syndrome is present, there is a further tendency for the terminal airways to collapse with subsequent atelectasis, loss of lung volume, ventilation-perfusion mismatch, and hypoxemia. This phenomenon is further exaggerated in preterm infants in whom collateral airflow cannot occur at the bronchoalveolar level because of the immaturity of the terminal airways and disturbed alveolarization [11, 12].

Thirdly, the neonatal respiratory system is challenged by the greater resistances of the upper airways and conducting airways of the lung compared with those in older children. The resistance in the upper airways can be substantive in neonates as the airflow is turbulent, and the resistance to airflow during turbulent flow increases with the fifth power of the decrease in radius. Hence, a 50 % reduction in the radius of the airway increases airflow resistance by 32-fold. In contrast, airflow in the smaller distal conducting airways of the lung (beyond the fourth or fifth bronchial division) is laminar. In these distal airways, resistance follows Poiseuille's equation for laminar flow and is inversely proportional to the fourth power of the radius of the airway). Thus, the radius of the airway is the most important variable in airway resistance, which explains the significant increase in the work of breathing in neonates when inflammatory disorders and thickened mucous membrane from respiratory infections or secretions are present. The gradual increase in airway resistance that occurs from the reductions in the airway radius from successive airway generations is offset by the greater cross-sectional area of the airways. In addition, studies have consistently demonstrated a reduction in airway resistance with increasing height [13, 14], whereas in neonates, airway resistance increases from airway closure and the loss in lung volume.

When considering the total respiratory system resistance, it is important to appreciate that the tracheal tube and the resistance from the forces generated by the viscoelastic component of the lung account for more than two-thirds of the total resistance. In neonates, the use of tracheal tubes with small diameters increases the respiratory resistance, and the relatively high elastic recoil of the lung may further exacerbate the resistive component of the respiratory system [13]. Thus, when ventilating the lungs of neonates, the pressure delivered to the lung must overcome both the frictional forces of the airway resistance as well as the tissue elastic recoil and the chest compliance. Many clinical conditions often observed in neonates alter ventilation and jeopardize our ability to successfully ventilate the lungs under anesthesia. Accordingly, positive-pressure ventilation of the lungs in the presence of decreased compliance such as after surfactant deficiency or congenital diaphragmatic hernia may become a serious challenge [15]. In addition, other congenital or acquired diseases (tracheomalacia, bronchial infection, and inflammation) may lead to increased resistance to air flow and require specific ventilation modes in order to obviate very high airway pressures that may contribute to ventilation-induced lung injury.

Ventilation Modes

Our expanding insight into neonatal respiratory pathophysiology combined with advances in ventilator technology has led to the introduction of a range of sophisticated ventilation modes, the impact of which has not yet been fully appreciated primarily because of the lack of randomized trials. Although a number of ventilation modes are used routinely in the neonatal intensive care unit (NICU), they have confusing terminology and are not available in anesthesia workstations. The available ventilation modes can be distinguished according to whether they are volumetric (e.g., flow generator), barometric (the pressure generator), or dual mode, a combination of both pressure and flow generators. Newer anesthetic ventilators allow the child to trigger the onset of the ventilator cycle, which further expands the number of ventilator strategies available [16].

Pressure-Controlled Ventilation

Pressure-controlled ventilation (PCV) is the most popular mode for use in neonates in clinical practice [16]. The basic and most frequently applied mode in NICU is the time-cycled, pressure-limited ventilation (also called intermittent positive-pressure ventilation: IPPV), a mode that is present on most anesthesia ventilators as PCV. The decelerating flow and the limited and constant inspiratory pressure that characterize this mode explain the reduced peak inspiratory pressure with attenuated tracheal and alveolar pressures. In addition, this mode compensates for a potential leak around an uncuffed tracheal tube, still routinely used in neonates. The combination of decelerating flow and constant airway pressure over time facilitates the equilibration of tracheal and alveolar pressures, which improves the distribution of ventilation and, thereby, improves gas exchange [17].

However, in PCV mode, three factors should be considered when selecting a tidal volume: (1) the pressure gradient between the maximum inspiratory set pressure (peak inspiratory pressure: PIP) and the end-expiratory positive pressure (PEEP); (2) the inspiratory time (T_i), which may depend and/or determine the ratio between the inspiratory and expiratory time as well as the respiration rate; and (3) the time constant, which depends on both the compliance and resistance of the total respiratory system and determines the time to equilibrate the pressures within the airways and alveoli. Therefore, when applying the PCV mode, in addition to limiting the peak inspiratory pressure (PIP) and the level of the PEEP, the settings for this mode require that the inspiratory and expiratory times (T_e) be adjusted in order to determine the respiration rate, irrespective of the child's own breathing, but usually at a level close to that observed physiologically. Whether T_i is large or small does not affect the incidence of chronic lung disease in neonates, although a brief T_i may decrease the risk of an air leak and decrease mortality [18]. Thus, T_i is usually adjusted to 0.35–0.5 s, with a greater T_e, the latter determining the respiration rate. However, during anesthesia, apart from increasing the level of PEEP, T_i can be increased if a greater mean airway pressure is required without causing asynchronous breathing between the child and the ventilator [19] that may occur in the absence of heavy sedation. Conversely, a smaller T_i during weaning is more advantageous in neonates. To overcome this limitation, synchronized ventilation with the neonate allowed to trigger the onset of inspiration is currently the most popular ventilation mode in the NICU. Among the different triggering techniques that have been developed, flow triggering via a flow sensor interposed between the tracheal tube and the ventilator's connection is the most sensitive trigger [20] and is therefore widely used in clinical practice. Synchronized intermittent mandatory ventilation (SIMV), pressure control mode, and assist-control (AC) modes have been introduced in the intensive care settings in order to assist the child's respiratory effort by securing a fixed respiration rate synchronized with the child's breathing (SIMV) or by assisting each breath on the basis of positive-pressure ventilation, but with a "control" of a minimum number of ventilator cycles (AC). If the child breathes rapidly, the initial T_i causes the ventilator to assist every triggered breath, which may decrease T_e and lead to air trapping from an inadequate expiratory time. This risk is also observed when using pressure-support ventilation (PSV), a mode that is present on most new anesthesia ventilators. In the PSV mode, both initiation and termination of ventilator assistance are controlled by the child's respiratory effort and changes in the airflow. Depending on the type of ventilator, inflation ceases when the inspiratory flow level decreases to between 10 % and 25 % of the maximum inspiratory flow [21]. This mode is very interesting in anesthesia and has been used in older children to reduce the work of breathing (WOB) associated with spontaneous respiration and to counteract the large resistance due to small diameter tracheal tubes. Because of the greater risk of patient-ventilator asynchrony in critically ill neonates with tachypnea, PSV may increase oxygen consumption and lead to ineffective respiratory efforts. A novel technique known as proportional assist ventilation (PAV) has been developed to prevent such phenomena from developing. This technique offers the advantage of further reducing the WOB. In this mode, the rate of lung inflation and thus the inspiratory pressure are controlled by the child and are proportional to the child's inspiratory effort [22]. Since the pressure applied depends on the inspiratory flow generated by the child, this mode assumes that neither hypopnea nor a leak around the tracheal tube is present [19]. However, this mode is not available on anesthesia machines. More interesting is the neurally adjusted ventilator assist (NAVA), which relies on the child's respiratory control and diaphragmatic activity [23, 16]. The inspiratory effort is detected via bipolar electrodes mounted on a nasogastric feeding tube, positioned at the level of the diaphragm. The level of ventilatory support is then proportional to the inspiratory effort. Although this mode is unaffected by the presence of a leak around the tracheal tube, its utility is still not defined in neonates, especially in premature infants with immature control of the respiration. In a retrospective study of NAVA compared with SIMV-PC in premature infants <1,500 g, NAVA resulted in better blood gas regulation, oxygen requirements, and reduced peak inspiratory pressure [24]. A recent prospective crossover study demonstrated that NAVA is associated with improved patient-ventilator synchrony and reduced peak airway pressure in comparison with PSV [25]. Moreover, a similar study demonstrated a reduced peak inspiratory pressure, inspired oxygen requirements, and respiratory rate to achieve a reduced carbon dioxide tension and better compliance after NAVA compared with PCV [26].

Volume-Controlled Ventilation

The major disadvantage of pressure-limited ventilation lies in the variable tidal volume (Vt). This results from changes in lung compliance and resistance that occur constantly in the neonate, particularly during general anesthesia. Thus, some anesthesiologists prefer volume-controlled ventilation (VCV), a mode that is based on the traditional delivery of a fixed preset Vt at a preestablished rate. This mode does not take into account the peak airway pressure that is needed to deliver the desired Vt and the magnitude of the tracheal pressures that may be encountered during ventilation, especially in the presence of reduced lung compliance or the increased airway resistance. Moreover, this mode of ventilation requires manual adjustment of the Vt to compensate for the compression of the gas within the ventilator circuit and gas leak around the uncuffed tracheal tube. These increased pressures may be attenuated by either setting the pressure pop-off valve or by adjusting the T_i in order to limit excessive pressures in neonates with chronic lung disease.

Volume-Targeted Ventilation

The increasing awareness of the usefulness of direct control of the PIP and the benefit of ventilation with a small constant Vt has led to the development of dual ventilation modes that guarantee Vt with a limited pressure [27]. Different ventilators with novel modes have been developed to permit the choice of both a target Vt and an adjustable pressure limit, the latter permitting the ventilator to autoregulate the inspiratory pressure (within the maximum limit set) or the T_i to guarantee the target Vt. These modalities are routinely used in NICU and are slowly finding their way into the operating room. These modes are known as volume-targeted ventilation modes that guarantee Vt by measuring the exhaled Vt and adjusting the peak inflation pressure to deliver the target Vt [28]. However, there is no evidence that volume-targeted ventilation offers any advantages over pressure-limited ventilation in terms of outcomes such as the risk of chronic lung diseases [29]. Nonetheless, volume-targeted ventilation has been associated with a significantly smaller duration of ventilation, a decreased rate of pneumothorax, and a decreased incidence of severe (grade 3 or 4) IVH when compared with pressure-limited ventilation [29, 30]. These modes are now available on some new anesthetic ventilators, but there is a dearth of studies on their clinical usefulness in anesthesia, despite their advantages.

Among these interesting novel ventilator modes, the volume guarantee (VG) ventilation mode is in fact a pressure-limited, volume-targeted time, or flow-cycled ventilator that merits further attention. The working pressure in this ventilation mode is adjusted to minimize the difference between the exhaled Vt (measured by the ventilator) and the desired Vt (set by the clinician) on a breath-by-breath basis. This mode can also be used in combination with other standard modes available for use in neonates including SIMV, AC, or PSV. When setting the parameters in this mode, not only should the desired Vt be taken into account but so should the T_i in order to determine the duration of insufflation based on the time-constant concept from pressure-controlled ventilation. In addition, the maximum peak inspiratory pressure should exceed the working pressure, but at a limit that protects the lungs from any risk of barotrauma should the lung compliance suddenly decrease. These ventilator characteristics are particularly interesting for the weaning period since the inspiratory pressure is adjusted in real time [27]. Other anesthesia machines have integrated the pressure-regulated volume control (PRVC) mode, where flow rate varies with the inspiratory pressure to deliver the targeted Vt [35]. Thus, this mode behaves in a manner similar to the pressure control modes in terms of the pressure and flow patterns but delivers the predetermined Vt by adjusting the PIP on the basis of the lung compliance. This ventilation mode has proven to be very effective in VLBW infants demonstrating a smaller duration of mechanical ventilation and less hemodynamic perturbations [32, 33] as well as in infants after congenital heart surgery in whom intratracheal pressure was reduced and the hemodynamics were stable [34]. When this mode is combined with other ventilator options that allow the infant to breathe spontaneously with pressure support, it is called "automode," which is now present on some anesthesia machines although again without studies in neonates.

High-Frequency Ventilation

High-frequency ventilation (HFV) has found application in the management of neonates with serious lung disease since it allows ventilation with small tidal volumes and a mean airway pressure (MAP) that is greater than that obtained with conventional ventilation. This strategy has been very effective in infants with severe respiratory failure since HFV improves the gas exchange by optimizing the lung volume while ventilating with small tidal volumes and reduced proximal airway pressures, thereby avoiding damage to the lungs [35]. HFV improves the gas exchange by enhancing both the convection and diffusion of the respiratory gases. The principle is based on the natural "resonant" frequency of the lung and the fact that less pressure is required to move the gas into and out of the lungs at this resonant frequency, which is approximately 10 Hz (1 Hz = 60 bpm) in neonates and even greater in premature infants than with conventional ventilation.

A number of different HFV ventilator strategies are available although, once again, no evidence distinguishes one strategy over another. The first strategy was high-frequency jet ventilation (HFJV), a very well-established technique in anesthesia that delivers short bursts of gas (with very short T_i) at very high frequencies (up to 600/min) superimposed on a constant flow that determines the level of PEEP. This strategy requires a specific tracheal tube. HFJV has failed to prove its usefulness in clinical practice, with conflicting results on the neurological and respiratory outcomes in neonates [36–38]. Another strategy for the provision of HFV is high-frequency flow interruption (HFFI), which consists of a continuous gas flow delivered by a high-pressure gas source that is interrupted at a high frequency (up to 20 Hz) [39]. However, this technique failed to demonstrate any beneficial advantage in terms of the pulmonary outcome, and some studies have even identified a greater incidence of air leaks in premature infants treated with HFFI [40, 41]. Currently, the most frequently used modality is high-frequency oscillatory ventilation (HFOV). This strategy is based on the presence of an electromagnetically driven piston or vibrating diaphragm that generates biphasic pressure waveforms at very high frequency (up to 15 Hz). HFOV has both an active inspiratory phase and an active expiratory phase (by inducing a negative proximal airway pressure during exhalation). With HFOV, the *I*/*E* ratio is adjusted to avoid gas trapping that results from inadequate time for exhalation [21]. HFOV provides very small oscillatory tidal volumes that are superimposed on an adjustable MAP. Theoretically, HFOV is particularly beneficial when an increased volume strategy is required to maintain FRC, as HFOV maintains FRC with a reduced MAP compared with other modes of ventilation. When HFOV is applied to premature infants with chronic lung disease, the oscillatory volumes are determined by the position of the tidal volume on the pressure–volume curve and the pressure amplitude [42]. It may offer some advantages as a ventilator strategy in neonates with congenital diaphragmatic hernia or severe respiratory distress with markedly reduced lung compliance. Nonetheless, a recent meta-analysis failed to demonstrate evidence that HFOV offers any advantages over conventional ventilation, when used as a primary or rescue mode to ventilate infants with an acute pulmonary dysfunction [43–45]. HFOV may be associated with a reduced incidence of chronic lung disease in premature infants [44, 46], but this requires confirmation.

Continuous Positive Airway Pressure and Noninvasive Ventilation

A large number of neonates benefit from a noninvasive respiratory support that allows the application of continuous positive airway pressure (CPAP) and/or the delivery of noninvasive ventilation (NIV). The aim of nasal CPAP (nCPAP) is to maintain FRC by recruiting and maintaining airway patency and lung expansion [47, 48]. It also decreases the WOB and reduces the frequency of apnea of prematurity [49]. As a result, it is routinely used in clinical practice to support the lungs in preterm infants whose airways were recently extubated and as an alternative to tracheal intubation and ventilation, to support those experiencing significant apnea of prematurity and those with respiratory distress soon after birth. Some techniques also provide a phasic positive increase in pressure (pressure support or pressure controlled) in addition to nCPAP that can be synchronized (SNIMV, synchronized nasal intermittent mandatory ventilation) or not (NIMV) to the infant's respiratory efforts [48]. This is also known as nasal intermittent positive-pressure ventilation (NIPPV) [49, 50]. During the past decade, the use of NIV for acute respiratory failure in neonates in NICUs has been expanding. Predictive factors for the successful use of NIV have recently been identified [51]. Meta-analyses have failed to demonstrate the benefit of NIV in the presence of respiratory distress syndrome [52], although it does prevent extubation failures in neonates [53, 48]. Accordingly in preterm infants, NIV reduces the need for reintubation, invasive mechanical ventilation, and surfactant during the first 72 h after birth [47, 50, 54–56]. For this purpose, NIV is often started after the minimal PEEP level is set to ~6 cm H_2O and the PIP to between 10 and 12 cm H_2O.

nCPAP can be delivered by two means: (1) a continuous flow and a device that varies exhalation either by modifying the expiratory orifice size or (2) by immersing the distal end under water to a depth that determines the level of CPAP. This latter is also termed bubble nCPAP. The bubbles create pressure oscillations that are transmitted to the airway. It has been suggested that this phenomenon may improve gas exchange by facilitating gas diffusion [57]. Evidence indicates that the regional distribution of ventilation with bubble nCPAP depends solely on anatomical ventilator patterns and is independent of the infant's position [58, 2]. A variable-flow mode that modifies the nCPAP uses nasal prongs that redirect the exhaled gas out the expiratory limb. The WOB with the variable-flow nCPAP is less than that with the bubble nCPAP [59]. Another approach that is based on the variable-flow setting is the bi-level nCPAP or BiPAP. BiPAP allows the child to trigger inspiration and to breathe between two levels of positive pressure, with some systems including an abdominal wall sensor to help synchronize the delivery of positive pressure with the child's inspiratory efforts. The BiPAP system appears to be superior to the nCPAP system in improving oxygenation and ventilation in LBW infants [60, 61].

The application and success of nCPAP and NIV rely on the airway interfaces and their ability to guarantee comfort and optimize the delivery of pressure. Of all the interfaces available to provide nCPAP, the binasal prongs appear to be the optimal design [62]. These nasal prongs are tight fitting in the nostrils, preventing an air leak. While prongs may be associated with a high incidence of nasal trauma in infants [21], leaks remain a major concern in NIV. Such leaks may reduce alveolar ventilation, lead to child-ventilator asynchrony, and increase nasal resistance. Nonetheless, when nCPAP is applied soon after birth, it may reduce the need for surfactant, the frequency of chronic lung disease, and sequelae including death in preterm infants [63].

High-flow nasal cannula (HFNC) (defined as an oxygen/air mixture flow rate >1 l/min) is used in preterm infants to support pulmonary function as well as deliver increased oxygen concentrations. The gas flow may or may not be heated and humidified [48]. The heated and humidified modes are commonly used to minimize nasal mucosal trauma, although unheated HFNC has also been used successfully. HFNC has found favor in preterm infants with apnea, chronic lung disease, and respiratory distress syndrome. This strategy may be effective as it flushes gas from the dead space of the nasopharyngeal cavity, facilitates improved alveolar ventilation, and promotes more efficient respiration [48]. In contrast to the nasal cannula used in nCPAP, these cannulas do not fit into the nasal passages snugly but have a large air leak. Although the presence of a leak was initially thought to reduce the incidence of nasal injury, nasal mucosal injury, nasal obstruction or bleeding, and even nosocomial infection have been reported [64, 65]. However, after tracheal extubation, HFNC may be associated with a greater frequency of tracheal intubation than nasal CPAP [55]. A recent review concluded there was insufficient evidence to determine whether HFNC is effective in preterm infants [64, 65].

Application of Ventilation Modes in the Operating Theater

Despite the great advances in the development of new anesthetic ventilators, which include a variety of modes of ventilation widely used in the intensive care setting, there is no evidence that any one of these ventilation strategies during general anesthesia improves clinical outcome. However, the application of these strategies to neonates helps the clinician to provide "lung protective ventilation" and optimize the distribution of ventilation. Since most neonates receive neuromuscular blocking drugs in the operating room, mandatory ventilation is often utilized with synchronized ventilation modes during induction and weaning from the ventilator.

The traditional mandatory VCV has been described as having several disadvantages in the neonatal anesthesia because it uses a constant flow and fails to take into account the compressible volume and the potential air leak around the tracheal tube. The constant flow characterizing the VCV strategy induces large PIPs with less time for equilibration between the airway (Paw) and the alveolar pressures (Palv), this being known as the time constant. The compressible volume within the breathing circuit is an important issue in the neonate. It is essential to know whether the ventilator corrects for this compressible volume loss. Most modern anesthesia ventilators correct for this compressible volume loss during the workstation check. However, if the anesthesia breathing circuits are changed between patients, it is important to recheck the workstation to correct for additional changes in the compressible volume loss of the breathing circuit. If an old ventilator or a ventilator with limited compensation for pressures in excess of 30 cm H_2O was used [66], then the compressible volume loss must be taken into account when adjusting the desired Vt. For instance, if the compressible volume reaches 1 ml/cm H_2O and the delivered Vt is set to 7 ml/kg for a 4 kg neonate, the ventilator may generate a PIP of 25 cm H_2O during ventilation and thus have 25 ml of compressible volume. The preset Vt should be adjusted to almost 13 ml/kg since 50 % or more may be lost in the delivery system (not taking into account the dead space and the potential gas leak). The adequacy of ventilation should be evaluated clinically by auscultating the chest, observing the chest movement with the phase of respiratory, and observing the capnogram. With VCV strategy, the overpressure valve must be set in order to protect the lung from excessive peak airway pressures that are associated with sudden reductions in lung compliance during surgery. In neonates, particularly those with less compliant lungs, the PCV is the preferred mode of ventilation.

The decelerating flow that characterizes the PCV mode offers a limited and constant inspiratory pressure with a plateau pressure that is reached rapidly, but at a reduced PIP. This mode improves the ventilation distribution, decreases the intrapulmonary shunt, and thus improves oxygenation. Additionally, the PCV mode compensates for a leak around the tracheal tube. Although PCV meets the criteria required by the protective-ventilation strategy, the Vt is variable in this strategy, particularly if the lung compliance decreases or respiratory resistance increases during the surgery. In the PCV mode, we already established (see above) that Vt depends on three variables: (1) the pressure gradient between the maximal set peak pressure and the PEEP level, (2) the T_i, and (3) the time constant. The time constant is characterized by the mechanical properties of the respiratory system, which include the total respiratory system compliance (Crs) and resistance (Rrs). Application of the time constant concept to the inspiratory phase implies that T_i is set in order to allow sufficient time to achieve pressure equilibration between the airways and the alveoli. Accordingly, if Rrs increases and/or Crs decreases, the equilibrium time increases. Further, it is important to provide sufficient time for complete exhalation, since the expiratory flow presents an exponential decelerating profile requiring up to 3–4 time constants of the respiratory system for complete deflation. Finally, it is important to note that anesthetic ventilators are not all equal in their abilities to generate a maximum insufflation flow. Accordingly, the Vt generated by a given pressure may vary among ventilators [67]. In terms of the variables T_i and the respiratory rate in the neonate, physiological T_i should not exceed 0.5 s. However, in an anesthetized neonate who is paralyzed pharmacologically, one may exceed this limit in order to augment alveolar recruitment. Nonetheless, increasing the T_i may jeopardize hemodynamic variables leading to asynchrony if a PSV mode has been selected. Therefore, the initial ventilator settings in PCV mode should include the pressure gradient established by a PEEP of 5 cm H_2O and a positive inspiratory pressure of 15 cm H_2O. The respiratory rate is determined by an initial T_i of 0.6 s. Selection of both the pressure gradient and T_i depends on both the compliance and the resistance of the respiratory system as well as the results of the blood gas analysis. In addition, it is also important to consider T_e, particularly in neonates with chronic lung disease (e.g., bronchopulmonary dysplasia), in whom the respiratory time constant must provide sufficient time to exhale completely in order to prevent auto-PEEP and alveolar overdistention.

Maintaining diaphragmatic activity decreases ventilation-perfusion mismatch during general anesthesia. Thus, the use of the PSV mode in routine practice is becoming very popular in pediatric anesthesia. The new ventilators include a flow trigger highly sensitive to minimal flow variations (similar to those observed with intensive care ventilators) and can therefore be applied in neonates since minimal WOB is required to activate the beginning of the inspiratory phase [68]. Pressure support is based on a decelerating flow, which generates a fixed insufflation pressure. As a consequence, Vt may vary with the infant's inspiratory efforts, the level of pressure support, and the mechanical characteristics of the lung. Currently, only some anesthetic ventilators include this strategy. In the case of ventilators with fixed cycling, insufflation stops when the flow is less than 25 % of the maximal inspiratory flow. This limitation may have a negative impact in a neonate with obstructive lung disease, for whom the cycling should occur later [69]. Although there have been no studies on the use of the PSV mode in neonates, it can be applied during anesthesia in clinical practice to compensate for the increase in the WOB, which is particularly great in neonates. For instance, application of a pressure support of 5 cm H_2O in addition to a PEEP level at induction will maintain patent airway, compensate for the WOB, and facilitate an inhalational induction by optimizing gas exchange. During the maintenance of anesthesia, increased pressure support may be necessary (up to 10 cm H_2O) to counteract the resistance from the tracheal tube and the circuit and to guarantee an optimal Vt for gas exchange [70]. At the end of an anesthetic, PSV allows a smoother recovery and weaning from the ventilator. In all cases, it is important to set a minimal default respiration rate should apnea occur. In addition, T_i should be adjusted to avoid asynchrony with the ventilator as a mismatch may even increase in the WOB. Finally, some anesthetic ventilators allow changes to the pressure slope (the time to achieve pressure support). By increasing this time (and thereby decreasing the pressure slope), we can limit the auto trigger activated by the cardiac activity, which is frequently observed in neonates at reduced trigger threshold [71]. To avoid this phenomenon, it is also possible to increase the trigger threshold, although this may increase the WOB.

Recently, the PRVC mode with automode (auto flow) has become part of the new anesthetic ventilators introduced in the operating theater. Volume-controlled ventilation with decelerating flow in combination with synchronization with a pressure support of the spontaneous ventilation offers the advantages of pressure modes but with the guarantee of a minimal Vt. Theoretically, this mode overcomes the inconvenience of both PCV and VCV in neonates, potentially offering a tremendous advantage in anesthetized neonates, particularly when faced with abrupt changes in lung compliance that occur during surgery (i.e., laparoscopy or abdominal or thoracic surgery). In order to determine the initial guaranteed volume, it is recommended to ventilate the lungs under pressure controlled and extract the tidal volume that ensures adequate alveolar ventilation. Thereafter, the determined tidal volume becomes the targeted tidal volume in PRVC mode while adapting the ventilator setting according to PCV mode and by applying a maximal inspiratory pressure of 30 cm H_2O in order to protect the alveoli from overdistention. Again, no data exists concerning the use of this strategy in the operating room, particularly in neonates, and hence its use is still anecdotal and based on the experience of different clinicians.

Ventilation Strategy in the Operating Theater

Maintenance of adequate ventilation is of particular importance in neonates who are especially vulnerable to hypoxemia when undergoing sedation or anesthesia. Inadequate bag and mask ventilation at induction of anesthesia may be associated with insufficient alveolar ventilation, gastric inflation, and regurgitation and aspiration of gastric contents. Furthermore, increasing amounts of air in the stomach may compromise respiratory function and gas exchange particularly in neonates whose resting lung volume is less than the closing volume. Although the use of an accessory circuit such as a modified T-piece breathing system (i.e., Jackson Rees) continues to be advocated as the best system to ensure both adequate ventilation and maintenance of FRC [72, 73], it is important to monitor airway pressure during manual ventilation in order to avoid both high-pressure inflation of the lungs and gastric air insufflations. The development of low resistance circle systems has rendered their use popular in routine practice [74, 75], but they may be less effective in applying a continuous positive airway pressure (CPAP) at end expiration in order to maintain upper airway patency and FRC. In this context, applying gentle mask ventilation with the use of a CPAP to maintain a mean airway pressure around 5–10 cm H_2O is becoming a popular ventilation strategy at the induction of anesthesia, even with full stomach, in order to avoid airway collapse and maintain adequate oxygenation [76, 77]. This so-called controlled induction technique meets the criteria for open-lung strategy that should be considered at all stages when a neonate is ventilated in the operating theater.

The open-lung strategy primarily targets atelectasis and the consequent ventilation inhomogeneity observed under general anesthesia, which can significantly impair pulmonary gas exchange. The physiological characteristics of the chest wall (high compliance) and the lung (increased static elastic recoil pressure) in neonates promote airway closure and a decrease in FRC. The decrease in ventilation induced by general anesthetics and the inactivation of the intercostal muscle activity associated with the cranial shift of the diaphragm are also responsible for the lung collapse and atelectasis formation. This latter is enhanced by the resorption of alveolar gas if the FiO_2 concentration is high. Thus, this "open-lung strategy" requires that recruitment maneuvers should be regularly performed and particularly after loss of positive end-expiratory level (at zero PEEP level). Such recruitment can be achieved by applying a vital capacity maneuver (or twice the Vt) after induction, after disconnection and suction, and thereafter every 30 min during the anesthetic procedure [78]. Alternately, alveolar recruitment may be achieved by maintaining a sustained peak inspiratory pressure of 20–30 cm H_2O pressure for 20–30 s, depending on the hemodynamic responses. In all cases, a minimum PEEP level of 5 cm H_2O is required to maintain recruitment of the distal airways [79] in combination with the minimum concentration of oxygen to maintain an adequate oxygen saturation. However, greater PEEP values may be required in the presence of poorly compliant and atelectatic lungs in order to maintain adequate alveolar recruitment.

In addition to this open-lung strategy, it is crucial to apply "protective ventilation" to protect against ventilator-induced lung injury [80]. Ventilation with low Vt at optimal FRC is therefore also essential in the operating theater. Optimization of the PEEP level increases the lung volume, while adapting T_i and T_e, will guarantee adequate lung inflation and deflation, respectively, especially if T_i/T_e is adjustable based on estimations of the time constants.

This ventilation strategy may lead to mild hypercapnia, which can be regarded as safe if maintained at approximately 6–7 kPa (or 45–52.5 mmHg) in the absence of increased intracerebral pressure and pulmonary hypertension. It has also been demonstrated that mild hypercapnia in this range improves both the cerebral oxygen saturation and the subcutaneous tissue oxygenation [81]. Pediatric anesthesiologists should appreciate the clinical relevance of the position of the oxygen–hemoglobin dissociation curve and its effect on oxygen release to tissues. The greater affinity of fetal hemoglobin for oxygen in comparison with that of adult hemoglobin explains the shift of the curve to the left yielding a very low P_{50}, which can be aggravated by hyperventilation (Bohr effect) and decrease oxygen delivery to tissues [82].

Monitoring of Ventilation

While real-time pulmonary monitoring is essential to interpret the changes in pulmonary function during mechanical ventilation of neonatal lungs, it is crucial to associate the information obtained from the different waveforms displayed by the ventilators with efficient gas exchange and tissue oxygenation. Applying the protective open-lung ventilation strategy requires adaptation of the ventilator settings according to this real-time pulmonary monitoring. Most ventilators available in the operating theater display continuous waveforms of pressure, volume, flow, and loops, and they also provide automatically derived respiratory mechanical variables. The classical pulmonary waveforms are represented by pressure, volume, and flow displayed versus time. The pressure and flow curves are specific for the ventilation mode used, and thus, while displaying the pressure curve is essential during VCV (since pressure is the dependent variable), it is crucial to focus on the flow versus time curve in the PCV mode since the efficacy of alveolar ventilation depends to a large extent on the flow waveform. The latter allows detection of the following features: (1) an interruption in the inspiratory waveform indicating insufficient time to equilibrate alveolar and airway pressures, with the risk of inadequate lung inflation, and (2) an incomplete deflation of the lung with the risk of auto-PEEP, overdistension of the lung, and an increased risk of barotrauma. Thus, in terms of the flow curve, it is essential to adjust both T_i and T_e (either by changing the ratio or by decreasing the respiratory rate) to ensure the waveform reaches the zero flow state before the transition to the next insufflation or exsufflation [83].

The pressure–volume and the flow–volume loops afford an insight into the respiratory mechanics during mechanical ventilation, namely, the respiratory system compliance and resistance. The flow–volume loop is very useful to detect changes in the inspiratory or expiratory resistances. For instance, increases in airway resistance may be identified in the flow–volume curve with a decrease in the expiratory flow peak that is expressed as a concave expiration loop. Moreover, an incomplete flow–volume loop indicates an air leak and may be very useful particularly in neonates in whom uncuffed tracheal tubes are routinely used. As cuffed tracheal tubes in neonates become more common practice, this finding may become infrequent. The dynamic pressure–volume (P–V) loop that is displayed by the ventilator describes the mechanical behavior of the respiratory system during inflation and deflation. It describes the resistive and convective acceleration components of the flow. Thus, the dynamic P–V curve provides essential information on the dynamic trends of the respiratory system compliance (defined by the slope of the loop) and also on the tidal volume. Although some information can be obtained from the curve to facilitate determining the optimal PEEP level, the beginning of the dynamic inspiration provides evidence on lung recruitment from tidal ventilation, independent of PEEP [84] particularly during PCV where the pressure remains constant. Conversely, when ventilating with a constant flow such as under VCV, the pressure–volume loop may detect lung overdistension as evidenced by a change in the slope of the inspiratory P–V curve, namely, the upper inflection point. The lower inflection point at the lower part of the loop corresponds to the beginning of alveolar recruitment and may give an insight on the importance of airway closure.

The derived respiratory values displayed on the ventilator monitor should be interpreted with caution as they reflect the determinations based on the infant's respiratory system as well as the equipment (breathing circuit, tracheal tube, and so on) [85]. These values are often obtained based on the interruption technique, which relies on the ratio of the decrease in airway pressure after an interruption to the inspiratory flow compared with the pressure before the interruption. In excess of 40 % of the measurements may be explained by the effects of the equipment itself. As a result, clinicians should be cautious when interpreting these values and not attribute the changes solely to the infant's respiratory physiology.

Conclusion

The literature has a surfeit of mounting evidence that supports the benefits of an open and protective lung strategy in neonates. Over the past 20 years, advances in technology have led to the development of novel ventilation modes that have exploited this strategy. However, there remains a dearth of evidence comparing these advances in ventilation modes in terms of neonatal pulmonary and neural outcomes. Without this evidence, clinicians have been left to base their choice of the optimal ventilation strategy for a particular infant on anecdotal experience and theory, a situation that appears to be changing as more randomized controlled trials are being published lately. The challenge that remains is to quantify the outcomes in premature and term neonates in order to select the ventilation strategy that optimizes lung volume and guarantees adequate tissue oxygenation without overdistending the alveoli, introducing acute and/or chronic lung injury and causing extreme fluctuations in hemodynamics that result in neurological and metabolic adverse outcomes.

References

1. Murat I, Constant I, Maud'huy H. Perioperative anaesthetic morbidity in children: a database of 24,165 anaesthetics over a 30-month period. Paediatr Anaesth. 2004;14:158–66.
2. Bhananker SM, Ramamoorthy C, Geiduschek JM, et al. Anesthesia-related cardiac arrest in children: update from the pediatric perioperative cardiac arrest registry. Anesth Analg. 2007;105:344–50.
3. Moloney ED, Griffiths MJ. Protective ventilation of patients with acute respiratory distress syndrome. Br J Anaesth. 2004;92:261–70.
4. Dreyfuss D, Saumon G. Ventilator-induced lung injury: lessons from experimental studies. Am J Respir Crit Care Med. 1998;157:294–323.
5. Wiswell TE, Graziani LJ, Kornhauser MS, et al. Effects of hypocarbia on the development of cystic periventricular leukomalacia in premature infants treated with high-frequency jet ventilation. Pediatrics. 1996;98:918–24.
6. Kaiser JR, Gauss CH, Pont MM, Williams DK. Hypercapnia during the first 3 days of life is associated with severe intraventricular hemorrhage in very low birth weight infants. J Perinatol. 2006;26:279–85.
7. Keens TG, Bryan AC, Levison H, Ianuzzo CD. Developmental pattern of muscle fiber types in human ventilatory muscles. J Appl Physiol. 1978;44:909–13.
8. Muller N, Volgyesi G, Becker L, et al. Diaphragmatic muscle tone. J Appl Physiol. 1979;47:279–84.
9. Nicolai T. The physiological basis of respiratory support. Paediatr Respir Rev. 2006;7:97–102.
10. Macklem PT, Proctor DF, Hogg JC. The stability of peripheral airways. Respir Physiol. 1970;8:191–203.
11. Hjalmarson O, Sandberg K. Abnormal lung function in healthy preterm infants. Am J Respir Crit Care Med. 2002;165:83–7.
12. Menkes H, Gardiner A, Gamsu G, et al. Influence of surface forces on collateral ventilation. J Appl Physiol. 1971;31:544–9.
13. Lanteri CJ, Sly PD. Changes in respiratory mechanics with age. J Appl Physiol. 1993;74:369–78.
14. Sly PD, Hayden MJ, Petak F, Hantos Z. Measurement of low-frequency respiratory impedance in infants. Am J Respir Crit Care Med. 1996;154:161–6.
15. Garcia A, Stolar CJH. Congenital diaphragmatic hernia and protective ventilation strategies in pediatric surgery. Surg Clin N Am. 2012;92:659–68.
16. Brown MK, DiBlasi RM. Mechanical ventilation of the premature neonate. Respir Care. 2011;56:1298–313.
17. Munoz J, Guerrero JE, Escalante JL, et al. Pressure-controlled ventilation versus controlled mechanical ventilation with decelerating inspiratory flow. Crit Care Med. 1993;21:1143–8.
18. Kamlin CO, Davis PG. Long versus short inspiratory times in neonates receiving mechanical ventilation. Cochrane Database Syst Rev 2004: CD004503.
19. Keszler M. State of the art in conventional mechanical ventilation. J Perinatol. 2009;29:262–75.
20. Dimitriou G, Greenough A, Cherian S. Comparison of airway pressure and airflow triggering systems using a single type of neonatal ventilator. Acta Paediatr. 2001;90:445–7.
21. Greenough A, Donn SM. Matching ventilatory support strategies to respiratory pathophysiology. Clin Perinatol 2007;34:35–53, v–vi.
22. Schulze A, Rieger-Fackeldey E, Gerhardt T, et al. Randomized crossover comparison of proportional assist ventilation and patient-triggered ventilation in extremely low birth weight infants with evolving chronic lung disease. Neonatology. 2007;92:1–7.
23. Sinderby C, Beck J, Spahija J, et al. Inspiratory muscle unloading by neurally adjusted ventilatory assist during maximal inspiratory efforts in healthy subjects. Chest. 2007;131:711–17.
24. Stein H, Howard D. Neurally adjusted ventilatory assist in neonates weighing <1500 grams: a retrospective analysis. J Pediatr. 2012;160:786–9.
25. Breatnach C, Conlon NP, Stack M, et al. A prospective crossover comparison of neurally adjusted ventilatory assist and pressure-support ventilation in a pediatric and neonatal intensive care unit population. Pediatr Crit Care Med. 2010;11(1):7–11.
26. Stein H, Alosh H, Ethington P, White DB. Prospective crossover comparison between NAVA and pressure control ventilation in premature neonates less than 1500 grams. J Perinatol. 2012. doi:10.1038/jp.2012.136 (Epub ahead of print).

27. Keszler M, Abubakar KM. Volume guarantee ventilation. Clin Perinatol. 2007;34:107–16, vii.
28. Singh J, Sinha SK, Clarke P, et al. Mechanical ventilation of very low birth weight infants: is volume or pressure a better target variable? J Pediatr. 2006;149:308–13.
29. McCallion N, Davis PG, Morley CJ. Volume-targeted versus pressure-limited ventilation in the neonate. Cochrane Database Syst Rev. 2005: CD003666.
30. Wheeler KI, Schmolzer GM, Morley CJ, Davis PG. High-frequency ventilation with the Drager Babylog 8000plus: measuring the delivered frequency. Acta Paediatr. 2011;100:67–70.
31. Singh J, Sinha SK, Donn SM. Volume-targeted ventilation of newborns. Clin Perinatol. 2007;34:93–105, vii.
32. Piotrowski A, Sobala W, Kawczynski P. Patient-initiated, pressure-regulated, volume-controlled ventilation compared with intermittent mandatory ventilation in neonates: a prospective, randomised study. Intensive Care Med. 1997;23:975–81.
33. D'Angio CT, Chess PR, Kovacs SJ, et al. Pressure-regulated volume control ventilation vs synchronized intermittent mandatory ventilation for very low-birth-weight infants: a randomized controlled trial. Arch Pediatr Adolesc Med. 2005;159:868–75.
34. Kocis KC, Dekeon MK, Rosen HK, et al. Pressure-regulated volume control vs volume control ventilation in infants after surgery for congenital heart disease. Pediatr Cardiol. 2001;22: 233–7.
35. Lampland AL, Mammel MC. The role of high-frequency ventilation in neonates: evidence-based recommendations. Clin Perinatol. 2007;34:129–44, viii.
36. Wiswell TE, Graziani LJ, Kornhauser MS, et al. High-frequency jet ventilation in the early management of respiratory distress syndrome is associated with a greater risk for adverse outcomes. Pediatrics. 1996;98:1035–43.
37. Carlo WA, Siner B, Chatburn RL, et al. Early randomized intervention with high-frequency jet ventilation in respiratory distress syndrome. J Pediatr. 1990;117:765–70.
38. Keszler M, Modanlou HD, Brudno DS, et al. Multicenter controlled clinical trial of high-frequency jet ventilation in preterm infants with uncomplicated respiratory distress syndrome. Pediatrics. 1997;100:593–9.
39. Cronin JH. High frequency ventilator therapy for newborns. J Intensive Care Med. 1994;9:71–85.
40. Thome U, Kossel H, Lipowsky G, et al. Randomized comparison of high-frequency ventilation with high-rate intermittent positive pressure ventilation in preterm infants with respiratory failure. J Pediatr. 1999;135:39–46.
41. Craft AP, Bhandari V, Finer NN. The sy-fi study: a randomized prospective trial of synchronized intermittent mandatory ventilation versus a high-frequency flow interrupter in infants less than 1000 g. J Perinatol. 2003;23:14–9.
42. Miedema M, de Jongh FH, Frerichs I, et al. The effect of airway pressure and oscillation amplitude on ventilation in preterm infants. Eur Respir J. 2012;40:479–84.
43. Henderson-Smart DJ, De Paoli AG, Clark RH, Bhuta T. High frequency oscillatory ventilation versus conventional ventilation for infants with severe pulmonary dysfunction born at or near term. Cochrane Database Syst Rev. 2009: CD002974.
44. Cools F, Henderson-Smart DJ, Offringa M, Askie LM. Elective high frequency oscillatory ventilation versus conventional ventilation for acute pulmonary dysfunction in preterm infants. Cochrane Database Syst Rev. 2009: CD000104.
45. Singh SN, Malik GK, Prashanth GP, et al. High frequency oscillatory ventilation versus synchronized intermittent mandatory ventilation in preterm neonates with hyaline membrane disease: a randomized controlled trial. Indian Pediatr. 2012;49:405–8.
46. Courtney SE, Durand DJ, Asselin JM, et al. High-frequency oscillatory ventilation versus conventional mechanical ventilation for very-low-birth-weight infants. N Engl J Med. 2002;347:643–52.
47. Courtney SE, Barrington KJ. Continuous positive airway pressure and noninvasive ventilation. Clin Perinatol 2007;34:73–92, vi.
48. Shaffer TH, Alapati D, Greenspan JS, Wolfson MR. Neonatal noninvasive respiratory support: physiological implications. Pediatr Pulmonol. 2012;47:837–47.
49. Davis PG, Lemyre B, de Paoli AG. Nasal intermittent positive pressure ventilation (NIPPV) versus nasal continuous positive airway pressure (NCPAP) for preterm neonates after extubation. Cochrane Database Syst Rev. 2001: CD003212.
50. Ramanathan R, Sekar KC, Rasmussen M, et al. Nasal intermittent positive pressure ventilation after surfactant treatment from respiratory distress syndrome in preterm infants <30 weeks' gestation: a randomized, controlled trial. J Perinatol. 2012;32: 336–43.
51. Bernet V, Hug MI, Frey B. Predictive factors for the success of noninvasive mask ventilation in infants and children with acute respiratory failure. Pediatr Crit Care Med. 2005;6:660–4.
52. Ho JJ, Henderson-Smart DJ, Davis PG. Early versus delayed initiation of continuous distending pressure for respiratory distress syndrome in preterm infants. Cochrane Database Syst Rev. 2002: CD002975.
53. Davis PG, Henderson-Smart DJ. Nasal continuous positive airways pressure immediately after extubation for preventing morbidity in preterm infants. Cochrane Database Syst Rev. 2003: CD000143.
54. Meneses J, Bhandari V, Alves JG. Nasal intermittent positive-pressure ventilation vs nasal continuous positive airway pressure for preterm infants with respiratory distress syndrome: a systematic review and meta-analysis. Arch Pediatr Adolesc Med. 2012; 166:372–6.
55. Kieran EA, Twomey AR, Molloy EJ, et al. Randomized trial of prongs or mask for nasal continuous positive airway pressure in preterm infants. Pediatrics. 2012;130:e1170–6.
56. Tapia JL, Urzua S, Bancalari A, et al. Randomized trial of early bubble continuous positive airway pressure for very low birth weight infants. J Pediatr. 2012;261:75–80.
57. Pillow JJ, Travadi JN. Bubble CPAP: is the noise important? An in vitro study. Pediatr Res. 2005;57:826–30.
58. Hough JL, Johnston L, Brauer SG, et al. Effect of body position on ventilation distribution in preterm infants on continuous positive airway pressure. Pediatr Crit Care Med. 2012;13:446–51.
59. Liptsen E, Aghai ZH, Pyon KH, et al. Work of breathing during nasal continuous positive airway pressure in preterm infants: a comparison of bubble vs variable-flow devices. J Perinatol. 2005; 25:453–8.
60. Migliori C, Motta M, Angeli A, Chirico G. Nasal bilevel vs. continuous positive airway pressure in preterm infants. Pediatr Pulmonol. 2005;40:426–30.
61. O'Brien K, Campbell C, Brown L, et al. Infant flow biphasic nasal continuous positive airway pressure (BP- NCPAPA) vs. infant flow NCPAP for the facilitation of extubation in infants' ≤1250 grams: a randomized controlled trial. BMC Pediatr. 2012;12:43.
62. De Paoli AG, Davis PG, Faber B, Morley CJ. Devices and pressure sources for administration of nasal continuous positive airway pressure (NCPAP) in preterm neonates. Cochrane Database Syst Rev. 2008: CD002977.
63. Carlo WA. Gentle ventilation: the new evidence from the SUPPORT, COIN, VON, CURPAP, Columbian network, and Neocosur Network trials. Early Human Dev. 2012;88(S2):S81–3.
64. Wilkinson D, Andersen C, O'Donnell CPF, et al. High flow nasal cannula for respiratory support in preterm infants. Cochrane Database Syst Rev. 2011: CD006405.

65. Manley BJ, Dold SK, Davis PG, et al. High-flow nasal cannulae for respiratory support of preterm infants: a review of the evidence. Neonatology. 2012;102:300–8.
66. Jaber S, Langlais N, Fumagalli B, et al. Performance studies of 6 new anesthesia ventilators: bench tests. Ann Fr Anesth Reanim. 2000;19:16–22.
67. Stayer SA, Bent ST, Skjonsby BS, et al. Pressure control ventilation: three anesthesia ventilators compared using an infant lung model. Anesth Analg. 2000;91:1145–50.
68. Aslanian P, El Atrous S, Isabey D, et al. Effects of flow triggering on breathing effort during partial ventilatory support. Am J Respir Crit Care Med. 1998;157:135–43.
69. Tassaux D, Michotte JB, Gainnier M, et al. Expiratory trigger setting in pressure support ventilation: from mathematical model to bedside. Crit Care Med. 2004;32:1844–50.
70. von Goedecke A, Brimacombe J, Hormann C, et al. Pressure support ventilation versus continuous positive airway pressure ventilation with the ProSeal laryngeal mask airway: a randomized crossover study of anesthetized pediatric patients. Anesth Analg. 2005;100:357–60.
71. Odin I, Nathan N. What are the changes in paediatric anaesthesia practice afforded by new anaesthetic ventilators? Ann Fr Anesth Reanim. 2006;25:417–23.
72. Nakae Y, Miyabe M, Sonoda H, et al. Comparison of the Jackson-Rees circuit, the pediatric circle, and the MERA F breathing system for pediatric anesthesia. Anesth Analg. 1996;83:488–92.
73. Von Ungern-Sternberg BS, Saudan S, Regli A, et al. Should the use of modified Jackson Rees T-piece breathing system be abandoned in preschool children? Paediatr Anaesth. 2007;17:654–60.
74. Spears RS, Yeh A, Fisher DM, Zwaas MS. The "educated hand": can anesthesiologists assess changes in neonatal pulmonary compliance manually? Anesthesiology. 1991;75:693–6.
75. Schily M, Koumoukelis H, Lerman J, Creighton RE. Can pediatric anesthesiologists detect an occluded tracheal tube in neonates? Anesth Analg. 2001;93:66–70.
76. Weiss M, Gerber AC. Induction of anaesthesia and intubation in children with a full stomach. Time to rethink! Anaesthesist. 2007;56:1210–16.
77. Eich C, Timmermann A, Russo SG, et al. A controlled rapid-sequence induction technique for infants may reduce unsafe actions and stress. Acta Anaesthesiol Scand. 2009;53:1167–72.
78. Rothen HU, Sporre B, Engberg G, et al. Prevention of atelectasis during general anaesthesia. Lancet. 1995;345:1387–91.
79. von Ungern-Sternberg BS, Regli A, Schibler A, et al. The impact of positive end-expiratory pressure on functional residual capacity and ventilation homogeneity impairment in anesthetized children exposed to high levels of inspired oxygen. Anesth Analg. 2007;104:1364–8.
80. Tobin MJ. Advances in mechanical ventilation. N Engl J Med. 2001;344:1986–96.
81. Akca O, Liem E, Suleman MI, et al. Effect of intra-operative end-tidal carbon dioxide partial pressure on tissue oxygenation. Anaesthesia. 2003;58:536–42.
82. Oski FA. Clinical implications of the oxyhemoglobin dissociation curve in the neonatal period. Crit Care Med. 1979;7:412–18.
83. Becker MA, Donn SM. Real-time pulmonary graphic monitoring. Clin Perinatol. 2007;34:1–17, v.
84. Adams AB, Cakar N, Marini JJ. Static and dynamic pressure-volume curves reflect different aspects of respiratory system mechanics in experimental acute respiratory distress syndrome. Respir Care. 2001;46:686–93.
85. Babik B, Petak F, Asztalos T, et al. Components of respiratory resistance monitored in mechanically ventilated patients. Eur Respir J. 2002;20:1538–44.

Thoracoabdominal and General Surgery

10

Kate Cross, Jonathan Smith, and Isabeau A. Walker

Introduction

Provision of anesthesia for thoracoabdominal surgery in the neonate presents a number of specific challenges to the anesthesiologist. Many neonates are born at term in good condition, with or without an antenatal diagnosis, but many others are born premature and/or of low birth weight with associated cardiac abnormalities, pulmonary hypertension, and/or complications relating to the specific surgical diagnosis. Many of the principles of neonatal surgery are discussed elsewhere—this chapter considers specific conditions that require thoracic or abdominal surgery in the neonatal period, and the anesthetic and surgical requirements for each. There are very few randomized controlled trials to guide management. Most management strategies are based on retrospective case reviews or expert opinion. The use of minimally invasive techniques is becoming increasingly common and these approaches are also discussed.

General Considerations

Anesthesia complications are more common in the neonatal period, so only essential surgery should be carried out in this period [1–4]. Conditions range from minor elective procedures such as neonatal inguinal hernia repair to emergency lifesaving procedures such as repair of abdominal wall defect or esophageal atresia. The anesthesiologist, surgeon, and neonatologist must collaborate to ensure that the neonate is optimally prepared for surgery, that every member of the team understands the surgical/anesthetic plan, and that the neonate is returned to the neonatal intensive care unit (NICU) in stable condition with appropriate IV access and monitors in place.

Preoperative Assessment and Preparation

Anesthetic evaluation includes a detailed history of the presenting condition and the current status, the birth history, gestational age, physical examination, and assessment of laboratory investigations and imaging. Cardiac defects are commonly associated with several congenital defects. A preoperative echocardiogram should be performed if a cardiac defect is possible or present, e.g., in esophageal atresia/tracheoesophageal fistula (EA/TEF) or omphalocele. A renal ultrasound should also be performed in neonates with abnormalities such as EA/TEF, and preoperative cranial ultrasound in those at risk of intraventricular hemorrhage, such as premature infants. For the acutely unwell neonate, or the extreme premature infant, it is useful to assess how the neonate responds to handling, in order to assess its physiological stability during transport to the operating room (OR).

Preoperatively, the anesthesiologist should review the coagulation profile to ensure that it is within normal limits for the local laboratory standards for age and for neonates and that vitamin K was administered postdelivery. Thrombocytopenia is common, particularly in neonates with sepsis, and should be corrected before undertaking surgery. Platelet concentrations <150,000/mm^3 are considered abnormal in neonates in many centers, but surgical bleeding is uncommon when the count is >50,000/mm^3 [5]. A platelet transfusion consisting of 10–20 ml/kg should be considered if the platelet count is <100 × 10^9/l before surgery, although in the case of necrotizing enterocolitis (NEC), the platelet count is often <100,000/mm^3 preoperatively and platelet transfusions have not been shown to be beneficial in the absence of bleeding [6]. Few would hesitate to transfuse platelets if the

K. Cross, FRACS
Great Ormond Street Hospital NHS Foundation Trust, Institute of Child Health, Unversity College London, Great Ormond Street, London WC1N 3JH, UK

J. Smith, FRCA • I.A. Walker, FRCA (✉)
Portex Department of Paediatric Anaesthesia, Great Ormond Street Hospital NHS Foundation Trust, Institute of Child Health, University College London, Great Ormond Street, London WC1N 3JH, UK
e-mail: isabeauwalker@mac.com

J. Lerman (ed.), *Neonatal Anesthesia*, DOI 10.1007/978-1-4419-6041-2_10,

platelet count was <50,000/mm^3 preoperatively. Prothrombin time (PT) and partial thromboplastin time (APTT) vary during the neonatal period, being prolonged immediately after birth due to reduced procoagulants and then decrease toward normal childhood values throughout the neonatal period [5]. Fresh frozen plasma (FFP) 15 ml/kg is recommended if the prothrombin time (PT) or activated partial thromboplastin time (APTT) ratio is >1.5 times normal. These indices should be rechecked once corrective actions are completed. One adult unit of CMV-negative leukodepleted blood should be crossmatched for all but minor procedures. Where possible, the mother's blood should be screened for atypical red cell antibodies; alternatively, the neonate's serum should be screened for antibodies of maternal origin [7, 8].

Sedative premedication is not required, but atropine or glycopyrrolate may be used to blunt vagal responses to intubation and to dry secretions if a bronchoscopy is planned. The plan for anesthesia and perioperative analgesia should be discussed with the parents, and informed consent for anesthesia and surgery obtained. All members of the theater team should be fully briefed before the start of surgery, and appropriate safety checks undertaken according to international recommendations [9].

Anesthesia Techniques

The anesthesia technique should be chosen with reference to the condition of the neonate, the surgical requirements, and postoperative management. For instance, epidural analgesia reduces the stress response to surgery, provides excellent analgesia, and reduces postoperative ventilatory requirements, whereas an opioid-based technique with fentanyl 10–50 mcg/kg may be more appropriate for the neonate who requires paralysis and controlled ventilation for 5 days after repair of a long-gap esophageal atresia [10]. Spinal anesthesia may reduce the need for postoperative ventilation in a premature neonate, but is not a suitable technique if the child is undergoing laparoscopic surgery.

The choice between inhalational and intravenous induction of anesthesia depends on personal preference and the condition of the neonate. Inhalational inductions are suited for neonates undergoing elective surgery or in those with poor venous access [11]. However, most surgeries in neonates are emergencies and/or involve a full stomach, both of which favor an IV induction of anesthesia. Propofol 2–3 mg/kg or ketamine 1–2 mg/kg may be used to induce anesthesia intravenously, with the latter preferred for cardiovascular stability. For the sick neonate with NEC, many prefer IV fentanyl. A nasogastric tube should be in place if there is a risk of aspiration and suctioned (and possibly removed) before induction of anesthesia. The debate to remove the nasogastric tube before induction or leave it in situ here favors the former, primarily to provide a clear view of the larynx with less concern for incompetence of the lower esophageal junction and potential regurgitation. A classic rapid sequence induction (RSI) is eschewed in neonates because desaturation is very common after even a brief apnea between induction of anesthesia and tracheal intubation and in spite of optimal preoxygenation [12]. In place of the classic RSI, a "modified" RSI is widely practiced. This differs from the classic RSI in that gentle mask ventilation (at the smallest peak inspiratory pressures possible) that continues after induction of anesthesia and paralysis until the airway is secured [13, 14]. Traditionally, cricoid pressure has been an essential element of the RSI, although recent evidence has cast doubts on its effectiveness [15]. Furthermore, the cricoid ring may be difficult to identify in neonates, the appropriate force is rarely applied, cricoid pressure may distort the airway, and tracheal intubation may be more difficult to perform [16, 17]. As a consequence, it is not used routinely by many anesthesiologists [13] (see Chaps. 4 and 5).

Secure vascular access should be obtained using an aseptic technique, including central access if required, with the aid of ultrasound guidance (4Fr or 5Fr catheter, internal jugular or femoral vein) (see Chap. 7). Arterial access is indicated for major surgery (22G or 24G cannula, with radial or femoral artery). An umbilical arterial catheter (UAC) or umbilical venous catheter (UVC) may be used for short-term access (<5 days). The tip of the UAC should ideally end in the thoracic region (above the diaphragm at the level of T6–T10), and the tip of the UVC or central line at the junction of the superior vena cava and right atrium. A peripherally inserted central line (PICC) or tunneled central line should be considered if total parenteral nutrition is required, for instance, after closure of gastroschisis.

Monitoring during anesthesia should be in accordance with international standards (see Chaps. 6 and 7). Invasive monitoring is indicated for major surgery and neonates with significant comorbidity such as congenital heart disease. Pre- and post-ductal oxygen saturation may be useful in the neonate at risk of pulmonary hypertensive crisis (saturation probe on right hand and either foot). Although transcutaneous CO_2 monitoring is commonplace in the NICU, it does not respond as rapidly as end-tidal pCO_2 monitoring on a breath-to-breath basis [18]. Provided non-HFOV ventilation strategies are used and the lung disease is not severe, capnography should be employed to monitor ventilation in preterm and full-term neonates [19–21]. Great care should be taken when removing adhesive ECG electrodes (and adhesive drapes) to avoid removing a layer of epidermis, particularly in very premature neonates.

Neonates are poikilotherms. They have limited ability to generate heat in a cold stress situation and as such should be maintained in a thermoneutral environment, 36.3–37.3 °C [22]. The neonate generates heat when stressed primarily using nonshivering thermogenesis via brown fat. To prevent hypothermia in the operating room, the temperature of the operating theater should be increased to 25–28 °C before the neonate enters the room to minimize radiation (39 %) and convective (34 %) heat losses. The other mechanisms for heat loss are evaporative (24 %) and conduction (3 %). A forced air-warming blanket should be placed on the operating room table and preheated before the neonate arrives [23]. Humidified gases and warmed fluids should be used intraoperatively. The temperature of surgical irrigation fluids should also be warmed, and exposed bowel covered to reduce evaporative losses. To monitor the effectiveness of these heating strategies, core temperature should be measured continuously from one of several sites. We recommend the mid-esophagus, immediately retrocardiac. Rectal temperature is not commonly used as it lags behind the central core temperature during changes in temperature and is best avoided in neonates with anal anomalies. Nasopharyngeal temperature may be cooled by ventilation gas and axillary temperature is often skewed by the temperature of the forced air warmer.

Fluid Management (See Chap. 8)

In the first few days of life, the serum concentrations of antidiuretic hormone (ADH) are increased, and fluid maintenance requirements are small (60 % of normal). Sodium requirements are small; hence, hyponatremic solutions are commonly used for maintenance. To prevent hypoglycemia, 10 % dextrose is commonly infused in neonates on the first day of life, and sodium should be added and fluids liberalized after the first few days when the postnatal diuresis occurs. It is important to monitor the serum electrolyte and glucose concentrations so that the fluid composition can be adjusted to suit the neonate. The volume of maintenance fluids is greater in premature neonates to compensate for their large insensible fluid losses.

Fluid management during surgery depends on the clinical condition of the child and the procedure. For example, the fluid requirements during elective inguinal hernia repair are vastly different from those in the neonate undergoing laparotomy for NEC. In both cases, there are limited studies to guide practice. Maintenance fluids should be continued at the same rates as preoperatively using isotonic fluids to replace intraoperative fluid losses [24, 25]. The aim of intraoperative fluid management is to replace preexisting fluid deficits and ongoing losses and to maintain cardiovascular stability. Modern fasting regimens before elective surgery minimize the preoperative deficit: no formula milk for 6 h, no breast milk for 4 h, and free clear fluids up to 2 h preoperatively [26]. Neonates scheduled for emergency surgery should be actively resuscitated with 10–20 ml/kg IV balanced salt solution preoperatively. Fluid replacement during surgery includes a balanced salt solution such as Ringer's lactate or PlasmaLyte, blood or colloid such as 5 % albumin, gelatin, or a third-generation starch solution, although the safety of starches in the neonatal population has not been fully established [25, 27]. Our practice is to give fluid boluses of 10–20 ml/kg lactated Ringer's solution, or an appropriate volume of albumin (or blood), and monitor fluid losses and clinical parameters such as heart rate, blood pressure, filling pressure, and capillary refill. Laboratory testing of hemoglobin, base excess, serum lactate, electrolytes, and blood glucose concentrations and the coagulation status is essential.

The volume of fluid required intraoperatively varies with the clinical condition of the child, from 10 to 20 ml/kg for a child undergoing an uncomplicated EA/TEF repair to 50–100 ml/kg for a critically ill neonate with NEC or ischemic gut due to malrotation/volvulus. 5 % albumin is commonly used in the septic neonate. The trigger for blood transfusion depends on the age of the neonate; a trigger of 12 g/dl on day 1 of life has been recommended due to the presence of fetal hemoglobin, 11 g/dl in a neonate with chronic oxygen dependency, and 7 g/dl in a stable neonate with chronic anemia in early infancy [7]. If blood is required, an infusion of 4 ml/kg of packed red blood cells increases the hemoglobin concentration by 1 g/dl (as an infusion of 6 ml/kg of whole blood increases the hematocrit 3 gm%); a generous target for the hemoglobin concentration should be set to minimize donor exposure. Neonates are susceptible to hypothermia and hyperkalemia after a rapid transfusion; all blood should be warmed and fresh and the neonates should be closely monitored. Clotting factors should be considered in large-volume blood transfusion (e.g., one circulating blood volume).

The question of intraoperative dextrose is controversial; some units suggest maintenance fluid with low-dose (0.9 %) dextrose in a balanced salt solution at 4 ml/kg/h (<10 kg) to maintain the blood sugar concentration and avoid lipid mobilization [9]. This fluid should not be used for volume replacement. Lactated Ringer's or PlasmaLyte solution should be used intraoperatively to maintain fluid homeostasis. If a child requires a dextrose-containing fluid to maintain blood sugar preoperatively, or is receiving TPN, this infusion should not be stopped; rather, it should be maintained at the same rate as preoperatively throughout the perioperative period and serial serum glucose concentration measured. Although some reduce the preoperative infusion rate of dextrose-containing solutions intraoperatively, such a strategy must account for the possibility that the increased insulin levels may lead to hypoglycemia. In such cases, the serum glucose concentrations should be monitored intraoperatively whenever the preoperative glucose infusion is manipulated. Some neonates such as those with Beckwith–Wiedemann syndrome are at risk for hypoglycemia.

Surgery in the Neonatal Intensive Care Unit

Most elective and major neonatal surgery is performed in the OR, but transfer from the NICU to the OR carries particular risks for critically ill neonates who require inotropic support or high-frequency oscillatory ventilation (HFOV) (see Chap. 12 Anesthesia Outside the Operating Room). Surgery can also be performed successfully in the neonatal intensive care unit (NICU) without an increase in infective or other complications, particularly for very low-birth-weight infants (<1,500 g) with NEC or intestinal perforation [28]. The use of a surgical headlight, thermal mattress, and transparent drapes improves operating conditions for the surgeon and access for the anesthesiologist. Total intravenous anesthesia (TIVA) and analgesia techniques are required (fentanyl or remifentanil, ± ketamine), although the need for a hypnotic agent in this age group has been questioned [29]. Most NICUs do not use end-tidal pCO_2 monitoring but prefer transcutaneous pCO_2 monitoring. To ensure rapid responses to changes in ventilation (provided the ventilation is not HFOV), a capnograph monitor may be transferred from the OR to the NICU. Portable screens should be in place to cordon off the surgical area and visitors should be excluded from the immediate vicinity in the NICU during surgery. Complex, endoscopic, or airway procedures are more appropriately performed in the OR, as are most procedures in neonates whose lungs are not ventilated before surgery.

Minimally Invasive Surgery

The benefits of minimally invasive surgery (MIS) are well known, and with improvements in technology, MIS is increasing in popularity in neonatal practice. There is a significant surgical and institutional learning curve to neonatal MIS, but it does speed recovery after procedures such as pyloromyotomy, accomplishes the surgery for reduced cost, and may reduce complications such as chest wall deformity after EA/TEF repair [30–33]. In expert hands, surgical complication rates are comparable to open surgery, although cardiac arrest has occurred in neonates [31, 34–37]. Thoracoscopy has been steadily gaining popularity as the approach for congenital thoracic lesions. A recent review of the published studies determined that thoracoscopic surgery is a reasonable alternative to thoracotomy in neonates [38].

It is essential that the anesthesiologist and surgeon work closely together to minimize complications during MIS. The physiological changes associated with laparoscopic surgery in neonates are substantive and depend on several variables including the intra-abdominal insufflation pressure, the neonate's position, and its fluid status. The physiological changes associated with a pneumoperitoneum in laparoscopic surgery in neonates and children are addressed in detail elsewhere [39]. Neonates with congenital heart defects, such as aortic stenosis and cyanotic heart disease, may experience very serious complications including cardiac arrest during laparoscopic surgery [40, 41]. These neonates should be screened preoperatively and only anesthetized by those with a thorough understanding of the cardiac pathophysiology and in an institution with adequate support [40–42]. Anesthetic complications relate to positioning, reduced access, and the effects of the pneumoperitoneum or pneumothorax. The neonate may be positioned head up, head down, or semiprone and will be surrounded by equipment and monitors, with limited access to intravenous lines or the tracheal tube after the surgical drapes are in place. It is essential that the tube and lines are checked and securely fixed at the start of the procedure.

Specific complications from MIS in neonates relate to hypercarbia, desaturation, hypotension, metabolic acidosis, and hypothermia and are seen more often during thoracoscopic procedures [43]. During laparoscopic surgery, the pneumoperitoneum or pneumothorax is created and maintained by insufflating carbon dioxide (CO_2), which results in significant absorption of CO_2 into the circulation. Insufflated CO_2 may contribute up to 30 % of the exhaled CO_2 during thoracoscopic procedures and up to 20 % during laparoscopic surgery [43]. As a result, high levels of arterial CO_2 may be reached [44–47]. End tidal CO_2 measurement does not give an accurate measurement of arterial CO_2 and it is important to monitor CO_2 absorption accurately with transcutaneous carbon dioxide monitoring or arterial blood gases, rather than end tidal measurements [13, 19]. The significance of severe hypercarbia in this context is unclear, but specific adverse effects have not been reported to date, although respiratory acidosis and cerebral oxygen desaturation have been demonstrated, and concerns remain about neuronal apoptosis in animal models [44, 45].

The CO_2 insufflation pressure should be limited to 8 mmHg and operative time to <100 min to minimize the adverse cardiorespiratory sequelae from insufflation [48–50]. Isolated cardiac arrests have occurred in several neonates undergoing abdominal insufflation with carbon dioxide. This should be suspected if sudden hemodynamic instability occurs during insufflation of the abdomen. Augmenting the preload with 10 ml/kg IV balanced salt solution before insufflation of the abdomen preserves circulatory homeostasis. Minute volume should be increased to compensate for increased arterial carbon dioxide ($PaCO_2$) [46, 51]. A range of procedures are now performed using MIS, although some, including repair of a congenital diaphragmatic hernia (CDH), have a high rate of conversion to open surgery [31, 34, 52, 53].

One-Lung Ventilation

One-lung ventilation (OLV) may be required for thoracic surgery in neonates. There are few absolute indications for OLV as the lung is generally easy to compress during open thoracotomy, and gentle insufflation of CO_2 is used to compress the lung and maintain the artificial pneumothorax during thoracoscopic surgery. Some authors recommend OLV for surgery for congenital thoracic malformations involving a bronchial connection, for instance, in congenital lobar emphysema (CLE) [54–56].

Double-lumen tubes are not available for neonates, and OLV is obtained by either selective endobronchial intubation or the use of a bronchial blocker [54–56].

Selective endobronchial intubation is relatively easy, although more so on the right than the left. The disadvantage is that tube must be withdrawn at the end of surgery to ventilate both lungs and check for air leaks, and there is a risk of accidental extubation at this time. Fiberoptic bronchoscopes with an external diameter as small as 2.0 mm are available, suitable for a 2.5 mm ID tracheal tube [57]. The following techniques have been described to achieve one-lung ventilation [54]:

Endobronchial Intubation

- Intubate the trachea in the normal way, check for bilateral breath sounds, and note the depth of the tracheal tube at the alveolar ridge.
- Selectively intubate the bronchus using a fiberoptic bronchoscope threaded through the tracheal tube. Advance the tube over the bronchoscope and withdraw the scope. Check if breath sounds have disappeared on the contralateral side. Note the depth of the tube. If the right bronchus was intubated, check for the presence of breath sounds in the right upper lobe. If not, withdraw the tube until the right upper lobe is ventilated. Although it may be more difficult to pass the tracheal tube into the left bronchus, there is no concern that a bronchus will be blocked inadvertently.
- At the end of surgery, carefully withdraw the tube to the original position to allow bilateral air entry (note length), and secure.

Bronchial Blocker

A balloon-tipped 3Fr Fogarty embolectomy catheter, atrioseptostomy catheter, pulmonary artery catheter, or 5Fr Arndt endobronchial blocker may be used to occlude the lung on the operative side. The last two have the advantage of a central lumen to decompress the lung. The bronchial blocker is placed alongside the tracheal tube, as the tracheal tube in a neonate is too small to accommodate the blocker within the lumen of the tube:

- Perform direct laryngoscopy; place the bronchial blocker into the lumen of the trachea.
- Intubate the trachea with the bronchial blocker alongside the tracheal tube, on the operative side.
- Place a fiberoptic bronchoscope into the lumen of the tracheal tube and advance the bronchial blocker into the bronchus on the operative side under direct vision.
- Inflate the balloon of the bronchial blocker with saline and check if breath sounds are absent on the operative side.

The primary disadvantage of the bronchial blocker is that it requires experience and expertise to place and is particularly difficult if the neonate has any degree of respiratory compromise. Another concern relates to the bronchial blocker becoming displaced during surgery and causing complete tracheal obstruction. This is thought to be less likely if the balloon is inflated with saline [54]. Oxygen saturation, arterial pCO_2, breath sounds, and airway pressures should be monitored continually during the surgery.

Specific Conditions

Congenital Thoracic Malformations

There are a number of congenital thoracic malformations that may require surgical intervention in the neonatal period. The three most common lesions described may represent a spectrum of disease rather than true separate entities [57].

Congenital Cystic Adenomatoid Malformation

This rare congenital lung lesion that occurs in 1:25–30,000 live births is the most common of the congenital thoracic malformations [58]. Congenital cystic adenomatoid malformation (CCAM) is a multicystic pulmonary mass usually affecting only one lobe of the lung, more commonly on

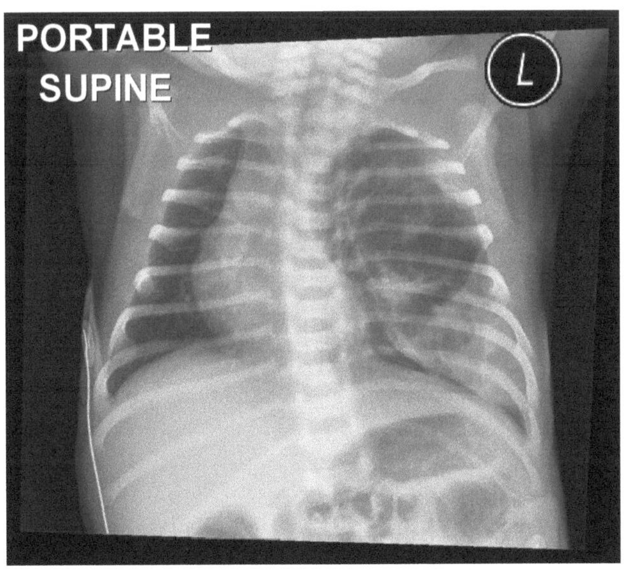

Fig. 10.1 Congenital cystic adenomatoid malformation. Chest radiograph in a neonate with a left-sided amorphous cystic mass filling most of the left hemithorax. The cardiac silhouette is shifted to the right. The right hemithorax is slightly opacified

Table 10.1 The Stocker classification of congenital cystic adenomatoid malformation (CCAM)

Stocker type 0 (rare). This is a fatal defect in which the lungs do not develop beyond the pseudoglandular level, resulting in small hypoplastic lungs bilaterally with a bronchial airway. Also known as acinar dysplasia
Stocker type I (macrocystic adenomatoid malformation) (60–70 %). Single or multiple large "cysts" (>2 cm diameter) are present, which communicate with the proximal airways and distal lung parenchyma. The lesion is relatively localized and most infants have a good prognosis after cyst resection. Good prognosis
Stocker type II (microcystic adenomatoid malformation) (10–15 %). Multiple small spongelike cysts (<1 cm) replace the distal lung parenchyma. This has a worse prognosis and is more commonly associated with other anomalies, such as renal agenesis and cardiac and chromosomal abnormalities
Stocker type III (solid cystic adenomatoid malformation) (5 %). The abnormality represents a severe end of the spectrum with multiple airless cysts involving an entire lobe or even lung. This has a poor prognosis, more commonly reported in stillbirths with CCAM
Stocker type IV (rare). This is an entirely alveolar pulmonary defect in which large cysts replace the numerous alveoli in the periphery of the lung. Good prognosis

the left, but may occur bilaterally in 5–15 % (Fig. 10.1). The etiology is unknown, although it may represent a hamartomatous process, focal pulmonary dysplasia, or a bronchiolar developmental anomaly [22]. Associated anomalies occur in up to 18 % of cases, involving renal agenesis and cardiac defects (see type II below) [58]. The prognosis depends on the size of the CCAM; small lesions may be asymptomatic, but large lesions may be associated with hypoplasia of the normal lung and pulmonary hypertension and, in severe cases, mediastinal shift causing cardiac compromise and nonimmune fetal hydrops [59, 60]. Fetal hydrops is the most serious harbinger of death [61]. The ratio of the CCAM volume to the head circumference on the first antenatal ultrasound predicts the fetus' perinatal course: a ratio <0.56 is consistent with a good postnatal outcome, whereas a ratio >1.6 is consistent with developing hydrops [62].

Classification of CCAM

Stocker originally classified CCAM based on cyst size and postnatal histology, yielding three types. Subsequently type 0 (tracheobronchial defect with small firm lungs and a bronchial airway) and type 4 (an entirely alveolar defect) were added to complete the current classification. Since types 1–3 are usually adenomatoid and types 1, 2, and 4 are cystic, Stocker proposed a broader term for these defects: congenital pulmonary airway malformations (CPAM) [58, 63]. However, CCAM remains the primary acronym for these defects. A simpler classification for this defect was proposed: macrocystic or microcystic (solid), based on anatomy and appearance on antenatal ultrasound, but Stocker's classification has persisted [58, 59, 63–65] (Table 10.1).

Diagnosis of CCAM

The diagnosis is usually made by antenatal ultrasound at approximately 20 weeks gestation [66–70]. The lesions are monitored throughout gestation following one of three courses: increase in size, remain unchanged, or undergo spontaneous resolution. In aggressive disease, the lesion may respond to maternal steroids. A few specialist centers offer fetal interventions for high-risk cases causing hydrops including thoracoamniotic shunt for isolated cysts, open fetal surgery, or an EXIT procedure at delivery (ex-utero intrapartum treatment), depending on gestational age, the size of the cyst, and the health of the mother [59, 68, 70].

Infants present with symptoms of respiratory distress in the neonatal period, with tachypnea, increased work of breathing, and desaturation in 30 % of cases, or occasionally with hyperinflation on the side of the CCAM. Some infants may appear to be relatively asymptomatic. Ten percent of the cases present with recurrent pneumonia or pneumothorax in later childhood. A significant number of infants remain asymptomatic and are only detected incidentally.

CCAM is evident on chest X-ray, especially if it is large. Microcystic lesions may be fluid filled, but macrocystic lesions are usually aerated and may be difficult to visualize. A CT scan with contrast is usually performed to delineate the limitations of the lesion. Ultrasound may be used to identify the blood supply and exclude an anomalous systemic artery.

Management of CCAM

Initial management involves respiratory support as needed and imaging to confirm and define the extent of the lesion. Neonates with hydrops have a very high perioperative mortality as a result of the pulmonary hypoplasia and pulmonary hypertension. These neonates should be medically stabilized before embarking on surgical interventions [61, 70]. Surgery may be beneficial for neonates with significant respiratory signs and symptoms and/or compression of adjacent cardiac or major vascular structures. Controversy exists regarding the appropriateness and timing of surgery in asymptomatic or smaller lesions [60, 71–74]. Resection in infancy or early childhood is increasingly advocated to preclude infectious complications and malignant transformation (rhabdomyosarcoma, squamous cell carcinoma, bronchoalveolar carcinoma, and pleuropulmonary blastoma in 2–4 % of cases) and to encourage compensatory lung growth. If surgery is not undertaken, ideally these neonates should be followed into adulthood to ensure a timely intervention should the lesion turn malignant [74].

Surgical Considerations

The aim of surgery is to preserve viable lung tissue and reduce the mediastinal shift. The standard approach is posterolateral thoracotomy and lobectomy. Segmental resection may be used for small lesions or multilobular disease but is associated with a greater incidence of postoperative air leak. Thoracoscopic resection can be performed but access may be difficult with large cystic lesions.

Anesthetic Considerations

Thoracotomy and lung resection are generally well tolerated in neonates; blood transfusions are not usually required. Full invasive monitoring should be used. CCAM are connected to the bronchial tree, and preoperative hyperinflation resulting in ball-valve effect is a possibility, although one-lung ventilation is not usually required. Nitrous oxide is best avoided.

Infants with severe respiratory distress may require HFOV preoperatively, but it is usually possible to wean to conventional ventilation in the early postoperative period [70]. Analgesia may be provided by intravenous opioids such as fentanyl or remifentanil or thoracic epidural analgesia with the catheter inserted via the caudal route [75, 76]. Most neonates require only a brief period of postoperative ventilation, although ventilation may be extended if pulmonary hypoplasia and/or pulmonary hypertension is present.

Lung Sequestration

This lesion consists of nonfunctioning lung tissue that does not have a tracheobronchial communication. There is anomalous systemic arterial supply, usually directly from the aorta, with more than one vessel in 15 % of lesions. Sequestrations may have a patent or non-patent connection to the gastrointestinal tract (bronchopulmonary foregut malformations) [70].

Classification of Lung Sequestration

- Intralobar sequestration (ILS) (75 %): the abnormal tissue is contained within normal lung predominantly within the lower lobes (often left sided). The child is generally asymptomatic but may present with hemoptysis, pneumothorax, or recurrent infections in later childhood. The venous drainage is often via the pulmonary veins. Right-sided ILS may be associated with anomalous pulmonary venous drainage characteristic of scimitar syndrome; care must be taken not to ligate pulmonary veins during surgical resection.
- Extralobar sequestration (ELS) (25 %): the sequestration is completely separated from the lung by visceral pleura. There is an infradiaphragmatic arterial supply in 20 % and the lesion itself is infradiaphragmatic in 3 % of cases. Venous drainage is to the azygous system in the majority. ELS affects males four times more commonly than females and is more often associated with other anomalies such as congenital diaphragmatic hernia (CDH) (16 %), CCAM (15 %), congenital heart disease, chest wall abnormalities, and hindgut duplications.

Diagnosis of Lung Sequestration

These lesions may be detected on antenatal ultrasound or postnatal chest X-ray. The systemic blood supply must be delineated using ultrasound, CT, or MRI.

ELS is generally asymptomatic but is often detected earlier than intralobar sequestrations. Both ILS and ELS may be detected antenatally and may resolve. Symptomatic infants with large sequestrations may present with respiratory distress, feeding difficulties, or cardiac failure if the sequestered lobe is associated with significant arteriovenous or left-to-right shunting [70]. Hydrops may result from severe cardiac failure in utero, and pulmonary hypoplasia and pulmonary hypertension may be associated with large lesions, as in CCAM.

Management of Lung Sequestration

Respiratory support should be instituted as required, and the systemic blood supply defined on imaging as the first step. Surgical excision is generally advocated. The timing of surgery depends on the clinical situation. Complications such as infection and cardiovascular compromise due to shunting should be treated before resection.

Surgical Considerations

As for CCAM, thoracotomy is the standard approach for pulmonary sequestrations. Thoracoscopic resection is a viable alternative due to the relatively smaller size of the lesions. A laparotomy or laparoscopic approach is required for infradiaphragmatic lesions. Additional therapeutic interventions have been reported anecdotally including radiofrequency ablation and coil embolization [77].

The anomalous systemic vessels can be fragile elastic vessels with significant blood flow. Careful dissection and meticulous control are required to prevent hemorrhage. Control of the systemic blood supply during surgery is critical especially when the origin of the vessel is on the opposite aspect of the diaphragm to the operative field (infradiaphragmatic vessel for intrathoracic lesions). A loss of control can result in retraction of the vessel out of the operative field and catastrophic hemorrhage. A crossmatch should be available for all of these neonates.

Anesthetic Considerations

These are similar to CCAM. Neonates with severe pulmonary hypertension should be optimized medically before surgery.

Congenital Lobar Emphysema

Congenital lobar emphysema (CLE) is an obstructive overinflation disorder, which may be due to defective bronchiolar development. The affected lobe is hyperinflated and compresses the adjacent normal lung. Hyperinflation becomes progressive after birth, although neonates usually present with respiratory distress in the first few days of life. Males are more commonly affected than females (3:1). The left upper lobe is involved in almost 50 % of cases followed by the right middle lobe (28 %) and the right upper lobe (20 %); bilateral involvement is rare (Fig. 10.2). Cardiac anomalies are present in 20 % of neonates with CLE [70].

Diagnosis of CLE

CLE may be detected antenatally but is difficult to distinguish from CCAM. Postnatally there is often early respiratory distress and clinical signs suggestive of pneumothorax. A CXR may show lobar hyperinflation, mediastinal shift, and flattening of the ipsilateral diaphragm. Ultrasound can help distinguish from a tension pneumothorax, or if stable enough, CT or MRI scan will confirm the diagnosis. If the neonate is stable, then a preoperative echocardiogram should be also performed.

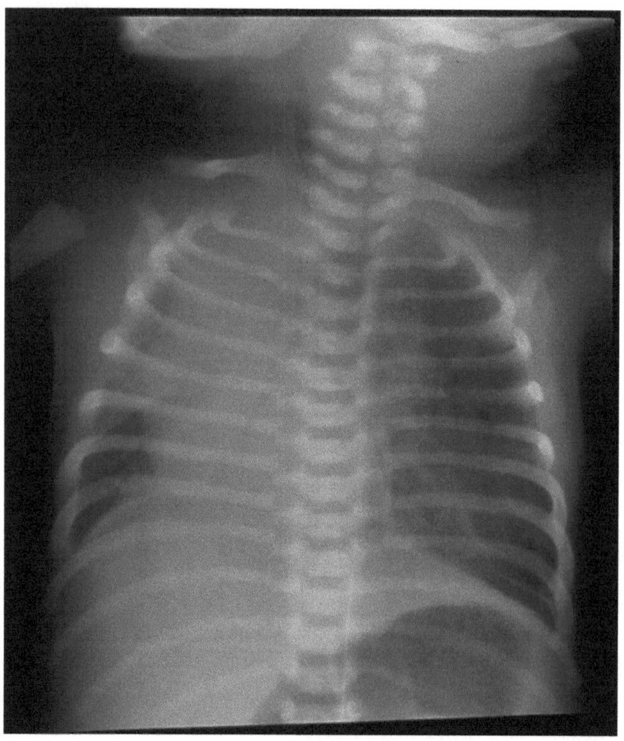

Fig. 10.2 Congenital lobar emphysema. Chest radiograph with hyperinflation of the left chest and displacement of the cardiac silhouette toward the right chest. A large gastric air bubble is present

Management of CLE

The primary treatment is lobectomy, which may be required on an emergent basis before a full preoperative workup can be performed. More recently, segmental lung resection has proven successful in preserving lung without an increased incidence of a recurrence [78]. Positive pressure ventilation worsens the hyperinflation, and if respiratory support is required preoperatively, then HFOV may be preferred. A chest drain should never be inserted as it may cause preferential ventilation of the abnormal lung leading to respiratory failure.

Surgical and Anesthetic Considerations

Induction of anesthesia with positive pressure ventilation may cause rapid deterioration due to air trapping. If possible, spontaneous ventilation should be maintained until one-lung ventilation has been achieved or until the chest is opened. Anesthesia should be introduced by inhalation, and lines placed while spontaneous ventilation is maintained. Muscle relaxants may be administered, but in these neonates, the inspiratory pressure should be minimized [79]. Alternatively, muscle relaxants may be avoided and intubation achieved using a combination of inhalational anesthesia, intravenous propofol with topical lidocaine (3 mg/kg) administered to the cords [54, 80]. The thoracotomy instruments and the surgeon must be ready in the event that urgent thoracotomy and decompression become necessary.

Esophageal Atresia/Tracheoesophageal Fistula

Esophageal atresia (EA) and tracheoesophageal fistula (TEF) occur in 1:3,000–1:4,500 live births [81–83]. The etiology is believed to be due to a defect in the separation of the trachea and esophagus from a common foregut, which normally occurs after 4 weeks gestation. The etiology and exact embryology remain unclear, although the theories put forth include failure of fusion of lateral tracheoesophageal folds or the tracheoesophageal septum, imbalance in epithelial proliferation and apoptosis, trifurcation of the lung bud, and a possible role of the notochord. Animal evidence suggests that a greater developmental role of the foregut in this defect as the fistula and distal esophagus may be respiratory in origin [58]. There is also evidence that specific targets in the molecular mechanisms responsible for complete separation of the trachea and the esophagus may be responsible for EA/TEF defects [84].

Classification

First classified in 1929, and modified in 1953, five common types of EA/TEF have been described, although it is probably more appropriate to describe the conditions anatomically [81, 82, 85] (see Fig. 10.3) (Table 10.2).

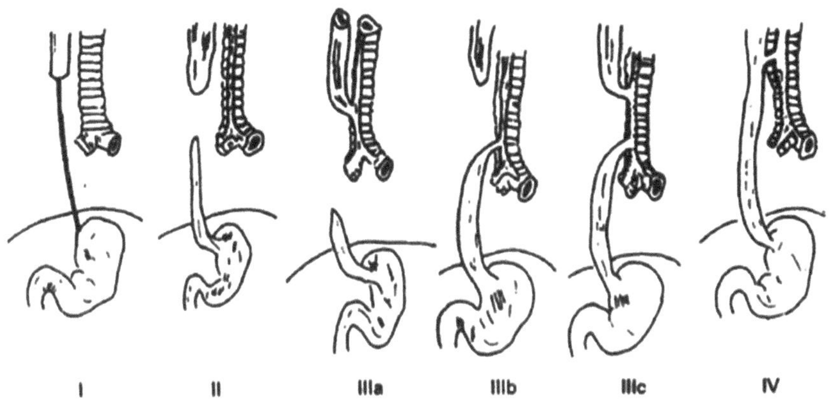

Fig. 10.3 Classification of esophageal atresia and tracheoesophageal fistula according to Vogt. Type 1: Obliteration of the esophagus. Type II: Atresia without fistula. Type IIIa: Atresia with proximal fistula. Type IIIb: Atresia with distal fistula. Type IIIc: Atresia with proximal and distal fistula. Type IV: Tracheoesophageal fistula (H-type fistula). *Adapted from: HolzKi J. Pediatric Anaesthesia 1992; 2: 297–303*

Table 10.2 EA/TEF classification and incidence in neonates

EA with distal TEF (80–85 %)
Pure EA (5–7 %)
Isolated TEF ("H"-type fistula) (3–6 %)
EA with proximal and distal TEF (3–5 %)
EA and proximal TEF (2 %)

The length of the gap between proximal and distal esophagus is variable, as is the position of fistula (or fistulae) within the trachea. These anatomical variations have important implications for surgical strategy and anesthesia management. In one series, the fistula was mid-tracheal in 61 %, at or just above the carina in 33 %, cervical in 8 %, and bronchial in 1 %. There was more than one fistula in 3 % of patients [85, 86]. In the "H"-type TEF, the fistula is typically in the cervical region, whereas in EA with a proximal fistula, the fistula is usually 1–2 cm from the blind-ending upper pouch [83].

Neonates with EA/TEF are often born premature, with low birth weight (Fig. 10.4) [82]. Approximately 50 % of neonates with EA/TEF have associated anomalies, an incidence that increases with decreasing birth weight (<2,500 g) and with pure EA. In contrast, anomalies are less common in those with an isolated H-type fistula [82, 83, 87, 88]. The most common anomalies associated with EA/TEF are cardiac anomalies (29 %), followed by duodenal atresia and anorectal anomalies (14 %), genitourinary anomalies (14 %), intestinal malrotation (13 %), chromosomal abnormalities (trisomies 21, 18, and 13q deletion) (4 %), vertebral and skeletal anomalies (10 %), and specific-named associations (see below). The most common cardiac defects are atrial or ventricular septal defects or tetralogy of Fallot [88, 89] (Fig. 10.5) [90]. A right-sided aortic arch is present in 2.5–5 % of infants with EA/TEF [91].

Several disorders have been associated with EA/TEF [82]. The VATER/VACTERL association, an association of unknown etiology, is defined by the presence of at least three of the following congenital malformations: *v*ertebral defects, *a*norectal anomaly, *c*ardiac defects, *T*EF, *r*enal anomalies, and *l*imb (radial) abnormalities [90, 92, 93]. Approximately 47 % of neonates with EA have VACTERL anomalies.

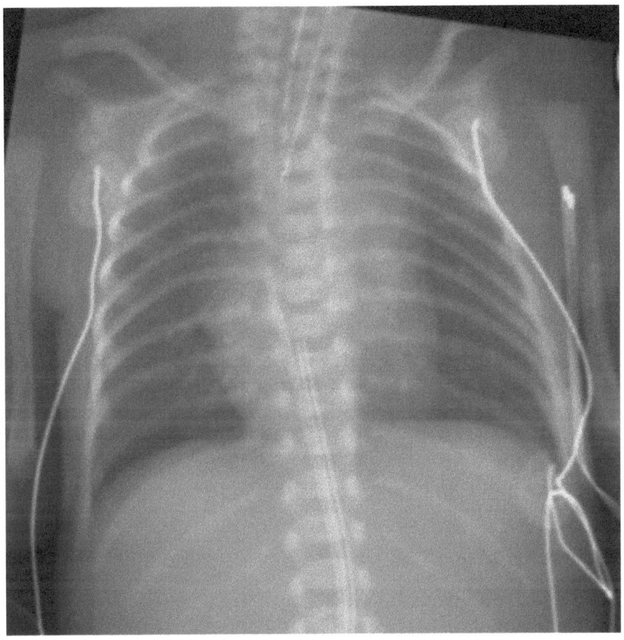

Fig. 10.4 Esophageal atresia in a neonate. This chest radiograph depicts a multi-orifice orogastric tube (with side holes) ending at the mid-thoracic level. A tracheal tube ends at the thoracic inlet. Umbilical vein and artery catheters enter radiograph from below; one terminates at T6–T7 and a second at T8–T9. A gastric air bubble is not visible here

VACTERL-H association is the VACTERL association with hydrocephalus, although hydrocephalus is often listed as a non-VACTERL anomaly (see above). CHARGE syndrome is an autosomal dominant disorder caused by a mutation on chromosome 7. It is associated with TEF, coloboma, cardiac defects, choanal atresia, neurocognitive and growth impairment, and genital, ear, and cranial nerve defects. Potter's syndrome, which is associated with renal agenesis, pulmonary hypoplasia, dysmorphic facies, and Schisis association, which is associated with omphalocele, cleft lip and/

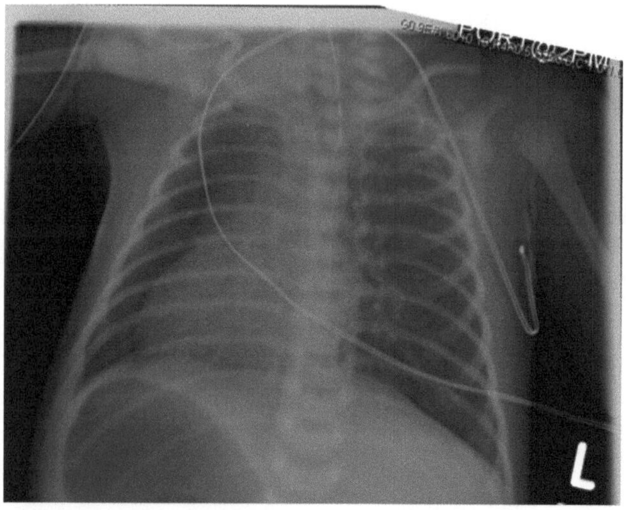

Fig. 10.5 EA/TEF with situs inversus. Chest radiograph of a neonate with EA/TEF. The multi-orificed orogastric tube (with side orifices) ends at T3–T4 reflecting EA. The cardiac silhouette and gastric bubble are reversed, present on the right side. Echocardiogram verified the presence of a ventricular septal defect. The large gastric air bubble is consistent with a distal tracheoesophageal fistula

or palate, and genital hypoplasia, may also be associated with EA/TEF. EA/TEF is also associated with CATCH syndrome (22q deletion that includes cardiac defects, abnormal facies, thymic aplasia, cleft palate, and hypocalcaemia). Of the trisomy syndromes [13, 20], EA/TEF is most often associated with Edwards syndrome (trisomy 18). Feingold syndrome (dominant inheritance) is similar to VACTERL syndrome but features microcephaly and learning difficulties [82]. Other syndromes associated with EA/TEF include DiGeorge sequence, Pierre Robin sequence, Fanconi syndrome, and polysplenia [58].

Non-VACTERL anomalies are being reported in association with EA/TEF with increasing frequency. Such anomalies include single umbilical arteries, genital defects, digital defects, neurologic anomalies, and respiratory tract defects [90, 94].

Diagnosis

EA may be suspected antenatally in the presence of polyhydramnios with a small or absent gastric bubble or associated abnormalities present in the fetus. Most cases, however, present after birth. A history of polyhydramnios should prompt the pediatrician to pass a size 8–10 Fr orogastric tube immediately after birth. The tube cannot pass the upper esophagus (EA). The diagnosis is strongly suspected in the first few hours after birth if an orogastric tube cannot be passed and mucous that accumulates in the upper airway cannot be cleared by swallowing. The neonate chokes or becomes cyanosed if it attempts to feed. Aspiration pneumonia due to delayed diagnosis was common decades ago but is quite uncommon in modern medicine.

The diagnosis of EA/TEF should be confirmed on plain X-ray of the chest and abdomen. A coiled nasogastric tube will be identified in the upper third of the esophagus (level T2–T4); air in the gastrointestinal tract indicates the presence of a distal TE fistula. A gasless gastrointestinal tract suggests the absence of a distal fistula, although a proximal fistula remains a possibility. Other abnormalities such as vertebral anomalies (usually in the lower thoracic region) or the "double bubble" of duodenal atresia can also be detected on preoperative films. A thorough clinical examination is important to exclude associated anomalies and the presence of coexisting problems, such as respiratory distress syndrome in premature infants. An echocardiogram is strongly recommended before surgery to identify cardiac defects and the position of the aortic arch. If the neonate has passed urine (thus excluding bilateral renal agenesis), then a renal US can be delayed until after surgery.

An H-type TEF is infrequently detected in the neonatal period but should be suspected with a history of recurrent chest infection due to repeated aspiration.

Risk Stratification

It is helpful to stratify neonates with EA/TEF according to risk. The original stratification by Waterson was based on birth weight, associated anomalies, and the presence of pneumonia [83]. Neonatal care has improved leading to a current risk stratification that is based solely on birth weight and the presence of cardiac anomalies [88, 89, 95]. Improved outcomes have resulted in survival rates exceeding 98 % in neonates with birth weights >1,500 g and without major cardiac anomalies, 82 % with birth weights <1,500 g or major cardiac anomalies, and 50 % with birth weights <1,500 g and major cardiac anomalies [95]. A four-part classification has been suggested more recently, with prediction of 100 % survival in neonates with birth weights >2,000 g without cardiac anomalies and 40 % survival in high-risk neonates with birth weights <2,000 g with major cardiac anomalies [89]. The premature infant with a major cardiac anomaly remains a high risk. Parents of infants with bilateral renal agenesis or major complications of prematurity such as grade IV intraventricular hemorrhage should be given the option of nonoperative treatment.

Medical Management

Initial management of neonates with EA/TEF is to prevent aspiration of oral secretions before definitive surgery. A 10Fr double-lumen oro-esophageal Replogle tube should be inserted into the upper pouch and placed on continuous suction, or secretions should be cleared frequently by naso-esophageal tube suction. The neonate should be given maintenance intravenous fluids and nursed 30° head up or in the decubitus position. Blood should be crossmatched and available for surgery. If preoperative ventilation is required, inspiratory pressures should be kept to a minimum, if possible placing the tip of the tracheal tube distal to the fistula (see below). Premature infants should receive surfactant according to standard protocols.

Surgical Considerations

The aim of surgery is to restore continuity of the esophagus and ligate the TE fistula, if present. Surgery is usually performed on the first or second day of life if the neonate is stable and does not require respiratory support. Primary esophageal anastomosis is usually possible in EA with distal TEF, although it may be preferable to divide the fistula and place a feeding gastrostomy in a neonate with severe comorbidities such as a duct-dependent cardiac anomaly. Primary esophageal repair can be performed 6–12 weeks after cardiac surgery.

Emergency surgery may be required if the child requires preoperative ventilation, as in the case of the preterm neonate with respiratory distress syndrome. If the lung compliance is poor, gas from the ventilator may preferentially enter the gastrointestinal tract via the fistula. This may lead to gastric distension, deteriorating cardiorespiratory status, and possible gastric rupture. Inadvertent intubation of the fistula must be excluded in cases of severe gastric distention with cardiorespiratory instability [96]. To prevent gastric distention from ventilation via the fistula, some have recommended clamping the distal esophagus as soon as the chest is opened [97]. Decompressive gastrostomy should not be undertaken as a primary intervention as it will lead to a torrential gas leak via the gastrostomy and worsening minute ventilation. The child should undergo emergency transpleural ligation of the fistula, with delayed division of the fistula and possible repair of EA at 8–10 days [83].

Neonates with pure EA or EA with a proximal TEF often have a long gap between proximal and distal ends of the esophagus. A feeding gastrostomy is inserted and the length of the gap estimated radiographically at the time of surgery. If the gap is greater than the vertical height of three vertebral bodies, upper pouch suction is continued postoperatively and delayed primary closure is usually possible by about 12 weeks of age; if the gap is greater than six vertebral bodies, a cervical esophagostomy is often fashioned and the esophagus repaired at a later date. Esophageal replacement surgery is occasionally required [83].

An esophagoscopy or bronchoscopy is often performed at the start of surgery to provide absolute confirmation of the diagnosis, to assess the position of the fistula if present, and to exclude multiple fistulae [86]. A variety of techniques have been described to identify fistulae in neonates: rigid bronchoscopy, esophagoscopy, or flexible fiberoptic bronchoscopy via the tracheal tube. The advantage of using a small flexible bronchoscope is that the scope may also be used to assess the position of the tip of tracheal tube, to pass through the fistula to assist the surgeon in identifying the fistula during surgery, and to assess the airway at the end of surgery to exclude a residual blind-ending tracheal pouch and the severity of the tracheomalacia near the fistula [98].

The traditional approach to repair of EA/TEF is extrapleural via a right posterolateral thoracotomy with the neonate placed in the lateral decubitus position with a roll under the chest to facilitate surgical access. The posterior mediastinum is approached via the 4th and 5th intercostal spaces and the extrapleural route, gently compressing the right lung. The approach is delicate and time consuming but reduces morbidity from an anastomotic leak, should one occur. If a right arch is confirmed on preoperative echo, a left-sided approach should be considered and a double aortic arch may be approached via the standard right thoracotomy [91]. If the child becomes unstable, a transpleural approach may be used.

Thoracoscopic repair has become popular in specialist centers in recent years and, in expert hands, has the same complication rate as open techniques, with comparable blood gases, operating times, and reduced time in intensive care postoperatively [99–101]. Currently recommendations are based on large case series, since no randomized controlled trials have compared the two techniques [34, 35, 102]. For thoracoscopic repair, the child is placed semiprone with the right side of the chest elevated at 45° so that the structures may be easily visualized. Lung deflation is produced by CO_2 insufflation, and care should be taken to minimize hypercarbia, as described previously.

Major concerns during open or thoracoscopic surgery include accurate identification of anatomical structures and cardiorespiratory instability due to OLV and distortion of the trachea. The anesthesiologist may be asked to push on the Replogle tube to help identify the proximal esophageal pouch. Test occlusion of the fistula is good practice to ensure that the right lung can still be inflated and that a vital structure (e.g., the pulmonary artery or main bronchus) has not been clamped in error. If the neonate does not tolerate OLV, surgery may have to proceed with intermittent two-lung ventilation once the neonate recovers. This requires good communication between the anesthesiologist and surgeon. Increased FiO_2 and hand ventilation may be required, but respiratory compromise usually improves after ligation of the fistula. The integrity of tracheal repair can be checked by instilling warm saline in the chest during a sustained inflation to identify an air leak by the presence of air bubbles. The lower esophagus should not be aggressively mobilized in order to avoid devascularization, as this may cause later problems with esophageal motility. A gas leak from the upper pouch during esophageal anastomosis should raise suspicion of an upper pouch fistula. Dissection of the upper pouch helps to identify a proximal fistula, if one is present, and allows mobilization of the esophagus to minimize tension of the repair. If there is significant tension at the anastomosis, the neonate should remain paralyzed and the lungs ventilated mechanically for approximately 5 days postoperatively [83]. A transanastomotic tube (TAT tube) placed under direct vision before the anastomosis is completed facilitates early feeding and should be clearly marked to preclude accidental removal postoperatively.

Early complications at EA/TEF repair include tracheobronchomalacia (20–40 %), anastomotic leak (15–20 %), anastomotic stricture (30–50 %), and recurrent fistula (10 %) [103]. Tracheomalacia is due to abnormal cartilage in the region of the fistula and often produces a typical barking cough. In severe cases, the child may develop recurrent chest infections or "near death" episodes due to acute airway collapse, and emergency aortopexy may be required in the first few months after repair [83]. An early anastomotic leak may cause a tension pneumothorax; a chest drain should be inserted and the leak explored and repaired. Late complications include gastroesophageal reflux (severe reflux in 40 %) and recurrent chest infections, probably related to gastroesophageal reflux [82]. Long-term respiratory complications including bronchiectasis may result from aspiration, GERD, and chest wall abnormalities [104]. Both the parents and their neonate are at risk for psychological and traumatic stress (including post-traumatic stress disorder) [105]. These are long-term issues centered around feeding difficulties, multiple painful procedures and surgeries, feeding, and airway issues.

Anesthetic Considerations

Anesthetic considerations include general factors relating to the thoracotomy or thoracoscopic surgery in neonates and the high incidence of comorbidity. Specific considerations include airway management and positioning the tracheal tube in the presence of a tracheal fistula. Selective OLV is not usually required as the surgeon can easily compress the lung to access the fistula. Every neonate should have a preoperative echocardiogram to identify the presence of a congenital heart defect that may range from a patent ductus arteriosus or ASD/VSD to a hypoplastic left heart. Failure to be aware of the presence of a congenital heart defect during one-lung anesthesia for an EA/TEF repair could lead to catastrophic complications including hypoxia, hypotension, and cardiac arrest.

The main anesthesia complications relate to inadvertent intubation of the fistula or preferential ventilation of the fistula causing gastric distension and desaturation [95, 106, 107]. As described above, the fistula may vary in position; two-thirds occur in the mid-trachea and one-third occur at or near the carina. The majority of complications have been described with large fistulae, particularly when they occur near the carina.

The traditional technique to secure the airway in these neonates has been to intubate the trachea while the neonate remains awake and maintain spontaneous respiration until the fistula was controlled. However, this is no longer recommended. A variety of anesthetic techniques and techniques of airway management have been described [82, 98, 106–109]. Most advocate inhalational or intravenous induction, according to personal preference, with muscle relaxant and gentle mask ventilation before intubating the trachea [98, 106–108].

Several approaches have been popularized to position the tracheal tube while avoiding intubating the tracheoesophageal atresia. One popular technique is to deliberately intubate the right main bronchus after general anesthesia is induced and then withdraw the tube until bilateral air entry is confirmed. This ensures the tracheal tube is below the fistula but does not prevent intubation of a large fistula at the carina [96]. Alternatively, rigid bronchoscopy (or flexible bronchoscopy after intubation) may be used to demonstrate the precise level of the fistula (or exclude multiple fistulae) and then plan the intubation strategy. If the fistula is mid-tracheal, the tip of the tracheal tube is ideally positioned just below the fistula, with the bevel facing anteriorly (to avoid ventilating the fistula since the origin of the fistula is the posterior tracheal wall) and gentle positive pressure ventilation used. If the fistula is at the carina, the tracheal tube may still be placed at the mid-tracheal level, provided the fistula is small. The tracheal tube should be fixed carefully and the position of the tube checked again after positioning for surgery to make sure that the dependent lung remains ventilated.

In the unusual situation of a large fistula at the level of the carina resulting in preferential gastric ventilation, some authors suggest passing a 2 or 3Fr Fogarty embolectomy catheter through the fistula into the stomach via the rigid bronchoscope; the balloon of the Fogarty catheter is then inflated to occlude the fistula. The tracheal tube is positioned alongside the Fogarty catheter [106]. This may not be a suitable technique if the child is very small or unstable. In such a case, the surgeon should proceed directly to thoracotomy to ligate the fistula as quickly as possible. Alternately, the chest may be opened rapidly and the distal esophagus ligated below the fistula [97]. If the stomach becomes very distended before the fistula is occluded, the tracheal tube should be disconnected intermittently to decompress the stomach via the airway.

Analgesia may be managed using an opioid-based technique such as fentanyl or remifentanil intraoperatively and morphine IV postoperatively, particularly for the child with long-gap EA who will remain ventilated postoperatively. Regional techniques using caudal catheters have been described and are most suitable for low-risk infants who are likely to be extubated in the immediate postoperative period. Many pediatric surgeons prefer a controlled extubation by anesthesia immediately postoperatively to reduce the risk/need for emergency reintubation that may damage the surgical closure.

Blood loss during surgery is usually minimal; intravenous crystalloid such as Ringer's is ideal and fluid volume of 10–20 ml/kg is usually required. The blood glucose concentration should be measured [24]. Broad-spectrum antibiotics should be given before skin incision and continued postoperatively. Secure intravenous access should be obtained, and some prefer arterial access to monitor blood pressure beat to beat and to sample the blood gases during one-lung ventilation, particularly in infants with significant comorbidity. Neonates with cardiac disease have a greater incidence of critical events such as desaturation or the need for new inotropic support compared with those without cardiac disease as well as a 57 % mortality during the hospitalization for those with ductal-dependent congenital heart disease [87]. These data underscore the need for a preoperative echocardiogram to identify a possible cardiac defect in all neonates with EA/TEF and, if a heart defect is present, to discuss the need for central venous access. Phenylephrine should be prepared to treat a "tet spell" in a neonate with an unrepaired tetralogy of Fallot.

Congenital Diaphragmatic Hernia

Congenital diaphragmatic hernia (CDH) occurs in 1:2,500 live births, with a slight predilection for males. There are two major types: Bochdalek (posterolateral defect) (Fig. 10.6a, b) and Morgagni (anterior) (Fig. 10.7a, b) [110]. The posterolateral defect accounts for 85–95 % cases of CDH and most are diagnosed antenatally. CDH is associated with herniation of the abdominal viscera into the affected hemithorax, with displacement of the mediastinum to the contralateral side (Fig. 10.6a, b). The lung on the side of the hernia is hypoplastic, whereas the lung on the contralateral side is usually normal (if survival is likely) or hypoplastic (if survival is unlikely). The degree of lung hypoplasia and associated pulmonary hypertension are the major determinants of outcome; surgical repair of the diaphragm has a relatively minor contribution to the long-term outcome. Anomalies occur in 40–60 % of neonates with CDH. These include cardiac, neural tube, chromosomal, renal, and genital anomalies and pulmonary sequestrations, as well as malrotation and duodenal atresia [111, 112]. The anterior (Morgagni) defect accounts for only 2 % of diaphragmatic hernias, located retrosternal (at the level of the xiphoid) or anteromedially in the diaphragm (Fig. 10.7a, b). These are often asymptomatic and may not be detected until adulthood [113].

Embryology

The diaphragm develops during weeks 4–8 from four embryological elements. A Bochdalek hernia results from failure of closure of the pleuroperitoneal canals during early embryonal life, often with early in-growth of the liver through the defect. The exact cause for CDH remains unknown but may be associated with genetic factors that lead to failure in cell migration, myogenesis and formation of connective tissue, or abnormalities of the retinoid signaling pathway, which is important in the development of the diaphragm. CDH may

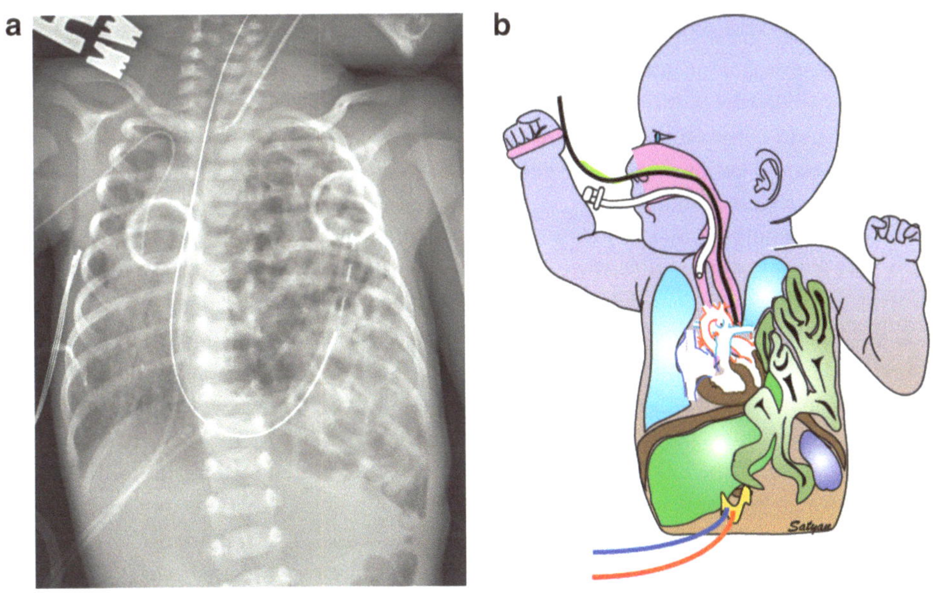

Fig. 10.6 Congenital diaphragmatic hernia (CDH): foramen of Bochdalek defect. (**a**) This chest radiograph depicts a neonate with congenital diaphragmatic hernia in the left (classic Bochdalek defect) chest with stomach and bowel in the chest, displacing the heart to the right chest. Note the multi-orificed orogastric tube (with side holes) in the esophagus, curving up and across the diaphragm and terminating in the stomach in the left chest. The tracheal tube ends at the thoracic inlet. PICC line enters the right chest and ends in the superior vena cava. (**b**) A schematic of a neonate with a CDH with bowel present in the left chest; the right lung is compressed and the heart is deviated toward the right chest (Courtesy of Dr. Satyan Lakshminrusimha, Division of Neonatology, Women and Children's Hospital of Buffalo, Buffalo, NY)

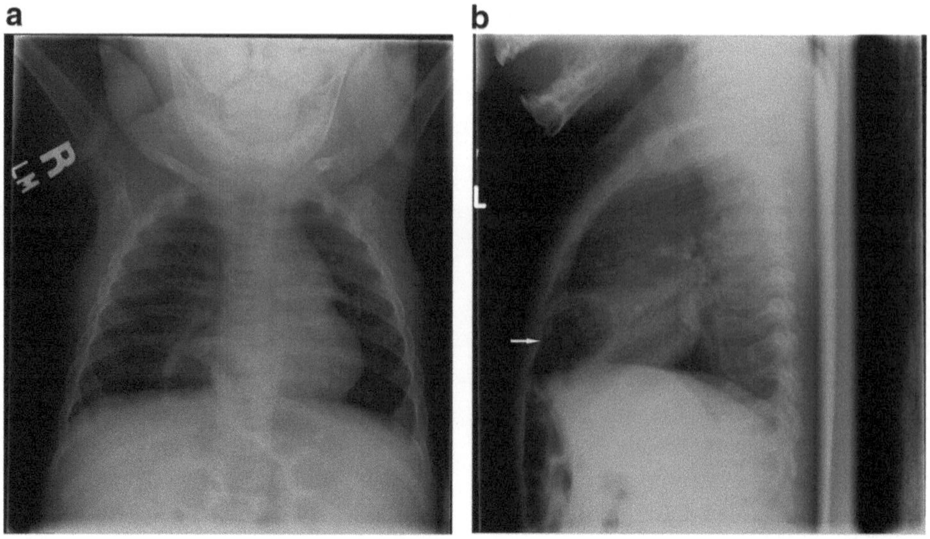

Fig. 10.7 (**a**, **b**). Congenital diaphragmatic hernia. Foramen of Morgagni defect. (**a**) This AP chest radiograph depicts a neonate with congenital diaphragmatic hernia with a loop of bowel that herniated through a defect in the anteromedial (retrosternal) area of the diaphragm (foramen of Morgagni). (**b**) This lateral chest radiograph depicts a loop of bowel in the immediate retrosternal space (see *arrow*), rising above the anterior aspect of the diaphragm (Courtesy of Dr. K. Valle, Division of Pediatric Surgery, Women and Children's Hospital of Buffalo, Buffalo, NY)

occur as an isolated abnormality (often associated with a mutation on chromosome 15q26) or occasionally associated with syndromes such as Pallister-Killian, Fryns syndrome, Cornelia De Lange, or Edwards syndrome [111]. Abnormal karyotyping has been reported in 16 % of neonates with CDH, in 4 % of those without anomalies, and 39 % of those with anomalies [114, 115].

Diagnosis

The diagnosis of CDH is made by antenatal ultrasound in ~70 % of cases, due to the presence of intrathoracic bowel loops or stomach, often signaled by a history of maternal polyhydramnios [114, 116]. All cases should be referred to a specialist center. The fetus should be screened for associated anomalies and the family provided with antenatal counseling, particularly if there are features associated with a poor prognosis (see below) [117, 118]. Antenatal MRI scans may provide further prognostic information about lung volume, liver herniation, left ventricular mass, and pulmonary diameter, but is not routine [111].

Postnatally, the neonate may present with an exacerbation of their respiratory distress. Symptoms may range from mild to severe, depending on severity of the CDH. The abdomen is scaphoid as the intestine is in the chest, and breath sounds are reduced on the affected side. The diagnosis is confirmed by X-ray of the chest and abdomen, which helps differentiate from other chest pathologies such as CCAM. A nasogastric tube should be placed before imaging as this may lie or curl above the diaphragm if the stomach is in the chest. An echocardiogram should be sought to delineate associated cardiac abnormalities and to estimate the severity of the pulmonary hypertension [119]. Serial cranial ultrasound should be performed to exclude an intracranial bleed.

Outcomes

Despite the advances in the medical and surgical management of this condition, the overall mortality remains at 21–48 %. However, specialist centers with a large number of cases have better survival rates of up to 80 % live births [120]. Mortality in nonsyndromic infants is primarily related to pulmonary hypoplasia and pulmonary hypertension and, as surrogate markers of severity, the need for ECMO/HFOV or for patch repair [121]. Right-sided, bilateral, or large defects, a lung to head ratio of 1.0 or less, and the presence of the liver in the chest portend worse outcomes, as do prematurity, chromosomal anomalies, severe cardiac defects (particularly transposition of the great arteries or single ventricle physiology), and spinal anomalies [122, 123]. In an effort to establish a standardized scoring system, an international consensus concluded that the size of the diaphragmatic defect (as a surrogate for the severity of pulmonary hypoplasia and hypertension) and the severity of the cardiac defect may predict outcome [124]. ECMO required for more than two weeks or associated with renal complications, or persistent pulmonary hypertension for more than 3 weeks are also associated with high mortality [117, 118, 120, 121].

Morbidity associated with CDH in the longer term includes ongoing respiratory problems with recurrent infections and reduced exercise capacity compared with age-matched peers, neurocognitive defects secondary to neonatal hypoxia or intracranial hemorrhage, and visual impairment and deafness, possibly related to intensive care management.

Gastroesophageal reflux is common and may require medical or surgical intervention. Recurrence rates of up to 50 % are reported in CDH especially if an initial patch repair is required. Scoliosis and chest wall deformity may also occur [111].

Prenatal Treatment

Prenatal treatment for CHD has been trialed with varying success. The most promising treatment is fetal endoscopic tracheal occlusion (FETO) with a balloon for babies with poor prognosis based on lung measurements. FETO prevents the egress of lung fluid from the fetal lung and improves lung growth and reduces vascular resistance. The tracheal balloon is either removed before delivery, by ex-utero intrapartum treatment (EXIT), or punctured immediately after delivery by tracheoscopy or percutaneous puncture [125, 126]. Promising results have been reported, but the complication rate is relatively high and may include previously unrecognized conditions such as tracheomegaly or bronchomegaly [127]. Premature delivery contributes to the poor outcomes of FETO [125]. In a randomized controlled trial of FETO, survival in neonates with isolated severe CDH is improved [125, 126, 128].

Medical Management

Medical management of CDH has changed dramatically over the last two decades, from a strategy of early emergency surgery with aggressive hyperventilation to reduce pulmonary hypertension to optimizing the cardiorespiratory status using a "gentle ventilation" strategy to minimize barotrauma that includes minimum peak inspiratory pressures, maintaining spontaneous ventilation and permissive hypercarbia followed by a planned, surgical intervention [129].

Delivery should be planned at or near a center with pediatric surgical and NICU expertise so that the optimal postnatal respiratory support and timely surgical intervention can be provided. The neonate should be allowed to mature to term to permit maximum maturation of the lung. A nasogastric tube should be passed after delivery to decompress the stomach, central and arterial access obtained, and the warming strategies commence with minimal handling. Pulmonary surfactant has not been shown to be beneficial [130].

Since most neonates require some level of ventilatory support after birth, it seems prudent to intubate their tracheas at delivery. The initial ventilation strategy (conventional or high-frequency oscillation) varies among centers in the absence of randomized controlled trials [131]. The aim should be to achieve pre-ductal SpO_2 85–95 %, post-ductal SpO_2 >70 %, arterial pCO_2 45–60 mmHg, and pH > 7.25. If a conventional ventilation strategy is used, the initial settings should include a peak inspiratory pressure (PIP) 20–25 cmH_2O, positive end-expiratory pressure (PEEP) 2–5 cmH_2O, and a frequency 40–60 breaths per minute with minimum required inspired oxygen to maintain the threshold oxygen saturation. Prolonged use of muscle relaxants is ideally avoided, and the neonate should be allowed to breathe spontaneously between assisted breaths. If HFOV is used, the initial settings should include a mean airway pressure 13–17 cmH_2O, frequency 10 Hz, amplitude (ΔP) 30–50 cmH_2O, and I:E ratio 1:1. Hyperinflation of the lungs should be avoided (<8 ribs on unaffected side on chest X-ray).

Echocardiography should be performed to estimate the pulmonary artery pressure, direction of shunting across the arterial duct/foramen ovale, myocardial contractility, the presence of a congenital heart/vascular defect, and the response to treatment. The oxygenation index (OI) should be calculated (OI = mean airway pressure (cmH_2O) × FiO_2 × 100/ PaO_2 (mmHg)). Inhaled nitric oxide (iNO) 10–20 ppm may be indicated if the OI is >20 or the pre-post-ductal oxygen saturation difference is >10 %. The use of iNO is controversial and response should be assessed using echocardiography. Prostacyclin or prostaglandin E1 (PGE1) should be considered if there is no response to iNO. Many units use PGE1 routinely to prevent closure of the arterial duct and to off-load the right ventricle. Sildenafil or milrinone may be indicated if pulmonary hypertension is refractory to treatment or persistent [132], but may cause systemic hypotension [130]. Endothelin receptor antagonists (bosentan) and tyrosine kinase inhibitors (imatinib) are currently under investigation. Fluid boluses may be required if peripheral perfusion is poor or hypotension is present. If cardiovascular instability persists, inotropes may be required to increase the mean arterial pressure to the upper normal range in order to reduce right to left shunting across the arterial duct.

Venoarterial extracorporeal membrane oxygenation (ECMO) may be offered in some centers as temporary stabilization and support in cases of severe cardiorespiratory failure. Specific ECMO criteria vary between centers; current European criteria for ECMO include inability to maintain pre-ductal saturation >85 % or post-ductal saturation >70 %, respiratory or metabolic acidosis with a pH < 7.15, need for aggressive ventilation, or refractory systemic hypotension [133]. The neonate should be >2 kg and >35 weeks gestation, have no lethal congenital abnormalities, have no irreversible organ dysfunction (including neurological injury), and have no contraindication to systemic anticoagulation.

Surgical Considerations

The objectives of surgery in the management of CDH are to reduce the herniated contents safely into the abdomen and repair the defect. Ideally, surgery should be delayed until the neonate is stable, that is, off inotropes (with the possible exception of dopamine) for 24 h. Some have used "stability" criteria to determine the neonate's eligibility for surgery; however these criteria may be more appropriate for determining the timing, rather than eligibility, for surgery [134]. Surgical intervention is possible while the neonate is on ECMO, although early studies suggested that the mortality was increased because of a greater risk of bleeding. Many centers undertake surgery only after weaning the neonate from ECMO, although some have achieved acceptable mortality rates repairing CDH on ECMO by limiting the use of anticoagulants and using antifibrinolytics [135]. For large defects, a patch repair may be required as a dome shape rather than a flat repair. Surgery may be performed by using an open technique (usually laparotomy) or a minimally invasive technique.

Laparotomy via an upper abdominal transverse incision allows good access to the length of the diaphragm and can be extended easily if further access is required. The abdominal contents are reduced into the abdomen and the defect is identified. The spleen may require gentle finger reduction rather than simple traction on the gastric and colonic attachments, to avoid damage and bleeding. A hernial sac, which is present in 10–20 % of cases, is usually excised during surgery. Pulmonary sequestrations may also be found, either supra- or subdiaphragmatic, and these are also excised. The hypoplastic ipsilateral lung may be seen via the defect in the chest. The diaphragmatic rim should be mobilized and, if possible, a primary repair performed without tension using nonabsorbable interrupted sutures. If the diaphragm is deficient laterally, then the sutures should incorporate a large bite of rib or muscle to prevent recurrence. If the defect cannot be closed without tension or is very large, a patch repair is required, although this technique is associated with worse short-term and long-term outcomes. A variety of nonabsorbable materials have been used, including Gore-Tex®, Marlex®, Dacron®, and Silastic®. Nonabsorbable materials have the advantage of cost, reduced bleeding, and easy handling; however they do not grow with the child and may actually shrink over time. These materials are associated with adhesions, increased recurrence, gastroesophageal reflux, and chest wall deformities [135]. Newer biosynthetic patch materials such as collagen lattices with embedded growth factors (Surgisis®, AlloDerm®) are under investigation, although they may increase the risk of postoperative small bowel obstruction. Techniques that involve muscular flaps have been described, but they are time-consuming and may be associated with increased bleeding and abdominal wall deformity. Myogenic patches may be developed in the future [135]. A chest drain is not used routinely as the underwater drain may cause overdistension of the hypoplastic lung. Such a drain may be inserted at a later date if a clinically significant effusion develops. The advantage of the abdominal approach is that a Ladd's procedure can be performed at the same time if the position of the duodenojejunal (D-J) flexure is consistent with malrotation and there is the potential for malrotation.

MIS for CDH has been reported using both laparoscopic and thoracoscopic approaches. The laparoscopic approach enables better instrument handling for the diaphragmatic repair. Reduction of contents against the pneumoperitoneum and the subsequent lack of intra-abdominal space after reduction can be challenging. The thoracoscopic approach is preferred by many and has the advantage that the pneumothorax encourages reduction and there is an excellent view of the diaphragm after reduction. The lateral suture placement can be very difficult due to the rigidity and shape of the thoracic cavity. Initial reports of thoracoscopic repair also suggested an early higher recurrence rate [136]. Right-sided CDH, CDH-associated liver herniation, and the need for patch closure may be better suited for an open procedure. As for thoracoscopic repair, carbon dioxide absorption and acidosis can be problematic during MIS [101]. For this reason, an open surgical approach is probably preferred for neonates with CDH and congenital heart disease, for those who required ECMO, or for those who have continuing systemic right ventricular pressures or require significant inotropic support [137].

It is important to avoid a "flat" diaphragmatic repair during primary or domed patch repair. When the herniated chest contents are reduced into the abdomen, the intra-abdominal pressures may increase to cause abdominal compartment syndrome. If there is evidence of significant venous congestion of lower limbs after closure, then an abdominal wall silo should be left as a laparotomy at the site of the abdominal incision, as for gastroschisis repair. This may be closed a few days later.

Anesthetic Considerations

Management of pulmonary hypertension and pulmonary insufficiency and the timing of surgery are primary considerations in these neonates. Surgical repair should only be performed in physiologically stable neonates, ideally when inotropic support is no longer required and the neonate has been weaned off ECMO, usually at 2–6 days after birth [120]. If the child becomes unstable on transfer to or in theater before surgery begins, then surgery should be postponed. Some units perform surgery in the NICU, but it remains a contentious issue (see Chap. 13) [135].

A balanced anesthesia technique that includes opioids such as high-dose fentanyl 20–50 mcg/kg [10], muscle relaxants, and an inhalational anesthetic should be used to preclude a pulmonary hypertensive crisis. Nitrous oxide should be avoided. The ventilatory strategy should be the same as in NICU; an intravenous technique will be required if the child is receiving HFOV or remains dependent on ECMO. Invasive monitoring should be continued from the NICU, with transcutaneous carbon dioxide monitoring to supplement direct measurement of arterial $PaCO_2$, particularly in MIS.

Surgical repair is usually uneventful and blood loss usually limited (special precautions are required if the child remains on ECMO). Hypotension usually responds to fluid boluses of 10–20 ml/kg balanced salt solution or an increase in the infusion rates of inotropes. Hypotension in the presence of an increasing difference between the pre- and postductal SpO_2 values may indicate an intraoperative pulmonary hypertensive crisis. Simple interventions include increasing FiO_2, increasing depth of anesthesia, opioid administration, and correction of the acidosis that are usually effective. iNO should be available in the event of a pulmonary hypertensive crisis unresponsive to these measures. If oxygenation deteriorates intraoperatively, a pneumothorax on the contralateral (good lung) side and an endobronchial intubation must be excluded. At the conclusion of surgery, the neonate should be transferred back to the NICU; the duration of postoperative ventilation is determined by the severity of pulmonary hypoplasia and pulmonary hypertension.

Abdominal Surgery

Inguinal Hernia

Inguinal hernias occur commonly with a childhood incidence of 0.8–4.4 %. Males are affected 8–10 times more than females. Premature infants have an increased risk of hernias with an incidence of 13 % in neonates born at <32 weeks gestational age (GA) and 30 % in infants <1 kg birth weight [138]. This group also has an increased risk of complications such as obstruction and incarceration. Inguinal hernia is also associated with cystic fibrosis, connective tissue disorders, and abdominal wall defects.

Pathophysiology

Inguinal hernias result from the failure of obliteration of the patent processus vaginalis (PPV), which develops during testicular descent. Up to 50–80 % of neonates may have a PPV and remain asymptomatic until bowel or other intra-abdominal contents enter this sac. When that occurs, it is classified as an inguinal hernia. The right side is more frequently affected (60 %) than the left, with 10–15 % of cases occurring bilaterally (with a greater incidence in infants).

Diagnosis

An inguinal hernia is diagnosed clinically with the history or presence of a groin swelling (Fig. 10.8). This may extend into the scrotum on the ipsilateral side. The testis should also be palpated during examination, separate to the groin swelling. The hernia may contain bowel, omentum, or the ovary in females. Examination should ensure that the hernia is reducible; if the hernia is irreducible (i.e., incarcerated), then the hernia immediately becomes a surgical emergency. The majority (60 %) of incarcerated inguinal hernias occur in the first 6 months of life.

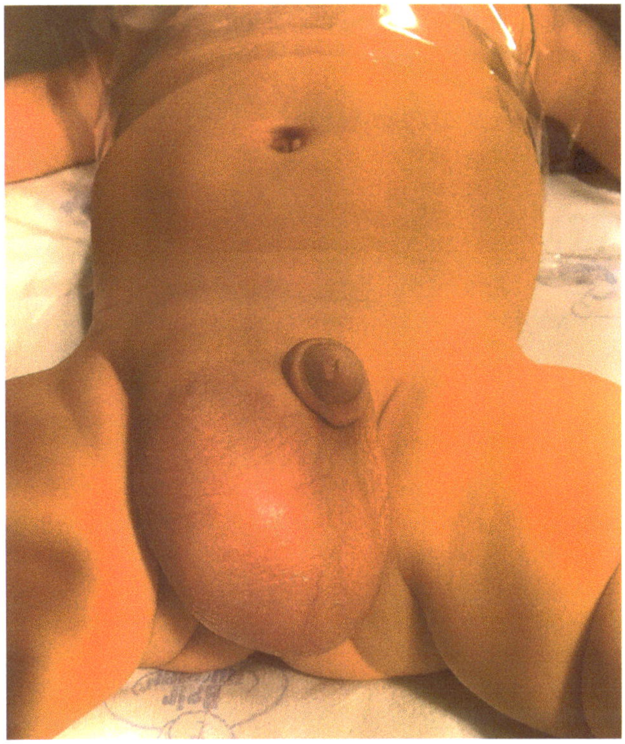

Fig. 10.8 Inguinal hernia in a neonate. Close-up of a right inguinal hernia (Courtesy of Dr. YH Lee, Division of Pediatric Surgery, Strong Hospital, University of Rochester, Rochester, NY)

Surgical Management

Inguinal hernias require surgical closure of the PPV. In many centers, hernia repair is performed as an open procedure via an inguinal incision with ligation of the sac after separating it from the vas and testicular vessels. Care must be taken to fully mobilize and ligate the sac to prevent recurrence, while preserving the vas and vessels with minimal surgical trauma. The duration of anesthesia and surgery for inguinal hernia repair in neonates is greater than in older children. The risks of recurrence or testicular atrophy are greater in neonates, particularly if the hernia has become incarcerated.

Laparoscopic repair may also be performed with closure of the internal ring with a nonabsorbable suture. This technique allows assessment of the contralateral side and bilateral repair if indicated, which may be particularly beneficial in infants as there is a 60 % incidence of bilateral hernia or contralateral PPV in infants. There is less dissection of the cord structures, which may result in less damage; laparoscopic hernia repair in infants is a safe procedure with a small complication rate, although long-term outcomes are not yet available [139]. The laparoscopic approach is feasible even in very small neonates, although the ability to tolerate carbon dioxide insufflation is an important factor, and the procedure may be more challenging technically in the very premature or low-birth-weight neonates. Instead of carbon dioxide insufflation, some advocate gasless laparoscopy in neonates thereby obviating the cardiorespiratory effects of a carboperitoneum [140].

Anesthetic Management

The timing of surgery in neonates who require hernia repair remains controversial, particularly in premature neonates; the younger the neonate, the more susceptible they are to postoperative apneas as well as surgical complications. This has to be balanced with the risk of incarceration if surgery is delayed. Many centers plan surgery for premature infants near the time of discharge from the hospital, and others delay surgery until after discharge to reduce the potential for postoperative apnea and the need for prolonged postoperative ventilation [141].

An analysis of data from prospective studies of former preterm infants undergoing hernia repair under general anesthesia in the mid-1980s and late 1990s suggested that the probability of postoperative apnea in premature infants was <1 % at PCA 56 weeks, with negligible risk of postoperative apnea at 60 weeks PCA. The risk factors for postoperative apnea were gestational age at birth, postconceptional age, ongoing preoperative apneas, and anemia (hematocrit<30 %) [142]. Factors that may reduce the frequency of apneas in premature infants after general anesthesia include regional block (spinal anesthesia) without sedation, an ilioinguinal/iliohypogastric nerve block, administration of intravenous caffeine 10mg/kg, and the avoidance of neuromuscular blockade or potent opioids [143, 144]. Respiratory events after sevoflurane and desflurane anesthesia occur with similar frequencies in premature neonates [145]. Current practice guidelines recommend postoperative apnoea monitoring for neonates/infants who are full term but less than 44 weeks PCA and infants who were premature at birth (e.g., ≤37 weeks gestation) and who are less than 60 weeks PCA, although it has been suggested that this guidance could be relaxed to 46 weeks for former preterm infants without other risk factors for postoperative apnea [146].

Spinal or caudal epidural anesthesia as a sole technique may be associated with fewer postoperative respiratory complications than general anesthesia but has a significant failure rate [146, 147]. The GAS study (general anesthesia versus spinal anesthesia for infants undergoing hernia repair) may yield further evidence to support the choice of anesthesia for hernia repair in this vulnerable group of infants [148].

Pyloric Stenosis

Pyloric stenosis occurs in 1–3:1,000 births and is four to five times more common in males than females and more commonly in firstborn males. The etiology of pyloric stenosis has been elusive, although there is some evidence for a genetic basis for the disease, feeding practices, erythromycin exposure postnatally (or prenatally), sleeping position (prone increases the risk), and possibly infectious moieties [149–152]. The age at which pyloric stenosis presents has been gradually decreasing. Currently, most cases present at 2–5 postnatal weeks, after several days of projectile vomiting [153–155]. Pathological hypertrophy of the inner layer of smooth muscle in the pylorus results in gastric outlet obstruction, which leads to the projectile nature of the vomiting.

Pyloric stenosis is usually an isolated defect. However, in many cases, it is associated with genetic syndromes including Cornelia de Lange and Smith–Lemli–Opitz syndromes as well as chromosome 8 and 17 translocations and (partial) trisomy 9 [150].

Diagnosis of Pyloric Stenosis

The classic symptom of pyloric stenosis is non-bilious projectile vomiting. Term infants are predominantly affected, although pyloric stenosis does occur in premature infants. The diagnosis may be confirmed by clinical examination with visible gastric peristalsis and a palpable pyloric "tumor." These signs may be more clearly demonstrated with a "test feed." The classical biochemical picture is one of dehydration with hypochloremic metabolic alkalosis due to loss of gastric acid. Total body potassium may be depleted due to the renal compensation and tubular reabsorption of hydrogen and sodium ions and water in exchange for potassium. However, mounting evidence suggests that neonates with pyloric stenosis present earlier in their disease process, resulting in less severe electrolyte imbalance in the past decade [155, 156]. As a result of the less severe electrolyte imbalance and the increasing reliability of ultrasound to delineate both the thickness and length of the pylori (with a sensitivity of 100 % and specificity of 98 %), ultrasound has supplanted the electrolyte panel as the cardinal criterion for diagnosis of pyloric stenosis [153–155, 157].

Medical Management

This disorder is a medical, not surgical, emergency. Initial management consists of rehydration and correction of any electrolyte imbalance. Depending on the severity of the fluid and electrolyte derangements, 24–48 h preparation may be required, although affected neonates are reaching pediatric surgeons earlier in the disease process currently, reducing the time required to correct electrolyte disturbances [155, 156]. Surgical intervention should not be undertaken until the neonates have been stable medically and the plasma bicarbonate is <28 mmol/l and plasma chloride >100 mmol/l. Infants with severe dehydration may require an initial fluid bolus of 20 ml/kg 0.9 % saline, followed by maintenance fluid with 5–10 % dextrose and 0.45 % saline, provided the plasma sodium is in the normal range. The stomach should be decompressed with a nasogastric tube, and gastric losses replaced ml for ml

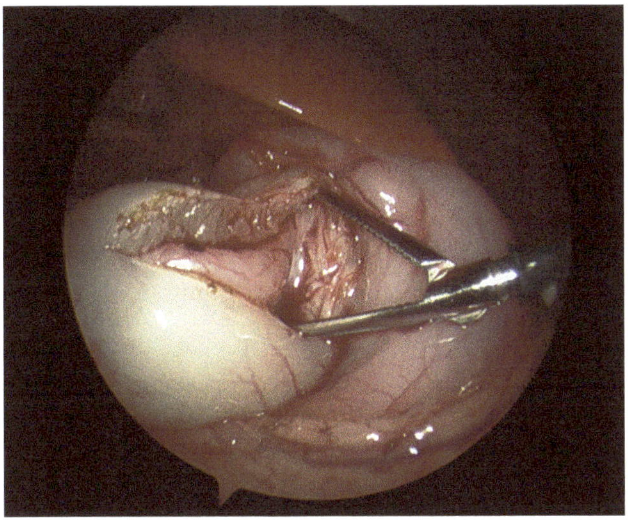

Fig. 10.9 Pyloromyotomy. The thickened muscle layer of the pylorus can be seen, incised down to the mucosa. To ensure the muscle has been completely incised, laparoscopic alligators distract the walls of the muscle layer. Note the very thick muscular wall that has been peeled off the pylorus. The liver edge is present immediately above the pylorus at the top of the figure (Courtesy of Dr. K. Bass, Division of Pediatric Surgery, Women and Children's Hospital of Buffalo, Buffalo, NY)

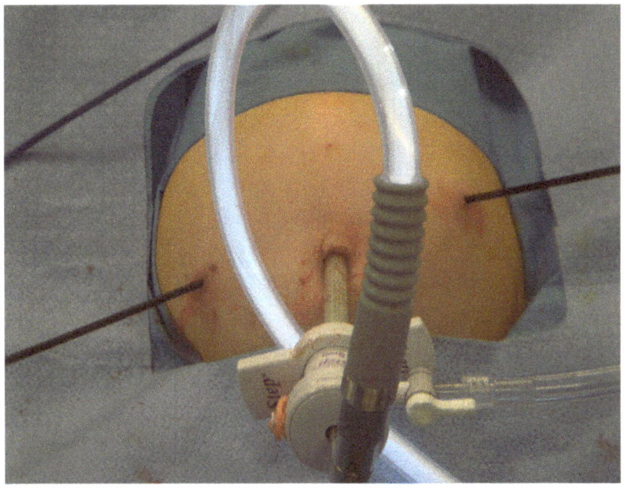

Fig. 10.10 Laparoscopic insufflation of the abdomen. The neonate's head is at the top of the figure and the legs are at the bottom. During laparoscopic pyloromyotomy, three ports are placed: the largest trocar (5 mm Mini Step) is inserted through the umbilicus, whereas the two smaller graspers are passed laterally through simple skin incisions. The peritoneal cavity is insufflated with carbon dioxide to ~8 mmHg pressure

with intravenous 0.9 % saline and 10 mmol KCL per 500 ml. Potassium should be added to maintenance fluids only after the child begins to pass urine [153].

Surgical Management

The traditional operation for pyloric stenosis is Ramstedt's pyloromyotomy, an extramucosal longitudinal splitting of the hypertrophied muscle (Fig. 10.9). This was originally described using an upper midline incision but many centers now use a supraumbilical approach to provide better cosmesis. Laparoscopic pyloromyotomy is also widely performed, and a recent randomized controlled study and meta-analysis have demonstrated some benefits from this approach (reduced time to full feed and length of stay), without an increase in postoperative complications although the debate continues regarding the superiority of the laparoscopic over the open approach for pyloric stenosis [158] (Fig. 10.10) [30]. Whether laparoscopic approach includes multiple incisions, a single incision, or a microlaparoscopic (<2 mm diameter instruments) approach [159], it would appear to be the evolving standard for pyloromyotomy.

Anesthetic Considerations

Surgery should only be scheduled after the fluid status and electrolyte concentrations (including pH) have been normalized; otherwise, the child will be at increased risk of postoperative apnea, arrhythmias, and circulatory instability. A nasogastric tube will be in situ before induction of anesthesia. After administering atropine 0.02 mg/kg IV, the nasogastric tube is replaced with a large red rubber catheter in some centers to suction the gastric contents in the supine and decubitus positions, before induction of anesthesia. When complete, the red rubber catheter is removed. The traditional induction technique for pyloromyotomy is a modified RSI, in which cricoid pressure is avoided after consciousness is lost, but gentle mask ventilation continues with 100 % oxygen until laryngoscopy begins. Surveys of experienced pediatric anesthesiologists reveal that fewer than 50 % apply cricoid pressure to infants with pyloric stenosis [160, 161]. In fact, cricoid pressure is difficult to apply correctly in young infants and may distort the airway, complicating laryngoscopy and tracheal intubation [16, 162, 163]. The modified RSI as described is commonly practiced in neonates and young infants with full stomachs to prevent desaturation during the interval between loss of consciousness and securing the airway.

The anesthetic regimen for pyloric stenosis in the neonate presents two offsetting conditions: to facilitate rapid tracheal intubation and recovery from anesthesia in ~30 min, the duration of surgery. IV induction of anesthesia is usually accomplished with IV propofol using a dose that depends on adjunctive medications. If succinylcholine (2 mg/kg) (preceded by atropine) is included in the regimen, then a dose of 2 mg/kg propofol may be used. Following the black box warning by the Food and Drug Administration, many clinicians in the US avoid succinylcholine in young males, so use either a non-depolarising muscle relaxant or other medications to facilitate intubation of the airway. If a nondepolarizing relaxant is used (most commonly rocuronium), then a small dose should be used to preclude difficulty antagonizing its effects after the brief surgery [164, 165]. Suggamadex may be effective for terminating the action of the relaxant, but it is expensive and not available in every country.

Faced with a male with pyloric stenosis, a fast surgeon, and reluctance to use a nondepolarizing muscle relaxant, several other regimens may be used. Some administer a short-acting IV opioid such as fentanyl 1–2 μg/kg or remifentanil followed by a large dose of propofol (3–5 mg/kg) to induce anesthesia and secure the airway. Alternately, others administer sevoflurane in oxygen while preoxygenating the neonate [166], judiciously timing a bolus of IV propofol (2–4 mg/kg) ± a short-acting opioid, to provide optimal intubating conditions.

In preparation for tracheal intubation, a hockey-stick curve to the tracheal tube (a 3.5 uncuffed or 3.0 Microcuff® tube) molded with a stylet to maintain its shape ensures a rapid and successful tracheal intubation, particularly in the absence of a muscle relaxant. Once the airway is secured, a gastric tube may be reinserted with a stopcock attached to permit inflation of the pylori with 20 ml boluses of air to test the integrity of the underlying mucosa.

Delayed emergence after pyloric stenosis is a common and perplexing problem. This has been attributed to several causes including the use of intraoperative opioids. Infiltration of the wounds with local anesthetic is usually sufficient to control the pain after pyloromyotomy, obviating the need for any opioid intraoperatively, although some prefer a short-acting opioid such as fentanyl or remifentanil [167]. Others advocate a regional block such as a rectus sheath block or epidural, depending on the surgical approach [168, 169]. IV or rectal acetaminophen may also provide mild pain relief intraoperatively and postoperatively, without slowing emergence [28]. However, despite avoiding opioids entirely, many continue to experience a very slow to emerge from anesthesia after this surgery. Some have attributed the slow emergence from anesthesia to the use of nondepolarizing muscle relaxants, although one retrospective study disputed this claim, noting that 0.7 mg/kg rocuronium minimally delayed the time to transport to recovery compared with succinylcholine, after a propofol/sevoflurane anesthetic [164, 165, 170]. Insufflating the abdomen in neonates and infants does not mandate the need for a nondepolarizing muscle relaxant. If relaxants were not used for tracheal intubation and are not part of the anesthetic regimen for surgery, then insufflation requires a deep level of anesthesia and controlled ventilation. This usually involves large concentrations of inhalational anesthetics, which could delay emergence unless the least soluble anesthetics, desflurane and nitrous oxide, were used for maintenance. At least one MAC of desflurane is required during insufflation, which corresponds to an end-tidal desflurane concentration of 9.6 % in this age group [171]. To reduce the concentration of inhalational anesthetic required, remifentanil may be added [167]. Antiemetics are not indicated in neonates as the incidence of postoperative vomiting in this age group is very small and surgeons may use ongoing vomiting as a sign of an incomplete repair or complication [172]. As soon as the surgeon desufflates the peritoneum, the inspired concentration of desflurane is reduced to 3 %. When the skin incisions are closed and dressed, all anesthetics are discontinued.

Intestinal Atresias

Congenital intestinal atresia or stenosis can occur at any point along the gastrointestinal tract. The neonate presents with intestinal obstruction, the timing and specific presenting features relating to the level of the obstruction [173, 174, 265].

Pyloric Atresia

Pyloric atresia is an extremely rare condition (1:100,000 live births) representing 1 % of intestinal atresias. Up to 30 % of patients have other associated anomalies including epidermolysis bullosa, aplasia cutis congenita, and esophageal atresia. Presentation is with non-bilious vomiting with a single gastric bubble on abdominal X-ray and no distal gas. Surgery involves a laparotomy to either excise the obstructing membrane or perform a bypass procedure (gastroduodenostomy or gastrojejunostomy) to restore intestinal continuity. The practical considerations are similar to those for duodenal atresia.

Duodenal Atresia

Duodenal atresia or stenosis occurs in 1:5,000–1:10,000 live births with a male preponderance. Half of the patients have associated anomalies, commonly trisomy 21 (30–40 %), malrotation (30–40 %), and cardiac anomalies (20 %). Anorectal and genitourinary anomalies, esophageal atresia, and Meckel's diverticulum are also associated with duodenal atresia and, more rarely, biliary anomalies. Up to 45 % of babies are born prematurely [173]. Duodenal atresia may be classified as follows (Table 10.3).

Embryology

Duodenal atresia may be due to abnormal embryological development of the duodenum, pancreas, and biliary tree.

Table 10.3 Classification of duodenal atresia

Type I—mucosal diaphragmatic membrane
Type II—short fibrous cord connecting two ends of the atretic duodenum
Type III—complete separation of the two ends of the duodenum

Proposed mechanisms include failure of recanalization of the duodenum during the 8–10th week and altered rotation of the ventral analogue of the pancreas resulting in an annular pancreas. The obstruction is distal to the ampulla in the majority of patients (60–85 %). An alternative theory common to all atresias is the possibility of a vascular accident (see jejunoileal atresia below).

Diagnosis

Polyhydramnios occurs in 33–60 % of pregnancies and antenatal ultrasound may demonstrate a "double bubble." Cardiac abnormalities may also be detected at this time. Postnatally the baby develops bilious vomiting in the majority, although vomiting may be non-bilious if the atresia is proximal to the ampulla. Abdominal X-ray shows the characteristic double bubble with an absence of gas distally. Distal gas may occasionally be seen if the atresia is periampullary with the main pancreatic and accessory duct opening on either side. Gas can then travel via the biliary tree into the distal intestine. The antenatal and abdominal X-ray findings are less clear in duodenal stenosis, which may present later depending on the degree of obstruction. The differential diagnosis of duodenal atresia is malrotation and volvulus, which can have catastrophic consequences if not detected. If there is any doubt about the diagnosis, for instance, if there is distal gas or no antenatal history, an urgent upper gastrointestinal contrast study should be performed to exclude malrotation. If doubt still remains, then an urgent laparotomy should be performed.

Management

Ultimate management is surgical; however the patient should be resuscitated and stabilized as required. A nasogastric tube should be passed with replacement of losses and maintenance fluids given intravenously. Preoperative workup includes a thorough clinical examination and echocardiography to exclude associated anomalies.

Outcomes

There is low reported mortality and morbidity associated with duodenal atresia. Early operative mortality is less than 5 %, predominantly due to complex cardiac anomalies, and long-term survival is 90 %. Morbidity associated with this condition includes gastroesophageal reflux disease, delayed gastric emptying, peptic ulcer disease, duodenal stasis and blind loop syndrome or megaduodenum, and adhesive small bowel obstruction. These complications may not be apparent until much later in life.

Surgical Considerations

A laparotomy and duodenostomy (either end-to-side or Kimura diamond anastomosis) are the primary procedures performed. Access is via a supraumbilical transverse or umbilical (Bianchi) incision. The minimally invasive laparoscopic approach is feasible and safe and is being introduced in some centers, although liver retraction and exposure of the duodenum can be difficult especially in a small infant or in the presence of hepatomegaly. It is important to check that a second duodenal web is not present (seen in 1–3 % of cases), and there are no distal atresias. Intestinal rotation should be checked and malrotation corrected if present. The gall bladder should be visualized for bile. Some surgeons choose to leave a transanastomotic tube in situ although full enteral feeds are usually achieved without this maneuver.

Anesthetic Considerations

Anesthetic considerations relate mainly to anesthesia for laparotomy in the presence of upper gastrointestinal obstruction and coexisting abnormalities, especially complex cardiac anomalies, and prematurity. If the child is otherwise well, the aim should be to extubate at the end of the procedure.

Jejunal/Ileal Atresia

Small bowel atresia or stenosis is a common cause of neonatal intestinal obstruction occurring in 1:3,000 live births [80]. A stenosis is due to a localized narrowing of the lumen without loss of continuity in the intestine or mesentery (Fig. 10.11). Small bowel atresias are classified into four major types [175, 176] (Table 10.4).

Types II and IIIa occur most commonly. There may be a family history especially in type IIIb atresia. Multiple atresias are not uncommon, with up to 67 % of jejunal atresias and 25 % of ileal atresias having further distal atresias. Chromosomal abnormalities are much less common in the

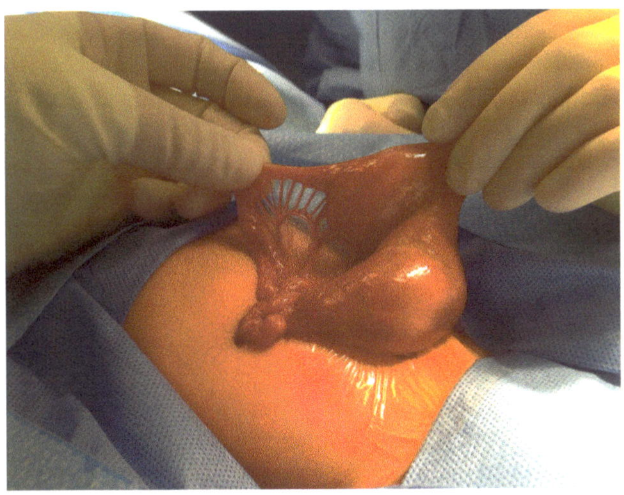

Fig. 10.11 Jejunal atresia. At laparotomy, normal jejunum is held up on the right side of the photo. The jejunal lumen narrows at the atresia in the middle of the photograph, with a very small lumen thereafter. The mesentery, which supplies blood to the bowel, is intact (Courtesy of Dr. YH Lee, Division of Pediatric Surgery, Strong Hospital, University of Rochester, Rochester, NY)

Table 10.4 Classification of small bowel atresias [175]

Type I—a membrane or web
Type II—blind ends separated by a fibrous cord
Type IIIa—disconnected blind ends
Type IIIb—absence of the superior mesenteric artery resulting in the "apple peel," "Xmas tree," or "Maypole" abnormality
Type IV—multiple segment atresia ("string of sausages")

more distal atresias compared to duodenal atresia although 12 % of patients with ileal atresia will also have cystic fibrosis. These patients should have genetic screening and a sweat test performed at an appropriate time postoperatively. There is an association between gastroschisis and small bowel atresias.

Embryology

The most popular theory is that the atresia is a result of an intrauterine "vascular accident." Interruption of the blood supply results in sterile necrosis and resorption of affected segments. Multiple causes of vascular interruption have been proposed including fetal intussusceptions, midgut volvulus, thromboembolic occlusions, transmesenteric internal hernias, and incarceration as the result of an abdominal wall defect. The use of methylene blue in amniocentesis for twin pregnancies has also been implicated. The insult is felt to occur late (after week 11), and this is supported by the findings of bile, lanugo hair, and squamous epithelial cells from swallowed amniotic fluid distal to the atresia.

Diagnosis

Polyhydramnios may be present prenatally although less common the more distal the obstruction. Dilated bowel lops may be seen on antenatal scans. Presentation after birth is with signs of intestinal obstruction including vomiting (usually bilious), abdominal distension, and failure to pass meconium. Respiratory compromise may occur if the distension is severe, and the baby may require preoperative respiratory support (and hence postoperative support). A plain abdominal X-ray will show dilated bowel loops (number depending on the level of the obstruction). A contrast enema may be performed preoperatively to exclude the differential diagnoses of meconium ileus, Hirschsprung's disease, and coexisting more distal atresias. Ten percent of neonates present with meconium peritonitis due to antenatal perforation; calcification or meconium pseudocyst may be seen on abdominal X-ray.

Outcomes

The long-term survival for patients with jejunoileal atresia is 84 %. The primary cause of morbidity and mortality is short bowel syndrome or intestinal failure requiring total parenteral nutrition, with associated risk of sepsis and liver disease.

Medical Management

As with all neonatal intestinal obstruction, the initial goal is to stabilize the neonate with nasogastric decompression, nil by mouth, intravenous resuscitation, and maintenance fluids. Investigations should be performed as above.

Surgical Considerations

The most common surgical procedure to localize the atresia is a laparotomy. Once it has been identified, the atresia is excised with a primary anastomosis. There may be significant discrepancy in size between the proximal and distal ends of the atresia, making an end-to-end primary anastomosis challenging. Despite this, a 7:1 discrepancy can be accommodated with meticulous technique and 7-0 suture material. If bowel length is not a problem, then the dilated bowel can be resected back to a more reasonable caliber. If a type IIIb "apple peel" atresia is discovered, particular care must be taken to avoid compromising the retrograde vascular supply from the marginal colic arteries to the remaining distal small bowel. Problems with absorption of feed and short bowel syndrome are also more common with this type of atresia. This has been attributed to the severity of the vascular insult. Given the high risk of multiple atresias, the continuity of the distal bowel should be confirmed by passing a small balloon catheter through the lumen and flushing with either air or saline before the anastomosis is performed. If the neonate is unstable or the distal bowel is significantly compromised, then a proximal stoma and mucous fistula are preferred as a temporizing measure, with restoration of bowel continuity restored when the neonate has fully recovered. The remaining length of small bowel should be measured and documented to help predict and manage neonates with possible short bowel syndrome.

Anesthetic Considerations

These are the same as for any neonate undergoing laparotomy. However, postoperative ventilation may be required after prolonged laparotomy and a significant fluid shift. Long term vascular access may be required for parenteral nutrition.

Colonic Atresia

This is a very rare cause of intestinal obstruction and represents <10 % of all intestinal atresias. A vascular insult is the likely cause of these atresias. These occur when closing abdominal wall defects especially gastroschises secondary to localized vascular interruption. Applying the Grosfeld classification, most are type IIIa or type I. Associated proximal atresias are common (22 %), and right-sided atresias are associated with Hirschsprung's disease.

Diagnosis

Colonic atresia presents with symptoms of distal obstruction, including abdominal distension, failure to pass meconium, and bilious vomiting. Multiple loops of distended bowel on plain abdominal X-ray confirm the presence of distal bowel obstruction. A hugely distended loop of bowel is often present because of the closed loop obstruction in the presence of a competent ileocecal valve. Contrast enema confirms the location of the most distal atresia.

Management

Preoperative management is the same as for all neonates with intestinal obstruction. This has been discussed above. Early surgical intervention is essential, as the mortality from perforation may reach 100 % if surgery is delayed for more than 4 days.

Surgical Considerations

Surgical options are laparotomy with either formation of decompressing colostomy or primary anastomosis. Although a high incidence of anastomotic leakage and sepsis has been reported previously in neonates undergoing primary anastomosis, more recent reports support this approach. Hirschsprung's disease should be considered if an anastomotic leak is detected. A stoma is preferred to direct anastomosis, if resection to bowel with a more appropriate caliber results in short bowel syndrome. As per jejunal/ileal atresias, the proximal bowel must be assessed intraoperatively by flushing with air or fluid to identify additional atresias.

Meconium Ileus

Meconium ileus results from the obstruction of the distal small bowel due to thick inspissated meconium. The majority (90 %) are due to intestinal and pancreatic dysfunction secondary to cystic fibrosis (CF). Up to 25 % of neonates with underlying cystic fibrosis will present with meconium ileus. Once the obstruction has been successfully treated, the infant must be tested for CF. The presence of meconium ileus does not predict a worse, long-term outcome from CF, although almost all children with meconium ileus develop pancreatic insufficiency and will require pancreatic enzyme replacement when feeds are introduced [177]. It is important to involve the respiratory physicians early, even though clinical lung disease is very uncommon in neonates.

Diagnosis

Simple meconium ileus presents with distal intestinal obstruction. Plain abdominal X-ray shows multiple loops of dilated bowel with a "soap bubble" appearance in the right lower quadrant (Neuhauser's sign). This results from the mixing of air and the tenacious meconium. A contrast enema will show a microcolon with pellets of meconium in the terminal ileum.

Complications occur in 50 % of cases. Perforation may occur in the antenatal period if the proximal bowel becomes ischemic or perforates secondary to a volvulus. This will lead to meconium peritonitis and possibly a giant pseudocyst. The neonate may present with a large abdominal mass or meconium may be passed vaginally or be evident in a patent processus vaginalis in the scrotum. Calcification is often evident on a flat plate (X-ray) of the abdomen. Intestinal volvulus or atresias may also occur.

Outcomes

Outcomes are slightly more favorable in simple meconium ileus with a 1-year survival of 92 % compared with 89 % in complicated meconium ileus [177].

Management

The usual resuscitative measures should be performed in conjunction with broad-spectrum intravenous antibiotics, and the neonate should remain nil by mouth. If the diagnosis is consistent with simple meconium ileus, the obstruction may be relieved by nonoperative measures using a hyperosmolar contrast enema (Gastrografin® or Omnipaque®), which may be repeated. Operative intervention is indicated for enema failures and complicated meconium ileus.

Surgical Considerations

Surgical options include manual disimpaction at laparotomy either via a proximal enterotomy or with the intraluminal injection of 4 % *N*-acetylcysteine. A combination of these two may be required to fully clear the impacted plugs. If this is not possible, a distal loop or double-barreled stoma should be performed, although this is rarely required. Primary laparotomy is performed in complicated meconium ileus; the options are resection and anastomosis or, alternatively, stoma formation. It is essential to ensure that the obstruction into the microcolon is relieved completely if a stoma is not performed. Additional *N*-acetylcysteine via a nasogastric tube is sometimes advocated. The stoma should be closed as soon as possible to avoid excessive sodium losses from the gastrointestinal tract and from sweat.

Anesthetic Considerations

Management is the same as for any neonatal laparotomy including fluid resuscitation and respiratory support according to clinical requirements. Hypertonic enemas increase the risk of hypovolemic shock in neonates as fluid becomes sequestered in the gut. Fluid may need to be replaced throughout the intra- and postoperative periods to replace the preoperative and intraoperative fluid losses. A sweat test should be performed early in the postoperative period to establish the diagnosis of cystic fibrosis. Fortunately, respiratory complications are uncommon in the neonatal period.

Malrotation and Volvulus

Malrotation is a congenital anomaly of the bowel in which an abnormal position and fixation of the midgut shortens the mesenteric base, predisposing to a volvulus [178]. The incidence

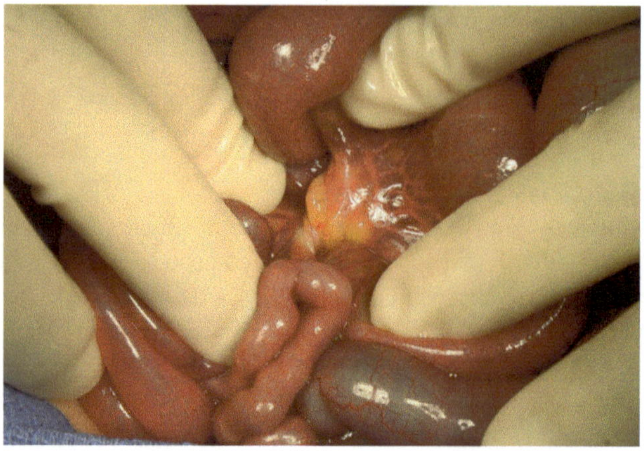

Fig. 10.12 Midgut volvulus. At the ends of the gloved fingers (center of the photo), a tightly twisted midgut (covered in yellow fat) volvulus is evident (Courtesy of Dr. YH Lee, Division of Pediatric Surgery, Strong Hospital, University of Rochester, Rochester, NY)

is 1:500–1:1,000 based on postmortem studies. The incidence based on symptomatic presentation is 1:6,000 live births or may be discovered incidentally. Other anomalies associated with malrotation include intestinal atresias, such as duodenal web, abdominal wall defects, congenital diaphragmatic hernia, imperforate anus, cardiac abnormalities, Meckel's diverticulum, and trisomy 21. Males are twice as likely to present in the neonatal period as females. Malrotation with midgut volvulus constitutes a true surgical emergency as the consequences are potentially catastrophic with loss of the entire small intestine (Fig. 10.12).

Embryology

The traditional theory of intestinal development has the small bowel undergoing a counterclockwise 270° rotation during the 6th–10th week of gestation as it returns to the abdomen from the physiological hernia. During weeks 10–12, the bowel undergoes fixation. Failure of these processes is termed "malrotation." This anomaly results in a shortened mesenteric base with the D-J flexure in an abnormal right-sided and low position, with a high position of the cecum, and a tendency of the small bowel to twist around the mesenteric base (volvulus). This causes obstruction of the blood supply and lymphatic drainage to the small bowel (as well as luminal bowel obstruction), which can lead to ischemia to ischemia with necrosis of the entire midgut. It is imperative that malrotation with volvulus is identified in a timely manner and corrected before necrosis of the bowel occurs.

Diagnosis

The majority of neonates with malrotation present in the first month of life (50–75 % of cases). The most common presenting symptom is bilious vomiting, although some may have non-bilious vomiting. Other signs including abdominal tenderness or distension, diarrhea or constipation, and lethargy present less commonly. Systemic compromise and blood in the stools are later signs of volvulus in which significant ischemia has already occurred. Abdominal X-ray may be deceptively normal. The gold standard for diagnosis is an upper GI contrast study, which demonstrates duodenal obstruction when volvulus has occurred. The appearance is that of a "bird's beak," coiled, or "corkscrew." The normal position of the D-J flexure is to the left of the midline, at or above the level of the pylorus. For uncomplicated malrotation in the absence of a volvulus, the contrast study demonstrates the abnormal position of the D-J flexure to the right of the midline. The position of the cecum is variable, rendering it an unreliable sign of a malrotation. CT or ultrasound may demonstrate reversal of the normal position of the superior mesenteric artery (SMA) relative to the superior mesenteric vein (SMV), with spiraling of these vessels if volvulus has occurred. Ultrasound can be used to track the course of the duodenum and D-J flexure. Urgent laparoscopy or laparotomy is required if the diagnosis remains in doubt [179].

Outcomes

Malrotation with volvulus may lead to ischemic necrosis of the entire midgut. Accordingly, it is essential that a pediatric surgeon assess all neonates with bilious vomiting in a timely manner to prevent ischemia of the bowel. The mortality rate is ≤10 %. Short bowel syndrome (see Gastroschisis for further discussion) occurs in 18 % of neonates with volvulus. Complications of surgery include adhesive bowel obstruction in up to 20 % and recurrent volvulus in 6 % of neonates. Those with a malrotation may develop intestinal dysmotility at a later date.

Management

A high level of clinical suspicion must be present when a neonate presents with bilious vomiting. The outcome after volvulus is time dependent so early diagnosis and intervention are critical. Initial resuscitation should be undertaken before an urgent upper GI contrast study. Immediate surgical intervention is indicated if a malrotation with volvulus is diagnosed. For those in whom a malrotation without volvulus is confirmed or suspected, the optimal management is controversial. Knowing there is a substantive risk for future volvulus, many surgeons advocate a semi-urgent surgical procedure to assess the mesenteric base and proceed to correction, if appropriate.

Surgical Considerations

The classic surgical approach is Ladd's procedure with derotation of the volvulus. In this procedure, the duodenum is mobilized, the mesenteric base is widened, and the D-J flexure and the small bowel are mobilized to the right of the abdomen and the cecum and large bowel to the left. If obstructing peritoneal bands (Ladd's bands) are identified, they are divided. Many surgeons also perform an appendicectomy as the cecum is abnormally located in the left upper quadrant. Ladd's procedure has been classically performed via laparotomy or more recently by laparoscopy, the latter providing a potentially less invasive means to assess the stability of the mesentery. If technical factors preclude the latter approach, then early conversion to an open technique must occur. The role of laparoscopy for correction of a volvulus in a neonate remains controversial: some do not endorse this approach, whereas others suggest it as not appropriate in an unstable neonate in whom necrotic bowel is likely [179, 180]. The long-term outcomes for the laparoscopic approach remain unclear. Despite a reduced risk of future adhesive bowel obstruction, the risk of recurrent volvulus remains uncertain.

Derotation of the bowel is often sufficient to restore the blood supply to the midgut and the viability of the bowel. However, if the diagnosis is delayed, the bowel may remain ischemic after derotation, possibly the result of vascular thrombosis in the mesenteric vessels. The surgical options to address the ischemic/necrotic bowel include excision of the necrotic segment, with or without anastomosis, or conservative management with a "second look" laparotomy after 36–48 h to determine whether perfusion of the ischemic bowel has improved. A technique that involves massage of the mesenteric vessels after derotation (to break up clot), and systemic thrombolysis using tissue recombinant tissue-type plasminogen activator (tPA), has recently been described in two neonates with severe intestinal ischemia due to thrombosis. This resulted in dramatic restoration of bowel perfusion, with subsequent complete recovery of bowel function [181]. If the small bowel is completely necrotic, then withdrawal of care should be explored with the parents.

Anesthetic Considerations

These cases are critical surgical emergencies that must be given priority over all other cases. Surgery must not be delayed. Preoperatively, the status of the neonate may range from relatively healthy to hypovolemic and/or septic shock. In the latter condition, preoperative resuscitation should occur concurrently with preparation and transfer of the neonate to the operating theater. Group "O"-negative blood should be available if necessary. A nasogastric tube should be passed to decompress the abdomen, and ventilatory support provided as required. If the neonate is in shock or extremis, then anesthesia should be induced using IV ketamine, fentanyl, and/or remifentanil and the airway secured after either rocuronium or atropine/succinylcholine [11]. Coagulopathy is common in the presence of necrotic bowel requiring platelets and fresh frozen plasma. Inotropic support with dopamine and/or adrenaline may be required. Invasive monitoring is very useful during this initial resuscitation phase.

If the neonate is stable, maintenance of anesthesia can include fentanyl or remifentanil or a low dose of inhalational anesthesia. Deep inhalational anesthesia must be avoided in critically ill neonates. The surgeon should inform the anesthesiologist when the volvulus is about to be reduced because derotation may lead to acute cardiovascular instability due to release of lactic acid and other vasoactive compounds. The anesthesiologist should be prepared to manage transient acidosis and hyperkalemia with IV calcium chloride (10–30 mg/kg), bicarbonate, and occasionally salbutamol.

Reperfusion of the bowel is the primary goal. Adequate fluid resuscitation with warmed boluses of lactated Ringer's solution, albumin, or packed red cells is required based on clinical assessment and monitoring. Fluid requirement may be substantial at this juncture; volumes as great as 50–100 ml/kg may be required. Inotropic support may also be required at this time to support the circulation, active warming of the neonate, and patience and time to assess recovery of the bowel.

If malrotation is identified early, and the child is in good condition preoperatively, it is reasonable to consider extubating the trachea at the end of surgery. The late-presenting infant with necrotic bowel may remain critically ill even after derotation, requiring full support in the intensive care unit until perfusion is restored. Long-term parenteral nutrition may be required in some cases to bridge until the bowel regains full functionality.

Hirschsprung's Disease

Hirschsprung's disease is congenital aganglionosis of the bowel of variable length extending from the anus proximally [182]. This results in a lack of propagation of the intestinal propulsive waves, failure of relaxation of the internal anal sphincter, and functional bowel obstruction. It occurs in 1:4,500–5,000 live births with males affected more than females. 80–90 % of those with Hirschsprung's disease present in the neonatal period.

Embryology

Hirschsprung's disease is one of the neurocristopathies with presumed failure of the craniocaudal migration of the neural crest-derived neuroblasts, which form the myenteric and submucosal enteric plexuses (which should reach the rectum by week 12 of development). Other theories include failure of neuroblast differentiation, defects in function, or cell death. Varying lengths of bowel are affected, the most frequent pattern being short-segment disease affecting the rectosigmoid region (80 %). Long-segment disease occurs when aganglionosis extends proximal to the rectosigmoid region, with total colonic disease in 3–8 % of cases. Total intestinal involvement is rare.

Genetics

Hirschsprung's disease is a multigenic disorder with ten different genes and five chromosomal loci currently implicated [183]. There appears to be a dysfunction in one of two signaling pathways, which are critical in the development of the enteric nervous system. There is low and sex-dependent penetrance, with variable phenotypic expression. 10 % of patients have a family history (more common in long-segment disease). The RET (receptor tyrosine kinase) proto-oncogene mutation 10q11.2 is involved in 50 % of familial and 15–20 % of sporadic cases and 70–80 % of long segment and up to 38 % of short-segment disease [182]. Currently, genetic profiles are not widely available to assess the disease risk in individuals.

Hirschsprung's disease occurs in isolation in 70 % of cases, but it may be associated with trisomy 21 (5–15 % of cases of Hirschsprung's disease), other neurocristopathies (Waardenburg–Shah syndrome (SW4), congenital central hypoventilation syndrome, multiple endocrine neoplasia (MEN) type 2, neuroblastoma, and neurofibromatosis I), other syndromes such as Shprintzen-Goldberg and Smith-Lemli-Opitz, and congenital anomalies such as cardiac, genital, gastrointestinal anomalies, facial dysmorphism, and cleft palate [182].

Diagnosis

In neonates, the most common presenting symptoms are bile-stained vomiting with failure to pass meconium in the first 24 h of life (94 % of normal term infants pass meconium <24 h). This may be associated with poor feeding, abdominal distension, and vomiting. Rectal examination may result in explosive stool and may temporarily relieve the symptoms. Signs of enterocolitis (fever, abdominal distension, and diarrhea) may also be present. Differential diagnoses include the other causes of neonatal distal bowel obstruction discussed in this chapter. Abdominal X-ray may show dilated loops of bowel with an absence of air in the rectum. A distal contrast study may show dilatation of the proximal colon with a change in caliber (transition zone) to normal bowel, but this is not reliable. Rectal biopsy provides a definitive diagnosis for Hirschsprung's disease when it fails to demonstrate ganglion cells, with altered acetyl cholinesterase staining with hypertrophied nerve trunks. It is performed using a suction rectal biopsy in the neonatal period or open biopsy in older children. Anorectal manometry is not usually performed in neonates.

Management

Initial management aims to relieve the functional bowel obstruction either with warm saline washouts or a defunctioning stoma into ganglionic bowel. A stoma is indicated if the neonate is unwell or has developed enterocolitis and perforation and has a grossly dilated colon or suspected long-segment disease. Hirschsprung's enterocolitis is a potentially fatal complication that must be identified early and managed aggressively to reduce the risk of sepsis, intestinal necrosis, and perforation. Treatment with fluid resuscitation and broad-spectrum antibiotics is required.

Definitive surgery consists of resection of the aganglionic segment, either after initial stoma formation or ideally as a primary procedure. Several "pull-through" techniques have been described, usually performed when the infant is approximately 3 months of age, 5–6 kg weight [184]. The timing and exact procedure performed varies among centers and according to the length of abnormal bowel. Each technique can be performed completely open, or with laparoscopically assisted intra-abdominal dissection and biopsies, or entirely laparoscopically [184, 185].

Surgical Procedures

The first surgical procedure described to address Hirschsprung's disease was the Swenson procedure. This procedure is a low anterior resection of the rectum and aganglionic bowel, with a low anastomosis performed by prolapsing the bowel outside the anus.

The Duhamel procedure was the first alternative operation proposed in which the native rectum remains unchanged and a side-to-side anastomosis is stapled to the ganglionic bowel, which is mobilized and brought down to the presacral space. This requires less rectal dissection and offers a better chance of continence in the long term. It is often the preferred technique for long-segment disease. A retrospective review of open and laparoscopic approaches yielded similar operative time and outcomes [185].

The Soave procedure further minimizes rectal dissection by performing a mucosal dissection in the rectum and leaving a rectal muscular cuff. The original description has been modified to include a formal anastomosis just above the level of the dentate line.

A pure anal pull-through without a laparotomy or laparoscopy has also been reported for Hirschsprung's disease but may not be appropriate for longer-segment disease. Long-segment disease is not always suspected preoperatively potentially complicating this approach. Other operations have been described, although less frequently reported.

Outcomes

Appropriately managed, Hirschsprung's disease is associated with low mortality, although up to 50 % of patients undergoing surgery develop a complication such as constipation, fecal incontinence, or enterocolitis. Enterocolitis, the most severe complication, can occur in all patients with Hirschsprung's disease, both before and after surgery. It occurs more frequently in those with long-segment disease and those with trisomy 21. Enterocolitis is the primary cause of mortality in children with Hirschsprung's disease and must be identified and managed aggressively. Constipation occurs more frequently after the Duhamel pull-through, whereas incontinence occurs more frequently after the Soave and Swenson procedures. To date, there are no prospective randomized controlled trials that compare the outcomes from the different surgical techniques, although overall complication rates appear to be similar among all approaches.

Surgical Considerations

The transition zone between ganglionic (normal) and aganglionic (abnormal) bowel can vary in length (up to 10 cm) and demonstrate an irregular margin. It is important to perform an anastomosis between bowel segments with adequate ganglion cells without tension or vascular compromise. Time must be allowed regardless of procedure for intraoperative frozen section results of serial biopsies at ascending levels to accurately assess the extent of affected bowel. If long-segment disease is discovered unexpectedly, then many recommend that the pull-through procedure be delayed until formal histology is available.

Anesthetic Considerations

A complete preoperative history should be completed including a history of existing syndromes and anomalies that are associated with Hirschsprung's disease. Definitive surgery, either open or laparoscopic, may take 1.5–4 h in experienced hands [185]. The anesthetic prescription should be designed to ensure tracheal extubation at the end of surgery. After anesthesia is induced, the trachea is intubated and the lungs are ventilated with positive pressure and positive end-expiratory pressure. For the laparoscopic approach, the neonate is supine but positioned in steep Trendelenburg. All of the airway fittings should be manually tightened and IV access points extended such that they are reachable once the neonate is draped. Blood loss is usually minimal obviating the need for blood transfusion. Caudal/epidural regional analgesia is well suited for perioperative analgesia after this surgery. Postoperatively, rectal analgesia is contraindicated.

Anorectal Anomalies

Anorectal anomalies occur on 1:4,000–1:5,000 neonates with a slight male preponderance. Associated abnormalities are present in 30–60 % of cases; the most common associations are listed below (Table 10.5).

Table 10.5 Conditions associated with anorectal anomalies

Genitourinary (renal dysplasia, vesicoureteric reflux, undescended testes, vaginal abnormalities)
Spinosacral (sacral agenesis, vertebral anomalies, tethered cord)
Cardiac (septal defects and tetralogy of Fallot)
Gastrointestinal (esophageal atresia, intestinal atresias, Hirschsprung's disease)
Chromosomal (trisomy 21, VACTERL association, Currarino triad)

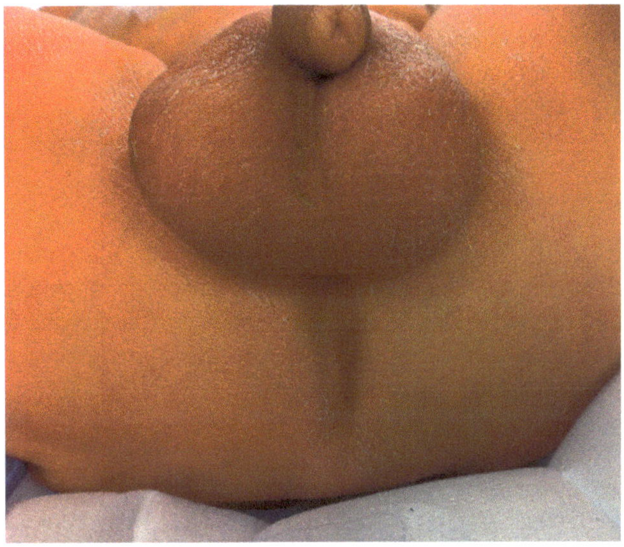

Fig. 10.13 Imperforate anus. A closeup photograph of the perineum in a male. Note that immediately inferior to the normal penis and scrotum, one observes the outline and pigmentation of the imperforate anus (Courtesy of Dr. YH Lee, Division of Pediatric Surgery, Strong Hospital, University of Rochester, Rochester, NY)

Embryology

During weeks 4–6, the pouch at the caudal end of the hindgut (the cloaca) is separated into the urogenital sinus (bladder, urethra, vagina) and rectum. Anorectal anomalies occur as the result of failure of this separation and usual subsequent degeneration (apoptosis of the membrane) resulting in a wide range of clinical abnormalities.

Classification

The Krickenbeck classification of anorectal anomalies is shown in Table 10.6 [186]. In males, imperforate anus with rectourethral fistula is the most common defect followed by rectoperineal fistulae (Fig. 10.13). In females the most common defect is imperforate anus with rectovestibular fistula [187].

Diagnosis

Anorectal anomalies are diagnosed clinically, requiring a thorough inspection of the perineum, sacrum, and buttocks to identify the anatomy. If the neonate's clinical condition permits, it is important to wait 16–24 h after birth to diagnose a fistula, especially in males, as it may take this time for meconium to reach the rectum [188].

Table 10.6 Krickenbeck classification of anorectal anomalies [186]

Major clinical groups
• Perineal (cutaneous) fistula
• Rectourethral fistula (prostatic, bulbar)
• Rectovesical fistula
• Vestibular fistula
• Cloaca
• No fistula
• Anal stenosis
Rare/regional variants
• Pouch colon
• Recta atresia/stenosis
• Rectovaginal fistula
• H fistula
• Others

Associated anomalies should be sought and further investigations may be required such as an echocardiogram, abdominal X-ray, and renal ultrasound. An "invertogram" was previously advocated, but this is not routinely performed in many centers.

Outcomes

Short-term complications after reconstructive surgery include anal stenosis, which may require repeated dilatation or formal revision and wound infection. Pelvic sepsis can occur as a life- and continence-threatening early complication of surgery, especially if a diverting stoma has not been performed.

Constipation is the most common long-term complication of anorectal surgery, occurring in 18–62 % of infants. Fecal incontinence is a second long-term complication, occurring in 25 % of infants. Social continence can often be achieved with a combination of modalities including antegrade enemas via an antegrade colonic enema (ACE) stoma. Urinary dysfunction may also occur, being attributable to the underlying urinary tract anomaly rather than the surgery.

Management

Initial management is supportive with intravenous fluids and gastric decompression with a nasogastric tube. Associated anomalies should be excluded and time allowed to detect a fistula, if clinically appropriate. Surgical decompression and reconstruction is required. Depending on the anatomy and associated anomalies, the neonate may undergo a primary anoplasty ("low" anomalies) with or without a diverting colostomy and distal mucous fistula or formation of colostomy/mucous fistula with later reconstructive surgery at 1–2 months of age ("high" anomalies). Several operative approaches have been proposed for reconstruction including posterior sagittal anorectoplasty (PSARP), an anterior sagittal approach, sacroperineal procedure, abdominosacral pull-through, abdominoperineal pull-through, and laparoscopic-assisted pull-through techniques. PSARP is the most common procedure, suitable for most females and 90 % of males. In the remaining males, a combined abdominal approach is required to mobilize the rectum.

Surgical Considerations

It is important to avoid damage to pelvic structures and their innervation during surgery. A muscle stimulator is essential to identify the sphincter complex and ensure correct placement of the neo-anus. For muscle function to be stimulated, muscle relaxants are avoided after induction of anesthesia. Dissection should be adequate to bring the rectum to the perineum without tension in order to minimize retraction after the repair and anal complications.

Anesthetic Considerations

An understanding of the associated anomalies, particularly cardiac and spinal anomalies, is important. Stoma formation is a relatively minor procedure in the neonatal period, and a single-shot caudal epidural provides excellent perioperative analgesia for primary anoplasty (provided there are no sacral abnormalities). Reconstructive surgery is usually performed in the prone position (PSARP) or occasionally as a combined abdominoperineal or laparoscopically assisted procedure. Intravenous access should be placed in the upper extremities to ensure that the fluids are infused into the circulation, not the surgical field. Blood transfusion is rarely required for this surgery. These reconstructive surgeries are usually several hours in duration, with the neonates in the Trendelenburg position. As a result, tracheal intubation is usually required. The anesthetic prescription should be designed to extubate the trachea at the end of surgery. Perioperative analgesia can be achieved with a continuous caudal/epidural infusion of local anesthetics (e.g., bupivacaine) [189] or IV morphine infusion [190–192].

Cloaca

This type of anorectal anomaly is uncommon, occurring in 1:50,000 live births.

Diagnosis

Careful clinical examination will reveal a single perineal opening. Further imaging studies such as contrast studies and CT scan with reconstruction can be very useful, as well as assessment of the common channel and structure via cystoscopy.

Management

Initial management is supportive as for other anorectal anomalies. Of note, hydrocolpos can result in urinary obstruction and pyocolpos can result in perforation. Both of these conditions may require urgent drainage.

Outcomes

The long-term results for cloacal repair in terms of continence are worse than for lower anorectal anomalies. Only 10 % of neonates with a common channel >3 cm in length will be continent.

Surgical Considerations

Recognition of the anomaly is important as a more proximal transverse colostomy is required to allow for adequate length for the reconstruction procedure. Assessment of the length of the common channel before reconstructive surgery is important for both prognostic reasons and to assess the need for a combined intra-abdominal approach.

Abdominal Wall Defects

Gastroschisis

Gastroschisis occurs in 1:4,000 live births, affecting males and females equally. The incidence of gastroschisis, which is increasing, is strongly associated with maternal age <20 years, smoking, use of recreational drugs, low maternal weight, maternal genitourinary infection, and low socioeconomic status [193–196].

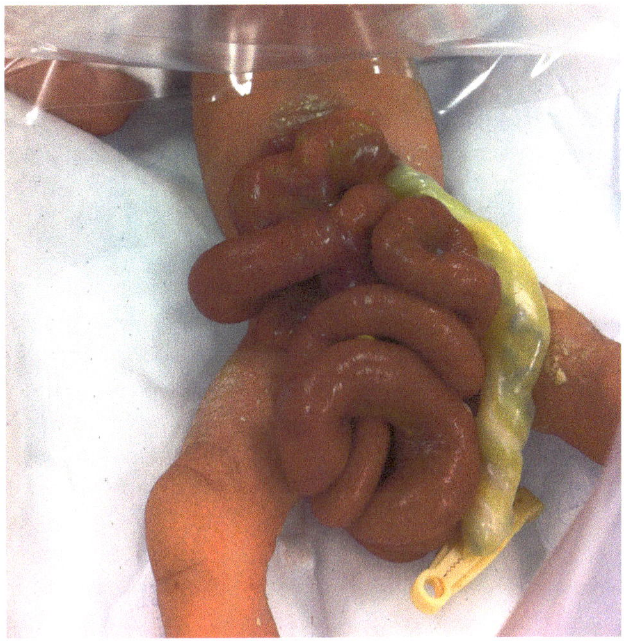

Fig. 10.14 Gastroschisis. In this preterm neonate, the thickened, red bowel from a gastroschisis lays open and exposed. Note that the gastroschisis arises from an anterior abdominal wall defect on the right side, lateral to the intact umbilical cord (Courtesy of Dr. YH Lee, Division of Pediatric Surgery, Strong Hospital, University of Rochester, Rochester, NY)

Pathophysiology

Gastroschisis is usually a small, right-sided (<10 % left) defect in the abdominal wall lateral to the intact umbilical cord, through which the intestines protrude, uncovered, and unprotected (Fig. 10.14). The exact embryological mechanism for this anomaly is still unclear. In utero, the eviscerated bowel floats uncovered and exposed in the amniotic fluid. This may contribute to thickening of the bowel wall and fibrinous "peel" that is often present on the bowel at delivery. The abdominal wall defect can narrow later in pregnancy, resulting in obstruction and ischemic changes to the gut. Associated anomalies are infrequent with this defect, but when they occur, they are usually gastrointestinal in origin. For example, intestinal atresias occur in 10–15 % of cases. The liver rarely herniates.

Diagnosis

The majority of neonates with gastroschisis are diagnosed on routine antenatal ultrasound. Blood testing shows increased maternal serum concentrations of alpha-fetoprotein in the absence of a myelomeningocele. "Complicated gastroschisis," as in the case of gastroschisis with intestinal atresia, may be predicted by the presence of dilated bowel on antenatal ultrasound [197]. Approximately 30–70 % of neonates have intrauterine growth retardation or small for gestational age. The mechanism for this latter effect is unclear but may be due to enteric loss of proteins or inadequate supply of fetal nutrients [198]. After delivery, the laterality of the defect, the absence of a sac, and an intact umbilical cord differentiate gastroschisis from omphalocele.

Management

Antenatal diagnosis allows prenatal planning and transfer of the parturient to a center where surgical management of the gastroschisis and a level-3 nursery are available [199]. There is insufficient evidence to determine the optimal management of these fetuses, for example, the age at which the fetus should be delivered and the delivery technique [200]. A survey of maternal-fetal medicine practitioners in Canada suggested that preterm (<36 weeks) delivery of fetuses with gastroschisis was associated with more complications, i.e., greater time requiring parenteral nutrition and greater length of stay in NICU, whereas delivery of fetuses ≥38 weeks was associated with increased bowel matting [201]. There is no evidence that cesarean section improves neonatal outcomes, although early induction of labor (from gestational week 36) may avoid the unexplained late fetal deaths that can occur with this condition.

Initial management at delivery is supportive, avoiding hypothermia, hypovolemia, and sepsis. The exteriorized bowel should be wrapped in clear plastic film and supported in the midline to minimize venous engorgement or placed in a preformed silo. Above all, care must be taken to avoid damaging the exposed bowel. A servo-controlled warm incubator should be used. Large volumes of intravenous fluids may be required to offset the large evaporative fluid loss from the exposed bowel. Broad-spectrum antibiotics should be given. A nasogastric tube should be placed to decompress the stomach and bowel.

Outcomes

Survival with gastroschisis is reported to be 90–95 %, with the majority of deaths due to massive bowel resection or necrosis [202]. Intestinal function may be slow to recover after closing the defect necessitating a long period of parenteral nutrition. A review of a gastroschisis database indicated that the time to achieve independence from parenteral nutrition, reduce length of stay, and achieve freedom from infection was optimized when enteral feeds were withheld for at least 7 days after closure of the defect [203]. However, these findings should be interpreted in the context of the neonate's status. Intestinal dysfunction and short bowel syndrome complicate gastroschisis. Gastroschisis accounts for approximately 20 % of the cases of short bowel syndrome, with the incidence of the latter inversely proportional to birth weight [204]. Surgical short bowel syndrome is defined as the need for parenteral nutrition for >3 months. Current advances in management strategies that involve a multidisciplinary team approach, parenteral nutrition, prophylaxis from infection, and ongoing surgical consultation have dramatically improved bowel function and survival in these neonates [204].

Surgical Considerations

The primary objective of surgery is to cover and protect the bowel. The secondary objective is to effect a staged return of the bowels to the abdomen, without causing an abdominal compartment syndrome. The latter is often identified by the onset of respiratory distress, ischemic or necrotic bowel, and renal insufficiency. For monitoring strategies to identify abdominal compartment syndrome, see Anesthetic Considerations below.

The surgical treatment of gastroschisis remains controversial. Primary closure may be undertaken in neonates with small-size gastroschises using general anesthesia in the operating theater. Complications such as intestinal atresia, perforation, necrosis, or volvulus may be addressed at the same time. Before attempting a primary closure, rectal decompression with possible rectal washouts may decrease intraluminal contents and facilitate a smooth reduction. Good long-term outcomes have also been reported using a "sutureless ward reduction" protocol with morphine sedation for carefully selected neonates with uncomplicated gastroschisis. The bowel is inspected carefully for intestinal anomalies and the neonate remains conscious during the procedure. The reduction should be abandoned if the neonate develops respiratory distress or the surgeon perceives the abdominal pressure is excessive [205].

A staged closure is required if primary closure is not appropriate or possible. This may be performed by surgical application of a hand-sewn Prolene mesh silo under general anesthesia or using a preformed spring-loaded silo. For neonates with uncomplicated gastroschisis who do not have significant viscero-abdominal disproportion, the preformed silo can be applied on the neonatal unit without the need for general anesthesia or routine intubation [206]. These techniques allow gradual compression of the bowel into the abdomen over a period of days and facilitate early extubation. The neonate undergoes planned surgical closure 3–5 days later, or closure of the defect using adhesive strips once the bowel is fully reduced, depending on the silo technique used [207]. Use of the preformed silo may be associated with reduced ventilator days in the NICU [97], but this approach may also be associated with specific technical complications leading to venous congestion of the intestine and bowel ischemia [208].

Anesthetic Considerations

Some centers do not use anesthesia for closure of gastroschisis if a sutureless or preformed silo technique is used, although others recommend routine anesthesia with paralysis to facilitate every attempt to reduce the bowel. An operative technique is required for complicated gastroschisis. A combination of general anesthesia with epidural anesthesia provides good postoperative analgesia and may reduce the need for postoperative ventilation [209]. The child must be kept warm and well hydrated with fluid blouses of 20 ml/kg Ringer's or albumin. Arterial access is useful for monitoring complex procedures. In neonates with otherwise uncomplicated gastroschisis, enteral feeding usually begins 7–10 days after delivery. In those who require long-term parenteral nutrition, it is important to preserve veins for chronic catheters for long-term parenteral feeding. Some units advocate placement of a tunneled feeding line at the time of initial surgery [210].

The major concern during closure is the development of abdominal compartment syndrome. If the reduction is performed under general anesthesia, care should be taken during face mask ventilation to avoid gaseous distention of the gastrointestinal tract and nitrous oxide should be avoided. Intra-abdominal pressures should be maintained <20 mmHg during primary closure of the defect [210]. Some centers advocate the use of a balloon-tipped catheter in the bladder or stomach, central venous pressure, or $P_{ET}CO_2$ to track changes in intra-abdominal pressure during the closure [211, 212]. The ventilator settings should be noted at the start of the procedure and followed throughout to identify any decreases in tidal volume due to upward movement and splinting of the diaphragm. If these occur, the reduction must stop and the approach reassessed. During closure the bowel must be constantly assessed for signs of venous congestion. Urine output can be used to reflect the adequacy of renal perfusion after completing the surgery. After closure but before leaving the operating room, the lower limbs should be examined for evidence of venous compromise and pulses.

Exomphalos (Omphalocele)

Exomphalos occurs in 1:4,000 live births, affecting males 1.5 times more frequently than females. It can be classified as major, minor, or giant, depending on the size of the defect and the presence of liver herniation. Major defects are greater than 4 cm in diameter or contain a herniated liver. Giant defects are greater than 6 cm in diameter or contain a herniated liver. Associated anomalies are common, occurring in more than 50 % of neonates, particularly those with a minor defect. Anomalies associated with exomphalos include chromosomal abnormalities (30 %) such as trisomies 13, 18, and 21, other midline defects (pentalogy of Cantrell, bladder and cloacal anomalies), and cardiac and musculoskeletal abnormalities. Beckwith–Wiedemann syndrome, an abnormality found on chromosome 11 associated with gigantism, macroglossia, exomphalos, pancreatic islet cell hyperplasia with hyperinsulinism, organomegaly, and hemihypertrophy, occurs in 12 % of cases. Pulmonary hypoplasia is associated with exomphalos major.

Pathophysiology

Exomphalos is a central defect of the umbilical ring. The herniated organs are covered with a membrane (sac) continuous with the umbilical cord (Fig. 10.15). This is thought to represent failure of the intestines to retract into the abdominal cavity from the umbilical stalk after the period of rapid growth of the intestines early in embryogenesis.

Diagnosis

As in gastroschisis, the diagnosis of exomphalos is confirmed antenatally using ultrasound imaging. Exomphalos is a midline abdominal wall defect with a sac that contains the herniated visceral contents. Antenatal chromosome testing is recommended. After delivery, the defect in the umbilical ring is visible, usually with an intact sac. It can be difficult to visualize externally whether the liver is herniated.

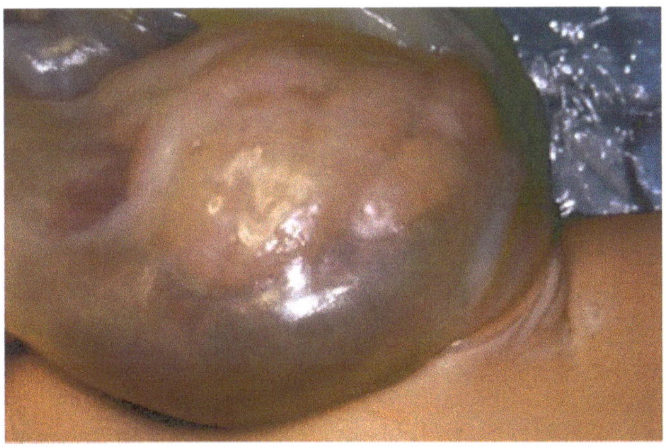

Fig. 10.15 Omphalocele. In this midline defect, the herniated bowels are covered by a thick membrane (Courtesy of Dr. YH Lee, Division of Pediatric Surgery, Strong Hospital, University of Rochester, Rochester, NY)

Outcomes

The mortality rate in neonates with exomphalos, 10–30 %, is substantively worse than it is for gastroschisis. However, unlike gastroschisis in which the severity of the bowel dysfunction and ischemia determines the morbidity and mortality in that condition, the severity of the associated anomalies determines the morbidity and mortality in exomphalos.

Management

Supportive management is the initial priority. If the sac remains intact, then the bowels are protected and urgent surgical intervention is unnecessary. The sac and its contents should be supported depending on its size. Time can be taken to delineate and stabilize the associated anomalies before proceeding with reduction. If the sac has ruptured, then surgical intervention becomes more urgent as in the case of gastroschisis.

Surgical Considerations

Primary reduction of the contents with excision of sac is usually achievable for small defects, but a staged closure is generally required for larger defects. A hand-sewn surgical silo is placed under general anesthesia, leaving the sac intact, with serial reductions performed in the neonatal unit, including after extubation. Once the visceral contents have been reduced, then the silo can be removed and the defect formally closed in theater. The likely success of primary closure should be assessed by gentle compression before excising the sac. If not favorable, then the sac should be left intact for silo placement. If the sac is excised, care must be taken superiorly to avoid damaging the hepatic veins, which may cause significant haemorrhage. Neonates with giant exomphalos are occasionally treated conservatively, particularly if there is marked disproportion between the viscera and the size of the abdominal cavity (typical "scaphoid" abdomen). The intact sac is allowed to epithelialize, with topical application of antibacterial sclerosing agents such as povidone-iodine or silver sulfadiazine, although systemic absorption of iodine or silver may themselves create a problem [213].

Anesthetic Considerations

The preoperative assessment should include an echocardiogram and appropriate investigations to fully define the severity of any other anomalies present. Otherwise, the anesthetic prescription is similar to that for gastroschisis repair. Neonates with exomphalos major are particularly at risk for abdominal compartment syndrome. Reduction of the liver into the abdomen can compress the inferior vena cava, acutely decreasing venous return and cardiac output. Intra-abdominal pressure can be monitored using either a bladder or gastric pressure transducer (see above) to provide an objective metric upon which to stage the reduction. As in the gastroschisis, close and clear communication between the surgeon and anesthesiologist will ensure a successful reduction.

Bladder Exstrophy/Cloacal Exstrophy

Bladder exstrophy occurs in 1:30–50,000 live births affecting males four times more frequently than females. Antenatal diagnosis occurs in only 25 % of cases [214]. This defect in the anterior bladder and abdominal wall exposes the bladder and urethra as part of the exstrophy–epispadias complex (Fig. 10.16).

Cloacal exstrophy occurs four to five times less frequently than bladder exstrophy, 1:200,000 live births. It occurs equally in both males and females. Cloacal exstrophy is a lower abdominal wall defect with two hemibladders separated by a midline cecum, exomphalos, and imperforate anus. Spinal malformations such as myelomeningocele may occur as part of the omphalocele–exstrophy–imperforate anus-spinal defects (OEIS) complex.

Outcomes

Optimal outcomes for these rare conditions are obtained by centralizing the care to specialist centers, with the involvement of a multidisciplinary team. Previously a commonly fatal condition, the dramatic advances in neonatal care have transformed the outcome from this defect to almost 100 % survival beyond the neonatal period, although long-term issues relating to function and psychological outcomes remain.

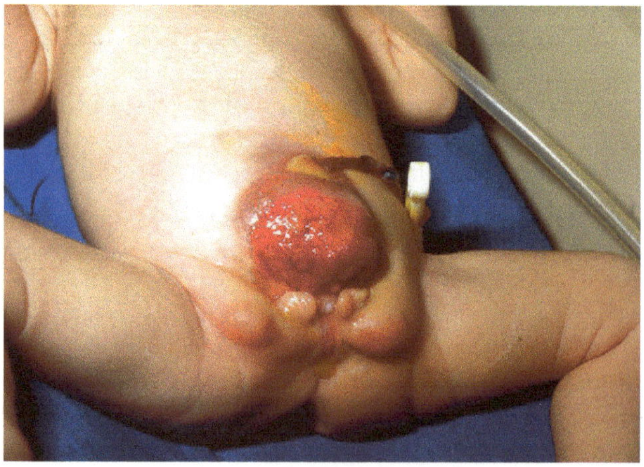

Fig. 10.16 Bladder exstrophy. This congenital defect in the anterior abdominal wall reveals the bladder wall, malformed genitalia, and widened pelvis with an absent symphysis pubis (Courtesy of Dr. RJ. Banchs, Children's Hospital, University of Illinois. Chicago, Ill)

Management

After delivery, care should be taken to avoid damage to the bladder plate. Moist nonadherent dressings should be applied prior to transfer of the child to the specialist center, and the umbilicus tied rather than clamped. In cloacal exstrophy, exomphalos is managed using the techniques described above.

Surgical Considerations in Bladder Exstrophy

The long-term aims of surgery are the reconstruction of the bladder for social urinary continence, treatment of vesicoureteric reflux, reconstruction of the genitalia to allow for cosmetic appearance, sexual and urinary function, and, in the case of cloacal exstrophy, reconstruction to obtain fecal continence. As a result of the wide diastasis of the pubic bones, pelvic osteotomies are often required in order to close the pelvic brim anteriorly and reduce the risk of wound dehiscence and bladder prolapse.

Surgery may be performed in staged procedures: the bladder is closed early in the neonatal period with or without pelvic osteotomies, depending on surgical preference; the genitalia is repaired at 3–6 months of age, in some centers with a radical bladder neck reconstruction at this stage (Kelly procedure) and a secondary hypospadias procedure at 3 years; and finally, bladder augmentation and ureteric reimplantation are performed if required in later childhood. If the bladder closure and osteotomies are performed in a single procedure, a multidisciplinary approach involving anesthesia, urology, and orthopedics is the prescription for success. In this case, the anticipated duration of surgery will be quite prolonged (see below). A single stage procedure of bladder closure, bladder neck reconstruction, and epispadias repair in the neonatal period has been described (Mitchell procedure), although concerns that urethral blood flow may be compromised with this technique must be considered [215]. The complication rate after single stage repair is reportedly similar to those after a staged repair, although soft tissue defects may be more common in the former [216].

Anesthetic Considerations

Neonates with bladder exstrophy are usually born at term without other associated anomalies. Surgery for primary bladder closure is ideally performed in the first few days of life, while the pelvic bones remain malleable. Blood loss is significant if pelvic osteotomies are performed, and a blood transfusion is often required. A plaster cast or external fixator may be applied at the end of surgery for support. Although systolic blood pressure remains a reliable metric for detecting hypovolemia in neonates, central venous access may be useful adjunct measure to monitor fluid status during this surgery as urine output is not easily quantified. Intravenous access should be placed in the upper extremities (or neck) to retain access to the lines and to ensure that all fluids remain in the circulation. With the prolonged duration of surgery and the need to monitor blood pressure, to perform laboratory tests (hemoglobin, electrolyte, and glucose concentrations), and to respond to sudden blood loss, arterial access should be considered. Surgery may be prolonged (4–6 h or greater). A combination of general anesthesia and epidural anesthesia allows many neonates to be extubated at the end of surgery. Some units advocate the use of tunneled epidural catheters to facilitate immobilization and reduce wound complications [217].

Posterior Urethral Valves

Posterior urethral valves (PUV) are the most common cause of lower urinary obstruction in males, occurring more commonly in non-Caucasians at a rate of 1:5,000 live births. Other less common causes of lower urinary obstruction include prune-belly syndrome and urethral stenosis or atresia. PUV is usually an isolated finding that causes severe obstructive uropathy, with 20–60 % of these neonates developing chronic kidney disease in childhood and 11–51 % progressing to end-stage renal failure in their lifetime [218]. Severe obstruction and oligohydramnios during lung development (16–24 weeks gestation) may cause pulmonary hypoplasia leading to substantial fetal and perinatal mortality (33–75 %) [219].

Diagnosis

PUV are frequently identified from the appearance of bilateral hydronephrosis during routine antenatal ultrasound (accounting for 10 % of cases of antenatal hydronephrosis), although many do not present until later in childhood, with urinary tract infection, failure to thrive, or continence. Late diagnosis is associated with less severe renal impairment and better long-term prognosis. At birth, renal ultrasound demonstrates a thick-walled bladder and hydronephrosis and provides an assessment of the degree of renal cortical damage. The urethral valves can be demonstrated in a voiding cystourethrogram or directly at cystoscopy.

Management

Definitive treatment for PUV in neonates is relief of the obstruction by catheterization and antibiotic prophylaxis, with cystoscopy and transurethral ablation. The results of antenatal treatment with vesicoamniotic shunt have been disappointing to date. Long-term follow-up is required, with active management of bladder dysfunction and reflux.

Anesthetic Considerations

Cystoscopy and resection of PUV during the neonatal period is a minor procedure that requires a brief general anesthetic. Nonetheless, most prefer to secure the airway in these neonates with a tracheal tube (rather than a supraglottic device) because the neonate may be positioned either cross-table or at the end of the operating room table and the duration of surgery is somewhat unpredictable, dependent on the extent of the pathology. Significant comorbidities such as pulmonary hypoplasia and renal dysfunction must be considered when planning the anesthetic prescription. Antibiotic prophylaxis is essential. A single-shot caudal epidural block can provide excellent perioperative analgesia depending on the extent of the surgery.

Sacrococcygeal Teratoma

Sacrococcygeal teratoma occurs in 1–2:40,000 live births, representing 35–60 % of all teratomas [220]. Females are more commonly affected than males by a 3–4:1 margin (Fig. 10.17). These tumors arise from an embryonic cell line in the pelvis that contains cells in different proportions from the ectoderm, mesoderm, and endoderm [221]. Structurally, sacrococcygeal teratomas are classified as cystic, solid, or a combination of the two. Cystic teratomas comprise 15 % of all sacrococcygeal teratomas, have more differentiated cells, and are usually benign. The majority of sacrococcygeal teratomas are solid or mixed (Fig. 10.18). The more solid the composition of the teratoma, the more likely it is to be malignant.

Perinatal mortality in neonates, whose tumors are diagnosed antenatally, is 25–37 %. Mortality is more likely in fetuses with rapidly growing vascular teratomas that act physiologically as arteriovenous malformations. These malformations lead to hydrops, polyhydramnios, high-output cardiac failure, preterm birth, and death. Two variables suggest a greater risk for a poor prognosis: the ratio of the tumor

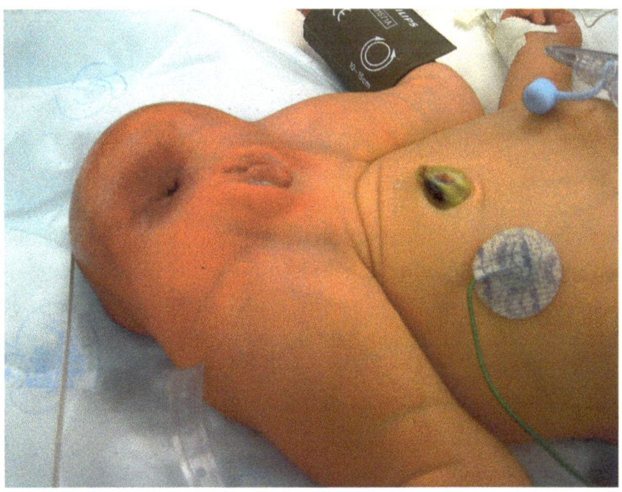

Fig. 10.17 Sacrococcygeal teratoma. This tumor was located on the outside of the sacrum, completely external to the pelvis. Consistent with the greater incidence of sacrococcygeal teratomas in females, this neonate was a female (Courtesy of Dr. W. Pegoli, Division of Pediatric Surgery, Strong Hospital, University of Rochester, Rochester, NY)

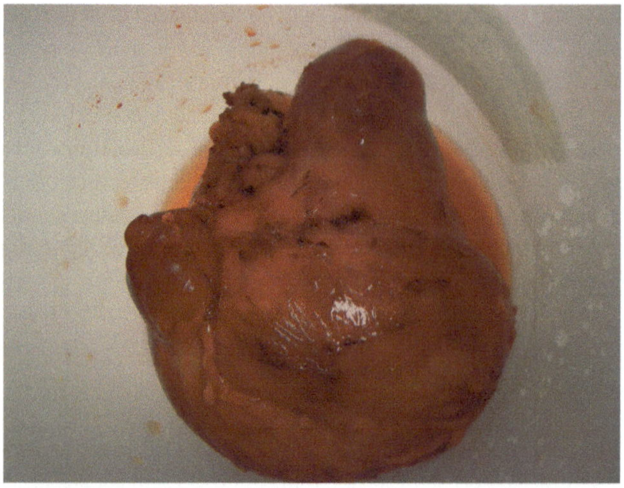

Fig. 10.18 Excised sacrococcygeal teratoma. The tumor appears to be multiloculated, but mostly solid in this case

volume to the fetal weight >0.11 determined before 32 weeks gestation and tumor morphology <60 % cystic [222].

At delivery, 90 % of sacrococcygeal teratomas are benign; the minority is malignant. However, the malignancy rate increases dramatically from 10 % at birth to 75 % by 1 year of age and 100 % by 5 years of age if the tumor is not resected. Hence, early detection and antenatal intervention or surgical excision of the tumor at birth is crucial to achieve long-term survival.

The Currarino triad, which is comprised of a presacral tumor, anorectal malformation, and sacral anomaly, follows an autosomal dominant familial inheritance pattern from a genetic defect on chromosome 7. Urogenital anomalies have been identified in females with sacrococcygeal teratomas and should be suspected in any female with voiding difficulties [223].

Diagnosis

Sacrococcygeal teratomas are often detected antenatally using ultrasound. Differential diagnoses include meningocele, lymphangioma, lipoma, or taillike remnant. At delivery, 85–95 % of these teratomas are external midline sacral masses. The skin covering the mass is usually normal, although hemangiomas, ulcers, and evidence of necrosis may be present [220]. Investigations should be performed preoperatively to define the borders of the mass within the pelvis. In older children, the tumor may be entirely intrapelvic, without external evidence of the tumor. The Altman classification of sacrococcygeal tumors is based on postnatal assessment of the external and internal elements of the teratomas (Table 10.7) [224].

Table 10.7 The Altman classification of sacrococcygeal tumors [224]

Type I—tumor is predominantly external with minimal presacral component
Type II—tumor presents externally, but with substantial intrapelvic extension
Type III—tumor is present externally, but the bulk of the tumor is intrapelvic with extension into the abdomen
Type IV—presacral tumor with no external component

Management

Complications associated with sacrococcygeal tumors relate to its vascularity, size, and position. In utero, the fetus should be monitored for the development of hydrops and placentomegaly. These occur in rapidly growing vascular teratomas that cause a vascular steal syndrome, which in turn may precipitate high-output cardiac failure necessitating an urgent in utero intervention to prevent premature delivery and/or death. These interventions may include amnioreduction, cyst aspiration, radiofrequency ablation, shunts, and surgical debulking [225, 226]. Outcomes after in utero interventions are similar to those who did not undergo interventions, despite the worsened features present in the intervention group, with a mortality between 25 and 45 % [226, 227]. Cesarean section is indicated for large tumors, that is, for those larger than the neonate's biparietal diameter [220]. Vaginal deliveries are best avoided in neonates with large tumors as the latter may rupture causing the neonate to rapidly exsanguinate. Rectal examination should be performed with great care to avoid rupturing the tumor. Imaging techniques including abdominal X-ray, echocardiogram, ultrasound, and/or MRI will help to define the anatomy, location, and vascularity of the tumor. Tumor markers should be monitored (alpha-fetoprotein and beta HCG): alpha-fetoprotein increases in the presence of a malignancy. These should be followed postoperatively to detect a malignant recurrence.

Outcomes

If the sacrococcygeal teratoma is identified as an incidental finding during the antenatal period, the expected survival rate is 90 %. Mortality approaches 60 % in complicated pregnancies, and 100 % in the presence of hydrops or placentomegaly, which reflects high-output heart failure due to shunting through the vascular teratoma.

The prognosis in terms of malignancy depends on the tumor type, stage, location (Altman classification), and completeness of excision, in addition to the child's age at the time of the operation. If the initial resection is performed after the neonatal period, the risk of a recurrence increases substantially, especially if the serum alpha-fetoprotein concentration is increased. Up to 7 % of tumors recur, mostly within the first 3 years. These tumors recur locally, although metastases are possible. The long-term prognosis in these children, including those with a malignant sacrococcygeal teratoma, exceeds 80 % due to platinum-based multimodal chemotherapy [220].

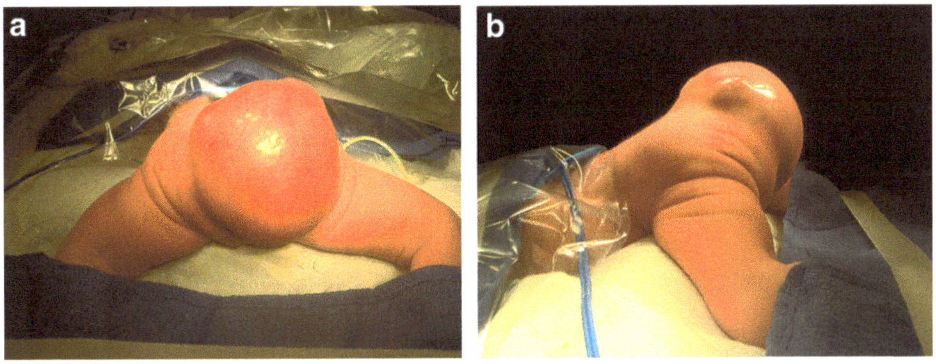

Fig. 10.19 Sacrococcygeal teratoma. (**a**) Caudal view. (**b**) Lateral view. The neonate was anesthetized, the tracheal intubated, and the neonate positioned prone for surgery. Note the large size of the tumor relative to the neonate (Courtesy of Dr. W. Pegoli, Division of Pediatric Surgery, Strong Hospital, University of Rochester, Rochester, NY)

Functional results are usually very good, although 17 % of patients develop a neuropathic bladder and 6 % develop complete fecal incontinence. This is possibly a tumor effect rather than surgical morbidity [225].

Surgical Considerations

Once the airway is secured, monitoring and vascular access (including arterial access) are established, and the bladder is catheterized, the neonate is turned prone (Fig. 10.19a, b). The coccyx should be removed with the tumor for a complete excision of the tumor. If the tumor has a small intrapelvic component, it should be resectable in this position. An abdominal approach may be indicated for larger intrapelvic tumors or in cases where early vascular control is required.

Anesthetic Considerations

Excision of sacrococcygeal teratoma is a high-risk procedure, with significant perioperative morbidity and mortality. In some cases, it may be prudent to have two experienced anesthesiologists to provide anesthesia for these cases as sacrococcygeal teratomas have been known to hemorrhage suddenly and massively. The perioperative risks relate primarily to a major hemorrhage from the highly vascular tumor, in the context of a neonate who may be premature and have pulmonary hypertension, renal and hepatic impairment, and a coagulopathy associated with high-output cardiac failure. Access to the neonate may be compromised if surgery is performed in the prone position. It is essential to make preparations for major blood loss with crossmatched fresh blood and blood products. Intraoperative cardiac arrest has been reported from hyperkalemia and hypocalcemia associated with a rapid, massive transfusion, especially when transfused rapidly through a central venous catheter, and hyperkalemia has been associated with surgical manipulation of a necrotic tumor [228]. Blood should be transfused slowly, preferably through peripheral IV access (not through a central line), especially if the blood is old.

At the conclusion of surgery, the neonate should be transferred to the intensive care unit in the prone position. The bladder catheter remains in situ for 24 h. The serum concentration of alpha-fetoprotein should be monitored on a regular basis to assess the risk of a malignant recurrence.

Biliary Atresia

Biliary atresia (BA) is the progressive obliteration and sclerosis of the extra- and intrahepatic bile ducts leading to liver fibrosis, cirrhosis, and death if untreated, occurring in 1:10,000–15,000 live births. Its etiology is unknown. It is associated with other anomalies in 15–20 % of cases. Biliary atresia splenic malformation syndrome (BASM) occurs in 10 % of cases, with polysplenia or asplenia, cardiac abnormalities, situs inversus, malrotation, preduodenal portal vein, and absent vena cava [229].

Classification

BA is classified according to the level of obstruction of the extrahepatic bile ducts (Table 10.8). Type III is further subdivided according to the pattern of obstruction of the common bile duct (CBD) and distal ducts. The most common type of BA is type IIIb.

Diagnosis

The key feature of BA is prolonged jaundice (conjugated hyperbilirubinemia) beyond the first 2 weeks of life with signs of biliary obstruction (pale stools and dark urine), in an otherwise healthy term neonate [229]. Infants who present later may show signs of failure to thrive due to fat malabsorption, with coagulopathy due to failure to absorb vitamin K, hepatosplenomegaly, and ascites [230]. The initial meconium is usually colored, as the obstructive jaundice develops postnatally. Diagnosis of BA is usually made by liver biopsy, or occasionally laparoscopic cholangiogram with direct

Table 10.8 Classification of biliary atresia

Type I—obstruction at common bile duct (5 % of cases)
Type II—obstruction at the common hepatic duct (2 % of cases)
Type III—obstruction the porta hepatis (>90 % of cases)
Subtype a. Patent CBD, atrophic gall bladder
Subtype b. Fibrous CBD, atrophic gall bladder
Subtype c. Absent common hepatic duct, mucocele of gall bladder
Subtype d. Miscellaneous

puncture of the gall bladder, or radioisotope scan to detect bile acid in the intestine (hepatobiliary iminodiacetic acid (HIDA) scan) [229].

The differential diagnosis of BA includes choledocal cyst, inspissated bile syndrome, and other infective/metabolic causes of neonatal hepatitis, which should be excluded with a TORCH screen, metabolic screen, and ultrasound. Choledocal cyst is a cystic disorder of unknown etiology affecting the pancreatobiliary system. Children may present with jaundice and an abdominal mass at any age from birth to adulthood. Without treatment, this disorder may progress to cholangitis or cirrhosis. The anesthetic considerations are similar to BA, although underlying hepatic function is usually normal, apart from obstructive jaundice.

Management

Once the diagnosis has been made, any coagulopathy should be corrected and surgery planned. Being a rare condition, best outcomes are usually obtained when these neonates are referred to a specialist center. In the UK, children with BA should be referred to one of three national specialist centers. Long-term prognosis is linked to the timing of operative correction of bile flow, so ideally, surgery should be performed as soon as possible, usually at age 1–2 months. Jaundice usually clears early in 50–60 % of patients. These children have a good 5-year prognosis, although liver transplantation may be required for those with persistent jaundice or clinically significant portal hypertension. Long-term survival is expected in 90 % of cases, although neonates may have significant long-term morbidity that is related to hepatic cirrhosis or the effects of immunosuppression after liver transplantation.

Surgical Approach

The initial surgery consists of an open Kasai procedure. Laparoscopic techniques do not appear to offer advantages such as fewer adhesions, over the open approach [231–235]. The Kasai procedure involves resection of the extrahepatic biliary tree including the portal plate and the fashioning of a Roux-en-Y jejunal anastomosis at this level to restore bile flow to the intestinal tract. If the diagnosis is not clear before the laparotomy, then an intraoperative cholangiogram can be performed before dissection [229]. Factors that predict success after a Kasai procedure include a preoperative direct bilirubin <2, absence of liver fibrosis, and limited episodes of cholangitis [230].

Anesthetic Considerations [230]

Coagulopathy should be corrected preoperatively using vitamin K. Platelets and fresh frozen plasma may occasionally be required as well. Oral neomycin and clear fluids should be given for 24 h preoperatively. Broad-spectrum prophylactic antibiotics are essential before skin incision and for 5 days postoperatively to prevent cholangitis (e.g., gentamicin and cefoxitin). Isotonic maintenance fluids containing dextrose are required to avoid intraoperative hypoglycemia, e.g., 1–5 % dextrose in lactated Ringer's solution or 5 % dextrose in PlasmaLyte. Transfusion is usual, although excessive blood loss is uncommon. Hepatorenal syndrome has not been reported in this age group. Ascites is uncommon, but if it develops, losses should be replaced with 5 % albumin. Active warming and invasive access are required as surgery usually takes 2–4 h. An opioid-based/muscle relaxant technique is ideal, avoiding nitrous oxide to prevent bowel distension. The surgeon may kink the inferior vena cava during mobilization of the liver resulting in unexpected hypotension, which may require the immediate infusion of additional intravenous fluids to restore circulatory homeostasis. At the end of surgery, the tracheas of most neonates can be extubated. These neonates are best managed in a high-dependency unit with morphine analgesia [236].

Necrotizing Enterocolitis

Necrotizing enterocolitis (NEC) is the most common surgical neonatal emergency affecting up to 0.5 % of all live births and 10 % of low birth weight (<1,500 g) live births [237]. Advances in neonatal care have improved survival rates for premature and low birth weight infants, as well as those affected by this disease.

Pathogenesis

The etiology of NEC remains unclear although risk factors include prematurity, early formula feeding, cardiac disease, low birth weight, transfusion in the preceding 48 h (transfusion-associated NEC), and sepsis [238, 239]. Breast milk appears to be protective, likely due to transferred immunoglobulins. Multiple gut factors predispose to the development of NEC in preterm neonates including dysmotility, abnormal microbiota, reduced mucin barrier, increased gut permeability, decreased immunoglobulins and gut immunity, increased risk of ischemia, and slow gastric emptying [240, 241]. This in turn may facilitate bacterial translocation across the bowel wall triggering an inflammatory cascade that results in ischemic damage to the bowel. The pathological organisms are often

Table 10.9 Bell classification for diagnosing NEC [242]

Stage IA—suspected disease: temperature instability, increased aspirates, mild distension; radiology normal or dilated loops
Stage IB—as above, with bright red blood per rectum
Stage IIA—proven NEC, mildly ill: as above with absent bowel sounds, ± abdominal tenderness; radiology shows intestinal dilatation, ileus, pneumatosis intestinalis.
Stage IIB—proven NEC, moderately ill: mild metabolic acidosis, mild thrombocytopenia, absent bowel sounds, abdominal tenderness +/– redness of abdominal wall or abdominal mass; radiology shows portal vein gas +/– ascites
Stage IIIA—advanced NEC, severely ill: as above with hypotension, bradycardia, metabolic acidosis, disseminated intravascular coagulation, neutropenia, generalized peritonitis, tenderness and distension; radiology as above with definite ascites
Stage IIIB—advanced NEC, severely ill with perforation: as above with pneumoperitoneum on abdominal X-ray

endogenous bowel flora suggesting an imbalance in the defensive mechanisms rather than a specific virulent organism, although clusters of cases have been known to occur.

Diagnosis

NEC is primarily a clinical diagnosis [237]. It is classified according to the criteria described by Bell (Table 10.9) [242].

Early signs include feeding intolerance, bilious vomiting or increased nasogastric aspirates, abdominal distension with or without tenderness, hemodynamic instability, and blood per rectum (Fig. 10.20). Thrombocytopenia, coagulation abnormalities, and increased inflammatory markers such as C-reactive protein are common. Radiological investigations are often helpful in confirming the presence of NEC. Pathognomonic findings of NEC on abdominal X-ray include distended loops of bowel, pneumatosis intestinalis, and portal venous gas with or without free perforation (Fig. 10.21). The value of ultrasound and other imaging modalities as diagnostic or prognostic tests has yet to be established. Recent laboratory investigations have identified several biomarkers that herald the onset of NEC/sepsis [243, 244]. Such insights may provide the basis for future studies to identify biomarkers that will identify a neonate's risk of developing NEC.

Outcomes

Despite early and aggressive therapy and support, the mortality from NEC remains substantial, in our local series ranging from 30 to 90 % with pan-intestinal disease [245]. In a large prospective study, perioperative mortality was 30 % for all neonates with NEC, compared with 6 % in those managed medically [245, 246]. The mortality rate in neonates who were treated with primary peritoneal drainage alone was 50 %. Significant morbidity occurs in up to 25 % of operative neonates, including stricture formation and failure to thrive, and in those who require extensive resection, short bowel syndrome, and long-term requirement for parenteral nutrition with associated risk of liver disease and sepsis [247]. Neonates with NEC may also experience worse neurological outcomes, particularly those with advanced disease that require surgical intervention [248].

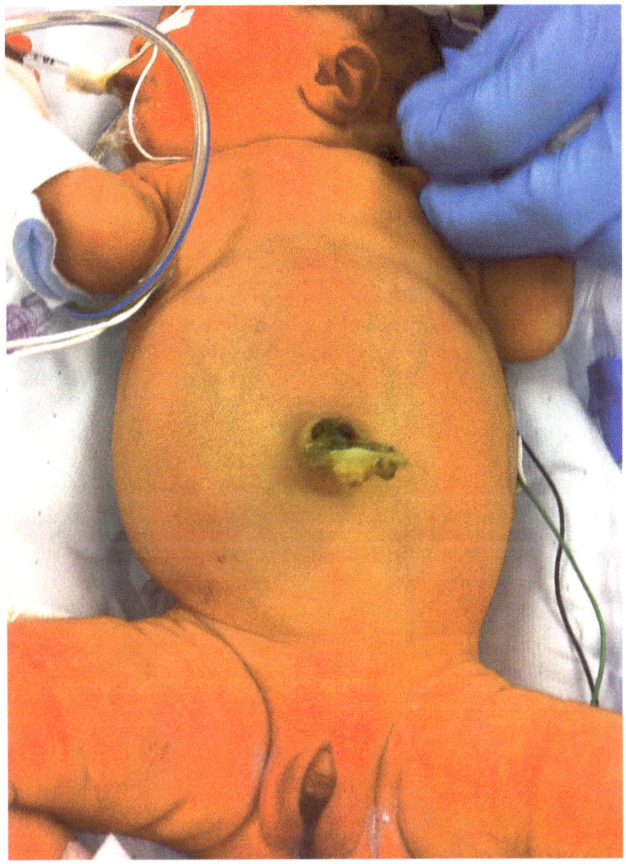

Fig. 10.20 NEC in a preterm neonate. This neonate developed NEC and a distended abdomen. Note the "rectus muscle-sparing" lines separated from the erythema of the anterior abdominal wall (Courtesy of Dr. YH Lee, Division of Pediatric Surgery, Strong Hospital, University of Rochester, Rochester, NY)

Management

The primary approach to NEC is to adopt strategies that prevent the disorder. Such strategies include standardized enteral feeding, exclusive use of human breast milk and milk-based fortifiers, minimal antibiotic exposure, minimal gastric acid blockade therapy, and the use of high-quality probiotics, if the preceding measures fail [240, 249, 250].

Definitive studies for managing NEC once it has occurred are lacking, and treatment has been determined by expert consensus and the neonate's clinical condition [251]. The

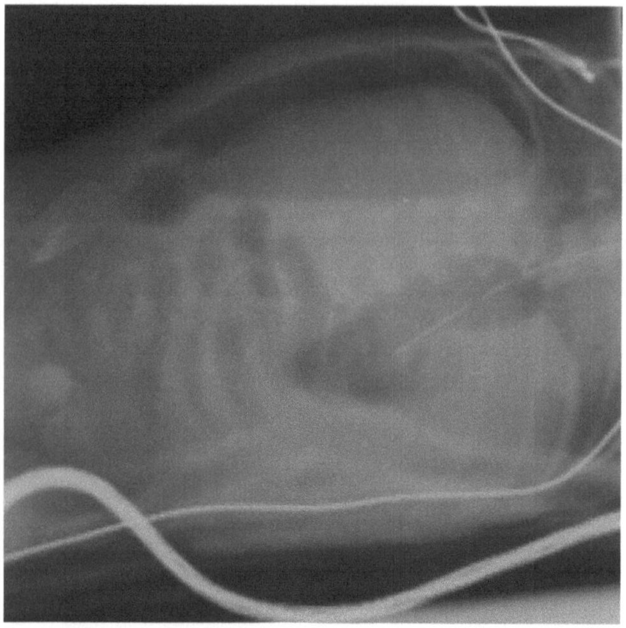

Fig. 10.21 Lateral radiograph of a neonate with NEC. The neonate was positioned in the left lateral decubitus position with a multi-orifice gastric tube in the stomach. Free air is evident against the right (*upper*) lateral abdominal wall, outlining the liver and falciform ligament (Courtesy of Dr. YH Lee, Division of Pediatric Surgery, Strong Hospital, University of Rochester, Rochester, NY)

first-line treatment is medical, targeting sepsis and preventing further intestinal damage. The neonate is kept nil by mouth for 7–10 days, with a nasogastric tube in situ to decompress the stomach, intravenous broad-spectrum antibiotics, and appropriate cardiorespiratory and hematological support. Nutritional challenges can be addressed using total parenteral nutrition (TPN).

It is important to appreciate a little known risk of red cell hemolysis when considering to transfuse with fresh frozen plasma or blood products with plasma [252]. The T antigen, also known as the Thomsen-Friedenreich (or T) cryptantigen, is a naturally occurring but concealed red cell antigen (cryptantigen) that becomes activated when bacteria (e.g., streptococcus, pneumococcus, and Clostridium perfringens) carrying neuraminidase activate the T antigen. Transfusion of plasma that contains immunoglobulin M anti-T antigen binds this activated T antigen causing polyagglutination and red cell hemolysis. Activated T antigen is present in approximately 11–27 % of neonates with NEC, with a greater frequency in more severe NEC (category III NEC 30 % vs. II 4 %) [253, 254]. The magnitude of the risk of T antigen in neonates with NEC is unclear, although many clinicians avoid transfusing plasma-rich blood products to these neonates and many blood banks screen plasma for antibodies to T antigen and release only plasma with low or no titers of T antigen to neonates with NEC. Nonetheless, any child with NEC who develops hemolysis after a transfusion should be investigated to identify the cause, not overlooking the possibility that activated T antigen is the putative agent [7].

Surgical intervention is required in 10–20 % of neonates with NEC, increasing to 50 % in very low birth weight neonates. The indications for surgery include serial examinations that indicate worsening physiological parameters or failure of medical treatment. The precise indications for surgery remain controversial; ideally, surgery is indicated for the presence of gangrenous bowel, before it has perforated [237]. However, there are no reliable metrics to define such a clinical scenario. Absolute indications for surgery include evidence of perforation, clinical deterioration despite maximal medical therapy, an abdominal mass with persistent obstruction or sepsis, and the presence of an intestinal stricture. Relative indications include abdominal tenderness, distension or discoloration where the clinical diagnosis may be in doubt, the finding of portal venous gas on plain abdominal X-ray, a fixed intestinal loop, and thrombocytopenia.

Surgical Approach

The surgical objectives are to control sepsis, to excise necrotic bowel, and to preserve intestinal length [237, 247]. A laparotomy remains the mainstay approach for most neonates with NEC. In the very low birth weight group (<1,000 g) with evidence of perforation, peritoneal drainage has been proposed as either an interim or definitive alternative to laparotomy, although a recent systematic review suggested that this approach is associated with increased morbidity [255]. Surgical options at laparotomy include resection with enterostomy, resection with primary anastomosis, a proximal diverting jejunostomy for extensive disease, and "clip and drop" or the watch and wait with possible "second look" laparotomy [237, 247]. The extent of the disease, the stability of the neonate, and the surgeons' experience/preference will determine which of these options are undertaken. For a stable neonate with focal or multifocal disease, a resection with anastomosis is appropriate. For an unstable neonate in whom the viability of the distal bowel is uncertain, a stoma may be fashioned. In the presence of pan-intestinal disease (>75 % of the small and large bowel involved), either a proximal diverting jejunostomy or the "clip and drop" approach requiring a repeat laparotomy in the next few days is performed. NEC is responsible for one-third of the cases of surgical short bowel syndrome in NICU. Although mortality has been substantial in these neonates, a multifaceted approach to resting and preserving bowel function, nutrition, infectious prophylaxis, and surgical consultation dramatically improved survival [204]. A general guide for the ability of the gut to support enteral feeds long term is the presence of 30 cm of bowel with the ileocecal valve or 50 cm without [237]. In extreme cases where the entire intestine is necrotic, withdrawal of care may be an important consideration.

The neonatal liver is fragile and often enlarged in these infants. Aggressive perioperative resuscitation can result in hepatic engorgement and may result in capsular rupture and life-threatening hemorrhage. Surgical handling can also have similar catastrophic consequences. The laparotomy incision may be performed more caudally or obliquely especially in extremely low birth weight infants, to lie below the liver edge. Strict avoidance of liver instrumentation can help decrease the risk of hemorrhage.

Laparoscopy may be used as a diagnostic tool in NEC if the neonate is stable, if there are signs of obstruction, and if the diagnosis is uncertain. Some have attempted gasless laparoscopic surgery to diagnose and manage NEC in neonates with limited success [256].

Anesthetic Considerations

Laparotomy for NEC in a premature neonate <1,000 g provides a significant challenge for the anesthesiologist. The potential for rapid blood loss in a neonate with cardiorespiratory instability, DIC, and sepsis requires meticulous preparation. In the operating theater, anesthesia may be induced using an opioid such as fentanyl in incremental IV doses of 5–10 mcg/kg up to 25–50 mcg/kg and/or ketamine 2–4 mg/kg and rocuronium [10, 257]. The clearance of fentanyl decreases with decreasing gestational age in neonates with normal intra-abdominal pressure [258]. Inhalational anesthetics are infrequently used in neonates with NEC. Balanced salt solution (10–20 ml/kg) should be administered before induction of anesthesia to prevent hypotension as anesthesia is induced. More recently, remifentanil has been investigated in preterm neonates [259, 260]. The duration of action of remifentanil in premature neonates between 24 and 41 weeks gestation and full-term neonates is similar, 5–10 min. This has been attributed to the similar activity of nonspecific tissues esterases throughout gestation [261]. Animal evidence also suggests that remifentanil may effectively attenuate ischemic-reperfusion injury in the intestines [262]. If true in humans, remifentanil may provide a salutary effect in neonates with potentially ischemic bowel. Before anesthesia is discontinued, a longer-acting opioid should be administered to provide postoperative analgesia.

Surgery may be performed in the operating room or in the NICU (see Anesthesia Outside the OR, Chap. 12). Indications for surgery in the NICU include minor procedures (insertion of a peritoneal drain); a very small, unstable neonate; and ventilation with HFOV. For anesthesia in the NICU, a TIVA technique is required. In such cases, incremental doses of IV fentanyl (10–20 mcg/kg) or a remifentanil infusion, together with ketamine and rocuronium, should provide hemodynamic stability and adequate surgical conditions. The extent of the procedure depends on the hemodynamic stability of the neonate, and close cooperation between surgeon, neonatologist/intensivist, and anesthesiologist is required at all times.

Inotropic support (dopamine, dobutamine, epinephrine, or norepinephrine) is often required, in neonates with NEC. In order to accurately monitor the responses to this support, arterial pressure monitoring is highly recommended. The inotropic support should be tailored to the neonate's requirements and titrated to the desired end point [263]. In addition, venous access large enough to rapidly deliver blood products should be secured. 5 % albumin, blood, platelets, and clotting factors may be required before or during surgery. Warmed IV fluid boluses of 10–20 ml/kg should be given depending on the clinical condition of the child and measured losses, guided by the results of arterial blood gas estimation. Since these neonates are often of very low birth weight, their albumin levels are low. Balanced salt solutions may be used to replace small fluid shifts but are best limited in volume administered to preclude exacerbating preexisting hypoalbuminemia and dilutional coagulopathy. If large volumes of fluid are required (up to 50 ml/kg), it is prudent to switch from balanced salt solutions to albumin and blood products early to maintain the hematological and coagulation profile. At the same time, care must be taken to avoid over transfusing the child, as this could open a ductus arteriosus or risk catastrophic bleeding from a distended liver. The neonate may remain critically ill after surgery requiring full intensive care support. Mild controlled hypothermia may be a therapeutic option in neonates with multiple organ dysfunction [264].

References

1. Morray JP, Geiduschek JM, Ramamoorthy C, et al. Anesthesia-related cardiac arrest in children: initial findings of the Pediatric Perioperative Cardiac Arrest (POCA) Registry. Anesthesiology. 2000;93:6–14.
2. Flick RP, Sprung J, Harrison TE, et al. Perioperative cardiac arrests in children between 1988 and 2005 at a tertiary referral center: a study of 92,881 patients. Anesthesiology. 2007;106:226–37.
3. Van der Griend BJ, Lister NA, McKenzie IM, et al. Postoperative mortality in children after 101,885 at a tertiary hospital. Anesth Analg. 2011;112:1440–7.
4. Thomas J. Reducing the risk in neonatal anesthesia. Pediatr Anesth. 2014;24:106–13.
5. Arnold PD. Coagulation and the surgical neonate. Pediatr Anesth. 2013;24:89–97.
6. Kenton AB, Hegemier S, Smith EO, et al. Platelet transfusions in infants with necrotizing enterocolitis do not lower mortality but may increase morbidity. J Perinatol. 2005;25:173–7.
7. Gibsen BE, British Committee for Standards in Haematology, et al. Transfusion guidelines for neonates and older children. Br J Haematol. 2004;124:433–53.
8. Sloan S. Neonatal transfusions. Pediatr Anesth. 2011;21:25–30.
9. Haynes AB, Weiser TG, Berry WR, et al. A surgical safety checklist to reduce morbidity and mortality in a global population. N Engl J Med. 2009;372:491–9.

10. Robinson S, Gregory GA. Fentanyl-air-oxygen anesthesia for ligation of patent ductus arteriosus in preterm infants. Anesth Analg. 1981;60:331–4.
11. Lonnquist PA. Major abdominal surgery of the neonate: anaesthetic considerations. Best Pract Res Clin Anaesthesiol. 2004; 18:321–42.
12. de Graaff JC, Bijker JB, Kappen TH, et al. Incidence of intraoperative hypoxemia in children in relation to age. Anesth Analg. 2013;117:169–75.
13. Weiss M, Gerber AC. Rapid sequence induction in children—it's not a matter of time! Paediatr Anaesth. 2008;18:97–9.
14. Eich C, Timmermann A, Russo SG, et al. A controlled rapid-sequence induction technique for infants may reduce unsafe actions and stress. Acta Anaesthesiol Scand. 2009;53:1167–72.
15. Lerman J. On cricoid pressure: "May the force be with you". Anesth Analg. 2009;109:1363–6.
16. Walker RWM, Ravi R, Haylett K. Effect of cricoid force on airway caliber in children: a bronchoscopic assessment. Br J Anaesth. 2010;104:71–4.
17. Oh J, Lim T, Chee Y, et al. Videographic analysis of glottic view with increasing cricoid pressure force. Ann Emerg Med. 2013; 61:407–13.
18. Hillier SC, Scamberger MS. Transcutaneous and end-tidal carbon dioxide analysis: complimentary monitoring strategies. J Intensive Care Med. 2005;20:307–9.
19. Trevisanuto D, Giuliotto S, Cavallin F, et al. End-tidal carbon dioxide monitoring in very low birth weight infants: correlation and agreement with arterial carbon dioxide. Pediatr Pulmonol. 2012;47:367–72.
20. Tingay DG, Mun KS, Perkins EJ. End tidal carbon dioxide is as reliable as transcutaneous monitoring in ventilated postsurgical neonates. Arch Dis Child Fetal Neonatal Ed. 2013;98:F161–4.
21. Singh BS, Gilbert U, Singh S, et al. Sidestream microstream end tidal carbon dioxide measurements and blood gas correlations in neonatal intensive care unit. Pediatr Pulmonol. 2013;48:250–6.
22. Freer Y, Lyon A. Temperature monitoring and control in the newborn baby. Paediatr Child Health. 2011;22:127–30.
23. Witt L, Dennhardt N, Eich C, et al. Prevention of intraoperative hypothermia in neonates and infants: results of a prospective multicenter observational study with a new forced-air warming system with increased warm air flow. Pediatr Anesth. 2013;23:469–74.
24. Murat I, Humblot A, Girault L, Piana F. Neonatal fluid management. Best Pract Res Clin Anaesthesiol. 2010;24:365–74.
25. O'Brien F, Walker IA. Fluid homeostasis in the neonate. Pediatr Anesth. 2014;24:49–59.
26. Apfelbaum JL, Caplan RA, Connis RT, et al. Practice guidelines for preoperative fasting and the use of pharmacologic agents to reduce the risk of aspiration: application to healthy patients undergoing elective procedures. Anesthesiology. 2011;114:495–511.
27. Sumpelmann R, Kretz F-J, Luntzer R, et al. Hydroxyethyl starch 130/0.42/6:1 for perioperative volume replacement in 1130 children: results of an European prospective multicenter observational postauthorization safety study (PASS). Paediatr Anaesth. 2012;22:371–8.
28. Hall NJ, Stanton MP, Kitteringham LJ, et al. Scope and feasibility of operating on the neonatal intensive care unit: 310 cases in 10 years. Pediatr Surg Int. 2012;28:1001–5.
29. Davidson AJ. Neurotoxicity and the need for anesthesia in the newborn. Does the Emperor have no clothes? Anesthesiol. 2012;116:507–9.
30. Hall NJ, Pacilli M, Eaton S, et al. Recovery after open versus laparoscopic pyloromyotomy for pyloric stenosis: a double blind multicentre randomised controlled trial. Lancet. 2009;373:390–8.
31. Sinha CK, Paramalingam S, Patel S, et al. Feasibility of complex minimally invasive surgery in neonates. Pediatr Surg Int. 2009;25:217–21.
32. Carrington EV, Hall NJ, Pacilli M, et al. Cost-effectiveness of laparoscopic versus open pyloromyotomy. J Surg Res. 2012; 179:315–20.
33. Dingemann J, Ure BM. Systematic review of level 1 evidence for laparoscopic pediatric surgery: do our procedures comply with the requirements of evidence-based medicine?? Eur J Pediatr Surg. 2013;23:474–9.
34. Rothenberg SS. Thoracoscopic repair of esophageal atresia and tracheo-esophageal fistula in neonates: evolution of a technique. J Laparoendosc Adv Surg Tech A. 2012;22:195–9.
35. Holcomb GW, Rothenberg SS, Klaas MA. Thoracoscopic repair of esophageal atresia and tracheoesophageal fistula. A multi institutional analysis. Ann Surg. 2005;242:422–30.
36. Chan IH, Lau CT, Chung PH, et al. Laparoscopic inguinal hernia repair in premature neonates: is it safe? Pediatr Surg Int. 2013;29:327–30.
37. Olsen M, Avery N, Khurana S, et al. Pneumoperitoneum for neonatal laparoscopy: how safe is it? Pediatr Anesth. 2013;23: 457–9.
38. Nasr A, Bass J. Thoracoscopic vs open resection of congenital lung lesions: a meta-analysis. J Pediatr Surg. 2012;47:857–61.
39. Lerman J, Kondo Y, Suzuki Y, et al. Chapter 27: General abdominal and urologic surgery. In: Coté CJ, Lerman J, Anderson B, editors. A practice of anesthesia for infants and children. Philadelphia, PA: Elsevier; 2012.
40. Groenewald CB, Latham GJ. An unexpected cause of cardiac arrest during laparoscopy in an infant with supravalvar aortic stenosis. Pediatr Anesth. 2013;23:91–3.
41. Gillory LA, Megison ML, Harmon CM, et al. Laparoscopic surgery in children with congenital heart disease. J Pediatr Surg. 2012;47:1084–8.
42. Slater B, Rangel S, Ramamoorthy C, et al. Outcomes after laparoscopic surgery in neonates with hypoplastic heart left heart syndrome. J Pediatr Surg. 2007;42:1118–21.
43. Pacilli M, Pierro A, Kinglsey C, et al. Absorption of carbon dioxide during laparoscopy in children measured using a novel mass spectrometric technique. Br J Anaesth. 2006;97:215–9.
44. Bliss D, Matar M, Krishnaswami S. Should intraoperative hypercapnea or hypercarbia raise concern in neonates undergoing thoracoscopic repair of diaphragmatic hernia of Bochdalek? J Laparoendosc Adv Surg Tech A. 2009;19:s55–8.
45. Bishay M, Giacomello L, Retrosi G, et al. Decreased cerebral oxygen saturation during thoracoscopic repair of congenital diaphragmatic hernia and esophageal atresia in infants. J Pediatr Surg. 2001;46:47–51.
46. McHoney M, Corizia L, Eaton S, et al. Carbon dioxide elimination during laparoscopy in children is age dependent. J Pediatr Surg. 2003;38:105–10.
47. Parelkar SV, Oak SN, Bachani MK, et al. Minimal access surgery in newborns and small infants; five years experience. J Minim Access Surg. 2013;9:19–24.
48. Kalfa N, Allal H, Raux O, et al. Tolerance of laparoscopy and thoracoscopy in neonates. Pediatrics. 2005;116:e785–91.
49. Ure BM, Suempelmann R, Metzelder M, et al. Physiological responses to endoscopic surgery in children. Semin Pediatr Surg. 2007;16:217–23.
50. Li LW, Zhang W, Ai YQ, et al. Influence of laparoscopic carbon dioxide pneumoperitoneum on neonate circulation and respiration. J Int Med Res. 2013;41:889–94.
51. McHoney M, Mackinlay G, Munro F, et al. Effect of patient weight and anesthetic technique on CO2 excretion during thoracoscopy in children assessed by end-tidal CO2. J Laparoendosc Adv Surg Tech A. 2008;18:147–51.
52. Kalfa N, Alla H, Raux O, et al. Multicentric assessment of the safety of neonatal videosurgery. Surg Endosc. 2007;21:303–8.
53. Kuebler JF, Ure BM. Minimally invasive surgery in the neonate. Semin Fetal Neonatal Med. 2011;16:151–6.

54. Tobias JD. Anesthesia for neonatal thoracic surgery. Best Pract Res Clin Anaesthesiol. 2004;18:303–20.
55. Hammer GB. Chapter 13: Anesthesia for thoracic surgery. In: Coté CJ, Lerman J, Anderson B, editors. A practice of anesthesia for infants and children. Philadelphia, PA: Elsevier; 2012.
56. Choudhry DK. Single-lung ventilation in pediatric anesthesia. Anesthesiol Clin North America. 2005;23:693–708.
57. Langston C. New concepts in the pathology of congenital lung malformations. Semin Pediatr Surg. 2003;12:17–37.
58. Guidry C, McGahren ED. Pediatric Chest 1. Developmental and physiologic conditions for the surgeon. Surg Clin N Am. 2012;92:615–43.
59. Adzick NS, Flake AW, Crombleholme TM. Management of congenital lung lesions. Semin Pediatr Surg. 2003;12:10–6.
60. Raychaudhuri P, Pasupati A, James A, et al. Prospective study of antenatally diagnosed congenital cystic adenomatoid malformations. Pediatr Surg Int. 2011;27:1159–64.
61. Kotecha S, Barbato A, Bush A, et al. Antenatal and postnatal management of congenital cystic adenomatoid malformation. Paediatr Respir Rev. 2012;13:162–70.
62. Yong PJ, Von Dadelszen P, Carpara D, et al. Prediction of pediatric outcome after prenatal diagnosis and expectant antenatal management of congenital cystic adenomatoid malformation. Fetal Diagn Ther. 2012;31:94–102.
63. Davenport M, Eber E. Long term respiratory outcomes of congenital thoracic malformation. Semin Fetal Neonatal Med. 2012;17:99–104.
64. Stocker JT, Madewell JE, Drake RM. Congenital cystic adenomatoid malformation of the lung. Classification and morphologic spectrum. Hum Pathol. 1977;8:155–71.
65. Stocker JT. Congenital pulmonary airway malformation-a new name for and an expanded classification of congenital cystic adenomatoid malformation of the lung. Histopathology. 2002;41 Suppl 2:424–58.
66. Fitzgerald DA. Congenital cyst adenomatoid malformations: resect some and observe all? Pediatr Respir Rev. 2007;8:67–76.
67. Khosa JK, Leong SL, Borzi PA. Congenital cystic adenomatoid malformation of the lung: indications and timing of surgery. Pediatr Surg Int. 2004;20:505–8.
68. Davenport M, Cacciaguerra S, Patel S, et al. Current outcome of antenatally diagnosed cystic lung disease. J Pediatr Surg. 2004;39:549–56.
69. Waszak P, Claris O, Lapillonne A, et al. Cystic adenomatoid malformation of the lung: neonatal management of 21 cases. Pediatr Surg Int. 1999;15:326–31.
70. Azizkhan RG, Crombleholme TM. Congenital cystic lung disease: contemporary antenatal and postnatal management. Pediatr Surg Int. 2008;24:643–57.
71. Colon N, Schlegel C, Pietsch J, et al. Congenital lung anomalies: can we postpone resection? J Pediatr Surg. 2012;47:87–92.
72. Peters RT, Burge DM, Marven SS. Congenital lung malformations: an ongoing controversy. Ann R Coll Surg Engl. 2013;95:144–7.
73. Delacourt C, Hadchouel A, Dunlop NK. Shall all congenital cystic lung malformations be removed? The case in favour. Paediatr Respir Rev. 2013;14:169–70.
74. Kotecha S. Should asymptomatic congenital cystic adenomatous malformations be removed? The case against. Paediatr Respir Rev. 2013;14:171–2.
75. Guruswamy V, Roberts S, Arnold P, et al. Anaesthetic management of a neonate with congenital cyst adenoid malformation. Br J Anaesth. 2005;95:240–2.
76. Nishimoto C, Inomata S, Kihara S, et al. Anesthetic management of four pediatric patients with CCAM for pulmonary lobectomy. Masui. 2002;51:162–5.
77. Baud D, Windrim R, Kachura JR, et al. Minimally invasive fetal therapy for hydropic lung masses: three different approaches and review of the literature. Ultrasound Obstet Gynecol. 2013;42:440–8.
78. Krivchenya DU, Rudenko EO, Dubrovin AG. Congenital emphysema in children: segmental lung resection as an alternative to lobectomy. J Pediatr Surg. 2013;48:309–14.
79. Iodice F, Harban F, Walker I. Anesthetic management of a patient with bilateral congenital lobar emphysema. Pediatr Anesth. 2008;18:340–1.
80. Arora MK, Karamchandani K, Bakhta P, et al. Combination of inhalational, intravenous, and local anesthesia for intubation in neonates with congenital lobar emphysema. Pediatr Anesth. 2006;16:997–1003.
81. Goyal A, Jones MO, Couriel JM, et al. Oesophageal atresia and tracheo-oesophageal fistula. Arch Dis Child Fetal Neonatal Ed. 2006;91:F381–4.
82. Knottenberlt G, Skinner A, Seefelder C. Tracheo-oesophageal fistula (TOF) and oesophageal atresia (OA). Best Pract Res Clin Anaesthesiol. 2010;24:387–401.
83. Spitz L. Oesophageal atresia. Orphanet J Rare Dis. 2007;2:24.
84. Jacobs IJ, Que J. Genetic and cellular mechanisms of the formation of esophageal atresia and tracheoesophageal fistula. Dis Esophagus. 2013;26:356–8.
85. Holzki J. Bronchoscopic findings and treatment in congenital tracheo-oesophageal fistula. Pediatr Anesth. 1992;2:297–303.
86. Passi Y, Sampathi V, Pierre J, et al. Esophageal atresia with double tracheoesophageal fistula. Anesthesiology. 2013;118:1207.
87. Diaz LK, Akpek EA, Radhika D, et al. Tracheoesophageal fistula and associated congenital heart disease: implications for anesthetic management and survival. Pediatr Anesth. 2005;15:862–9.
88. Stringer MD, McKenna K, Goldstein RB, et al. Prenatal diagnosis of esophageal atresia. J Pediatr Surg. 1995;30:1258–63.
89. Okamoto T, Takamizawa S, Hiroshi A. Esophageal atresia: prognostic classification revisited. Surgery. 2009;145:675–81.
90. La Placa S, Giuffre M, Gangemi A, et al. Esophageal atresia in newborns: a wide spectrum from the isolated forms to a full VACTERL phenotype? Ital J Pediatr. 2013;39:45.
91. Babu R, Pierro A, Spitz L, et al. The management of oesophageal atresia in neonates with right-sided aortic arch. J Pediatr Surg. 2000;35:56–8.
92. Solomon BD. VACTERL/VATER Association. Orphanet J Rare Dis. 2011;6:56.
93. Solomon BD, Baker LA, Bear KA, et al. An approach to the identification of anomalies and etiologies in neonates with identified or suspected VACTERL (vertebral Defects, anal atresia, tracheoesophageal fistula with esophageal atresia, cardiac anomalies, renal anomalies, and limb anomalies) Association. J Pediatr. 2014;164:451–7.e1.
94. De Jong EM, Felix JF, Deurloo JA, et al. Non-VACTERL-type anomalies are frequent in patients with esophageal atresia/tracheoesophageal fistula and full or partial VACTERL association. Birth Defects Res A Clin Mol Teratol. 2008;82:92–7.
95. Lopez PJ, Keys C, Pierro A, et al. Oesophageal atresia: improved outcome in high-risk groups? J Pediatr Surg. 2006;41:331–4.
96. Alabbad SI, Shaw K, Puligandla PS, et al. The pitfalls of endotracheal intubation beyond the fistula in babies with type C esophageal atresia. Semin Pediatr Surg. 2009;18:116–8.
97. Ni Y, Yao Y, Liang P. Simple strategy of anesthesia for the neonate with tracheoesophageal fistula: a case report. Int J Clin Exp Med. 2014;7(1):327–8.
98. Deanovic D, Gerber A, Dodge-Khatatami A, et al. Tracheoscopy assisted repair of tracheo-esophageal fistula (TARTEF): a 10-year experience. Pediatr Anesth. 2007;17:557–62.

99. Huang J, Tao J, Chen K, et al. Thoracoscopic repair of oesophageal atresia: experience of 33 patients from two tertiary referral centres. J Pediatr Surg. 2012;47:2224–7.
100. Rothenberg SS. Thoracoscopic repair of esophageal atresia and tracheoesophageal fistula in neonates, first decade's experience. Dis Esophagus. 2013;26:359–64.
101. Bishay M, Giacomello L, Retrosi G, et al. Hypercapnia and acidosis during open and thoracoscopic repair of congenital diaphragmatic hernia and esophageal atresia: results of a pilot randomized controlled trial. Ann Surg. 2013;258:895–900.
102. McKinnon G. Esophageal atresia surgery in the 21st century. Semin Pediatr Surg. 2009;18:20–2.
103. Delacourt C, Hadchouel A, Toelen J, et al. Long term respiratory outcomes of congenital diaphragmatic hernia, esophageal atresia, and cardiovascular anomalies. Semin Fetal Neonatal med. 2012;17:105–11.
104. Kovesi T. Long-term respiratory complications of congenital esophageal atresia with or without tracheoesophageal fistula: an update. Dis Esophagus. 2013;26:413–6.
105. Caplan A. Psychological impact of esophageal atresia: review of the research and clinical evidence. Dis Esophagus. 2013;26:392–400.
106. Andropoulos DB, Rowe RW, Betts JM. Anaesthetic and surgical airway management during tracheo-oesophageal fistula repair. Pediatr Anesth. 1998;8:313–9.
107. Knottenbelt G, Costi D, Stephens P, et al. An audit of anesthetic management and complications of tracheo-esophageal fistula and esophageal atresia repair. Pediatr Anesth. 2012;22: 268–74.
108. Krosnar S, Baxter A. Thoracoscopic repair of esophageal atresia with tracheoesophageal fistula: anesthetic and intensive care management of a series of eight neonates. Pediatr Anesth. 2005; 15:541–6.
109. Broemling N, Campbell F. Anaesthetic management of congenital tracheoesophageal fistula. Pediatr Anesth. 2011;21:1092–9.
110. Haroon J, Chamberlain RS. An evidence-based review of the current treatment of congenital diaphragmatic hernia. Clin Pediagtr (Phila). 2013;52:115–24.
111. Tovar JA. Congenital diaphragmatic hernia. Orphanet J Rare Dis. 2012;7:1.
112. Bosenberg A, Brown RA. Management of congenital diaphragmatic hernia. Curr Opin Anaesthesiol. 2008;21:323–31.
113. Seydel B, Detry O. Morgagni's hernia. NEJM. 2010;362:e61.
114. Samangaya RA, Choudhri S, Murphy F, et al. Outcomes of congenital diaphragmatic hernia: a 12-year experience. Prenat Diagn. 2012;32:523–9.
115. Veenma DCM, de Klein A, Tibboel D. Developmental and genetic aspects of congenital diaphragmatic hernia. Pediatr Pulmonol. 2012;47:534–5.
116. Garne E, Haeusler M, Barisic I, et al. Congenital diaphragmatic hernia: evaluation of prenatal diagnosis in 20 European regions. Ultrasound Obstet Gynecol. 2002;19:329–33.
117. The Congenital Diaphragmatic Hernia Study Group. Defect size determines survival in infants with congenital diaphragmatic hernia. Pediatrics. 2007;120:e651–7.
118. Hedrick HL, Danzer E, Merchant A. Liver position and lung-to-head ratio for prediction of extracorporeal membrane oxygenation and survival in isolated left congenital diaphragmatic hernia. Am J Obstet Gynecol. 2007;197:422.e1–4.
119. Suda K, Bigras JL, Bohn D, et al. Echocardiographic predictors of outcome in newborns with congenital diaphragmatic hernia. Pediatrics. 2000;105:1106.
120. Garriboli M, Duess JW, Ruttenstock E, et al. Trends in the treatment and outcome of congenital diaphragmatic hernia over the last decade. Pediatr Surg Int. 2012;28:1177–81.
121. Chiu PPL, Ijsselstijn H. Morbidity and long term follow-up in CDH patients. Eur J Pediatr Surg. 2012;22:384–92.
122. Congenital Diaphragmatic Hernia Study Group, Morini F, Valfre L, Capolupo I, et al. Congenital diaphragmatic hernia: defect size correlates with developmental defect. J Pediatr Surg. 2013;48:1177–82.
123. Takahashi S, Sago H, Kanamori Y, et al. Prognostic factors of congenital diaphragmatic hernia accompanied by cardiovascular malformation. Pediatr Int. 2013;55:492–7.
124. Lally KP, Lasky RE, Lally PA, et al. Standardized reporting for congenital diaphragmatic hernia—an international consensus. J Pediatr Surg. 2013;48:2408–15.
125. Harrison MR, Sydorak RM, Farrell JA, et al. Fetoscopic temporary tracheal occlusion for congenital diaphragmatic hernia: prelude to a randomized, controlled trial. J Pediatr Surg. 2003;38:1012–20.
126. Jani JC, Nicolaides KH, Gratacos E, et al. Severe diaphragmatic hernia treated with endoscopic tracheal occlusion. Ultrasound Obstet Gynecol. 2009;34:304–10.
127. Speggiorin S, Fierens A, McHugh K, et al. Bronchomegaly as a complication of fetal endoscopic tracheal occlusion. A caution and a possible solution. J Pediatr Surg. 2011;46:e1–3.
128. Ruano R, Yoshisaki CT, Da Silva MM, et al. A randomized controlled trial of fetal endoscopic tracheal occlusion versus postnatal management of severe isolated congenital diaphragmatic hernia. Ultrasound Obstet Gynecol. 2012;39:20–7.
129. Boloker J, Bateman DA, Wung JT, et al. Congenital diaphragmatic hernia in 120 infants treated consecutively with permissive hypercapnea/spontaneous respiration/elective repair. J Pediatr Surg. 2002;37:357–66.
130. Logan JW, Rice HE, Goldberg RN, Cotten CM. Congenital diaphragmatic hernia: a systematic review and summary of best-evidence practice strategies. J Perinatol. 2007;27:535–49.
131. Van den Hout L, Tinbboel D, Vifhuize S, et al. The VICI trial: high frequency oscillation versus conventional mechanical ventilation in newborns with congenital diaphragmatic hernia: an international multicentre randomized controlled trial. BMC Pediatr. 2011;11:98.
132. Bialkowski A, Moenkemeyer F, Patel N. Intravenous sildenafil in the management of pulmonary hypertension associated with congenital diaphragmatic hernia. Eur J Pediatr Surg. 2013 Oct 25. [Epub ahead of print].
133. Vijfhuize S, Schaible T, Kraemer U, et al. Management of pulmonary hypertension in neonates with congenital diaphragmatic hernia. Eur J Pediatr Surg. 2012;22:374–83.
134. Beres AL, Puligandla PS, Brindle ME, et al. Stability prior to surgery in congenital diaphragmatic hernia: is it necessary? J Pediatr Surg. 2013;48:919–23.
135. Morini F, Bagolan P. Surgical techniques in diaphragmatic hernia. Eur J Pediatr Surg. 2012;22:355–63.
136. Congenital diaphragmatic hernia group. Minimally invasive repair of congenital diaphragmatic hernia. J Pediatr Surg. 2011;46: 11158–64.
137. Ellinas H, Seefelder C. Congenital thoracoscopic repair in neonates: is thoracoscopy feasible? Pediatr Anesth. 2010;20:967–8.
138. Peevy KJ, Speed FA, Hoff CJ. Epidemiology of inguinal hernia in preterm neonates. Pediatrics. 1986;77:246–7.
139. Choi W, Hall NJ, Garriboldi M, et al. Outcomes following laparoscopic inguinal hernia repair in infants compared with older children. Pediatr Surg Int. 2012;28:1165–9. doi:10.1007/s00383-012-3188-1.
140. Pennant JH. Anesthesia for laparoscopy in the pediatric patient. Anesthesiol Clin North America. 2001;19:69–88.
141. Lee SL, Gleason JM, Sydorak RM. A critical review of premature infants with inguinal hernias: optimal timing of repair, incarceration risk, and postoperative apnea. J Pediatr Surg. 2011;46:217–20.
142. Cote CJ, Zaslavsky A, Downes JJ, et al. Postoperative apnea in former preterm infants after inguinal herniorrhaphy. A combined analysis. Anesthesiology. 1995;82:809–22.

143. Lacrosse D, Pirotte T, Veyckmans F. Caudal block and light sevoflurane mask anesthesia in high-risk infants: an audit of 98 cases. Ann Fr Anesth Reanim. 2012;31:29–33.
144. Walther-Larsen S, Rasmussen LS. The former preterm infant and risk of postoperative apnoea: recommendations for management. Acta Anaesthesiol Scand. 2006;50:888–93.
145. Sale SM, Read JA, Stoddart PA, Wolf AR. Prospective comparison of sevoflurane and desflurane in formerly premature infants undergoing inguinal herniotomy. Br J Anaesth. 2006;96:774–8.
146. Craven PD, Badwani N, Henderson-Smart D-J, O'Brien M. Regional (spinal, epidural, caudal) versus general anesthesia in preterm infants undergoing inguinal herniorrhaphy in early infancy (review). Cochrane Database Syst Rev. 2003;3, CD003669.
147. Welborn LG, Hannallah RS, Fink R, et al. High-dose caffeine suppresses postoperative apnea in former preterm infants. Anesthesiology. 1989;71:347–9.
148. Davidson A, McCann ME, Morton N, et al. Protocol 09PRT/9078: a multi-site randomised controlled trial to compare regional and general anaesthesia for effects on neurodevelopmental outcome and apnoea in infants: the GAS study (ACTRN12606000441516, NCT00756600). The Lancet protocol reviews. http://www.thelancet.com/protocol-reviews/09PRT9078. Accessed 6 Dec 2012.
149. Modarressi T. The question of an infectious etiology or contribution to the pathogenesis of infantile hypertrophic pyloric stenosis. J Pediatr Gastroenterol Nutr. 2014;58:546–8. doi:10.1097/MPG.
150. Georgoula C, Gardiner M. Pyloric stenosis a 100 years after Ramstedt. Arch Dis Child. 2012;97:741–5.
151. McAteer JP, Ledbetter DJ, Goldin AB. Role of bottle feeding in the etiology of hypertrophic pyloric stenosis. JAMA Pediatr. 2013;167:1143–9.
152. Krogh C, Biggar RJ, Fischer TK, et al. Bottle-feeding and the risk of pyloric stenosis. Pediatrics. 2012;130:e943–9.
153. Aspelind G, Langer JC. Current management of hypertrophic pyloric stenosis. Semin Pediatr Surg. 2007;16:27–33.
154. Glatstein M, Carbell G, Boddu SK, et al. The changing clinical presentation of hypertrophic pyloric stenosis: the experience of a large tertiary care pediatric hospital. Clin Pediatr. 2011;50:192–5.
155. Taylor ND, Cass DT, Holland AJ. Infantile hypertrophic pyloric stenosis: has anything changed? J Paediatr Child Health. 2013;49:33–7.
156. Tutay GJ, Capraro G, SPirko B, et al. Electrolyte profile of pediatric patients with hypertrophic pyloric stenosis. Pediatr Emerg Care. 2013;29:465–8.
157. Iqbal CW, Rivard DC, Mortellaro VE, et al. Evaluation of ultrasonographic parameters in the diagnosis of pyloric stenosis relative to patient age and size. J Pediatr Surg. 2012;47:1542–7.
158. Oomen MWN, Hoekstra LT, Bakx R, et al. Open versus laparoscopic pyloromyotomy for hypertrophic pyloric stenosis: a systematic review and meta-analysis focusing on major complications. Surg Endosc. 2012;26:2104–10.
159. Turial S, Enders J, Schier F. Microlaparoscopic pyloromyotomy in children: initial experiences with a new technique. Surg Endosc. 2011;25:266–70.
160. Bissonnette B, Sullivan PJ. Pyloric stenosis. Can J Anaesth. 1991;38:668–76.
161. Stoddart PA, Brennan L, Hatch D-J, Bingham R. Postal survey of paediatric practice and training among consultant anaesthetists in the UK. Br J Anaesth. 1994;73:559–63.
162. Black SJ, Carson EM, Doughty A. How much and where: assessment of knowledge level of the application of cricoid pressure. J Emerg Nurs. 2012;38:370–4.
163. Landsman I. Cricoid pressure: indications and complications. Paediatr Anaesth. 2004;14:43–7.
164. Rapp HJ, Altenmueller CA, Waschke C. Neuromuscular recovery following rocuronium bromide single dose in infants. Pediatr Anesth. 2004;14:329–35.
165. Driessen JJ, Robertson EN, Booij LHDJ. Acceleromyography in neonates and small infants: baseline calibration and recovery of the responses after neuromuscular blockade with rocuronium. Eur J Anaesthesiol. 2005;22:11–5.
166. Hassid S, Nicaise C, Michel F, et al. Randomized controlled trial of sevoflurane for intubation in neonates. Pediatr Anesth. 2007;17:1053–8.
167. Davis PJ, Galinkin J, McGowan FX, et al. A randomized multicenter study of remifentanil compared with halothane in neonates and infants undergoing pyloromyotomy. 1. Emergence and recovery profiles. Anesth Analg. 2011;93:1380–6.
168. Breschan C, Jost R, Stettner H, et al. Ultrasound-guided rectus sheath block for pyloromyotomy in infants: a retrospective analysis of a case series. Pediatr Anesth. 2013;23:1199–204.
169. Willschke H, Machata AM, Rebhandl W, et al. Management of hypertrophic pylorus stenosis with ultrasound guided single shot epidural anaesthesia—a retrospective analysis of 20 cases. Paediatr Anaesth. 2011;21:110–5.
170. Ghazal E, Amin A, Wu A, et al. Impact of rocuronium vs succinylcholine neuromuscular blocking drug choice for laparoscopic pyloromyotomy: is there a difference in tine to transport to recovery? Pediatr Anesth. 2013;23:316–21.
171. Taylor RH, Lerman J. Minimum alveolar concentration of desflurane and hemodynamic responses in neonates, infants, and children. Anesthesiology. 1991;75:975–9.
172. Lerman J. Surgical and patient factors involved in postoperative nausea and vomiting. Br J Anaesth. 1992;69 Suppl 1:24S–32.
173. Hajivassiliou CA. Intestinal obstruction in neonatal/pediatric surgery. Semin Pediatr Surg. 2003;12:241–53.
174. Best KE, Tennant PW, Addor MC, et al. Epidemiology of small intestinal atresia in Europe: a register-based study. Arch Dis Child Fetal Neonatal Ed. 2012;97:F353–8.
175. Grosfeld JL, Ballantine TVN, Shoemaker R. Operative management of intestinal atresia and stenosis based on pathologic findings. J Pediatr Surg. 1979;14:368–75.
176. Vecchia LKD, Grosfeld JL, West KW, et al. Intestinal atresia and stenosis. A 25-year experience with 277 cases. Arch Surg. 1998;133:490–7.
177. Carlyle BE, Borowitz DS, Glick PL. A review of pathophysiology and management of fetuses and neonates with meconium ileus for the pediatric surgeon. J Pediatr Surg. 2012;47:772–81.
178. Kumar N, Curry I. Bile-stained vomiting in the infant: green is not good! Arch Dis Child Educ Pract Ed. 2008;93:84–6.
179. Hagendoorn J, Viera-Travassos D, van der Zee D. Laparoscopic treatment of intestinal malrotation in neonates and infants: retrospective study. Surg Endosc. 2001;25:217–20.
180. Hsiao M, Langer JC. Surgery for suspected rotation abnormality: selection of open vs laparoscopic surgery using a rational approach. J Pediatr Surg. 2012;47:904–10.
181. Kiely EM, Pierro A, Pierce C, Cross K, De Coppi P. Clot dissolution: a novel treatment of midgut volvulus. Pediatrics. 2012;129: e1601–4.
182. Kenny S, Tam PKH, Garcia-Barcelo M. Hirschsprung's disease. Semin Pediatr Surg. 2010;19:194–200.
183. Saeed A, Barreto L, Neogii SG, et al. Identification of novel genes in Hirschsprung disease pathway using whole genome expression study. J Pediatr Surg. 2012;47:303–7.
184. Georgeson KE, Cohen RD, Hebra A, et al. Primary laparoscopic-assisted endorectal pull-through for Hirschsprung's disease. A new gold standard. Ann Surg. 1999;229:678–83.
185. Nah SA, De Coppi P, Kiely EM, et al. Duhamel pull-through for Hirschsprung's disease: a comparison of open and laparoscopic techniques. J Pediatr Surg. 2012;47:308–12.
186. Holscheneider A, Hutson J, Pena A. Preliminary report on the international conference for the development of standards for the treatment of anorectal malformations. J Pediatr Surg. 2005;40:1521–6.

187. Levitt MA, Pena A. Anorectal malformations. Orphanet J Rare Dis. 2007;2:33.
188. Rintala RJ. Congenital anorectal malformations: anything new? J Pediatr Gastroenterol Nutr. 2009;48:s79–82.
189. Berde CB. Convulsion associated with pediatric regional anesthesia. Anesth Analg. 1992;75:164–6.
190. Kart T, Chrisrup LL, Rasmussen M. Recommended use of morphine in neonates, infants and children based on a literature review: Part 1-Pharmacokinetcs. Pediatr Anaesth. 1997;7:5–11.
191. Hall RW, Kronsberg SS, Barton BA, et al. Morphine, hypotension, and adverse outcomes among preterm neonates: who's to blame? Secondary results from the NEOPAIN trial. Pediatrics. 2005;115:1351–9.
192. Anand KJS, Anderson BJ, Holford NHG, et al. Morphine pharmacokinetics and pharmacodynamics in preterm and term neonates: secondary results from the NEOPAIN trial. Br J Anaesth. 2008;101:680–9.
193. Mastrolacovo P. Risk factors for gastroschisis. BMJ. 2008; 336:1386–7.
194. Gill SK, Broussard C, Devine O, et al. Association between maternal age and birth defects of unknown etiology—United States 1997-2007. Birth Defect Res A Clin Mol Teratol. 2012;94: 1010–18.
195. Kirby RS, Marshall J, Tanner JP, et al. Prevalence and correlates of gastroschisis in 15 states, 1995-2005. Obstet Gynecol. 2013; 122:275–81.
196. Kim K, Wang Y, Kirby RS, et al. Prevalence and trends of selected congenital malformations in New York state, 1983 to 2007. Birth Defects Res A Clin Mol Teratol. 2013;97:619–27.
197. Ghionzoli M, James CP, David AL, et al. Gastroschisis with intestinal atresia—predictive value of antenatal diagnosis and outcome of postnatal treatment. J Pediatr Surg. 2012;47:322–8.
198. Horton AL, Powell MS, Wolfe HM. Intrauterine growth patterns in fetal gastroschisis. Am J Perinatol. 2010;27:211–7.
199. Nasr A, Langer JC. Canadian paediatric surgery network. J Pediatr Surg. 2012;47:2022–5.
200. Grant NH, Dorling J, Thornton JG. Elective preterm birth for fetal gastroschisis. Cochrane Database Syst Rev. 2013 (6): CD009394.pub2.
201. Nasr A, Wayne C, Bass J, et al. Effect of delivery approach on outcomes in fetuses with gastroschisis. J Pediatr Surg. 2013; 48:2251–5.
202. Ledbetter DJ. Congenital abdominal wall defects and reconstruction in pediatric surgery: gastroschisis and omphalocele. Surg Clin N Am. 2012;92:713–27.
203. Aljahdali A, Mohajerani N, Skarsgard ED, et al. Effect of timing of enteral feeding on outcome in gastroschisis. J Pediatr Surg. 2013;48:971–6.
204. Amin SC, Pappas C, Iyengar H, et al. Short bowel syndrome in the NICU. Clin Perinatol. 2013;40:53–68.
205. Choi WW, McBride CA, Bourle C, et al. Long-term review of sutureless ward reduction in neonates with gastroschisis in the neonatal unit. J Pediatr Surg. 2012;47:1516–20.
206. Pastor AC, Phillips JD, Fenton SJ, et al. Routine use of a SILASTIC spring-loaded silo for infants with gastroschisis: a multicenter randomized controlled trial. J Pediatr Surg. 2008;43: 1807–12.
207. Mayhew JF, Mychaskiew G. Gastroschisis. Pediatr Anesth. 2009;19:54.
208. Lobo JD, Kim AC, Davis RP, et al. NO free ride? The hidden costs of delayed operative management using a spring-loaded silo for gastroschisis. J Pediatr Surg. 2010;45:1426–32.
209. Raghavan M, Montgomerie J. Anesthetic management of gastroschisis—a review of our practice over the past 5 years. Pediatr Anesth. 2008;18:1055–9.
210. Vegunta RK, Wallace LJ, Leonardi MR, et al. Perinatal management of gastroschisis: analysis of a newly established clinical pathway. J Pediatr Surg. 2005;40:528–34.
211. Yaster M, Schere TL, Stone MM, et al. Prediction of successful primary closure of congenital abdominal wall defects using intraoperative measurements. J Pediatr Surg. 1989;24:1217–20.
212. Puffinbarger NK, Taylor DV, Tuggle DW, et al. End-tidal carbon dioxide for monitoring primary closure of gastroschisis. J Pediatr Surg. 1996;31:280–2.
213. Mortellaro VE, St Peter SD, Fike FB, Islam S. Review of the evidence on the closure of abdominal wall defects. Pediatr Surg Int. 2011;27:391–7.
214. Siffel C, et al. Bladder exstrophy: an epidemiologic study from the International Clearinghouse for Birth Defects Surveillance and Research, and an overview of the literature. Am J Med Genet C Semin Med Genet. 2011;157C(4):321–32.
215. Purves T. Modern approaches in primary exstrophy closure. Semin Pediatr Surg. 2011;20:79–84.
216. Gearhart JP, Baird AD. The failed complete repair of bladder exstrophy: insights and outcomes. J Urol. 2005;174:1669–73.
217. Kost-Byerly S, Jackson EV, Yaster M, et al. Perioperative anesthetic and analgesic management of newborn bladder exstrophy repair. J Pediatr Urol. 2008;4:280–5.
218. Ansari MS, Gulia A, Srivastava A, Kapoor R. Risk factors for progression to end-stage renal disease in children with posterior urethral valves. J Pediatr Urol. 2010;6:261–4.
219. Morris RK, Kilby MD. Long-term renal and neurodevelopmental outcome in infants with LUTO, with and without fetal intervention. Early Hum Dev. 2011;87:607–10.
220. Davenport KP, Blanco FC, Sandler AD. Pediatric malignancies: neuroblastoma, Wilm's tumor, hepatoblastoma, rhabdomyosarcoma, and sacrococcygeal teratoma. Surg Clin N Am. 2012;92:745–67.
221. Winderl LM, Silverman RK. Prenatal identification of a completely cystic internal sacrococcygeal teratoma (Type IV). Ultrasound Obstet Gynecol. 1997;9:425–8.
222. Shue E, Bolouri M, Jelin EB, et al. Tumor metrics and morphology predict poor prognosis in prenatally diagnosed sacrococcygeal teratoma: a 25-year experience at a single institution. J Pediatr Surg. 2013;48:12225–31.
223. Shalaby MS, O'Toole S, Driver C, et al. Urogenital anomalies in girls with sacrococcygeal teratoma: a commonly missed association. J Pediatr Surg. 2012;47:371–4.
224. Altman RP, Randolph JG, Lilly JR. Sacrococcygeal teratoma: American Academy of Pediatrics Surgical Section Survey 1973. J Pediatr Surg. 1974;9:389–98.
225. Ledrick H, Flake AW, Crombleholme TM, et al. Sacrococcygeal teratoma: prenatal assessment, fetal intervention, and outcome. J Pediatr Surg. 2004;39:430–8.
226. Lee MY, Won HS, Hyun MK, et al. Perinatal outcome of sacrococcygeal teratoma. Prenat Diagn. 2011;31:1217–21.
227. Van Mieghem T, Al-Ibrahim A, Deprest J, et al. Minimally invasive therapy for fetal sacrococcygeal teratomas: case series and systematic review of the literature. Ultrasound Obstet Gynecol. 2014;43:611–9. doi:10.1002/uog.13315.
228. Kim J-W, Gwak M, Park J-Y, et al. Cardiac arrest during excision of a huge sacrococcygeal teratoma. A report of two cases. Korean J Anesthesiol. 2012;63:80–4.
229. Davenport M. Biliary atresia: clinical aspects. Semin Pediatr Surg. 2012;21:175–84.
230. Jacob R. Anesthesia for biliary atresia and hepatectomy in paediatrics. Indian J Anesthesial. 2012;56:479–84.
231. Chan KW, Lee KH, Tsui SY, et al. Laparoscopic versus open Kasai portoenterostomy in infant with biliary atresia: a retrospective review on the 5-year native liver survival. Pediatr Surg Int. 2012;28:1109–13.

232. Yamataka A, Lane GJ, Cazares J. Laparoscopic surgery for biliary atresia and choledochal cyst. Semin Pediatr Surg. 2012;21:201–10.
233. Diao M, Li L, Cheng W. Initial experience of single-incision laparoscopic hepaticojejunostomy using conventional instruments for correctable biliary atresia. J Laparoendosc Adv Surg Tech A. 2012;22:615–20.
234. Oetzmann von Sochaczewski C, Petersen C, Ure BM, et al. Laparoscopic versus conventional Kasai portoenterostomy does not facilitate subsequent liver transplantation in infants with biliary atresia. J Laparoendosc Adv Surg Tech A. 2012;22: 408–11.
235. Wong KK, Chung PH, Chan KL, et al. Should open Kasai portoenterostomy be performed for biliary atresia in the era of laparoscopy? Pediatr Surg Int. 2008;24:931–3.
236. Green DW, Howard ER, Davenport M. Anaesthesia, perioperative management and outcome of correction of extrahepatic biliary atresia in the infant: a review of 50 cases in the King's College Hospital series. Pediatr Anaesth. 2000;10:581–9.
237. Kastenberg Z, Sylvester KG. The surgical management of necrotizing enterocolitis. Clin Perinatol. 2013;40:135–48.
238. Gordon PV, Swanson JR. Necrotizing enterocolitis is one disease with many origins and potential means of prevention. Pathophysiology. 2014;21:13–9. doi:10.1016/j.pathophys.2013.11.015.
239. Wan-Huen P, Bateman D, Shapiro DM, Parravicini E. Packed red blood cell transfusion is an independent risk factor for necrotizing independent risk factor for necrotizing enterocolitis in premature infants. J Perinatol. 2013;33:786–90.
240. Kim JH. Necrotizing enterocolitis: the road to zero. Semin Fetal Neonatal Med. 2014;19:39–44.
241. Stewart CJ, Marrs ECL, Nelson A, et al. Development of the preterm gut microbiome in twins at risk of necrotizing enterocolitis and sepsis. PLoS One. 2013;8(8):e73465.
242. Lee JS, Polin R. Treatment and prevention of necrotizing enterocolitis. Semin Neonatol. 2003;8:449–59.
243. Ng PC, Chan KYY, Poon TCW. Biomarkers for prediction and diagnosis of necrotizing enterocolitis. Clin Perinatol. 2013;40:149–59.
244. Ng PC. Biomarkers of necrotising enterocolitis. Semin Fetal Neonatal Med. 2014;19:33–8.
245. Thyoka M, de Coppi P, Eaton S, et al. Advanced necrotizing enterocolitis Part 1: mortality. Eur J Pediatr Surg. 2012;22:8–12.
246. Hull MA, Fisher JG, Gutierrez IM, et al. Mortality and management of surgical necrotizing enterocolitis in very low birth weight neonates: a prospective cohort study. J Am Coll Surg. 2014;218:1148–55.
247. Pierro A. The surgical management of necrotizing enterocolitis. Early Hum Dev. 2005;81:79–85.
248. Rees C, Pierro A, Eaton S. Neurodevelopmental outcomes of neonates with medically and surgically treated necrotizing enterocolitis. Arch Dis Child Fet Neonatal Ed. 2007;92:F193–8.
249. Huda S, Chaudhery S, Ibrahim H, et al. Neonatal necrotizing enterocolitis: clinical challenges, pathophysiology and management. Pathophysiology. 2014;21:3–12.
250. Patel RM, Denning PW. Therapeutic use of prebiotics, probiotics, and postbiotics to prevent necrotizing enterocolitis. Clin Perinatol. 2013;40:11–25.
251. Downward CD, Renaud E, St Peter SD, et al. Treatment of necrotizing enterocolitis: an American Pediatric Surgical Association Outcomes and Clinical Trials Committee systematic review. J Pediatr Surg. 2012;47:2111–22.
252. Wong MP, Droubatchevskaia N, Chipperfield KM, et al. Guidelines for frozen plasma transfusion. B C Med J. 2007;49:311–9.
253. Osborn DA, Lui K, Pussell P, et al. T and Tk antigen activation in necrotizing enterocolitis: manifestations, severity of illness, and effectiveness of testing. Arch Dis Child Fetal Neonatal Ed. 1999;80:F192–7.
254. Hall N, Ong EGP, Ade-Ajayi N, et al. T cryptantigen activation is associated with advanced necrotizing enterocolitis. J Pediatr Surg. 2002;37:791–3.
255. Rao SC, Basani L, Simmer K, et al. Peritoneal drainage versus laparotomy as initial surgical treatment for perforated necrotizing enterocolitis or spontaneous intestinal perforation in preterm low birth weight infants. Cochrane Database Syst Rev. 2011: CD006182.
256. Leva E, Di Cesare A, Canazza L, et al. The role of laparoscopy in newborns affected by NEC. J Laparoendosc Adv Surg Tech A. 2010;20:187–9.
257. Pani N, Panda CK. Anaesthetic consideration for neonatal surgical emergencies. Indian J Anaesth. 2012;56:463–9.
258. Saarenmaa E, Neuvonen PJ, Fellman V. Gestational age and birth weight effects on plasma clearance of fentanyl in newborn infants. J Pediatr. 2000;136:767–70.
259. Sammartino M, Garra R, Sbaraglia F, et al. Experience of remifentanil in extremely low-birth-weight babies undergoing laparotomy. Pediatr Neonatol. 2011;52:176–9.
260. Penido MG, Garra R, Sammartino M, et al. Remifentanil in neonatal intensive care and anaesthetic practice. Acta Paediatr. 2010;99:1454–63.
261. Welzing L, Evenfeld S, Dlugay V, et al. Remifentanil degradation in umbilical cord blood of preterm infants. Anesthesiology. 2011;114:570–7.
262. Cho SS, Rudloff I, Berger PJ, et al. Remifentanil ameliorates intestinal ischemia-reperfusion injury. BMC Gastroenterol. 2013;13:69.
263. Cox DJ, Groves AM. Inotropes in preterm infants—evidence for and against. Acta Paediatr. 2012;101 Suppl 464:17–23.
264. Hall NJ, Eaton S, Peters MJ, et al. Mild controlled hypothermia in preterm neonates with advanced necrotizing enterocolitis. Pediatrics. 2010;125:e300–8.
265. Dalla Vechia LK, Grosfield JL, West KW, et al. Intestinal atresia: a 25 year experience with 277 cases. Arch Surg. 1998;133:490–7.

Anesthesia for the Neonate: Neurosurgery and Ophthalmology

11

Andrew J. Davidson, Reema Nandi, and Susan M. Carden

Both major intracranial and intraocular procedures tend to be avoided wherever possible in neonates due to the technical difficulties of the surgery and high risk of surgical complications. Nevertheless, such surgery is not uncommon and it provides a great challenge for the pediatric anesthesiologist. Lesser procedures, such as examination of the eye, are common and they too can present many challenges to the anesthesiologist.

Neurosurgery

Neonatal neurosurgery requires an understanding of the general principles of both surgery in a neonate and neurosurgery in general. The anesthesia is particularly challenging due to the paucity of data about normal neurophysiology in the neonate.

Anatomy and Physiology

Anatomy of the Cranium

Neuroanatomy and neurophysiology vary with age. At birth, the calvarium or skull cap is composed of ossified plates that cover the dura mater. The plates are separated by fibrous sutures and fontanelles. The posterior fontanelle closes between 2 and 3 months and the anterior fontanelle between 10 and 18 months of age. The dura mater is relatively noncompliant and unable to accommodate an acute increase in intracranial pressure (ICP) even when the fontanelles are open. An acute increase in intracranial volume will therefore cause a rapid increase in ICP that will compress and displace vital CNS tissue and cause cerebral dysfunction. A slow increase in pressure may be accommodated to a limited extent, by expansion of the fontanelles and separation of the fibrous sutures. The fontanelles tend to remain open in the presence of any chronic process that increases the intracranial volume including tumors and hydrocephalus. Intracranial pressure can be monitored clinically in the infant by palpation of open fontanelles or by the application of skin surface pressure transducers [1, 2]. At birth, the brain weighs about 335 g or 10–15 % of the total body weight. It doubles its weight by 6 months of age and weighs 900 g by 1 year. By 12 years of age, the brain reaches adult weight of 1,200–1,400 g. In a meta-analysis of studies, the volume of the brain in infants who are born very premature was very much less than in those born full term and was associated with reduced cognitive function in childhood and adolescence [3]. Such cognitive impairment was exacerbated by the presence of reduced volume of the cerebellum and reduced size of the corpus callosum.

The intracranial space is separated into the supratentorial and infratentorial compartments by a horizontal layer of the dura mater, the tentorium cerebelli. The tentorium is tent shaped and forms a roof over the posterior cranial fossa.

The Supratentorial Compartment

This is the largest compartment of the intracranial space and contains the cerebrum and all structures formed from the diencephalon (see below). The cerebrum is separated into 2 hemispheres by the longitudinal cerebral fissure and falx cerebri. Each hemisphere is further divided into frontal, temporal and parieto-occipital lobes. This physical division correlates with the division of function.

The diencephalon is the most rostral part of the brainstem. It is located in the central portion of the supratentorial compartment and consists predominantly of the thalamus

A.J. Davidson, MBBS, MD, FABZCA (✉)
Anesthesia and Pain Management, Murdoch Children's Research Institute, Royal Children's Hospital,
Flemington Road, Parkville, VIC 3052, Australia
e-mail: andrew.davidson@rch.org.au

R. Nandi
Great Ormond Street Hospital for Children,
London WC1N3JH, UK

S.M. Carden, MBBS, FRANZCO, FRACS, PhD
Department of Ophthalmology, Royal Children's Hospital,
Flemington Road, Parkville, VIC 3052, Australia

J. Lerman (ed.), *Neonatal Anesthesia*, DOI 10.1007/978-1-4419-6041-2_11,

together with some epithalamic, subthalamic, and hypothalamic regions. The brainstem is continuous with the spinal cord. It passes through the tentorial notch of the tentorium cerebelli where its anterior surface lies on the body of the sphenoid bone.

If a primary lesion or injury involves gross expansion by hemorrhage or edema, then structures near to the tentorium and the falx become sites of secondary injury. This secondary injury is caused by both direct pressure and shearing forces and by ischemia from anterior cerebral artery compression. If the pressure continues to increase within the supratentorial compartment, the diencephalon, cerebral peduncles, oculomotor nerves, posterior communicating artery and the uncus of the temporal lobe may eventually herniate through the incisura tentorii resulting in contralateral hemiplegia, ipsilateral pupil signs (dilated, irregular, poor reaction to light) and abnormal posturing.

The Infratentorial Compartment

The infratentorial compartment is located within the posterior cranial fossa and contains the cerebellum, pons and medulla oblongata. The cerebellum is a dorsal expansion of the brainstem with a function that is expressed ipsilaterally and predominantly regulates motor functions. The medulla oblongata lies inferior to the pons and contains the nuclei of the cranial nerves VII to XII as well as the ascending sensory and descending motor pathways.

The Spinal Canal Compartment

The spinal cord and CSF are contained within the cylindrical vertebral canal. The spinal cord is the continuation of the brainstem. Its caudal tip reaches the intervertebral space of L3 at birth and the adult level of L1–L2 by 8 years of age.

Vascular Anatomy

In neonates, the brain comprises 2 % of the body weight but receives 15 % of the cardiac output. Cerebral blood flow is supplied by an extensive network of arteries originating from paired internal carotid and vertebral arteries. The vertebral arteries join to form a single midline basilar artery that divides again at the junction of the pons and the midbrain into the paired posterior cerebral and superior cerebellar arteries. The posterior cerebral arteries become interconnected with the vessels originating from the carotid arteries to form the circle of Willis. The communicating arteries are effective anastomoses that reduce the risk of clinical ischemia if a contributing vessel is occluded.

Cerebral veins run in the pia mater and into collecting veins within the subarachnoid layer. They eventually traverse the subdural space and open into venous sinuses that lie between the dura mater and the cranial periosteum. The cerebral venous system is valveless and its walls are thin and lacking smooth muscle. The brain is insensitive to pain but the cerebral dura mater has nociceptive receptors particularly around the venous sinuses.

The superior sagittal sinus is clinically important because it is superficial and midline in location. This makes it vulnerable to damage during surgery. This sinus empties into a confluence of sinuses that drains into bilateral transverse sinuses. The occipital sinus that lies along the foramen magnum also ends in the confluence of sinuses. The cavernous sinus, which surrounds the sella turcica, joins the superior petrosal sinuses and drains into the transverse sinus. The transverse sinuses then course laterally along the attachment line of the tentorium to the occipital bone and become continuous with the sigmoid sinus located within the posterior cranial fossa finally to form the jugular venous bulbs.

Spinal Cord Vascular Anatomy

The arterial supply to the spinal cord primarily arises from a single anterior spinal artery and 2 posterior spinal arteries both originating from the vertebral arteries. The anterior spinal artery supplies the ventromedial aspect of the spinal cord, which contains the corticospinal tracts and motor neurons. The 2 posterior spinal arteries form a plexus-like network on the posterior cord surface and supply the dorsal and lateral aspects of the spinal cord, which contain the sensory tracts responsible for proprioception and light touch.

The anterior spinal artery does not supply the whole length of the spinal cord. Supplemental blood supply is also received from radicular arteries originating from the spinal branches of the ascending cervical, deep cervical, intercostal, lumbar, and sacral arteries. A large anterior radicular artery called the artery of Adamkiewicz is responsible for supplying blood to as much as the caudal two-thirds of the spinal cord. It arises most commonly between T9 and L5 on the left side, although it may originate beyond these limits. All the other radicular arteries provide important collateral supply to the thoracic and lumbar spinal cord.

The venous drainage of the spinal cord consists of 2 median veins, 2 anterolateral veins, and 2 posterolateral longitudinal veins that empty via the anterior and posterior radicular veins into the internal vertebral venous plexus. This plexus lies between the dura mater and the vertebral periosteum. All the veins are thin walled and valveless. The internal plexus communicates with an external plexus that then drains via the vertebral, intercostal, lumbar, and lateral sacral veins into ascending lumbar, azygous, or hemizygous veins. At the cervical levels, the internal plexus connects to a basivertebral vein, which communicates through the foramen magnum with the occipital and basilar sinuses.

Physiology

Cerebral Blood Flow and Cerebral Blood Volume

Global CBF is approximately 15 % lesser in neonates (42 mL/100 g/min) than it is in adults (50 mL/100 g/min). CBF increases during infancy, reaching 90 mL/100 g/min by 6 months postnatal age, and peaks at 100–110 mL/100 g/min by 3–4 years of age. CBF decreases gradually thereafter, reaching 80 mL/100 g/min by 9 years of age. The greater CBF in infants and children reflects the greater energy requirements of the developing brain. As a consequence, cerebral oxygen consumption varies with age. In anesthetized neonates and infants, $CMRO_2$ is 2.3 mL O_2/100 g/min. $CMRO_2$ peaks at 5.2 mL O_2/100 g/min in children 3–12 years of age and gradually decreases thereafter, reaching 3.5 mL O_2/100 g/min in adults. This change again is attributed substantially to the greater energy requirements in the brains of children compared with adults [4].

Cerebral blood flow (CBF) depends on the pressure gradient within the vascular system, known as the cerebral perfusion pressure (CPP). CPP is defined as the mean arterial pressure (MAP) minus either ICP or central venous pressure (CVP), whichever is greater:

$$\mathrm{CPP} = \mathrm{MAP} - (\mathrm{ICP\,or\,CVP})$$

While the MAP remains within a specific range, cerebral perfusion is under autoregulatory control. Autoregulation of cerebral blood flow is the intrinsic ability of the cerebral vasculature to maintain constant cerebral blood flow (CBF) despite changes in cerebral perfusion pressure (CPP). In the stressed neonate or preterm infant, loss of autoregulation or perturbations in CBF has been associated with periventricular hemorrhage, hence the importance of understanding cerebral autoregulation and its variables. Myogenic, neurogenic and metabolic factors have been hypothesized as mechanisms responsible for the control of this intrinsic function. If excessive hypotension, hypertension, hypoxia, hypercapnia or cerebral ischemia occurs, these mechanisms may begin to fail, rendering CBF pressure passive. In addition to physiologic variables, pharmacologic therapeutics such as inhalational anesthetic agents may blunt autoregulation via a dose-dependent cerebral vasodilatation (see above).

CBF is autoregulated to maintain oxygen delivery over a wide range of perfusion pressures. Three factors affect CBF: MAP, CO_2, and O_2. CBF remains constant between MAPs of 50 and 150 mmHg in older children. However, thresholds for autoregulation in infants have not been fully elucidated. Recent concepts in the autoregulation of CBF in stressed neonates have shifted from the notion of "loss of autoregulation" during stress (e.g., hypoxia) to a flattening of the autoregulation curve [5]. In addition, evidence has shown that cerebral autoregulation waxes and wanes with time [6].

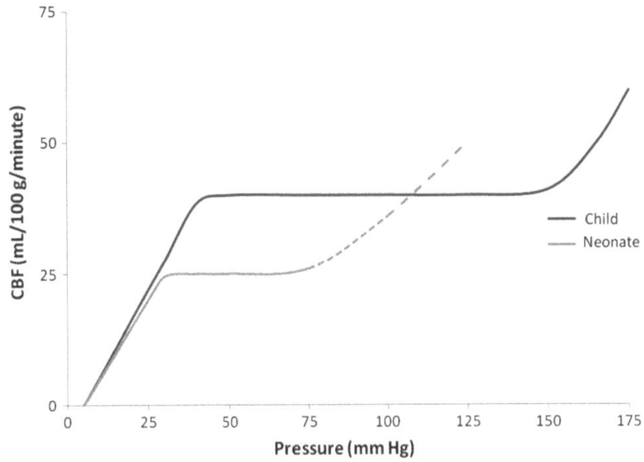

Fig. 11.1 Cerebral blood flow and cerebral perfusion pressure in a neonate and older child. Note that the relationship between flow and pressure is poorly defined in the neonate especially at higher pressures

Studies in neonatal animals suggest that the limits for autoregulation in this age group lie between 25 and 75 mmHg MAP (Fig. 11.1). Once the limits of autoregulation have been exceeded, CBF changes more passively with MAP [7]. Neonates in severe physiological distress may have blunted autoregulation, demonstrated by a minimal change in CBF in response to varying $PaCO_2$ levels or a direct pressure-passive CBF [8]. The nadir of autoregulation in awake preterm infants 24–34 weeks gestation is 23 mmHg [9, 10]. Studies using more recent technology such as near-infrared spectroscopy have demonstrated that autoregulation is a dynamic phenomenon. For example, CBF is pressure passive 20–50 % of the time in sick preterm infants <1,500 g during the first 5 days after birth [6]. Cerebral autoregulation was maintained despite fluctuations in MAP in normotensive preterm infants weighing ~1,000 g whose lungs were ventilated, although their response to CO_2 was blunted. In contrast, cerebral autoregulation to MAP was blunted in hypotensive preterm infants, and their response to CO_2 was markedly attenuated or absent [11]. Clinical evidence suggests that fluctuating CBF as in preterm infants with impaired or abolished autoregulation may be at increased risk for IVH [12, 13].

Change in $PaCO_2$ exerts a profound effect on cerebral perfusion. Hypercapnia impairs cerebrovascular autoregulation, while hypocapnia increases vascular tone and hence cerebrovascular resistance, thus decreasing CBF. Changes in ventilation and intrathoracic pressure rather than $PaCO_2$ may be the primary cause of the observed changes in cerebrovascular autoregulation [14]. These observations are in conflict with an understanding of interaction between $PaCO_2$ and cerebrovascular autoregulation but may result from the technique by which cerebral autoregulation was quantified. In adults, CBF decreases 3 % with every 0.75 mmHg (0.1 kPa) decrease in $PaCO_2$ between 20 mmHg (2.7) and 80 mmHg

(10.7 kPa). In contrast, the immature brain is relatively unresponsive to small changes in $PaCO_2$ [15]. In infants and children, cerebral vasoconstriction occurs at a much reduced $PaCO_2$ compared with that in adults [16]. Although hyperventilation minimally increases cerebral vasculature resistance in neonates, a sudden increase in $PaCO_2$ after chronic hyperventilation of more than 24 h may cause cerebral vasodilatation and increased ICP [17]. Mild hypothermia decreases, whereas hyperthermia increases dynamic cerebrovascular autoregulation, although these effects are small. Hemodilution reduces blood viscosity and vascular resistance, thereby increasing CBF [18]. This decrease in vascular resistance can decrease autoregulatory capacity, and the lower limit of autoregulation has been shown to increase with anemia [19].

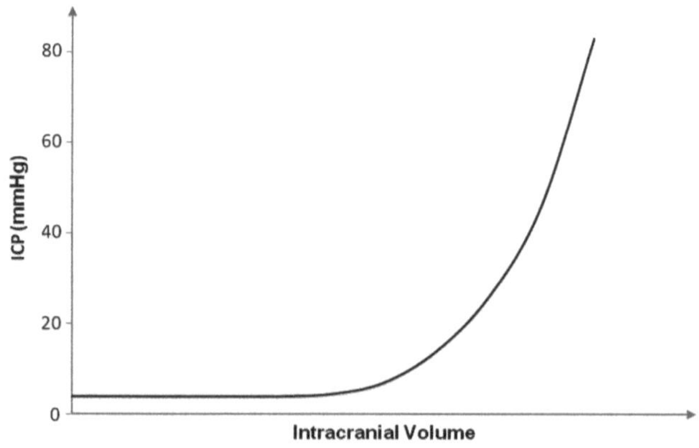

Fig. 11.2 Idealized intracranial compliance curve in a neonate

Spinal Cord Blood Flow

Animal data suggest that spinal cord blood flow is influenced by the same factors that influence CBF, although the flow rate is less, reflecting the reduced metabolic rate of the spinal cord. Perfusion of the spinal cord is determined by an equation similar to that for CBF:

$$\mathrm{SCPP} = \mathrm{MAP} - (\mathrm{CSF\ or\ extrinsic\ pressure})$$

This highlights the importance of extrinsic pressure on the integrity of the spinal cord, an effect that occurs in the presence of tumors, hematomas, or spinal venous congestion.

CSF and ICP

Between 50 and 80 % of the cerebrospinal fluid (CSF) surrounding the brain and spinal cord is produced by the choroid plexus, which lines the floor of the lateral ventricles and the roof of the third and fourth ventricles. Up to 30 % of the CSF can be formed in other sites such as ependyma, the brain parenchyma and endothelium of cerebral capillaries. The CSF produced by the choroid plexus flows from the lateral ventricles, through the interventricular foramen of Monro into the third ventricle, then into the cerebral aqueduct of Sylvius to the fourth ventricle. It emerges from the interior of the brain through the two lateral foramina of Luschka and the single medial foramen of Magendie to enter the subarachnoid space. The CSF is absorbed by the arachnoid villi. The mean production rate of CSF in children is about 0.35 mL/min. CBF and CBV are much more important determinants of ICP than is the volume of the CSF.

Controlling ICP is critically important in maintaining CPP. Normal ICP is 8–18 mmHg in adults and 2–4 mmHg in children. The ICP in neonates is positive on the day of birth but then becomes negative, probably because of salt and water loss. Intracerebral volume also acutely and briefly decreases and is matched by a reduction in head size.

Neonates can compensate for slow increases in ICP because their fontanelles and suture lines are open. However, acute changes in intracranial volume are not tolerated because the fibrous connective tissue connecting the fontanelles and sutures is relatively difficult to separate. A small change in volume may result in an insignificant increase in ICP in a neonate with a normal baseline ICP, but once the noncompliant point on the intracranial compliance curve is reached, a small increase in volume causes a greater increase in ICP. Ultimately, the brainstem and cerebellar peduncles may herniate through the foramen magnum (coning), causing coma and death (Fig. 11.2).

Blood-Brain Barrier

The blood-brain barrier (BBB) is a lipid membrane interface between the endothelial cells of the brain blood vessels and the ECF of the brain. It acts as a barrier to water-soluble drugs. Research from animals suggests that the BBB in the neonate has restrictive properties that are similar to those in the adult. At birth, saturable, carrier-mediated transport mechanisms are present, regulating the entry of glucose, amino acids, organic acids, purines, nucleosides, and choline. No difference in brain uptake of glucose has been observed between adults and neonates in a rabbit model. In contrast to the early suggestion that the BBB in young animals is an immature barrier, studies indicate that the BBB at birth is sophisticated and selective, with carrier systems that have a vital function in regulating the concentrations of metabolites within the neonatal brain [20].

Embryology and the Pathology of Neural Tube Defects

The CNS is the first organ system to develop in the fetus. Development of the CNS involves the 3 major phases of neurulation, canalization and retrogressive differentiation. Neurulation is the process by which the neural plate, derived from the neuroectodermal layer, folds upon itself to make a groove and then fuses to form the neural tube. Differentiation of the neural tube occurs within the first 60 days after fertilization of the ovum. The nervous system appears in the second week of gestation.

Differentiation of the cortex takes place during the third trimester.

Canalization is the formation of the caudal neural tube including the development of the lower lumbar, sacral and coccygeal segments. Within the neural tube, groups of cells with their corresponding vertebrae proliferate and produce an excess number of segments. These excess segments degenerate in a process called retrogressive differentiation, and the filum terminale and cauda equina remain. The growth of the spinal column brings the conus medullaris to its adult level. Neural tube defects occur during neurulation. Failure of neurulation in early development results in total dysraphism within the brain and spinal cord. Anencephaly occurs only if the brain fails to close. Abnormal neuronal migration results in cortical malformations. Failure of canalization results in spina bifida: a myelocele exposes only neural tissue, a myelomeningocele exposes meninges in addition to neural tissue and a meningocele contains only meninges.

General Principles of Neuroanesthesia in the Neonate

There are general principles and issues that apply to anesthesia in neonates for any surgical procedure. These have been discussed in other chapters. There are also general principles that apply to anesthesia for all neurosurgical procedures, regardless of age. What follows is a discussion of the latter principles as they apply to the neonate.

Access and Positioning

Access to the patient is limited during most types of neonatal surgery. Neurosurgery is no exception and indeed access to the airway may be particularly fraught. Great care must be taken that the tracheal tube is well secured and ideally located in the mid-trachea to avoid extubation or migration into a main bronchus. Nasal tubes are easier to firmly secure than oral tubes, particularly for posterior fossa surgery. The anesthesiologist must remain vigilant for the occurrence of dislodged or kinked tracheal tubes throughout the surgery.

Intravenous and arterial lines should also be placed before surgery begins and carefully secured. Attempting to establish new intravenous access during surgery is very difficult in the neonate, so if there is any question regarding the patency of the vascular access, then access must be established before surgery commences. For major neurosurgery, central venous access should be considered in order to provide a secure intravenous line, a line for vasopressor support and a means to measure central venous pressure and hence ensure optimal filling pressures. However, femoral or subclavian access is preferred over jugular venous access to preclude jugular venous obstruction.

ECG and noninvasive blood pressure and temperature monitoring should also be secured before the baby is covered. The eyes should be taped closed to prevent injury. Some neurosurgeons use paraffin and other elaborate means to protect the eyes from pressure and alcoholic skin preparation. Before the drapes cover the neonate, there should be a final check to ensure that pressure areas are well padded, that the tracheal tube is not at risk of being kinked and that all intravenous lines are free of excess tension.

Temperature

Cooling is neuroprotective and may reduce brain injury, whereas hyperthermia can exacerbate brain injury. Although mild hypothermia may be beneficial in terms of brain protection, it is also associated with cardiovascular instability, apnea, coagulopathy, and reduced immune resistance. If hypothermia is used to reduce potential brain injury, it must be undertaken cautiously with adequate cardiovascular and ventilatory support. Neonates can both lose heat and become overheated very quickly. Hyperthermia must be strictly avoided.

Neurosurgical procedures may involve exposure of relatively large areas as the head is relatively larger in neonates compared with that in adults. Particular care must be taken that heat loss is not excessive during antiseptic skin preparation. A forced air warmer should be used whenever possible and may be complemented with an overhead heating device to maintain thermoneutrality. All neonates need careful temperature monitoring during neurosurgery. Monitoring the temperature via the esophagus or pharynx is preferable to the skin and rectal sites.

Blood Pressure

Blood pressure control is crucial to maintain an adequate CPP during neurosurgery. With CPP depending on the venous pressure and ICP, the head must be carefully positioned to preclude any obstruction to venous drainage from the brain. Hypotension may lead to underperfusion and ischemia, whereas hypertension may lead to an increased capillary flow, transudation of fluid, and interstitial edema. Evidence suggests that hypotension may impair autoregulation as well as the reactivity to changes in $PaCO_2$. Such edema increases the oxygen gradient between capillaries and neurons, thereby increasing the risk of hypoxic injury. In normal brain and under normal conditions, autoregulation ensures flow matches demand over a range of blood pressures. It reduces the risk of hypertension leading to edema or hypotension leading to ischemia. However, in the injured brain, this autoregulation may be impaired, and thus the range of blood pressures that avoids either excess or insufficient perfusion is much narrower.

Hypotension is poorly defined in both awake and anesthetized neonates and varies with specialists.

In neonates born 26–30 weeks gestation, a MAP <30 mmHg has been associated with IVH. This led to the general principle that the MAP should be ≥gestational age in weeks [21]. Some advocate the use of vasopressors to maintain an adequate MAP, although these have been associated with sequelae. In a survey, the majority of pediatric anesthesiologists defined hypotension in neonates during general anesthesia as a MAP >20–30 % below than awake values [22].

The range of CPP in which autoregulation can be maintained is poorly defined in neonates. In the absence of better data, good practice is to maintain a normal blood pressure for a neonate—though even this is unclear. Certainly excessive hypotension and hypertension must be avoided. To maintain adequate blood pressure, the neonate should be volume replete first, but there should also be a low threshold for vasopressor support. This is best given as an infusion rather than by intermittent boluses as the latter may lead to large fluctuations in blood pressure. To ensure prompt and appropriate responses, blood pressure should be accurately monitored. For critical cases, intra-arterial blood pressure monitoring is ideal.

Many anesthetic drugs also reduce the capacity of autoregulation or lead to a mismatch of flow and demand. All inhalational anesthetics impair autoregulation in a dose-dependent manner, although this effect is limited at concentrations <1 MAC. Nitrous oxide tends to increase flow. Propofol affects autoregulation the least of all drugs, although there are few data describing total intravenous anesthesia dosing regimens for propofol in neonates. Opioids can be used to provide stable hemodynamics and to supplement anesthesia, with limited impact on the autoregulation of CBF. Fentanyl at 5–10 mcg/kg/min may be used, provided there is capacity to continue to provide ventilatory support postoperatively. There is limited experience with remifentanil in neurosurgery in neonates, but it may have a very promising role, given its rapid metabolism and fast recovery. (See section on neuropharmacology below.)

Ventilation

The primary aim of ventilation is to prevent hypoxia and strive to maintain normocapnia. Hypercapnia increases ICP, possibly causing cerebral edema and making operating conditions difficult. Hypocapnia may lead to hypoperfusion and ischemia. Similarly, hypoxia may exacerbate brain injury. In theory, excessive PEEP increases ICP, although if such a PEEP level optimizes oxygenation and ventilation, then this must take priority. Muscle relaxation may be used to prevent straining and the resultant increase in ICP.

Fluids, Glucose, and Electrolytes

Extreme fluctuations in blood glucose concentration may exacerbate brain injury. Hypoglycemia may itself lead to brain injury. Hyperglycemia may worsen existing brain injury, although in neonates, there is evidence that this risk is not as great as in older children and adults [23, 24]. Intravenous dextrose should be continued during major neurosurgery in neonates and the blood concentration of glucose checked regularly for extreme shifts in the concentration.

Hyponatremia reduces plasma tonicity, thereby exacerbating cerebral edema. During neurosurgery, isotonic fluids should be administered and the plasma sodium concentration measured regularly. Excessive amounts of sodium chloride may lead to hyperchloremic metabolic acidosis as the immature kidney is unable to excrete the excess chloride. If there is a risk of diabetes insipidus or increased ADH secretion, then the plasma concentration of electrolytes must be checked frequently.

With relatively large heads that receive a disproportionate fraction of the cardiac output, blood loss during neurosurgery in a neonate may be more significant than in older children. A coagulation profile and full blood count should be obtained before all major neurosurgeries. Packed red blood cells should be available for any neurosurgical procedure that may result in bleeding. In neonates, fresh blood is preferable to aged stored blood since rapid transfusion of the latter may lead to acidosis and hyperkalemia, for both of which the neonate has limited buffering capacity. The ideal hematocrit to trigger transfusion in the setting of acute blood loss in neonates is unknown. Not only is it very easy to underestimate ongoing blood loss, but acute losses can occur very rapidly and lead to hemodynamic instability. Therefore, if significant blood loss is occurring, red cells should be given earlier rather than later. During major neurosurgery, platelets and fresh frozen plasma should be available and given early before a coagulopathy develops.

Analgesia Postoperatively

Neonates have well-developed systems of nociception; they feel and respond to pain as do older children. Furthermore, failure to alleviate pain in neonates can lead to changes in spinal cord morphology and increase postoperative complications. Analgesia should be provided after neurosurgery. Minor procedures may require only simple analgesics such as paracetamol, whereas more involved procedures will require parenteral opioids.

Neuropharmacology

The effects of anesthetic agents on cerebrovascular autoregulation vary. Inhaled anesthetics exert a dose-dependent uncoupling effect on autoregulation. Sevoflurane, however, impairs cerebrovascular autoregulation the least of all of the inhaled anesthetics. In healthy children, cerebral pressure autoregulation is preserved up to 1.5 MAC of sevoflurane, a finding similar to that in adults [25]. Although regional CBF varies with inhaled anesthetics, global CBF remains unaffected [26]. CBF increases to the greatest extent during halothane anesthesia, followed by enflurane, isoflurane and then desflurane.

Hypercapnia impairs cerebrovascular autoregulation. Furthermore, this effect of hypercapnia compounds the effects of inhaled anesthetics on the loss of autoregulation. Propofol preserves cerebrovascular autoregulation at $PaCO_2$ values as great as 56 mmHg (7.5 kPa), whereas a similar level of hypercapnia abolishes cerebrovascular autoregulation during sevoflurane anesthesia. Importantly, hypocapnia reverses isoflurane-induced impairment of cerebrovascular autoregulation.

The effects of the non-inhaled anesthetics on cerebral autoregulation vary. Nitrous oxide increases CBF alone and when given with other anesthetic agents. Propofol preserves cerebral autoregulation at both large and small doses in healthy adults. When remifentanil is combined with propofol, it induces a dose-dependent metabolism-coupled reduction in CBF with preserved cerebrovascular autoregulation in adults. Comparable data in neonates are lacking. Opioids have little or no effect on CBF and ICP and cerebral autoregulation remains intact. Benzodiazepines and barbiturates decrease CBF and thus ICP. Barbiturates cause vasoconstriction in the cerebral vasculature and preserve autoregulation. Ketamine may increase CBF by up to 60 % under normocapnia and is therefore contraindicated in patients with increased ICP.

Neurosurgical Conditions

Neural Tube Defects

Neural tube defects (NTDs) (also known as spinal dysraphism) include all congenital anomalies that involve failure of the neural tube to close during the fourth week of embryogenesis and can occur anywhere along the formation of the spinal cord, from the brain to the sacrum. The two most common forms of NTDs are spina bifida and anencephaly.

Spina bifida is almost always compatible with survival, although severe physical and cognitive impairments are common. Spina bifida lesions are classified depending on whether or not neural tissue is exposed. Myelomeningocele is the most common and most severe form of spinal dysraphism. It is an open spina bifida lesion in which the spinal cord and meninges protrude through a defect in the vertebral arches and are either uncovered or covered with only a thin membrane. The defect can occur anywhere along the spinal column but is most common in the lumbar region. It can result in marked neurological deficit caudal to the level of the protruding sac.

In contrast to spina bifida, anencephaly is almost always fatal before or soon after birth. In this defect, there is partial or complete absence of the skull bones with only a minimal remnant of a brain.

Occult spinal dysraphism refers to a spina bifida lesion with intact skin covering. This form of dysraphism includes lipomeningocele, meningocele (when the sac contains meninges and cerebrospinal fluid but the spinal cord and spinal root are in their normal position), myelocystocele, dermal sinus, tight filum terminale, and diastematomyelia. With encephalocele, the brain and its covering membranes with CSF protrude through the skull, most often in the occipital region (Fig. 11.3). Spina bifida occulta is a benign and common abnormality in which the spinous processes of the lower lumbar or sacral spine fail to fuse. With these lesions, individuals are asymptomatic. The diagnosis is usually an incidental finding on plain radiographs of the spine/abdomen.

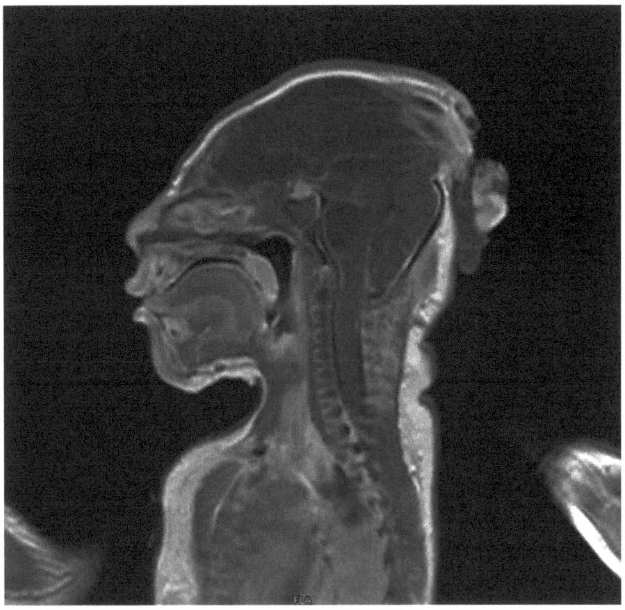

Fig. 11.3 Sagittal T1 MRI scan of a child with severe cranial dysraphism, with a pronounced brain malformation and encephalocele

The birth frequency of NTDs varies among countries and regions within countries but, in general, is approximately 1 in 1,000. In the UK, the prevalence is around 3 per 1,000 live births compared with 1 in 10,000 in sub-Saharan Africa. Worldwide, the prevalence of NTDs at birth appears to be decreasing. The prevalence in the UK was about 4 per 1,000 in the 1970s and has decreased to 3 per 1,000 live births. There is a significant genetic component to the development of NTDs. If either parent has had an affected child or is affected by the condition, the risk of further offspring having an NTD is approximately 10 %. If 2 affected pregnancies occur, the risk to a further pregnancy is increased by about 20-fold. Nevertheless, at least 90 % of NTDs occur to women without a family history. Since the 1970s, maternal nutrition, particularly regarding folate, has been linked to the occurrence of NTDs. In 1991, a large randomized trial determined that the recurrence risk of NTDs in mothers who consumed folic acid before conception was reduced by 72 % [27]. Two other controlled trials also showed similar reductions in the recurrence risk, with a pooled reduction in risk among those who were compliant of 87 % [28]. A definitive randomized controlled trial that compared the frequency of NTD in a multivitamin-supplemented group (containing 0.8 mg of folic acid) with a non-supplemented group showed no occurrences in the supplemented group (n=2,104 pregnancies) and six in the non-supplemented group (n=2,052). It is now recommended that a daily dietary supplement of 5 mg of folic acid before conception will prevent a recurrence of NTD. All women should be advised to take 400 mg of folic acid daily prior to conception to prevent a first occurrence of NTD as well as increasing consumption of folic-rich foods, such as green vegetables and fortified breakfast cereals, until the 12th week of pregnancy. However, because the compliance in taking these supplements is poor, the USA and several other countries instituted folic acid fortification of foods. In 1998, a US policy was drafted to require that enriched grain products be fortified with folic acid. Since this policy was adopted, the frequency of NTDs in the USA has been reduced to about 31 % for spina bifida and 16 % for anencephaly [29]. In addition, infants with spina bifida who were born after the fortification policy had a significantly better first-year survival rate than did those who were born before the policy [30]. However, many countries have not been as willing to embrace fortification. For example, in Finland, mandatory fortification is not permitted over concerns of possibly masking megaloblastic anemia caused by vitamin B12 deficiency in women older than 65 years, a possible small increase in the risk of wheeze and respiratory tract infections in offspring whose mothers took folic acid supplements during pregnancy and a possible increased incidence of lung cancer. However, there is no clear evidence confirming these concerns. The American College of Medical Genetics recommends that all women who are capable of becoming pregnant should strive for an intake of 0.4 mg of folic acid daily, and women who have had a previous NTD-affected pregnancy, who are themselves affected or have a first- or second- degree relative with an NTD, should ingest 4 mg of folic acid, commencing 3 months before conception and continuing throughout the first trimester.

Myelomeningocele

This is the most common and severe form of spinal dysraphism resulting from a failure of closure of the neural tube around day 21 of development (Fig. 11.4).

Open myelomeningocele is immediately apparent at birth as a defect on the back with a neural placode, which is the open spinal cord. Abnormal nerve roots emerge from it ventrally. It is surrounded by arachnoid adhesions, an incomplete dura and associated paravertebral soft tissues. Antenatal diagnosis is usual. Maternal serum alpha-fetal protein is used to establish the diagnosis, and ultrasound will demonstrate the contents of the lesion as well as other congenital abnormalities. The defect may be covered by a thin epithelial or arachnoid layer, but in some cases, this may have ruptured and CSF can be seen leaking from the defect. Most infants will develop hydrocephalus and a Chiari II malformation (disorganization of brainstem topography, a small posterior fossa, and herniation of the cerebellum through the foramen magnum) is very common. Abnormalities of cerebral gyration, the posterior fossa contents and agenesis of the corpus callosum as well as vertebral anomalies may also be present.

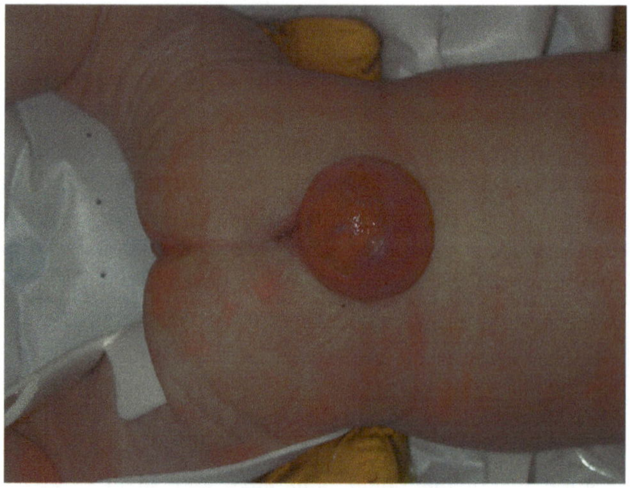

Fig. 11.4 A child with a lumbar myelomeningocele

The infant with an open myelomeningocele is preferably delivered by Cesarean section to avoid acquiring a CNS infection during passage through the birth canal. The baby should be nursed prone or in the lateral decubitus with a sterile moist dressing covering the defect. Surgery cannot restore neurological function but will protect existing neural structures and prevent infection. Neural tube lesions are investigated with ultrasound, CT and/or MRI scanning. The open myelomeningocele should be closed within 48 h of birth since the risk of infection increases with the more time the defect is exposed.

Two less common forms of dysraphism occur in relation to skull defects. Cephaloceles involve herniation of either meninges (cranial meningocele) or brain and meninges (encephalocele) into the cele. These neural tube defects occur in ~1–3:10,000 live births [31]. Occipital encephaloceles occur two to three times more commonly than nasal (or anterior), parietal, and temporal encephaloceles, with a geographic distribution in which occipital cephaloceles are more common in Western countries, whereas anterior cephaloceles are more common in Asian countries [32, 33]. Occipital cephaloceles more commonly include brain tissue in addition to CSF (which may have to be excised) and are more commonly complicated by hydrocephalus and seizures and thus carry a poorer prognosis than anterior celes [32]. Neurological defects most commonly associated with dysraphism include brainstem hypoplasia, cerebellar dysplasia, Arnold-Chiari defect, Dandy-Walker syndrome, and lissencephaly (smooth gyri and sulci) [31, 32]. Cephaloceles may also be associated with other congenital defects including cleft lip and palate, syndactyly, ocular defects, and congenital heart defects [31, 34]. Although surgery is usually undertaken in older infants and children, 20–30 % of neonates with cephaloceles undergo surgery in the neonatal period [32, 33].

Anesthetic Considerations for Neonates with Neural Tube Defects

During the preoperative anesthetic assessment, the presence of any associated congenital anomalies should be excluded and the degree of the neurological deficit confirmed. With cervical encephalocele, the neck is often short and rigid which can make tracheal intubation difficult. These neonates may have feeding difficulties due to the neurological deficit and be volume depleted secondary to evaporative and third space losses from the exposed area. Consequently, preoperative intravenous fluids may be required. Induction of anesthesia may be accomplished using either an inhalational or intravenous induction. In the past, tracheal intubation has been recommended in the left lateral position, but this is not necessary if the spinal defect is first padded to prevent pressure from being applied to the layers covering the spinal cord. The head and body can be raised and supported using foam pads. Surgery is usually performed with the neonate in the prone position. Tracheal intubation is usually accomplished with a reinforced orotracheal tube. However, some anesthesiologists prefer nasotracheal intubation as it may better secure the tube fixation in the prone position because these tubes are less likely to become dislodged by secretions and loose tape than orotracheal tubes. In the case of cephaloceles, tracheal intubation may be difficult. For occipital celes, the airway is often secured with the neonate in the left lateral decubitus position as it is difficult to stabilize the large CSF-filled cephalocele with the neonate supine. With anterior cephaloceles, the child may be positioned supine with the airway secured using orotracheal intubation.

Large-bore intravenous access should be secured, and for cephaloceles that require a craniotomy, an arterial line should also be secured. Blood loss is usually small unless a large skin flap or a craniotomy (in the case of cephaloceles) is planned [32, 34]. However, if brisk blood loss is anticipated (as in the case of cephaloceles), packed red blood cells should be in the operating room at the time of skin incision. Additional monitoring includes core temperature and urine output. In the prone position, particular attention should be paid to the eyes, which should be padded and protected from pressure. Pressure on the abdomen should also be avoided to prevent compression of the IVC and engorgement of the paraspinal vessels as well as to allow free abdominal movement with respiration. This can be achieved by placing "jellies" under the chest and hips. Large lesions may require rotational flaps or tissue expanders to allow skin closure. Analgesia should be multimodal with small doses of intraoperative opioids, intravenous paracetamol, and wound infiltration with local anesthetics. Postoperative analgesia should be paracetamol for smaller defects. Nurse-controlled analgesia using morphine may be required when larger defects are closed. In this case, a high-dependency postoperative bed is needed for the monitoring of respiration and oxygen saturation. Preterm infants are at increased risk of postoperative apnea, especially after neurosurgery [35].

Hydrocephalus and Shunts

Hydrocephalus occurs as a result of impaired circulation or absorption of CSF. In addition, hydrocephalus can occur as a result of the overproduction of CSF, e.g., in association with choroid plexus papillomas, although these tumors are rare.

Between 70 and 80 % of CSF is produced from the choroid plexus and the remainder of the ependyma and brain parenchyma. Production occurs by filtration across the capillary endothelium and active secretion of sodium by the choroidal epithelium. CSF production is mainly independent of ICP, although production is reduced somewhat in the presence of increased ICP and reduced CPP. CSF absorption is linearly related to ICP. Most CSF is absorbed at the arachnoid villi, which are herniations of arachnoidal tissue into the dural venous sinuses. The precise mechanism of CSF absorption remains unclear.

In adults, CSF is produced at a rate of about 550 mL/day. The total volume of CSF is 100–150 mL, of which 15–25 mL is contained within the ventricular system.

Etiology and Pathophysiology of Hydrocephalus

An obstruction at any point along the CSF pathway can result in hydrocephalus. Obstructive or noncommunicating hydrocephalus is an obstruction within the ventricular system or at the fourth ventricular outflow. Communicating hydrocephalus is impaired circulation through the subarachnoid spaces or impaired absorption into the venous system.

Posthemorrhagic Hydrocephalus

Intraventricular hemorrhage is detected in 40–45 % of preterm neonates with a birth weight less than 1,500 g. In this weight range, the hemorrhages often occur in the germinal matrix because the blood vessels there are irregular, have immature connective tissue architecture and lack the ability to autoregulate [12]. About 20 % of neonates who suffer an IVH, which usually occurs within the first few days after birth, require a shunt because of increased ICP. In addition to prematurity, vigorous resuscitation, respiratory distress syndrome, pneumothorax and seizures are associated with an increased risk of IVH [36].

IVHs can be identified using cerebral ultrasound and graded according to the location of the hematoma and its effect on the size of the ventricles. The presence of blood and its breakdown products may lead to hydrocephalus by obstructing the subarachnoid space and arachnoid villi. In addition, it leads to an ependymal reaction with blockage at the aqueduct or outlet foramina of the fourth ventricle. Increasing head circumference and progressive ventricular enlargement require intervention. Preterm, low-birth-weight neonates are at increased risk of shunt infection, and the presence of heavy blood staining or excessive cellular debris in the CSF precludes shunt insertion due to an increased risk of blockage. A shunt can be inserted once the CSF is clear of blood products.

Hydrocephalus and Myelomeningocele

85–95 % of children with open spina bifida develop hydrocephalus. This is due to the development of the Chiari II malformation which is the disorganization of brainstem topography, a small posterior fossa, and herniation of the cerebellum through the foramen magnum and up through the incisura (Fig. 11.5). This causes obstruction to CSF flow at a number of sites including the cerebral aqueduct and the fourth ventricular outlet, resulting in hydrocephalus.

Other causes of hydrocephalus include aqueduct stenosis, Dandy-Walker syndrome, obstructive hydrocephalus due to tumors and post-meningitic hydrocephalus. Aqueductal stenosis is responsible for about 10 % of cases of childhood hydrocephalus and can present at any time from birth to adulthood. Dandy-Walker syndrome comprises agenesis of the cerebellar vermis with cystic dilatation of the fourth ventricle, enlargement of the posterior fossa and hydrocephalus, which is usually present by 3 months of age. Additional brain malformations are present in over half of the cases, and neurodevelopmental delay is reported in up to 70 %.

Midline tumors, particularly those of the pineal gland and posterior fossa, commonly result in obstructive hydrocephalus, and this is one of the principal ways in which these conditions present. In a case series of posterior fossa tumors with hydrocephalus, 20 % required shunting. Chronic inflammation can produce obstruction to CSF flow especially after bacterial, parasitic, and granulomatous infection.

Clinical Presentation of Hydrocephalus

Hydrocephalus results in disproportionate head growth before closure of the cranial sutures and fontanelles. Clinical symptoms are often subtle. In the neonate, symptoms include general irritability and poor feeding. Signs include increased head circumference, bulging fontanelles, separation of the cranial sutures, prominence of the scalp veins and sunsetting of the eyes. The presence of bradycardia, hypertension, and irregularities in breathing suggests critically increased ICP and requires urgent treatment. In the neonate, cranial ultrasound

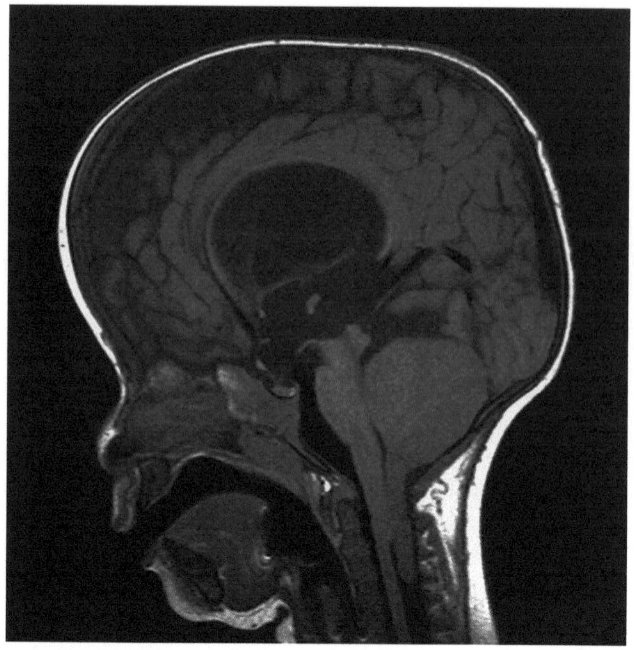

Fig. 11.5 Sagittal T1 MRI scan of a child with a severe Chiari II malformation and hydrocephalus

scanning is widely used to confirm the diagnosis of hydrocephalus, which can also be investigated by CT and MRI scanning for full evaluation of the ventricular system (Fig. 11.6).

Treatment of Hydrocephalus

The treatment of hydrocephalus involves bypassing the site of obstruction of CSF flow or diversion of CSF from the ventricular cavity to a site where it can be more readily absorbed. This is usually achieved by inserting a ventricular shunt but to a lesser degree also by using neuroendoscopic techniques, such as endoscopic third ventriculostomy. The shunt consists of a proximal catheter, the tip of which is located within the cerebral ventricle, and a distal catheter that drains to an alternative site of CSF absorption, most commonly to the peritoneal cavity but also to the pleural cavity or right atrium. In addition to the tubing that connects the origin of the accumulated CSF with the drainage location, shunts include a valve and reservoir. A variety of valve designs are available. Numerous shunt systems have been devised and marketed over the years, suggesting that the perfect shunt system has yet to be manufactured, although great strides have been made towards perfecting shunt technology.

Some children have a reservoir incorporated into the shunt, e.g., a Rickham reservoir, which is a shunt system reservoir that collects CSF or permits the injection of medications. It is used if frequent collection of CSF is required such as for infection or if injection of medications directly into the CSF is necessary. Its use is uncommon.

If only a brief period of CSF diversion is required, a subgaleal or an external ventricular drain may be used.

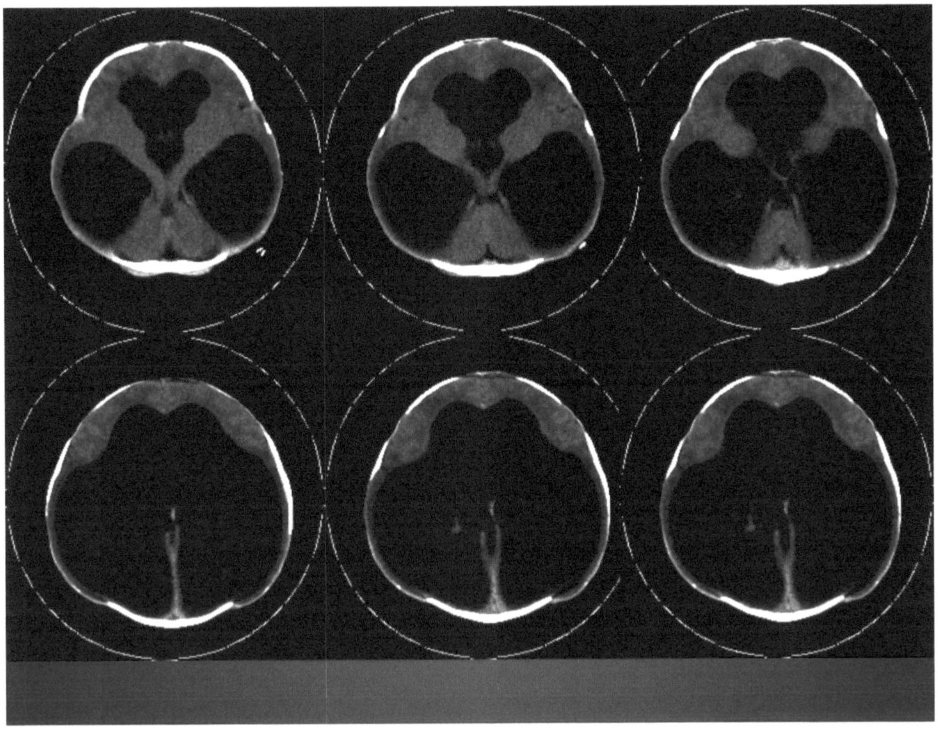

Fig. 11.6 MRI images of a child with hydrocephalus

The ventriculosubgaleal shunt drains CSF from the ventricles to the space between the skull and the scalp. They are used as a temporizing measure, for weeks to several months in preterm infants [36, 37]. For preterm infants, particularly those <2,000 g, these shunts appear to be most effective to bridge until the infant is large enough for a ventriculoperitoneal shunt. The external ventricular drain consists of a ventricular catheter connected to an external reservoir for the accumulation of drained CSF. They may be placed as a temporary measure, for example, if an infection is present in the CSF, while CSF flow is restored via the normal anatomic pathways or via a peritoneal shunt. Hydrocephalus related to tumor, infection, or hemorrhage may require external drains, at least temporarily.

Insertion of the distal catheter into the peritoneal cavity for a ventriculoperitoneal (VP) shunt is either by mini laparotomy or the use of an abdominal trocar. The VP shunt is the most common surgical CSF shunt procedure offering the advantage of reducing the need for repeated shunt revisions as the child grows. The most common complications are infection and obstruction of the shunt, requiring shunt revision. Mechanical failure and infection account for the majority of shunt complications, although these occur far less frequently today than in the past.

Ventriculoatrial shunts from the lateral ventricle to the right atrium are much less common. The incidence of complications with these shunts including infection, obstruction, pulmonary thromboembolism and air embolism is greater than with VP shunts. Ventriculoatrial shunts require revisions as the child grows. These shunts are generally used when VP shunts are contraindicated, e.g., adhesions or abdominal sepsis. Ventriculopleural shunt, from the lateral ventricle to pleural cavity, is rarely used.

Anesthetic Considerations

Preoperative assessment should include a general assessment of the infant and a neurological examination for increased intracranial pressure. Any associated conditions should be optimized. Sedative premedication should not be prescribed. Preoperative preparation includes planning for the positioning of the infant, particularly if the head is large (Fig. 11.7). Achieving the optimal position is essential for tracheal intubation, which could otherwise be difficult due to head size.

Induction of anesthesia may be achieved via either the intravenous or inhalational route. Oxygenation and hemodynamic stability should be maintained throughout and acute increases in ICP avoided. The trachea may be intubated with a reinforced or regular uncuffed tracheal tube and/or a nasal tube as the head is heavily draped and access to the airway during surgery is almost impossible. The lungs should be ventilated throughout as spontaneous ventilation is contraindicated when the cranium is open. Bradycardia or other arrhythmias may occur when the ventricular catheter is

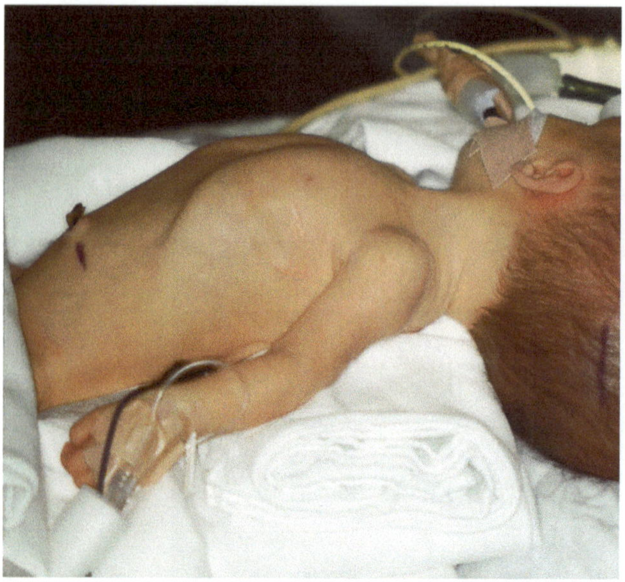

Fig. 11.7 Position of a neonate with hydrocephalus for a ventriculoperitoneal shunt

inserted. Insertion of the distal end of the VP shunt into the peritoneum requires that a passageway be tunneled under the skin from the head to the abdomen to accommodate the shunt catheter. This is usually a very stimulating maneuvre, requiring small doses of an opioid such as fentanyl. Paracetamol may be used for postoperative analgesia. It is also helpful to infiltrate the abdominal wound with local anesthetic. The abdominal component can be quite painful as access to the peritoneum requires a mini laparotomy.

Thermoregulation can be problematic as a large proportion of the neonate is washed with antiseptic prep and surgery requires a large amount of exposure. To prevent hypothermia, the room must be warmed before the neonate arrives (≥26°C) and a forced air warmer used. Central temperature should be monitored (e.g., esophageal) throughout surgery and the trachea extubated only if the neonate is normothermic.

Vein of Galen Malformations

Vein of Galen aneurysmal malformation (VGAM) is a rare congenital abnormality (less than 1/25,000 deliveries), in which multiple arteriovenous shunts drain into the median prosencephalic vein of Markowski (not into the vein of Galen itself). Typically, this malformation presents in the neonatal period with high-output cardiac failure and, in severe cases, with brain destruction resulting in serious morbidity and mortality. In the neonatal period, the presentation is usually with high-output cardiac failure, which in the past was often associated with rapid progression to multisystem organ failure (MOF) and death. Endovascular treatment has emerged as the treatment of choice for VGAM presenting in infancy with heart failure. Embolization, both of feeding arteries and draining veins, can substantially reduce aneurysmal blood flow. In many series, however, neonates have not been treated because of perceived poor outcome. A 21-point scale predicts the therapeutic efficacy of endovascular embolization in neonates based on several factors, including cardiac, cerebral, hepatic, respiratory, and renal functions [38]. A score <8 suggests that endovascular therapy would be futile, and thus treatment is not indicated, whereas a score between 8 and 12 suggests emergency embolization is indicated. A score >12 supports medical management until endovascular treatment can be performed when the infant is between 5 and 6 months of age. Although it is desirable to obtain complete occlusion of the lesion in the fewest procedures possible, endovascular treatment often entails multiple sessions.

After birth, with the loss of the low-resistance uteroplacental unit, up to 70 % of cardiac output is directed to the cerebral circulation. Pulmonary arterial pressures remain increased, and the ductus arteriosus remains open, directing right ventricular output through the patent ductus arteriosus and into the descending aorta. The right ventricle becomes distended and noncompliant because of the chronic pressure load. Subsequent right to left shunting at atrial and ductal levels causes arterial hypoxemia and increases the likelihood of ventricular failure. The left ventricle is hyperkinetic with a shortening fraction greater than 40 %. A large shunt through the VGAM occurs during diastole. The increased diastolic flow to the VGAM reduces coronary blood flow and, in combination with increased ventricular pressure, reduces subendocardial perfusion. This may produce myocardial ischemia and potentially exacerbate right heart failure. Stabilization of neonates before neurointervention or neurosurgery is difficult, and the cardiac failure is often resistant to treatment. The use of beta-adrenergic agents (dobutamine, dopamine, or adrenaline) in this setting often worsens cardiac output. Shortening of diastolic coronary filling time induced by tachycardia worsens diastolic dysfunction. The combination of low-dose dopamine and a vasodilator can substantially improve systemic perfusion and reduce the severity of metabolic acidosis [39]. The use of systemic arterial vasodilators or phosphodiesterase inhibitors may be effective in neonates with VGAM who fail to respond to conventional inotropic support since extracranial systemic vascular resistance is increased despite a reduction in total systemic vascular resistance. Arterial vasodilators (especially nitroprusside, glyceryl trinitrate, and milrinone) used to treat severe cardiac failure may reduce neurological injury before, during, and after surgery and are important to stabilize the hemodynamics before intervention. During surgery, they offset rapid changes in systemic vascular resistance induced by coil occlusion of feeding vessels of the AVM. After surgery, they may reduce the incidence of cerebral hyperemia. Prevention of hypertension during and after AVM embolization also theoretically reduces the incidence of AVM rupture secondary to increased intravascular pressure proximal to the site of occlusion or rerouting of blood flow and pressure away from the AVM.

Effective anesthetic management for AVM interventions involves aggressive cardiovascular monitoring and avoiding hypotension, hypovolemia, and low diastolic blood pressure. Excellent communication and teamwork are required between the interventional neuroradiologist and the anesthetist. Embolization of the aneurysm results in an acute increase in ventricular afterload and may exacerbate cardiac failure. The use of inotropes and vasodilators as discussed above is required to mitigate the effects of increased afterload.

Tumors

Brain tumors in infants under the age of 1 year are extremely rare. Surgery can be technically challenging, if possible at all, and the sensitivity of the developing nervous system to the side effects of radio- and chemotherapy limits their usefulness. These tumors are often histologically benign, of large dimensions, but are often situated in locations within the brain that preclude surgical intervention and lead to a fatal outcome. In a case series of 250 tumors in the neonatal period, the most common tumors diagnosed in the fetus/neonate were teratomas (29 %), followed by astrocytomas (18 %), primitive neuroectodermal tumors (13 %) and choroid plexus papillomas (13 %) [40, 41].

Brain tumors can be detected on antenatal scans as an intracranial space-occupying lesion, abnormal echogenicity in the head, macrocephaly, and hydrocephalus. The diagnosis can be confirmed and further information gained by performing magnetic resonance imaging. 50–60 % of neonates with tumors present with an isolated increase in head circumference. Tumors can also present with increased intracranial pressure, as evidenced by bulging fontanelle, failure to thrive, apneic episodes, irritability, drowsiness, vomiting, neurological deficits, intraventricular hemorrhage and hydrocephalus. Seizures are present in a minority of cases, 10–15 %. The overall 5-year survival rate of neonatal tumors is in the range of 23–36 %, despite treatment. Postoperative mortality can be as great as 7.3–33 %. The choice of technique and the extent of resection depend on the size, position, histology, and anatomical relationships of the tumor to contiguous structures. Many neonatal and childhood tumors present with hydrocephalus, and it is often this that is immediately life threatening rather than the tumor itself. The neonate may therefore require emergency insertion of a VP shunt or an EVD.

Anesthetic Considerations for Tumor Resection

Preanesthetic assessment should be as for any neonate undergoing major surgery. Ideally the neonate should have intravenous access and IV fluid hydration preinduction. The site of the craniotomy will depend on the location of the tumor and will determine the position of the neonate during surgery. This should be discussed with the surgeon. Anesthesia can be inhalational or intravenous. Tracheal intubation should be accomplished with either an oral or nasal (reinforced) tracheal tube, depending on the position required during surgery. Craniotomy in a neonate requires invasive monitoring—arterial access is essential and central venous access is desirable. Surgery should not be undertaken without large-bore intravenous access as there is an increased risk of intraoperative bleeding. A urinary catheter should be inserted. Surgery is likely to take place in the prone position as many neonatal tumors are located in the posterior, third ventricle/pineal region. In the prone position, some prefer nasotracheal intubation. After tracheal intubation and before turning the neonate prone, the position of the tip of the tracheal tube is evaluated by maximally flexing the neck to verify that the tip does not impinge on the carina or lodge endobronchially when the surgeon maximally flexes the neck to expose the posterior fossa in the prone position. If the tube is too far down the trachea, then it should be withdrawn and retaped so that it does not cause or trigger airway reflex responses. The usual precautions should be taken when turning the neonate prone with padding. Warming devices should be used. Intraoperative analgesia should be provided with opioids. Blood gases, hemoglobin, and blood sugar as well as urine output should be regularly monitored. This monitoring will give an indication of the condition of the neonate and how long surgery can continue. Again, excellent communication with the surgeon is required in these high-risk procedures. He or she should be informed if the baby's condition is deteriorating so that surgery can be curtailed if necessary. Blood should be present in the operating room before tumor surgery begins in the event sudden and unexpected massive bleeding occurs. Postoperatively, the baby may be extubated, depending on the duration of surgery and the nature of any difficulties encountered. Postoperative care should be in a monitored neurosurgical high dependency or intensive care area. Posterior fossa tumor resections are more painful postoperatively, and analgesia should be with regular paracetamol and IV morphine.

Hemorrhage and Trauma

In the neonate, surgery is occasionally needed after a trauma or intracranial hemorrhage. The most frequent cause of trauma is birth trauma, and the most frequent complication requiring neurosurgery is evacuation of a subdural hematoma. Intracerebral bleeds may occur due to a rupture of AVMs or in the setting of thrombocytopenia or other form of severe perinatal coagulopathy. Often, attempts are made to treat such hemorrhages conservatively. Neurosurgery for hemorrhage in the neonate is fraught as the brain is soft and easily damaged during retraction or if the brain herniates through the craniotomy. If surgery is performed, the anesthetist should note that blood loss might have been substantial, and they should check that any preoperative hypovolemia or anemia has been corrected. Similarly, any coagulopathy or thrombocytopenia should be corrected. Intraoperative blood loss may also be substantial. Therefore, large-bore intravenous access is essential and invasive pressure monitoring is preferable. Packed red cells, platelets and plasma must be available and given early in the event of serious bleeding.

Fetal Neurosurgery

Human prenatal myelomeningocele repair by hysterotomy was first performed in 1997, and by 2003, more than 200 fetuses had undergone the procedure. In studies in animals, prenatal coverage of a spina bifida-like lesion preserved neurological function and improved hindbrain herniation, suggesting the final neurological deficit in spina bifida is a consequence of 2 factors—a failure of neural tube formation as well as spinal cord injury resulting from prolonged exposure of neural elements to the intrauterine environment. The Management of Myelomeningocele Study (MOMS) to compare the safety and efficacy of prenatal repair of myelomeningocele with that of standard postnatal repair has recently been published [42]. In this study, eligible women were randomly assigned to undergo either prenatal surgery before 26 weeks of gestation or standard postnatal repair. Of the 158 women whose children were evaluated at 12 months, shunt placement was required in 40 % of the prenatal surgery group compared with the 82 % of the postnatal surgery group. Prenatal surgery resulted in improvement in the composite score for mental development and motor function at 30 months and improvement in hindbrain herniation by 12 months and ambulation by 30 months. However, prenatal surgery was associated with an increased risk of preterm delivery and uterine dehiscence at delivery. One-third of women who underwent prenatal surgery had an area of dehiscence or a very thin prenatal uterine surgery scar at the time of delivery. Fetuses that were treated prenatally were born at an average gestational age of 34.1 weeks, and 13 % were delivered before 30 weeks of gestation, whereas those in the postnatal surgery group were born at an average of 37.3 weeks of gestation with none delivered before 30 weeks. Thus, although prenatal surgery for myelomeningocele reduced the need for shunting and improved motor outcomes at 30 months, it was associated with maternal and fetal risks.

Surgery for Craniosynostosis

Craniosynostosis occurs when one or more of the sutures of the skull fuse prematurely (Fig. 11.8a, b). This results in an abnormally shaped skull. If uncorrected, craniosynostosis may lead to hydrocephalus, neurological impairment, and a cosmetic deformity. The most common sutures involved are the sagittal, coronal, and metopic sutures. Craniosynostosis may occur in isolation or in association with a syndrome [43]. Although craniosynostosis may be diagnosed in the

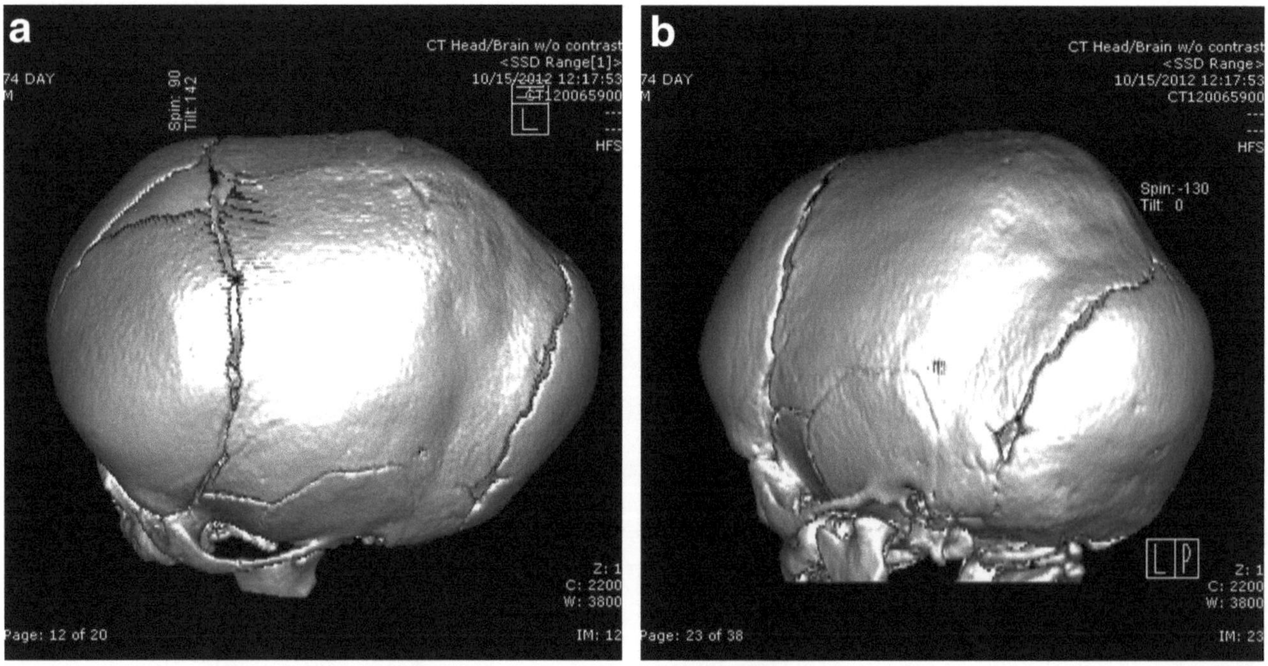

Fig. 11.8 (**a**, **b**) CT scan of a 2-month-old infant with sagittal synostosis preoperatively

neonatal period and the best results obtained during early correction in infancy, such large procedures are generally not performed in neonates. A variety of procedures have been described for this condition including strip craniectomies, where the fused suture is excised, and larger procedures where extensive areas of the skull are removed, remodeled and replaced [43]. The inner and outer tables may be split to provide more bone areas. These later operations are large procedures that are lengthy and may involve considerable blood loss. If neonatal surgery is undertaken, blood must be available at the time of skin incision to preclude severe hypovolemia and cardiac arrest.

Ophthalmology

Introduction

Neonates are subject to ophthalmic conditions such as retinopathy of prematurity (ROP), cataracts, infections, trauma and a variety of developmental conditions. The ophthalmologist has become an integral part of the neonatal intensive care unit, participating in weekly ward rounds to screen for ROP in preterm infants. Optimal anesthesia care is important for surgery in the operating room as well as on the ward and in other off-site locations for the ophthalmic examinations.

Anatomy, Physiology, and Development

The globe has three layers: the sclera, uveal tract, and retina. The sclera is the fibrous outer covering that maintains the shape of the globe; anteriorly, it is continuous with the cornea, which is transparent and avascular. The uveal tract comprises the iris, ciliary body, and choroid. The iris divides the eye into the anterior and posterior chambers. The ciliary body secretes aqueous humor for the anterior chamber and contains muscles that alter the shape of the lens. The choroid is a highly vascular tissue that supplies blood to the retina. The retina is the thin tissue layer located posteriorly within the globe, where light generates nerve potentials.

At birth, the globe is relatively large, about half the size of that in the adult. The anterior structures are relatively larger at birth compared with those in the adult. The shape of the globe becomes more spherical as the posterior structures grow with age. The sclera is thin at birth and appears translucent with a bluish tinge. The iris is blue in Caucasian neonates with the final adult coloring developing over the first 6 months of age. The eyes appear divergent in as many as 75 % neonates, but this resolves with time.

The eye becomes reactive to light at about 7 months gestation with the full-term neonate capable of following moving targets, albeit slowly. Visual acuity is poor at birth (about 20/400) but this improves rapidly during infancy.

The globe is filled with vitreous humor and aqueous humor. The vitreous humor is the more viscous component. The volume of the vitreous humor remains fairly constant as the neonate matures. The aqueous humor is formed by the ciliary body, flows through the pupil, and is absorbed via the trabecular meshwork (pores of Fontana) and the canal of Schlemm into the venous system in the anterior chamber. Changes in aqueous humor absorption can change intraocular pressure (IOP). IOP increases with increases in venous pressure such as with coughing, vomiting, and valsalva maneuvres as the episcleral veins drain through a valveless system. Hypercapnia and hypoxia also increase IOP; systemic hypertension only increases IOP, about 30 % of the increase in blood pressure.

The oculocardiac reflex is a reflex bradycardia that mediated through the third cranial nerve and the vagus. It occurs after either brisk traction on an extraocular muscle or with direct pressure on the globe. The reflex is enhanced in neonates. Release of the traction by the surgeon immediately resolves the bradycardia. Alternately, atropine (10–20 mcg/kg) or glycopyrrolate (5 mcg/kg) IV can be administered to treat the bradycardia. Both the severity and the incidence of an anticipated bradycardia may be attenuated by pretreatment with an anticholinergic [44]. It remains unclear whether any particular anesthetic regimen significantly affects either the severity or risk of an oculocardiac reflex, although there is some evidence that ketamine may attenuate the bradycardia and propofol may augment the bradycardia [45]. It is important to note that these latter studies were conducted in older children, and little is known about the optimal management of the reflex during anesthesia in neonates. Traction on the muscles and pressure on the globe may also lead to apnea.

Principles of Ophthalmic Anesthesia

Neonates who require ophthalmic procedures frequently present with other medical conditions such as prematurity, and/or pathological or congenital conditions that might impact the anesthetic care. Careful preoperative assessment is important. Anesthesia in the premature and ex-premature infant is covered in another chapter; however, particular care must be taken to assess the respiratory and cardiac systems. The infant may have chronic lung disease and/or apnea of prematurity. In the case of the latter condition or if the neonate was premature at birth, postoperative admission for 12 h of apnea monitoring should be anticipated and planned before embarking on any anesthetic including sedation. Cardiac diseases such as pulmonary hypertension and cyanotic congenital heart disease should be considered, particularly in the premature infant.

Neonates with syndromes may present with a host of medical issues that warrant our consideration preoperatively.

The incidence of cataracts, glaucoma, and nasolacrimal duct obstruction is greater in neonates with trisomy 21. These infants may also require a smaller-diameter tracheal tube than comparable infants at the same age (due to subglottic airway narrowing, congenital heart defects, and hypothyroidism). Ophthalmic conditions are also associated with Apert and Crouzon syndromes, Goldenhar syndrome, Hunter syndrome, Marfan syndrome, CHARGE syndrome and homocystinuria.

Many of the principles of anesthesia during ophthalmic surgery are similar to those for other operations in the neonate. Access to the infant may be limited, so the airway and intravenous lines must be reliable and secure. Care must be taken to prevent hypothermia or hyperthermia, and glucose and fluids should be given during surgery.

All general anesthetics decrease IOP except ketamine, which may raise IOP although this remains controversial. Succinylcholine causes a transient increase in IOP, but in neonates, this response has not been specifically studied. Brief procedures such as examinations under anesthetic or tear duct probing may be performed with spontaneous ventilation via face mask or with a laryngeal mask airway. Some examinations are performed under sedation. Procedures of greater duration require a tracheal tube. For intraocular surgery, immobility is paramount and hence tracheal tubes and neuromuscular blocking agents are recommended. Some anesthesiologists extubate the trachea during a deep level of anesthesia to avoid coughing. This should only be attempted where the airway is not compromised and staff competent in airway support is in continuous attendance until the infant is fully awake.

Ophthalmic Conditions in the Neonate

Retinopathy of Prematurity

In 1988, the landmark multicenter trial of Cryotherapy for Retinopathy of Prematurity ("Cryo-ROP") study was published [46]. Cryo-ROP found that ablative treatment for retinopathy of prematurity almost halved the rate of blindness in severe cases. Before the publication of that study, there was little evidence that treatment for ROP decreased poor visual outcomes, and hence ophthalmic procedures were rarely performed in neonatal units. Infants were sent to ophthalmologists' offices for examinations once they were well enough. Today, the commonest ophthalmic procedure in a neonatal ward is an ROP screening examination.

Severe ROP can lead to a lifetime of blindness. ROP is caused by abnormal neovascularization of the developing retina. Soon after World War II ended, an epidemic of the ROP appeared in the USA, the UK, Australia, and other developed countries. This was due in part to the improved technologies that improved the survival of extremely premature infants (as young as 24 weeks gestation) and allowed the delivery of greater concentrations of inspired oxygen to young infants, particularly those who were premature and who survived to reach childhood and older. It soon became evident that many of the premature infants were blind. In 1952, the landmark Gallinger trial suggested that the administration of excessive concentrations of oxygen was responsible for the blindness [47]. In the subsequent 15 years, the prevalence of ROP decreased from 50–4 % of premature infants, although early neonatal death and cerebral palsy increased dramatically. Currently, approximately 65 % of infants <1,250 g develop ROP [48]. ROP accounts for 13 % of childhood blindness. Although oxygen increases the risk of ROP, reduced oxygen levels have been associated with a greater risk of neonatal death and cerebral palsy. As a result, the dose and delivery of oxygen to premature infants have been debated, resulting in the current position that oxygen saturations should be maintained between 90 and 95 % as saturations >95 % increase the risk of ROP, whereas those <90 % increase the early mortality rate [49, 50].

The notion that gestational age and weight at birth and excessive oxygen levels were the sole determinants of the prevalence and severity of ROP and blindness in premature infants has proven to be oversimplistic. A multitude of factors interact to trigger the retinal vascularization that leads to ROP. Temporally, the pathogenesis and treatment of ROP are regarded in two phases: the first is an avascular phase that results from hyperoxia-induced arrest of retinal vascularization, whereas the second is a proliferative period of neovascularization. The initial trigger for ROP may occur in utero period with a systemic inflammatory response that renders infants susceptible to excess oxygen concentrations. Oxygen modulates the activities of hypoxia-inducing factor 1 and vascular endothelial growth factor, both of which regulate neuroangiogenesis in the retina. A shift in the concentrations of these factors may arrest the initial vascularization of the retina. Additionally, insulin-like growth factor 1 and erythropoietin may modulate the proliferation of retinal angiogenesis. Two further mechanisms may impact on the pathogenesis of ROP. The first is a genetic component that is associated with differential responses to nitric oxide, adenosine, apelin and beta-adrenergic receptors [51]. Indeed, the differential prevalence of ROP in Caucasians and African American infants suggests that single nucleotide polymorphisms in, for example, beta-adrenergic receptors may affect the susceptibility to ROP and its treatment. The second is an inflammatory response that may expose the retina to infectious or inflammatory mediators or to oxidative stress in utero, thereby priming the retina for ROP later [52]. Understanding the relative importance of these mechanisms in the pathogenesis of ROP has led to several innovative therapeutic interventions that may prove to be widely effective [53, 54].

Treatment needs to be a timely evaluation of the vascularity of the neonatal retina to prevent a retinal detachment or dragging of the macula. The macula is the area of the retina devoted to central vision. Any distortion of the macula leads to poor central vision. Several innovative, targeted interventions have been investigated that in the future may hold promise for preventing blindness from developing in these infants [54].

ROP Screening Procedures

Pupil Dilation

The use of topical medication to dilate the pupil is crucial to permit examination of the peripheral retina where ROP occurs. Refinements to topical anesthesia regimens have ensured that the pupil can be well dilated, without increasing the risks of drug toxicity to the infants (Table 11.1).

To prevent toxicity from topical ophthalmic medication, the doses should be meticulously calculated a priori. Medications that dilate the pupils are known as mydriatics. Examination of the eyes of infants with possible ROP requires good mydriasis in order to visualize the entire retina, all the way to the ora serrata. Mydriatic drop regimens vary from nursery to nursery. A common combination is cyclopentolate 0.25 % combined with phenylephrine 2.5 %, one drop to each eye, followed by another dose 10–15 min later. The initial dose is given approximately 30–60 min before the examination.

Atropine is also a potent mydriatic. However, like tropicamide, it produces adverse gastrointestinal effects. In the neonate, these effects can be severe. Atropine is an anticholinergic/parasympatholytic (anti-muscarinic) that, in addition to causing tachycardia, flush, and fever, can also cause gastrointestinal effects that minimize bowel sounds. This can imitate necrotizing enterocolitis.

Analgesia

A screening procedure can be very painful in some situations, e.g., with an inexperienced screener or on an infant with significant periorbital edema from prolonged assisted ventilation. Infants with small palpebral fissures can also be difficult to examine. Steps should be taken to minimize all pain in neonates.

Examination is usually performed under topical anesthesia. Pain can be caused by (a) the bright light of the indirect ophthalmoscope, (b) an eyelid speculum, and (c) the use of an instrument for scleral indenting. Various protocols have been developed to minimize the pain from examination, and each will have been developed for individual nurseries. Topical anesthetic agents are given immediately before an examination. Corneal and conjunctival discomfort is decreased significantly as is the sensitivity to the brightness of the indirect ophthalmoscope's light. Agents including proxymetacaine, tetracaine, oxybuprocaine, and proparacaine are useful topical ophthalmic local anesthetics. However, excessive doses to the eye can weaken the intercellular attachments of the corneal epithelium, which can cause haziness of the cornea or sometimes sloughing of epithelial cells. Some nurseries administer paracetamol or oral sucrose for additional analgesia. However, strong repeated sucking actions by the infant can make the procedure more difficult.

Anesthesia for Laser Surgery of ROP

During the 1990s, the standard treatment for ROP changed from cryotherapy to laser surgery. Cryotherapy is painful, requiring general anesthesia. Furthermore, postoperative pain after cryotherapy is significant because there is considerable swelling of the conjunctiva. Alternatively, laser surgery causes much less pain and is brief, lasting approximately 30–40 min per eye. Laser burns are applied to the peripheral retina, usually to a full 360°. A lens loupe is used to gently move the eye to the appropriate positions. Occasionally, infants are sensitive to the burns themselves, but more often, the distress from the surgery is associated with physical maneuvring of the globe, the intensity of the light from the indirect ophthalmoscopic delivery system of the laser, the swaddling of the infant and the length of the procedure.

Table 11.1 Eye drops commonly used in neonates and their possible complications

Drug	Action	Side effects
Cyclopentolate	Anticholinergic (similar action to atropine but faster onset of action and shorter half-life)	Grand mal seizure [31–33]; psychotic reactions (in children) [34–37]; gastrointestinal toxicity including death from necrotizing enterocolitis after 6 drops of 1 % (in an infant) [38]
Phenylephrine	Sympathomimetic/adrenergic	Increased blood pressure in any age group
Tropicamide	Anticholinergic/parasympatholytic	Gastrointestinal (more pronounced in children) [39]
Atropine	Anticholinergic/parasympatholytic (anti-muscarinic)	Increased heart rate (in any age group but more pronounced in children) [39]; gastrointestinal [39]; atropine flush/fever (more pronounced in children), acute confusional psychosis
Homatropine	Anticholinergic/parasympatholytic similar effects to atropine but weaker	

The type of anesthesia required for the laser treatment of ROP varies depending on the ophthalmologist and the stability of the infant.

Many ophthalmologists prefer the infants to be paralyzed. This reduces the duration of the procedure as the surgeon can apply the burns more rapidly. Infant eyes can be lasered with sedation (e.g., with chloral hydrate) and a dose of morphine (0.5 mg/kg), but with sicker and smaller infants requiring laser, the risk of oxygen desaturation, apnea, and requirement for emergent intubation during the procedure increases. The heart rate and respiratory rate should be monitored to identify episodes of bradycardia and apnea during the procedure, and this should be communicated to the ophthalmic surgeon.

Congenital Cataracts

Congenital cataracts may occur in isolation or be associated with many congenital conditions. Cataract surgery is generally delayed until the infant is older than 6 weeks to minimize the risk of aphakic glaucoma. Aphakic glaucoma is a condition that can be catastrophic to vision and has a much greater incidence in infants with cataracts that are extracted before the first month of age. The onset of aphakic glaucoma can occur at any time during childhood.

Congenital Glaucoma

Congenital glaucoma, as opposed to aphakic glaucoma, sometimes requires surgical treatment in the first few weeks of life to minimize damage from an increased intraocular pressure. Infants with congenital glaucoma may receive antiglaucoma medication as eye drops that could impact on anesthesia. Medication includes

1. Prostaglandin analogues, e.g., latanoprost, travoprost and bimatoprost
2. Beta blockers, e.g., timolol and betaxolol
3. Alpha(2)-adrenoreceptor agonists, e.g., brimonidine and apraclonidine
4. Carbonic anhydrase inhibitors (CAI), e.g., brinzolamide, dorzolamide and acetazolamide

Beta Blockers

Timolol 0.25 % is widely used. Systemic absorption can lead to side effects relating to beta-adrenergic receptor blockage, including bradycardia and respiratory compromise. Beta-blocking drugs are avoided in premature infants, although on occasion, they may be used in full-term infants with glaucoma.

A new use of beta-blocking agents in ophthalmology in infants and children is to treat capillary hemangiomas [55]. Orbital and periorbital hemangiomas can cause astigmatism and lead to amblyopia. Systemic and topical beta-blocking agents are being used with increasing frequency to treat hemangiomas.

Alpha(2)-Adrenoreceptor Agonists

Alpha(2)-adrenoreceptor agonists, e.g., brimonidine, are avoided in infants because they may cause drowsiness and CNS depression. Just one drop of topical brimonidine can lead to sleepiness that can be quite prolonged [56].

Carbonic Anhydrase Inhibitors

Carbonic anhydrase inhibitors such as acetazolamide are used to treat open-angle glaucoma and intracranial hypertension. However, these compounds can lead to significant side effects in neonates, the most serious being metabolic acidosis, dehydration, and renal stones. Paresthesia, which is a problem in adults who ingest acetazolamide, is an uncommon problem in children.

Tear Duct Obstruction

Neonates may be born with a congenital stenosis or obstruction of the nasolacrimal duct. If the obstruction remains unresolved by the end of the first year, a lacrimal probing may be indicated. During general anesthesia, the duct is dilated with a blunt metal probe passed from either the upper or lower lacrimal punctum. Success is confirmed by the metal probe making contact with another metal probe placed at the inferior meatus in the nose and/or by injecting fluorescein into the punctum and detecting a patent duct by the presence of fluorescein on a pipe cleaner inserted into the nostril. If fluorescein is injected, it may be prudent to place a roll under the infant's shoulders and position the child in slight Trendelenburg. A face mask or laryngeal mask airway may be used; however, if a nasendoscopy is performed, the duration of the procedure may be extended and a tracheal tube required. At the conclusion, it is prudent to suction the oropharynx to remove any blood or fluorescein in the hypopharynx before the infant is awakened.

References

1. Hill A. Intracranial pressure measurements in the newborn. Clin Perinatol. 1985;12(1):161–78.
2. Wayenberg JL. Non-invasive measurement of intracranial pressure in neonates and infants: experience with the Rotterdam teletransducer. Acta Neurochir Suppl. 1998;71:70–3.
3. de Kieviet JF, Zoetebier L, van Elburg RM, et al. Brain development of very preterm and very low-birthweight children in child-

hood and adolescence: a meta-analysis. Dev Med Child Neurol. 2012;54:313–23.

4. Settergren G, Lindblad BS, Persson B. Cerebral blood flow and exchange of oxygen, glucose ketone bodies, lactate, pyruvate and amino acids in anesthetized children. Acta Paediatr Scand. 1980;69(4):457–65.
5. Greisen G. To autoregulate or not autoregulate – that is no longer the question. Semin Pediatr Neurol. 2009;16:207–15.
6. Soul JS, Hammer PE, Tsuji M, et al. Fluctuating pressure-passivity is common in the cerebral circulation of sick premature infants. Pediatr Res. 2007;61:467–73.
7. Liem KD, Greisen G. Monitoring of cerebral haemodynamics in newborn infants. Early Hum Dev. 2010;86(3):155–8.
8. Tweed A, et al. Impairment of cerebral blood flow autoregulation in the newborn lamb by hypoxia. Pediatr Res. 1986;20(6):516–19.
9. Tyszczuk L, Meek J, Elwell C, et al. Cerebral blood flow is independent of mean arterial blood pressure in preterm infants undergoing intensive care. Pediatrics. 1998;102:337–41.
10. Cayabyab R, McLean CW, Seri I. Definition of hypotension and assessment of hemodynamics in preterm neonate. J Perinatol. 2009;29 Suppl 2:S58–62.
11. Jayasinghie D, Gill AB, Levene M. CBF reactivity in hypotensive and normotensive preterm infants. Pediatr Res. 2003;54:848–53.
12. Ballabh P. Intraventricular haemorrhage in premature infants: mechanism of disease. Pediatr Res. 2010;67:1–8.
13. Alderliesten T, Lemmers PMA, Smarius JJM, et al. Cerebral oxygenation, extraction, and autoregulation in very preterm infants who develop peri-ventricular haemorrhage. J Pediatr. 2013;162: 698–704.
14. Ainslie PN, et al. Dynamic cerebral autoregulation and baroreflex sensitivity during modest and severe step changes in arterial PCO2. Brain Res. 2008;1230:115–24.
15. Yamashita N, Kamiya K, Nagai H. CO2 reactivity and autoregulation in fetal brain. Childs Nerv Syst. 1991;7(6):327–31.
16. Pilato MA, Bissonnette B, Lerman J. Transcranial Doppler: response of cerebral blood-flow velocity to carbon dioxide in anesthetized children. Can J Anaesth. 1991;38(1):37–42.
17. Muizelaar JP, et al. Pial arteriolar vessel diameter and CO2 reactivity during prolonged hyperventilation in the rabbit. J Neurosurg. 1988;69(6):923–7.
18. Todd MM. Cerebral blood flow during isovolemic hemodilution: mechanistic observations. Adv Pharmacol. 1994;31:595–605.
19. Vavilala MS, et al. Cerebral autoregulation before and after blood transfusion in a child. J Neurosurg Anesthesiol. 2001;13(3):233–6.
20. Braun LD, Cornford EM, Oldendorf WH. Newborn rabbit blood-brain barrier is selectively permeable and differs substantially from the adult. J Neurochem. 1980;34(1):147–52.
21. McCann ME, Soriano SG. Perioperative central nervous system injury in neonates. Br J Anaesth. 2012;109:i60–7.
22. Nafiu OO, Voepel-Lewis T, Morris M, et al. How do pediatric anesthesiologists define intraoperative hypotension? Paediatr Anaesth. 2009;19:1048–53.
23. Loepke AW, Spaeth JP. Glucose and heart surgery: neonates are not just small adults. Anesthesiology. 2004;100(6):1339–41.
24. Vannucci RC, Yager JY. Glucose, lactic acid, and perinatal hypoxic-ischemic brain damage. Pediatr Neurol. 1992;8(1):3–12.
25. Wong GT, et al. The effect of sevoflurane on cerebral autoregulation in young children as assessed by the transient hyperemic response. Anesth Analg. 2006;102(4):1051–5.
26. Schlunzen L, et al. Effects of dose-dependent levels of isoflurane on cerebral blood flow in healthy subjects studied using positron emission tomography. Acta Anesthesiol Scand. 2006;50(3): 306–12.
27. MRC Vitamin Study Research Group. Prevention of neural tube defects: results of the medical research council vitamin study. Lancet. 1991;338(8760):131–7.
28. Grosse SD, Collins JS. Folic acid supplementation and neural tube defect recurrence prevention. Birth Defects Res A Clin Mol Teratol. 2007;79(11):737–42.
29. Williams LJ, et al. Prevalence of spina bifida and anencephaly during the transition to mandatory folic acid fortification in the United States. Teratology. 2002;66(1):33–9.
30. Bol KA, Collins JS, Kirby RS. Survival of infants with neural tube defects in the presence of folic acid fortification. Pediatrics. 2006;117(3):803–13.
31. Alexiou GA, Sfakianos G, Prodromou N. Diagnosis and management of cephaloceles. J Craniofac Surg. 2010;21:1581–2.
32. Mahajan C, Rath GP, Dash HH, Bithal PK. Perioperative management of children with encephalocele: an institutional experience. J Neurosurg Anesthesiol. 2011;23:352–6.
33. Mahapatra AK. Giant encephalocele: a study of 14 patients. Pediatr Neurosurg. 2011;47:406–11.
34. Leelanukrom R, Wacharasint P, Kaewanuchit A. Perioperative management for surgical correction of frontoethmoidal encephalomeningocele in children: a review of 102 cases. Pediatr Anesth. 2007;17:856–62.
35. Steward DJ. Preterm infants are more prone to complications following minor surgery than are term infants. Anesthesiology. 1982;56(4):304–6.
36. Robinson S. Neonatal posthemorrhagic hydrocephalus from prematurity: pathophysiology and current treatment concepts. J Neurosurg Pediatr. 2012;9:242–58.
37. Koksal V, Oktem S. Ventriculosubgaleal shunt procedure and its long-term outcomes in premature infants with post-hemorrhagic hyrodcephalus. Childs Nerv Syst. 2010;26:1505–15.
38. Lasjaunias PL, et al. The management of vein of Galen aneurysmal malformations. Neurosurgery. 2006;59(5 Suppl 3):S184–94. discussion S3–13.
39. Frawley GP, et al. Clinical course and medical management of neonates with severe cardiac failure related to vein of Galen malformation. Arch Dis Child Fetal Neonatal Ed. 2002;87(2):F144–9.
40. Isaacs Jr H. I. Perinatal brain tumors: a review of 250 cases. Pediatr Neurol. 2002;27(4):249–61.
41. Isaacs Jr H. II. Perinatal brain tumors: a review of 250 cases. Pediatr Neurol. 2002;27(5):333–42.
42. Engelhardt T, Crawford MW, Subramanyam R, Lerman J. Plastic and reconstructive surgery. In: Coté CJ, Lerman J, Anderson BA, editors. A practice of anesthesia for infants and children. Philadelphia: Saunders; 2013. Chap. 33.
43. Adzick NS, et al. A randomized trial of prenatal versus postnatal repair of myelomeningocele. N Engl J Med. 2011;364(11): 993–1004.
44. Chisakuta AM, Mirakhur RK. Anticholinergic prophylaxis does not prevent emesis following strabismus surgery in children. Paediatr Anaesth. 1995;5(2):97–100.
45. Hahnenkamp K, et al. Effect of different anesthetic regimes on the oculocardiac reflex during paediatric strabismus surgery. Paediatr Anaesth. 2000;10(6):601–8.
46. Cryotherapy for Retinopathy of Prematurity Cooperative Group. Multicenter trial of cryotherapy for retinopathy of prematurity. Preliminary results. Arch Ophthalmol. 1988;106(4):471–9.
47. Patz A, Hoeck L. Studies on the effect of high oxygen administration in retrolental fibroplasia. I. Nursery observations. Am J Ophthalmol. 1952;35:1248–53.
48. Rubaltelli DM, Hirose T. Retinopathy of prematurity update. Int Ophthalmol Clin. 2008;48:225–35.

49. SUPPORT Study Group of the Eunice Kennedy Shriver NICHD Neonatal Research Network. Target ranges of oxygen saturation in extremely preterm infants. NEJM. 2010;362:1959–69.
50. Askie LM. Optimal oxygen saturations in preterm infants: a moving target. Curr Opin Pediatr. 2013;25:188–92.
51. Cavallaro G, Filippi L, Bagnoli P, et al. The pathophysiology of retinopathy of prematurity: an update of previous and recent knowledge. Acta Ophthalmol. 2014;92:2–20.
52. Lee J, Dammann O. Perinatal infection, inflammation, and retinopathy of prematurity. Semin Fetal Neonatal Med. 2012;17:26–9.
53. Markhoul IR, Peleg O, Miller B, et al. Oral propranolol versus placebo for retinopathy of prematurity: a pilot, randomised, double-blind prospective study. Arch Dis Child. 2013;98:565–7.
54. Hartnett ME, Penn JS. Mechanisms and management of retinopathy of prematurity. NEJM. 2012;367:515–26.
55. Leaute-Labreze C, et al. Propranolol for severe hemangiomas of infancy. N Engl J Med. 2008;358(24):2649–51.
56. Bowman RJ, Cope J, Nischal KK. Ocular and systemic side effects of brimonidine 0.2 % eye drops (Alphagan) in children. Eye. 2004; 18(1):24–6.

Anesthesia for Cardiac Surgery in Neonates

12

Wanda C. Miller-Hance, Erin A. Gottlieb, and Pablo Motta

Introduction

Cardiac surgery in the neonate usually is indicated for treatment of congenital malformations of the heart or cardiovascular system. Extremely rare is the need for surgical intervention for pathologies such as endocarditis, cardiac tumors, rhythm disturbances, or pericardial disease. Thus, the focus of this chapter is on anesthesia for cardiac surgery in the neonate with congenital heart disease (CHD).

This chapter begins with a brief overview of the cardiovascular physiology of the fetus and neonate, followed by a discussion of CHD that includes the epidemiology, clinical features, and diagnosis in the neonate. Selected anomalies of particular relevance in this age group are reviewed, with emphasis on anatomic features, pathophysiology of the defect, perioperative management, and specific considerations during anesthetic care. This is followed with an in-depth discussion on the important aspects of anesthetic practice in the neonate with CHD undergoing cardiac surgery. Finally, several specific perioperative problems and concerns in the neonate are highlighted.

W.C. Miller-Hance, MD (✉)
Divisions of Pediatric Anesthesiology and Pediatric Cardiology, Departments of Anesthesiology and Pediatrics, Baylor College of Medicine, Texas Children's Hospital, 6621 Fannin Street, Suite W 17417, Houston, TX 77030, USA
e-mail: wmh@bcm.tmc.edu

E.A. Gottlieb, MD • P. Motta, MD
Division of Pediatric Anesthesiology, Department of Anesthesiology, Baylor College of Medicine, Texas Children's Hospital, Houston, TX USA
e-mail: eagottli@texaschildrens.org; pxmotta@texaschildrens.org

Cardiovascular Physiology

An understanding of important features of the fetal and neonatal circulations, including their distinct blood flow patterns, distribution of blood flow, transition of the circulations, and changes at birth, in addition to clinically relevant developmental aspects of cardiac physiology, is essential for those who care for the neonate with heart disease [1, 2]. The section that follows provides a brief review of our current understanding of the subject. It should be noted that much of the data regarding the fetal circulation has been derived from the fetal lamb model, with the information extrapolated to the human fetus.

Types of Circulation

Fetal Circulation

The placenta is the organ for exchange of oxygen and carbon dioxide between the fetus and the mother, serving the role of the pulmonary system in utero. It is also the site of nutrient uptake for developing fetus. Oxygenated blood from the placenta is transferred to the fetus via a single umbilical vein (Fig. 12.1) and has the greatest oxygen tension (pO_2) in the fetus (range, ~30 to 35 mmHg). Blood from the umbilical vein courses through the liver; the left lobe receives blood from the umbilical vein, whereas the right lobe receives blood from both the umbilical and portal venous systems. A significant amount of umbilical venous blood (~50 to 60 %) bypasses the hepatic circulation by midterm gestation and enters the inferior vena cava (IVC)-right atrial (RA) junction through the ductus venosus. Thus, blood in the IVC during fetal life originates from the liver, the lower body, and the placenta (via the ductus venosus). Approximately 30 % of IVC blood is directed across the foramen (or fossa) ovale into the left atrium (LA). Preferential streaming blood flow patterns in the fetal heart allow the more saturated venous blood from the umbilical

J. Lerman (ed.), *Neonatal Anesthesia*, DOI 10.1007/978-1-4419-6041-2_12,

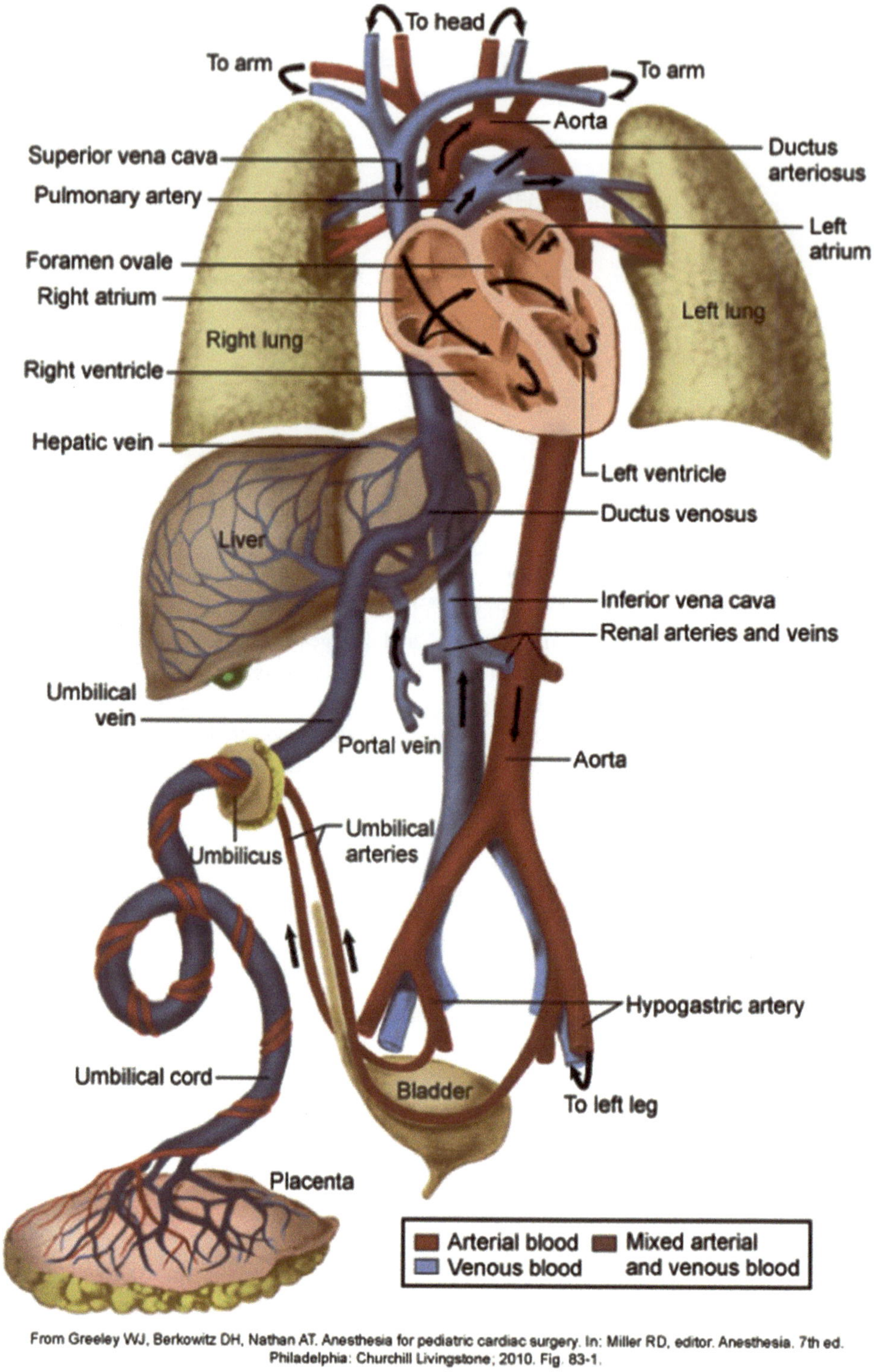

Fig. 12.1 Course of the fetal circulation in late gestation. Note the selective blood flow patterns across the foramen ovale and ductus arteriosus. From Greeley WJ, Berkowitz DH, Nathan AT. *Anesthesia for pediatric cardiac surgery*. In: Miller RD, editor. Anesthesia. 7th ed. Philadelphia: Churchill Livingstone; 2010; with permission

vein (via the ductus venosus) and left hepatic vein to be diverted into the LA across the limbus of the foramen ovale. Thus, this anatomic structure represents an important site of shunting in the fetal heart. The direction of blood flow across the foramen ovale in utero, normally from the RA to the LA, deserves mention. In the LA, blood mixes with the small amount of return from the pulmonary veins and is ejected by the left ventricle (LV) into the ascending aorta (Asc Ao). From there, the relatively "highly" oxygenated blood is distributed to the coronary arteries, cerebral circulation, and upper extremities. The remaining blood from the IVC (mostly from the lower body and liver) mixes in the RA with blood from the superior vena cava (SVC) and coronary sinus, which has a relatively low pO_2 (~12 to 14 mmHg). Mixed blood then courses across the tricuspid valve and enters the right ventricle (RV; pO_2 ~ 18 to 19 mmHg), where it is ejected into the main pulmonary artery (MPA). A state of high pulmonary vascular resistance associated with the airless collapsed lungs and fetal low pO_2 limits pulmonary blood flow, and most of the ejected RV blood courses through the ductus arteriosus into the descending aorta (Desc Ao). Desaturated blood from the Desc Ao reaches the placenta via the umbilical arteries. The fetal circulation in this fashion is extremely efficient, allowing for the least saturated blood to be directed into the RV and via the ductus arteriosus into the Desc Ao in order for oxygen and substrate uptake to take place in the placenta; the most saturated blood is directed into the LV to be ejected into the Asc Ao for distribution to highly metabolic active organs (the heart and brain) for oxygen and substrate delivery.

In summary, the fetal circulation possesses a physiology characterized by parallel circulations, the presence of shunts (intracardiac and extracardiac), and an increased pulmonary vascular resistance (Table 12.1). Although structural heart disease in the fetus can be associated with hemodynamic alterations and abnormal blood flow patterns, the presence of shunts to a great extent compensates for these changes, ensuring fetal viability until delivery in most cases.

Table 12.1 Characteristic features of the fetal and neonatal circulations

Feature	Fetal circulation	Neonatal circulation
Arrangement of the circulation	In parallel	In series
Shunts	Present (essential)	Absent
Pulmonary vascular resistance	High	Low
Cardiac output	Low	High
Site of gas exchange	Placenta	Lungs

Transitional Circulation

At birth, major changes occur as follows: (1) with ligation of the umbilical cord, the placenta is excluded from the circulation and the lungs assume the function of gas exchange, (2) expansion of the lungs results in a large reduction in pulmonary vascular resistance, (3) an associated significant increase in pulmonary blood flow occurs, and (4) removal of the low-resistance placental vascular bed leads to an increase in systemic vascular resistance, a rise in LV afterload, and a decrease in the volume of blood returning to the IVC. At this time, the shunts between the pulmonary and systemic circulations during fetal life (ductus venosus, foramen ovale, and ductus arteriosus) normally close. The ductus venosus usually closes within 24 h of birth. Although the mechanisms involved in this process are incompletely understood, it is thought to occur primarily as a passive process. Postnatal functional closure of the foramen ovale occurs as the LA pressure exceeds RA pressure. An increase in LA pressure is a consequence of the marked augmentation of pulmonary venous return associated with increased pulmonary blood flow. A reduction in RA pressure is due to the concomitant decrease in IVC pressure/flow. Patency of the foramen ovale can result in atrial level shunting, the direction being influenced by the atrial pressures. It is not unusual for occasional right-to-left shunting or bidirectional shunting across the foramen to occur during the first few hours or days of life; this normally has no hemodynamic consequence. A change in the direction of shunting across the ductus arteriosus occurs, from right-to-left in fetal life to left-to-right postnatally. This change in flow fills the ductus with blood having a greater oxygen tension, which stimulates ductal closure. Constriction of the ductus arteriosus is linked to the local effect of increased oxygen tension plus the reduction in plasma concentrations of circulating prostaglandins that ensues at birth. Functional closure of the ductus arteriosus occurs within 10–25 h after birth, whereas complete obliteration of the ductal lumen occurs in the first few weeks of postnatal life. If the normal increase in the arterial pO_2 does not take place, because of either pulmonary or cardiac disease, or the constrictor response to oxygen is diminished (i.e., prematurity), the ductus can remain open.

It is important to recognize that all these changes that take place at birth, essential to the normal infant, may significantly compromise the circulation of the neonate with structural heart disease [1]. A reduction or lack of shunting across anatomic fetal structures in the neonate with CHD at birth, for example, can be catastrophic postnatally until restoration of these communications is established.

Postnatal Circulation

In the neonate, the adult pattern of the blood flow through the heart is established; RV output (pulmonary blood flow) and LV output (systemic blood flow) are equal and, normally, no shunts are present. In summary, in contrast to that of the fetus, the circulation operates in series, lacks shunts, and is characterized by a progressive decrease in pulmonary vascular resistance (Table 12.1).

Cardiac Output and Distribution of Blood Flow

In the fetus, both the RV and the LV eject into the systemic circulation, denoting that cardiac output of the two ventricles is in parallel. The total volume of blood ejected by both ventricles in the fetus is referred to as the combined ventricular output (CVO). The RV contributes two-thirds of the CVO, whereas the LV ejects only one-third. A small amount of the CVO, in the range of 5 to 10 %, reaches the pulmonary circulation, and 55 to 60 % crosses the ductus arteriosus into the Desc Ao. Approximately 3 % of the CVO reaches the heart and 22 % the upper body. Only 10 % of the CVO courses through the Ao isthmus into the Desc Ao. Throughout gestation, a gradual reduction occurs in the fraction of CVO that is distributed to the placenta as the ventricular output increases to meet the increased demands of developing fetal organs [3]. Cardiac output increases immediately after birth to meet the metabolic demands of the neonate, with associated significant increases in blood flow to the lungs, kidneys, and gastrointestinal system; the LV output increases to approximate that of the RV.

Developmental Aspects in the Myocardium

The fetal myocardium is structurally and functionally immature and has limited potential to increase cardiac output. The ultrastructure of the neonatal myocardium is not well organized. The neonatal heart has fewer myocytes, the organization of the myofibrils is relatively poor, and the proportion of contractile elements is less than that of the adult myocardium [4]. In essence, the neonatal heart operates with an incompletely developed contractile system. Additional characteristics of the neonatal myocardium include the following: (1) control of contractility is more dependent on adrenal function and circulating catecholamines than on direct autonomic influences, (2) the sarcoplasmic reticulum, the primary source of calcium storage for excitation-contraction coupling, is poorly developed, and (3) deficient T tubules result in a significant dependence on transmembrane calcium fluxes [5, 6]. The neonatal heart is, therefore, not able to increase contractility under conditions of demand.

Other important aspects of the neonatal myocardium that impacts its ability to augment cardiac output include: (1) less compliant ventricles that are less able to augment stroke volume, (2) a greater dependence upon the heart rate to increase cardiac output, (3) limited tolerance to changes in preload and less ability to recruit the Frank-Starling mechanism, (4) less ability to significantly increase the contractile state, and (5) poor compensation for changes in afterload. These characteristics dictate many of the principles of neonatal cardiac perioperative practice including the frequent need for inotropic support, the value of calcium boluses/infusions, and the use of cardiac pacing. These factors also explain the greater sensitivity of the neonatal myocardium to anesthetic drugs [7]. The major differences between the neonatal and adult myocardium are summarized in Table 12.2.

An important aspect of neonatal cardiac function is the interdependence of ventricular function. Failure of one ventricle is likely to impact the filling and hence the function of the other.

Table 12.2 Summary of major differences between neonatal and mature myocardium

Parameters	Neonatal heart	Mature heart
Physiology		
Contractility	Limited	Normal
Heart rate dependence	High	Low
Contractile reserve	Low	High
Preload tolerance	Limited	Better
Afterload tolerance	Low	High
Ventricular interdependence	Significant	Less
Ca^{++} handling		
Predominant site of Ca^{++} flux	Sarcolemma	Sarcoplasmic reticulum
Dependence on normal iCa^{++}	High	Lower
Circulating catecholamines	High	Lower
Adrenergic receptors	Downregulated insensitive β_2, β_1 predominant	Normal β_1 predominant
Innervation	Parasympathetic predominates; sympathetic incomplete	Complete
Cytoskeleton	High collagen and water content	Lower collagen and water content
Cellular elements	Incomplete SR, disorganized myofibrils	Mature SR organized myofibrils

From Andropoulos DB. Physiology and molecular biology of the developing circulation. In Andropoulos DB, Stayer SA, Russell I, and Mossad EB, editors. *Anesthesia for Congenital Heart Disease*. Hoboken: Wiley-Blackwell; 2010; with permission

Ca^{++} calcium, *iCa^{++}* ionized calcium, *SR* sarcoplasmic reticulum

Epidemiology of Congenital Heart Disease

CHD is the most common type of birth defect in humans. In the United States, these defects affect approximately 8 out of 1,000 live births (Table 12.3) [8]. A recent systematic review and meta-analysis comprising a large study population reported that the worldwide prevalence of CHD has increased substantially over time, from <1 per 1,000 live births in 1930 to 9 per 1,000 live births in recent years, corresponding to 1.35 million worldwide live births affected with CHD every year [9]. The prevalence may be even greater than previously thought as a recent study in a large cohort of neonates undergoing echocardiographic screening revealed a live birth prevalence of CHD of 26.6 per 1,000 [10]. To further complicate the epidemiology of CHD in neonates, a large regional variation in the prevalence has been reported in various countries [11]. The prevalence of CHD in preterm infants is twice that in infants born full term [12]. Approximately 16 % of infants presenting with CHD were born preterm. CHD may also be associated with a genetic pattern of inheritance (10 %) (e.g., trisomy 18, 21, 4p deletion, and 22q11 deletion) and epigenetic and/or a syndromic pattern (as in omphalocele and Holt-Oram syndrome) [13–15].

CHD is a predominant cause of death in the first year of life [16]. Without treatment, the pathology is fatal in many neonates. Increased mortality is observed in preterm infants [12]. Twenty-five percent of infants with CHD require intervention in the first year of life in order to limit mortality [17]. Neonates account for nearly 20 % of patients included in the Congenital Heart Surgery Database (The Society of Thoracic Surgeons) that undergo cardiothoracic surgical interventions each year (6,571 of 33,979 patients as per the Fall 2013 report, mostly from North American Centers), emphasizing the need to appreciate the considerations for anesthetic care in neonates.

Table 12.3 Annual birth prevalence of congenital cardiovascular defects in the United States

Type of presentation	Rate per 1,000 live births	Estimated number (variable with yearly birth rate)
Fetal loss	Unknown	Unknown
Invasive procedure during the first year	2.4	9,200
Detected during the first year[a]	8	36,000
Bicuspid aortic valve	13.7	54,800

From Go et al. [8], with permission
[a]Includes stillbirths and pregnancy termination at <20 weeks of gestation; includes some defects that resolve spontaneously or do not require treatment

Clinical Presentation and Diagnosis of Congenital Heart Disease in the Neonate

The presentation of CHD in the neonate depends upon the nature and severity of the pathology [18]. Although in many cases, CHD is detected during fetal screening or immediately after birth, in some instances the diagnosis is made at a later age. A particularly ominous presentation is that of the apparently healthy neonate who develops life-threatening symptoms after discharge from the nursery, which require urgent medical attention. Early recognition and appropriate management of the infant with critical CHD are essential to maximize outcome [19].

The neonate with significant CHD varies in his/her manifestations of the heart disease from no signs immediately after birth to the gradual onset of signs as their physiology changes (i.e., ductal closure, changes in pulmonary vascular resistance). The most common clinical manifestations of CHD in the neonate are respiratory distress, cyanosis, a heart murmur, and signs of reduced cardiac output [18, 20]. Respiratory distress (i.e., tachypnea, labored breathing, retractions) usually is associated with lesions that result in an increased LA volume/pressure. These symptoms may reflect pulmonary over-circulation (left-to-right shunts), obstructed pulmonary venous drainage, or pathology that leads to increased LV end-diastolic volume/pressure. Clinical cyanosis is usually apparent when the concentration of reduced hemoglobin exceeds 5 g/dL. Although often due to lung disease, cyanosis may indicate cardiac disease and is secondary to reduced pulmonary blood flow, right-to-left shunting, or mixing physiology. The presence of a heart murmur in the neonate is sometimes, but not always, associated with CHD. Conversely, serious CHD can be present in the absence of a murmur. Hypotension may indicate impending or frank hemodynamic decompensation and often implies serious pathology requiring immediate intervention, aimed at stabilization of the infant and prevention of vital organ damage.

In the neonate with suspected CHD, physical examination should include four extremity blood pressure determinations and pulse oximetry measurement in pre- and post-ductal regions. A hyperoxia test may be performed in an effort to distinguish cardiac disease from other causes of cyanosis. It consists of measuring the arterial oxygen tension (PaO_2) in the right radial artery (pre-ductal site) and in a lower extremity/umbilical artery (post-ductal site) during the administration of room air and 100 % oxygen. If the cyanosis is related to pulmonary disease, supplemental oxygen can be expected to increase the $PaO_2 > 150$ mmHg. In contrast, in the case of CHD, supplemental oxygen will have no or minimal effect, and the PaO_2 will typically remain less than 100 mmHg. This response in the neonate with CHD is referred to as *failure of the hyperoxia test.* Additional studies such as a chest radiograph and a complete electrocardiogram that includes right-sided leads (V_3R and V_4R) are routinely obtained. Echocardiography is the primary modality for the initial evaluation and serial assessment of most types of CHD. It is diagnostic in most neonates, and in only selected cases are additional studies such as chest computed tomography, magnetic resonance imaging, or cardiac catheterization and angiography required to further delineate the anatomical or functional abnormalities.

Classification of Congenital Heart Disease

Numerous classification schemes have been proposed for CHD [21, 22]. These categorize malformations based on (1) complexity of the lesion as simple versus complex pathology, (2) presence or absence of cyanosis, (3) whether pulmonary blood flow is increased or decreased, (4) whether an obstruction affects the RV or LV, and (5) the direction of shunting patterns (i.e., left-to-right, right-to-left). Other classification schemes consider the underlying physiologic alterations or common features of the anomalies. An alternate approach that facilitates differential diagnosis in the neonate with CHD considers the clinical presentation and categorizes defects based on the presence of cyanosis, congestive heart failure, or murmur [23]. Yet another scheme relevant to newborn screening for CHD suggests three main categories in terms of clinical significance as follows [24]:

- *Life-threatening congenital heart defects:* those in which collapse is likely (e.g., transposition of the great arteries, coarctation/interrupted aortic arch, aortic stenosis, pulmonary atresia, and hypoplastic left heart/mitral atresia)
- *Clinically significant congenital heart defects:* those with effects on heart function but where collapse is unlikely (e.g., ventricular septal defect, complete atrioventricular septal defect, atrial septal defect, tetralogy of Fallot)
- *Clinically nonsignificant congenital heart defects:* those with no functional clinical significance (e.g., ventricular septal defect only detectable by echocardiography and requiring no treatment)

This scheme is useful for determining the gravity of the situation and the immediate action needed once the diagnosis is made. Life-threatening lesions, often because of ductal dependency for pulmonary or systemic blood flow or other reasons, require prompt attention (Table 12.4). Clinically significant CHD, although important, may not have major hemodynamic manifestations within the first few weeks of life and is less likely to necessitate urgent care. Defects considered clinically insignificant have little to no potential of impacting the physiology in the neonate.

Table 12.4 Ductal-dependent congenital heart disease in the neonate

Ductal-dependent lesions for pulmonary blood flow	Ductal-dependent lesions for systemic blood flow
Critical pulmonary stenosis	Coarctation of the aorta
Pulmonary atresia with intact ventricular septum	Critical aortic stenosis
Complex lesions associated with severe pulmonary outflow tract obstruction or pulmonary atresia	Hypoplastic left heart syndrome Interrupted aortic arch
Severe form of Ebstein anomaly with anatomic or functional pulmonary atresia	Complex lesion associated with systemic outflow tract obstruction or aortic atresia
d-Transposition of the great arteries[a]	

[a]Patency of the ductus arteriosus in *d*-transposition increases pulmonary blood flow and augments pulmonary venous return, leading to stretching of the interatrial communication and enhancing intercirculatory mixing

Although any cataloging system has limitations, a pathophysiological classification is particularly helpful in the practice of anesthesia, as it allows for the formulation of hemodynamic goals based on the main consequences of the defect. One such classification system of CHD is presented in Table 12.5 [25].

Congenital Cardiovascular Anomalies of the Neonate: Anatomy, Pathophysiology, and Management, with Anesthetic Considerations

The progressive advances in perioperative care that have taken place during the last 50 years have allowed the evolution of neonatal congenital heart surgery and resulted in increased survival rates and greatly improved outcomes [26]. These advances have permitted new approaches for many lesions; early corrective surgery is now preferred to initial palliation and later repair. The rationale for early correction is based on the premise that by restoring the anatomy and physiology towards normal early in life, subsequent morbidity will be minimized, thus permitting the most favorable long-term outlook. As a consequence, the volume of neonatal corrective surgery has markedly increased.

Patent Ductus Arteriosus

Anatomic Features

The ductus arteriosus is a vascular communication between the pulmonary artery (PA) and the Desc Ao (Fig. 12.2). This structure is an essential component of fetal life, serving as a conduit for RV output into the Desc Ao. In some cases, normal

Table 12.5 Physiologic classification of congenital heart defects and respective salient features

Lesions characterized by volume overload
• Due to communications at the atrial, ventricular, and/or arterial level
• Frequently the result of physiologic left-to-right shunting
• If communication proximal to the mitral valve (i.e., atrial septal defects, partial anomalous pulmonary venous return, or unobstructed total anomalous pulmonary venous return), right heart dilation is present; if the shunt is distal to the mitral valve (i.e., ventricular septal defect, patent ductus arteriosus), dilation of left-sided cardiac structures is seen
• Symptoms related to magnitude of the shunt and pulmonary to systemic blood flow ratio
• Shunting influenced by the pulmonary vascular tone and relationships between the pulmonary and systemic vascular resistances
• Diuretic therapy and afterload reduction are main medical management strategies
Lesions characterized by obstruction to systemic blood flow
• Include those with ductal-dependent systemic blood flow (i.e., critical aortic stenosis, severe aortic coarctation, aortic arch interruption, hypoplastic left heart syndrome)
• Prostaglandin E_1 therapy required to maintain ductal patency and systemic blood flow until an intervention is undertaken
• Diuretic therapy and manipulation of the systemic and pulmonary vascular resistances may be required to control increased pulmonary blood flow
• Inotropic and/or mechanical ventilatory support frequently necessary
Lesions characterized by obstruction to pulmonary blood flow
• Include those with ductal-dependent pulmonary blood flow (i.e., critical pulmonary valve stenosis and pulmonary atresia with intact ventricular septum)
• Prostaglandin E_1 therapy is indicated for the treatment of arterial hypoxemia until obstruction can be relieved or alternate sources of pulmonary blood flow are established
Parallel circulation
• Classic lesion is that of *d*-transposition of the great arteries where the pulmonary and systemic circulations run in parallel
• Associated with cyanosis
• Intercirculatory mixing is essential for survival
Single ventricle lesions
• Include those with atrioventricular valve atresia (i.e., tricuspid atresia), severe ventricular hypoplasia (i.e., double-inlet left ventricle), or anomalies where a biventricular repair is not feasible (i.e., unbalanced atrioventricular septal defect)
• Common among these lesions is complete mixing of the systemic and pulmonary venous blood at the atrial or ventricular level, and aortic or pulmonary outflow tract obstruction, accounting for the presence of cyanosis
• An important goal of early management involves optimization of the balance between the pulmonary and systemic circulations

closure does not take place, resulting in persistent ductal patency. Prematurity and respiratory distress syndrome are risk factors for developing a patent ductus arteriosus (PDA). This lesion affects nearly a 33 % of infants weighing less than 1,500 grams at birth. PDA occurs with increased frequency in certain genetic disorders (e.g., Holt-Oram syndrome), in association with in utero viral infections (Rubella) and within utero drug ingestion (sodium valproate) [27].

A PDA may be found in isolation or in association with other forms of CHD. In the isolated form, it accounts for nearly 10 % of all congenital heart defects. It is important to recognize that in some cardiovascular malformations, ductal patency may be essential for either pulmonary or systemic blood flow and, therefore, survival. The following discussion addresses the isolated defect.

Pathophysiology

Communication at the level of the great arteries permits shunting between the systemic and pulmonary circulations. Two factors determine the direction and magnitude of the shunting: the relative vascular resistances of the pulmonary and systemic vascular beds and the size of the communication. The pulmonary vascular resistance significantly affects the direction of shunting. As the resistance decreases postnatally, the typical direction of blood flow through an isolated PDA is left-to-right, resulting in increased pulmonary blood flow and volume loading of the heart.

The clinical manifestations of a PDA depend on the magnitude of the shunt and the pulmonary and cardiac responses to the shunt. Some shunts are restrictive (small diameter) in nature and limit the blood flow to some extent. Other shunts are large communications that permit a large blood flow from the Ao to the PA. In the latter case, the neonate may develop signs of pulmonary overload (labored breathing, radiologic evidence of increased interstitial lung water, LA/LV dilation, cardiomegaly) and overt congestive heart failure. The preterm neonate is particularly vulnerable to the hemodynamic effects of a left-to-right shunt, and pulmonary edema can develop [28]. Frequently, a PDA is associated with respiratory impairment, a requirement for mechanical ventilatory support, and/or failure to wean from support. PDA in preterm infants is a risk factor for bronchopulmonary dysplasia and intracranial hemorrhage. The diastolic runoff, (left-to-right shunt) also called *pulmonary steal*, causes

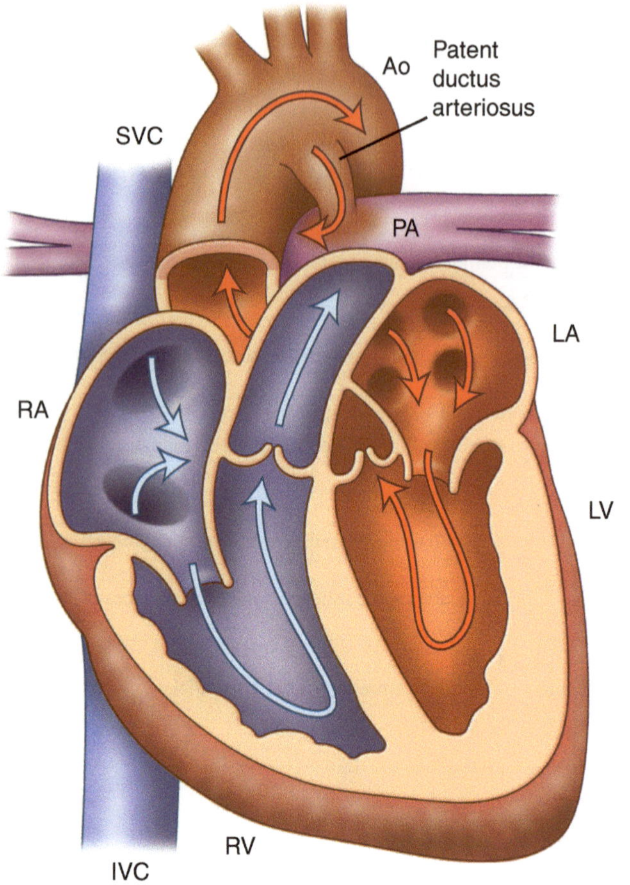

Fig. 12.2 Graphic representation of a patent ductus arteriosus. The communication between the aorta (Ao) and pulmonary artery (PA) is shown. The usual direction of shunting, from left-to-right, in the isolated lesion is noted. *IVC* inferior vena cava, *LA* left atrium, *LV* left ventricle, *RA* right atrium, *RV* right ventricle, *SVC* superior vena cava

hypoperfusion of systemic vascular beds with potential end-organ complications (i.e., impaired myocardial perfusion, necrotizing enterocolitis). The lack of significant ductal restriction and the increased pulmonary blood flow leads to pulmonary hypertension, imposing a further pressure load on the RV.

Management

The goals of medical therapy are designed to control pulmonary over-circulation and ventricular volume overload. In most cases, this includes fluid restriction and diuretic therapy [29]. The administration of indomethacin or ibuprofen in an effort to alter prostaglandin metabolism and promote ductal closure in the premature infant is a well-established clinical practice [30]. Drug therapy may not be effective in the very low-birth-weight infant. It may actually be contraindicated due to side effects affecting renal, gastrointestinal, and cerebral perfusion. Surgical management usually consists of placing a clip on the communication, most commonly via a small posterior lateral thoracotomy. Although ductal closure using video-assisted thoracoscopy has been reported in the neonate and even in preterm infants, this approach is more likely to be considered for the older infant or child [31, 32]. A catheter-based procedure to occlude the PDA is an option in the term infant.

Anesthetic Considerations

The need for intervention for a hemodynamically significant PDA in the full-term neonate is extremely rare and is more likely to occur if other coexisting disease is present. Infants undergoing catheter-based therapies may suffer vascular injury, rhythm disturbances, and hemodynamic instability. These problems result from factors such as difficulty with vascular access, catheter manipulations, or blood loss. In the neonate undergoing surgical ductal ligation, standard anesthetic practice for thoracotomy procedures in the small infant should be followed. The use of regional anesthesia techniques can improve perioperative pain management. If the premature infant requires surgical ligation, a left thoracotomy is often performed in the neonatal intensive care unit in many centers, obviating the need to transport the infant to the operating room, thereby decreasing the risk of problems such as hypothermia and accidental tracheal extubation. This is particularly useful if the infant requires high-frequency oscillating ventilation. An opioid-muscle relaxant-based intravenous anesthetic technique is the most common practice.

Specific Issues

- *Intravascular volume.* Fluid restriction and diuretic therapy in the neonate with a PDA can result in intravascular volume depletion in the presence of congestive symptoms. This problem alone or in combination with surgical manipulations that impair ventricular filling can predispose the infant to hemodynamic alterations during the ligation procedure, necessitating fluid administration or other acute interventions.
- *Ventilation.* Ductal ligation requires manual manipulation of thoracic structures and retraction of the non-dependent lung to achieve optimal surgical exposure. These maneuvers frequently impair gas exchange to some extent. Therefore, vigilance is of outmost importance combined with monitoring the arterial saturation measured by pulse oximetry (SpO_2) continuously and assiduously. Preoperative placement of additional "reserve" oximetry probes may be considered advisable! Frequent adjustments to the ventilation parameters, guided by variables being monitored to optimize gas exchange, may be necessary.
- *Pulmonary blood flow.* An important hemodynamic goal prior to surgical ligation is to minimize increases in pulmonary blood flow that can compromise systemic output or myocardial function. Although limiting the inspired oxygen concentration is desirable in this instance, in addition to the

concern of the risk of retinopathy of prematurity (refer to Chap. 10), this objective should be balanced with that of providing adequate systemic oxygen delivery during the procedure [33].

- *Blood loss.* Even a small amount of blood loss can have a major hemodynamic impact in the preterm or term neonate due to the relatively small blood volume. Thus, as in any major vascular surgery, appropriate vascular access and immediate availability of blood products is imperative. Blood loss is usually minimal, but disastrous hemorrhage can occur.
- *Anemia.* Many preterm infants are anemic and this increases the risk of congestive heart failure. In many infants, red cell transfusion to correct anemia will significantly improve the cardiac status.
- *Inadvertent ligation of other structures.* Unintentional ligation of adjacent thoracic structures such as the left pulmonary artery (LPA), left mainstem bronchus, and Desc Ao is a well-known complication during ductal ligation [34]. Pre- (right upper extremity) and post-ductal (lower extremity) monitoring with a pulse oximeter/blood pressure cuff in some cases can permit early recognition of these complications. Ductal closure is associated with narrowing of the pulse pressure and an increase in diastolic and, frequently, systolic blood pressures. Confirmation of these changes during ductal ligation is reassuring.
- *Postoperative problems.* Other important issues that are associated with ductal ligation deserve mention. One is the potential for nerve injury and related morbidity. The recurrent laryngeal nerve courses around the ductus arteriosus and can be injured during the procedure, resulting in vocal cord paralysis [35]. Diaphragmatic paralysis secondary to phrenic nerve injury leading to significant ventilator dependency also has been reported [36]. Chylothorax due to thoracic duct injury is a rare complication. Other concerns after ductal ligation in the preterm infant relate to the effects of obliteration of the left-to-right shunt on cardiopulmonary function. In some cases, the acute increase in LV afterload can be detrimental to myocardial performance, particularly in the presence of preexistent ventricular dysfunction, [37] which can manifest as a low cardiac output state and hypotension. Others may have a potential immediate need for increased mechanical ventilatory support due to changes in pulmonary compliance.

Coarctation of the Aorta

Anatomic Features

Coarctation of the aorta (CoA) represents 5 to 8 % of all congenital cardiovascular defects. The anomaly is characterized by narrowing of the lumen of the thoracic Ao near the region of the ductus arteriosus or ligamentum, resulting in obstruction to the systemic blood flow (Fig. 12.3). The constriction can be discrete or diffuse. In the neonate, this lesion can be part of a complex setting with hypoplasia of the transverse Ao arch and Ao isthmus (region proximal to the coarctation between the left subclavian artery and the ductus arteriosus). This constellation of findings is less likely to occur in older infancy or later in life.

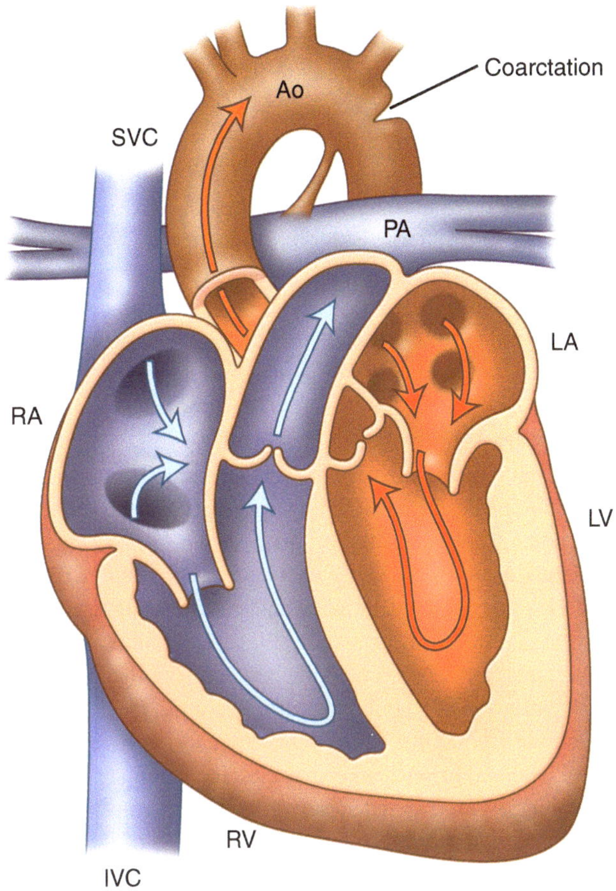

Fig. 12.3 Graphic representation of coarctation of the aorta. The posterior shelf in the descending thoracic aorta (Ao) in this lesion is shown. *IVC* inferior vena cava, *LA* left atrium, *LV* left ventricle, *PA* pulmonary artery, *RA* right atrium, *RV* right ventricle, *SVC* superior vena cava

Associated pathology in CoA may include a PDA, bicuspid Ao valve, aortic stenosis (AS), subaortic obstruction, and ventricular septal defect (VSD). CoA also can be part of the group of defects identified in Shone's complex, characterized in addition by subaortic obstruction, parachute mitral valve, and supravalvar mitral ring [38].

Pathophysiology

This lesion has a spectrum of severity, as is the case in many other forms of CHD; presentation in a young infant usually implies more severe obstruction or the presence of coexisting anomalies. The hemodynamic consequences of CoA relate to obstruction of the systemic blood flow and inadequate distal perfusion. When the PDA provides most or essentially all of the entire distal systemic perfusion via the

RV, CoA is considered a ductal-dependent lesion for systemic blood flow. Ductal constriction will have profound repercussions in this setting. In the case of less severe obstruction, ductal closure results in increased LV afterload and end-diastolic pressure, myocardial work, and wall tension, which assumes a potential for myocardial ischemia. Increased LA pressures may lead to left-to-right shunting at the atrial level and increased pulmonary blood flow. Pulmonary hypertension results from increased pulmonary venous pressures related to LA hypertension and from the increased pulmonary blood flow. Coexistent defects can contribute to the volume or pressure load of the myocardium.

Management

Neonates with severe obstruction frequently require treatment for congestive heart failure and possible ventricular dysfunction. A presentation of poor cardiac output is more ominous as manifested by decreased peripheral perfusion, metabolic acidosis, lactic acidemia, renal insufficiency, poor ventricular function, or shock [39]. This condition requires immediate intervention with tracheal intubation and mechanical ventilation in addition to prostaglandin E_1 (PGE_1) therapy to reestablish/maintain ductal patency and improve systemic perfusion. Additional care includes inotropic support and, potentially, cautious afterload reduction. In most cases of moderate to severe narrowing, surgical relief of the obstruction is the treatment of choice. Selection of the surgical approach, median sternotomy versus lateral thoracotomy (discussed later in the chapter), is influenced by the associated pathology, particularly the presence of arch hypoplasia. The goal of the surgical procedure, regardless of the details of the specific technique or approach, is to resect the narrowed segment and remove adjacent ductal tissue that can be part of the pathology and carries the potential for recurrence of the obstruction. Aortic continuity in the neonate is established preferably using native tissue. Associated significant Ao arch hypoplasia requires more extensive reconstruction [40, 41].

Endovascular balloon dilation has been performed in the neonate, even in those with significant transverse arch hypoplasia [42]. Many centers, however, favor surgical intervention to achieve the most effective long-term outcome.

Anesthetic Considerations

Adequate vascular access is essential. Related to Ao cross-clamping is a potential for acidosis and end-organ dysfunction (the spinal cord, kidneys, gut) due to hypoperfusion of respective vascular beds. This concern is usually less for older children because of the development of collateral circulation. Several strategies have been used in the neonate and young infant in efforts to minimize the potential for spinal cord injury [43]. Inducing mild hypothermia to 34–35 °C before applying the Ao clamp is standard of care at some centers, although the incidence of spinal cord injury in the absence of hyperthermia is exceedingly rare [44]. Hemodynamic changes during CoA surgery via thoracotomy include hypertension upon application of the Ao cross-clamp, hypotension associated with its release, and paradoxical or rebound hypertension after the repair is complete. This latter problem has been linked to altered baroreceptor responses and abnormalities in the renin-angiotensin system [45]. Recent data also suggest that underlying pathological adjustment of autonomic cardiovascular homeostasis occurs in these infants [46].

Specific Issues

- *Arterial pressure monitoring.* The selection of monitors (sites and types) varies according to the surgical plan and specific approach (e.g., lateral thoracotomy versus median sternotomy; resection with end-to-end repair, extended Ao arch repair, Ao arch advancement, and the need for cardiopulmonary bypass). Monitoring of arterial blood pressure at sites proximal and distal to the obstruction should be considered. Right radial artery blood pressure monitoring is ideal in most cases. A blood pressure cuff in a lower extremity can also be helpful.
- *Surgical considerations.* In view of the fact that associated Ao arch hypoplasia requires more extensive reconstruction aimed not only at immediately relieving the obstruction but also at providing the best long-term outcome, cardiopulmonary bypass (CPB) is frequently needed that may include the use of special bypass techniques (e.g., selective cerebral perfusion). Depending on these strategies, additional monitors (e.g., neuromonitors) may enhance the safety of these interventions.

d-Transposition of the Great Arteries

Anatomic Features

d-Transposition of the great arteries (*d*-TGA) accounts for 6 % of all CHD. This malformation is identified in 10 % of neonates with critical heart disease and represents the most common cause of cardiac cyanosis during the neonatal period. A male predominance is seen among affected infants.

In *d*-transposition the Ao arises from the anatomic RV and the PA from the LV (Fig. 12.4). In most cases, the Ao is spatially oriented anterior and to the right of the PA, in contrast to the posterior location of the Ao in the normal heart. This malformation is thought to result from abnormal rotation and septation of the conotruncus, resulting in discordant ventriculoarterial connections.

In the most common form of the defect, an intact ventricular septum or a small VSD is present. *d*-Transposition is associated with a VSD in 10 to 25 % of cases. In complex forms of the defect, a large VSD and various degrees of pulmonary stenosis (PS) or left ventricular outflow tract (LVOT)

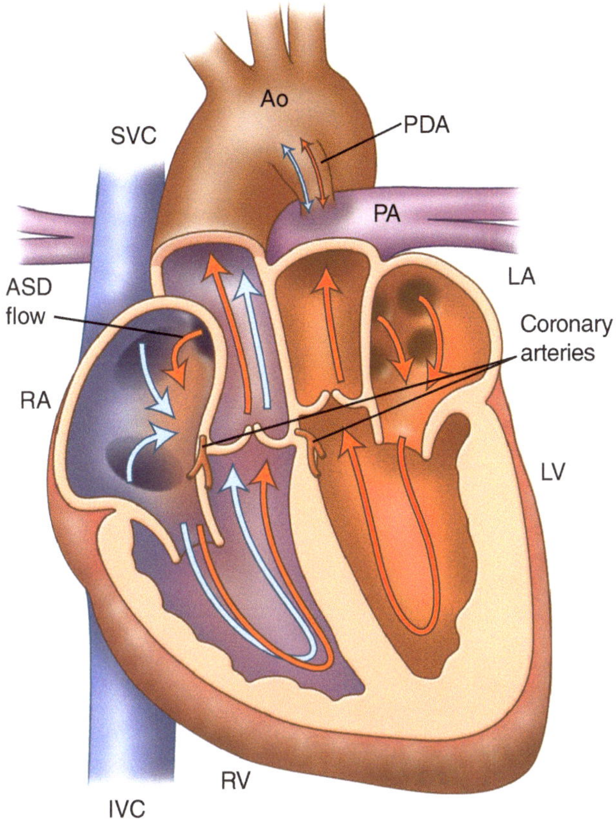

Fig. 12.4 Graphic representation of *d*-transposition of the great arteries. The discordant connections between the ventricles and great arteries in this lesion are depicted. Intercirculatory mixing is essential for survival in this lesion and is allowed for by flow across a patent ductus arteriosus (PDA) and atrial septal defect (ASD). *Ao* aorta, *IVC* inferior vena cava, *LA* left atrium, *LV* left ventricle, *PA* pulmonary artery, *RA* right atrium, *RV* right ventricle, *SVC* superior vena cava

obstruction is seen. Other anomalies include additional VSDs, coronary artery variants, and Ao arch obstruction.

Pathophysiology

In *d*-TGA, the systemic and pulmonary circulations operate in parallel (separate) rather than in series. This anomaly results in recirculation of blood, deoxygenated blood in the systemic circulation and oxygenated blood in the pulmonary circulation. Intercirculatory mixing is essential for survival. The typical presentation is that of cyanosis shortly after birth as the ductus closes in an otherwise healthy-appearing neonate. There is minimal or no response to the administration of oxygen. A restrictive foramen ovale can result in poor mixing and profound arterial hypoxemia, potentially progressing to metabolic acidosis and severe shock due to compromised tissue oxygenation. Less commonly, a high pulmonary vascular resistance accounts for severe cyanosis despite ductal patency and an adequate anatomic interatrial communication.

Symptoms of congestive heart failure are not likely to occur even in the presence a PDA, VSD, or CoA within the first few days of life. In the case of concomitant shunts such as at the ventricular or ductal levels, the relative high pulmonary vascular resistance limits significant shunt volume.

Management

Without intervention, this defect is almost uniformly fatal. Preoperative management is determined by the adequacy of mixing between the parallel circulations. PGE_1 therapy frequently is used to enhance intercirculatory mixing. The goal of maintaining ductal patency is to increase the pulmonary blood flow and the volume of pulmonary venous blood returning to the LA, which in turn raises the LA pressure to the extent that it stretches the interatrial communication, enhancing intercirculatory mixing. Balloon atrial septostomy is required to enlarge a restrictive interatrial communication in the presence of significant hypoxemia.

The arterial switch operation (Jatene procedure) is the surgical procedure of choice for uncomplicated *d*-transposition (Fig. 12.5). The intervention achieves anatomic correction and restores normal physiology. The operation involves transection of the great arteries above their semilunar valves, anastomotic connections to their appropriate respective outflows, translocation of the coronary arteries to the neoaortic root, closure of existing intracardiac communications, and repair of additional defects, as indicated. Early in the surgical experience, certain coronary patterns were considered to preclude this type of surgery, given the need to mobilize and reimplant these tiny vessels. Today, however, the concern is much less, and, in fact, many centers do not regard abnormal coronary patterns a contraindication for the arterial switch operation. Timing of the operation is relevant as it is undertaken before pulmonary vascular resistance falls in order to prevent deconditioning of the LV, given that it will become the systemic ventricular chamber upon completion of the operation [47]. Hence, in most cases, this type of surgery is performed within the first few weeks of life while the LV afterload is high. Beyond the neonatal period, the approach to this lesion depends on numerous factors, but importantly on the ability of the LV to support the systemic circulation based on the presence or absence of associated defects and their impact on LV "preparedness."

Anesthetic Considerations

If balloon atrial septostomy is required prior to performing corrective surgery, it can be undertaken at the bedside or in the cardiac catheterization laboratory. Frequently, the intervention is of an urgent nature due to profound arterial hypoxemia. In this situation, the main goal is to maintain cardiovascular stability while an atrial communication is enlarged or created. Marked clinical improvement is seen with adequate atrial mixing. Access to emergency equipment, medications, and blood products is essential in this setting. Some centers routinely perform balloon atrial septostomy in most affected neonates to allow for adequate mixing while awaiting surgical intervention.

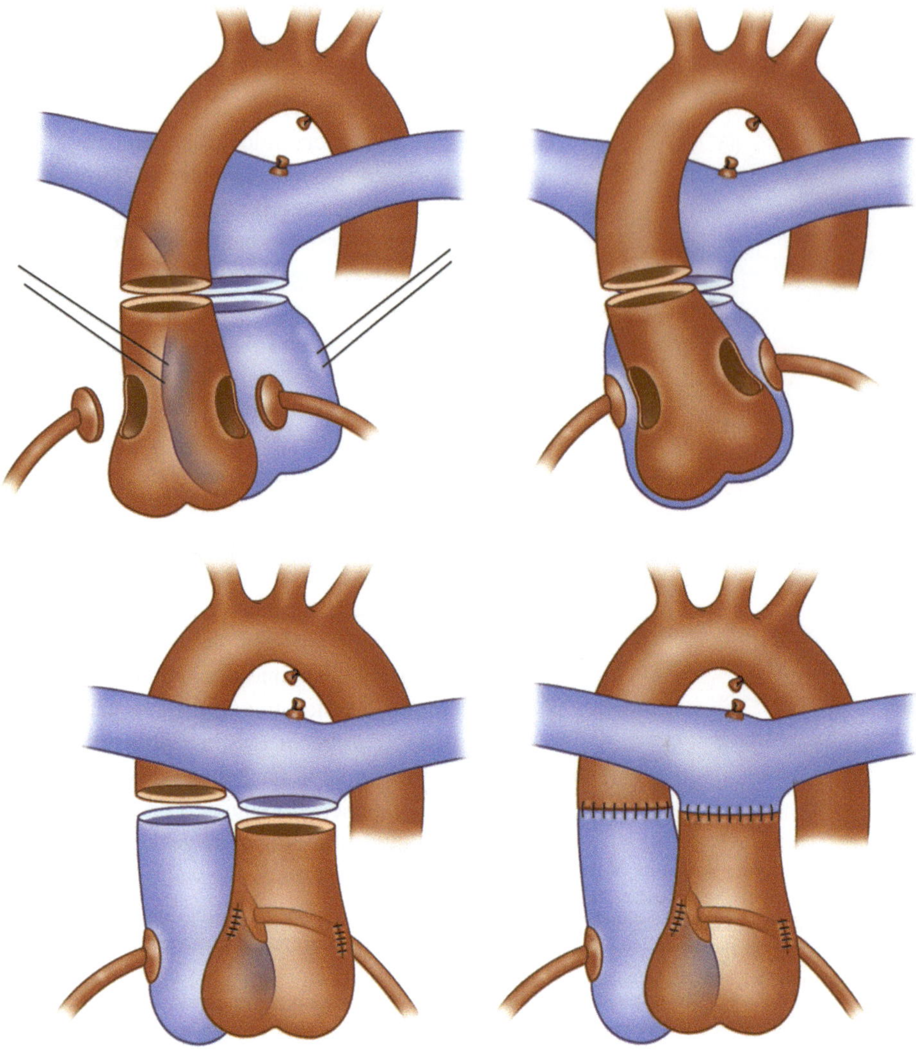

Fig. 12.5 Graphic representation of the arterial switch operation in *d*-transposition of the great arteries. *Upper left panel*, the ductus arteriosus/ligamentum is divided, and the great arteries are transected above the level of their native semilunar valves and roots. Coronary artery buttons are then removed from the typically anterior and rightward aorta. *Upper right panel*, the coronary arteries are translocated to the posterior "neoaortic" root (native pulmonary root). *Left lower panel*, the *Lecompte maneuver* is performed allowing for the main pulmonary artery to be mobilized in front of the neoaorta. *Right lower panel*, the aortic anastomosis is completed and after repairing the defects in the native aorta ("neopulmonary artery") where the coronary buttons were removed, the pulmonary arterial anastomosis is completed

Specific Issues

- *Myocardial ischemia.* Translocation of the coronary arteries involves manipulation, probing, and, in some cases, potential stretching or distortion of the vessels. These maneuvers in addition to other aspects of the repair can predispose the neonate to coronary artery spam and/or myocardial ischemia. Thus, these cases require careful surveillance for potential compromise of myocardial blood flow (electrocardiographic monitoring of ST segments, regional wall motion assessment by transesophageal echocardiography, or TEE) and a low threshold to consider inadequate coronary blood flow as the etiology of ventricular dysfunction, failure of separation from CPB, or intractable ventricular arrhythmias. At some centers, the postoperative administration of a nitroglycerine infusion in these neonates is routine.
- *Left ventricular compliance.* The LV in the neonate with *d*-transposition is relatively "stiff" or noncompliant immediately after surgery, which is manifested by extreme sensitivity to the administration of volume, resulting in a significant increase in LA pressure and a fall in cardiac output. Chamber overdistension is poorly tolerated, so fluids should be administered cautiously and guided by LA pressure, systemic arterial blood pressure, and qualitative echocardiographic assessment of LV size.

- *Pulmonary hypertension.* Because surgical correction is performed early in infancy prior to the normal fall in pulmonary vascular resistance, pulmonary hypertension can be a problem in the immediate post-bypass period and postoperatively. Strategies that support the RV, as well as the use of pulmonary vasodilators, should be considered.

Tetralogy of Fallot

Anatomic Features

Tetralogy of Fallot (TOF) is the most common cause of cyanotic heart disease in childhood, accounting for approximately 6 to 11 % of CHD. The absence of cyanosis or the failure to recognize mild cyanosis immediately after birth explains why TOF is often diagnosed beyond the neonatal period and is not recognized as the most common cyanotic heart defect in the neonate.

The four components of TOF in the classic lesion include a large VSD, right ventricular outflow tract (RVOT) obstruction, Ao override, and RV hypertrophy (Fig. 12.6). The wide spectrum of clinical manifestations in this lesion is due to the variable anatomic features, particularly the severity of the RVOT obstruction. Associated pathology includes an atrial communication, additional VSDs, a persistent connection from a left superior vena cava (LSVC) to the coronary sinus, coronary artery anomalies, and variants of Ao arch laterality or branching pattern. Concomitant lesions such as that of a complete atrioventricular septal defect can be present in some cases (colloquially referred to as "tet-canal" defect). Pulmonary atresia with a VSD is considered to represent an extreme form of TOF.

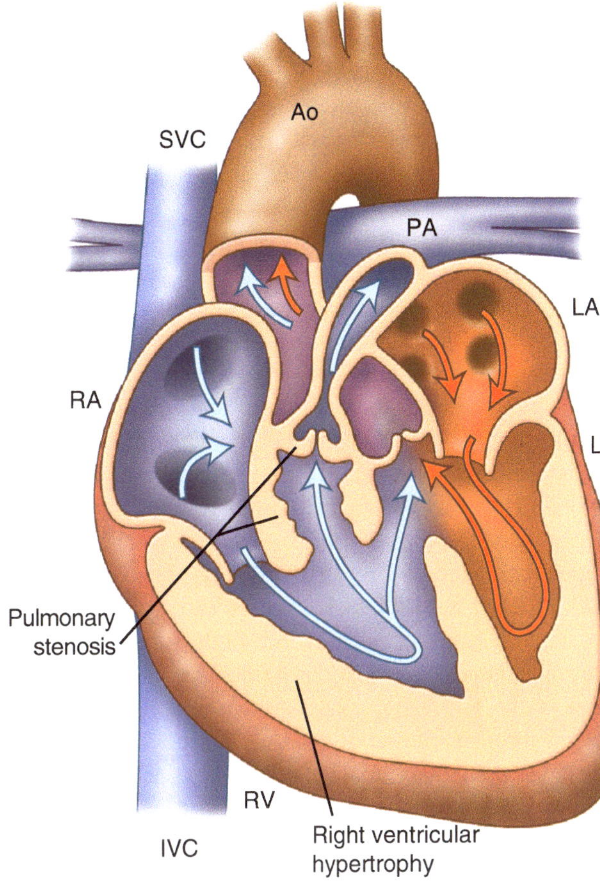

Fig. 12.6 Graphic representation of tetralogy of Fallot showing the classic features of this lesion: ventricular septal defect, pulmonary stenosis, overriding aorta (Ao), and right ventricular hypertrophy. The potential various levels of right ventricular outflow tract obstruction are noted (subvalvar, valvar, and supravalvar). The right-to-left shunt across the ventricular septal defect (shown by the *arrow*) accounts for the presence of cyanosis in this defect. *IVC* inferior vena cava, *LA* left atrium, *LV* left ventricle, *PA* pulmonary artery, *RA* right atrium, *RV* right ventricle, *SVC* superior vena cava

Pathophysiology

The RVOT obstruction in TOF, which is often found at multiple levels, is characterized by variable dynamic and fixed components. The dynamic obstruction occurs only in the muscular infundibular region. In contrast, the fixed component occurs at the subvalvar, valvar, and supravalvar regions and/or the branch pulmonary arteries. Cyanosis is caused by decreased pulmonary blood flow and right-to-left shunting across the VSD, implying lower pulmonary blood flow relative to systemic blood flow. The nonrestrictive nature of the VSD together with the RVOT obstruction account for equalization of RV and LV pressures. Hypercyanotic episodes ("tet spells") result from increases in RVOT obstruction and right-to-left intracardiac shunting, which can lead to significant morbidity or even death. Fortunately, it is a very unusual occurrence during the neonatal period.

TOF has a spectrum of clinical presentations. At one end is the large VSD and minimal RVOT obstruction. In this case, shunting across the ventricular communication is typically in the left-to-right direction and the neonate is acyanotic. In fact, some degree of heart failure from pulmonary over-circulation often is present, accounting for the "pink" form of tetralogy. At the other end of the spectrum is the neonate with severe pulmonary stenosis/near pulmonary atresia who is quite cyanotic, ductal dependent, and in need of an intervention to establish a reliable source of pulmonary blood flow. In the middle of this continuum is the "classic" form of TOF, characterized by moderate pulmonary outflow tract obstruction and associated mild cyanosis at rest (systemic oxygen saturation ~ 80 to 90 %). This condition is the case in most neonates, although increasing cyanosis can occur with crying, agitation, or pain.

A particular variant of TOF with potential significant clinical implications in the neonatal period is that associated with absent pulmonary valve syndrome. This pathology is characterized by a dysplastic pulmonary valve, various degrees of valvar stenosis, and regurgitation, in addition to the usual findings in TOF. Massive dilation of the main and branched pulmonary arteries in this defect accounts for abnormalities of the tracheobronchial tree. These abnormalities can result in severe respiratory compromise due to air trapping and are frequently associated with significant morbidity related to poor lung mechanics.

Management

Ongoing controversy exists regarding the favored surgical approach in the neonate or very young infant with TOF associated with severe RVOT obstruction and significant cyanosis [48–50]. Some centers advocate initial palliation consisting of a systemic-to-PA shunt, most frequently in the form of a modified Blalock-Taussig shunt (graft between subclavian artery and PA), via a lateral thoracotomy or median sternotomy approach, followed by corrective surgery later in infancy. Others prefer, even in very young infants, a single-stage definitive repair consisting of closure of the VSD, relief of the RVOT obstruction, and repair of associated defects. Many technical aspects of the surgical intervention are variable and surgeon/institution dependent [51]. The relief of the RVOT/pulmonary obstruction can be accomplished through transatrial and/or PA access. An incision across the pulmonary annulus and placement of a transannular patch is necessary in some cases, usually related to annular hypoplasia, which is more likely to be the case in younger infants. With regard to closure of the VSD, the approach can be a transatrial, transventricular, or combined, based on the surgeon's preference. In view of the fact that ventriculotomy, or the need for a transannular patch, can impact on the long-term outcome, some prefer palliation rather than total correction in very young infants [52]. Alternative medical temporizing measures at some centers include the use of beta-adrenergic receptor antagonists to minimize the risk of infundibular "spasm" and associated hypercyanotic events. In selected cases, cardiac catheterization procedures such as percutaneous balloon pulmonary valvuloplasty or stenting of the ductus arteriosus can be beneficial while the infant awaits corrective surgery.

Anesthetic Considerations

During anesthetic care, the main concern in the unrepaired neonate with TOF is the potential for hypercyanotic episodes that can result in profound hypoxemia and significant morbidity. These episodes can be triggered by crying, light anesthesia, hypovolemia, sympathetic stimulation (or sympathomimetic drugs), or anesthetic-related decreases in systemic vascular tone with augmentation of the right-to-left shunting. Immediate management of an acute spell usually requires titration of a systemic vasoconstrictor drug (phenylephrine, norepinephrine, or vasopressin). Augmenting the cardiac preload by administering fluids to facilitate forward flow across the obstructed RVOT can also help. Beta-blockers (e.g., esmolol or propranolol) can be given in an effort to decrease heart rate and enhance diastolic filling time, while also relaxing the dynamic RVOT, but should be used with caution in the neonate. A measure that is usually considered once the neonate has been stabilized is blunting of the sympathetic tone by increasing the anesthetic depth by the administration of a sedative, opioid, or inhalational agent. Carefully titrated inhalational agents can be especially advantageous in view of their cardiac depressant effects, especially as exerted on the RVOT. Halothane was ideal for the child with TOF but is not readily available now. Isoflurane is a good second best! Rarely during cardiac surgery, a hypercyanotic episode is refractory to treatment and emergent initiation of CPB is required. The main goals of anesthetic care of the neonate with TOF are to preserve myocardial function, promote forward pulmonary blood flow, and minimize the potential for further increases in right-to-left shunting. Even issues that may not significantly influence the physiology of other forms of CHD can impact that of the neonate with TOF. An example is the potential detrimental effect of mechanical ventilation on intrathoracic pressure, further limiting pulmonary blood flow.

Specific Issues

- *Pulmonary vascular resistance.* Although, in general, pulmonary vascular tone does not play a major role in this lesion, the normally increased pulmonary vascular resistance in the neonate can impede forward flow across the outflow tract. It can have important implications regarding perioperative management and surgical decision-making as it complicates the assessment of the severity of the RVOT obstruction. Therefore, a reasonable anesthetic goal is to minimize acute increases in pulmonary vascular tone.
- *Coronary artery anomalies.* These anomalies are present in 5 to 12 % of patients with TOF and potentially impact the surgical procedure. The left coronary artery, for example, can originate anomalously from the right coronary artery and course across the RVOT, near or at the location of a planned transannular incision, requiring a change in the surgical plan [53].
- *Arterial pressure monitoring.* The presence of an aberrant subclavian artery, a relatively common associated lesion, should be considered in the selection of sites for arterial line placement. In this setting, insertion and manipulation of a TEE probe during complete repair may compress the retroesophageal vessel leading to blunting or disappearance of the arterial pressure tracing. When palliation in the form of a modified Blalock-Taussig shunt is anticipated, the arterial catheter is best placed in a vessel other than the one in which the vascular graft is planned to allow for uninterrupted assessment of arterial blood pressure throughout the case.

- *Arch laterality.* During palliative surgery via thoracotomy, Ao arch sidedness can influence the site of shunt placement and, hence, the surgical approach (right versus left thoracotomy). Although Ao arch anatomy is determined preoperatively, it is a matter of consideration during surgical positioning.
- *Effects of surgery.* It is important to highlight the impact of the surgical intervention on the physiology and influence on perioperative care as follows:
  - Transannular incision and patch in the definitive surgical repair of TOF invariably lead to pulmonary regurgitation because the intervention violates the integrity of the annulus and valve. In some cases, the relatively "stiff" RV limits the regurgitant volume, and this restrictive physiology is well tolerated initially [54]. However, in other infants, the acute RV volume load exacerbates an underlying element of diastolic dysfunction. This issue, compounded by some degree of systolic impairment related to myocardial edema, ischemic time, mechanical effects of the manipulations of the heart, and injury to the anterior RV wall resulting from the ventriculotomy/transannular patch, can complicate the postoperative course. The consequence is a low cardiac output state manifested in the first 24 h postoperatively. In patients with severe low cardiac output syndrome, spontaneous or negative pressure pulmonary ventilation may improve cardiac output and cerebral oxygenation [55, 56].
  - After complete repair, RV function can be impaired as previously described, and inotropic support may be required. However, it should be emphasized that inotropic agents can influence the postoperative assessment of the adequacy of the repair, because tachycardia and increased inotropy can exacerbate any residual RVOT gradient.
  - Pathology such as residual VSDs or RVOT obstruction, or significant tricuspid regurgitation may not be well tolerated in this particular patient group.
  - An intentional atrial communication, in the form of a patent foramen ovale, might be created during corrective surgery to facilitate postoperative care in anticipation of decreased RV compliance. This communication allows for maintenance of cardiac output at the expense of a small amount of right-to-left shunting at the atrial level and a mild degree of hypoxemia.
- *Junctional ectopic tachycardia.* This rhythm disturbance can occur in the immediate postoperative period following corrective interventions in children, including those with TOF repair [57]. The arrhythmia is characterized by a narrow QRS tachycardia (heart rate greater than 170 beats per minute), atrioventricular dissociation, and a ventricular rate faster than the atrial rate. The loss of the atrial contribution to ventricular filling and shortened diastolic filling time can have significant hemodynamic effects in this vulnerable patient group. Strategies applied in the management of this arrhythmia include sedation (to reduce sympathetic tone), decrease in the level of inotropic support, surface cooling, correction of electrolyte disturbances, various forms of pacing, and administration of magnesium. Pharmacological treatment with intravenous amiodarone or procainamide may be indicated in some cases [58]. In the extremely unstable neonate, circulatory support may be necessary. Pretreatment with a beta-blocker may reduce the incidence of JET [59].

Total Anomalous Pulmonary Venous Return

Anatomic Features

Total anomalous pulmonary venous return (TAPVR) accounts for 2 % of all CHD. It is characterized by drainage of all pulmonary venous blood back into the pulmonary circulation through remnants of vascular connections normally present during fetal life. The lesion represents an obligatory shunt as oxygenated blood from the pulmonary veins is diverted to the RA. This anomaly is classified into several types according to the main pathway of drainage of the anomalous pulmonary veins (Fig. 12.7): *supracardiac*, via a vertical vein to innominate vein or right SVC; *cardiac*, into the coronary sinus or RA; *infracardiac*, via a common pulmonary vein into the portal system, from there through the ductus venosus to the IVC; or *mixed*, a combination of the various types. In two-thirds of the cases, it is an isolated lesion. An atrial communication and PDA almost always are present. The remaining one-third of cases is associated with other defects (VSD, CoA, and complex CHD such as heterotaxy syndromes).

Pathophysiology

Anomalous pulmonary venous return is well tolerated in the fetus because of the limited pulmonary blood flow associated with the high pulmonary vascular resistance. In the first few days/weeks of life, the presence or absence of obstruction along the pulmonary venous pathway plays a major role in the physiologic consequences of the defect. In the absence of pulmonary venous obstruction and high pulmonary blood flow, a nonrestrictive ASD is associated with a relatively high systemic arterial oxygen saturation and adequate systemic cardiac output. Over time, however, RV volume overload and congestive symptoms ensue. This physiology can result in a late presentation. In contrast, a restrictive atrial communication leads to a greater degree of arterial hypoxemia and compromised systemic output. Pulmonary venous obstruction almost always is the norm in infradiaphragmatic TAPVR related to constriction of the ductus venosus. This condition is characterized by profound hypoxemia caused by

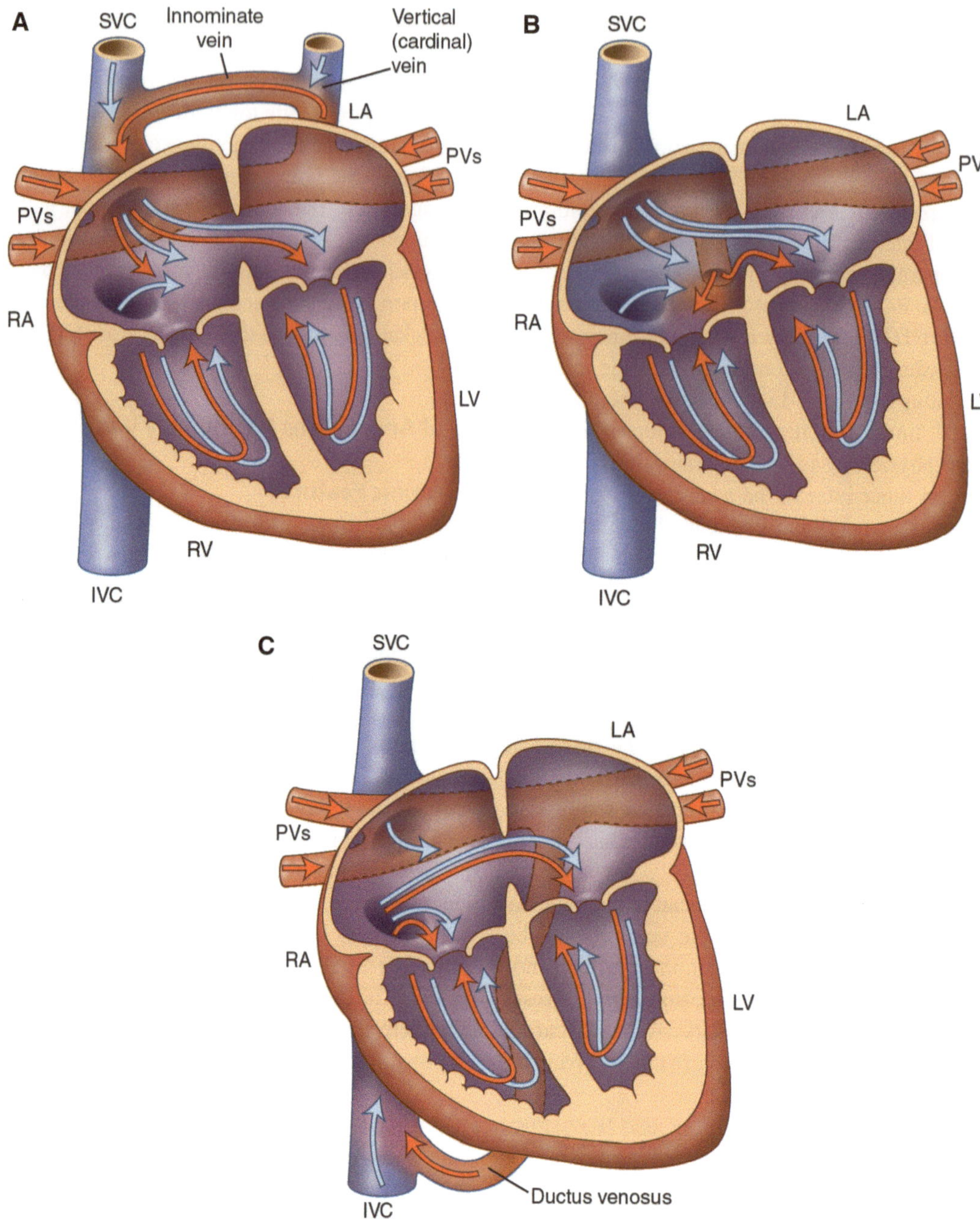

Fig. 12.7 Graphic representation of total anomalous pulmonary venous return. *Panel a*, supracardiac drainage. In this lesion the path of pulmonary venous drainage is from a vertical vein to the innominate vein into the right atrium (RA). In most defects an associated atrial septal defect is present. *Panel b*, cardiac drainage. In this pathology, the pulmonary veins (PVs) typically empty into the coronary sinus, draining into the RA. *Panel c*, infracardiac drainage. In this setting, PVs drain through the ductus venosus to the RA. Frequently this anomaly is associated with pulmonary venous obstruction. *IVC* inferior vena cava, *LA* left atrium, *LV* left ventricle, *RV* right ventricle, *SVC* superior vena cava

decreased pulmonary blood flow and pulmonary venous congestion, pulmonary hypertension, and respiratory compromise. Relative "hypoplasia" of left-sided cardiac structures can be seen in the affected neonate with TAPVR.

All forms of this lesion have complete mixing of systemic and pulmonary venous returns at the level of the RA. Right-to-left atrial shunting allows mixed blood to enter the LA, which is then ejected by the LV into the systemic circulation. The degree of hypoxemia depends on the severity of the pulmonary venous obstruction; it can be mild, mimicking, respiratory distress syndrome, or profound, in the case of a moribund infant with obstructed pulmonary venous drainage.

Management

Initial efforts are directed at stabilization of the neonate and respiratory/hemodynamic support as necessary. Surgical intervention can be undertaken on an elective basis if minimal to no pulmonary venous obstruction is present and the infant is doing well clinically. Most cases with obstruction require urgent surgery. The neonate with obstructed pulmonary venous return represents an emergency because profound hypoxemia generally is the case. Some providers consider the administration of PGE_1 potentially detrimental in the presence of severe obstruction as it further increases pulmonary blood flow, aggravating the obstruction and worsening oxygenation. Others regard PGE_1 beneficial as it influences vascular smooth muscle tone and may maintain patency of the ductus venosus, relieving the obstruction. Regardless of the details of the anatomy in TAPVR, the surgical correction aims at rerouting the drainage of the anomalous pulmonary veins to the LA.

Anesthetic Considerations

The main issues regarding anesthetic care in these neonates before the pathology is addressed center around respiratory and hemodynamic support. In the presence of pulmonary venous obstruction and severe hypoxemia, relatively high ventilatory settings that include the use of high peak inspiratory and positive end-expiratory pressures usually are required. The repair is performed frequently under deep hypothermic circulatory arrest (DHCA) or using low-flow perfusion. Upon separation from CPB, support of the RV with inotropic agents and pulmonary vasodilators is important in order to maintain forward flow in the face of potentially increased ventricular afterload resulting from an elevated pulmonary vascular resistance. This management aims at limiting the likelihood of negative ventricular interactions. In addition, the LV in this lesion is relatively noncompliant and subject to failure, with increases in blood volume resulting in reductions in stroke volume. Thus, the administration of fluid deserves caution to prevent LV wall overdistension.

Specific Issues

- *Pulmonary vascular reactivity.* There is a propensity in these infants to develop acute *pulmonary hypertensive crises in the post-bypass or postoperative period* due to a reactive pulmonary vascular bed. These episodes are prevented/managed by deep sedation, measures to decrease pulmonary vascular tone, and the administration of pulmonary vasodilators, including inhaled nitric oxide, as required. In cases at risk, PA pressure monitoring via a direct transthoracic catheter facilitates management.
- *Partial anomalous pulmonary venous drainage.* Defects that include anomalous drainage of only a few pulmonary veins are not uncommon in association with other forms of CHD, but usually this is of little physiological consequence during the neonatal period.

Truncus Arteriosus

Anatomic Features

Truncus arteriosus (TA) is a relatively uncommon malformation, representing only 1 to 2 % of congenital cardiac defects. Approximately one-third of infants with this anomaly have deletions of chromosome 22 (e.g., DiGeorge syndrome). In TA, also referred to as *persistent truncus arteriosus* or *common arterial trunk*, a single arterial root emerges from the heart, giving rise to the Asc Ao, PA, and coronary arteries (Fig. 12.8). An unrestrictive outlet, VSD, almost always is present, and the origin of the common arterial trunk characteristically straddles the defect. This defect is thought to be caused by failure of the normal process of conotruncal septation that results in two great arteries.

TA is subdivided into several subtypes (types I, II, III) based on the anatomical origin of the pulmonary arteries from the truncal vessel as described by Collett and Edwards [60]. The most common variant is one somewhere between types I and II, colloquially referred to as *truncus arteriosus type 1½*.

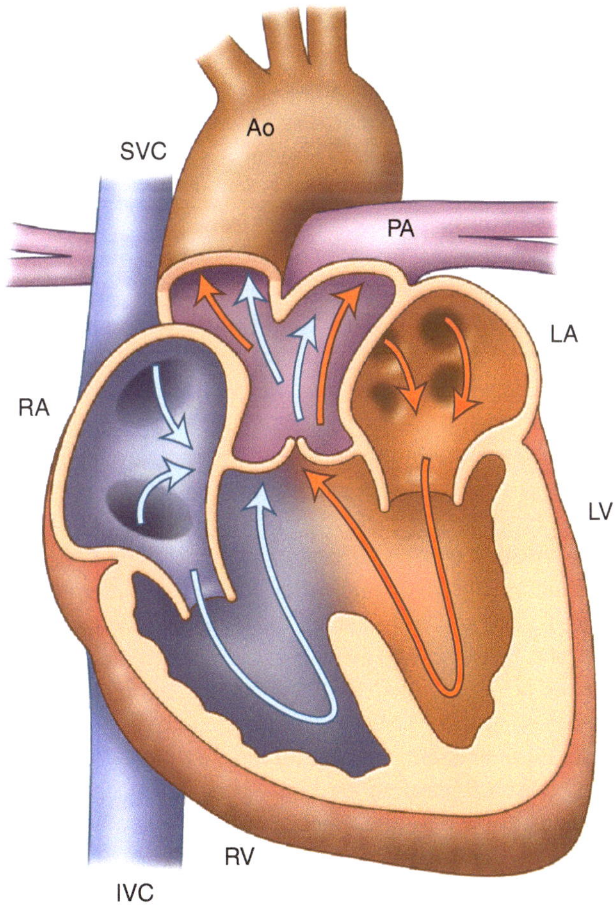

Fig. 12.8 Graphic representation of truncus arteriosus demonstrating the common truncal root with a biventricular origin. In this lesion, there is obligatory mixing of the systemic and pulmonary venous returns. *Ao* aorta, *IVC* inferior vena cava, *LA* left atrium, *LV* left ventricle, *PA* pulmonary artery, *RA* right atrium, *RV* right ventricle, *SVC* superior vena cava

Associated lesions include truncal valve issues (abnormal number of cusps, dysplasia, stenosis, regurgitation), abnormal origin and course of the coronary arteries, and Ao arch anomalies (right Ao arch and Ao arch interruption).

Pathophysiology

Hypoxemia associated with this anomaly is due to complete admixture of systemic and pulmonary venous blood as it emerges from both ventricles into the single arterial vessel. The hemodynamic repercussions of the defect relate to the direct physical communication between the systemic and pulmonary circulations at the level of the truncal root. This arrangement imposes a pressure and volume load to both ventricles further exacerbated by truncal valve pathology (stenosis or regurgitation), if present. The clinical features depend largely on two factors: the pulmonary vascular resistance and the presence of any intrinsic stenosis in the pulmonary arteries. These variables determine the volume of blood that enters the pulmonary vascular bed from the truncal root.

The neonate usually is well compensated immediately after birth due to the normal relatively high pulmonary vascular resistance. As the resistance decreases, symptoms related to pulmonary over-circulation and congestive heart failure ensue. In the presence of branched PA stenosis, the neonate can remain clinically stable to the degree that pulmonary blood flow is adequately restricted. If the obstruction is severe, cyanosis can be significant.

Management

Anticongestive therapy is indicated preoperatively in most cases and in some instances, inotropes. The current preferred approach is surgical repair during the neonatal period consisting of removal of the PA(s) from the truncal root, repair of the ensuing defect, patch closure of the VSD, RVOT reconstruction, and repair of associated pathology. Early correction is undertaken in view of the potential for rapid development of pulmonary vascular obstructive disease in this lesion.

Anesthetic Considerations

A major challenge in the perioperative care of the neonate with TA pertains to balancing the pulmonary and systemic vascular resistances to achieve cardiovascular stability during the pre-bypass period. A low pulmonary vascular resistance results in hemodynamic compromise because pulmonary over-circulation is associated with a steal phenomenon characterized by high systemic arterial oxygen saturation, low diastolic arterial pressures, and a wide pulse pressure. This runoff condition leads to impaired systemic output, hypotension, compromised oxygen transport caused by hypoperfusion of distal beds, and potential for myocardial ischemia, implying a high likelihood for morbidity and critical events. In fact, this defect is considered one of the congenital lesions associated with a very high risk of adverse perioperative events [61].

The anesthetic management of the neonate with unrepaired TA therefore focuses largely on controlling pulmonary blood flow and maintaining adequate systemic output. Increasing pulmonary vascular resistance by decreasing the inspired oxygen concentration, if possible to near room air, and increasing arterial carbon dioxide tension ($PaCO_2$) are the most common strategies for limiting pulmonary blood flow. Due to anesthetic effects, positive pressure ventilation, and changes in intravascular volume, managing pulmonary over-circulation during the pre-bypass period can be difficult and systemic arterial blood pressure can decrease. In fact, electrocardiographic changes associated with myocardial ischemia may occur. Care should be taken in the administration of agents that depress the myocardium. Potential strategies to address hypotension include volume administration, increasing the hematocrit level, and the use of inotropes for ventricular support/vasoconstrictors as required. During cardiac surgery, a temporary snare can be placed around one of the PA branches to mechanically restrict pulmonary blood flow and augment systemic output. As would be expected, this approach is associated with systemic arterial desaturation, and frequently the inspired oxygen concentration needs to be increased.

Specific Issues

- *Residual lesions.* After surgery, volume loading the LV, as imposed by a residual VSD or truncal valve regurgitation, may not be well tolerated. The post-repair TEE examination plays a major role in this assessment as well as being able to exclude hemodynamically significant truncal valve stenosis and RVOT obstruction, to interrogate for atrioventricular valve regurgitation, and to evaluate ventricular function.
- *Pulmonary hypertension.* Affected neonates are particularly vulnerable to the development of acute increases in PA pressures during the post-bypass period and in the intensive care unit. This vulnerability can lead to acute decompensation, significant morbidity, and even death. The perioperative management of pulmonary hypertensive crises is addressed in subsequent sections of this chapter (refer to page x).

Critical Aortic Stenosis

Anatomic Features

Congenital AS is present in 3 to 6 % of all patients with CHD; however, symptomatic disease in the neonate or infant accounts for fewer than 10 % of cases of Ao valve stenosis consistent with the rare nature of the lesion. The valve in critical AS is characterized by leaflet fusion, frequently exhibiting a unicuspid appearance, or might be severely thickened and dysplastic (Fig. 12.9). The Ao annulus, root, and Asc Ao typically display some element of hypoplasia. In

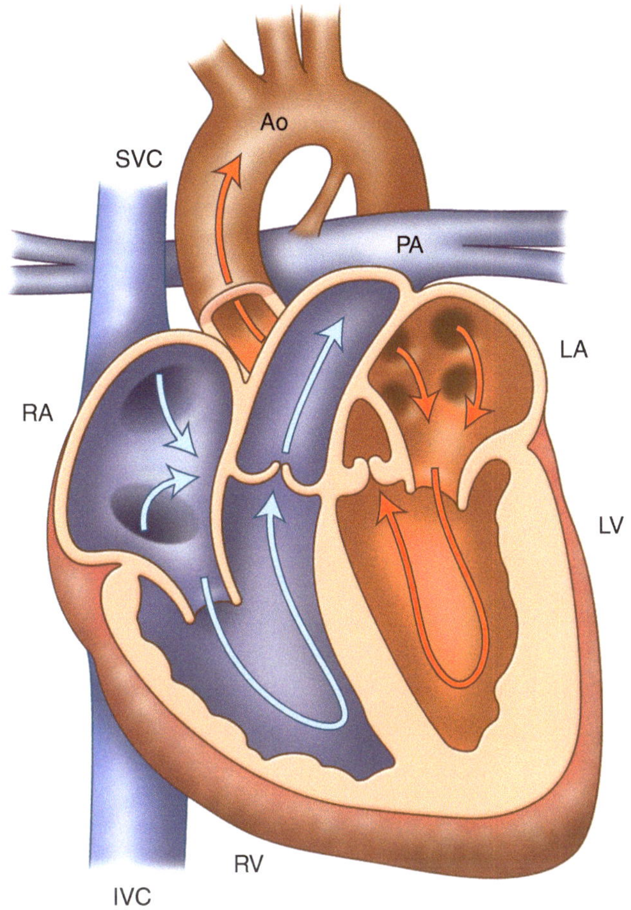

Fig. 12.9 Graphic representation of critical aortic stenosis. *Ao* aorta, *IVC* inferior vena cava, *LA* left atrium, *LV* left ventricle, *PA* pulmonary artery, *RA* right atrium, *RV* right ventricle, *SVC* superior vena cava

many cases, LV dilation in combination with poor function and mitral regurgitation is present. This condition is frequently associated with atrophy and infarction of papillary muscles as well as endocardial fibroelastosis (EFE). Various degrees of LV hypoplasia and mitral and Ao arch hypoplasia also can be present in some infants.

Pathophysiology

Obstruction to LV ejection due to a restricted aortic valvar orifice leads to increased LV systolic pressure, a transvalvular pressure gradient, increased myocardial force, and LV wall stress. The thickened myocardium is at risk for developing subendocardial ischemia as a consequence of an imbalance in the ratio of myocardial oxygen supply and demand. LV EFE results from compromised subendocardial oxygen delivery secondary to myocardial ischemia. Fibrotic myocardial changes lead to severe ventricular functional impairment and associated marked increases in LV end-diastolic and LA pressures. The presence of EFE along with LV dilation/dysfunction carries a poor prognosis. A large gradient across the Ao valve places a severe stress on systemic function of the LV.

Critical AS in the fetus can lead to hydrops caused by ongoing subendocardial ischemia and severe myocardial dysfunction. In most cases of critical disease in the neonate, antegrade flow through the Ao is inadequate to maintain cardiac output, and right-to-left shunting through the ductus arteriosus accounts for most of the systemic blood flow. In fact, retrograde flow through the arch via the ductus may in some cases be responsible for coronary and cerebral perfusion.

The neonate can exhibit signs and symptoms of severe heart failure or frank shock, usually related to ductal constriction or closure. Clinical evidence of congestive heart failure in the neonate includes tachypnea, poor feeding, diaphoresis with feeds, failure to thrive, hepatomegaly, and a gallop rhythm. A low cardiac output state is associated with severe ventricular dilation and dysfunction characterized by poor peripheral perfusion, paleness, cool extremities, and lactic acidemia. Papillary muscle infarction can be part of a grim presentation. In the neonate, systemic compensatory responses consist of systemic vasoconstriction, increased blood volume, and increased heart rate. The physiologic alterations are complex and impact not only the cardiovascular system but also other major organs.

Management

Fetal congestive heart failure and hydrops present a unique challenge. Transplacental digitalization has been used to manage fetal heart failure. In recent years, fetal interventions for critical AS have been attempted at specialized centers in hopes of altering the natural history of the condition in utero and potentially obviating progression of the disease [62]. Critical AS without intervention carries a high mortality rate in the neonate. PGE_1 therapy maintains systemic perfusion and is life saving. Concomitant therapy in the critically ill neonate consists of mechanical ventilatory support to reduce the work of breathing, diuretic therapy, and infusion of inotropic agents to augment systemic output as needed.

Options for management include percutaneous balloon valvuloplasty and surgery. In some cases, catheter interventions are favored; however, this is controversial. If surgery is undertaken, the approach is influenced by factors such as size of the Ao annulus, root, subaortic area, adequacy of the mitral valve and LV, and coexisting defects. Options include aortic valvotomy (open/closed), commissurotomy, aortic homograft placement, Ross procedure, Ross-Konno operation or other root-enlargement procedures, Damus-Kaye operation, and Norwood palliation. In some infants, cardiac transplantation may be the only feasible option. Mechanical circulatory support may be considered at several points along the care of the affected neonate as a bridge to an intervention, for postoperative failure, or while awaiting cardiac transplantation.

Anesthetic Considerations

The care of the neonate with critical AS can be extremely challenging. Concerns relate to anesthesia as well as the procedure itself. Hemodynamic decompensation can occur during induction of anesthesia or at any time during either a catheter or surgical intervention. Even the most careful induction can result in cardiovascular instability because sedatives/anesthetic agents expectedly decrease sympathetic tone, which may represent the main compensatory mechanism in the neonate. Cardiac massage may not be effective because of the restrictive Ao valve orifice; therefore, one should recognize the potential for untoward events and proceed extremely cautiously. Having immediate access to emergency drugs and defibrillation therapy is vital. In addition, these cases require advanced discussions regarding the potential need for urgent circulatory support during either the catheter-based intervention or the pre-bypass phase.

Regardless of the management or stage of a given intervention, it is important to optimize ventricular filling and function without overlooking the potential detrimental effects of volume overload in the failing heart or the increased myocardial work and decreased ventricular filling times associated with the use of inotropic drugs. The potential myocardial depressant effects of drugs, anesthetic agents, and other perioperative interventions must be carefully considered.

Specific Issues

- *Transcatheter interventions*. Complication rates for transcatheter procedures are greater in the neonate. Potential problems include bleeding, ventricular arrhythmias, transient myocardial ischemia during balloon inflation, development of or increase in the severity of aortic regurgitation, and arterial compromise due to vascular access.
- *Post-bypass problems*. In the post-bypass setting, major issues include residual systemic outflow obstruction, aortic regurgitation resulting from or exacerbated by the intervention, hemodynamic perturbations due to associated defects, and myocardial dysfunction.

Hypoplastic Left Heart Syndrome

Anatomic Features

It is estimated that hypoplastic left heart syndrome (HLHS) accounts for 2 % of CHD. The morphologic features of this malformation include aortic atresia or stenosis, mitral atresia or stenosis, Ao arch hypoplasia, CoA, PDA, and an atrial level communication (Fig. 12.10). Although HLHS is considered a spectrum of disease and the degree of LV hypoplasia varies, the LV in the classic lesion (aortic and mitral atresia) is significantly underdeveloped and the Asc Ao is markedly hypoplastic [63].

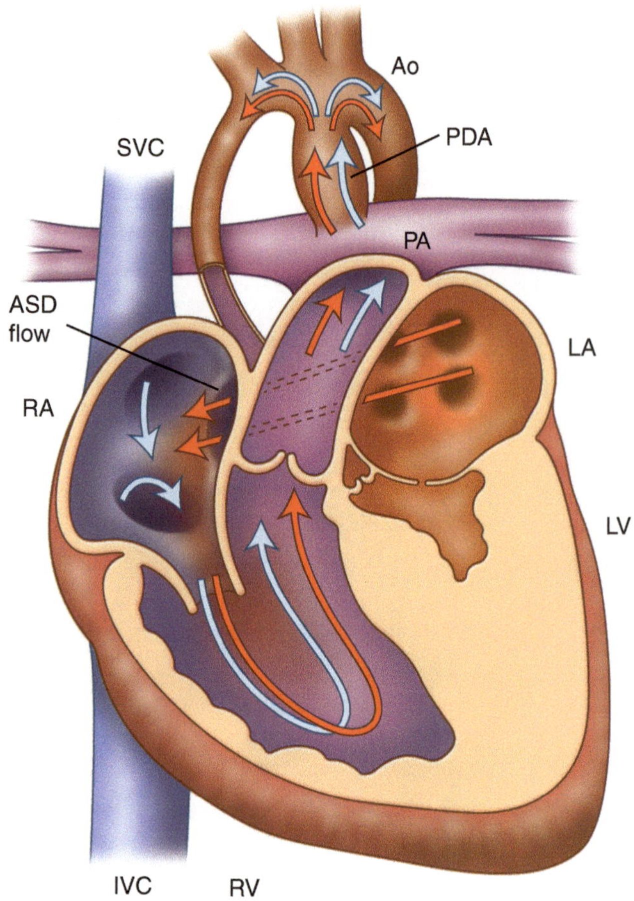

Fig. 12.10 Graphic representation of hypoplastic left heart syndrome. Note the small left-sided cardiac structures and direction of flow across the ductus arteriosus (right-to-left shunting). The ductus allows for antegrade blood flow into the descending aorta (Ao) and retrograde flow around the aortic arch. An atrial communication allows for unobstructed egress of left atrial blood. *ASD*, atrial septal defect, *IVC* inferior vena cava, *LA* left atrium, *LV* left ventricle, *PA* pulmonary artery, *PDA* patent ductus arteriosus, *RA* right atrium, *RV* right ventricle, *SVC* superior vena cava

Physiology

The diagnosis of HLHS usually is made either in utero, immediately or very soon after birth. Most affected neonates are born at term and appear normal at birth. Because right-to-left shunting across the ductus arteriosus provides for the entire systemic blood flow in the case of aortic atresia, it is considered a "ductal-dependent circulation." The atrial communication allows for egress of pulmonary venous return into the RA, where it mixes with the systemic venous blood entering the RV and MPA.

The clinical presentation in HLHS varies; some infants display cyanosis and/or features of pulmonary venous congestion and others present with ominous signs of low cardiac output and impending or frank cardiovascular collapse. The acute decompensation is associated with ductal constriction and hypoperfusion of systemic vascular beds, resulting in metabolic acidosis and lactic acidemia. The shunted blood across the ductus arteriosus in most cases not only serves as the entire source of systemic cardiac output but also provides coronary blood flow because there is absent (aortic atresia) or virtually no antegrade flow through the Ao valve (severe AS). An aspect of the pathology that influences the clinical presentation is the degree of severe restriction across the interatrial communication or in some patients, an intact atrial septum. On occasion, a decompressing vein can be present, allowing for the egress of LA blood elsewhere in the circulation. If this is not the case, the critically ill neonate displays profound hypoxemia and acidosis requiring immediate attention. This condition represents a major clinical problem associated with a poor outcome [64].

Management

The initial management of HLHS includes optimization of the clinical status of the neonate and maintenance of ductal patency with an infusion of PGE_1 [65]. Mechanical ventilation, correction of acid–base status, and inotropic support may be necessary. Strategies to manipulate the ratio of pulmonary to systemic blood flow (Qp/Qs) and to optimize oxygen delivery are the mainstay of management (Fig. 12.11) [66]. Commonly, steps are taken to maintain a relatively high pulmonary vascular resistance, thereby limiting pulmonary blood flow and increasing systemic blood flow. In most cases, maintaining normocarbia or allowing mild hypercarbia, and/or limiting the fraction of inspired oxygen concentration, can achieve this goal. The administration of nitrogen to deliver a hypoxic gas mixture also has been used as has carbon dioxide in an effort to increase pulmonary vascular tone and balance the Qp/Qs [67, 68]. In a study that assessed the effects of inspired gas mixtures to reduce pulmonary over-circulation and improve systemic perfusion, inspired carbon dioxide (3 %) improved cerebral oxygenation and mean arterial pressure, whereas a hypoxic mixture (17 % inspired oxygen) affected neither [69]. The neonate with a high PaO_2 caused by pulmonary over-circulation may have inadequate systemic blood flow. This condition will be associated with severe metabolic acidosis and with problems secondary to decreased perfusion of metabolically active organs (e.g., necrotizing enterocolitis resulting from impaired splanchnic blood flow).

Various approaches have been utilized in the management of this lesion and reflect the ongoing challenges in the care of these infants even today [70]. Options include comfort care and no intervention, in which case death is almost assured; a stepwise palliative surgical strategy; an initial combined

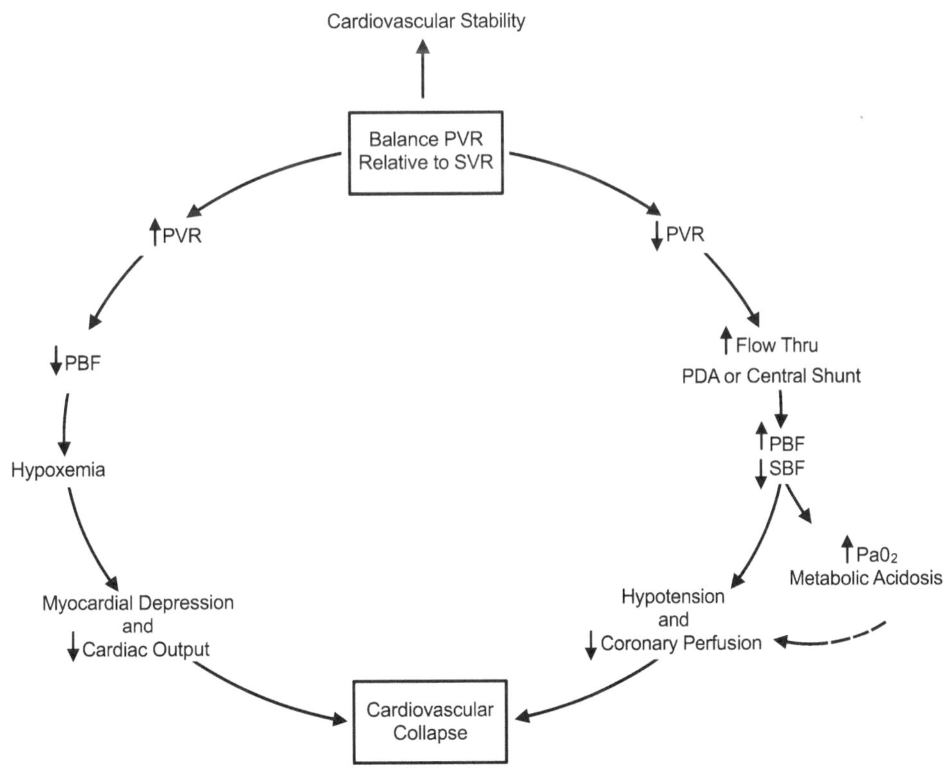

Fig. 12.11 Physiologic balance between the systemic and pulmonary circulations required for hemodynamic stability in the infant with hypoplastic left heart syndrome prior to and following palliation. Reproduced with permission from Hansen DD, Hickey PR. Anesthesia for hypoplastic left heart syndrome: use of high-dose fentanyl in 30 neonates. *Anesth Analg* 1986,65:127–132. *PBF* pulmonary blood flow, *PVR* pulmonary vascular resistance, *SBF* systemic blood flow, *SVR* systemic vascular resistance

catheter-surgical approach (hybrid procedure) and subsequent step palliation; and cardiac transplantation [71, 72].

The initial surgical strategy for HLHS during the neonatal period is referred to as *Stage I palliation* or the *Norwood procedure*. It involves neoaortic reconstruction using the native pulmonary root and homograft material to relieve the systemic outflow tract obstruction, an atrial septectomy to allow for unobstructed drainage of the pulmonary venous return into the RA, and creation of a reliable source of pulmonary blood flow through either a modified Blalock-Taussig shunt (Fig. 12.12) or an RV to PA conduit (Sano modification; Fig. 12.13) [73]. The RV becomes the chamber that supports both circulations at this stage of surgical palliation. Complications after this operation are associated with significant morbidity and risk of mortality [74].

The *hybrid procedure* for HLHS represents an alternate palliative option to Stage I reconstruction during the neonatal period (Fig. 12.14) [72]. This approach involves a combined catheter-based and surgical strategy wherein a stent is deployed by the interventionalist across the ductus arteriosus to maintain patency and bilateral bands are placed across the PA branches by the surgeon to restrict pulmonary blood flow. Enlargement of the interatrial communication (via balloon atrial septostomy) usually is performed during or within a few days after this procedure. The hybrid approach delays Ao reconstruction until later in infancy and is considered of potential benefit, as the fragile neonate is not subject to CPB or associated techniques such as DHCA. In these infants, the Norwood reconstruction is subsequently combined with the creation of a *superior cavopulmonary connection or Glenn anastomosis (Stage II palliation)*, thus effectively merging the first two stages of the palliative pathway. Depending on institutional preference, the hybrid approach is either reserved for high-risk neonates with HLHS or used liberally as the favored strategy.

Anesthetic Considerations

As initial interventions in HLHS are very high risk, it is essential to procure absolutely reliable vascular access and ensure excellent function of all monitors at the outset of the procedure. In the operating room, the same management principles discussed previously to maintain systemic output, oxygen delivery, and balance of the pulmonary and systemic blood flows are followed. Partial occlusion of a branch PA by

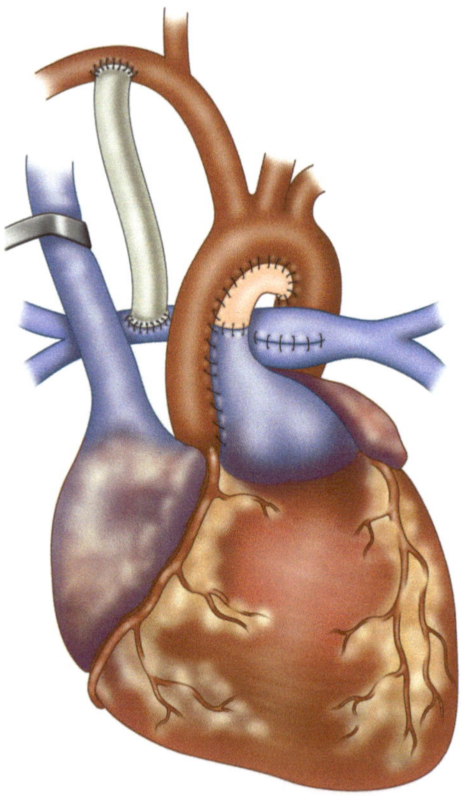

Fig. 12.12 Graphic representation of the Norwood procedure with a systemic to pulmonary artery shunt (modified Blalock-Taussig shunt)

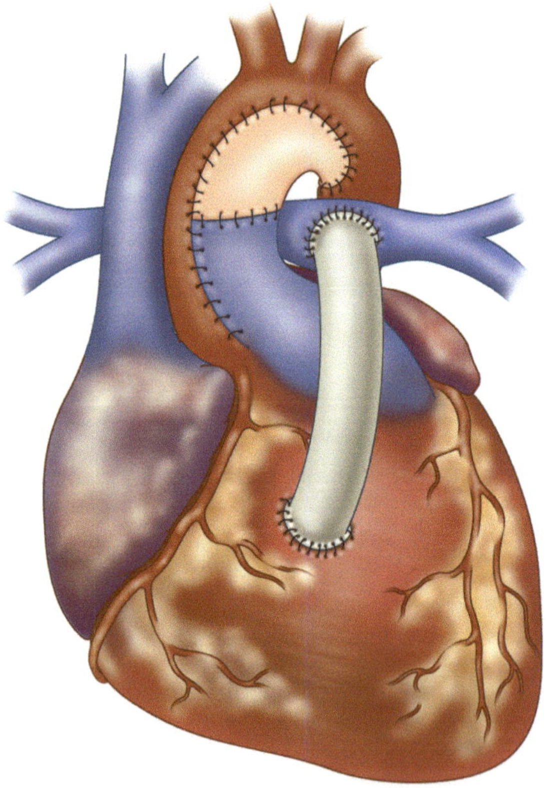

Fig. 12.13 Graphic representation of the Sano modification of the Norwood procedure with a right ventricular to pulmonary artery conduit. *Ao* aorta, *IVC* inferior vena cava, *LA* left atrium, *LPA* left pulmonary artery, *LV*, left ventricle, *PDA*, patent ductus arterious, *RA*, right atrium, *RPA* right pulmonary artery, *RV* right ventricle, *SVC* superior vena cava

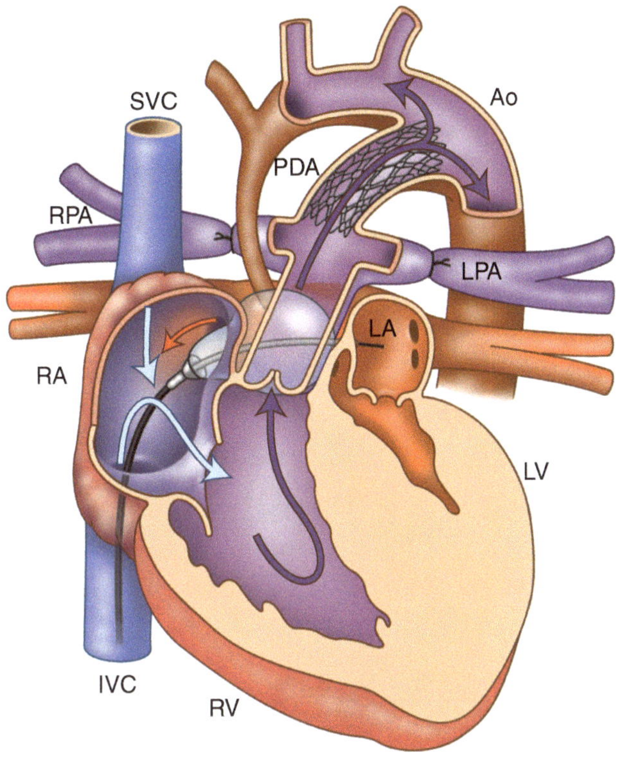

Fig. 12.14 Graphic displaying hybrid palliation for hypoplastic left heart syndrome. The approach consists of ductal stenting, banding of both branch pulmonary arteries, and enlargement of an interatrial communication

the surgeon to mechanically limit pulmonary blood flow also can be of benefit in this setting. The anesthetic technique varies among centers; in some, a high-opioid-muscle relaxant technique is preferred, whereas in others the use of opioid is more limited and volatile anesthetic is favored.

The use of an alpha-adrenergic blocking agent (phentolamine) has been advocated as a means to optimize peripheral vasodilation during the cooling phase of CPB. Long-acting blockade with phenoxybenzamine has been shown to improve systemic oxygen delivery [75]. This is secondary to minimizing regional variations in SaO_2-induced vascular resistance, thereby allowing the use of greater oxygen concentrations to improve systemic oxygen delivery in the post-operative period [76].

Specific Issues

- *Surgical palliative approach.* The particular surgical approach for Stage I palliation (systemic to PA shunt or RV to PA conduit), as well as the favored perfusion strategy (circulatory arrest or antegrade cerebral perfusion), remains dependent on the surgeon and the center where the procedure is performed [77]. These factors impact the selection of arterial blood pressure-monitoring sites and may favor the use of additional monitors, including those that allow for monitoring of the brain. In some patients special bypass strategies may be used (refer to page x), and in these cases, additional monitoring may be required (refer to monitoring section, page x). Whereas a modified Blalock-Taussig shunt allows for pulmonary blood flow to occur during the entire cardiac cycle, in a Sano connection, most of this flow occurs during systole. The narrower pulse pressure and relatively greater diastolic blood pressure allowed by the Sano conduit as compared with the modified Blalock-Taussig shunt is regarded as an advantage for end-organ and coronary perfusion. The Sano strategy is preferred at some centers in order to improve the immediate postoperative course. This relatively more stable circulation is also thought to potentially limit the rates of interstage mortality that occurs in these infants while they await a second palliative procedure [78]. In a study that included a large number of infants with HLHS undergoing the Norwood procedure, the transplantation-free survival rate at a year post-operation was better with the RV to PA shunt than with the modified Blalock-Taussig shunt. After that time period, no significant difference in transplantation-free survival was evident between the two groups [77].
- *Right ventricular optimization.* With the RV operating as the systemic pump in HLHS, all efforts to maintain/enhance RV function during the perioperative period should be considered.
- *Balancing the circulations.* After separation from CPB, care is taken to optimize the balance between the pulmonary and systemic blood flows. A conventional management strategy has been to monitor the arterial oxygen saturation for this assessment and to guide this balance by targeting a value between 75 and 80 %. If the arterial oxygen saturation is less than expected after separation from CPB and potential factors such as inappropriate shunt size and shunt occlusion/distortion have been excluded, steps are undertaken to decrease the pulmonary vascular resistance and increase the systemic arterial blood pressure in an attempt to improve the pulmonary blood flow. A relatively high hemoglobin concentration is important in this setting to enhance the delivery of oxygen and to prevent anemia-related low peripheral vascular tone. At the same time, the deleterious effects of overtransfusion and polycythemia should be considered, particularly in view of the potential negative impact on blood flow across the systemic to PA shunt and patency of this connection. If maneuvers that decrease the pulmonary vascular tone are unsuccessful, administration of inhaled nitric oxide as a selective pulmonary vasodilator should be considered. If the arterial oxygen saturation is greater than expected, it is reasonable to reduce the inspired oxygen concentration and ensure normocarbia or mild hypercarbia. If there is evidence of

adequate systemic output and tissue perfusion, a relatively high arterial oxygen saturation may be acceptable.

- *Mixed venous oxygen saturation monitoring.* An approach proposed in the neonate with single ventricle physiology following Stage I palliation to ensure systemic oxygenation is the use of continuous mixed venous oxygen saturation (SvO_2) monitoring, using transthoracic catheters with oximetric capabilities placed directly by the surgeon at the time of surgery [78]. A reported strategy is to target an SvO_2 value over 50 %, a mean arterial pressure over 45 mmHg, normocarbia, and to administer oxygen as required to maintain the SpO_2. Relying on SvO_2 as an indicator of systemic oxygen delivery and an SvO_2-directed strategy has been associated with favorable outcomes in neonates with HLHS [79, 80].
- *Postoperative issues.* Regardless of the surgical technique, patients with HLHS present major challenges of bleeding, myocardial dysfunction, and hemodynamic instability during the post-bypass period. Other potential problems include renal dysfunction and hepatic impairment [81]. As a result of these concerns, sternal closure may be delayed and some may need postoperative mechanical circulatory support. Routine use of circulatory support immediately after the Norwood procedure to facilitate postoperative management has been reported; however, this is not the standard of care at most centers [82].
- *Hybrid procedure.* Deferring the risks associated with the Norwood operation to a later time in infancy, as allowed by a hybrid procedure, can offer potential advantages to the neonate. Although caring for a neonate with a critical lesion, such as HLHS, outside the typical surgical setting can present major challenges, a report on the anesthetic management of neonates undergoing the hybrid procedure documented relatively stable intraoperative and early postoperative hemodynamics [83]. In addition, this experience indicated that most neonates did not require blood transfusions or inotropic support and performing endotracheal extubation was feasible either at the end of the procedure or soon after the infant was admitted to intensive care.

Interrupted Aortic Arch

Anatomic Features

Interrupted aortic arch (IAA), a discontinuity of the Ao arch, is an uncommon lesion representing only 1 % of all CHD. Affected children have a high incidence of DiGeorge syndrome (22q11 microdeletion).

This anomaly is defined in terms of the site of interruption as follows: *type A*, if distal to the left subclavian artery; *type B*, if between the left carotid and left subclavian arteries (most common variant; Fig. 12.15); and *type C*, if between the carotid arteries. The pathology frequently is associated with a posteriorly malaligned VSD, resulting in obstruction of the LVOT. Coexisting anomalies include a right Ao arch, aberrant origin of a subclavian artery, truncus arteriosus, and aortopulmonary window.

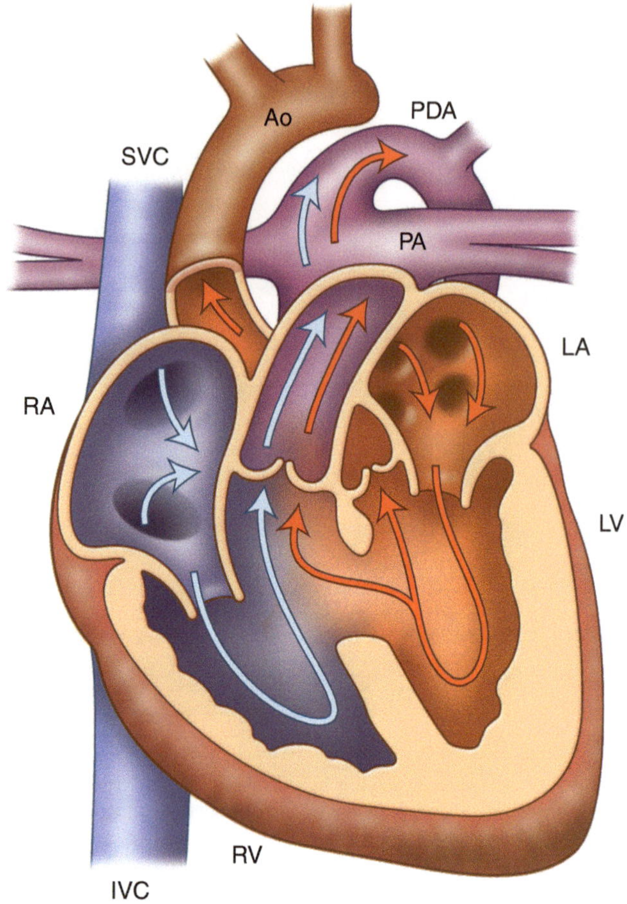

Fig. 12.15 Graphic representation of type B interrupted aortic arch. Note the site of interruption between the left carotid and left subclavian arteries. The patent ductus arteriosus (*PDA*) supplies the systemic circulation beyond the level of interruption. *Ao* aorta, *IVC* inferior vena cava, *LA* left atrium, *LV* left ventricle, *PA* pulmonary artery, *RA* right atrium, *RV* right ventricle

Pathophysiology

Patency of the ductus arteriosus is essential for survival in this anomaly, as it allows for perfusion of systemic beds distal to the interruption. The presentation of IAA in the neonate is characterized by congestive heart failure, poor perfusion, cardiovascular collapse/shock as the ductus arteriosus closes, and, occasionally, differential cyanosis. In this regard, the physiology resembles that of severe CoA. The presence of a VSD can cause pulmonary over-circulation and the associated consequences.

Management

After the diagnosis is established, stabilization of the infant is critical; PGE_1 therapy should be initiated to maintain ductal patency. Anticongestive therapy and inotropes should be administered as needed. Surgery is undertaken in the neonatal period, typically soon after the diagnosis is made. Aortic arch reconstruction, closure of the VSD, and possible resection of subaortic obstruction are performed. Much less commonly, an initial palliative approach is undertaken with Ao arch repair and pulmonary artery banding (PAB), followed by delayed complete repair later in infancy. If the LVOT obstruction is severe (marked subaortic narrowing, annular/Ao root/Asc Ao hypoplasia), alternate approaches, including Ao root-enlargement, replacement, or other complex interventions, may be necessary. A single ventricle strategy is required in some cases.

Anesthetic Considerations

Although echocardiography is diagnostic in most neonates with IAA, additional preoperative studies may be needed to further define the details of the arch anatomy. These examinations in most cases require care of the neonate at remote locations, adding to the management considerations for the sick infant.

Maintenance of the PGE_1 infusion is critical before reconstructing the Ao arch. An adequate response generally implies no significant pressure gradient between proximal and distal areas of the interruption. In view of the common association between PGE_1 therapy and apnea, and other clinical issues, these neonates frequently are intubated and mechanically ventilated in the critical care unit.

Specific Issues

- *Monitoring*. Selection of the sites for monitoring systemic arterial blood pressure and pulse oximetry is an important consideration in IAA. It is dictated by the Ao arch anatomy and the presence of coexistent anomalies. In the case of a type B interruption with left Ao arch and aberrant right subclavian artery, for example, none of the vessels that supply the limbs are proximal to the interruption site. Thus, the arterial blood pressure proximal to the site of interruption cannot be measured in any extremity. This issue can have implications for the surgical intervention, as the perfusion pressure cannot be recorded while on CPB during the period of Ao arch reconstruction. Neuromonitoring can be reassuring in this setting. With regard to pulse oximetry, an oxygen saturation differential would be expected in the unrepaired neonate, with greater values in the beds supplied proximal to the site of interruption by the Asc Ao and reduced values distally reflecting flow from the ductus arteriosus.
- *Concerns related to DiGeorge syndrome*. In view of the potential for developing hypocalcemia in neonates with DiGeorge syndrome, calcium levels should be measured frequently. In such cases, calcium infusions may be required. The presence of coexisting noncardiac anomalies in this syndrome must be considered including immune deficiency. Irradiated blood products should be used to prevent potentially fatal transfusion-associated graft-versus-host disease.
- *Surgical considerations.* Interventions for IAA can be quite complicated, requiring considerable bypass and myocardial ischemic times, particularly when concomitant LVOT obstruction is present. This can be a very challenging condition to treat.

Critical Pulmonary Stenosis and Pulmonary Atresia with Intact Ventricular Septum

Anatomic Features

Pulmonary stenosis is the most common form of RVOT obstruction among infants, accounting for more than 80 % of the cases. This lesion is reported in approximately 10 % of patients with CHD. In the classic isolated pathology, leaflet tethering/thickening and commissural fusion lead to the formation of peripheral raphes and narrowing of the valve lumen. Systolic valvar doming is usually identified on cardiac imaging.

Critical PS (Fig. 12.16) and *pulmonary atresia with intact ventricular septum* (Fig. 12.17) represent lesions characterized by pulmonary valve/RVOT obstruction. The pulmonary valve in the neonate with *critical PS,* the most severe form of valvar obstruction in infancy, displays fused raphes with a restrictive, eccentric pin-size opening. In the uncomplicated or pure form of critical PS, the ventricular septum is intact and an interatrial communication (patent foramen ovale or secundum atrial septal defect) is present. *Pulmonary atresia with intact ventricular septum* is a lesion characterized by membranous or muscular atresia of the RVOT and wide diversity in the size of the RV cavity, infundibular region, and pulmonary arteries. This defect is the third most common cyanotic congenital pathology in the neonate and accounts for approximately 3 to 4 % of all congenital lesions diagnosed in infancy [84].

The tricuspid valve, RV, and pulmonary arteries frequently display abnormalities in both of these defects (abnormal tricuspid valve leaflets, tricuspid annular hypoplasia, reduced size of the RV cavity, main and branch pulmonary arteries), but they are likely to be of a more severe nature in the neonate with pulmonary atresia and intact ventricular septum.

Pathophysiology

Cyanosis is a common presentation in both of these congenital heart anomalies. The severity of the hypoxemia is determined

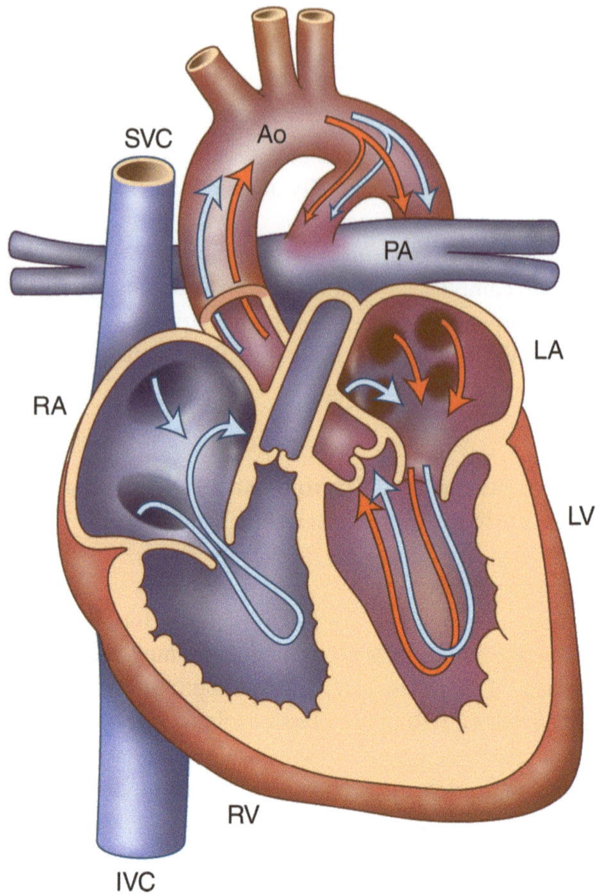

Fig. 12.16 Graphic representation of critical pulmonary stenosis. In this defect, the ductus arteriosus serves as the main source of pulmonary blood flow. *Ao* aorta, *IVC* inferior vena cava, *LA* left atrium, *LV* left ventricle, *PA* pulmonary artery, *RA* right atrium, *RV* right ventricle, *SVC* superior vena cava

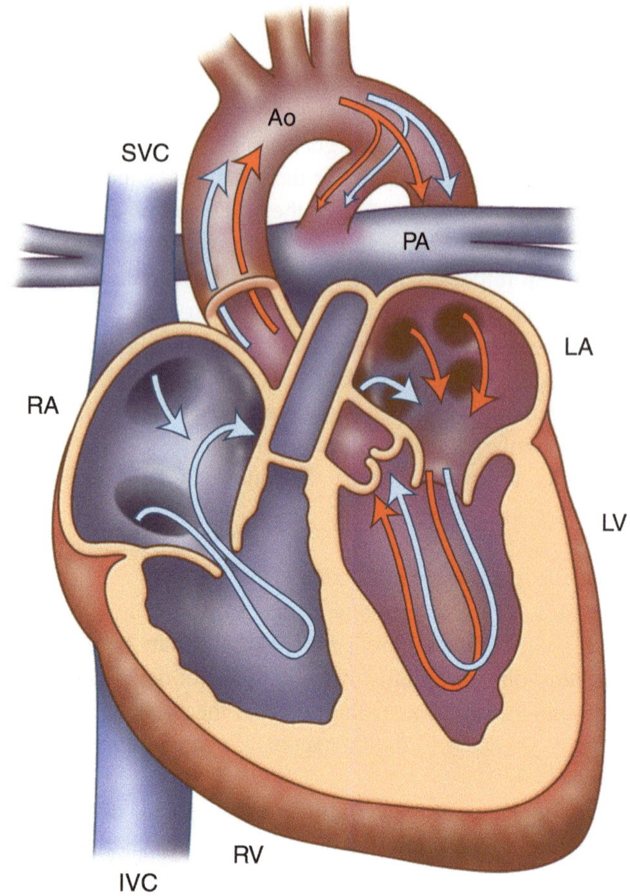

Fig. 12.17 Graphic representation of pulmonary atresia and intact ventricular septum. Note the associated findings in this defect that usually include a patent ductus arteriosus, hypoplastic right ventricle, atrial septal defect, and, in some cases, some degree of tricuspid regurgitation. The ductus arteriosus provides the source of pulmonary blood flow in this lesion prior to an intervention. The atrial communication allows for right-to-left shunting. *Ao* aorta, *IVC* inferior vena cava, *LA* left atrium, *LV* left ventricle, *PA* pulmonary artery, *RA* right atrium, *RV* right ventricle, *SVC* superior vena cava

by the decrease in pulmonary blood flow and the extent of interatrial right-to-left shunting. Affected neonates have ductal-dependent pulmonary blood flow. The severity of the obstruction in critical PS is determined by the extent of valvar narrowing. In pulmonary atresia with intact ventricular septum, no antegrade flow is feasible across the valve, as the outflow is completely obstructed. The main physiologic consequence of these pathologies is an increase in the RV systolic pressure that can exceed systemic pressures.

In infants with critical PS, the infundibular region (subpulmonary area) participates in the hypertrophic response, aggravating the outflow obstruction and contributing to the reduction in RV cavity size. Right ventricular hypertrophy serves as a compensatory mechanism to maintain ventricular output over time. However, it is associated with diminished RV compliance and diastolic dysfunction. Subendocardial ischemia resulting in myocardial infarction and fibrosis accounts for systolic impairment, eventual chamber dilation, and congestive heart failure.

In pulmonary atresia with intact ventricular septum, unusual communications between the coronary arteries and the RV can be present, as may a number of coronary abnormalities. When this is the case, the myocardium may rely on coronary perfusion directly from the RV (RV-dependent coronary circulation) [85]. This condition is a vulnerable situation that can predispose the infant to the development of myocardial ischemia and infarction.

In both of these lesions, critical PS and pulmonary atresia with intact ventricular septum, the structural abnormalities of the tricuspid valve frequently are associated with regurgitation, particularly in the presence of RV hypertension, leading to RA dilation.

Management

The mainstay of therapy in lesions with severe RVOT obstruction is stabilization of the neonate and PGE_1 therapy to provide for pulmonary blood flow. Options for management are catheter-based or surgical. Unfavorable anatomy or suboptimal results from a catheter intervention may require surgery. In infants with critical PS, the most common cardiac catheterization interventions are percutaneous balloon valvuloplasty and ductal stenting. Surgical options include pulmonary valvotomy with splitting of the commissures and/or partial valvectomy. Concomitant resection of infundibular obstruction or placement of a transannular patch may be necessary. In a minority of cases, valve replacement with an RV to PA conduit is the most suitable option. In rare instances, a systemic to PA shunt is required.

In the neonate with pulmonary atresia and intact ventricular septum, angiographic data are obtained before any intervention to determine the presence/absence of communications between the RV and coronary arteries [86]. Potential significant coronary artery abnormalities (stenosis, interruptions) also need to be characterized for planning interventional strategies. The concern when RV decompression or pulmonary valve perforation is performed is the potential for myocardial ischemia or infarction related to reductions in RV pressure in the case of RV-dependent coronary circulation. If a patent infundibulum is present and other aspects of the anatomy are favorable, radiofrequency valve perforation and balloon dilation may be considered. This procedure has been performed successfully in affected neonates, allowing antegrade flow into the pulmonary arteries [87]. In some cases, however, the amount of pulmonary blood flow is inadequate, as manifested by significant arterial desaturation upon weaning or discontinuation of PGE_1 therapy, and the infant benefits from a surgical intervention to augment pulmonary blood flow (i.e., systemic to PA shunt, valvotomy). An approach that combines transventricular valvotomy with a systemic to PA shunt has been reported to promote growth of right-sided structures, increasing the likelihood of an eventual biventricular repair [88]. Ductal stenting also has been performed in these lesions. Another procedure that may be considered, depending on the size of the RV and likelihood of a future biventricular circulation, is reconstruction of the RVOT. If anatomic factors such as severely hypoplastic pulmonary arteries preclude a definitive intervention, palliation consisting of a systemic to PA shunt is performed in order to promote vessel growth. Conditions such as severe coronary obstruction, myocardial ischemia/infarction, and LV dysfunction warrant consideration for cardiac transplantation because of the likely fatal nature of this lesion.

Anesthetic Considerations

An important aspect of the care in the neonate affected by these lesions is to ensure patency of the ductus arteriosus by the continuous intravenous infusion of PGE_1. Catheter-based therapy can lead to effective relief of the obstruction, but factors such as abnormal ventricular morphology/geometry, relatively small pulmonary/tricuspid annulus, hypoplasia of the pulmonary arteries, and interatrial right-to-left shunting may not allow for immediate improvement in the arterial oxygen saturation in some infants. It is not unusual for the PGE_1 infusion to be continued after the procedure is completed. Hemodynamic changes that occur during catheter-based interventions aimed at relieving the RV obstruction are reasonably well tolerated, provided the ductus arteriosus remains patent and the interatrial communication is adequate to maintain LV filling, particularly during the period of balloon dilation. In infants with pulmonary atresia and intact ventricular septum, the potential coronary abnormalities leading to a predisposition for myocardial ischemia warrant monitoring for this problem. As in the case of all other neonatal cardiac interventions, adequate preparation for these cases is of outmost importance.

After surgery that involves relief of the RVOT obstruction, inotropic support should be used judiciously as it can exacerbate the dynamic RVOT gradient, complicating the assessment of the results of the repair. Additional anesthetic considerations apply depending on the planned procedure, approach, and need for CPB.

Specific Issues

- *Suicide right ventricle*. A potential post procedure problem is that adequate relief of the valvar obstruction, either by a catheter intervention or surgery, can result in a physiology referred to as *suicide right ventricle*. This results as the hypertrophied infundibulum contracts vigorously and creates significant post-procedural dynamic outflow tract obstruction, in the absence of fixed obstruction. In the case of severe obstruction and associated low cardiac output, therapy with volume expansion and/or beta-blockade may be required. An important goal is to preserve RV function by avoiding significant myocardial depression or increases in RV afterload.
- *Circular shunt physiology*. Another major problem that can occur after these procedures is a *circular shunt*. This condition represents a morbid state in which the presence of a large PDA (or ductal stent) or placement of a systemic to pulmonary shunt after a pulmonary valve intervention is associated with pulmonary regurgitation. This leads to retrograde shunt flow into the RV, which proceeds to the RA due to an incompetent tricuspid valve. Blood then courses across the atrial communication into the LA, LV, and Ao, thus reentering the shunt. This situation is very precarious because it may lead to significant RV volume overload and a pulmonary steal phenomenon. The unsustainable hemodynamic state requires immediate attention, frequently consisting of escalating support and/or immediate intervention, for survival.

Aortopulmonary Window

Anatomic Features

Aortopulmonary (AP) window, also known as *aortopulmonary septal defect*, is a rare defect, accounting for only 0.1 % of all CHD. This anomaly is characterized by a defect in the wall between the Asc Ao and the PA, creating a communication between these structures (Fig. 12.18) [89]. From an anatomic and physiologic standpoint, this defect resembles truncus arteriosus; however, unlike truncus arteriosus, two distinct semilunar valves are present. The size and location of the communication varies, and thus the defect has been classified into various types [90]. The lesion can occur in isolation but in most cases is associated with other cardiovascular malformations (PDA, intracardiac communications, TOF, double outlet right ventricle, IAA).

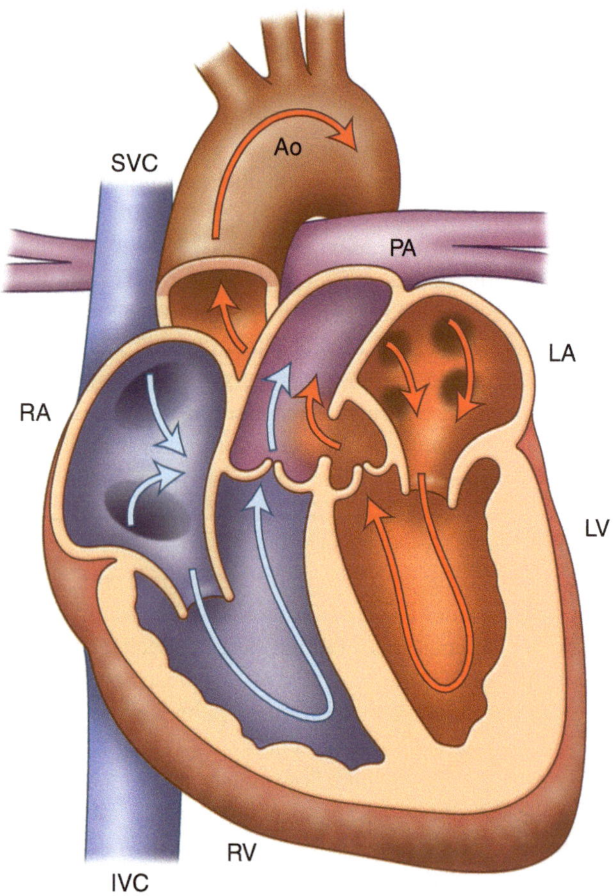

Fig. 12.18 Graphic representation of an aortopulmonary window demonstrating the defect that allows for left-to-right shunting between the great arteries. *Ao* aorta, *IVC* inferior vena cava, *LA* left atrium, *LV* left ventricle, *PA* pulmonary artery, *RA* right atrium, *RV* right ventricle, *SVC* superior vena cava

Pathophysiology

The magnitude of the shunt across an AP window depends on the size of the communication, PA pressures, and relative resistances of the pulmonary and systemic vascular beds. Left-to-right shunting across the defect and the increased pulmonary blood flow are associated with elevated PA pressures, left-sided volume overload, and congestive symptoms. An uncorrected communication can lead to pulmonary vascular disease relatively early in life.

Management

The preferred approach to this lesion is considered to be surgical, although successful transcatheter closure of the communication has been reported [91]. In most cases, a patch is required to obliterate the defect and associated pathology is also addressed at the time of surgery.

Anesthetic Considerations

The same anesthetic principles that apply to the management of the neonate with any large vascular communication (i.e., PDA) or any other cardiac defect for which further increases in pulmonary blood flow are detrimental and for which a balance between pulmonary and systemic blood flow should be maintained also apply in this lesion.

Ebstein Anomaly

Anatomic Features

Ebstein anomaly represents the most common congenital malformation of the tricuspid valve, but, overall, is a rare lesion accounting for 0.3 to 0.7 % of CHD. It is characterized by apical displacement of the septal and posterior leaflets of the tricuspid valve towards the RV apex and a redundant, "sail-like" anterior leaflet (Fig. 12.19). The severity of valve displacement and dysplasia varies, accounting for different degrees of tricuspid regurgitation and the diversity of clinical manifestations. The lesion results in an atrialized RV, referring to the region of the RV proximal to the abnormal tricuspid valve attachments. The distal portion of the RV represents the functional cavity. An interatrial communication is present in the majority of affected neonates, and some degree of RV dysplasia and or dysfunction is usually seen. Other potential associated defects include severe pulmonary stenosis/valve atresia and PDA. In some cases, the RV output is decreased to such an extent that it is difficult to distinguish between functional and anatomic pulmonary stenosis/atresia. An association with Wolff-Parkinson-White syndrome is well recognized.

Pathophysiology

Tricuspid regurgitation in this anomaly results in increased RA pressure and right-sided volume overload. As the RA

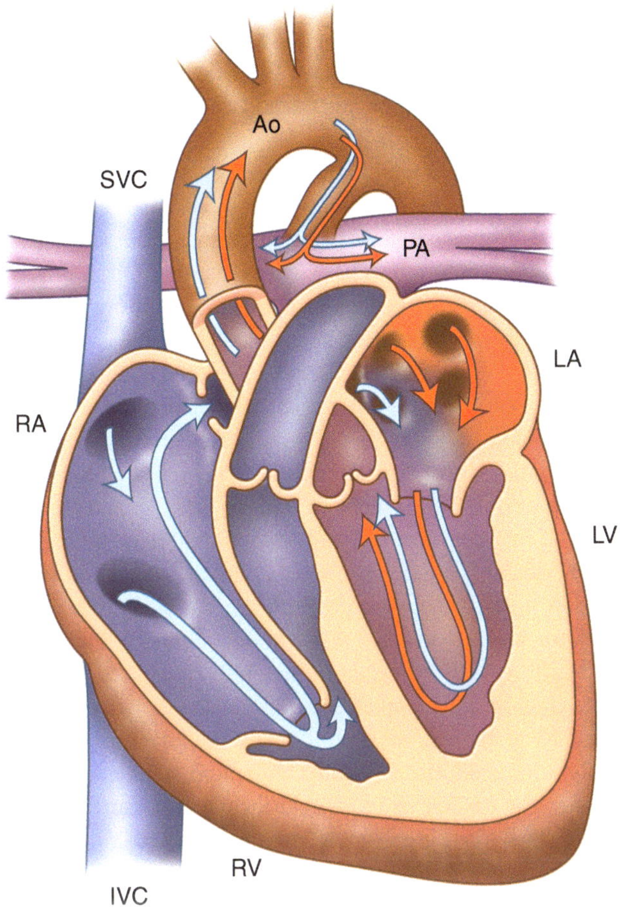

Fig. 12.19 Graphic representation of Ebstein anomaly displaying the displaced tricuspid valve leaflets, associated tricuspid regurgitation, and right-to-left atrial level shunting. In the neonate with anatomic of functional pulmonary stenosis/atresia, a patent ductus arteriosus is the source of pulmonary blood flow. *Ao* aorta, *IVC* inferior vena cava, *LA* left atrium, *LV* left ventricle, *PA* pulmonary artery, *RA* right atrium, *RV* right ventricle, *SVC* superior vena cava

pressure increases, it exceeds LA pressure, stretching an existing interatrial communication. This process allows for right-to-left shunting and results in decreased pulmonary blood flow and clinical cyanosis. The redundant anterior tricuspid valve leaflet can cause functional obstruction to the RV. Another frequently found feature of the pathology is abnormal RV systolic function. These factors can have detrimental effects on the LV because (1) the dilated and/or dysfunctional RV can impair LV filling and (2) the abnormal interventricular septum can affect LV geometry and function (ventricular interdependence).

Ebstein anomaly represents a wide clinical spectrum that ranges from minimal or no symptomatology to intractable congestive heart failure and even death. In utero, it can result in fetal hydrops. The hemodynamic status of the neonate is influenced by factors such as the severity of tricuspid regurgitation, presence/degree of RVOT obstruction, size and function of the RV, and associated structural defects. Cyanosis caused by right-to-left atrial shunting under conditions of elevated pulmonary vascular resistance is the most common presentation. Severe tricuspid regurgitation almost invariably results in congestive heart failure; if intractable in nature, it can lead to circulatory collapse. A neonatal presentation implies a major clinical problem and generally portends a poor prognosis.

In the neonate with Ebstein anomaly, several additional cardiac problems can complicate the clinical course. Atrial arrhythmias related to atrial dilation or abnormal conduction pathways can occur, and pulmonary stenosis or atresia (either functional or anatomic) can further compromise pulmonary blood flow.

Management

Some infants require only conservative treatment and follow-up. In the symptomatic neonate, the main issues requiring intervention are congestive heart failure and hypoxemia. Diuretic therapy and inotropic support are instituted as needed. Initial hypoxemia in the neonate can improve as pulmonary vascular resistance falls, allowing for forward pulmonary blood flow. In cases of severe pulmonary stenosis or atresia, an intervention is required. Distinguishing hypoxemia related to increased pulmonary vascular resistance from that resulting from anatomic RVOT obstruction can be difficult. Hence, PGE_1 therapy frequently is instituted to maintain ductal patency until the nature of the hypoxemia can be ascertained or the expected decrease in pulmonary vascular resistance occurs. Initiating other measures aimed at decreasing pulmonary vascular tone and supporting the overall critically ill neonate are warranted.

During the neonatal period, a catheter-based intervention and/or cardiac surgery may be necessary. Catheter therapy targets the relief of RV outflow obstruction and/or to increase pulmonary blood flow (pulmonary valve dilation/perforation, ductal stenting). The choice of surgical procedure is influenced by factors such as details of the anatomy, associated defects, RV size and function, and the clinical status of the neonate. Approaches range from creation of a systemic to PA shunt, tricuspid valve repair, palliative surgery anticipating a future single ventricle strategy, and cardiac transplantation. The overall success of the various surgical interventions in the neonatal period has generally been poor in the presence of severe disease.

Anesthetic Considerations

Anesthetic care, when required, is usually for cardioversion, cardiac catheterization, or surgery. The neonate with Ebstein anomaly presents a challenge to the provider of anesthetic care because of the typically poor clinical status frequently characterized by severe tricuspid regurgitation, cyanosis, congestive heart failure, lactic acidosis, and impending circulatory collapse.

Specific Issues

- *Respiratory status.* In the sick neonate, pulmonary mechanics can be compromised by factors such as prematurity, interstitial lung edema, and lung hypoplasia. The management of mechanical ventilatory support needs consideration of these factors while balancing the need to enhance antegrade pulmonary blood flow.
- *Pulmonary vascular resistance.* Increased RV afterload leads to right heart distention and compromises LV performance. Thus, it is important to optimize not only RV contractility but also to aggressively avoid increases in pulmonary vascular tone that will impair the function of both ventricles.
- *Rhythm disturbances.* Numerous rhythm abnormalities have been reported in these children. Although supraventricular arrhythmias predominate, other abnormalities include atrioventricular block and ventricular arrhythmias. These rhythm disturbances usually are poorly tolerated and require aggressive therapy that may include cardioversion, the administration of antiarrhythmic drug therapy, and/or cardiac pacing.
- *Circular shunt.* This physiology can also occur after interventions in this lesion, as described in a preceding section (refer to page x).

Preoperative Assessment of the Neonate with Congenital Heart Disease

History and Physical Examination

It is important for the anesthesiologist to perform a comprehensive preoperative evaluation to identify and anticipate factors that could influence the perioperative management in the neonate with CHD. This evaluation begins with a review of the prenatal history that includes details of the pregnancy such as maternal illnesses (e.g., diabetes, hypertension), medications, and drug use, as well as a family history. Data regarding fetal studies, if available, should be reviewed as in many cases today the diagnosis of cardiovascular disease is established "in utero." Specific issues of interest, in addition to the details of the anatomy, include functional assessment of the cardiovascular system, presence of extracardiac abnormalities, genetic syndromes or other disorders of potential impact, as well as an impression of the overall well-being of the fetus. Relevant information to be obtained regarding the delivery includes gestational age, Apgar scores, events related to the neonatal resuscitation, and need for interventions immediately after birth. If the diagnosis of heart disease is made postnatally, details such as clinical presentation, hospital course, results of all diagnostic studies obtained to define the cardiovascular abnormalities, interventions performed, and response to these interventions should be reviewed. It is essential to gather information regarding coexistent medical problems or conditions that could potentially affect other organ systems and impact on the anesthetic management.

The physical examination should note the neonate's weight and length. General appearance should include the level of distress, if any, presence/degree of cyanosis, and overall clinical status. Vital signs, including blood pressure measured in the upper and lower limbs and any gradients between the limbs, should be recorded. The measured SpO_2 at both pre- and post-ductal levels should be noted. A careful examination of the airway and the respiratory and cardiovascular systems should be performed. Respiratory evaluation should note rate and breathing patterns, quality of the breath sounds noting the presence of rales or rhonchi, and the presence of intercostal retractions. If the infant is receiving supplemental oxygen, the inspired oxygen concentration should be recorded. If the airway is intubated, the date the current endotracheal tube (ETT) was inserted should be noted; any difficulties with blockage of the ETT identified, a recent chest radiograph should be reviewed as well as the depth of the ETT at the lips/nose. Similarly, if the lungs are mechanically ventilated, the ventilator mode and settings should be noted. The cardiac exam should include assessment of precordial activity, heart sounds, murmurs, and gallop rhythms. The presence of any existing vascular access, patency of the catheter(s), and appropriateness of catheter tip position should be recorded. The abdomen should be examined for the presence of hepatosplenomegaly. Assessment of the extremities should include examination of pulses, capillary refill, skin temperature and color, and overall perfusion.

A significant number of infants with CHD (1 out of 8) are known to have chromosomal abnormalities. Dysmorphic features or any other noncardiac anomalies that can impact anesthetic care should be noted. Medications being administered, including indications, doses, and route, need to be reviewed.

Ancillary Studies and Laboratory Data

The preoperative electrocardiogram in the neonate with heart disease should be examined to assess for evidence of chamber dilation and/or ventricular hypertrophy, rhythm disturbances, and myocardial ischemia (Fig. 12.20). A recent chest radiograph provides information regarding cardiac size and shape, chamber enlargement, and pulmonary vascularity (Fig. 12.21). In addition, it serves to document the position of the ETT tube, stomach tube, and indwelling vascular catheters. The echocardiogram and additional imaging studies as required (magnetic resonance imaging, computed chest

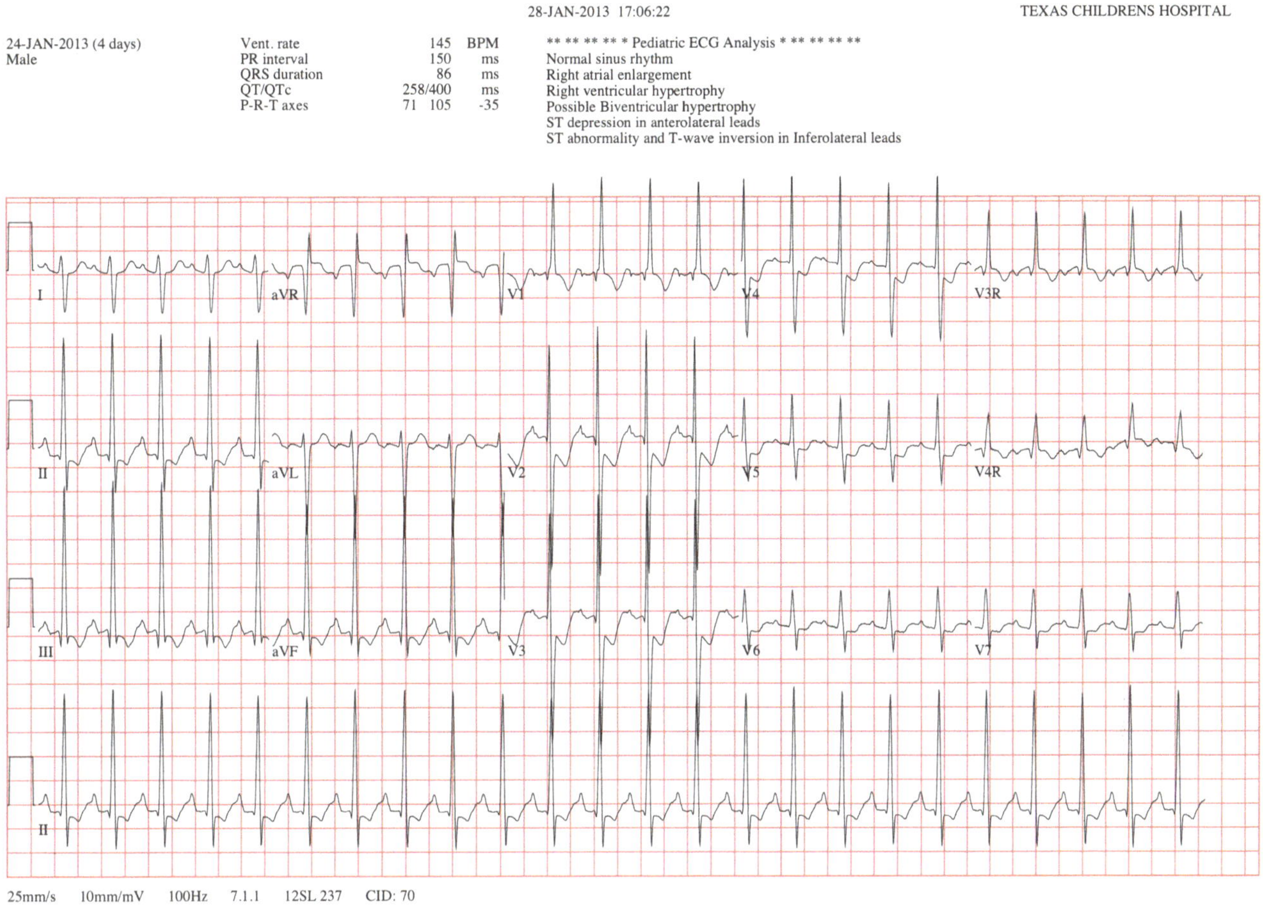

Fig. 12.20 Preoperative electrocardiographic recording in a newborn infant with diagnosis of truncus arteriosus. Note the peaked P waves in lead II indicative with right atrial enlargement, the prominent precordial voltages suggestive of biventricular hypertrophy, and the diffuse ST-T wave changes consistent with compromised myocardial blood flow

tomography, cardiac catheterization) are instrumental in delineating the structural and functional abnormalities. All of these studies should be reviewed carefully and the findings documented.

A complete blood count, electrolyte levels, blood glucose, renal/hepatic function tests, and coagulation studies (prothrombin time, partial thromboplastin times, and international normalized ratio [INR]) should be available. The most recent blood gas analysis should be reviewed to assess oxygenation, ventilation, and acid–base status. The results of any other investigations that may have been performed (head ultrasound, renal ultrasound) also should be reviewed.

Informed Consent

The preoperative visit allows the anesthesiologist an opportunity to meet the family, discuss the anesthetic plan, and address questions in preparation for the procedure. A surgical intervention in a neonate with cardiac disease may imply a substantive risk of morbidity and even mortality. In addition, the anesthetic care for cardiac surgery also entails greater risks when compared with other neonatal surgeries [61, 92]. Although it may not be possible to specify the contribution of anesthesia itself to the overall risks of the procedure, it is reasonable to discuss the most likely potential anesthetic problems that may be encountered perioperatively.

Cardiac surgery in the neonate is a major undertaking regardless of the nature of the procedure, and one must always expect the parents to be apprehensive and concerned. In some cases, particularly those with a postnatal cardiac diagnosis or if the infant had been previously discharged from a well-baby nursery, significant parental stress may be present. The preoperative consultation provides an opportunity to defuse parental anxiety, answer questions, and reassure the parents regarding the unwavering commitment of the entire perioperative team towards a good perioperative outcome.

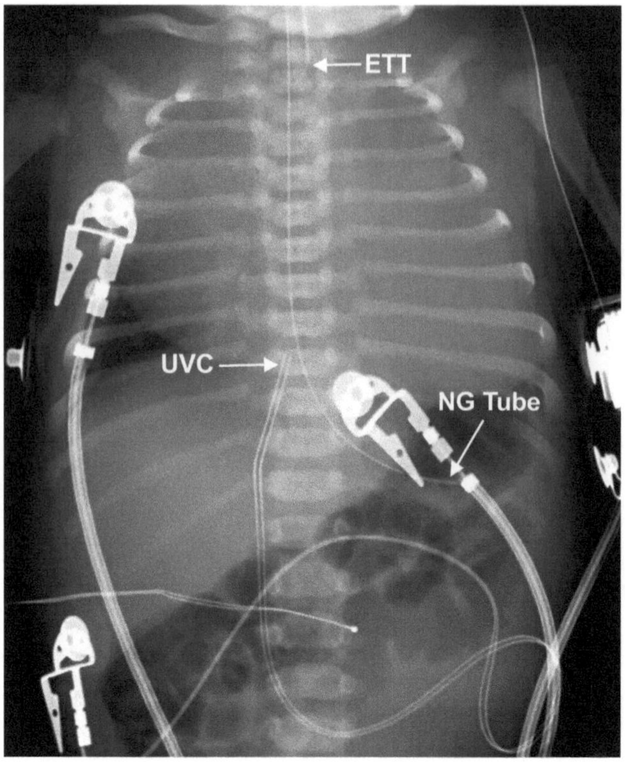

Fig. 12.21 Radiograph in a neonate with congenital heart disease displaying massive cardiomegaly. The tip of the endotracheal tube (ETT) appears just above the level of the clavicles prompting readjustment. The nasogastric (NG) tube is the stomach and the tip of the umbilical venous catheter (UVC) is in good position

Fasting Period

The established preoperative fasting guidelines for surgery in neonates should be followed [93]. Gastric emptying times can be prolonged in those with CHD [94]. A significant number of infants receive maintenance intravenous fluids preoperatively. Adequate hydration is particularly important in the presence of obstructive pathology, cyanotic disease, or single ventricle physiology, as optimization of ventricular preload can limit potential detrimental hemodynamic changes associated with anesthesia and surgery.

Perioperative Considerations in the Neonate Undergoing Cardiac Surgery

Anesthesia Care Provider

Anesthesia for cardiac surgery in the neonate should be delivered by highly skilled individuals with expertise in the various forms of pediatric heart disease. This requires knowledge of the wide spectrum of anatomic and physiologic abnormalities involved, the natural history of the defects, possible management strategies, and overall short- and long-term outcomes. A comprehensive understanding of the disease process, hemodynamic perturbations, and how they are influenced by the anesthetic and surgical procedure are of outmost importance. Familiarity with the anticipated perioperative course, including potential problems and complications, is essential. In addition to these cognitive skills, the treatment of small infants with critical heart disease requires the technical proficiencies that are essential for the care of small infants. The ability to communicate clearly and work effectively with other members of the team is extremely important to ensure the best possible outcome.

Transport to the Operating Room

Most infants who require cardiac surgery within the first few weeks of life are cared for in a critical care setting, either in a neonatal or cardiac unit. The collaborative effort of members of the unit's multidisciplinary team strives to maintain and optimize vital organ function until the planned intervention. At the time of transport, good communication between the care providers and the operating room team must be assured in order to address any recent changes in the neonate's clinical status, current therapy, and any other relevant issues. During transport, the main considerations include temperature homeostasis, adequate airway support/ventilation, careful maintenance of essential infusions, and availability of emergency airway equipment and drugs. Be aware that essential drug infusions can be compromised by kinking of the lines or alterations in the height of the delivery systems. In some cases, a self-inflating bag, air tank, or oxygen/air blender system is needed to deliver room air or a specific inspired oxygen concentration between room air and 100 % oxygen. Monitoring the vital signs and systemic oxygen saturation is essential.

Premedication

The need for premedication is rarely, if ever, indicated in the neonate because this age group is not at risk to experience separation or other forms of anxiety. On rare occasion, premedication can be useful to minimize metabolic stresses and facilitate placement of intravenous access in the agitated or struggling infant. Specific concerns, such as the potential for hypercyanotic spells in tetralogy, also may warrant the judicious use of premedication. Close observation with pulse oximetry and oxygen administration as indicated are recommended after premedication [95].

Intravenous Access

Absolutely reliable intravenous access is mandatory for the administration of fluids, blood products, and medications during anesthetic care. In most neonates with heart disease, a peripheral or indwelling intravenous catheter is already in place, facilitating an intravenous induction of anesthesia. In the neonate without intravenous access, consideration should be given for securing peripheral access before induction of anesthesia. The size of the catheter and need for more than a single site of access should be determined by the infant's clinical status and nature of the intervention. Never rely solely on the integrity of an intravenous access route that arrives with the child!

In all neonates, the potential for right-to-left shunting across a patent foramen ovale or the presence of any intracardiac communication mandates the meticulous removal of air from all injections and the intravenous infusion tubing. Air filters can be difficult to use in the intraoperative setting because they can limit how fast intravenous fluids, propofol, and blood products can be administered, but they may be useful for drug infusions and in the preoperative and postoperative periods.

Availability of Emergency Medications

In view of the potential for hemodynamic compromise in the neonate with CHD, drugs for emergency situations should be prepared in anticipation of the procedure and be immediately available to the anesthesiologist delivering the care. It is essential for these drugs to be available during transport to and from the operating room or any other setting where anesthetic care may be provided.

Physiologic Monitoring

The selection of monitors is guided by the child's clinical status and the nature of the planned procedure. In addition to routine monitors, the intricate nature of cardiac surgery mandates the need for additional monitors as outlined in the sections that follows.

Electrocardiography

Five-lead electrocardiography during cardiac surgery is used to assess heart rate, cardiac rhythm, and ST segments. In most cases, leads II and V5 are displayed on a monitor, and tracings from other leads can be examined as needed. Changes in heart rate can be caused by hypoxia, light anesthesia, stimulation, hypovolemia, or the surgical dissection. Abnormalities in cardiac rhythm can occur as a result of hypoxia, electrolyte imbalance, acid–base abnormalities, intravascular/intracardiac catheters, and surgical manipulations near or around the thorax. Ischemia may be evident on direct examination of the electrocardiographic tracing or ST-segment analysis.

Pulse Oximetry

Monitoring the arterial oxygen saturation is essential during cardiac surgery. The need for sampling at various sites is dictated by the anatomy and pathophysiology. Oxygen saturation monitoring serves as an indicator of intracardiac or great artery level shunting and of pulmonary blood flow. In addition to providing continuous assessment of oxygen saturation and heart rate, the pulse oximeter waveform can be used as a surrogate of the adequacy of peripheral perfusion and cardiac output [96, 97]. It is wise to place backup sensors, which can be used if the primary sensors fail.

Capnography

Capnography confirms proper placement of the ETT, the adequacy of ventilation, and pulmonary blood flow. It also facilitates the recognition of acute problems that can influence lung compliance. End-tidal carbon dioxide ($ETCO_2$) monitoring provides a gross index of pulmonary blood flow and can be useful during cases in which it may be altered. A specific example of its use is during PAB, at which time the $ETCO_2$ can be a useful guide of optimal occlusion. A caveat in interpreting capnography occurs in cyanotic heart disease, during which $ETCO_2$ measurements can underestimate $PaCO_2$ values owing to altered pulmonary blood flow and ventilation-perfusion mismatch [98, 99].

Temperature Monitoring

Temperature is monitored routinely during all cardiac procedures. In cases requiring CPB, temperature is sampled at multiple sites. The most common sampling locations include the nasal, rectal, bladder, esophageal, tympanic membrane, and skin. The goal is to have an indicator of core (central), peripheral, and, possibly, brain temperature, given that hypothermia used during bypass plays a major role in organ preservation. Temperature monitoring is also essential to ensure that a suitable period of cooling has taken place before initiation of circulatory arrest or related bypass strategy. Likewise, temperature assessment is necessary during warming. Although hypothermia is part of most neonatal interventions, an unwanted low body temperature can increase oxygen consumption, and cause acidosis, as well as detrimental changes in hemodynamics, and coagulation status.

Arterial Blood Pressure Monitoring

Noninvasive Monitoring

A blood pressure cuff of appropriate size is used in all neonates undergoing cardiac surgery to allow automated measurements, regardless of the presence of an indwelling arterial catheter, because it offers an alternate option for blood pressure assessment in case of a malfunction of the arterial line. A second site also enables determination of gradients between upper and lower extremities, depending on the pathology or surgical procedure. The selection of suitable monitoring sites is influenced by the underlying anatomic abnormalities and the history of prior surgical interventions (e.g., Blalock-Taussig shunt, arterial cutdown, subclavian flap aortoplasty).

Indwelling Arterial Monitoring

Because of the involved nature of cardiac surgery in the neonate, invasive arterial pressure monitoring almost always is warranted. In addition to providing for blood pressure assessment on a continuous, beat-to-beat basis, it allows for frequent blood sampling to determine the hematocrit, acid–base status, PaO_2 and $PaCO_2$, blood glucose, calcium levels, and electrolyte values.

Sites for Invasive Monitoring

A variety of different sites are available for invasive arterial blood pressure monitoring in the neonate, each with specific advantages and disadvantages. *Umbilical artery* blood pressure monitoring is unique to the neonate. Catheter placement in this vessel often is possible during the first few days of life. Ideal umbilical arterial catheter position is between T6 and T10 (high position) or between L3 and L5 (low position). Advantages of umbilical artery access include relative ease of placement and reliability of access as there is a low likelihood for a catheter in the Ao to be "positional" or subject to the problems that can affect peripheral arterial catheters (vasospasm upon placement, vasoconstriction following CPB). In general, umbilical artery catheters provide optimal tracings of arterial blood pressure and facilitate blood sampling. Complications include potential obstruction of blood flow to specific beds (e.g., renal), distal emboli, thrombotic complications (e.g., mesenteric, Ao, renal artery), and infection. Associations with necrotizing enterocolitis and problems during enteral feedings in the neonate with an indwelling catheter are other concerns [100]. Monitoring the blood pressure via an umbilical arterial catheter is not recommended beyond 7–10 days of life.

The *radial artery* is the most usual site for monitoring invasive arterial blood pressure in the neonate. It can be accessed percutaneously, and a 22 gauge catheter can be placed, often using a Seldinger technique. This can be facilitated by ultrasound guidance if necessary [101, 102]. Radial arterial tracings are very occasionally dampened after CPB, rendering blood pressure assessment during this critical period somewhat challenging. This situation can be resolved by having the surgeon place a small recording needle into the Asc Ao and transducing the root pressure or, alternatively, attaching a pressure-monitoring catheter to a stopcock integrated into the arterial cannula tubing. Vasospasm also can hinder obtaining accurate blood pressure measurements throughout the case. This issue may respond to the administration of lidocaine or papaverine through the catheter.

Before inserting a radial arterial catheter for cardiac surgery, one should review the anatomy and planned operation. In the case of a CoA, right radial artery catheter placement is preferred, as it reflects proximal Ao pressure perfusing the brain and coronary arteries, and the tracing will not be lost if the surgeon has to clamp the left subclavian artery. Monitoring at this site also can guide management of regional cerebral perfusion if this strategy is used (discussed later in the chapter). If an aberrant or retroesophageal right subclavian artery is present and the use of TEE is planned, cannulation of the right radial artery is discouraged; the tracing will likely be dampened or flat after the imaging probe is inserted into the esophagus due to compression of the vessel. If the surgical plan involves placing a modified Blalock-Taussig systemic to PA shunt, an arterial catheter in the ipsilateral side of the graft would not be advised because the blood pressure may not be measurable during portions of the procedure as the vessel is temporarily occluded. Furthermore, measurements obtained after opening of the shunt may not be accurate.

The ulnar and the radial arteries constitute the dual blood supply to the hand. The *radial artery* usually is preferred over the ulnar because avoiding the ulnar artery allows preservation of a larger contributor of blood supply to the hand. The *ulnar artery* often is the larger vessel, and it alternatively can be cannulated for monitoring invasive arterial blood pressure. Allen's test to assess the distal circulation to the hand is difficult to apply, inconclusive, and not generally performed in neonates.

Some practitioners find that cannulation of the ulnar artery is easier than accessing the radial artery, particularly in infants with Down syndrome. This group, known to have a high incidence of congenital heart defects, can present challenges during percutaneous radial artery cannulation [103]. Because of the risk of ischemia to the hand, placement of a catheter in the ulnar artery is contraindicated if the radial artery is thrombosed or after attempts at cannulation have been made. Despite concerns of distal ischemia, a literature report indicates a similar risk for ulnar, radial, and femoral arterial lines [104].

The *brachial artery* has been considered an end artery without collateral circulation. Because of concerns for distal limb ischemia, it is not usually a recommended site to establish arterial access. However, it has been used extensively in some centers without consequences. For example, in one institution where the brachial artery was the second choice for arterial cannulation (after the radial artery) in neonates and infants, there were no major complications in 386 patients who underwent brachial artery cannulation [105].

The foot arteries (*dorsalis pedis* and *posterior tibial vessels*) can be considered as alternate sites for monitoring blood pressure. Although they may not be the first option for arterial cannulation, they can be quite useful during surgery when bypass/hypothermia is not planned or for monitoring in the intensive care unit. Disadvantages of these sites include a high incidence of failure of the catheter to reliably display central Ao pressure after hypothermic CPB and a somewhat greater pressure recorded from these sites as compared with central pressure due to pulse wave amplification. The latter issue can confound the interpretation of blood pressure gradients in some cases.

The right *temporal artery* historically was used for monitoring arterial pressure in neonatal intensive care units [106]. The only time it should be considered for arterial access in the modern era, after the risk-benefit ratio has been carefully assessed, is when all other sites do not allow for the arterial blood pressure of interest to be monitored (i.e., CoA or IAA with an aberrant subclavian artery that arises distal to the coarctation or interruption). In these situations, the temporal artery provides the only monitoring site that reflects the Asc Ao pressure perfusing the brain and coronary arteries. The very serious concern related to temporal artery catheterization is the fact that emboli can be introduced into the cerebral and ophthalmic circulations by even minute volumes of flush fluid. Serious neurologic injury and/or blindness are well-documented complications of the use of this site [107].

Cutdown for Arterial Cannulation

If percutaneous arterial line placement is unsuccessful, arterial cannulation via surgical exposure of the vessel can be performed. At some centers, a cutdown is performed primarily or very early in the process of gaining arterial access. Advantages of a surgical cutdown include speed of placement and direct visualization of the artery/catheter during cannulation, minimizing trauma to the vessel, creation of a false lumen, or formation of a hematoma. Disadvantages include possible damage to the vessel caused by scarring. If the radial artery is accessed by cutdown, the time for Doppler-detected flow to resume in the vessel after decannulation is prolonged. It can also be difficult to cannulate the same vessel during future interventions.

Central Venous Pressure Monitoring

Central venous access provides for monitoring of the central venous pressure (CVP) but also for delivery of vasoactive agents safely and expeditiously into the central circulation, intravascular volume replacement, and the administration of blood products. Caution should be exercised in delivering blood products/fluids rapidly via a central line as this route leads directly to the heart! Complications may arise if the fluids are inadequately warmed or if the potassium concentration is increased. In addition, the venous pressure tracing can facilitate the recognition of an abnormal rhythm (i.e., junctional rhythm, Fig. 12.22), the "fine-tuning of pacemaker" settings, and the recognition of inadequate venous

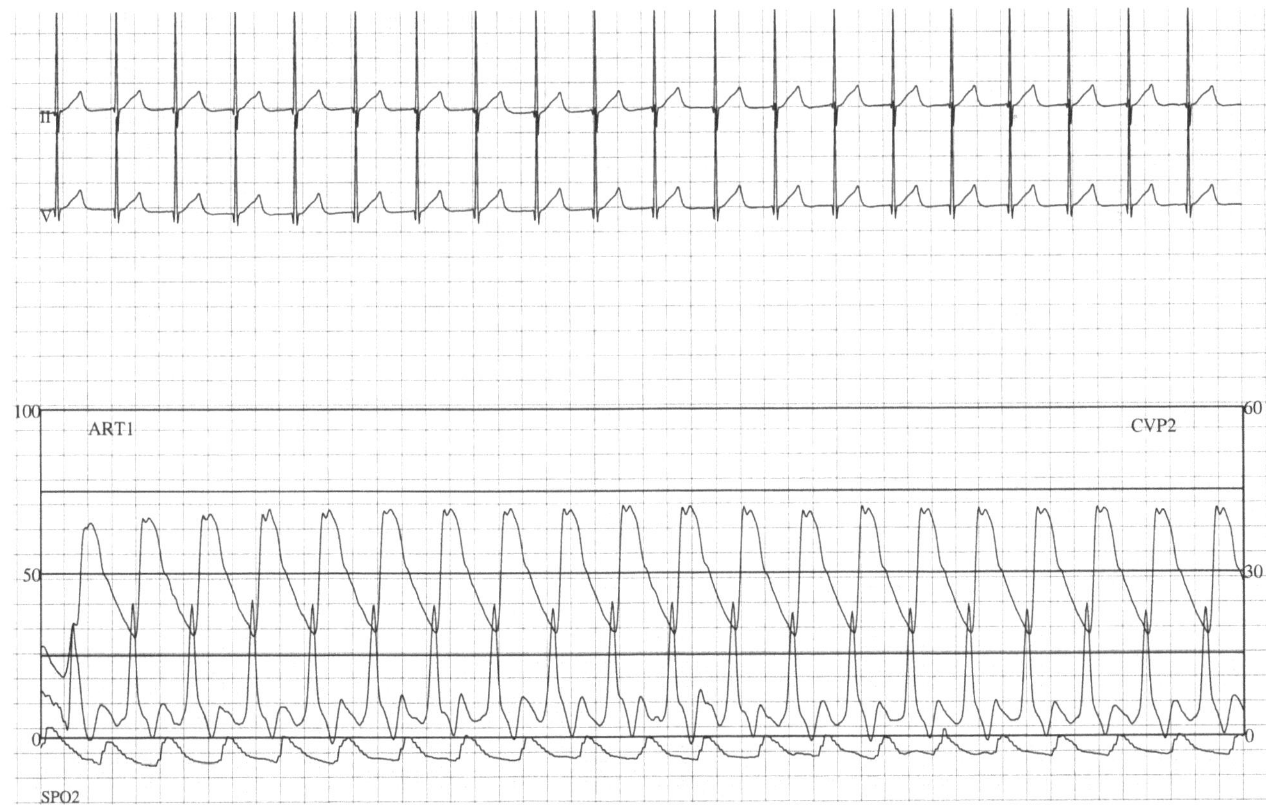

Fig. 12.22 Intraoperative recording in a neonate during junctional rhythm. Note the absence of normal P waves on the electrocardiographic leads II and V in the *upper panel*. The *lower panel* displays superimposed systemic arterial and central venous pressure tracings. Tall cannon atrial waves ("A" waves) are seen in the central venous pressure tracing corresponding to atrial contraction during ventricular systole against a closed tricuspid valve. The bottom tracing in the *lower panel* corresponds to the pulse oximeter tracing

drainage (e.g., SVC drainage in the case of a catheter in the internal jugular vein). Sampling from the SVC also can be obtained to measure mixed venous oxygen saturation, serving as a surrogate of cardiac output and oxygen delivery. In general, the catheter with the smallest diameter possible should be used for percutaneous access. The length of insertion varies according to the site of placement [108]. In some cases, direct transthoracic placement of catheters may be favored (see below). The position of the tip of the CVP catheter should always be assessed on the postoperative radiograph. It should not extend beyond the junction of either the SVC or IVC with the atrium to avoid the possibility of cardiac perforation and tamponade (since the junction is the limit of the pericardium).

Ultrasound Guidance

The success rate and safety of central venous cannulation can be markedly improved by the use of imaging techniques [102, 109]. Various ultrasound modalities that include audio Doppler and two-dimensional imaging assisted by color flow/spectral Doppler have been applied with good success. Real-time ultrasound guidance has been shown to improve the success rate, decrease the procedural time, and reduce the rate of complications of internal jugular vein cannulation [110, 111].

Percutaneous Sites for Central Venous Access

Several sites in the neonate are available for central venous access. In addition to the challenges imposed by the small size of the vessels in the young infant, factors such as venous anatomy, vessel patency/prior attempts, hydration status, and operator skill/experience all influence the success of cannulation. Preferred sites vary according to institutional preference; in most cases, the femoral vein and internal jugular vein are favored.

The *umbilical vein* can be cannulated during the first few days after birth and can provide useful access to the central circulation. As the catheter is advanced, it can be threaded either into the hepatic veins or through the ductus venosus into the IVC. It is important to document the position of the catheter tip. If the catheter has entered the IVC, its tip can be seen above the level of the diaphragm on a radiograph. This is the optimal position as the catheter can be used to monitor CVP and deliver medications directly to the heart. If the tip of the catheter is located within the liver, it may not provide an accurate measurement of the CVP, and delivery of vasoactive medications can result in complications (liver necrosis and portal vein thrombosis). In this case, an alternate site should be considered for placement of the central venous catheter. A clear advantage of umbilical venous cannulation is the preservation of other venous sites for future interventions that require vascular access. This consideration is especially important for the neonate with planned staged palliation and anticipated serial cardiac catheterizations, for which venous cannulation is paramount. Umbilical venous catheters may be left in place for less than 2 weeks.

The *femoral vein* also can be used as a site for placement of a central venous catheter in the neonate. In fact, the femoral site is favored at many centers over the internal jugular vein in infants less than 4 kg in weight. Femoral venous cannulation obviates the need to place a catheter in the SVC and decreases the likelihood of problems such as stenosis and/or thrombosis that can result from cannulation of the internal jugular vein in small infants. Patency of the SVC is crucial in infants with single ventricle physiology for whom a superior cavopulmonary anastomosis is part of the palliation pathway. Infection is a rare complication of femoral venous cannulation, and the rate of infection is comparable to that of other sites in children [112].

The *internal jugular vein* is a very common site for central line placement in children undergoing cardiac surgery and is also commonly used in neonates. The main advantage of the internal jugular route is the direct path between the vessel and the RA. However, disadvantages of this site in the neonatal age group include (1) difficult cannulation due to the small size of the vessels, which are relatively small structures in a tiny infant, with little margin for error; (2) increased risk of carotid artery puncture; (3) the possibility of SVC complications (thrombus, narrowing) as mentioned; (4) potential for vessel or cardiac puncture and less tolerance for hemodynamic compromise as compared to older children; and (5) risk of lung puncture and development of pneumothorax. The routine use of ultrasound to locate the vessel is strongly recommended. In some cases, the right internal jugular vein can be quite small compared with the left internal jugular vein. This may indicate the presence of a persistent LSVC.

The *external jugular vein* is sometimes very easy to visualize and to puncture. It is often possible to pass a catheter centrally through the external jugular vein with a small diameter "J wire." This route tends to be overlooked but is often successful and less likely to result in complications than repeated attempts at a difficult internal jugular puncture [113, 114].

The *subclavian vein* also can be used for central venous access in the neonate. Cannulation of the left subclavian vein generally is preferred over the right because the angle taken as the vessel continues into the innominate vein and enters the SVC is less acute than the right, and, therefore, the end of the catheter is less likely to be against the wall of the vessel causing potential injury [102]. This site might be preferred over the internal jugular approach as it may be more stable. Disadvantages of subclavian venous line placement include a greater potential for pneumothorax, inability to hold pressure at the vascular entry site, and tendency for malposition (contralateral brachiocephalic vein or the ipsilateral internal jugular vein) [115]. A catheter in the subclavian vein also is more likely than a catheter in another site to kink or malfunction with placement of a sternal retractor.

Direct Transthoracic Pressure Monitoring

In some cases, transthoracic pressure-monitoring catheters (e.g., in the RA, LA, PA), as well as those with oximetric capabilities, are placed by the surgeon under direct vision while the sternum is open, usually near or after separation from CPB. This route offers the only approach in some cases for monitoring pressure in a structure of interest (e.g., LA, PA). Assessment of LA pressure can assist in the setting of anticipated poor LV function, decreased ventricular compliance, or mitral regurgitation. The use of transthoracic PA pressure monitoring has decreased over the years, but certain cardiac pathologies in the neonate continue to have a significant potential for acute pressure increases after repair (e.g., obstructed TAPVR, TA). In these types of settings, the presence of a PA pressure catheter can be useful for postoperative management. In addition to serving as a means to monitor pressure, depending on the location of the catheter, it can also be used for infusion of drugs, volume administration, and mixed venous saturation monitoring. Extreme care must be taken to ensure that emboli (air or otherwise) are not introduced to LA catheters.

A benefit of transthoracic-placed catheters is that they preserve other sites for future percutaneous vascular access and reduce complications associated with placement. The main concerns of these types of lines, however, are bleeding, particularly upon removal, and inability to compress the site. Chest tubes usually are maintained in place well after the catheter is removed to avoid the potential to accumulate blood, resulting in cardiac tamponade. In rare cases, the presence of the catheter against the endocardial surface of the heart can result in ectopy or sustained arrhythmias.

Urinary Output Measurements

Cardiac surgery involves fluid shifts, blood loss, and alterations in systemic perfusion that can impact renal blood flow/function. Therefore, output of urine is measured routinely in most cases, particularly when the intervention is anticipated to take place over the course of several hours. Measurements of urine output provide a useful index of the adequacy of renal perfusion and cardiac output. For infants, the use of a miniature-graduated burette in the urine line makes it possible to record small urinary volumes. Although the presence of urine output is reassuring, no specific value is necessarily predictive of good renal function postoperatively. In some cases, the neonate taking diuretic therapy chronically may need intraoperative dosing to promote the output of urine. Factors such as the use of cardioplegic solutions that may include agents such as mannitol or furosemide also can influence urine output.

Transesophageal Echocardiography

Intraoperative TEE is recommended to provide real-time information about cardiac anatomy and function during surgery (Fig. 12.23) [116–118]. It is particularly valuable to confirm the adequacy of surgical repair, detect residual shunts, evaluate valvar competence, determine outflow patency, and examine ventricular function [119]. If significant hemodynamic abnormalities are identified in the immediate bypass period, revision of the repair can then be undertaken [120].

At the time of this writing, two multiplane imaging probes of differing transducer tip size are available for use in the neonate. Both devices incorporate full capabilities for two-dimensional imaging, spectral and color Doppler, and M-Mode echocardiography. Data regarding the safety of TEE in the pediatric age group demonstrate a large margin of safety and a small incidence of complications, in the range of

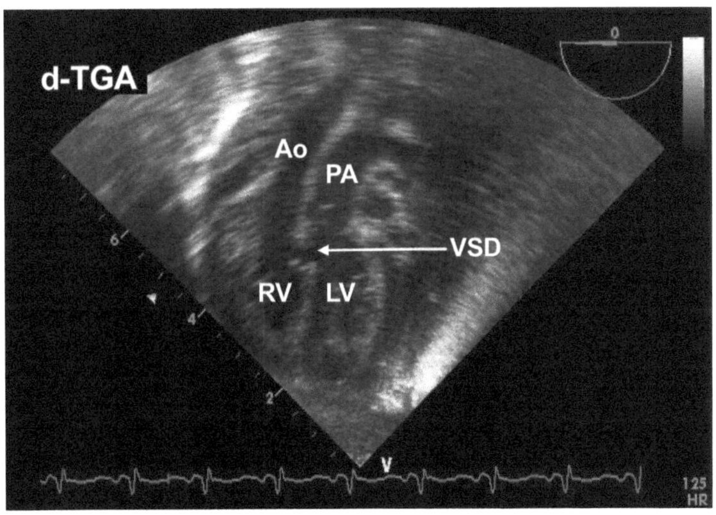

Fig. 12.23 Preoperative transesophageal echocardiographic image in a neonate with *d*-transposition of the great arteries (d-TGA) and ventricular septal defect (VSD) undergoing complete repair. *Ao* aorta, *LV* left ventricle, *PA* pulmonary artery, *RV* right ventricle

1 to 3 % [121]. However, the infant should be very carefully monitored for cardiorespiratory compromise during passage and manipulation of the probe [122, 123]. The successful use of TEE in tiny infants, less than 3.0 kilograms in weight, has been reported [124, 125].

Neurologic Monitoring

Infants and children undergoing congenital heart surgery are at risk for neurologic and behavioral impairment [126–132]. In contrast to embolic episodes, which affect adults undergoing cardiac surgery, global cerebral hypoxia and/or ischemia is the primary etiology of neurologic dysfunction in infants and children, explaining the interest in multimodal brain monitoring in the form of near-infrared spectroscopy (NIRS), transcranial Doppler ultrasound, and bispectral index electroencephalography (BIS) that can potentially minimize neurologic morbidity and optimize outcome [75, 133–138]. Specific applications of neurologic monitors in this regard include the determination of maximum acceptable duration of circulatory arrest and minimum acceptable bypass flow rates.

Near-Infrared Spectroscopy

NIRS is a noninvasive technology used to monitor regional cerebral tissue oxygenation (rSO_2; (Fig. 12.24) [139]. When the NIRS probe is placed on the forehead, it directs a light source through the skull and brain tissue that is then sensed by different detectors (shallow and deep). The optical principle relies on the distinct absorption spectra of hemoglobin species. The various wavelengths of infrared light are able to measure the concentrations of oxygenated and deoxygenated hemoglobin in order to determine rSO_2. Online trend monitoring of this parameter then provides indirect information on the adequacy of cerebral oxygenation, a surrogate of cerebral perfusion, allowing opportunities for intervention if critical values are detected. In contrast to pulse oximetry values which reflect saturation in the arterial component of the circulation, the measured rSO_2 represents the combined saturation in both the arterial and venous blood, an issue considered a limitation of the technology.

NIRS monitoring of cerebral oxygenation has been advocated for most neonatal cardiac cases but particularly when Ao arch reconstruction is performed using bypass techniques that involve regional cerebral perfusion [140–142]. This type of monitoring also has been reported to aid in the recognition of problems such as bypass cannula malposition that can result in neurologic injury if not detected [143]. Treatment algorithms for low NIRS have been developed for use during congenital heart surgery [144]. Ongoing experience continues to be accumulated regarding the contributions of this technology to perioperative care [133, 136, 137, 145].

Although NIRS monitoring is increasingly being used, its value is as yet uncertain, and it may not be standard of care

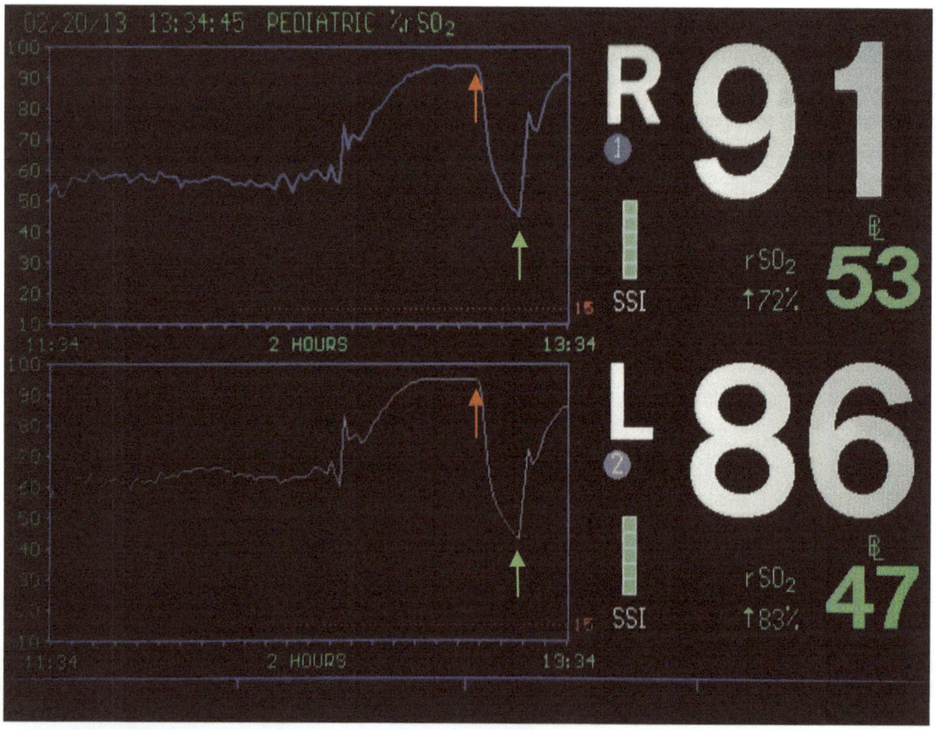

Fig. 12.24 Photograph of near-infrared monitor displaying *right* (*R*) and *left* (*L*) cerebral oxygen saturation (rSO_2) during neonatal cardiac surgery. The *red arrow marks* the initiation of a period of circulatory arrest and the associated decrease in cerebral oxygenation as recorded from both hemispheres. As pump flows are reestablished (*green arrow*), the cerebral saturation increases. A very brief period of low pump flows results in a transient minimal drop in the rSO_2

at all centers that specialize in the care of infants and children with heart disease [146]. Cerebral oximetry also has been recommended for routine use in the postoperative period after cardiac surgery in view of the observation that infants with prolonged low rSO_2 demonstrate a greater incidence of periventricular leukomalacia [138, 144, 147]. This finding can contribute to impaired neurodevelopment [138, 148].

Transcranial Doppler Ultrasound

Transcranial Doppler ultrasonography (TCD) has been used as a monitor of cerebral blood flow velocity and microemboli during cardiac surgery [149, 150]. The technique for flow assessment uses pulsed-wave ultrasound at 2 MHz and provides peak systolic and mean flow velocities (expressed in cm/s) (Fig. 12.25). Cerebral blood flow velocity in the neonate

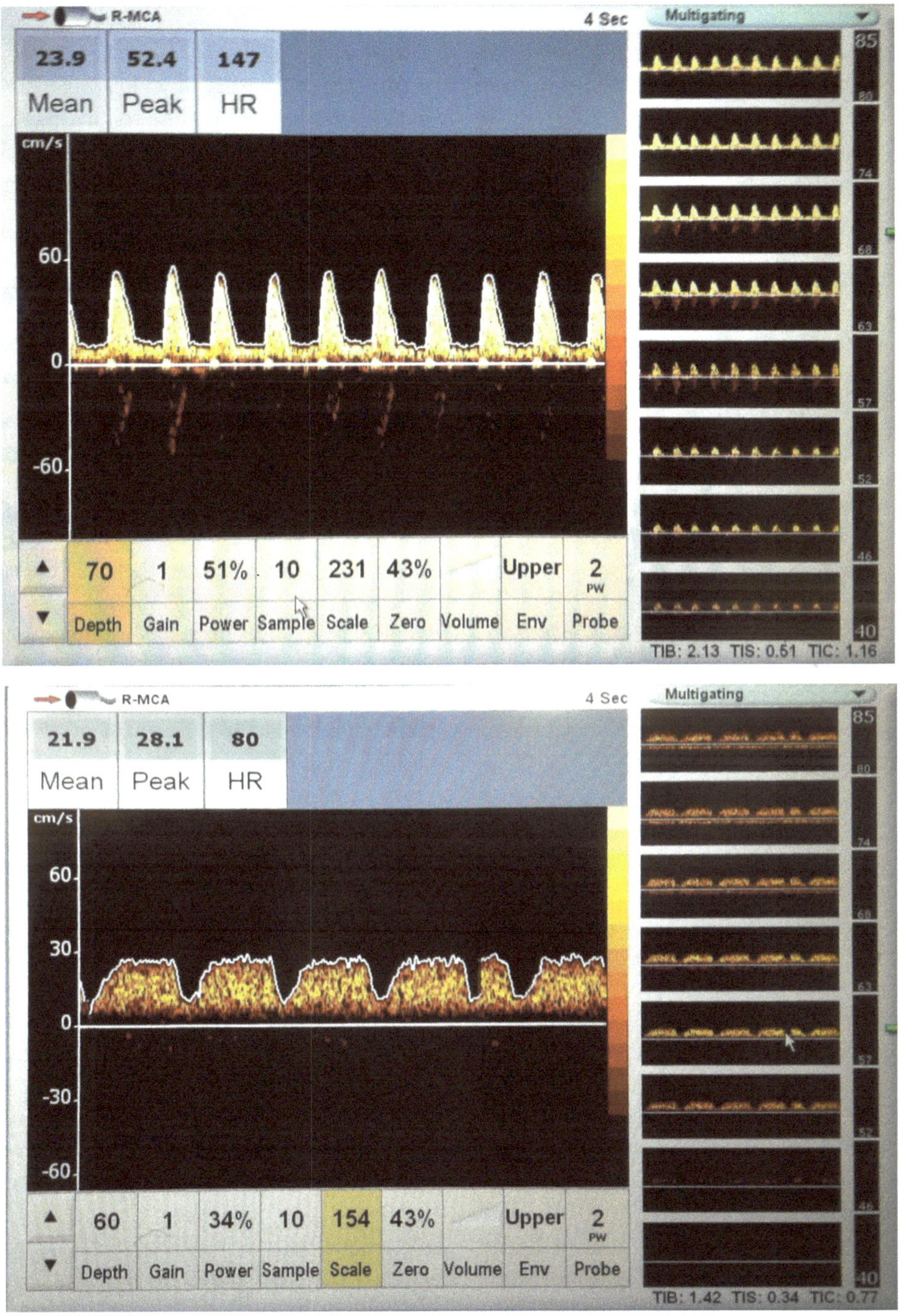

Fig. 12.25 Transcranial Doppler ultrasonography of the right middle cerebral artery obtained with probe placement over the anterior fontanelle in a neonate undergoing cardiac surgery. The *upper panel* displays the tracing during the pre-bypass period and the *lower panel* during cardiopulmonary bypass. Note the different characteristics of the flow patterns

is monitored using a temporal window or open anterior fontanelle with insonation of the middle cerebral artery.

In neonates, TCD has been used to determine the threshold for detectable cerebral blood flow during low-flow bypass. During the arterial switch operation using alpha-stat arterial blood gas management, 30 mL/kg/min was the threshold for detectable cerebral perfusion in this population [151]. In neonatal Ao arch reconstruction during the Norwood operation, a mean bypass flow of 63 mL/kg/min maintained both rSO_2 (using cerebral oxygenation) and blood flow velocities (using TCD) within 10 % on the baseline [152]. This represented sufficient but not excessive cerebral perfusion.

Transcranial Doppler can detect and quantify cerebral emboli, the latter identified as high intensity signals (HITS) on a display. Data regarding the use of this modality in the detection of cerebral emboli during cardiac surgery in infants and children are somewhat limited, although one study demonstrated that microemboli could be detected in the carotid arteries of children during congenital heart surgery, particularly immediately after Ao unclamping [153]. However, the interpretation of the Doppler signals was confounded by a variety of artifacts. No correlation was identified between the number of emboli detected and acute postoperative neurologic injuries. Currently, TCD monitoring is reserved by some centers for special indications and is not recognized as a standard procedure for routine use.

Intraoperative Management of the Neonate Undergoing Cardiac Surgery

Induction of Anesthesia

Induction of anesthesia in the neonate usually is accomplished via the intravenous route, which is preferred over the inhalational route because the former enables the airway to be rapidly secured without the use of cardiac depressant drugs and, hence, provides a greater margin of safety. The presence of shunts can impact the kinetics of intravenous agents; a large left-to-right shunt may prolong induction of anesthesia because the drugs are recirculated through the lungs. Hence, a less concentrated amount of anesthetic agent reaches the brain, delaying the onset of anesthesia. In contrast, a large right-to-left shunt speeds an intravenous induction because a significant portion of the drug bypasses the pulmonary circulation and directly enters the systemic circulation, rapidly reaching the brain.

In the neonate, intravenous access usually is present preoperatively. If this is not the case, access can be established before induction, or, less frequently, a carefully titrated inhalation induction and early placement of an intravenous catheter can be performed. Inhalational anesthetics dilate vascular beds and reduce sympathetic tone. Although these are desirable goals in general, the effects can be detrimental in the neonate with decreased myocardial performance who requires an increased resting sympathetic tone to maintain systemic output.

Two factors, the presence of a shunt and a decrease in cardiac output, may independently and substantively affect the uptake and distribution of inhalational anesthetics in neonates. These effects depend on the solubilities of the inhalational anesthetics. In the cyanotic neonate, a right-to-left shunt with a soluble anesthetic such as halothane (blood/gas partition coefficient 2.4) will only minimally slow the increase in the arterial partial pressure of anesthetic in blood because soluble anesthetics depend on alveolar ventilation for their delivery and, thus, their washin. Maintaining a constant alveolar ventilation (normal $PaCO_2$) increases the washin of soluble inhalational anesthetics in the blood that perfuses the lungs, thus offsetting the lack of anesthetic in the shunted blood. The net effect is a washin that is similar to that in neonates without a shunt. In contrast, with an insoluble anesthetic such as sevoflurane (blood/gas coefficient 0.66) or desflurane (blood/gas coefficient 0.42), a right-to-left shunt profoundly limits the increase in arterial partial pressure because less soluble anesthetics are minimally affected by alveolar ventilation for their delivery and, thus, their washin. Maintaining a constant alveolar ventilation (normal $PaCO_2$) does not change the washin of insoluble anesthetics in the blood perfusing the lungs and thus cannot offset the lack of anesthetic in bypassed blood. The net effect is a reduced anesthetic partial pressure in blood when the perfused and bypassed blood combine, a speed of washin that is less than that in neonates without a shunt (refer to Pharmacology Chapter). A left-to-right intracardiac shunt has limited effects on the speed of washin and, thus, induction of anesthesia of inhalational anesthetics. In contrast to the profound effects of a right-to-left shunt on the washin of less soluble anesthetics, changes in cardiac output profoundly affect the washin of more soluble anesthetics because these anesthetics depend on delivery for the speed of washin. With soluble anesthetics such as halothane, a reduced cardiac output and therefore reduced pulmonary blood flow speed the washin of anesthetic partial pressure in blood because less anesthetic is removed from the alveoli. This is a potentially dangerous situation, which may be compounded by a further decrease in cardiac output from administration of a soluble inhalational anesthetic. In contrast, the washin of less soluble anesthetics such as sevoflurane and desflurane does not depend significantly on delivery and, thus, on cardiac output for their washin. Thus, their washin is relatively unaffected by even substantive decreases in cardiac output (refer to Pharmacology Chapter).

An important goal of the anesthetic management in the neonate with heart disease undergoing surgery is the selection of drugs that have the least impact on the cardiovascular system in order to maintain adequate cardiac function and ensure systemic oxygen delivery. A technique that combines several agents (balanced technique) with minimal myocardial depressant effects traditionally has been used for induction of anesthesia in order to limit the extent of cardiac depression. Titrated doses of an opioid and non-depolarizing muscle relaxant are commonly used. A benzodiazepine also can be added. It is important to emphasize that even the smallest dose of an opioid can depress cardiac function in the critically ill neonate as a result of a reduction in the release of endogenous catecholamines. Therefore, it is imperative to monitor carefully and intervene promptly if decompensation occurs.

Maintenance of Anesthesia

After induction, anesthesia may be maintained with an inhalation anesthetic, an intravenous technique, or a combination. For many years, a large-dose, synthetic opioid-muscle relaxant technique was used because it minimally decreases cardiovascular function and offers significant benefits in blunting the physiologic stress response [154]. Over the years, however, practice has changed; many centers now favor inhalational anesthetics as the primary agents and a limited opioid dose. Contemporary data support this approach. The use of large-dose opioids with the goal of providing "stress free" anesthesia is not an important determinant of early postoperative outcome [155]. At the same time, when inhalational anesthetics are properly used (e.g., isoflurane or sevoflurane), they do not significantly reduce the cardiac index in children with CHD [156]. The potential benefit of anesthetic preconditioning of the heart is currently being investigated, with no particular anesthetic agent as yet proven to be superior in this role. Moreover, no regimen or combination of anesthetics has been shown to be suitable or superior for all neonates with CHD. Each infant and lesion must be considered individually and the most appropriate technique administered. The main goals of the anesthetic management are to optimize systemic oxygen delivery, maintain ventricular function, and ensure the adequacy of cardiac output.

Cardiopulmonary Bypass in the Neonate

Pre-Bypass Period

After monitors have been applied and anesthesia induced, the neonate is positioned for the procedure. In most cases, after arterial access is established, a blood sample is obtained for initial assessment of blood gases, acid–base status, hematocrit, glucose, and calcium levels, and a baseline value of the activated clotting time (ACT) is recorded. This is the optimal time for transesophageal imaging in order to avoid interference from electrocautery once the operation is initiated. Vigilance is of outmost importance during this phase of surgery because of the potential for blood loss, rhythm abnormalities, compression of cardiac and vascular structures, and several other factors that can impact hemodynamic stability.

The neonate should be very carefully monitored during dissection around the heart. Sometimes it is necessary to alert the surgeon to pause his activities and allow the heart to recover if function appears compromised. On the other hand, minor changes in cardiac function have to be accepted if the procedure is to be performed!

Perfusion Equipment, Tubing, Circuits, and Bypass Prime

Neonatal cardiac surgery frequently requires the use of CPB [157]. During full bypass, all the systemic venous blood is directed to the extracorporeal circuit; in contrast, during partial bypass, only a portion of the systemic venous return is captured in the venous reservoir and the remainder reaches the beating heart. Ventilation is required during partial bypass for gas exchange of the blood that enters the pulmonary circulation. Full bypass is almost always required in neonates and small infants.

Over the years, the sophisticated CPB system has been modified and miniaturized to make it suitable for use in the smallest of infants and to minimize morbidity [158]. Many elements are common to all perfusion circuits used for bypass in the neonate (Fig. 12.26). The following sections describe the various components of a CPB circuit:

Heart-lung machine (pump). Most are non-pulsatile. Occlusive roller pumps are favored because of their accuracy at very low-flow rates as well as their smooth revolutions at very low speed (revolutions per minute). Most machines incorporate a servo regulating reservoir level sensor and high-pressure alarm, plus a bubble detector.

Heat exchanger unit. These devices provide for blood cooling and warming. In the neonatal age group, an important feature of these units is their ability to change temperatures very slowly and precisely, thereby providing for adequate equilibration of temperature between blood and tissues, allowing for even cooling or warming.

Membrane oxygenator. This unit provides for gas exchange. The optimal device should be efficient, require a low priming volume, provide appropriate flow capabilities, and be dependable. A coating material may be added, variable among manufacturers, which aids in decreasing platelet aggregation as blood flows through the oxygenator.

Arterial filter. Various arterial filters are available aimed at avoiding the introduction of particulate matter into the

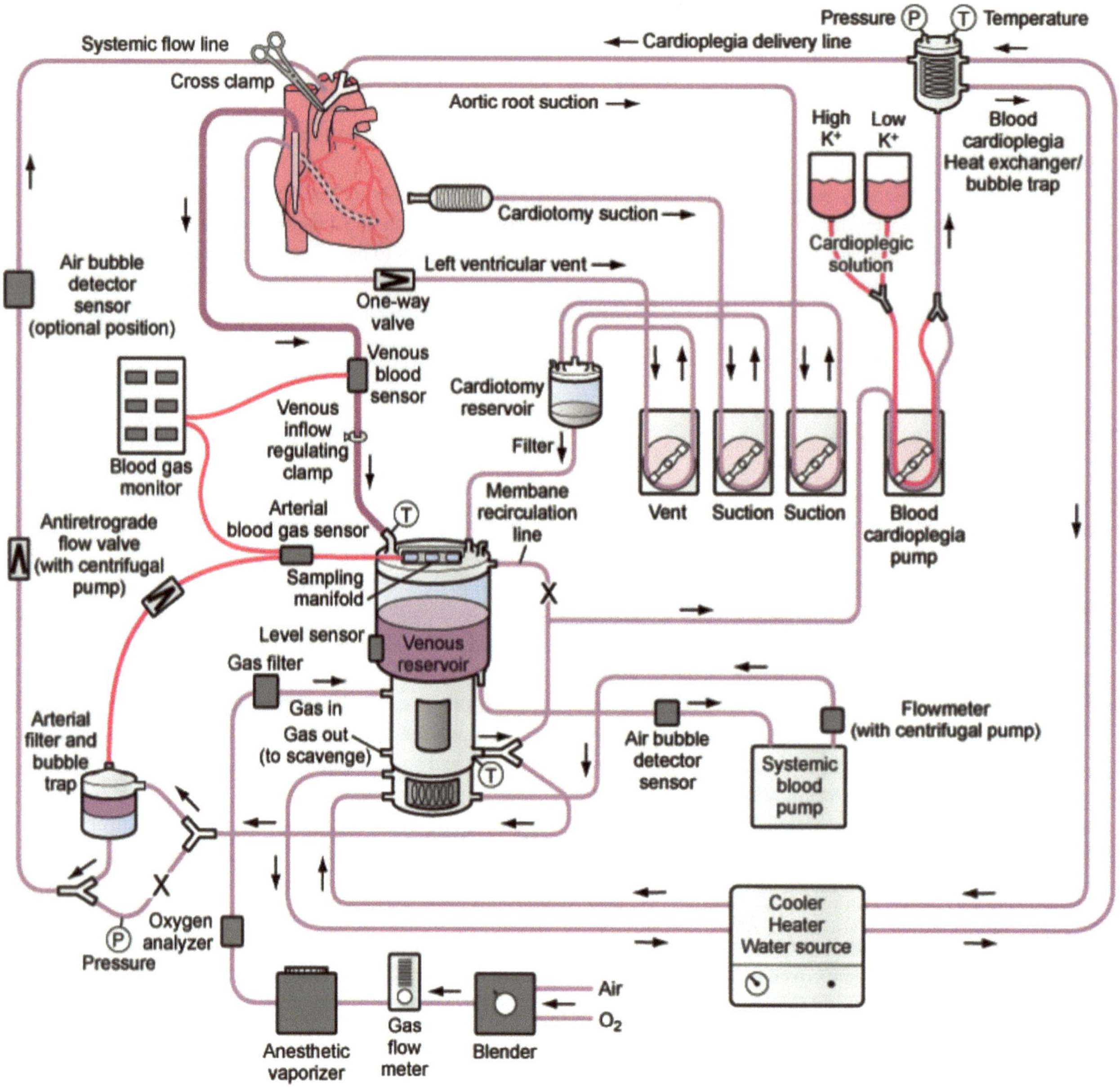

Fig. 12.26 This schematic diagram depicts a cardiopulmonary bypass circuit. Note the venous reservoir with integrated membrane oxygenator. Other components of the circuit include the cardioplegia solution and pump, water heater/cooler, safety devices, and monitors. The flow is driven by either a roller head or centrifugal pump. Bicaval cannulation may be required during pediatric cardiac surgery for venous drainage, in contrast to a single cannula as depicted here. Carbon dioxide can be added to the inspired gas mixture to facilitate pH-stat blood gas management. *Arrows* indicate direction of flow, *P* pressure sensor, *T* temperature sensors, *X* placement of tubing clamps. From Hessel EA. *Circuitry and cannulation techniques*. In: Gravlee GP, Davis RF, Stammers AH, Ungerleider RM, editors. Cardiopulmonary Bypass: Principles and Practice. 3rd ed. Philadelphia: Lippincott Williams & Wilkins; 2007; with permission

arterial return line. Desirable features are a low priming volume, suitable flow capabilities, and ease of debubbling. A coating, as described for the membrane oxygenator, provides similar benefits.

Cannulas and tubing. The selection of cannulas and tubing is based primarily on flow requirements. Selecting cannulas of the appropriate size is extremely important for proper arterial flow and venous drainage in pediatric patients. The size of the neonate/anatomic structures (systemic veins, RA, Ao) influences the selection of bypass cannulas. Drainage of venous return can be accomplished in some cases by a single RA cannula, although frequently the need for intracardiac surgery requires bicaval cannulation as an alternative to circulatory arrest. Abnormal venous anatomy may require the use of additional cannulas. The arterial cannula, which returns blood to the neonate, typically is placed in the Asc Ao. However, depending on the bypass strategy, this site might be altered to a more distal location. Also based on the nature of the intervention, additional arterial cannula sites may be considered, such as is required for antegrade cerebral perfusion (graft in innominate artery) or when maintenance of distal systemic blood flow is planned (ductal cannulation).

Venous reservoir. The reservoir functions as the temporary storage site for venous blood during extracorporeal circulatory support. Venous drainage generally is passive, relying on gravity. Vacuum-assisted venous drainage can be an option to facilitate the egress of blood from the patient into the venous reservoir; however, this procedure can result in trauma to blood elements.

Air/oxygen blender, carbon dioxide tank, high-/low-flow meter. These instruments provide capabilities for controlling pO_2 and pCO_2 precisely at all temperatures, facilitating blood gas management on bypass.

Cardioplegia circuit. This circuit is designed to deliver cardioplegic solution and frequently incorporates the ability for cooling.

Blood hemoconcentrator. This unit allows for ultrafiltration to be performed during CPB aimed at removing free water and inflammatory mediators.

Venous saturation and hematocrit monitor. These monitors, once appropriately calibrated, serve to enhance the overall safety of the CPB process and allow for less frequent blood sampling.

Activated clotting time machine. This machine is able to provide point-of-care testing of the heparin activity that is monitored by measuring the activated clotting time (ACT) and facilitates anticoagulation management. Various agents can be used as activators of the coagulation system. Kaolin is favored because it is much less influenced by the presence of antifibrinolytic agents.

Arterial blood gas machine. Sampling of gas exchange, acid–base status, hematocrit, and other chemistries is mandatory during CPB. Having immediate accessibility to a machine with those capabilities is essential during cases that require bypass.

Cell saver. This system is used for processing of the sequestered blood aspirated from the operative field, allowing it to be reinfused to the patient in an effort to decrease blood product exposure in some cases.

Miniaturization of bypass circuit. The miniaturized bypass apparatus provides a simple and safe method to reduce autologous blood transfusions in the neonate [159, 160]. The small components can significantly reduce priming volumes, thus reducing the enormous disproportion between the extracorporeal volume and small blood volume of the neonate. A small prime volume circuit consisting of only a rotary blood pump head and a membrane oxygenator is used. The venous blood returns to the pump through active drainage. No venous reservoir or cardiotomy suction device is used, minimizing hemodilution and mechanical blood trauma but at the expense of safety features. Recent studies demonstrate that the use of the miniaturized circuit was associated with significant reduction in blood transfusions but no difference in short-term outcomes [161].

Pump prime. During the pre-bypass period, the pump prime is adjusted to a physiologically balanced solution, with a desirable hematocrit, procoagulant levels, and oncotic pressure [162]. Other additives may include antibiotics, antifibrinolytic agents, and corticosteroids.

Stages of Cardiopulmonary Bypass

Before CPB, multiple steps are followed including systemic anticoagulation, placement of purse-string sutures, and cannulation of arterial and venous sites. After initiation of CPB, core cooling, Ao clamping, and myocardial protection, the surgical procedure, followed by warming, release of the Ao clamp, reperfusion of the heart, separation from support, reversal of anticoagulation, and removal of the cannulas, occurs in sequence. The following sections highlight selected aspects of the bypass period.

Anticoagulation

Before placing the cannulas for CPB, heparin is administered and anticoagulation is confirmed. Most neonates require relatively large doses of heparin (~400 units/kg) due to a relative heparin "resistance" as compared with older children [163]. The optimal ACT for CPB is controversial, but most centers consider a value above 400 s acceptable (480 s at some institutions). A subtherapeutic ACT can result from inadequate dosing, low concentrations of antithrombin III, or relative heparin "resistance." Measurements of heparin concentrations provide an alternative to ACT testing [164, 165]. Heparin is also added to the bypass circuit before the initiation of CPB and at regular intervals thereafter, with subsequent repeated monitoring of the ACT. Conditions such as hypothermia and renal dysfunction delay the elimination of heparin.

Cannulation and Initiation of Cardiopulmonary Bypass

Transient decreases in blood pressure, mild arterial desaturation, and transient arrhythmias frequently occur during purse-string and cannula placement in the neonate. These changes are to be expected, and usually no treatment or only a minor intervention such as volume replacement is required. Any blood lost into venous cannulas during their insertion and priming should be immediately replaced via the arterial cannula. The objective should be to avoid any immediate pre-bypass hypotension or cardiac compromise. Before initiating CPB, satisfactory arterial cannula position can be assessed by comparing the mean arterial pressures recorded from the arterial line with that of the arterial inflow cannula of the bypass circuit to the patient.

Once CPB is established, the adequacy of venous drainage should be confirmed. This can be achieved by direct inspection of the heart, confirmation of a low CVP measurement, and assessment of NIRS values. In addition, venous distension of head structures (e.g., bulging of fontanels), which could suggest obstruction of SVC drainage, should be excluded. Be aware that even modest increases in SVC pressure can compromise cerebral blood flow during CPB. Despite priming of the bypass circuit with banked blood in the neonate, low arterial pressures related to hemodilution are sometimes seen upon initiation of CPB, especially in infants with cyanotic lesions. In most cases, this situation is associated with a transient decrease in rSO_2 as documented by NIRS monitoring. Increasing pump flows for a brief period of time or early surgical control of runoff connections (i.e., ductus arteriosus, aortopulmonary collaterals, shunts) frequently restores perfusion pressures to acceptable levels. The use of vasoconstricting agents is undesirable, as an important goal at this stage is the homogeneous cooling of systemic vascular beds.

The adequacy of perfusion should be assessed carefully throughout the entire period of extracorporeal support. This assessment is based on the pump flow rate, mean arterial pressure on bypass, and measurements of mixed venous saturation. Additional indirect indices include arterial blood gas analysis (pH, lactate, base deficit), regional oxygenation measurements by NIRS, and urine output.

Maintaining adequate anesthesia during CPB is important; light anesthesia, particularly during the cooling or warming phases of the procedure, can lead to a significant increase in metabolic rate and oxygen consumption, with an increase in systemic vascular tone, compromising organ perfusion.

Cooling and Temperature Management

Active cooling using the CBP circuit is initiated once it is confirmed that bypass is satisfactorily established. The goal of hypothermia is to supplement the preservation of vital organ function by decreasing the metabolic rate during CPB [166]. Various levels of hypothermia are utilized based on the nature of the intervention. These levels are mild (30–36 °C), moderate (22–30 °C), and deep hypothermia (18–22 °C). Extensive or complex surgery that requires low-flow perfusion or circulatory arrest is more likely to be performed under the lower temperatures. Surface cooling of the brain by applying ice bags to the neonatal head is still used in clinical practice, particularly during conditions of low-flow or circulatory arrest. An important aspect of cooling is for it to be uniform across body structures and without temperature gradients. The use of vasodilators (phentolamine, phenoxybenzamine, nitroprusside) during the initial phase of cooling, particularly when deep hypothermia is planned, helps to accomplish this goal [167–169]. Slow cooling is favored, as rapid cooling has been linked to neurologic impairment [170].

Aortic Cross-Clamping and Myocardial Protection

If myocardial arrest is planned, Ao clamping is performed in order to deliver a cardioplegic solution into the Ao root or, in some cases, into the coronary arteries directly. The goal of cardioplegia is to preserve the myocardium while the heart is ischemic. The Ao clamp usually is placed between the arterial cannula and Ao root. The catheter used to deliver cardioplegia into the root in antegrade fashion typically is placed just below the Ao clamp. Various cardioplegic preparations are used in clinical practice, and the optimal combination of ingredients is the subject of ongoing debate. The advantages of blood cardioplegic solutions have led to its increasing use in neonatal patients. After the initial infusion of cardioplegia, additional doses can be given at regular intervals, as needed, depending on the duration of the ischemic time. A good general guide for the perfusionist is to deliver cardioplegic solution at a pressure near the diastolic blood pressure of each individual patient before bypass. This delivery usually is coupled with surface cooling of the heart for added myocardial protection. A venting catheter (vent) is placed in the LV to decompress it. The distribution of cardioplegic solutions throughout the infant myocardium may be compromised by hypertrophy and abnormal coronary artery distribution or other pathology.

Release of Aortic Clamp and Myocardial Reperfusion

Once all extraneous air has been removed from the heart, the Ao clamp is released, allowing for reperfusion of the myocardium, initiation of electrical activity, and spontaneous cardiac beating soon thereafter. TEE can be useful to detect residual air. In some cases, cardioversion/defibrillation and/or pacing is required during this phase of CPB. Warming is initiated around this time as a gradual, slow process. Several temperature targets have been proposed and vary according to monitoring site (nasopharyngeal end point>35 °C, skin>30 °C, bladder>35 °C, rectal>35.5 °C) [171, 172]. The temperature of the perfusate should not exceed 37 °C, as cerebral hyperthermia at this stage can be very detrimental to the neonatal brain [173]. In fact, a mild degree of hypothermia is more desirable.

Separation from CPB, Reversal of Anticoagulation, and Removal of Cannulas

After the Ao clamp has been removed and during the period of active rewarming, vasoactive/inotropic infusions are initiated as required. The preference for agents varies among institutions. Some centers favor dopamine as the first-line inotrope, whereas others prefer epinephrine and yet others, dobutamine. An important consideration is that all these drugs increase heart rate, have arrhythmogenic potential, and increase oxygen consumption [174]. In recent years, vasopressin has been reported increasingly as an agent to enhance systemic vascular tone [175, 176]. A study in a group of neonates who had undergone the Norwood procedure or arterial switch operation demonstrated that low-dose vasopressin was associated with decreased fluid resuscitation and catecholamine requirements in the first postoperative day [177]. Milrinone has inotropic properties in addition to pulmonary and systemic vasodilatory effects and has been found to be of benefit after neonatal cardiac surgery [178, 179]. The drug was demonstrated to be particularly useful in reducing the risk of a postoperative low cardiac output state and, thus, is used frequently [180]. During the rewarming phase, consideration should be given to the administration of additional doses of muscle relaxants and sedatives. Blood components can be added to the circuit during this time in order to optimize hematocrit and coagulation factors. Weaning from CPB is initiated once the target temperature is reached and ventilation is established. It is a critical intraoperative time period. As the myocardium has suffered a major stress, this process takes place slowly, over several minutes, guided by factors such as the appearance of the heart on direct inspection, TEE monitoring, and hemodynamic parameters (filling pressures, arterial blood pressure). The administration of calcium as an infusion and/or as intermittent boluses often is necessary during separation from CPB in the neonate to address the dependence on free cytosolic ionized calcium for contractility and in order to offset the effects of citrated blood products on serum ionized calcium levels. If other than sinus rhythm is present, pacing wires should be placed and sequential pacing initiated. Once circulatory support has been discontinued and hemodynamics are optimized, results of the intervention are evaluated. TEE is of significant benefit in this regard. If the results of the intervention are deemed satisfactory, anticoagulation is reversed by the administration of protamine, cannulas are removed, and efforts towards establishing hemostasis are initiated. If significant hemodynamic residua are identified, a return to bypass may be necessary. In most infants undergoing open-heart interventions, temporary epicardial pacing wires are placed. In addition to being used for pacing as needed, atrial wires facilitate the identification of rhythm disturbances as they allow for an atrial electrogram to be obtained. At the conclusion of the surgical procedure, after the mediastinal drainage tubes are placed, chest closure is undertaken. Delayed sternal closure may be considered in the presence of severe cardiac dysfunction requiring significant inotropic support, myocardial edema resulting from extensive/complex surgery, pulmonary impairment, bleeding, sustained arrhythmias, or any other concerns regarding the neonate's clinical status [181].

Transport to the Intensive Care Unit

Although early extubation has been performed successfully in neonates after major cardiac surgery, it is a rare practice, particularly in view of the underlying pathology, nature of the intervention, and concerns for an untoward event [182]. Therefore, with few exceptions, most neonates remain intubated postoperatively, even for a few hours. Preparation of the neonate for transport from the operating room to the intensive care unit represents an important time period. Although it can be a distracting time, continuing surveillance of vital signs and hemodynamics during this process is of essence as termination of surgical stimulation in some cases is associated with undesirable changes in blood pressure. Extreme care must be taken to ensure that monitoring and infusion lines are safeguarded during transfer from the OR table. Note that vertical displacement of some infusion pumps may disturb the flow rates. Adequate oxygenation and ventilation, as well as ongoing hemodynamic monitoring, must be ensured during transport. Hypoventilation during this time can negatively affect pulmonary vascular tone and overall clinical status in the fragile neonate. Adequate analgesia and, in most cases, sedation are important postoperative requirements [183]. Upon the neonate's arrival at the intensive care unit, a chest radiograph and blood sampling usually are obtained, and ideally the anesthesia provider should review these results. A comprehensive report of the intraoperative course should be given to the team involved in the postoperative care. This report should include airway management (ETT size, ease of tracheal intubation), location of vascular access and invasive monitors, presence/numbers of chest draining tubes, pacing wires and other surgical hardware, duration of bypass, ischemic time, and active infusions of drugs. Highlights of the procedure and problems should be discussed, as should TEE findings and plan, in addition to specific concerns. The hemodynamic management of the neonate with CHD in the postoperative setting assumes many of the same physiologic principles applicable to intraoperative care.

Special Cardiopulmonary Bypass Techniques: Deep Hypothermic Circulatory Arrest and Selective Antegrade Cerebral Perfusion

Deep hypothermic circulatory arrest (DHCA) and selective antegrade cerebral perfusion (SACP; also referred to as *antegrade cerebral perfusion* [ACP], *regional low-flow cerebral perfusion* [RLFP], or *regional cerebral perfusion*) are techniques used in association with CPB during neonatal cardiac surgery. DHCA commonly is used for specific cardiac interventions including Ao arch reconstructive procedures, such as the Norwood operation. It involves lower levels of hypothermia (<20 °C) and complete cessation of bypass flow while the procedure is undertaken. This technique allows for a surgical field free of hardware and blood, facilitating the surgery. Not surprisingly, prolonged duration of DHCA has been associated with increased neurologic morbidity [184]. Hence, alternate modalities, such as in SACP, have been developed to maintain continuous cerebral circulation and to minimize or avoid the need for circulatory arrest and potentially to prevent hypoxic ischemic injury [185–188]. However, the specific technique for SACP varies among centers. In some cases, a cannula is advanced into the Asc Ao so as to provide for flow to the brain, whereas in others, a graft is sewn into the base of the innominate or subclavian artery to maintain the arterial cannula away from the surgical field (Fig. 12.27) [189]. At the time of SACP, after the nasopharyngeal temperature has reached a target value of ~ 18 to 20 °C or the rectal temperature has reached 20 to 22 °C (these temperatures may vary among institutions), snares are placed around the arch/arch vessels and flow is reduced to approximately 30 % of the predicted full flow, allowing for selective blood flow to the brain. The adequacy of brain perfusion during this period is guided by neuromonitoring [140, 152]. After Ao arch reconstruction is completed, full bypass flow is reestablished. A recent study using magnetic resonance imaging and examining 12-month neurodevelopmental outcomes in neonates undergoing Ao arch reconstruction demonstrated that the technique was effective and safe in supporting the brain [190].

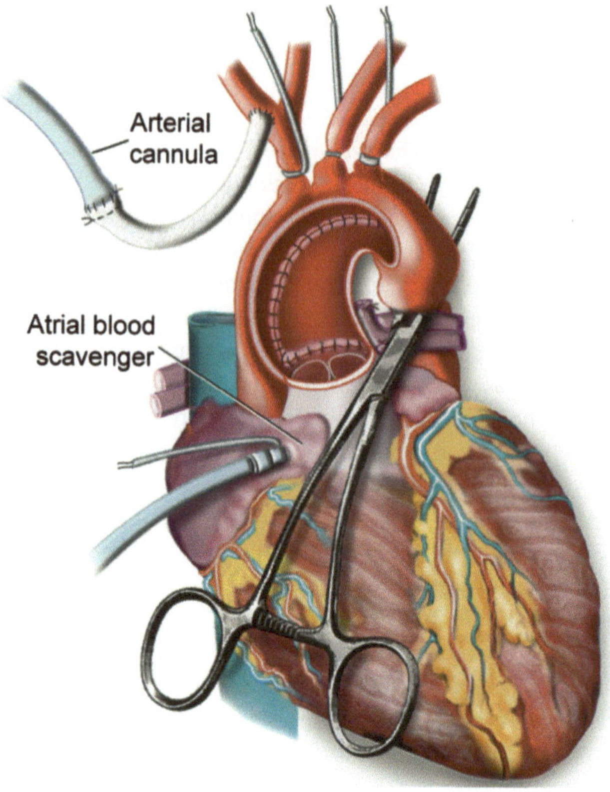

Fig. 12.27 The figure depicts the technique for selective (antegrade) cerebral perfusion. Note the polytetrafluoroethylene graft that has been sewn into the base of the right innominate artery and attached to the arterial inflow cannula of the cardiopulmonary bypass circuit. This allows for flow to the brain and a bloodless operative field while aortic arch reconstruction is undertaken. From Gertler R, Andropoulos DB. Cardiopulmonary Bypass and Management. In: Cote CJ, Lerman J, Anderson B, editors. A Practice of Anesthesia for Infants and Children. Philadelphia: Saunders; 2013; with permission

Unique Aspects of Neonatal Cardiopulmonary Bypass and Differences from the Adult

Notable differences exist between CPB in the neonate and CPB in the adult (Table 12.6). Different techniques are used in the two age groups, and the effects of these techniques on the infant's physiology also differ. Whereas in all age groups hypothermia is used, the neonate is more likely to undergo lower levels of hypothermia during cardiac surgery. Strategies such as total circulatory arrest, low-flow bypass, and SACP are used frequently during complex neonatal surgery. Associated with these strategies is the more likely administration of vasodilating agents such as alpha-blocking drugs in the neonate. Flow requirements and perfusion pressures also differ among patients according to age, weight, and body surface area. Recommended flow rates in the neonate (2.6–3.2 L/min/m^2) are greater than in infants (2.4–2.6 L/min/m^2). During neonatal surgery, a wide variation of bypass flow rates are used, ranging from no flow during DHCA to up to large flow rates of 200 ml/kg/min, depending on the particular strategy utilized. The need for variable flow rates is less likely in older children or adults. Perfusion pressures usually are reduced in the neonate (~30 mmHg), due to the reduced impedance systemic circulation.

Blood gas management during hypothermic bypass in the neonate has been controversial in the past. Recently the pH-stat acid-based strategy is used more frequently in the neonate/child, in contrast to alpha-stat management in the adult.

Table 12.6 Differences between pediatric and adult cardiopulmonary bypass

Parameter	Pediatric	Adult
Temperature	Commonly 18–20 °C	Rarely below 32 °C
Use of deep hypothermic circulatory arrest	Common	Rare
Pump prime components	Blood products and albumin	Crystalloid solutions
Dilution effect of pump prime	Up to 200 %	25–33 %
Perfusion pressure	30–50 mmHg	50–80 mmHg
Cannulation sites	Variable (arterial may include ductus arteriosus, main pulmonary artery; venous, mostly bicaval, may require additional cannulas)	Standardized, mostly ascending aorta and single venous cannula
Flow rates	0–250 ml/kg/min	2.5 L/min/m^2 or 50–65 ml/kg/min
Blood gas management	pH-stat favored	Alpha-stat preferred
Hypoglycemia	Common, due to low hepatic glycogen stores	Rare, seen with severe hepatic dysfunction
Hyperglycemia	Less common	Frequent, increases mortality

Modified from Gertler R and Andropoulos DB. Cardiopulmonary bypass. In Andropoulos DB, Stayer SA, Russell I, and Mossad EB, editors. Anesthesia for Congenital Heart Disease. Hoboken: Wiley-Blackwell; 2010; with permission

The pH-stat acid–base strategy maintains the blood pH constant at any temperature; in other words, pH management is temperature-corrected and aims for a $PaCO_2$ of 40 and pH of 7.40 at the patient's actual temperature. Often, carbon dioxide is introduced into the oxygenator in order to maintain these parameters within a desirable range during hypothermic CPB. The proposed benefits of the temperature-corrected pH-stat management approach in pediatric patients are to favor tissue oxygenation and cerebral vasodilation, thereby allowing for even cooling and better brain protection [191]. Data suggest that pH-stat management results in better outcomes with shorter ventilation times and intensive care unit stays [192]. [In contrast, alpha-stat management corrects the blood gas results to 37 °C irrespective of the patient's actual body temperature. In other words, alpha-stat maintains the uncorrected $PaCO_2$ and pH values at normal levels.]

Cannulation for CPB in the pediatric age group frequently differs from that in the adult. In the young, placement of cannulas in both caval veins (bicaval cannulation) sequesters all the venous return and facilitates intracardiac interventions. In contrast, this procedure is rarely necessary in the adult. In some cases, even additional venous cannulas are required in congenital surgery due to abnormal systemic venous anatomy. The site of arterial cannulation also may vary in pediatric versus adult patients. In fact, during neonatal cardiac surgery, multiple sites of arterial cannulation (e.g., Asc Ao and ductus arteriosus during repair of IAA) may be required. The use of ultrafiltration is standard in the neonate but is rarely used in adults [193]. Conventional ultrafiltration (CUF) during bypass or modified ultrafiltration (MUF) at the completion of bypass allows for the removal of body water and reduces the plasma concentration of circulating cytokines and vasoactive substances [194]. Ultrafiltration hemoconcentrates the infant's blood and removes excess fluid together with inflammatory mediators. This decreases blood transfusion requirements, improves coagulation status, and confers additional significant benefits involving major organ function [195]. A recent meta-analysis demonstrated that MUF after pediatric cardiac surgery significantly increased the hematocrit and mean arterial pressure after CPB as compared with CUF. However, postoperative outcome parameters, including chest tube drainage, ventilator time, and duration of intensive care unit stay, were unchanged [196].

Many physiologic effects of CPB differ between children and adults. In neonates there is a larger disproportion of the pump prime volume to the blood volume. Thus, there is the need for whole blood or packed cells and plasma in the prime to achieve a target hematocrit and thus ensure adequate oxygen carrying capacity. In the past, the target during hypothermic CPB was a low hematocrit, but more recently, the target has increased from 20 % to 30 % as evidence has demonstrated better short-term outcomes and 1-year neurodevelopmental scores with a greater hematocrit [197].

Glucose homeostasis is important in neonates undergoing cardiac surgery. Although the neonate is prone to hypoglycemia, there is a tendency towards hyperglycemia during periods of stress. Both of these glucose perturbations have been associated with adverse clinical outcomes. The reduced hepatic glycogen stores, particularly during physiologic stress, increase the risk for hypoglycemia in the neonate, which supports the routine use of glucose-containing intravenous solutions to prevent related morbidity in this population. Furthermore, CPB can lead to hyperglycemia by activating the stress response, through the use of components that contain large amounts of glucose (e.g., blood products and cardioplegic solution) and the use of steroids.

The perioperative management of glucose during pediatric cardiac surgery remains a controversial issue, largely the result of limited and conflicting data [198]. Some studies have shown a link between hyperglycemia and poor outcomes after cardiac surgery in children [199, 200]. Postoperative hyperglycemia upon arrival at the intensive care unit has been associated with a younger patient age, reduced body weight, and decreased bypass temperature [201]. Conversely, a recent investigation using tight glycemic control with the use of insulin in children (similar to that shown to be beneficial during adult cardiac surgery) failed to significantly affect the infection rate, mortality, duration of stay, or measures of organ failure after pediatric cardiac surgery, questioning the utility of this strategy [202]. This latter finding is consistent with previous data that suggested that post-bypass and postoperative hyperglycemia were not risk factors for morbidity and mortality after cardiac surgery in the infant [203].

Effects of Cardiopulmonary Bypass and Related Strategies

Cardiopulmonary bypass, though essential for the correction of many lesions, does have some significant adverse physiological effects. These effects represent major challenges in the postoperative neonate [174].

Systemic Inflammatory Response Syndrome

The systemic inflammatory response syndrome (SIRS) [204, 205] is characterized by a capillary leak state, body edema, hemodynamic instability, and multisystem organ dysfunction. Although the mechanisms involved in this syndrome are not fully understood, it is thought that activation of humoral cascades due to contact of blood components and endothelial cells with the plastic circuit surfaces plays a major role [206, 207]. Other systems activated during CPB include the complement system, coagulation, and fibrinolytic cascades. SIRS has been linked to major morbidity and mortality rates in the pediatric age group [204, 208, 209]. Several bypass strategies have been devised to ameliorate the inflammatory response and its associated morbidity including heparin coating of circuits, ultrafiltration, the administration of corticosteroids, the use of protease inhibitors (aprotinin), and other pharmacologic approaches (complement inhibitors, thromboxane antagonists, anticytokine therapy) [210–213].

Effects on Bleeding and Coagulation

Bleeding represents a major clinical problem after cardiac surgery in the neonate. Risk factors include low birth weight, use of profound hypothermia, increased preoperative hematocrit, cyanosis, and complex surgery [214]. The increased risk of bleeding in the neonate is due to immaturity of the coagulation system, characterized by reduced plasma concentrations of both procoagulant and anticoagulant proteins (30–70 % of adult values) [215]. The neonate is known to have decreased levels of factors II (prothrombin), V, VII, X, XI, XII, and XIII until approximately 6 months of age. Reduced levels of fibrinogen or dysfunctional fibrinogen also have been documented in neonates [216]. All of these factors are compounded by the relative large volume of the pump prime and the resultant dilutional effect. The fact that the liver is not completely functional at birth, given that hepatic maturation continues throughout the first few weeks of life, also contributes to the issue. Hypoperfusion states can delay the timing of hepatic maturation, adding further to the bleeding risk.

Many neonatal surgical procedures are complex, requiring extensive surgical dissection, extracardiac suture lines, prolonged periods of CPB, and low levels of hypothermia. Cyanotic CHD is associated with hemostatic abnormalities that include polycythemia, thrombocytopenia, platelet functional abnormalities, disseminated intravascular coagulation, decreased production of coagulation factors (due to impaired liver function and vitamin K deficiency), and fibrinolysis [216, 217]. These factors when combined with a dilutional coagulopathy and platelet dysfunction related to CPB contribute to the tendency for bleeding and the greater likelihood for bleeding in the neonate.

The need for large volumes of blood and blood components has been associated with poor outcomes. The detrimental effects of blood transfusion include activation of the inflammatory cascade, hemodynamic alterations requiring infusion of vasoactive agents, prolonged duration of mechanical ventilation, and extended duration of intensive care stay and hospitalization [218–221]. Therefore, early detection and treatment of bypass-related coagulopathy, as well as transfusion strategies, are essential [222].

An individualized strategy that includes patient-specific heparin and protamine management to optimize anticoagulation and minimize bleeding problems in infants [223] has been advocated. For many years, the approach to bleeding during neonatal cardiac surgery was the early prophylactic administration of blood components. Today, several technologies are available to manage coagulation/bleeding in a more objective fashion. These point-of-care testing devices provide immediate or rapid results for partial thromboplastin time and prothrombin time, thromboelastography (TEG), rotating thromboelastometry (ROTEM), and specific assays of platelet function (Sonoclot analyzer, PFA-100, and Multiplate platelet aggregometer) [224–226]. TEG is a widely available technology that allows for a live graphic display of the coagulation process. This can detect residual anticoagulant or deficiency of clotting factors, poor clot strength, or fibrinolysis. This technology has already been found to be useful in assessing post-bypass coagulopathies and in guiding blood component therapy [227–229].

Antifibrinolytic agents have been used in an effort to minimize bleeding [230]. Agents such as ε-aminocaproic acid and tranexamic acid are analogs of the amino acid lysine and exert their antifibrinolytic effects by interfering with the binding of plasminogen to fibrin, which is necessary for activation to plasmin. Aprotinin causes inhibition of kallikrein and plasmin. In addition to having hemostatic properties (decreased hemostatic activation, antifibrinolysis, and preservation of platelet adhesiveness), the drug also has favorable properties on inflammation [231]. The literature reveals significant support for the efficacy of all three drugs for decreasing bleeding, with current data suggesting no significant difference in efficacy among these drugs [232]. Aprotinin was withdrawn from the market in 2008 due to the risk of renal dysfunction and death in adult cardiac surgery [233]. These detrimental effects have not been reproduced in children. Retrospective studies in neonates with renal dysfunction who received aprotinin when the drug was available have indicated either the duration of CPB or blood product transfusion as more likely etiologies for the kidney injury over the drug itself [234, 235].

Despite advances, empiric treatment of excessive bleeding after reversal of heparin may sometimes be needed in the absence of point-of-care testing devices; waiting for the results of coagulation studies can only lead to delay in treatment and additional bleeding. In many cases, components such as platelets, plasma, and cryoprecipitate are still used based on clinical judgment. Most recently, recombinant factor VII also has been administered in selected cases [236–238].

Neurologic Effects

Neurologic morbidity has received increasing attention during the last several years as survival after neonatal cardiac surgery continues to improve [126, 132, 186, 239–241]. Injury to the central nervous system during surgery for CHD can be manifested in acute fashion during the postoperative period as seizures, stroke, and coma [129]. The incidence of seizures, as documented by electroencephalographic monitoring, is 14–20 % when bypass included strategies such as either DHCA or low-flow but to be infrequent when high-flow bypass is used [186, 242]. Seizures are more likely to occur after prolonged duration of DHCA. However, a history of seizures after surgery did not predict worse developmental outcome on short-term follow-up (1 year) of 178 neonates and infants with complex congenital heart defects [243]. With regard to stroke, a study of 122 infants undergoing cardiac surgery reported a prevalence of 10 %, half of which was found to exist preoperatively [244]. Most strokes were clinically silent and undetected without neuroimaging. Significant factors associated with stroke identified in multivariate analysis were reduced birth weight, preoperative intubation, reduced intraoperative hematocrit, and greater blood pressure at the time of postoperative admission to the intensive care unit.

A significant concern is the substantial incidence (>50 %) of periventricular leukomalacia reported in neonates after cardiac surgery [245]. This finding of cerebral white matter necrosis that results from injury to immature neurons has been linked to an increased incidence of developmental delay and attention deficit/hyperactivity disorder [246]. Neurodevelopmental deficiencies after cardiac surgery include problems such as cognitive impairment, speech and language abnormalities, impaired visual and spatial motor skills, impaired attention and executive function, and learning disabilities [247]. In recent years, there has been intense interest and investigation in this complex area, given the relatively high incidence of neurodevelopmental sequelae among children with CHD [128, 130, 132, 248–250]. Thus far, it is known that patient-specific factors play a significant role [251] and, at the same time, potentially modifiable perioperative factors can influence neurologic outcomes [190, 252, 253].

Techniques such as DHCA and low-flow bypass have been considered major contributors to these sequelae [186, 254]. In addition, other factors associated with CPB, such as the rate of cooling and rewarming, arterial blood gas management strategy (alpha- versus pH-stat), and hematocrit levels during this period, also have been demonstrated to impact neurologic outcome [191, 197, 255–258]. The neonate with CHD may have an abnormal and, in many cases, immature central nervous system, potentially also increasing the risk of neurologic injury [226, 259–263]. A younger gestational age has been associated with worse neurodevelopmental outcomes after cardiac surgery during infancy [264]. Preoperative structural brain abnormalities and abnormal cerebral blood flow are present in neonates with severe CHD [265]. These neurologic abnormalities may be exacerbated by a concomitant genetic syndrome or chromosomal abnormality unrelated to the cardiovascular pathology [266].

Fetuses with left-sided obstructive cardiac lesions have abnormal cerebrovascular physiology, the brain being perfused via retrograde flow through the ductus arteriosus with blood that has a less-than-usual oxygen content. This can affect brain development. For example, microcephaly has been associated with a small Asc Ao [131, 267]. In infants with *d*-TGA, preoperative brain injury has been linked to preoperative balloon atrial septostomy, [268] although others dispute this association [269, 270]. To confound matters further, recent data in young animals suggest a potential association between exposure to a number of anesthetic/sedative agents and deficits in the areas of learning and memory, in addition to degenerative changes in the central nervous system, [271] although these effects have been shown to be reversible [272]. This subject is now at the forefront of pediatric anesthesia research [273, 274]. The issue of anesthesia-induced neurologic morbidity is a complex one, with the evidence suggesting that the etiology is likely multifactorial.

In addition to the previously discussed neuroprotective strategies, other approaches have been explored in an effort to limit neurologic morbidity after cardiac surgery [275]. These strategies include specific anesthetic regimens (e.g., ketamine, dexmedetomidine), administration of drugs (e.g., erythropoietin, anti-inflammatory agents, free radical scavengers, and neurotrophic factors), preconditioning (hypoxia-ischemia and remote ischemia), and stem cell treatment [276]. This field continues to evolve, with no definitive results that would merit a change in clinical practice.

Pulmonary Effects

Lung injury in the neonate after bypass is manifested by impaired pulmonary function characterized by arterial hypoxemia, carbon dioxide retention, and inability to wean from ventilatory support. The insult likely is the result of ischemic-reperfusion injury and the inflammatory process [277]. Preexisting causes or other issues also contribute to postoperative pulmonary dysfunction. Phrenic nerve injury leading to diaphragmatic paralysis should be excluded by radiological or other type of screening. Additional factors involved in the impairment include atelectasis, pulmonary edema, decreased functional residual capacity, altered total lung capacity, ventilation-perfusion mismatch, and increased dead space [278, 279]. Given that pulmonary complications are one of the most frequent contributors of adverse perioperative outcomes, several approaches that may moderate pulmonary dysfunction (e.g., leukocyte-depleted lung reperfusion) have been explored with variable results [280–282].

Myocardial Effects

An element of myocardial dysfunction after cardiac surgery that requires bypass is present in most, if not all, neonates. The mechanisms appear to be related to ischemia-reperfusion and the inflammatory response [283]. These alterations affect the ability of the myocardium not only to contract (systolic function) but also to relax (ventricular compliance or diastolic function). Thus, inotropes and vasoactive drugs are commonly required.

Renal and Gastrointestinal Effects

Several studies reported an 11 to 17 % incidence of acute kidney injury (AKI) in children undergoing CPB [284–287]. AKI during cardiac surgery in infancy portends a poor clinical outcome [288]. The vulnerability of the neonate to AKI is well known and is due to loss of autoregulation and ischemia [284, 289]. In recent years, there has been growing interest to elucidate the risk factors for AKI in infants undergoing cardiothoracic procedures with CPB. Five factors have been shown to predict AKI including younger age, weight <10 kg, myocardial dysfunction, sepsis, and duration of CPB >90 min [286]. Another study reported multiple perioperative risk factors for acute kidney risk or injury, failure, and mortality in children undergoing CPB [290]. The perioperative use of milrinone, particularly in young infants, and furosemide independently predicted poor renal outcomes. In recognition of the risk of AKI, peritoneal dialysis catheters are routinely placed at some centers after separation from CPB. These catheters can be connected in a sterile manner to a bag and passively allowed to drain or can be used for dialysis as needed for removal of fluid or in the event of reduced renal function in the postoperative period [291, 292].

Postoperative gastrointestinal complications associated with CPB are relatively rare. They have been mostly attributed to alterations in splanchnic blood flow and have been linked to high mortality rates in adults [293, 294]. Factors such as hemodynamic instability and the use of vasoactive agents are believed to contribute, although the data are limited. In view of ductal dependency in many congenital lesions and the potential for pulmonary steal, it is not unreasonable to consider the presence of this physiology as a potential perioperative risk. CHD is a risk factor for necrotizing enterocolitis in term infants [295, 296].

A study evaluating serum transaminases as a prognostic factor in children after cardiac surgery determined that increases in transaminases occur more frequently than previously reported, more commonly in the setting of right heart failure [297]. Significant increases in transaminases-alanine aminotransferase (ALT) and aspartate aminotransferase (AST), and lactate dehydrogenase (LDH) correlated with decreased postoperative survival.

Surgery Without Cardiopulmonary Bypass

Some cardiac surgery is undertaken without CPB. These surgeries can be performed through a lateral thoracotomy or median sternotomy incision. The most common palliative operations are PAB and systemic to pulmonary shunt placement. Corrective procedures include PDA ligation (discussed earlier in this chapter), CoA repair, and vascular ring division. More complex operations, either palliative or corrective, may also be undertaken (e.g., unifocalization of aortopulmonary artery collaterals). From an anesthetic standpoint, these cases require many of the same considerations as outlined above for procedures requiring CPB, reliable vascular access and intraoperative monitoring, as well as planning for postoperative care.

Pulmonary Artery Banding

A palliative approach to mechanically limit excess pulmonary blood flow is to apply a PAB (Fig. 12.28). This intervention may be indicated for pulmonary over-circulation in the neonate with single ventricle physiology, for lesions where the anatomy precludes a definitive repair, or when delaying a corrective procedure is beneficial. The goal of the surgery to restrict pulmonary blood flow is to alleviate congestive symptoms and prevent the development of pulmonary vascular disease. Frequently, the procedure is performed via a median sternotomy approach. The adequacy of the PAB can be assessed by direct measurement of the distal PA pressure or by estimation of the band gradient by TEE. A PA pressure between 25 and 30 % of systemic values or peak PAB flow velocity near 3.5 m/s (estimated band gradient of ~ 50 mmHg) is considered satisfactory. The systemic arterial oxygen saturation and PaO_2 values are very helpful in guiding band adjustments, as is the $ETCO_2$. Therefore, it is advisable during this period to mimic conditions of room air or minimal inspired oxygen supplementation and normocarbia. In most cases, a PAB improves the symptoms and allows for later staged palliation or corrective repair.

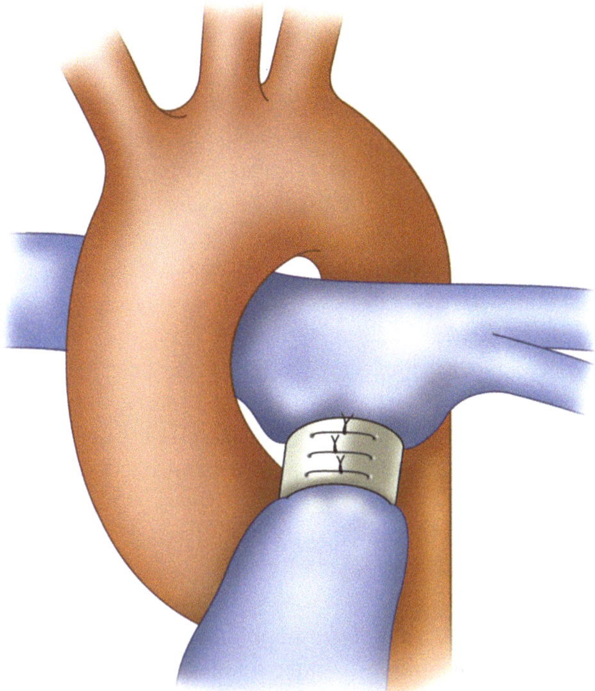

Fig. 12.28 Graphic representation of a pulmonary artery band

Systemic to Pulmonary Artery Shunt Placement

When pulmonary blood flow is inadequate or ductal dependent, a procedure to increase pulmonary blood flow is indicated. Creation of a systemic to PA shunt is usually performed by placement of a graft between the innominate or subclavian artery and a branch PA (modified Blalock-Taussig shunt; Fig. 12.29). In many cases, a central shunt to the MPA may be preferred as this encourages more general growth of the branch pulmonary arteries. The surgical approach to this shunt consists of either a median sternotomy or lateral thoracotomy, whereas other extracardiac shunts in most cases require a sternotomy. Specific issues of the intervention regarding anesthetic care include the selection of appropriate sites for monitoring blood pressure and pulse oximetry, as this is influenced by the site of the shunt placement; the need to continue PGE_1 infusion intraoperatively; and the administration of low-dose heparin before performing the shunt placement. The problems with this procedure are that the partially occluding clamp on the PA will further restrict pulmonary blood flow and that once the anastomosis is commenced, the clamp cannot be removed until it is completed. On rare occasions, it may be necessary to administer inotropes to support the patient until the clamps can be removed. It is important to oxygenate the patient well before allowing the surgeon to place the clamps and maintain the FiO_2 near 1.0 during shunt placement. Occasionally the position of the

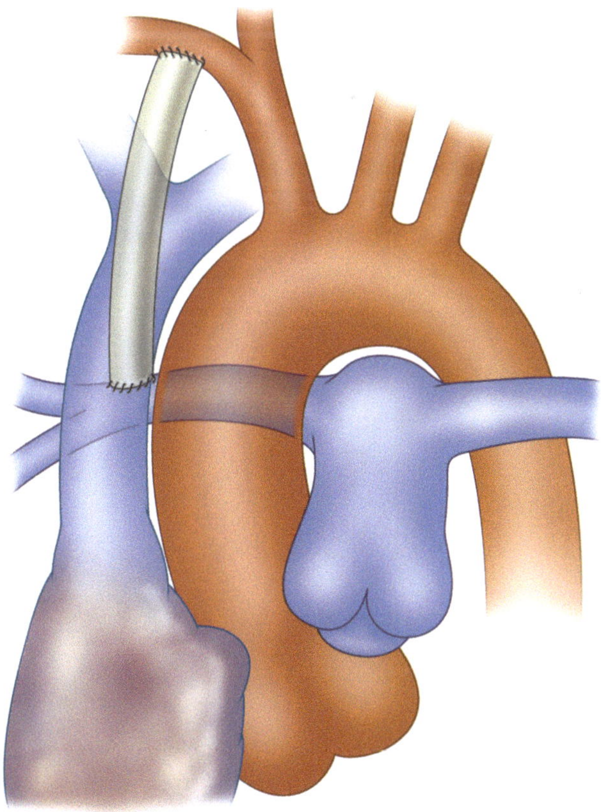

Fig. 12.29 Graphic representation of modified Blalock-Taussig shunt

clamps needs to be modified to correct significant further reductions in pulmonary blood flow. Before and after shunt placement, fluctuations in the level of systemic arterial oxygen saturation parallel changes in systemic arterial pressure as it represents the driving force at the Ao end of the ductus arteriosus (preoperatively) or shunt (postoperatively). It is important to confirm the expected changes at the time of shunt unclamping, namely, an increase in SpO_2 and a decrease in diastolic and, possibly, systolic blood pressures, in addition to a widening of the pulse pressure. In some cases, the decreased diastolic pressure may adversely affect myocardial perfusion leading to ventricular failure; this may respond to inotrope therapy. After the intervention, if the shunt is too large, an important concern may relate to balancing the systemic and pulmonary circulations.

Coarctation of the Aorta Repair

CoA represents one of the most common congenital defects requiring intervention within the first few weeks of life. The surgical approach to this lesion depends on the status of the Ao arch and associated pathology. These factors determine whether the repair is undertaken via a thoracotomy approach usually as resection of the diseased segment and end-to-end anastomosis (Fig. 12.30) or a more complex procedure through a median sternotomy incision using CPB. The main considerations for providing care for the neonate during thoracotomy repair include continuation of the PGE_1 infusion (if ongoing), adequate vascular access (may include central venous access depending on clinical status and institutional preference), and availability of blood products. In terms of arterial monitoring, a right radial arterial line is preferred. The Ao clamp site can impact rSO_2 as assessed by NIRS; thus, this type of monitoring has been recommended as a clinical practice [298]. The need for inotropic support usually is established preoperatively based on factors such as the clinical presentation, patient status, and echocardiographic assessment of LV systolic function. Continuing the infusion of these drugs perioperatively is appropriate in most cases. Concerns specific to the procedure include the need for ventilatory adjustments during the dissection phase, as lung isolation is accomplished by manual compression of the non-dependent lung by the surgeon, and the potential for blood loss. The administration of low-dose heparin (100 units/kg) to obtain a target ACT value near 200 s may be part of the center-specific protocol before applying the Ao cross-clamp. Mild hypothermia (~34–35 °C) is a standard strategy at some centers for spinal cord protection due to the risk of ischemia; however, as previously stated, overt evidence of spinal cord injury in this setting is extremely rare. Transient changes in blood pressure associated with application and removal of the Ao clamp usually are managed by altering the anesthetic depth and administering intravascular volume and/or calcium. Controlling the blood pressure is a key aspect of postoperative management. Agents such as esmolol, nitroprusside, and nicardipine have all been utilized to control post-repair rebound hypertension. Adequate pain control is an important aspect of the perioperative care.

Vascular Ring Division

Vascular rings are anomalies of the great arteries/their branches that can cause extrinsic compression of the tracheobronchial tree and/or esophagus. The presentation usually is with airway or feeding difficulties [299]. The most common anatomic causes of a vascular ring are double Ao arch (50–60 %)

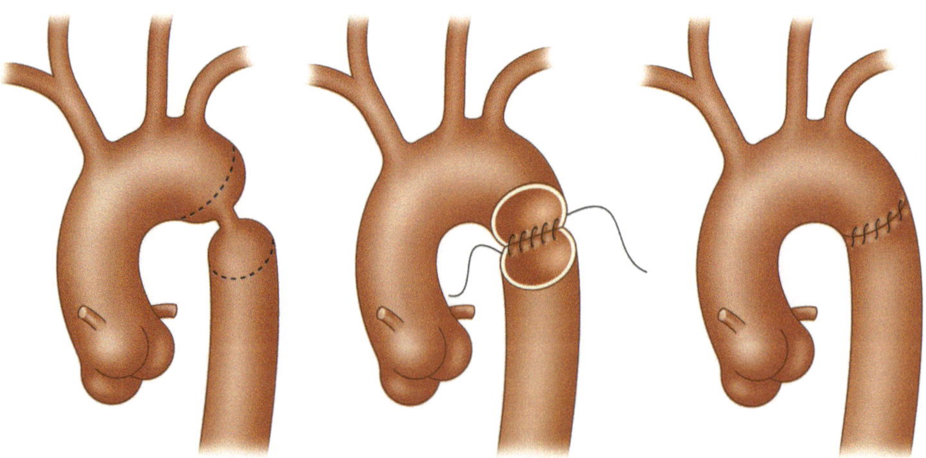

Fig. 12.30 Graphic representation of coarctation of the aorta repair. The figure demonstrates resection of the diseased, narrowed aortic segment and end-to-end anastomosis of the proximal and distal aortic arch segments

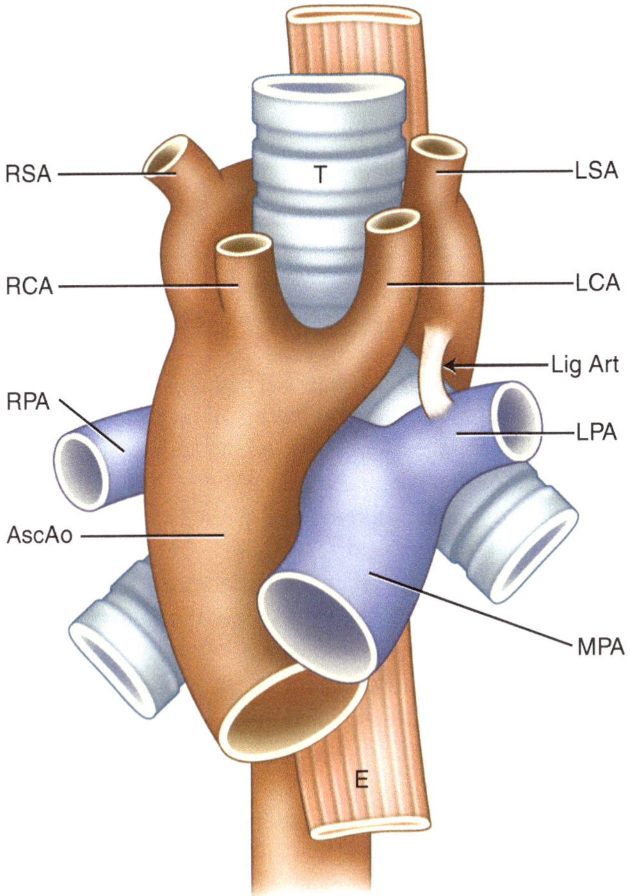

Fig. 12.31 Graphic representation of a vascular ring-double aortic arch. Note the relationship of the right and left aortic arches around the trachea and esophagus. *AscAo* ascending aorta, *E* esophagus, *LCA* left carotid artery, *LPA* left pulmonary artery, *LSA* left subclavian artery, *Lig Art* ligamentum arteriosus, *MPA* main pulmonary artery, *RCA* right carotid artery, *RPA* right pulmonary artery, *RSA* right subclavian artery, *T* trachea

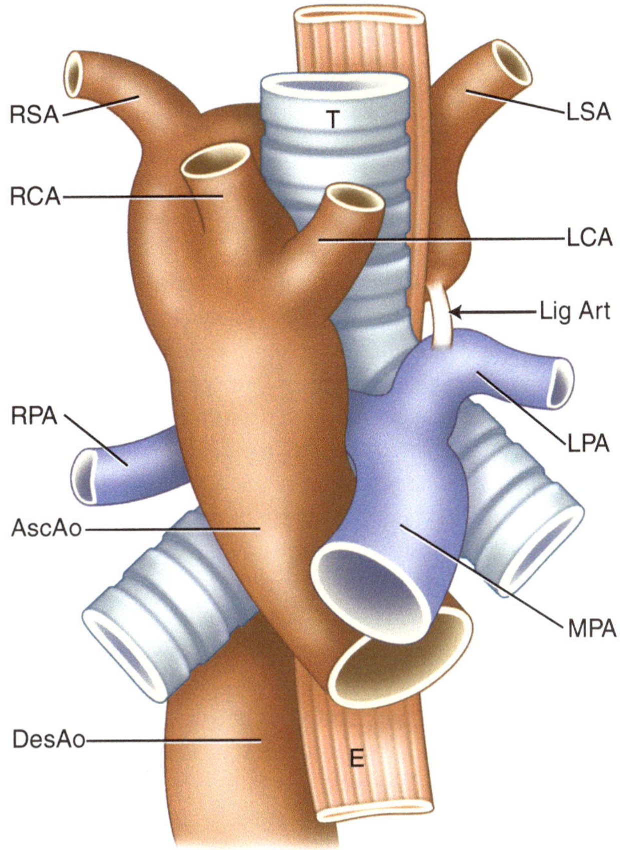

Fig. 12.32 Graphic representation of a vascular ring-right aortic arch and aberrant subclavian artery. In this anomaly, a left ductus arteriosus arises from a bulbous region at the base of the left subclavian artery (Kommerell diverticulum) and attaches to the left pulmonary artery. *AscAo* ascending aorta, *DesAo* descending aorta, *E* esophagus, *LCA* left carotid artery, *LPA* left pulmonary artery, *LSA* left subclavian artery, *Lig Art* ligamentum arteriosus, *MPA* main pulmonary artery, *RCA* right carotid artery, *RPA* right pulmonary artery, *RSA* right subclavian artery, *T* trachea

(Fig. 12.31) and right Ao arch with retroesophageal left subclavian artery and left ligamentum arteriosum (12–25 %) (Fig. 12.32) [300, 301]. The evaluation of these anomalies frequently requires multimodality imaging [302]. A double Ao usually is an isolated anomaly not associated with CHD. A report indicated that a right-sided Ao arch was dominant in 75 % of cases, a left-sided Ao arch in 18 %, and arches were of equal size in 7 % [303]. Surgical treatment consists of division of the non-dominant arch via thoracotomy. The ligamentum arteriosum or any other constricting bands are also released. Right Ao arch with retroesophageal left subclavian artery and intact ligamentum arteriosum is more likely to be associated with CHD. The approach to this lesion varies, but division of the ligamentum arteriosum is the primary intervention. Passage of an esophageal stethoscope or TEE probe can cause airway obstruction in these patients.

Vascular rings frequently are associated with tracheobronchomalacia and other abnormalities of the airway. Anesthetic care may be required for diagnostic evaluation as well as surgical treatment. In some cases, a formal bronchoscopic examination is performed as part of the overall evaluation. The airway should be assessed during spontaneous ventilation, examining the trachea for pulsatile compression(s). Recognizing that preexisting tracheobronchomalacia persists postoperatively, influencing postoperative patient management, also is important.

Mechanical Circulatory Support in the Neonate with Congenital Heart Disease

Circulatory support may be required for cardiac or cardiopulmonary failure [304–306]. The history typically is that of a reversible cause of circulatory failure or a condition that is untreatable/end stage for which the patient awaits heart

Table 12.7 Indications for mechanical circulatory support in the neonate with congenital heart disease

Stabilization prior to cardiac surgery or catheter-based intervention
Inability to wean from cardiopulmonary bypass
Postoperative low cardiac output state
Acute cardiopulmonary decompensation resulting from cardiac surgery

transplantation. In most cases, there is acute or impending hemodynamic decompensation. When mechanical support is instituted before circulatory collapse occurs, the goal is to prevent irreversible end-organ damage. Indications for mechanical circulatory support associated with cardiac surgery in the neonate are listed in Table 12.7. This therapy can be applied in the preoperative, intraoperative, or postoperative period. Preoperatively, the indication for support usually is related to either the need for stabilization or due to circulatory compromise. In the intraoperative setting, the use of mechanical support is more likely related to failure to wean from CPB, which may be due to the effects of surgery, bypass, and/or preoperative impairment of myocardial function. This clinical problem is referred to as *postcardiotomy failure*. More unusual in the intraoperative setting is the unanticipated need for acute circulatory support during procedures that do not require bypass. In the postoperative period, the indication usually is related to a low cardiac output state or cardiopulmonary arrest [307–309]. Contraindications to supporting the circulation mechanically include multisystem organ dysfunction, sepsis, severe coagulopathy, neurologic impairment, or intracranial hemorrhage.

Mechanical support in the neonate can be performed using venoarterial extracorporeal membrane oxygenation (ECMO) or a ventricular assist device (VAD). These strategies vary somewhat in their abilities to support body functions. ECMO provides isolated support of the respiratory system or full cardiopulmonary support; in contrast, VAD only supports the circulation. The components of an ECMO circuit include a centrifugal or roller pump, hollow fiber membrane oxygenator, oxygen blender, pump console, and heat exchanger. ECMO is the form of mechanical circulatory support used most frequently. This choice is due to the extensive clinical experience with the use of ECMO in neonates with respiratory failure from meconium aspiration, persistent pulmonary hypertension, and congenital diaphragmatic hernia. ECMO also has been shown to be extremely valuable in the neonate suffering from a cardiopulmonary arrest, serving as rescue therapy [310]. This form of therapy, also referred to as *extracorporeal support during cardiopulmonary resuscitation* (ECPR) or ECMO during cardiac arrest or rapid response, lead to an overall survival of 40 % in the near 600 patients who received this type of therapy as part of their resuscitation [310]. As indicated, ECMO is also of benefit when cardiopulmonary or pulmonary function is compromised. In the less likely case of the neonate with isolated ventricular impairment and good pulmonary function, a VAD may be a better option. In postcardiotomy heart failure, however, numerous considerations come into play. The presence of biventricular dysfunction, hypoxemia, and pulmonary hypertension, common findings in the neonate with CHD, favor the use of ECMO in this patient group. The overall survival of cardiac patients on ECMO ranges from 33 % to 43 % [310].

When ECMO is required, cannulation is performed using the neck or via a sternotomy. Neck access to the central circulation is via the jugular vein and carotid artery. When the sternum is open, cannulas are placed in the RA and Ao, and left-sided decompression is performed if needed. This is referred to as central cannulation.

There are several different types of VADs that can support the left, right, or both ventricles [304, 311]. A biventricular assist device (BIVAD), when necessary, is more likely to be used in the older child. The selection of the form of support depends on many factors, including the nature of the problem, the clinical situation, details of the anatomy (e.g., presence of intracardiac shunts), and pulmonary function. Other issues such as availability of equipment, training of personnel, familiarity among practitioners, and institutional preference also influence the selection of technology. Each support strategy has definitive benefits and limitations, which also have an important impact on decision-making.

Placement of a VAD is accomplished via a sternotomy; a temporary centrifugal LVAD, for example, requires an inflow cannula in the LA and an outflow cannula in the Ao. The use of a long-term LVAD in the neonate involves placement of an inflow cannula in the LV apex and an outflow cannula in the Asc Ao. At the time of this writing, paracorporeal pulsatile devices, meaning those placed outside the body, are the only option for long-term VAD support in the neonate, in contrast to intracorporeal or implantable devices available in older age groups. The Berlin Heart Excor Pediatric VAD® (Fig. 12.33) was the first device to become commercially available specifically for use in children [312]. This air-driven device is available in a variety of pump sizes including one suitable for the newborn (10 ml pump). Already in use in numerous countries for several years, this device recently was granted regulatory approval by the Food and Drug Administration for pediatric use as bridge to cardiac transplantation in the Unites States [312, 313]. The Berlin Heart has been used as an aid to myocardial recovery in the pediatric age group in other countries. The MEDOS HIA® device is also a pneumatic paracorporeal VAD available in Europe for infants and children [314]. It should be emphasized that while all these forms of support are lifesaving and offer the only option for survival in many infants, they are associated with significant morbidity and even death. Major complications usually are of a hemorrhagic, thromboembolic,

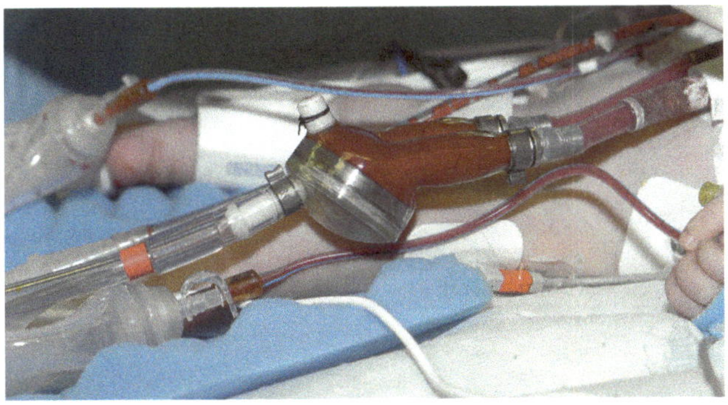

Fig. 12.33 Photograph depicts a neonate with a Berlin Heart Excor Pediatric VAD® left ventricular assist device

or infectious nature [315]. They can produce devastating consequences to the central nervous system. Although good neurological outcomes have been documented after mechanical circulatory support, a number of questions, including long-term neurocognitive outcomes and other important issues that impact quality of life, remain unanswered [316]. Therefore, the deployment of these sophisticated circulatory support modalities requires a careful risk-benefit assessment in recognition of the significant potential complications associated with these treatments.

The choice of mechanical support depends on the anticipated duration of therapy (short versus long term). Both ECMO and VAD are suitable support strategies in the short term. This is the case when the goal is used as a bridge to immediate survival, to recovery, to decision-making, or to a prolonged type of support (bridge-to-bridge). A greater period of circulatory support as a bridge to transplantation requires a different hardware that among its many desirable properties allows for a greater level of patient functionality [317–319]. Technological innovations over the years have resulted in miniaturization of pumps and cannulas, rendering the use of specialized long-term VAD feasible in the neonate [311].

Anesthetic care of the neonate who requires mechanical support is greatly influenced by factors such as the neonate's clinical condition, situation, and the type of therapy being instituted. During an acute event when ECMO is being applied for immediate survival, management is similar to that involving any cardiopulmonary resuscitation effort in the neonate. Additional considerations include the underlying structural cardiovascular abnormalities, need for anticoagulation, and administration of volume/blood components as needed [320]. Vasodilators are required on occasion upon initiation of support in order to be able to deliver full flows, particularly after vasoconstrictive agents have been administered as part of the resuscitation effort. Although ECMO has been applied on a routine basis in neonates with HLHS after the Norwood procedure to facilitate postoperative management, as previously noted, this is not common practice [82].

The use of any form of short-term circulatory support for postcardiotomy failure usually is in the setting of a long operative procedure and after several failed attempts at weaning from CPB. An extended bypass period is by default associated with problems such as bleeding, a heightened inflammatory response, potential pulmonary dysfunction, and many other factors that complicate management. All these issues come into play in the intraoperative and postoperative settings. The need for operative procedures such as mediastinal exploration for bleeding, adjustments of cannula, or weaning of support requires adequate planning, preparation, and communication among all team members.

Data regarding anesthetic care in children with long-term devices are extremely limited. A study in children with a Berlin Heart, including infants undergoing anesthesia for noncardiac procedures, demonstrated poor tolerance for reductions in systemic vascular resistance due to the relatively fixed cardiac output of the device. Preoperative stability was not predictive of the intraoperative hemodynamic course. The study recommended the administration of volume and alpha-agonists for the treatment of hypotension in this patient group [321]. Lastly, caring for these infants involves greater knowledge than just the technology (e.g., hardware, settings) but also the physiologic aspects of the various circulatory support modalities and anticoagulation algorithms that may be in use [322]. This knowledge implies an understanding of how device parameters can be affected and what types of interventions may be indicated to address any unfavorable hemodynamic effects. For example, an important issue in these patients relates to factors that can influence LV preload and, consequently, filling of the device and stroke volume. Increases in pulmonary vascular tone or acute alterations in RV function may be detrimental. Therefore, strategies that maintain low pulmonary vascular resistance and promote RV performance are essential for successful management of these infants [323].

Perioperative Issues and Specific Considerations in the Neonate Undergoing Cardiac Surgery

Many issues related to the specific cardiac defect, pathophysiology of the disease process, or other factors present challenges in the care of the neonate with heart disease. Some of these potential problems and intraoperative considerations are addressed briefly below.

Pulmonary Hypertension

Pulmonary hypertension in the neonatal period can be due to a number of different etiologies including persistent pulmonary hypertension of the newborn (PPHN), lung disease such as bronchopulmonary dysplasia, congenital anomalies including congenital diaphragmatic hernia, and CHD. Increased PA pressure is a common feature among many congenital cardiovascular defects. It is usually the result of increased pulmonary blood flow caused by a pressure unrestrictive direct communication between the great arteries, ventricles, or an obstruction to pulmonary venous flow [324, 325]. Pulmonary arterial hypertension develops over a variable period of time depending on the amount of pulmonary blood flow and the level of the shunt. Lesions associated with excessive pulmonary blood flow in the neonatal period or early infancy include, for example, a large PDA, VSD, complete atrioventricular septal defect, and over-circulated HLHS. Over time, high-flow lesions can lead to remodeling of the pulmonary arterial smooth muscle and vascular changes. Defects such as TA and AP window are associated with accelerated development of pulmonary vascular disease. Down syndrome also is considered a risk factor for pulmonary vascular disease [326]. Perioperative management of infants with lesions resulting in excessive pulmonary blood flow includes avoiding decreases in pulmonary vascular resistance that will increase the left-to-right shunt. Pulmonary venous hypertension associated with pulmonary venous obstruction, LV failure, or left heart lesions with impedance to blood flow results in reflex pulmonary arterial hypertension. It can be secondary to defects such as TAPVR, mitral stenosis, cor triatriatum, congenital pulmonary vein stenosis, and HLHS with a restrictive atrial septum. Over a period of time and depending on the degree of obstruction, the lungs become congested and pulmonary arterial hypertension develops. A benefit of early interventions in CHD is limitation of pulmonary blood flow and repair of obstruction to pulmonary venous blood flow. The end result is a reduction in PA pressures and less likelihood of pulmonary vascular reactivity [327]. Reduced PA pressures and vascular resistance are critically relevant in the infant with a single ventricle, as they are prerequisites for future palliative strategies that rely on passive pulmonary blood flow.

In the neonate, predisposing factors for a reactive pulmonary vascular bed during the perioperative period include the underlying increased pulmonary vascular tone, effects of CPB, and physiologic consequences of the cardiac pathology. In neonates with increased pulmonary blood flow or obstruction to pulmonary venous return, the potential for pulmonary hypertension to be present immediately after bypass and in the postoperatively setting should be recognized. Pulmonary hypertensive crises are a consequence of acute increases in pulmonary vascular tone, triggered by a variety of factors (Table 12.8). Hemodynamic decompensation during these events is due to acute right heart failure, decreased LV preload related to resistance of the egress of blood across the pulmonary bed, and unfavorable leftward shift of the interventricular septum, compromising LV filling and decreasing cardiac output. Prevention and management of these crises include sedation and measures that favor a low pulmonary vascular resistance (e.g., hyperventilation, hyperoxygenation, and alkalosis) [328]. Treatment focuses on optimization of RV function using inotropic support as necessary [329]. Milrinone also can be quite helpful in decreasing pulmonary vascular tone and enhancing RV function [330]. The use of selective pulmonary vasodilators such as inhaled nitric oxide may also be indicated [330, 331].

Table 12.8 Factors that may increase pulmonary vascular tone

Hypoxemia
Hypercarbia
Acidemia
Hypothermia
Atelectasis
Transmitted positive airway pressure
Agitation, pain, stimulation, light anesthesia, stress response

Systemic Hypotension

Intraoperative hypotension can be secondary to factors such as hypovolemia (due to fluid restriction, diuretic therapy, or blood loss), the effects of sedatives/anesthetic agents, rhythm abnormalities, ventricular dysfunction, or mechanical influences of the surgical intervention. A helpful management algorithm to determine cause and initiate appropriate therapy is to consider the contributions of ventricular preload, contractility, afterload, and factors related to the physiology of the defect, to the hemodynamic problem. In addition, the electrocardiogram should be evaluated for evidence of rhythm disturbances or myocardial ischemia. Treatment should focus on the cause and consider whether it represents an unavoidable transient occurrence related to the procedure itself or an event of more concern. If an acute intervention is necessary to increase blood pressure, it can be accomplished by the administration of volume, calcium, or other pharmacologic agent while definitive therapy is instituted.

Congestive Heart Failure

In the neonate, congestive heart failure can be caused by volume overload resulting from a physiologic left-to-right shunt, severe valvar regurgitation, obstructive pathology, and imbalance between the pulmonary and systemic circulations favoring pulmonary blood flow. Heart failure also can be seen in conditions associated with poor myocardial contractility. Severe heart failure is a known risk factor for perioperative complications in children [332].

Cyanosis

Cyanosis related to CHD is the result of limited pulmonary blood flow and/or intracardiac mixing. Delayed surgery, palliation, or staged correction of CHD usually is associated with some element of cyanosis. In the neonate and young infant, the effects of cyanosis may not be as pronounced as in older children with long-standing hypoxemia. Chronic hypoxemia affects all major organ systems and invokes compensatory mechanisms to enhance systemic oxygen delivery. Despite the favorable effects of these adaptive responses, they can also be detrimental due to increased blood viscosity, red cell sludging, and alterations in the coagulation system [333, 334]. Important perioperative considerations in cyanotic infants include the need for adequate preoperative hydration (refer to section on fasting period) and meticulous care of venous lines in order to avoid the potential risk of paradoxical embolization (discussed to follow).

Ventricular Pressure Overload

Outflow tract obstruction or increased PA pressure/vascular resistance imposes a pressure load on the ventricle, resulting in increased wall tension. This condition implies a susceptibility of the myocardial supply-and-demand relationship, reduced tolerance for factors that can alter this fine balance, and potential increased risk of ischemia. In addition, an important consideration is the fact that RV pressure in some defects can exceed systemic values and negatively impact the function of the LV. The negative effect of the RV on the LV is explained based on a principle of direct mechanical interaction between the ventricles referred to as *ventricular interdependence* [335].

Ventricular Volume Overload

A volume load to the LV is characterized by increased LA pressure, LV end-diastolic volume, and stroke volume. This physiology is associated with LA and LV dilation, and cardiomegaly. In the postoperative neonate, residual valvar regurgitation can be associated with altered loading conditions that, if significant, can result in congestive symptoms and ventricular dysfunction. The palliated single ventricle patient can be particularly vulnerable to conditions associated with ventricular volume overload (e.g., systemic to PA shunts).

Myocardial Ischemia

Anomalies associated with increased systolic and diastolic wall stress and those with decreased coronary perfusion, secondary to low diastolic pressures, have the potential for myocardial ischemia in the neonate. Lesions, such as anomalous origin of the left coronary artery from the pulmonary artery (ALCAPA) and large coronary fistula(s), are known to have a propensity to develop myocardial ischemia. Although the clinical manifestations of these anomalies usually become evident beyond the neonatal period in association with a decline in pulmonary vascular resistance (ALCAPA) or RV pressure (coronary fistula(s) to the RV), an element of ongoing ischemia can be present in the neonate. For the neonate undergoing a surgical intervention for any type of CHD, the negative effects of CPB, Ao cross-clamp, coronary manipulations, and the procedure itself should also to be considered as potential etiologies for myocardial compromise.

Altered Respiratory Mechanics

Many congenital defects associated with increased pulmonary blood flow and vascular pressures result in increased LA pressure, leading to interstitial pulmonary edema and compression of small airways. These alterations in lung mechanics are characterized by increased airway resistance and decreased lung compliance [336, 337]. These abnormalities, in addition to inadequate palliation or residual shunts and the effects of surgery, all have detrimental consequences in the already vulnerable respiratory status of the neonate [338].

Systemic Air Embolization

An important recognition is the potential for right-to-left shunting and paradoxical systemic air embolization in the neonate due to the presence of shunts or even across a patent foramen ovale. The risk is magnified by increased right-sided pressures or pulmonary vascular resistance associated with CHD. This potential mandates meticulous de-airing of all vascular lines.

Conduction Disturbances and Arrhythmias

Infants, particularly those with Down syndrome, can develop bradycardia during induction of anesthesia in association with the administration of drugs (e.g., opioids) and at the time of laryngoscopy, endotracheal intubation, or placement of a TEE probe. Usually, the bradycardia is self-limited and requires no treatment; however, if it persists, the administration of drugs such as atropine or glycopyrrolate or, less likely, a small dose of epinephrine if the low heart rate is a concern, should be considered. Placement of central venous access occasionally can trigger cardiac arrhythmias. Usually, they are of a transient nature and require no intervention unless sustained, in which case either pharmacologic treatment or cardioversion/defibrillation is indicated. Because it may not be well tolerated in the critically ill neonate, caution must be exercised to minimize stimulation of the heart during central catheter placement.

Perioperative Stress Response

The typical physiologic response to painful stimuli in normal children consists of an increase in heart rate and blood pressure, in addition to a transient decrease in PaO_2. These normal patterns, however, can be detrimental to infants with CHD. Tachycardia shortens diastolic filling time, whereas hypertension increases ventricular afterload, thus decreasing stroke volume. The reduced ability of the neonate with CHD to increase cardiac output in response to the many perioperative stresses is well recognized.

Although the use of regional anesthesia in the neonate undergoing major surgery is well documented, with benefits that include blunting of the stress response and pain control, the application of these techniques during cardiac surgery remains the subject of debate [339–341] because, in many cases, there is already an anticipated need for postoperative sedation and mechanical ventilation that frequently includes the use of opioids [342]. Furthermore, there is a paucity of data regarding increased benefits of regional anesthesia over standard management, and concerns of complications after neuroaxial anesthesia remain despite the lack of reported adverse events or serious complication when applied in this setting. The use of these techniques is more likely during thoracic surgery [343].

Post-cardiac Transplant Recipients

Cardiac disease not amenable to palliation or correction may leave heart transplantation as the only option [21]. The post-transplanted infant has a denervated heart; the lack of external nerve supply implies that the usual autonomic regulatory mechanisms are not operational, increasing the potential for hemodynamic alterations. In addition, compensatory responses may be delayed, further augmenting the likelihood for compromise [344]. Critical determinants of cardiac output include an adequate heart rate and blood volume. In the immediate posttransplant period, heart rate is supported by exogenous chronotropes or pacing. Subsequently, circulating endogenous catecholamines drive the heart rate. Regardless of the time interval from transplantation, when caring for these neonates, the following considerations are suggested: (1) have drugs with chronotropic properties immediately available, (2) use agents with a direct action on the myocardium and vasculature, and (3) prepare emergent cardiac pacing modalities. Several additional issues are important in the anesthetic care of the transplanted patient [345]. Immunosuppressant agents, which may need to be given during the perioperative period, may have secondary effects on various organ systems (particularly the heart, liver, and kidney) and interact with anesthetic agents (muscle relaxants). Other considerations include the potential need for "stress"-dose corticosteroids (a controversial subject), the requirement for strict aseptic technique, and the adequate preparation of blood products (irradiated, leukocyte reduced, and cytomegalovirus negative/safe).

Summary

The management of the neonate with congenital cardiac malformations presents significant challenges. The ability to provide optimal care for affected neonates relies heavily on an understanding of the structural abnormalities, hemodynamic consequences of the defects, strategies available to each patient, and the impact of anesthetic/surgical interventions on the physiology. This wealth of knowledge allows for the application of many important principles, with the ultimate goal being to maintain hemodynamic stability, systemic output, and oxygen delivery in the neonate with heart disease throughout the perioperative period. Successful management of these challenging patients is most likely to be achieved in those specialized units that have a dedicated comprehensive team and a large volume of neonates who require cardiac surgery.

References

1. Rudolph AM. The changes in the circulation after birth. Their importance in congenital heart disease. Circulation. 1970;41:343–59.
2. Friedman AH, Fahey JT. The transition from fetal to neonatal circulation: normal responses and implications for infants with heart disease. Semin Perinatol. 1993;17:106–21.
3. Rudolph AM. Fetal and neonatal pulmonary circulation. Annu Rev Physiol. 1979;41:383–95.
4. Friedman WF. The intrinsic physiologic properties of the developing heart. Prog Cardiovasc Dis. 1972;15:87–111.
5. Nakanishi T, Seguchi M, Takao A. Development of the myocardial contractile system. Experientia. 1988;44:936–44.
6. Chin TK, Friedman WF, Klitzner TS. Developmental changes in cardiac myocyte calcium regulation. Circ Res. 1990;67:574–9.
7. Prakash YS, Seckin I, Hunter LW, Sieck GC. Mechanisms underlying greater sensitivity of neonatal cardiac muscle to volatile anesthetics. Anesthesiology. 2002;96:893–906.
8. Go AS, Mozaffarian D, Roger VL, et al. Heart disease and stroke statistics–2013 update: a report from the American Heart Association. Circulation. 2013;127:e6–e245.
9. van der Linde D, Konings EE, Slager MA, et al. Birth prevalence of congenital heart disease worldwide: a systematic review and meta-analysis. J Am Coll Cardiol. 2011;58:2241–7.
10. Zhao Q, Ma X, Jia B, Huang G. Prevalence of congenital heart disease at live birth: an accurate assessment by echocardiographic screening. Acta Paediatr. 2013;102:397–402.

11. Bernier PL, Stefanescu A, Samoukovic G, Tchervenkov CI. The challenge of congenital heart disease worldwide: epidemiologic and demographic facts. Semin Thorac Cardiovasc Surg Pediatr Card Surg Annu. 2010;13:26–34.
12. Tanner K, Sabrine N, Wren C. Cardiovascular malformations among preterm infants. Pediatrics. 2005;116:e833–838.
13. Pierpont ME, Basson CT, Benson DW, et al. Genetic basis for congenital heart defects: current knowledge: a scientific statement from the American heart association congenital cardiac defects committee, council on cardiovascular disease in the young: endorsed by the American academy of pediatrics. Circulation. 2007;115:3015–38.
14. Zaidi S, Choi M, Wakimoto H, et al. *De novo* mutations in histone-modifying genes in congenital heart disease. Nature. 2013; 498:220–3.
15. Fahed AC, Nemer GM. Genetic causes of syndromic and non-syndromic congenital heart disease. In: Cooper DN, Chen JM, editors. Mutations in human genetic disease. Open Access; 2012.
16. Wren C, Irving CA, Griffiths JA, et al. Mortality in infants with cardiovascular malformations. Eur J Pediatr. 2012;171:281–7.
17. Moller JH. Prevalence and incidence of cardiac malformations. Perspectives in pediatric cardiology: surgery for congenital heart disease 1984–1995. Armonk, NY: Futura Publishing Company; 1998. p. 6:19–6:26.
18. Silberbach M, Hannon D. Presentation of congenital heart disease in the neonate and young infant. Pediatr Rev. 2007;28:123–31.
19. Yun SW. Congenital heart disease in the newborn requiring early intervention. Korean J Pediatr. 2011;54:183–91.
20. Lee JY. Clinical presentations of critical cardiac defects in the newborn: decision making and initial management. Korean J Pediatr. 2010;53:669–79.
21. Sauvage LR, Mansfield PB, Stamm SJ. Physiologic classification of congenital heart disease. AORN J. 1973;18:61–83.
22. Thiene G, Frescura C. Anatomical and pathophysiological classification of congenital heart disease. Cardiovasc Pathol. 2010; 19:259–74.
23. Rowe RD, Freedom RM, Mehrizi A, Bloom KR. The neonate with congenital heart disease. Major Probl Clin Pediatr. 1981;5: 137–65.
24. Knowles R, Griebsch I, Dezateux C, Brown J, Bull C, Wren C. Newborn screening for congenital heart defects: a systematic review and cost-effectiveness analysis. Health Technol Assess. 2005;9:1–152, iii–iv.
25. Gertler R, Miller-Hance WC. Essential cardiology. In: Cote CJ, Lerman J, Anderson BJ, editors. A practice of anesthesia for infants and children. Philadelphia: W. B. Saunders; 2013. p. 291–326.
26. Welke KF, Komanapalli C, Shen I, Ungerleider RM. Advances in congenital heart surgery. Curr Opin Pediatr. 2005;17:574–8.
27. Schneider DJ, Moore JW. Congenital heart disease for the adult cardiologist: patent ductus arteriosus. Circulation. 2006;114: 1873–82.
28. El-Khuffash AF, Jain A, McNamara PJ. Ligation of the patent ductus arteriosus in preterm infants: understanding the physiology. J Pediatr. 2013;162:1100–6.
29. Reese J. Patent ductus arteriosus: mechanisms and management. Semin Perinatol. 2012;36:89–91.
30. Johnston PG, Gillam-Krakauer M, Fuller MP, Reese J. Evidence-based use of indomethacin and ibuprofen in the neonatal intensive care unit. Clin Perinatol. 2012;39:111–36.
31. Burke RP, Wernovsky G, van der Velde M, Hansen D, Castaneda AR. Video-assisted thoracoscopic surgery for congenital heart disease. J Thorac Cardiovasc Surg. 1995;109:499–507 (discussion 508).
32. Laborde F, Folliguet T, Da Cruz E, Batisse A, Carbognani D, Dibie A. Video surgical technique for interruption of patent ductus arteriosus in children and neonates. Pediatr Pulmonol Suppl. 1997;16:177–9.
33. Wolf AR. Ductal ligation in the very low-birth weight infant: simple anesthesia or extreme art? Paediatr Anaesth. 2012;22:558–63.
34. Harris LL, Krishnamurthy R, Browne LP, Morales DL, Friedman EM. Left main bronchus obstruction after patent ductus arteriosus ligation: an unusual complication. Int J Pediatr Otorhinolaryngol. 2012;76:1855–6.
35. Rukholm G, Farrokhyar F, Reid D. Vocal cord paralysis post patent ductus arteriosus ligation surgery: risks and co-morbidities. Int J Pediatr Otorhinolaryngol. 2012;76:1637–41.
36. Hsu KH, Chiang MC, Lien R, et al. Diaphragmatic paralysis among very low birth weight infants following ligation for patent ductus arteriosus. Eur J Pediatr. 2012;171:1639–44.
37. El-Khuffash AF, Jain A, Dragulescu A, McNamara PJ, Mertens L. Acute changes in myocardial systolic function in preterm infants undergoing patent ductus arteriosus ligation: a tissue Doppler and myocardial deformation study. J Am Soc Echocardiogr. 2012;25:1058–67.
38. Shone JD, Sellers RD, Anderson RC, Adams PJ, Lillihei CW, Edwards JE. The developmental complex of "parachute mitral valve," supravalvular ring of left atrium, subaortic stenosis, and coarctation of aorta. Am J Cardiol. 1963;11:714–25.
39. Fesseha AK, Eidem BW, Dibardino DJ, et al. Neonates with aortic coarctation and cardiogenic shock: presentation and outcomes. Ann Thorac Surg. 2005;79:1650–5.
40. Elgamal MA, McKenzie ED, Fraser CDJ. Aortic arch advancement: the optimal one-stage approach for surgical management of neonatal coarctation with arch hypoplasia. Ann Thorac Surg. 2002;73:1267–72. discussion 1272–1273.
41. Wright GE, Nowak CA, Goldberg CS, Ohye RG, Bove EL, Rocchini AP. Extended resection and end-to-end anastomosis for aortic coarctation in infants: results of a tailored surgical approach. Ann Thorac Surg. 2005;80:1453–9.
42. Rao PS, Singh GK, Balfour IC, Jureidini SB, Fiore AC. Balloon angioplasty of long-segment aortic coarctation in the neonate. J Invasive Cardiol. 1999;11:734–8.
43. Keen G. Spinal cord damage and operations for coarctation of the aorta: aetiology, practice, and prospects. Thorax. 1987;42:11–8.
44. Ungerleider RM, Pasquali SK, Welke KF, Wallace AS, Ootaki Y, Quartermain MD, Williams DA, Jacobs JP. Contemporary patterns of surgery and outcomes for aortic coarctation: an analysis of the society of thoracic surgeons congenital heart surgery database. J Thorac Cardiovasc Surg. 2013;145:150–7 (discussion 157–158).
45. Rosenthal E. Coarctation of the aorta from fetus to adult: curable condition or life long disease process? Heart. 2005;91:1495–502.
46. Polson JW, McCallion N, Waki H, et al. Evidence for cardiovascular autonomic dysfunction in neonates with coarctation of the aorta. Circulation. 2006;113:2844–50.
47. Bisoi AK, Sharma P, Chauhan S, et al. Primary arterial switch operation in children presenting late with d-transposition of great arteries and intact ventricular septum. When is it too late for a primary arterial switch operation? Eur J Cardiothorac Surg. 2010;38:707–13.
48. Van Arsdell GS, Maharaj GS, Tom J, et al. What is the optimal age for repair of tetralogy of Fallot? Circulation. 2000;102: III123–129.
49. Mulder TJ, Pyles LA, Stolfi A, Pickoff AS, Moller JH. A multicenter analysis of the choice of initial surgical procedure in tetralogy of Fallot. Pediatr Cardiol. 2002;23:580–6.
50. Kanter KR, Kogon BE, Kirshbom PM, Carlock PR. Symptomatic neonatal tetralogy of Fallot: repair or shunt? Ann Thorac Surg. 2010;89:858–63.
51. Morales DL, Zafar F, Fraser CDJ. Tetralogy of Fallot repair: the right ventricle infundibulum sparing (RVIS) strategy. Semin Thorac Cardiovasc Surg Pediatr Card Surg Annu. 2009;54–58.

52. Padalino MA, Vida VL, Stellin G. Transatrial-transpulmonary repair of tetralogy of Fallot. Semin Thorac Cardiovasc Surg Pediatr Card Surg Annu. 2009:48–53.
53. Kalfa DM, Serraf AE, Ly M, Le Bret E, Roussin R, Belli E. Tetralogy of Fallot with an abnormal coronary artery: surgical options and prognostic factors. Eur J Cardiothorac Surg. 2012;42:e34–39.
54. Rajagopal SK, Thiagarajan RR. Perioperative care of children with tetralogy of fallot. Curr Treat Options Cardiovasc Med. 2011;13:464–74.
55. Shekerdemian LS, Schulze-Neick I, Redington AN, Bush A, Penny DJ. Negative pressure ventilation as haemodynamic rescue following surgery for congenital heart disease. Intensive Care Med. 2000;26:93–6.
56. Bronicki RA, Herrera M, Mink R, Domico M, Tucker D, Chang AC, Anas NG. Hemodynamics and cerebral oxygenation following repair of tetralogy of Fallot: the effects of converting from positive pressure ventilation to spontaneous breathing. Congenit Heart Dis. 2010;5:416–21.
57. Makhoul M, Oster M, Fischbach P, Das S, Deshpande S. Junctional ectopic tachycardia after congenital heart surgery in the current surgical era. Pediatr Cardiol. 2013;34:370–4.
58. Bar-Cohen Y, Silka MJ. Management of postoperative arrhythmias in pediatric patients. Curr Treat Options Cardiovasc Med. 2012;14:443–54.
59. Mahmoud AB, Tantawy AE, Kouatli AA, Baslaim GM. Propranolol: a new indication for an old drug in preventing postoperative junctional ectopic tachycardia after surgical repair of tetralogy of Fallot. Interact Cardiovasc Thorac Surg. 2008;7:184–7.
60. Collett RW, Edwards JE. Persistent truncus arteriousus: a classification according to antomic types. Surg Clin N Am. 1949; 29:1245–70.
61. Odegard KC, DiNardo JA, Kussman BD, et al. The frequency of anesthesia-related cardiac arrests in patients with congenital heart disease undergoing cardiac surgery. Anesth Analg. 2007;105:335–43.
62. Oepkes D, Moon-Grady AJ, Wilkins-Haug L, Tworetzky W, Arzt W, Devlieger R. 2010 Report from the ISPD Special Interest Group fetal therapy: fetal cardiac interventions. Prenat Diagn. 2011;31:249–51.
63. Hickey EJ, Caldarone CA, McCrindle BW. Left ventricular hypoplasia: a spectrum of disease involving the left ventricular outflow tract, aortic valve, and aorta. J Am Coll Cardiol. 2012;59: S43–54.
64. Vlahos AP, Lock JE, McElhinney DB, van der Velde ME. Hypoplastic left heart syndrome with intact or highly restrictive atrial septum: outcome after neonatal transcatheter atrial septostomy. Circulation. 2004;109:2326–30.
65. Villa CR, Marino BS, Jacobs JP, Cooper DS. Intensive care and perioperative management of neonates with functionally univentricular hearts. World J Pediatr Congenit Heart Surg. 2012;3: 359–63.
66. Hansen DD, Hickey PR. Anesthesia for hypoplastic left heart syndrome: use of high-dose fentanyl in 30 neonates. Anesth Analg. 1986;65:127–32.
67. Tabbutt S, Ramamoorthy C, Montenegro LM, et al. Impact of inspired gas mixtures on preoperative infants with hypoplastic left heart syndrome during controlled ventilation. Circulation. 2001; 104:I159–164.
68. Stayer S, Gouvion J, Evey L, Andropoulos D. Subambient gas delivery. Anesth Analg. 2002;94:1674–5.
69. Ramamoorthy C, Tabbutt S, Kurth CD, et al. Effects of inspired hypoxic and hypercapnic gas mixtures on cerebral oxygen saturation in neonates with univentricular heart defects. Anesthesiology. 2002;96:283–8.
70. Feinstein JA, Benson DW, Dubin AM, et al. Hypoplastic left heart syndrome: current considerations and expectations. J Am Coll Cardiol. 2012;59:S1–42.
71. Bailey LL, Nehlsen-Cannarella SL, Doroshow RW, et al. Cardiac allotransplantation in newborns as therapy for hypoplastic left heart syndrome. N Engl J Med. 1986;315:949–51.
72. Galantowicz M, Cheatham JP, Phillips A, et al. Hybrid approach for hypoplastic left heart syndrome: intermediate results after the learning curve. Ann Thorac Surg. 2008;85:2063–70 (discussion 2070–2071).
73. Sano S, Ishino K, Kawada M, Honjo O. Right ventricle-pulmonary artery shunt in first-stage palliation of hypoplastic left heart syndrome. Semin Thorac Cardiovasc Surg Pediatr Card Surg Annu. 2004;7:22–31.
74. Hornik CP, He X, Jacobs JP, et al. Complications after the Norwood operation: an analysis of the society of thoracic surgeons congenital heart surgery database. Ann Thorac Surg. 2011;92:1734–40.
75. Tweddell JS, Hoffman GM, Fedderly RT, et al. Phenoxybenzamine improves systemic oxygen delivery after the Norwood procedure. Ann Thorac Surg. 1999;67:161–7 (discussion 167–168).
76. Hoffman GM, Tweddell JS, Ghanayem NS, et al. Alteration of the critical arteriovenous oxygen saturation relationship by sustained afterload reduction after the Norwood procedure. J Thorac Cardiovasc Surg. 2004;127:738–45.
77. Ohye RG, Sleeper LA, Mahony L, et al. Comparison of shunt types in the Norwood procedure for single-ventricle lesions. N Engl J Med. 2010;362:1980–92.
78. Ghanayem NS, Allen KR, Tabbutt S, et al. Interstage mortality after the Norwood procedure: results of the multicenter single ventricle reconstruction trial. J Thorac Cardiovasc Surg. 2012;144:896–906.
79. Tweddell JS, Hoffman GM, Mussatto KA, et al. Improved survival of patients undergoing palliation of hypoplastic left heart syndrome: lessons learned from 115 consecutive patients. Circulation. 2002;106:I82–9.
80. Tweddell JS, Ghanayem NS, Mussatto KA, et al. Mixed venous oxygen saturation monitoring after stage 1 palliation for hypoplastic left heart syndrome. Ann Thorac Surg. 2007;84:1301–10 (discussion 1310–1311).
81. Wernovsky G, Kuijpers M, Van Rossem MC, et al. Postoperative course in the cardiac intensive care unit following the first stage of Norwood reconstruction. Cardiol Young. 2007;17: 652–65.
82. Shen I, Ungerleider RM. Routine use of mechanical ventricular assist following the Norwood procedure. Semin Thorac Cardiovasc Surg Pediatr Card Surg Annu. 2004;7:16–21.
83. Naguib AN, Winch P, Schwartz L, et al. Anesthetic management of the hybrid stage 1 procedure for hypoplastic left heart syndrome (HLHS). Paediatr Anaesth. 2010;20:38–46.
84. Ferencz C, Rubin JD, McCarter RJ, et al. Congenital heart disease: prevalence at livebirth. The Baltimore-Washington Infant Study. Am J Epidemiol. 1985;121:31–6.
85. Gittenberger-de Groot AC, Sauer U, Bindl L, Babic R, Essed CE, Buhlmeyer K. Competition of coronary arteries and ventriculo-coronary arterial communications in pulmonary atresia with intact ventricular septum. Int J Cardiol. 1988;18:243–58.
86. Freedom RM, Anderson RH, Perrin D. The significance of ventriculo-coronary arterial connections in the setting of pulmonary atresia with an intact ventricular septum. Cardiol Young. 2005;15:447–68.
87. Justo RN, Nykanen DG, Williams WG, Freedom RM, Benson LN. Transcatheter perforation of the right ventricular outflow tract as initial therapy for pulmonary valve atresia and intact ventricular septum in the newborn. Cathet Cardiovasc Diagn. 1997;40: 408–13.

88. Shaddy RE, Sturtevant JE, Judd VE, McGough EC. Right ventricular growth after transventricular pulmonary valvotomy and central aortopulmonary shunt for pulmonary atresia and intact ventricular septum. Circulation. 1990;82:IV157–63.
89. Neufeld HN, Lester RG, Adams PJ, Anderson RC, Lillehei CW, Edwards JE. Aorticopulmonary septal defect. Am J Cardiol. 1962;9:12–25.
90. Ho SY, Gerlis LM, Anderson C, Devine WA, Smith A. The morphology of aortopulmonary windows with regard to their classification and morphogenesis. Cardiol Young. 1994;4:146–55.
91. Tulloh RM, Rigby ML. Transcatheter umbrella closure of aortopulmonary window. Heart. 1997;77:479–80.
92. Ramamoorthy C, Haberkern CM, Bhananker SM, et al. Anesthesia-related cardiac arrest in children with heart disease: data from the pediatric perioperative cardiac arrest (POCA) registry. Anesth Analg. 2010;110:1376–82.
93. Practice guidelines for preoperative fasting and the use of pharmacologic agents to reduce the risk of pulmonary aspiration: application to healthy patients undergoing elective procedures: a report by the American Society of Anesthesiologist Task Force on Preoperative Fasting. Anesthesiology. 1999;90:896–905.
94. Cavell B. Gastric emptying in infants with congenital heart disease. Acta Paediatr Scand. 1981;70:517–20.
95. DeBock TL, Davis PJ, Tome J, Petrilli R, Siewers RD, Motoyama EK. Effect of premedication on arterial oxygen saturation in children with congenital heart disease. J Cardiothorac Anesth. 1990;4:425–9.
96. Barker SJ, Tremper KK. Pulse oximetry: applications and limitations. Int Anesthesiol Clin. 1987;25:155–75.
97. Tremper KK, Barker SJ. Pulse oximetry. Anesthesiology. 1989;70:98–108.
98. Burrows FA. Physiologic dead space, venous admixture, and the arterial to end-tidal carbon dioxide difference in infants and children undergoing cardiac surgery. Anesthesiology. 1989;70:219–25.
99. Lazzell VA, Burrows FA. Stability of the intraoperative arterial to end-tidal carbon dioxide partial pressure difference in children with congenital heart disease. Can J Anaesth. 1991;38:859–65.
100. Tiffany KF, Burke BL, Collins-Odoms C, Oelberg DG. Current practice regarding the enteral feeding of high-risk newborns with umbilical catheters in situ. Pediatrics. 2003;112:20–3.
101. Schwemmer U, Arzet HA, Trautner H, Rauch S, Roewer N, Greim CA. Ultrasound-guided arterial cannulation in infants improves success rate. Eur J Anaesthesiol. 2006;23:476–80.
102. Detaille T, Pirotte T, Veyckemans F. Vascular access in the neonate. Best Pract Res Clin Anaesthesiol. 2010;24:403–18.
103. Sulemanji DS, Donmez A, Akpek EA, Alic Y. Vascular catheterization is difficult in infants with Down syndrome. Acta Anaesthesiol Scand. 2009;53:98–100.
104. Kahler AC, Mirza F. Alternative arterial catheterization site using the ulnar artery in critically ill pediatric patients. Pediatr Crit Care Med. 2002;3:370–4.
105. Schindler E, Kowald B, Suess H, Niehaus-Borquez B, Tausch B, Brecher A. Catheterization of the radial or brachial artery in neonates and infants. Paediatr Anaesth. 2005;15:677–82.
106. Prian GW. Temporal artery catheterization for arterial access in the high risk newborn. Surgery. 1977;82:734–7.
107. Prian GW. Complications and sequelae of temporal artery catheterization in the high-risk newborn. J Pediatr Surg. 1977;12:829–35.
108. Andropoulos DB, Bent ST, Skjonsby B, Stayer SA. The optimal length of insertion of central venous catheters for pediatric patients. Anesth Analg. 2001;93:883–6.
109. Lamperti M, Bodenham AR, Pittiruti M, et al. International evidence-based recommendations on ultrasound-guided vascular access. Intensive Care Med. 2012;38:1105–17.
110. Verghese ST, McGill WA, Patel RI, Sell JE, Midgley FM, Ruttimann UE. Ultrasound-guided internal jugular venous cannulation in infants: a prospective comparison with the traditional palpation method. Anesthesiology. 1999;91:71–7.
111. Hosokawa K, Shime N, Kato Y, Hashimoto S. A randomized trial of ultrasound image-based skin surface marking versus real-time ultrasound-guided internal jugular vein catheterization in infants. Anesthesiology. 2007;107:720–4.
112. Reyes JA, Habash ML, Taylor RP. Femoral central venous catheters are not associated with higher rates of infection in the pediatric critical care population. Am J Infect Control. 2012;40:43–7.
113. Mitto P, Barankay A, Spath P, Kunkel R, Richter JA. Central venous catheterization in infants and children with congenital heart diseases: experiences with 500 consecutive catheter placements. Pediatr Cardiol. 1992;13:14–9.
114. Malik M, et al. A comparison of external and internal jugular venous pressures to monitor pulmonary artery pressure after superior cavopulmonary anastomosis. Interact Cardiovasc Thorac Surg. 2011;13:566–8.
115. Andropoulos DB, Stayer SA, Bent ST, et al. A controlled study of transesophageal echocardiography to guide central venous catheter placement in congenital heart surgery patients. Anesth Analg. 1999;89:65–70.
116. Stevenson JG, Sorensen GK, Gartman DM, Hall DG, Rittenhouse EA. Transesophageal echocardiography during repair of congenital cardiac defects: identification of residual problems necessitating reoperation. J Am Soc Echocardiogr. 1993;6:356–65.
117. Lee HR, Montenegro LM, Nicolson SC, Gaynor JW, Spray TL, Rychik J. Usefulness of intraoperative transesophageal echocardiography in predicting the degree of mitral regurgitation secondary to atrioventricular defect in children. Am J Cardiol. 1999;83:750–3.
118. Ayres NA, Miller-Hance W, Fyfe DA, et al. Indications and guidelines for performance of transesophageal echocardiography in the patient with pediatric acquired or congenital heart disease: report from the task force of the pediatric council of the American society of echocardiography. J Am Soc Echocardiogr. 2005;18:91–8.
119. Muhiudeen Russell IA, Miller-Hance WC, Silverman NH. Intraoperative transesophageal echocardiography for pediatric patients with congenital heart disease. Anesth Analg. 1998;87:1058–76.
120. Kamra K, Russell I, Miller-Hance WC. Role of transesophageal echocardiography in the management of pediatric patients with congenital heart disease. Paediatr Anaesth. 2011;21:479–93.
121. Stevenson JG. Incidence of complications in pediatric transesophageal echocardiography: experience in 1650 cases. J Am Soc Echocardiogr. 1999;12:527–32.
122. Andropoulos DB, Stayer SA, Bent ST, Campos CJ, Fraser CD. The effects of transesophageal echocardiography on hemodynamic variables in small infants undergoing cardiac surgery. J Cardiothorac Vasc Anesth. 2000;14:133–5.
123. Andropoulos DB, Ayres NA, Stayer SA, Bent ST, Campos CJ, Fraser CD. The effect of transesophageal echocardiography on ventilation in small infants undergoing cardiac surgery. Anesth Analg. 2000;90:47–9.
124. Mart CR, Fehr DM, Myers JL, Rosen KL. Intraoperative transesophageal echocardiography in a 1.4-kg infant with complex congenital heart disease. Pediatr Cardiol. 2003;24:84–5.
125. Zyblewski SC, Shirali GS, Forbus GA, et al. Initial experience with a miniaturized multiplane transesophageal probe in small infants undergoing cardiac operations. Ann Thorac Surg. 2010;89:1990–4.
126. Ferry PC. Neurologic sequelae of cardiac surgery in children. Am J Dis Child. 1987;141:309–12.
127. Ferry PC. Neurologic sequelae of open-heart surgery in children. An 'irritating question'. Am J Dis Child. 1990;144:369–73.

128. Fallon P, Aparicio JM, Elliott MJ, Kirkham FJ. Incidence of neurological complications of surgery for congenital heart disease. Arch Dis Child. 1995;72:418–22.
129. Menache CC, du Plessis AJ, Wessel DL, Jonas RA, Newburger JW. Current incidence of acute neurologic complications after open- heart operations in children. Ann Thorac Surg. 2002; 73:1752–8.
130. Wernovsky G, Newburger J. Neurologic and developmental morbidity in children with complex congenital heart disease. J Pediatr. 2003;142:6–8.
131. Dominguez TE, Wernovsky G, Gaynor JW. Cause and prevention of central nervous system injury in neonates undergoing cardiac surgery. Semin Thorac Cardiovasc Surg. 2007;19:269–77.
132. Marino BS, Lipkin PH, Newburger JW, et al. Neurodevelopmental outcomes in children with congenital heart disease: evaluation and management: a scientific statement from the American heart association. Circulation. 2012;126:1143–72.
133. Andropoulos DB, Stayer SA, Diaz LK, Ramamoorthy C. Neurological monitoring for congenital heart surgery. Anesth Analg. 2004;99:1365–75.
134. Ghanayem NS, Mitchell ME, Tweddell JS, Hoffman GM. Monitoring the brain before, during, and after cardiac surgery to improve long-term neurodevelopmental outcomes. Cardiol Young. 2006;16 Suppl 3:103–9.
135. Williams GD, Ramamoorthy C. Brain monitoring and protection during pediatric cardiac surgery. Semin Cardiothorac Vasc Anesth. 2007;11:23–33.
136. Kussman BD, Wypij D, DiNardo JA, et al. Cerebral oximetry during infant cardiac surgery: evaluation and relationship to early postoperative outcome. Anesth Analg. 2009;108:1122–31.
137. Kussman BD, Wypij D, Laussen PC, et al. Relationship of intraoperative cerebral oxygen saturation to neurodevelopmental outcome and brain magnetic resonance imaging at 1 year of age in infants undergoing biventricular repair. Circulation. 2010;122: 245–54.
138. Hoffman GM, Brosig CL, Mussatto KA, Tweddell JS, Ghanayem NS. Perioperative cerebral oxygen saturation in neonates with hypoplastic left heart syndrome and childhood neurodevelopmental outcome. J Thorac Cardiovasc Surg. 2013;146:1153–64.
139. Jobsis FF. Noninvasive, infrared monitoring of cerebral and myocardial oxygen sufficiency and circulatory parameters. Science. 1977;198:1264–7.
140. Fraser CDJ, Andropoulos DB. Neurologic monitoring for special cardiopulmonary bypass techniques. Semin Thorac Cardiovasc Surg Pediatr Card Surg Annu. 2004;7:125–32.
141. Hoffman GM. Neurologic monitoring on cardiopulmonary bypass: what are we obligated to do? Ann Thorac Surg. 2006; 81:S2373–2380.
142. Hoffman GM. Pro: near-infrared spectroscopy should be used for all cardiopulmonary bypass. J Cardiothorac Vasc Anesth. 2006;20:606–12.
143. Gottlieb EA, Fraser CDJ, Andropoulos DB, Diaz LK. Bilateral monitoring of cerebral oxygen saturation results in recognition of aortic cannula malposition during pediatric congenital heart surgery. Paediatr Anaesth. 2006;16:787–9.
144. Nelson DP, Andropoulos DB, Fraser CDJ. Perioperative neuroprotective strategies. Semin Thorac Cardiovasc Surg Pediatr Card Surg Annu. 2008:49–56.
145. Andropoulos DB, Diaz LK, Fraser CDJ, McKenzie ED, Stayer SA. Is bilateral monitoring of cerebral oxygen saturation necessary during neonatal aortic arch reconstruction? Anesth Analg. 2004;98:1267–72.
146. Kasman N, Brady K. Cerebral oximetry for pediatric anesthesia: why do intelligent clinicians disagree? Paediatr Anaesth. 2011;21: 473–8.
147. Hoffman GM, Stuth EA, Jaquiss RD, et al. Changes in cerebral and somatic oxygenation during stage 1 palliation of hypoplastic left heart syndrome using continuous regional cerebral perfusion. J Thorac Cardiovasc Surg. 2004;127:223–33.
148. Dent CL, Spaeth JP, Jones BV, et al. Brain magnetic resonance imaging abnormalities after the Norwood procedure using regional cerebral perfusion. J Thorac Cardiovasc Surg. 2006;131: 190–7.
149. Burrows FA. Transcranial Doppler monitoring of cerebral perfusion during cardiopulmonary bypass. Ann Thorac Surg. 1993;56:1482–4.
150. Doblar DD. Intraoperative transcranial ultrasonic monitoring for cardiac and vascular surgery. Semin Cardiothorac Vasc Anesth. 2004;8:127–45.
151. Zimmerman AA, Burrows FA, Jonas RA, Hickey PR. The limits of detectable cerebral perfusion by transcranial Doppler sonography in neonates undergoing deep hypothermic low-flow cardiopulmonary bypass. J Thorac Cardiovasc Surg. 1997;114: 594–600.
152. Andropoulos DB, Stayer SA, McKenzie ED, Fraser CDJ. Novel cerebral physiologic monitoring to guide low-flow cerebral perfusion during neonatal aortic arch reconstruction. J Thorac Cardiovasc Surg. 2003;125:491–9.
153. O'Brien JJ, Butterworth J, Hammon JW, Morris KJ, Phipps JM, Stump DA. Cerebral emboli during cardiac surgery in children. Anesthesiology. 1997;87:1063–9.
154. Anand KJ, Hickey PR. Halothane-morphine compared with high-dose sufentanil for anesthesia and postoperative analgesia in neonatal cardiac surgery. N Engl J Med. 1992;326:1–9.
155. Gruber EM, Laussen PC, Casta A, et al. Stress response in infants undergoing cardiac surgery: a randomized study of fentanyl bolus, fentanyl infusion, and fentanyl-midazolam infusion. Anesth Analg. 2001;92:882–90.
156. Rivenes SM, Lewin MB, Stayer SA, et al. Cardiovascular effects of sevoflurane, isoflurane, halothane, and fentanyl-midazolam in children with congenital heart disease: an echocardiographic study of myocardial contractility and hemodynamics. Anesthesiology. 2001;94:223–9.
157. Shen I, Giacomuzzi C, Ungerleider RM. Current strategies for optimizing the use of cardiopulmonary bypass in neonates and infants. Ann Thorac Surg. 2003;75:S729–734.
158. Hickey E, Karamlou T, You J, Ungerleider RM. Effects of circuit miniaturization in reducing inflammatory response to infant cardiopulmonary bypass by elimination of allogeneic blood products. Ann Thorac Surg. 2006;81:S2367–2372.
159. Koster A, Huebler M, Boettcher W, Redlin M, Berger F, Hetzer R. A new miniaturized cardiopulmonary bypass system reduces transfusion requirements during neonatal cardiac surgery: initial experience in 13 consecutive patients. J Thorac Cardiovasc Surg. 2009;137:1565–8.
160. Redlin M, Habazettl H, Boettcher W, et al. Effects of a comprehensive blood-sparing approach using body weight-adjusted miniaturized cardiopulmonary bypass circuits on transfusion requirements in pediatric cardiac surgery. J Thorac Cardiovasc Surg. 2012;144:493–9.
161. Bojan M, Constanza Basto Duarte M, Lopez Lopez V, Tourneur L, Pouard P, Vouhe P. Use of a miniaturized cardiopulmonary bypass circuit in neonates and infants is associated with fewer blood product transfusions. ASAIO J. 2011;57:527–32.
162. Golab HD, Scohy TV, de Jong PL, Kissler J, Takkenberg JJ, Bogers AJ. Relevance of colloid oncotic pressure regulation during neonatal and infant cardiopulmonary bypass: a prospective randomized study. Eur J Cardiothorac Surg. 2011;39:886–91.
163. Markarian M. Heparin resistance in newborn infants. [letter]. J Pediatr. 1983;103:175.

164. Guzzetta NA, Bajaj T, Fazlollah T, et al. A comparison of heparin management strategies in infants undergoing cardiopulmonary bypass. Anesth Analg. 2008;106:419–25.
165. Guzzetta NA, Monitz HG, Fernandez JD, Fazlollah TM, Knezevic A, Miller BE. Correlations between activated clotting time values and heparin concentration measurements in young infants undergoing cardiopulmonary bypass. Anesth Analg. 2010;111:173–9.
166. Jonas RA. Neurological protection during cardiopulmonary bypass/deep hypothermia. Pediatr Cardiol. 1998;19:321–30.
167. Motta P, Mossad E, Toscana D, Zestos M, Mee R. Comparison of phenoxybenzamine to sodium nitroprusside in infants undergoing surgery. J Cardiothorac Vasc Anesth. 2005;19:54–9.
168. Guzzetta NA. Phenoxybenzamine in the treatment of hypoplastic left heart syndrome: a core review. Anesth Analg. 2007;105: 312–5.
169. Mossad E, Motta P, Sehmbey K, Toscana D. The hemodynamic effects of phenoxybenzamine in neonates, infants, and children. J Clin Anesth. 2008;20:94–8.
170. Bellinger DC, Wernovsky G, Rappaport LA, et al. Cognitive development of children following early repair of transposition of the great arteries using deep hypothermic circulatory arrest. Pediatrics. 1991;87:701–7.
171. Muravchick S, Conrad DP, Vargas A. Peripheral temperature monitoring during cardiopulmonary bypass operation. Ann Thorac Surg. 1980;29:36–41.
172. Ramsay JG, Ralley FE, Whalley DG, DelliColli P, Wynands JE. Site of temperature monitoring and prediction of afterdrop after open heart surgery. Can Anaesth Soc J. 1985;32:607–12.
173. Shum-Tim D, Nagashima M, Shinoka T, et al. Postischemic hyperthermia exacerbates neurologic injury after deep hypothermic circulatory arrest. J Thorac Cardiovasc Surg. 1998;116: 780–92.
174. Bronicki RA, Chang AC. Management of the postoperative pediatric cardiac surgical patient. Crit Care Med. 2011;39:1974–84.
175. Mastropietro CW. Arginine vasopressin in neonates after surgery for congenital heart disease: right from the start? Pediatr Crit Care Med. 2012;13:360–1.
176. Noori S, Seri I. Neonatal blood pressure support: the use of inotropes, lusitropes, and other vasopressor agents. Clin Perinatol. 2012;39:221–38.
177. Alten JA, Borasino S, Toms R, Law MA, Moellinger A, Dabal RJ. Early initiation of arginine vasopressin infusion in neonates after complex cardiac surgery. Pediatr Crit Care Med. 2012; 13:300–4.
178. Chang AC, Atz AM, Wernovsky G, Burke RP, Wessel DL. Milrinone: systemic and pulmonary hemodynamic effects in neonates after cardiac surgery. Crit Care Med. 1995;23:1907–14.
179. Hoffman TM, Wernovsky G, Atz AM, et al. Efficacy and safety of milrinone in preventing low cardiac output syndrome in infants and children after corrective surgery for congenital heart disease. Circulation. 2003;107:996–1002.
180. Hoffman TM, Wernovsky G, Atz AM, et al. Prophylactic intravenous use of milrinone after cardiac operation in pediatrics (PRIMACORP) study. Prophylactic intravenous use of milrinone after cardiac operation in pediatrics. Am Heart J. 2002;143: 15–21.
181. Ozker E, Saritas B, Vuran C, Yoruker U, Ulugol H, Turkoz R. Delayed sternal closure after pediatric cardiac operations; single center experience: a retrospective study. J Cardiothorac Surg. 2012;7:102.
182. Heinle JS, Diaz LK, Fox LS. Early extubation after cardiac operations in neonates and young infants. J Thorac Cardiovasc Surg. 1997;114:413–8.
183. Wolf AR, Jackman L. Analgesia and sedation after pediatric cardiac surgery. Paediatr Anaesth. 2011;21:567–76.
184. Wypij D, Newburger JW, Rappaport LA, et al. The effect of duration of deep hypothermic circulatory arrest in infant heart surgery on late neurodevelopment: the Boston circulatory arrest trial. J Thorac Cardiovasc Surg. 2003;126:1397–403.
185. Pigula FA. Surgery for aortic arch disease in the neonate. Pediatr Cardiol. 2007;28:134–43.
186. Newburger JW, Jonas RA, Wernovsky G, et al. A comparison of the perioperative neurologic effects of hypothermic circulatory arrest versus low-flow cardiopulmonary bypass in infant heart surgery. N Engl J Med. 1993;329:1057–64.
187. Kilpack VD, Stayer SA, McKenzie ED, Fraser CDJ, Andropoulos DB. Limiting circulatory arrest using regional low flow perfusion. J Extra Corpor Technol. 2004;36:133–8.
188. Algra SO, Kornmann VN, van der Tweel I, Schouten AN, Jansen NJ, Haas F. Increasing duration of circulatory arrest, but not antegrade cerebral perfusion, prolongs postoperative recovery after neonatal cardiac surgery. J Thorac Cardiovasc Surg. 2012;143: 375–82.
189. Fraser CDJ, Andropoulos DB. Principles of antegrade cerebral perfusion during arch reconstruction in newborns/infants. Semin Thorac Cardiovasc Surg Pediatr Card Surg Annu. 2008;61–68.
190. Andropoulos DB, Easley RB, Brady K, et al. Neurodevelopmental outcomes after regional cerebral perfusion with neuromonitoring for neonatal aortic arch reconstruction. Ann Thorac Surg. 2013;95:648–55.
191. Duebener LF, Hagino I, Sakamoto T, et al. Effects of pH management during deep hypothermic bypass on cerebral microcirculation: alpha-stat versus pH-stat. Circulation. 2002;106:I103–108.
192. Griffin DA. Blood gas strategies and management during pediatric cardiopulmonary bypass. ASAIO J. 2005;51:657–8.
193. Montenegro LM, Greeley WJ. Pro: the use of modified ultrafiltration during pediatric cardiac surgery is a benefit. J Cardiothorac Vasc Anesth. 1998;12:480–2.
194. Elliott MJ. Ultrafiltration and modified ultrafiltration in pediatric open heart operations. Ann Thorac Surg. 1993;56:1518–22.
195. Journois D, Pouard P, Greeley WJ, Mauriat P, Vouhe P, Safran D. Hemofiltration during cardiopulmonary bypass in pediatric cardiac surgery. Effects on hemostasis, cytokines, and complement components. Anesthesiology. 1994;81:1181–9 (discussion 26A–27A).
196. Kuratani N, Bunsangjaroen P, Srimueang T, Masaki E, Suzuki T, Katogi T. Modified versus conventional ultrafiltration in pediatric cardiac surgery: a meta-analysis of randomized controlled trials comparing clinical outcome parameters. J Thorac Cardiovasc Surg. 2011;142:861–7.
197. Jonas RA, Wypij D, Roth SJ, et al. The influence of hemodilution on outcome after hypothermic cardiopulmonary bypass: results of a randomized trial in infants. J Thorac Cardiovasc Surg. 2003;126:1765–74.
198. Steven J, Nicolson S. Perioperative management of blood glucose during open heart surgery in infants and children. Paediatr Anaesth. 2011;21:530–7.
199. Yates AR, Dyke PC, Taeed R, et al. Hyperglycemia is a marker for poor outcome in the postoperative pediatric cardiac patient. Pediatr Crit Care Med. 2006;7:351–5.
200. Polito A, Thiagarajan RR, Laussen PC, et al. Association between intraoperative and early postoperative glucose levels and adverse outcomes after complex congenital heart surgery. Circulation. 2008;118:2235–42.
201. Scohy TV, Golab HD, Egal M, Takkenberg JJ, Bogers AJ. Intraoperative glycemic control without insulin infusion during pediatric cardiac surgery for congenital heart disease. Paediatr Anaesth. 2011;21:872–9.
202. Floyd TF, Horak J. Con: tight perioperative glycemic control. J Cardiothorac Vasc Anesth. 2009;23:906–8.

203. DeCampli WM, Olsen MC, Munro HM, Felix DE. Perioperative hyperglycemia: effect on outcome after infant congenital heart surgery. Ann Thorac Surg. 2010;89:181–5.
204. Rubens FD, Mesana T. The inflammatory response to cardiopulmonary bypass: a therapeutic overview. Perfusion. 2004;19 Suppl 1:S5–12.
205. Kozik DJ, Tweddell JS. Characterizing the inflammatory response to cardiopulmonary bypass in children. Ann Thorac Surg. 2006;81:S2347–2354.
206. Hall RI, Smith MS, Rocker G. The systemic inflammatory response to cardiopulmonary bypass: pathophysiological, therapeutic, and pharmacological considerations. Anesth Analg. 1997;85:766–82.
207. Laffey JG, Boylan JF, Cheng DC. The systemic inflammatory response to cardiac surgery: implications for the anesthesiologist. Anesthesiology. 2002;97:215–52.
208. Seghaye MC, Grabitz RG, Duchateau J, et al. Inflammatory reaction and capillary leak syndrome related to cardiopulmonary bypass in neonates undergoing cardiac operations. J Thorac Cardiovasc Surg. 1996;112:687–97.
209. Seghaye MC. The clinical implications of the systemic inflammatory reaction related to cardiac operations in children. Cardiol Young. 2003;13:228–39.
210. Bronicki RA, Backer CL, Baden HP, Mavroudis C, Crawford SE, Green TP. Dexamethasone reduces the inflammatory response to cardiopulmonary bypass in children. Ann Thorac Surg. 2000;69:1490–5.
211. Schroeder VA, Pearl JM, Schwartz SM, Shanley TP, Manning PB, Nelson DP. Combined steroid treatment for congenital heart surgery improves oxygen delivery and reduces postbypass inflammatory mediator expression. Circulation. 2003;107:2823–8.
212. Checchia PA, Bronicki RA, Costello JM, Nelson DP. Steroid use before pediatric cardiac operations using cardiopulmonary bypass: an international survey of 36 centers. Pediatr Crit Care Med. 2005;6:441–4.
213. Heying R, Wehage E, Schumacher K, et al. Dexamethasone pretreatment provides antiinflammatory and myocardial protection in neonatal arterial switch operation. Ann Thorac Surg. 2012;93:869–76.
214. Eaton MP, Iannoli EM. Coagulation considerations for infants and children undergoing cardiopulmonary bypass. Paediatr Anaesth. 2011;21:31–42.
215. Guzzetta NA, Miller BE. Principles of hemostasis in children: models and maturation. Paediatr Anaesth. 2011;21:3–9.
216. Kern FH, Morana NJ, Sears JJ, Hickey PR. Coagulation defects in neonates during cardiopulmonary bypass. Ann Thorac Surg. 1992;54:541–6.
217. Mauer HM, McCue CM, Caul J, Still WJ. Impairment in platelet aggregation in congenital heart disease. Blood. 1972;40:207–16.
218. Kneyber MC, Hersi MI, Twisk JW, Markhorst DG, Plotz FB. Red blood cell transfusion in critically ill children is independently associated with increased mortality. Intensive Care Med. 2007;33:1414–22.
219. Szekely A, Cserep Z, Sapi E, et al. Risks and predictors of blood transfusion in pediatric patients undergoing open heart operations. Ann Thorac Surg. 2009;87:187–97.
220. Kipps AK, Wypij D, Thiagarajan RR, Bacha EA, Newburger JW. Blood transfusion is associated with prolonged duration of mechanical ventilation in infants undergoing reparative cardiac surgery. Pediatr Crit Care Med. 2011;12:52–6.
221. Salvin JW, Scheurer MA, Laussen PC, et al. Blood transfusion after pediatric cardiac surgery is associated with prolonged hospital stay. Ann Thorac Surg. 2011;91:204–10.
222. Guzzetta NA. Benefits and risks of red blood cell transfusion in pediatric patients undergoing cardiac surgery. Paediatr Anaesth. 2011;21:504–11.
223. Gruenwald CE, Manlhiot C, Chan AK, et al. Randomized, controlled trial of individualized heparin and protamine management in infants undergoing cardiac surgery with cardiopulmonary bypass. J Am Coll Cardiol. 2010;56:1794–802.
224. Andreasen JB, Hvas AM, Christiansen K, Ravn HB. Can RoTEM(R) analysis be applied for haemostatic monitoring in paediatric congenital heart surgery? Cardiol Young. 2011;21: 684–91.
225. Hofer A, Kozek-Langenecker S, Schaden E, Panholzer M, Gombotz H. Point-of-care assessment of platelet aggregation in paediatric open heart surgery. Br J Anaesth. 2011;107:587–92.
226. Abdel Raheem MM, Mohamed WA. Impact of congenital heart disease on brain development in newborn infants. Ann Pediatr Cardiol. 2012;5:21–6.
227. Miller BE, Guzzetta NA, Tosone SR, Levy JH. Rapid evaluation of coagulopathies after cardiopulmonary bypass in children using modified thromboelastography. Anesth Analg. 2000;90: 1324–30.
228. Romlin BS, Wahlander H, Berggren H, et al. Intraoperative thromboelastometry is associated with reduced transfusion prevalence in pediatric cardiac surgery. Anesth Analg. 2011;112:30–6.
229. Gautam NK, Schmitz ML, Harrison D, et al. Impact of protamine dose on activated clotting time and thromboelastography in infants and small children undergoing cardiopulmonary bypass. Paediatr Anaesth. 2013;23:233–41.
230. Eaton MP. Antifibrinolytic therapy in surgery for congenital heart disease. Anesth Analg. 2008;106:1087–100.
231. Hill GE, Pohorecki R, Alonso A, Rennard SI, Robbins RA. Aprotinin reduces interleukin-8 production and lung neutrophil accumulation after cardiopulmonary bypass. Anesth Analg. 1996;83:696–700.
232. Pasquali SK, Li JS, He X, et al. Comparative analysis of antifibrinolytic medications in pediatric heart surgery. J Thorac Cardiovasc Surg. 2012;143:550–7.
233. Coleman CI, Rigali VT, Hammond J, Kluger J, Jeleniowski KW, White CM. Evaluating the safety implications of aprotinin use: the retrospective evaluation of aprotinin in cardio thoracic surgery (REACTS). J Thorac Cardiovasc Surg. 2007;133:1547–52.
234. Guzzetta NA, Evans FM, Rosenberg ES, et al. The impact of aprotinin on postoperative renal dysfunction in neonates undergoing cardiopulmonary bypass: a retrospective analysis. Anesth Analg. 2009;108:448–55.
235. Bojan M, Vicca S, Boulat C, Gioanni S, Pouard P. Aprotinin, transfusions, and kidney injury in neonates and infants undergoing cardiac surgery. Br J Anaesth. 2012;108:830–7.
236. Kylasam S, Mos K, Fijtin S, Webster B, Chard R, Egan J. Recombinant activated factor VII following pediatric cardiac surgery. J Intensive Care Med. 2009;24:116–21.
237. Pychynska-Pokorska M, Pagowska-Klimek I, Krajewski W, Moll JJ. Use of recombinant activated factor VII for controlling refractory postoperative bleeding in children undergoing cardiac surgery with cardiopulmonary bypass. J Cardiothorac Vasc Anesth. 2011;25:987–94.
238. Guzzetta NA, Russell IA, Williams GD. Review of the off-label use of recombinant activated factor VII in pediatric cardiac surgery patients. Anesth Analg. 2012;115:364–78.
239. del Nido PJ. Developmental and neurologic outcomes late after neonatal corrective surgery. J Thorac Cardiovasc Surg. 2002; 124:425–7.
240. Hovels-Gurich HH, Seghaye MC, Schnitker R, et al. Long-term neurodevelopmental outcomes in school-aged children after neonatal arterial switch operation. J Thorac Cardiovasc Surg. 2002;124:448–58.
241. Walker K, Holland AJ, Winlaw D, Sherwood M, Badawi N. Neurodevelopmental outcomes and surgery in neonates. J Paediatr Child Health. 2006;42:749–51.

242. Gaynor JW, Nicolson SC, Jarvik GP, et al. Increasing duration of deep hypothermic circulatory arrest is associated with an increased incidence of postoperative electroencephalographic seizures. J Thorac Cardiovasc Surg. 2005;130:1278–86.
243. Gaynor JW, Jarvik GP, Bernbaum J, et al. The relationship of postoperative electrographic seizures to neurodevelopmental outcome at 1 year of age after neonatal and infant cardiac surgery. J Thorac Cardiovasc Surg. 2006;131:181–9.
244. Chen J, Zimmerman RA, Jarvik GP, et al. Perioperative stroke in infants undergoing open heart operations for congenital heart disease. Ann Thorac Surg. 2009;88:823–9.
245. Galli KK, Zimmerman RA, Jarvik GP, et al. Periventricular leukomalacia is common after neonatal cardiac surgery. J Thorac Cardiovasc Surg. 2004;127:692–704.
246. Gaynor JW. Periventricular leukomalacia following neonatal and infant cardiac surgery. Semin Thorac Cardiovasc Surg Pediatr Card Surg Annu. 2004;7:133–40.
247. Kirkham FJ. Recognition and prevention of neurological complications in pediatric cardiac surgery. Pediatr Cardiol. 1998; 19:331–45.
248. Kaltman JR, Jarvik GP, Bernbaum J, et al. Neurodevelopmental outcome after early repair of a ventricular septal defect with or without aortic arch obstruction. J Thorac Cardiovasc Surg. 2006;131:792–8.
249. Schultz AH, Jarvik GP, Wernovsky G, et al. Effect of congenital heart disease on neurodevelopmental outcomes within multiple-gestation births. J Thorac Cardiovasc Surg. 2005;130:1511–6.
250. Tabbutt S, Nord AS, Jarvik GP, et al. Neurodevelopmental outcomes after staged palliation for hypoplastic left heart syndrome. Pediatrics. 2008;121:476–83.
251. Gaynor JW, Wernovsky G, Jarvik GP, et al. Patient characteristics are important determinants of neurodevelopmental outcome at one year of age after neonatal and infant cardiac surgery. J Thorac Cardiovasc Surg. 2007;133:1344–53, 1353.e1-3.
252. Andropoulos DB, Easley RB, Brady K, et al. Changing expectations for neurological outcomes after the neonatal arterial switch operation. Ann Thorac Surg. 2012;94:1250–5 (discussion 1255–1256).
253. Tabbutt S, Gaynor JW, Newburger JW. Neurodevelopmental outcomes after congenital heart surgery and strategies for improvement. Curr Opin Cardiol. 2012;27:82–91.
254. Bellinger DC, Wypij D, Kuban KC, et al. Developmental and neurological status of children at 4 years of age after heart surgery with hypothermic circulatory arrest or low-flow cardiopulmonary bypass. Circulation. 1999;100:526–32.
255. Groom RC, Hill AG, Akl B, Lefrak EA, Kurusz M. Rapid cooling: a potentially dangerous practice.[letter]. Perfusion. 1994;9: 142–3.
256. Laussen PC. Optimal blood gas management during deep hypothermic paediatric cardiac surgery: alpha-stat is easy, but pH-stat may be preferable. Paediatr Anaesth. 2002;12:199–204.
257. Newburger JW, Jonas RA, Soul J, et al. Randomized trial of hematocrit 25 % versus 35 % during hypothermic cardiopulmonary bypass in infant heart surgery. J Thorac Cardiovasc Surg. 2008;135:347–54, 354.e1-4.
258. Wypij D, Jonas RA, Bellinger DC, et al. The effect of hematocrit during hypothermic cardiopulmonary bypass in infant heart surgery: results from the combined Boston hematocrit trials. J Thorac Cardiovasc Surg. 2008;135:355–60.
259. Limperopoulos C, Majnemer A, Shevell MI, Rosenblatt B, Rohlicek C, Tchervenkov C. Neurologic status of newborns with congenital heart defects before open heart surgery. Pediatrics. 1999;103:402–8.
260. Miller SP, McQuillen PS, Hamrick S, et al. Abnormal brain development in newborns with congenital heart disease. N Engl J Med. 2007;357:1928–38.
261. Andropoulos DB, Hunter JV, Nelson DP, et al. Brain immaturity is associated with brain injury before and after neonatal cardiac surgery with high-flow bypass and cerebral oxygenation monitoring. J Thorac Cardiovasc Surg. 2010;139:543–56.
262. McQuillen PS, Miller SP. Congenital heart disease and brain development. Ann N Y Acad Sci. 2010;1184:68–86.
263. Clouchoux C, du Plessis AJ, Bouyssi-Kobar M, et al. Delayed cortical development in fetuses with complex congenital heart disease. Cereb Cortex. 2013;23:2932–43.
264. Goff DA, Luan X, Gerdes M, et al. Younger gestational age is associated with worse neurodevelopmental outcomes after cardiac surgery in infancy. J Thorac Cardiovasc Surg. 2012; 143:535–42.
265. McQuillen PS, Goff DA, Licht DJ. Effects of congenital heart disease on brain development. Prog Pediatr Cardiol. 2010;29: 79–85.
266. Zeltser I, Jarvik GP, Bernbaum J, et al. Genetic factors are important determinants of neurodevelopmental outcome after repair of tetralogy of Fallot. J Thorac Cardiovasc Surg. 2008;135:91–7.
267. Licht DJ, Shera DM, Clancy RR, et al. Brain maturation is delayed in infants with complex congenital heart defects. J Thorac Cardiovasc Surg. 2009;137:529–36 (discussion 536–7).
268. McQuillen PS, Hamrick SE, Perez MJ, et al. Balloon atrial septostomy is associated with preoperative stroke in neonates with transposition of the great arteries. Circulation. 2006;113:280–5.
269. Petit CJ, Rome JJ, Wernovsky G, et al. Preoperative brain injury in transposition of the great arteries is associated with oxygenation and time to surgery, not balloon atrial septostomy. Circulation. 2009;119:709–16.
270. Beca J, Gunn J, Coleman L, et al. Pre-operative brain injury in newborn infants with transposition of the great arteries occurs at rates similar to other complex congenital heart disease and is not related to balloon atrial septostomy. J Am Coll Cardiol. 2009;53:1807–11.
271. Mintz CD, Wagner M, Loepke AW. Preclinical research into the effects of anesthetics on the developing brain: promises and pitfalls. J Neurosurg Anesthesiol. 2012;24:362–7.
272. Shih J, May LDV, Gonzalez HE, Lee EW, et al. Delayed environmental enrichment reverses sevoflurane-induced memory impairment in rats. Anesthesiology. 2012;116:586–602.
273. Ramsay JG, Roizen M. SmartTots: a public-private partnership between the United States food and drug administration (FDA) and the international anesthesia research society (IARS). Paediatr Anaesth. 2012;22:969–72.
274. Vutskits L, Davis PJ, Hansen TG. Anesthetics and the developing brain: time for a change in practice? A pro/con debate. Paediatr Anaesth. 2012;22:973–80.
275. Hirsch JC, Jacobs ML, Andropoulos D, et al. Protecting the infant brain during cardiac surgery: a systematic review. Ann Thorac Surg. 2012;94:1365–73 (discussion 1373).
276. Andropoulos DB, Brady KM, Easley RB, Fraser CDJ. Neuroprotection in pediatric cardiac surgery: what is on the horizon? Prog Pediatr Cardiol. 2010;29:113–22.
277. Chai PJ, Williamson JA, Lodge AJ, et al. Effects of ischemia on pulmonary dysfunction after cardiopulmonary bypass. Ann Thorac Surg. 1999;67:731–5.
278. Hachenberg T, Tenling A, Nystrom SO, Tyden H, Hedenstierna G. Ventilation-perfusion inequality in patients undergoing cardiac surgery. Anesthesiology. 1994;80:509–19.
279. von Ungern-Sternberg BS, Petak F, Saudan S, Pellegrini M, Erb TO, Habre W. Effect of cardiopulmonary bypass and aortic clamping on functional residual capacity and ventilation distribution in children. J Thorac Cardiovasc Surg. 2007;134:1193–8.
280. Friedman M, Sellke FW, Wang SY, Weintraub RM, Johnson RG. Parameters of pulmonary injury after total or partial cardiopulmonary bypass. Circulation. 1994;90:II262–268.

281. Apostolakis EE, Koletsis EN, Baikoussis NG, Siminelakis SN, Papadopoulos GS. Strategies to prevent intraoperative lung injury during cardiopulmonary bypass. J Cardiothorac Surg. 2010;5:1.
282. Kagawa H, Morita K, Nagahori R, Shinohara G, Kinouchi K, Hashimoto K. Prevention of ischemia/reperfusion-induced pulmonary dysfunction after cardiopulmonary bypass with terminal leukocyte-depleted lung reperfusion. J Thorac Cardiovasc Surg. 2010;139:174–80.
283. Blatchford JWr, Barragry TP, Lillehei TJ, Ring WS. Effects of cardioplegic arrest on left ventricular systolic and diastolic function of the intact neonatal heart. J Thorac Cardiovasc Surg. 1994;107:527–35.
284. Skippen PW, Krahn GE. Acute renal failure in children undergoing cardiopulmonary bypass. Crit Care Resusc. 2005;7:286–91.
285. Kist-van Holthe tot Echten JE, Goedvolk CA, Doornaar MB, et al. Acute renal insufficiency and renal replacement therapy after pediatric cardiopulmonary bypass surgery. Pediatr Cardiol. 2001;22:321–326.
286. Sethi SK, Goyal D, Yadav DK, et al. Predictors of acute kidney injury post-cardiopulmonary bypass in children. Clin Exp Nephrol. 2011;15:529–34.
287. Aydin SI, Seiden HS, Blaufox AD, et al. Acute kidney injury after surgery for congenital heart disease. Ann Thorac Surg. 2012;94:1589–95.
288. Blinder JJ, Goldstein SL, Lee VV, et al. Congenital heart surgery in infants: effects of acute kidney injury on outcomes. J Thorac Cardiovasc Surg. 2012;143:368–74.
289. Jetton JG, Askenazi DJ. Update on acute kidney injury in the neonate. Curr Opin Pediatr. 2012;24:191–6.
290. Chiravuri SD, Riegger LQ, Christensen R, et al. Factors associated with acute kidney injury or failure in children undergoing cardiopulmonary bypass: a case-controlled study. Paediatr Anaesth. 2011;21:880–6.
291. Sorof JM, Stromberg D, Brewer ED, Feltes TF, Fraser CDJ. Early initiation of peritoneal dialysis after surgical repair of congenital heart disease. Pediatr Nephrol. 1999;13:641–5.
292. Bojan M, Gioanni S, Vouhe PR, Journois D, Pouard P. Early initiation of peritoneal dialysis in neonates and infants with acute kidney injury following cardiac surgery is associated with a significant decrease in mortality. Kidney Int. 2012;82:474–81.
293. Allen KB, Salam AA, Lumsden AB. Acute mesenteric ischemia after cardiopulmonary bypass. J Vasc Surg. 1992;16:391–5 (discussion 395–396).
294. Ott MJ, Buchman TG, Baumgartner WA. Postoperative abdominal complications in cardiopulmonary bypass patients: a case-controlled study. Ann Thorac Surg. 1995;59:1210–3.
295. Carlo WF, Kimball TR, Michelfelder EC, Border WL. Persistent diastolic flow reversal in abdominal aortic Doppler-flow profiles is associated with an increased risk of necrotizing enterocolitis in term infants with congenital heart disease. Pediatrics. 2007;119:330–5.
296. Stapleton GE, Eble BK, Dickerson HA, Andropoulos DB, Chang AC. Mesenteric oxygen desaturation in an infant with congenital heart disease and necrotizing enterocolitis. Tex Heart Inst J. 2007;34:442–4.
297. Shteyer E, Yatsiv I, Sharkia M, Milgarter E, Granot E. Serum transaminases as a prognostic factor in children post cardiac surgery. Pediatr Int. 2011;53:725–8.
298. Farouk A, Karimi M, Henderson M, Ostrowsky J, Siwik E, Hennein H. Cerebral regional oxygenation during aortic coarctation repair in pediatric population. Eur J Cardiothorac Surg. 2008;34:26–31.
299. Shah RK, Mora BN, Bacha E, et al. The presentation and management of vascular rings: an otolaryngology perspective. Int J Pediatr Otorhinolaryngol. 2007;71:57–62.
300. Kussman BD, Geva T, McGowan FX. Cardiovascular causes of airway compression. Paediatr Anaesth. 2004;14:60–74.
301. Dillman JR, Attili AK, Agarwal PP, Dorfman AL, Hernandez RJ, Strouse PJ. Common and uncommon vascular rings and slings: a multi-modality review. Pediatr Radiol. 2011;41:1440–54 (quiz 1489–90).
302. Hernanz-Schulman M. Vascular rings: a practical approach to imaging diagnosis. Pediatr Radiol. 2005;35:961–79.
303. Backer CL, Mavroudis C, Rigsby CK, Holinger LD. Trends in vascular ring surgery. J Thorac Cardiovasc Surg. 2005;129: 1339–47.
304. Duncan BW. Mechanical circulatory support for infants and children with cardiac disease. Ann Thorac Surg. 2002;73:1670–7.
305. Morales DL, Zafar F, Rossano JW, et al. Use of ventricular assist devices in children across the United States: analysis of 7.5 million pediatric hospitalizations. Ann Thorac Surg. 2010;90:1313–8.
306. Checchia PA. Perioperative mechanical circulatory support in children with critical heart disease. Curr Treat Options Cardiovasc Med. 2011;13:414–24.
307. del Nido PJ, Dalton HJ, Thompson AE, Siewers RD. Extracorporeal membrane oxygenator rescue in children during cardiac arrest after cardiac surgery. Circulation. 1992;86:II300–4.
308. Walters HLr, Hakimi M, Rice MD, Lyons JM, Whittlesey GC, Klein MD. Pediatric cardiac surgical ECMO: multivariate analysis of risk factors for hospital death. Ann Thorac Surg. 1995;60:329–36 (discussion 336–7).
309. Aharon AS, Drinkwater DCJ, Churchwell KB, et al. Extracorporeal membrane oxygenation in children after repair of congenital cardiac lesions. Ann Thorac Surg. 2001;72:2095–101 (discussion 2101–2102).
310. Dalton HJ, Rycus PT, Conrad SA. Update on extracorporeal life support 2004. Semin Perinatol. 2005;29:24–33.
311. Adachi I, Fraser CDJ. Mechanical circulatory support for infants and small children. Semin Thorac Cardiovasc Surg Pediatr Card Surg Annu. 2011;14:38–44.
312. Hetzer R, Alexi-Meskishvili V, Weng Y, et al. Mechanical cardiac support in the young with the Berlin Heart EXCOR pulsatile ventricular assist device: 15 years' experience. Semin Thorac Cardiovasc Surg Pediatr Card Surg Annu. 2006:99–108.
313. Fraser CDJ, Jaquiss RD, Rosenthal DN, et al. Prospective trial of a pediatric ventricular assist device. N Engl J Med. 2012;367:532–41.
314. Konertz W, Hotz H, Schneider M, Redlin M, Reul H. Clinical experience with the MEDOS HIA-VAD system in infants and children: a preliminary report. Ann Thorac Surg. 1997;63: 1138–44.
315. Fragasso T, Ricci Z, Grutter G, et al. Incidence of healthcare-associated infections in a pediatric population with an extracorporeal ventricular assist device. Artif Organs. 2011;35:1110–4.
316. Joffe AR, Lequier L, Robertson CM. Pediatric outcomes after extracorporeal membrane oxygenation for cardiac disease and for cardiac arrest: a review. ASAIO J. 2012;58:297–310.
317. Brancaccio G, Amodeo A, Ricci Z, et al. Mechanical assist device as a bridge to heart transplantation in children less than 10 kilograms. Ann Thorac Surg. 2010;90:58–62.
318. Gazit AZ, Gandhi SK, Canter CC. Mechanical circulatory support of the critically ill child awaiting heart transplantation. Curr Cardiol Rev. 2010;6:46–53.
319. Brancaccio G, Filippelli S, Michielon G, et al. Ventricular assist devices as a bridge to heart transplantation or as destination therapy in pediatric patients. Transplant Proc. 2012;44:2007–12.
320. Yuki K, Sharma R, DiNardo J. Ventricular-assist device therapy in children. Best Pract Res Clin Anaesthesiol. 2012;26:247–64.
321. Cave DA, Fry KM, Buchholz H. Anesthesia for noncardiac procedures for children with a Berlin heart EXCOR pediatric

ventricular assist device: a case series. Paediatr Anaesth. 2010;20:647–59.
322. Pratap JN, Wilmshurst S. Anesthetic management of children with in situ Berlin heart EXCOR. Paediatr Anaesth. 2010;20: 812–20.
323. Haynes S, Cassidy J, Murphy T, McClintock J, Smith J, McCheyne A. Pratap JN, Wilmhurst S: Anesthetic management of children with in situ Berlin heart EXCOR: pediatric anesthesia: 2010: 20: 812–820. Paediatr Anaesth. 2010;20:1137–8.
324. Tulloh RM. Congenital heart disease in relation to pulmonary hypertension in paediatric practice. Paediatr Respir Rev. 2005;6:174–80.
325. Tulloh R. Etiology, diagnosis, and pharmacologic treatment of pediatric pulmonary hypertension. Paediatr Drugs. 2009;11: 115–28.
326. Suzuki K, Yamaki S, Mimori S, et al. Pulmonary vascular disease in Down's syndrome with complete atrioventricular septal defect. Am J Cardiol. 2000;86:434–7.
327. Bando K, Turrentine MW, Sharp TG, et al. Pulmonary hypertension after operations for congenital heart disease: analysis of risk factors and management. J Thorac Cardiovasc Surg. 1996;112:1600–7. discussion 1607–1609.
328. Friesen RH, Williams GD. Anesthetic management of children with pulmonary arterial hypertension. Paediatr Anaesth. 2008; 18:208–16.
329. Bronicki RA. Perioperative management of pulmonary hypertension in children with critical heart disease. Curr Treat Options Cardiovasc Med. 2011;13:402–13.
330. Khazin V, Kaufman Y, Zabeeda D, et al. Milrinone and nitric oxide: combined effect on pulmonary artery pressures after cardiopulmonary bypass in children. J Cardiothorac Vasc Anesth. 2004;18:156–9.
331. Checchia PA, Bronicki RA, Goldstein B. Review of inhaled nitric oxide in the pediatric cardiac surgery setting. Pediatr Cardiol. 2012;33:493–505.
332. Murphy TW, Smith JH, Ranger MR, Haynes SR. General anesthesia for children with severe heart failure. Pediatr Cardiol. 2011;32:139–44.
333. Suarez CR, Menendez CE, Griffin AJ, Ow EP, Walenga JM, Fareed J. Cyanotic congenital heart disease in children: hemostatic disorders and relevance of molecular markers of hemostasis. Semin Thromb Hemost. 1984;10:285–9.
334. Tempe DK, Virmani S. Coagulation abnormalities in patients with cyanotic congenital heart disease. J Cardiothorac Vasc Anesth. 2002;16:752–65.
335. Haddad F, Hunt SA, Rosenthal DN, Murphy DJ. Right ventricular function in cardiovascular disease, part I: anatomy, physiology, aging, and functional assessment of the right ventricle. Circulation. 2008;117:1436–48.
336. Bancalari E, Jesse MJ, Gelband H, Garcia O. Lung mechanics in congenital heart disease with increased and decreased pulmonary blood flow. J Pediatr. 1977;90:192–5.
337. Yau KI, Fang LJ, Wu MH. Lung mechanics in infants with left-to-right shunt congenital heart disease. Pediatr Pulmonol. 1996;21:42–7.
338. Stayer SA, Diaz LK, East DL, et al. Changes in respiratory mechanics among infants undergoing heart surgery. Anesth Analg. 2004;98:49–55.
339. Holtby H. Con: regional anesthesia is not an important component of the anesthetic technique for pediatric patients undergoing cardiac surgical procedures. J Cardiothorac Vasc Anesth. 2002; 16:379–81.
340. Rosen DA, Rosen KR, Hammer GB. Pro: regional anesthesia is an important component of the anesthetic technique for pediatric patients undergoing cardiac surgical procedures. J Cardiothorac Vasc Anesth. 2002;16:374–8.
341. Bosenberg AT, Johr M, Wolf AR. Pro con debate: the use of regional vs systemic analgesia for neonatal surgery. Paediatr Anaesth. 2011;21:1247–58.
342. Hammer GB, Golianu B. Opioid analgesia in neonates following cardiac surgery. Semin Cardiothorac Vasc Anesth. 2007;11: 47–58.
343. Golianu B, Hammer GB. Pain management for pediatric thoracic surgery. Curr Opin Anaesthesiol. 2005;18:13–21.
344. Martin RD, Parisi F, Robinson TW, Bailey L. Anesthetic management of neonatal cardiac transplantation. J Cardiothorac Anesth. 1989;3:465–9.
345. Blasco LM, Parameshwar J, Vuylsteke A. Anaesthesia for noncardiac surgery in the heart transplant recipient. Curr Opin Anaesthesiol. 2009;22:109–13.

13 Anesthesia Outside the Operating Room

Christopher Heard, Satyan Lakshminrusimha, and Jerrold Lerman

Neonates Are Not Small Children

In the same way children are not just small adults, neonates (especially premature neonates) are not small children. There are a number of unique physiological features in term and premature neonates that hold great importance to the anesthesiologist. Some of these features are shown in Fig. 13.1 and described below:

1. Oxygen toxicity: Human fetuses are hypoxemic with PO_2 values ranging between 20 and 32 mmHg. The antioxidant mechanisms are not well developed in neonates [1] and premature infants are even more susceptible to oxygen toxicity after exposure to excessive levels of oxygen [2]. The association between oxygen exposure and retinopathy of prematurity (ROP) and bronchopulmonary dysplasia (BPD) is well established [3–7]. Several animal and human studies have also reported increased pulmonary arterial contractility [8], biochemical oxidative stress [9], and increased risk of cancer [10] after even brief exposure to 100 % oxygen in the delivery room at birth. In the past, anesthesiologists routinely used 100 % oxygen to ventilate the lungs of neonates with during surgery to avoid hypoxia or due to a lack of air. Increased awareness of oxygen toxicity has led to changes in this practice. In the OR, all neonates undergoing emergent surgery with a rapid sequence induction are still preoxygenated for several minutes to prevent desaturation while the airway is secured, although most neonates do not tolerate a face mask without objection. This practice continues today. A recent survey of 247 anesthetists in the United Kingdom demonstrated that <40 % oxygen is used during neonatal anesthesia by 52 % of respondents and >40 % oxygen is used by <16 % [11]. Few anesthesiologists administer 100 % oxygen to neonates and premature infants [11]. However, 10 % of the respondents suggested that they do not make a conscious effort to avoid 100 % oxygen during neonatal anesthesia. The use of 100 % oxygen is also associated with pulmonary atelectasis. The potential risks of desaturation during anesthesia and concern over the need for a margin of safety in light of the evidence that the incidence of desaturation including severe desaturation (<80 %) increases with decreasing age [12] have led to the use of 30–40 % oxygen during neonatal anesthesia (in the absence of significant lung disease) to maintain a target preductal oxygen saturation of ~90 % (see Complication chapter 16). The pulse oximeter should be sited on the right hand (preductal) to display the oxygen saturation. Oxygen saturations of 99–100 % are often associated with supraphysiological PaO_2 and potential toxicity to the retina and lungs in neonates and, in particular, in very low birth weight (VLBW) infants. Oxygen saturations of 85–89 % have been associated with an increased mortality when compared with 91–95 % in infants <28 weeks gestation at birth, although this notion remains contentious and unresolved (see Complication chapter). Oxygen saturations should be closely monitored during mechanical ventilation of both premature and full-term neonates under anesthesia with target saturations set to ~90 %, to limit ROP and lung disease while avoiding an increase in mortality [5–7].
2. Similarly, the use of 100 % oxygen for transport from the NICU to the OR is also contentious. The use of 100 % oxygen delays the time to serious desaturation in

C. Heard, MD (✉)
Department of Anesthesiology, Division of Pediatrics, Women and Children's Hospital of Buffalo, 219 Bryant Street, Buffalo, NY 14222, USA
e-mail: gazzzman13@gmail.com

S. Lakshminrusimha
Division of Neonatology, Department of Pediatrics, Women and Children's Hospital of Buffalo, 219 Bryant Street, Buffalo, NY 14222, USA

J. Lerman
Department of Anesthesiology, Women and Children's Hospital of Buffalo, State University of New York, Buffalo, NY USA

University of Rochester Medical Center, Rochester, NY USA

J. Lerman (ed.), *Neonatal Anesthesia*, DOI 10.1007/978-1-4419-6041-2_13,

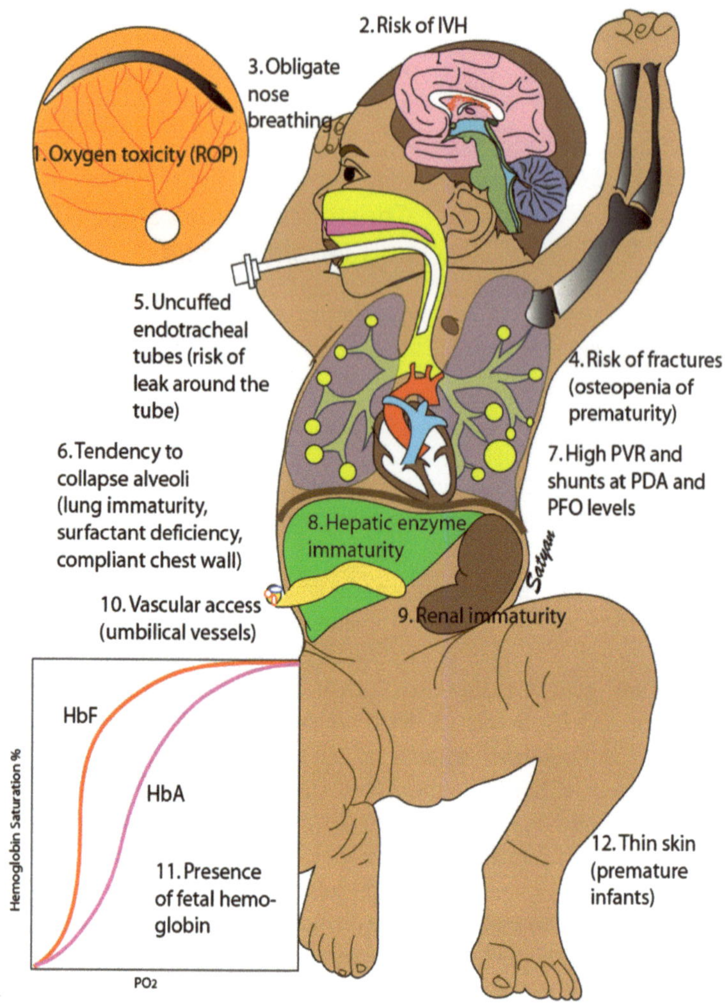

Fig. 13.1 Physiologic factors in the full-term and premature infants that can influence their management during anesthesia and surgery. See text for details

both infants [13] and critically ill patients during transport [14]. This allows more time for corrective action before cardiac and neurologic sequelae from hypoxia may occur. The notion of using 100 % oxygen for high-risk procedures balances the potential of a possible long-term risk of ROP and lung disease against the immediate potentially lifesaving benefits of delayed desaturation and cardiac arrest.

3. Lung development continues during fetal life with limited surfactant production until almost 34 weeks gestation [15]. The combination of a lack of surfactant and a compliant chest wall increases the risk that the small bronchioles will collapse during expiration. Positive end expiratory pressure (PEEP) is crucial during ventilation in premature infants. Furthermore, if BPD is present, airway resistance is increased leading to an increased risk of air trapping. The use of appropriate PEEP, low rates, and prolonged expiratory times may be necessary to optimize ventilation (see Ventilation chapter 9).
4. Respiratory control is immature in premature infants resulting in episodes of apnea and bradycardia. The risk of postoperative apnea (of prematurity) increases with infants of younger gestational and/or postconceptional age and anemia [16].
5. Premature and full-term neonates are considered obligate nose breathers, although they are capable of mouth breathing during nasal occlusion [17]. The shift to mouth breathing in response to nasal occlusion becomes more automatic with advancing postconceptional age [18]. Nonetheless, infants with choanal stenosis and atresia and some craniofacial anomalies (e.g., Pierre Robin sequence, Crouzon syndrome) remain at risk for apnea. It is important to suction the nares and ensure the patency of the nasal passages before extubating the trachea in these infants.
6. Uncuffed tracheal tubes (TTs) have been the standard for premature and term neonatal infants. Issues associated with the use of uncuffed TTs during anesthesia include difficulties in maintaining targeted tidal volumes

during mechanical ventilation (particularly in infants with poorly compliant lungs), multiple tracheal intubations to achieve a properly sized tube, and expiratory gas leak and OR pollution [19, 20]. Two manufacturers currently supply small-diameter cuffed TTs: the Lo-Pro/Lo-Contour 3.0 mm internal diameter TT (Mallinckrodt© USA) and the 3.0 mm Microcuff© TT (Kimberly Clark, USA). These TTs have similar outer diameters as the comparable uncuffed TTs although the latter tubes have been modified to include an elliptical-shaped, more caudally placed, thin-walled cuff without a Murphy eye. Few studies have documented the safety and long-term use of these TTs in premature and full-term neonates [21]. A recent report cited three cases of stridor in young infants whose weights were less than those recommended for the 3.0 mm Microcuff TT, 3 kg, suggesting that even high-compliance cuffed TTs may cause stridor [22]. Preliminary retrospective data from the NICU support such a concern [23]. The use of cuffed TTs in premature and full-term neonates warrants further study (see Airway chapter 5).

7. Premature and term infants may have increased pulmonary vascular resistance (PVR). When PVR increases as in the presence of hypoxia or acidosis, right-to-left shunting of blood at the patent foramen ovale (PFO) or Patent Ductus Arteriosus (PDA) may occur, resulting in cyanosis [24, 25]. Since the pCO_2 may directly increase the PVR, one strategy to reduce the PVR is to reduce the pCO_2. However, hypocarbia from overventilation decreases cerebral perfusion and may lead to periventricular leukomalacia (PVL) in premature infants [26].
8. Intraventricular hemorrhage (IVH) is common in extremely low birth weight (ELBW) premature infants [27]. Friable vasculature in the subependymal region of the lateral ventricles is prominent during early gestation and involutes with advancing gestational age. Several risk factors increase the risk of IVH including wide fluctuations in $PaCO_2$ or hypercapnia, rapid infusion of fluids and sodium bicarbonate, and increases in intrathoracic pressure (e.g., as a result of pneumothorax) [28]. Studies in ELBW infants (<1,000 g at birth) suggest that wide fluctuation in $PaCO_2$ (i.e., difference between maximum and minimum $pCO_2 > 42$ mmHg) during the first 4 days of life is an important risk factor for IVH [29]. Wide swings in monitored variables should be avoided during anesthesia as well, although this presents a great challenge in infants with BPD.
9. Immaturity of the hepatic enzyme systems increases the neonate's risk for toxicity from medications. Neonates receiving parenteral alimentation for prolonged periods are at risk for cholestatic liver disease [30] resulting in further compromise to hepatic function.
10. Fetal accretion rates for calcium and phosphorus are high. Many growing premature infants cannot maintain similar bone mineralization after birth because of low calcium and phosphorus absorption from parenteral and enteral nutrition [31]. In addition, many extremely premature infants receive medications such as diuretics, methylxanthines, and steroids that interfere with calcium metabolism. These infants may develop osteopenia of prematurity [32] and are susceptible to pathological fractures. The risk of osteopenia and fractures increases as gestational age decreases. These fractures can occur during routine limb manipulations such as placement of an intravenous catheter. Anesthesiologists should be aware of the existence of previous pathological fractures and the current serum alkaline phosphatase levels [31, 33]. Alkaline phosphatase levels >750 IU/L may be associated with radiological features of osteopenia in some premature infants. In the 1980s, the incidence of osteopenia was 50 % in premature infants <1,000 g birth weight. Fractures were detected in as many as 24 % of these infants. With better nutrition, the incidence of osteopenia and fractures has decreased in recent years [31], although this problem persists.
11. Glomerular filtration rate (GFR) is reduced in premature and term neonates, but improves postnatally reaching adult rates by 1–2 years of age. The use of nephrotoxic medications such as indomethacin and vancomycin may compromise renal function in some cases requiring blood sampling to determine concentrations at increased intervals between doses.
12. During the first few postnatal days, umbilical vessels provide arterial and venous access to sick neonates. Anesthesiologists should be familiar with the location of these lines (see below).
13. Term infants at birth have approximately 70 % fetal hemoglobin (HbF). HbF has increased affinity for oxygen resulting in a greater oxygen saturation compared with adult hemoglobin (HbA). For example, a pulse oximeter reading of 90 % is associated with a PaO_2 close to 60 mmHg with HbA but maybe as low as 50 mmHg in premature infants with increased levels of HbF. Some infants receive multiple packed RBC transfusions, thereby increasing the HbA content. The oxygen dissociation curve in such infants with multiple blood transfusions resembles that of adults resulting in a reduced oxygen saturation (e.g., PaO_2 of 50 mmHg will result in an oxygen saturation of 85 % in a baby that has received multiple transfusions).
14. Premature infants have thin permeable skin and are prone to increased heat and water loss by evaporation during the first few days of life. This thin fragile skin is vulnerable to accidental loss from peeling tape.

15. The ratio of surface area to body weight in neonates exceeds that in adults. As a consequence, the neonate is at increased risk for heat loss by radiation (39 %), convection (37 %), evaporation (21 %), and conduction (3 %) [34]. During surgery, appropriate measures to maintain thermal homeostasis must be used including a servo-controlled or thermal-neutral incubator to the suite in which the procedure/investigation will take place, increasing the room temperature, using an overhead heat lamp, thermal mattress, and forced-air warmer. Some or all of these devices may not be MRI compatible and cannot be used in that environment. The skin should remain dry and contact with wet linens should be avoided to prevent heat loss. Direct contact with the heating sources must also be avoided to minimize the risk of skin injury.

Benefits of Performing Surgery in the NICU

The most common reason for performing surgery in the NICU is to avoid comorbidities that may occur during transport of the critically ill neonate to another unit, such as the operating room (OR). There are several potential risks from transporting these infants (Table 13.1). The transport may require a change in the mode of ventilation [35]. Transporting a neonate whose lungs are ventilated with a high-frequency oscillatory ventilator (HFOV) or high-frequency jet ventilator (HFJV) is difficult and very challenging. Often, the lungs must be ventilated manually during transport and HFOV reinstituted only upon arrival in the OR. The transport incubator should be designed to maintain the neonate's temperature [36]. The neonate requires four transfers [37] during the trip to the OR (NICU bed to the transport incubator, incubator to the OR table, OR table back to the transport incubator, and lastly from the incubator back to the NICU bed). The risks are increased with the distance to be traveled and the need to use an elevator [36]. In a report of neonatal surgical practices from the United Kingdom [38], more than one-third of the transports to the OR involve transfer to a separate building from the NICU, whereas only 3 % of the responders provide anesthesia for surgical procedures in the NICU. Furthermore, the neonate is difficult to observe during the transport. Monitors during the transport often suffer from interference or movement artifact rendering the measurements unreliable, and the frequency of false alarms may mask true critical events. This, along with the fact that it is more difficult to clinically assess the neonate in the closed incubator, may cause a delay in the diagnosis and management of complications such as hypoxia, bleeding, pneumothorax, and cardiac arrest.

Table 13.1 Risks of transporting neonate

Disrupting of stable ventilation parameters
Loss of the airway or movement of the endotracheal tube
Loss of IV or central line access and interruption of infusions
Hypothermia
Requirement for 4 transfer episodes
Distance to operating room
Cardiovascular instability
The postoperative patient usually more fragile
Difficulty in examining the neonate during transport
Incompatibility of monitoring systems between the NICU and the OR

Hypothermia is more common after a procedure in the OR than one in the NICU. In a comparison of 80 infants undergoing laparotomy or diaphragmatic hernia repair, the core temperature decreased by 2.2 C° in those who underwent surgery in the OR compared with 0.6 C° in those who underwent surgery in the NICU [39]. Extreme hypothermia (30 °C) has also been reported in neonates after surgery in the OR [35]. The risk of extreme hypothermia (33 °C) is more common in VLBW neonates <1,500 g. Interestingly, there are also reports of hyperthermia (>37.5 °C) in neonates who underwent surgery in the OR [24]. Hyperthermia in the perioperative period should be eschewed. Hyperthermia in the immediate postnatal period in infants with hypoxic-ischemic encephalopathy has been associated with worse outcomes [40]. Although similar data are not available for normal neonates after surgery, hyperthermia is best avoided.

Patient Indications for Surgery in the NICU

There are several patient indications for performing surgery in the NICU (Table 13.2). Neonates who are too unstable to transfer either within the hospital or between hospitals and those in whom the risk of mortality is very high with or without the operative procedure (ASA class 5) are good candidates to undergo surgery in the NICU. Performing surgery in VLBW neonates <1,500 g in the NICU has resulted in more stable clinical situation with less disruption of physiologic parameters [35]. Transporting neonates who require high-frequency (HFJV or HFOV) ventilation is difficult, requiring the presence of a respiratory therapist and neonatologist in the OR for the duration of the surgery to assist with the ventilation management as well as the transport back to the NICU. In contrast, the ventilator in the OR may be incapable of ventilating the neonate's lungs with the same mode and parameters as were used with the NICU ventilator. Additionally, when emergent surgery is required and the OR is fully occupied, the surgery can be performed in the NICU without delay, assuming OR personnel is available.

Table 13.2 Indications for neonatal surgery in the NICU

Too unstable for transfer
Weight <1,000 g or <1,500 g
High-frequency oscillatory ventilation
Jet ventilation
Inhaled nitric oxide
Complex conventional ventilatory requirements
Surgical team willing to do "out-of-OR surgery"
Emergency procedure and delay in the OR

Table 13.3 Logistics of performing operative procedure in the NICU

Availability of surgical equipment and lighting
Availability of anesthesia equipment
Location for operative procedure
Consideration for other NICU patients
Infection control
Communication
Team concept

Logistics of Performing Surgery in the NICU

In order to provide anesthesia and perform operative procedures in the NICU, several logistic considerations need to be appreciated (Table 13.3). Consent must be obtained for the anesthetic and surgery from the parents or guardians. A thorough discussion of risks and benefits of anesthesia and surgery in very unstable infants must be completed in advance, in order to prepare for all possible options that may ensue including the need for changes in ventilation, blood transfusion, up to and including cardiopulmonary resuscitation. Although parents may be present at the infant's bedside during routine care, we do not allow parents to be present during surgery.

The surgeon and surgical team require a complete sterile surgical equipment tray, gowns, gloves, and masks. Appropriate surgical lighting must also be available, including portable overhead lights as well as surgical optical headlights and light sources [41]. Appropriate suction and cautery equipment must also be available. A full array of surgical instruments must be immediately available in the NICU in the event additional instruments are unexpectedly required urgently.

The anesthesiologist requires access to pharmacological, airway, and fluid supplies. An anesthetic workstation is usually neither available in the NICU nor required as inhalational anesthetics are infrequently used for several reasons including the absence of waste gas scavenging in the NICU. As a result, anesthesia in the NICU usually involves a total intravenous technique that consists of intermittent boluses of opioids and muscle relaxants. Infusion pumps are generally not used unless inotropes are required. Most monitors that we require are present in the NICU, although they may be difficult to access. One monitor that historically has been absent in the NICU is a capnogram. Many NICUs are now routinely using end-tidal CO_2 monitors, especially in VLBW infants. If a capnogram is not present, a portable capnogram may be brought from the OR, unless the neonate is ventilated with HFO, in which case the capnogram will be of limited value. A fluid warming device is recommended if large volumes of fluids or blood are required. Emergency equipment should also be available in the NICU including a resuscitation cart.

When surgery is performed in the NICU, it occurs in the neonate's bedside location. During surgery, all visitors and nonessential staff are cleared from the procedural area before the OR staff arrive. This should limit the risk of airborne contamination and microbial shedding resulting in infections. The use of barriers will also discourage inadvertent access to the operative procedure by unauthorized persons. Many new neonatal units have single-patient room design. Space constraint may necessitate transfer to a larger room. Some NICUs have a fully equipped procedure room with a high airflow exchange or a "twin room" with a larger area that may be utilized in the NICU unit. Using such a room requires that the infant be transferred from the incubator to the procedure room, which is usually a short distance.

Good communication among the NICU and the OR staff, the surgical team, and the anesthesiologist is very important. Moreover, establishing a close liaison with the NICU bedside nurse before anesthesia and surgery commence is very helpful to ensure that the latest laboratory values are available and within acceptable limits, that vascular access is available at a distance from the neonate, and that blood products are available. Since anesthesiologists have a limited knowledge of the layout of the NICU, it is imperative that the bedside nurse is available to provide syringes, needles, and other supplies during the surgery. Similarly, the presence of the neonatologist is extremely important in order to ensure that changes in management strategies of the neonate, such as ventilation changes, are undertaken with a thorough understanding of the child's preexisting conditions. A cooperative environment will increase the efficiency and safety of the anesthetic and surgery. An efficient and organized surgical service for the NICU minimizes disruption of the care the nurses must provide to the other infants in the room and minimizes the time that family members of other neonates in the room are barred from visiting their infants.

Vascular Access: Establishing adequate vascular access in neonates may be challenging. This is particularly challenging in ELBW infants (<1,000 g birth weight). In addition to peripheral venous access, some neonates may have umbilical lines and percutaneous PICC lines (peripherally inserted central catheters). Anesthesiologists should be comfortable using these access lines and should be capable of inserting lines in emergency situations. A brief review of umbilical venous and arterial lines and PICC lines is given below:

1. *Umbilical venous catheter*: The umbilical vein is large and easily accessible in neonates. Many infants in the NICU have an indwelling umbilical venous line for the first 5–7 days of life. It is important to document the exact location of the tip of the umbilical venous catheter on a recent X-ray before using it during anesthesia. The optimal location of the catheter tip should be in the inferior vena cava at or just above the level of the diaphragm (see Fig. 13.2). If the catheter tip is caudal (in hepatic veins), hepatic necrosis can occur in response to the infusion of hypertonic or vasospastic solution into the liver tissue [42]. If the catheter tip is too rostral, it may be located in the right atrium, superior vena cava, foramen ovale, left atrium, pulmonary veins (Fig. 13.3), right ventricle, or pulmonary artery. These locations may be associated with complications such as pericardial effusion, pleural effusion, and cardiac arrhythmias. Umbilical venous catheters are usually 5 Fr in diameter (occasionally 8 Fr in large term infants), consisting of either single-lumen or double-lumen catheters. These catheters should not be left open to atmosphere (because of the risk of an air embolus) [42]. For emergency vascular access, vital infusions (not hypertonic solutions) may be administered slowly through an umbilical venous catheter placed in the umbilical vein (usually 2–4 cm below the skin) [42] and checking for blood return. The umbilical venous catheters traverse the falciparum ligament and are usually removed before laparotomy.
2. *Umbilical arterial catheter*: An umbilical arterial catheter is often placed in a sick neonate to monitor blood pressure and to sample blood (especially arterial blood gas samples). The catheter is usually a 3.5 Fr or a 5 Fr single-lumen catheter placed in the umbilical artery and advanced into the aorta. The catheter tip is usually located either high (at the level of thoracic vertebrae 6–9) or low (at the level of lumbar vertebrae 3–4). Locating the catheter tip between thoracic vertebra 10 and lumbar vertebra 2 is best avoided because this region includes the origins of the celiac, mesenteric, and renal arteries (Fig. 13.4). If the catheter tip is located above

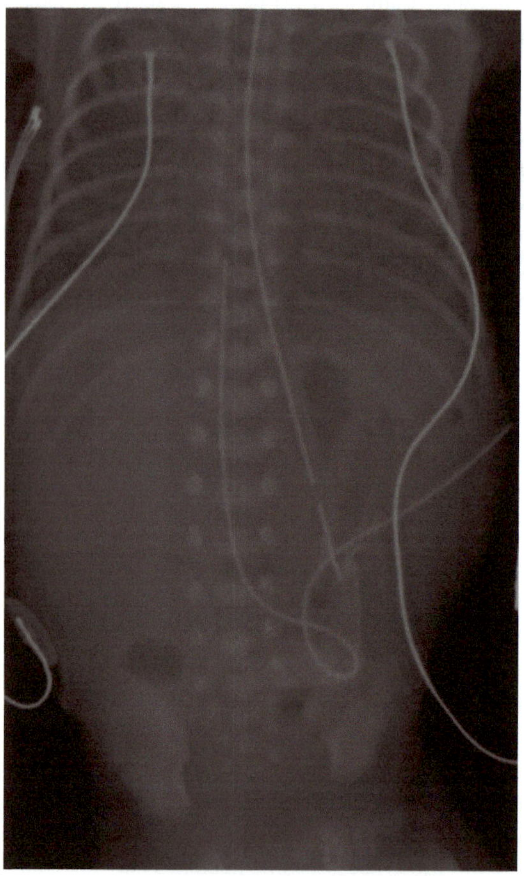

Fig. 13.2 Optimal position of the umbilical venous line. The tip of the umbilical venous catheter should be located in the inferior vena cava just above the level of the diaphragm

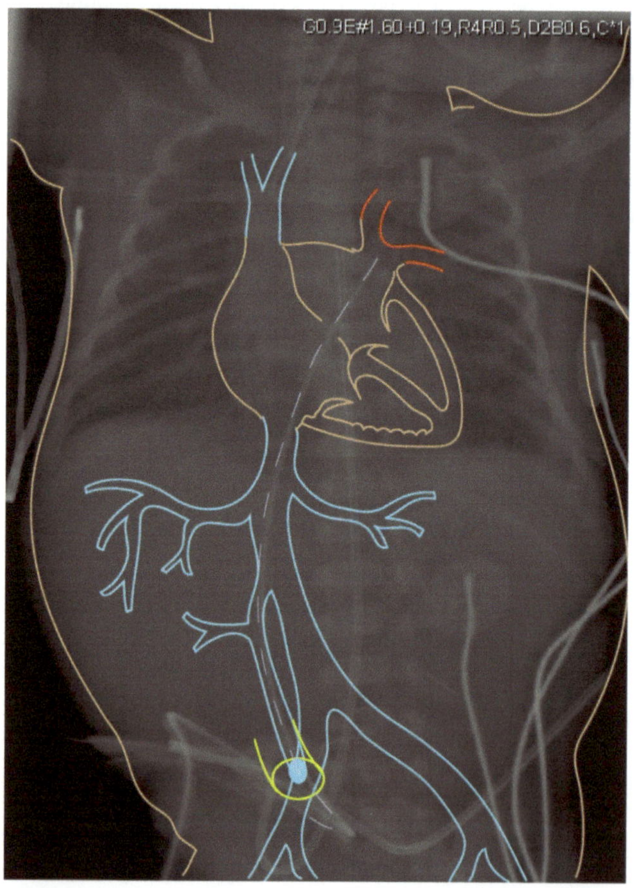

Fig. 13.3 Umbilical venous catheter advanced into the right atrium, patent foramen ovale, left atrium, and pulmonary veins (shown by *dashed lines*). This is an inappropriate location for an umbilical venous catheter

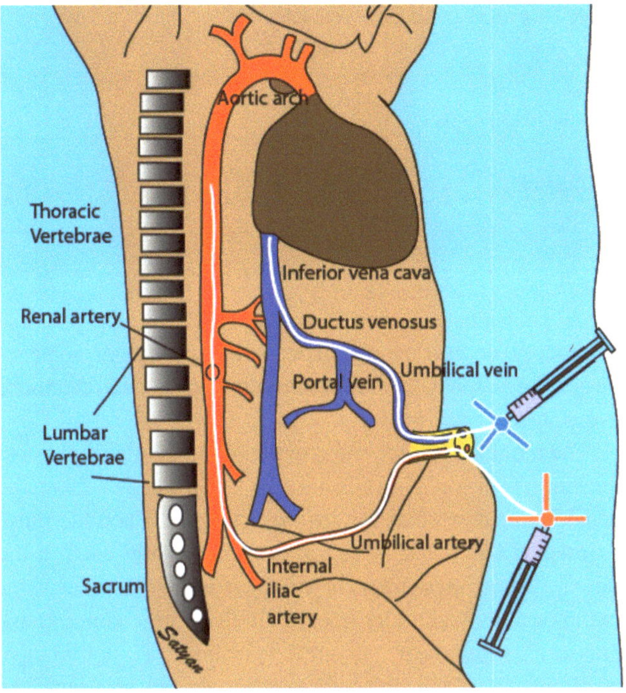

Fig. 13.4 Appropriate locations of the umbilical venous and arterial catheters from a lateral view. The umbilical venous catheter traverses the umbilical and portal veins and enters the inferior vena cava through the ductus venosus. The optimal location of the tip is in the inferior vena cava just below the right atrium. The umbilical arterial catheter is advanced through the umbilical, internal iliac, and common iliac arteries and advanced into the aorta. The celiac axis, superior and inferior mesenteric arteries, and renal arteries arise from the abdominal aorta at the level of thoracic vertebra T12 to lumbar vertebra L3. The umbilical arterial catheter can be positioned below this region (low line L3–L4) or above this region (T6–9, as shown in this figure)

thoracic vertebra 6, there is a risk of embolization to the carotid and subclavian arteries. Umbilical arterial catheters can also be used to deliver parenteral fluids, although vasospastic agents such as dopamine are best avoided. If there is evidence of vascular compromise (pallor in the lower limbs and buttocks), the umbilical line should be removed immediately. In neonates in whom abdominal emergencies such as spontaneous intestinal perforation (SIP) are developing, the umbilical arterial catheter should be removed before surgery. To remove an umbilical arterial catheter, the catheter should be withdrawn slowly until approximately 5 cm remains in the vessel and then tightened using an umbilical tie around the base of the umbilical cord (and not on the skin). The remainder of the catheter should be pulled out of the vessel at a slow rate of 1 cm/min (to allow vasospasm of umbilical artery). If bleeding occurs once the catheter has been removed, lateral pressure should be applied to the cord by compressing it between the thumb and first finger [43].

3. *Peripheral arterial cannulation*: The most peripheral artery with good collateral flow, with low infectious risk, and that is large enough to measure systemic blood pressure should be selected for cannulation [44]. Ongoing bacteremia and fungal infections are relative contraindications to arterial cannulation because of the risk of colonization of the catheter. Common sites for peripheral cannulation include the radial, ulnar, dorsalis pedis, and posterior tibial arteries, with the right radial artery selected the most in one retrospective review of infants <5 kg [45]. Evidence for collateral flow must be checked before cannulation. This can be done by using a modified Allen test or by Doppler ultrasound [46]. Transillumination of the wrist is helpful in identifying the location of radial, ulnar, dorsalis pedis, and posterior tibial arteries. Care should be taken not to injure the ulnar nerve during ulnar arterial cannulation as it runs along the medial side of the artery. Sedation and analgesia with fentanyl are usually provided before arterial cannulation. Some also infiltrate the site before arterial cannulation with 0.5 ml of lidocaine. After aseptic precautions are followed, an Angiocath is inserted into the artery by direct puncture and advanced at a 10–15° angle to the skin with the bevel facing down [47]. When blood appears in the stylet, the cannula is advanced off the stylet and into the artery. Alternately, the needle stylet may be inserted at a 30–40° angle to the skin with the bevel facing up through the artery. The stylet is removed and the cannula is withdrawn slowly until pulsatile arterial flow is established. The cannula is then advanced into the lumen of the artery [44]. Transparent semipermeable dressing is often used to cover the site of insertion to facilitate early detection of bleeding at the site. All fingers/toes should be clearly visible to monitor for signs of vascular insufficiency. Complications of peripheral arterial cannulation in neonates include thrombosis, vasospasm, infection, hematoma, damage to peripheral nerves, and air embolism [45, 48, 49].
4. *Central venous catheterization*: Placing a peripherally inserted central catheter (PICC) is a common procedure in the NICU to establish long-term central venous access in neonates. PICC lines are 1.1–5 Fr catheters of varying lengths, with the smallest single-lumen size being 1.1 Fr and the smallest double lumen being 2 Fr. In general, 1.1–2 Fr catheters are used in infants <2,500 g and those 1.9–3 Fr in those >2,500 g (http://www.nann.org/pdf/pdf/PICCGuidelines.pdf). The PICC tip should be located in the superior or inferior vena cava, outside the pericardial reflection [50]. Common indications for PICC placement include parenteral nutrition and need for long-term IV medication (antibiotics for bacterial, fungal, or viral infections). PICC has significant risks and complications (such as sepsis) and must be avoided when peripheral

venous access is adequate and possible [50]. Many neonatologists prefer to place a PICC after 24 h of parenteral antibiotics or when the blood culture is no longer positive for infection. Strict aseptic precautions must be followed when placing the catheter.

A central venous catheter is usually inserted percutaneously in neonates. A cutdown or surgical technique is used only when percutaneous insertion has been unsuccessful. Adequate sedation and analgesia should be provided before beginning to insert the catheter. A slow infusion of 2–4 mcg/kg of fentanyl is preferred, although larger doses may be required for infants who have been receiving opioids and in infants whose lungs are mechanically ventilated. Infants who do not require significant respiratory support may receive non-pharmacologic comfort measures such as sucrose-dipped pacifier in addition to fentanyl. For catheter insertion by surgical cutdown, local infiltration with lidocaine is recommended.

It is important to check the position of the catheter tip before commencing surgery. The use of radio-opaque contrast improves localization of the catheter tip. The most recent chest radiograph should be evaluated for catheter position. Migration of catheters associated with complications is known to occur after insertion.

Most indwelling catheters are made of silicone or polyurethane to minimize the risk of perforation and fracture. In neonates, small gauges (1.1, 1.9, 2, and 3 Fr) are commonly used for percutaneous insertion. These catheters often cannot be used for withdrawing blood or rapidly infusing fluid boluses or anesthetic induction drugs (such as propofol) or blood products during surgery. Sterile precautions should be observed when breaking into a PICC circuit during surgery.

Anesthesia Requirements

There are several important issues that the anesthesiologist should establish when planning to provide anesthesia in the NICU (Table 13.4). First, dedicated IV access should be available to the anesthesiologist for drug and fluid administration. Drugs such as antibiotics or vasopressors pressors not be co-infused in that dedicated line. Second, the anesthesia regimen most frequently used for neonates is an (high-dose) opioid technique with neuromuscular blockade. Fentanyl is the most widely used opioid in neonates and vecuronium or rocuronium the most commonly used neuromuscular blocking agent. All medications should be flushed through the line as medications are often administered at a site remote from the infant and may cause an unexpected delayed effect when the IV line is later flushed. All fluid boluses, flushes, and infusions should be carefully documented to prevent fluid overdoses. There have been some reports of the adjunct use of midazolam and propofol [61] in neonates during surgery in the NICU. The potential circulatory depression associated with the use of some of these drugs, especially in the compromised neonate, cannot be overstated.

Table 13.4 Anesthesia requirements

IV access
Drugs
Anesthetic technique
Monitoring
Ventilation
Fluids

The monitoring equipment in the NICU is often foreign to the anesthesiologist. Assistance is often needed from the bedside nurse or neonatologist to activate the audible pulse oximetry/ECG tones, which are not frequently used in the NICU. Blood pressure may be measured invasively via a radial or umbilical artery line, but in those in whom invasive pressure monitoring is not present, a noninvasive oscillometric blood pressure monitor should be used. The reliability of noninvasive measures of blood pressure monitoring in premature infants has been affirmed by some and questioned by others [51, 52]. Recent evidence supports applying the blood pressure cuff in either the upper or lower extremity in infants >1,000 g but may provide more accurate readings from the lower extremities in infants <1,000 g [53]. Mean and systolic blood pressures in premature and full-term neonates increase with gestational age, birth weight, and postnatal age [54]. Of importance is the observation that the systolic and mean blood pressures measured noninvasively in premature and full-term neonates asleep is 10–20 % less than the corresponding awake values [54]. This is consistent with the expected decrease in systolic blood pressure of 20–30 % after induction of anesthesia. Because complex ICU ventilators or HFOV/ HFJV is often used in the NICU, a neonatologist and respiratory therapist should be present throughout the procedure [37] to assist with ventilation, oxygenation, and ventilator-related issues. Changes in oxygenation and ventilation may occur as a result of increases in the abdominal pressure and/or decreases in lung compliance associated with surgery. Persistent changes in oxygenation and ventilation may require compensatory changes in PEEP, PIP, and mean airway pressure depending on the mode of ventilation as well as the inspired fraction of oxygen. If conventional ventilation cannot maintain adequate blood gases, it is possible that the strategy will have to be changed to perhaps HFOV [67]. Neonates whose lungs require HFOV are often monitored using transcutaneous CO_2 monitoring. This monitor tracks the $PaCO_2$ [55] although it requires recalibration periodically; the response lags compared with end-tidal capnography and its accuracy should be confirmed by comparing the results to an arterial blood gas before commencing surgery. Capnography is not routinely available in most NICUs, but the anesthesiologist should ensure that capnography is available for those neonates and VLBW infants with reasonable lung function and whose lungs are ventilated with conventional ventilators [55, 56, 99]. End-tidal CO_2 does not provide accurate estimates of $PaCO_2$ in neonates whose lungs are ventilated with HFOV (see discussion on high-frequency ventilation below).

Thermoregulation is a vital function in the neonate that may prove challenging during surgery in the NICU. Surgery is often performed in open radiant warmers with overhead radiant heaters in the NICU. However, these heaters may be less effective at maintaining thermoneutrality during surgery as the surgeons cover the neonate blocking the infants from the heat source. In the OR, the ambient temperature is often increased to 26 °C [57, 58] to prevent radiation and, to a lesser extent, convective heat losses. This is not usually possible in the NICU setting unless a designated procedure room is used. A forced-air heating blanket, which is a very effective method to prevent intraoperative hypothermia [59] better than most other strategies during surgery, is usually unavailable in the NICU. However, if it is available, it should be placed under the infant before surgery commences. A fluid warmer should be used to warm all fluids, especially if blood products are required. Often, a fluid warmer must be supplied from the OR. Hypothermia during neonatal surgery has been associated with reduced OR ambient temperature as well as with major surgical procedures [60], e.g., open abdominal procedure. Similar data from the NICU have not been forthcoming.

One major controversy regarding surgery in the NICU when this subject was initially considered was the potential risk for increased infections and sepsis. However, several small studies failed to demonstrate any increased risk associated with operating in the NICU. One study that involved repair of congenital diaphragmatic hernia in the NICU [61] reported an increased but not statistically significant change in the infection rate. However, they did demonstrate a significant increase in the inflammatory marker C-reactive protein (CRP) in the NICU operative group, suggesting that inflammation was present. Because critically ill neonates are more prone to infections as well as a greater morbidity and mortality from infection than healthy neonates, it is imperative to adhere to OR infection control policies including the use of appropriately timed (pre-incision) surgical site antibiotics irrespective of the location of the surgery [41].

There have been several published reports of neonates undergoing a variety of different operative procedures in the NICU. Most of these studies included small sample sizes, most were retrospective, and none were randomized trials evaluating outcomes. A review of the publications to date suggests that the neonates in the NICU operative group had a greater mortality than those operated in the OR [35, 39, 61, 62], although selection bias limits the external validity of these data: these neonates were sicker and required more ventilatory and inotropic support. The extent to which these differences of pre-procedural morbidity were responsible for the increased mortality is difficult to determine. A retrospective study [35] utilizing the score for neonatal acute physiology (SNAP) demonstrated that neonates undergoing surgery in the NICU had a greater preoperative SNAP score than those undergoing surgery in the OR, but that SNAP increased by 20 % in both groups during the initial 24 h post-procedure.

Despite the lack of evidence concerning improved outcomes after surgery in the NICU, it is difficult to determine whether the challenges associated with undertaking surgery in a foreign environment offset those associated with transferring the neonate to the OR [35]. As surgery is performed more frequently in the NICU on more stable neonates, the mortality rate is decreasing significantly [35]. In many centers today, surgery in the NICU is regarded as routine and safe.

Sedation and Analgesia for Common Procedures in the NICU

Critically ill neonates in the NICU undergo frequent painful procedures such as blood draws, heel sticks, and intravenous catheter placement daily [63]. Other procedures that may cause discomfort in some neonates include tracheal intubation, mechanical ventilation, and tracheal suctioning [64, 65]. Neonates who require mechanical ventilation are often sedated with a combination of fentanyl and midazolam. The American Academy of Pediatrics (AAP) recently published guidelines for premedicating neonates who require nonemergent tracheal intubation [66]. They recommended atropine, fentanyl as a slow infusion, and vecuronium/rocuronium. These guidelines recommend avoiding midazolam in premature neonates because of its prolonged half-life, hypotension, reduced cerebral blood flow, and the presence of benzyl alcohol as a preservative.

High-Frequency Ventilation: Critically ill neonates, especially premature infants, may develop hypoxemic respiratory failure as a result of small lung volumes, poor compliance, increased intra- and extrapulmonary shunts, and ventilation perfusion mismatch. High-frequency ventilation is a commonly used lung-protection strategy that benefits oxygenation and ventilation [67]. Two types of high-frequency ventilators are used in neonates in the United States:

(a) High-frequency oscillatory ventilation (HFOV, Sensor Medics 3100A, CareFusion Corporation, San Diego CA) utilizes a piston pump to generate oscillations.

This is the only mode of ventilation in which inspiration and expiration are active. A constant distending pressure is applied to the lungs (mean airway pressure), over which small tidal volumes (amplitude) are superimposed at a rapid respiratory frequency (6–15 Hz). Typically a frequency range between 10 and 15 Hz is used in neonates. Greater frequencies are commonly used in premature infants. The frequency of oscillation influences the CO_2 removal in a direction opposite to that of conventional ventilation. Greater frequencies decrease tidal volume and increase $PaCO_2$. Decreasing the frequency and increasing the amplitude independently increase tidal volume and decrease $PaCO_2$. The following factors should be considered if a critically ill infant who depends on HFOV requires surgery:

1. Performing surgery while the lungs are ventilated using a HFOV may be technically difficult for the surgeon.
2. Mean airway pressure recruits alveoli and is closely related to oxygenation. When an infant is switched from conventional ventilation to HFOV, it is recommended that the starting mean airway pressure be 2 cmH_2O above the mean airway pressure on conventional ventilation.
3. If a neonate is weaned from HFOV to conventional ventilation for surgery, adequate PEEP must be provided to maintain alveolar recruitment and oxygenation.
4. Increased mean airway pressure can impede venous return and decrease blood pressure. If hypotension is encountered during HFOV, fluid boluses may be required. If hypotension persists, the mean airway pressure should be decreased providing the respiratory status of the neonate remains stable.
5. Wide fluctuations in $PaCO_2$ (especially hypocarbia) can occur during HFOV. Frequent blood gases and/or transcutaneous pCO_2 monitoring provide useful indices of ventilation with HFOV; end-tidal pCO_2 monitor is unreliable. The skin at the site of transcutaneous monitor application must be frequently checked to avoid burns. The site may have to be changed frequently particularly in premature infants.

(b) High-frequency jet ventilation (HFJV, Life Pulse, Bunnell Incorporated, Salt Lake City, UT) is the second form of high-frequency ventilation in the Unites States. HFJV is particularly effective for early intervention and treatment of pulmonary interstitial emphysema. The jet ventilator provides small, high-velocity breaths and fast rates with passive exhalation. A conventional ventilator operates in tandem with the jet ventilator to maintain optimal PEEP. The conventional ventilator is attached to the regular connector of the tracheal tube, and the HFJV is connected through a special adaptor to the side port of the tube. Mean airway pressure is adjusted primarily by changing the PEEP on the conventional ventilator. Just as in the case of conventional ventilation, faster respiratory rates and greater PIP with the HFJV reduces the $PaCO_2$. See Chapter 9 for further information [68].

Transport: The majority of births in the United States occur in hospitals without tertiary level neonatal intensive care units. Neonates who are born extremely premature outside a tertiary hospital may require transport to a tertiary hospital (interhospital transport) soon after birth because of respiratory distress, congenital anomalies, and/or surgical problems. A transport incubator should be used for all interhospital transports. Once inside the tertiary hospital, these neonates may require transport within the facility for diagnostic or special procedures such as radiography, cardiac catheterization, or surgery [69] (intrahospital transport). Many of these neonates are critically ill, require mechanical ventilation, and are at increased risk for cardiorespiratory instability. Increased stimulation during transport can destabilize a critically ill infant. Accordingly, appropriate sedation and analgesia during transport will prevent cardiorespiratory instability.

For short transports within the hospital, critically ill infants are transported on radiant warmer beds. In these instances, the infant's head should be covered with a hat, and the body wrapped in a plastic/vinyl insulated bag to prevent heat loss. In neonates with abdominal wall defects (gastroschisis or omphalocele) or large neural tube defects (meningomyelocele and encephalocele), sterile vinyl bags should be applied to prevent infection, hypothermia, and hypovolemia. Intrahospital transports are best managed by manually ventilating the lungs. Hand ventilation enables the operator to continuously evaluate the compliance of the lungs including early detection of accidental extubation, a tube disconnect or tracheal tube kinking, or occlusion to be detected earlier although this depends on the fresh gas flow and operator experience [70]. However if the lungs are ventilated manually, it is imperative that the operator remains focused on the ventilation (rather than steering the incubator) to ensure the respiratory rate and peak inspiratory pressure are appropriate.

It is recommended that the neonatal transport team carry medications for analgesia, sedation, and paralysis [69] including analgesics and sedatives (fentanyl, morphine, midazolam), neuromuscular blocking drugs (pancuronium and vecuronium) and reversal agents (flumazenil to reverse benzodiazepines, naloxone to reverse opioid-induced respiratory depression, neostigmine to antagonize neuromuscular blocking agents). In addition, they must have equipment to manage a sudden airway emergency including an appropriately sized laryngoscope, tracheal tubes, stylet, and ventilation circuit (Ambu bag or T-piece).

Specific Conditions Requiring Surgery in the NICU (For Further Details See Chap. 9 Thoracoabdominal Surgery)

Closure of Patent Ductus Arteriosus (PDA)

Failure of the PDA to close spontaneously or in response to medical management with indomethacin or ibuprofen is common in ELBW premature infants. Medical management appears to fail in up to two-thirds of ELBW infants [71]. When medical treatment was compared with surgical closure of the PDA as first-line therapy in premature infants, the incidence of mortality and post-closure complications were similar [72]. In some, medical treatment may be contraindicated because of intraventricular hemorrhage or renal failure. A PDA results in significant left-to-right shunting of blood causing pulmonary over-circulation, respiratory failure, prolonged ventilator dependence, congestive cardiac failure and chronic lung disease, and NEC (necrotizing enterocolitis). In these patients, surgical ligation of the PDA may be performed [71]. More recently, percutaneous closure of the PDA has been performed successfully in young neonates and may point to another approach to open surgical ligation [73].

Surgical ligation of a PDA in neonates has a low morbidity and mortality. The CXR may indicate fluid overload or evidence or a respiratory distress syndrome. The echocardiogram establishes the size of the ductus and the degree and direction of blood flow. Although surgical closure of the PDA is routinely performed in the OR, it has also been performed in the NICU [74]. The outcome from surgical ligation appears to be related to the underlying degree of pulmonary and cardiovascular disease. In a nonrandomized study of PDA ligation in the OR and NICU, it demonstrated that postoperative mortality (17 %) was due to respiratory failure and sepsis, with risk factors being surgery in the NICU and low birth weight [75]. The overall outcome of PDA ligation was early extubation (<10 days) in 30 % of neonates, late extubation (no chronic lung disease, CLD) in 22 %, and late extubation with CLD in 31 %. There was no difference between the groups in terms of early incidence of extubation suggesting that the outcome after PDA closure in neonates without severe cardiorespiratory disease is similar whether it is done in the OR or NICU. In another study of 41 PDA ligations in neonates <1500 g with a mean gestational age of 27 weeks in the NICU, no complications were attributable to anesthesia, and 5 deaths were all related to prematurity and congestive heart failure [74]. In some institutions ligation of a PDA in the NICU is considered standard. Some regional centers have a team comprising of a pediatric cardiac surgeon, pediatric anesthesiologist, and pediatric OR nurses traveling to pediatric hospitals to perform PDA ligation in the referring hospital's NICU to avoid the interhospital transfer of the neonate [76]. There was no difference in either the preoperative complication rate or mortality between these neonates and those operated on at the surgical institution. Most importantly, by not transferring the neonates, the same neonatal team that is most familiar with the infant's medical and social history could provide the infant's care, and the family is minimally inconvenienced.

Necrotizing Enterocolitis (NEC)

Is the most common gastrointestinal surgical emergency in premature neonates [77] affecting approximately 6–7 % of VLBW infants. Full-term infants rarely present with NEC. The pathogenesis of NEC remains unknown, but it is quite likely a multifactorial disease. Risk factors include prematurity, enteral feeding (especially formula), infection, and ischemia (Fig. 13.5). Classic radiographic findings include

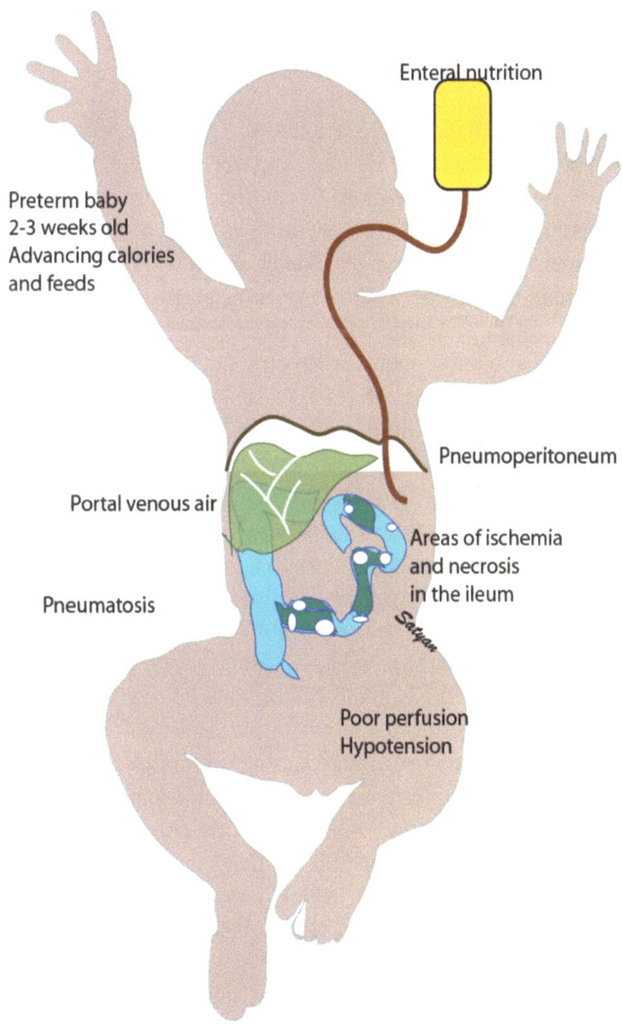

Fig. 13.5 Pathophysiology of necrotizing enterocolitis (NEC) requiring surgery. A typical patient is a premature infant on advancing feeds at approximately 2–3 weeks of age. The terminal ileum is commonly involved. Areas of ischemic necrosis and pneumatosis (intramural collection of air) are observed in the ileum. Portal venous air can be visible on abdominal X-ray. Pneumoperitoneum is the most common indication for surgery in NEC

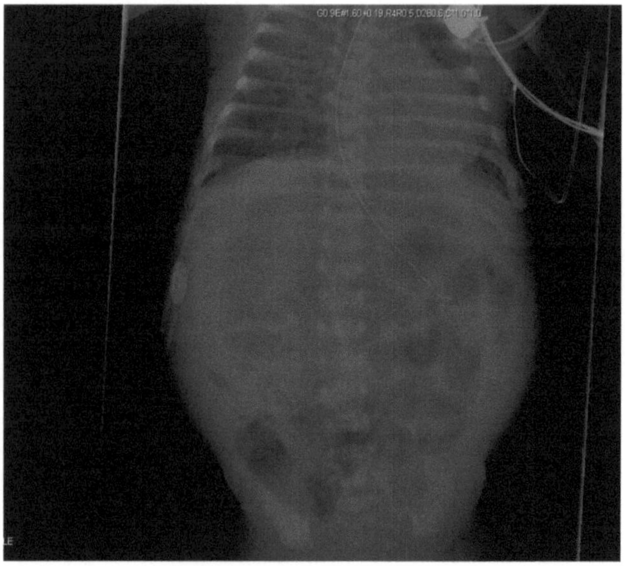

Fig. 13.6 X-ray showing pneumoperitoneum (anterior to the liver), pneumatosis in a patient with NEC prior to surgery

Table 13.5 Average perioperative resuscitation requirements for NEC patients in the NICU

Inotropes eg., Dopamine	Increased dose by 4 mcg/kg/min
Bicarbonate	2.5 mmol/kg
Blood	32 ml/kg
Platelets	12 ml/kg
Fresh frozen plasma	15 ml/kg
5 % albumin	35 ml/kg

gas in the intestinal wall (pneumatosis), air in the branches of the portal vein and biliary tract, and free air within the abdomen (Fig. 13.6). Indications for surgical exploration include intestinal perforation with pneumoperitoneum or continued clinical deterioration despite maximal medical management. Surgical management with a peritoneal drainage is often favored in an unstable, critically ill premature infant with the caveat that a subsequent laparotomy may be required if the condition deteriorates.

Neonates who require surgery for NEC are usually critically ill and require intensive resuscitation before surgery. Preoperative management before exploratory laparotomy should address the following issues:

(a) Blood pressure—Hypotension is common in NEC and is secondary to third spacing of fluids in the abdomen, capillary leak, high peak inspiratory pressures, sepsis with poor vascular tone, and low cardiac output. Fluid boluses (both crystalloids and colloids) may be required repeatedly until the vital signs stabilize. Many infants require inotropic support with dopamine and/or epinephrine.
(b) Respiratory failure—Pulmonary edema and acute respiratory distress syndrome (ARDS) are commonly associated with fulminant NEC. Infants require high peak inspiratory pressures during conventional ventilation. Some infants may be so ill that their lungs require HFO (see discussion above).
(c) Electrolyte and acid–base disturbances—Fulminant NEC results in respiratory and metabolic acidosis. Hyponatremia is common secondary to third spacing and hyperkalemia due to acidosis occurs in some infants and may need to be corrected either before or during surgery. Hypocalcemia secondary to multiple blood product infusion may exacerbate hypotension and should be avoided.
(d) Hematologic disturbances—A review of 25 neonates who required surgery for NEC in the NICU required many blood products perioperatively (Table 13.5) [35]. This report illustrates the need to have blood products immediately available for the anesthesiologists to administer during the procedure. Thrombocytopenia occurs commonly in NEC. NEC associated with ischemic or necrotic bowel may also present with disseminated intravascular coagulation (DIC). PT, PTT, fibrinogen, and fibrin split products should be frequently monitored along with complete blood counts in neonates with NEC. Transfusions with packed red blood cells (PRBC), fresh frozen plasma (FFP), and platelets are often required.
(e) Many neonates with NEC may have received systemic glucocorticoids for hypotension or management of bronchopulmonary dysplasia (BPD). Such patients may need a stress dose of glucocorticoids before surgery.
(f) Vascular access—At least two peripheral intravenous catheters are recommended during surgery for NEC. A central venous catheter is useful to infuse inotropic agents (since most neonates will require support) and an arterial catheter to monitor blood pressure continuously and sample arterial blood.

General tracheal anesthesia with neuromuscular blockade is the preferred anesthetic technique for NEC surgery [78]. Lung ventilation is commonly managed with a standard neonatal ventilator, rendering an intravenous anesthetic approach preferable over inhalational anesthetics. A high-dose opioid technique with intravenous fentanyl (20–50 mcg/kg), midazolam (0.1 mg/kg), and a muscle relaxant is often used. Hypotension is common after induction of anesthesia but can be prevented in most infants by preinfusing 10–20 mL/kg of balanced salt solution, normal saline, or lactated Ringer's solution. Persistent hypotension may necessitate the use of inotropes such as dopamine and stress dose glucocorticoids. Third space losses are common during surgery in NEC and many infants require 50–100 mL/kg of fluid during surgery. Depending on what the infant received preoperatively, this may include balanced salt solution, colloid, or blood products (PRBCs, FFP, and platelets). Infants with NEC continue to require large fluid volumes during the postoperative period because of ongoing third space losses.

The mortality for NEC surgery in the NICU has been reported to be as great as 50 %. Mortality is affected by several variables including the location and extent of the disease (Table 13.6) [109]. Neonates with extensive NEC are those in whom surgery is undertaken preferentially in the NICU, and it is in those neonates that the mortality is significantly greater. In neonates with NEC who are the most unstable, placement of a peritoneal drain in the right lower quadrant is usually sufficient [36].

Table 13.6 Location, extent of disease, and mortality for NEC [109]

Location	% Bowel involved	% Mortality
Ileum	15	15
Large bowel	20	35
Jejunum-ileum	65	80
Large bowel–ileum	35	40
Large bowel–jejunum–ileum	85	95

Spontaneous Intestinal Perforation

A subset of premature neonates who present with intestinal perforation without signs of NEC, such as pneumatosis intestinalis, are classified as focal or spontaneous intestinal perforation (SIP). This condition presents early (7–10 days of age) in ELBW infants [79, 80]. Prior exposure to early postnatal steroids and indomethacin may be risk factors for SIP [110, 111]. Although these neonates are not as sick as those with advanced NEC, they tend to be much younger, their lungs are often mechanically ventilated, and they have umbilical lines secondary to their respiratory distress syndrome (RDS) at birth (Fig. 13.7). Surgery for SIP often involves resection of the perforated site and reanastomosis or ileostomy. This procedure is often done at the bedside in the NICU because of the young gestational age.

Gastroschisis

Gastroschisis is an anterior abdominal defect resulting from an occlusion of the omphalomesenteric artery. Gastroschisis is located in the periumbilical region usually on the left side. The intestines are not covered and are exposed to amniotic fluid during fetal life resulting in inflammation and edema

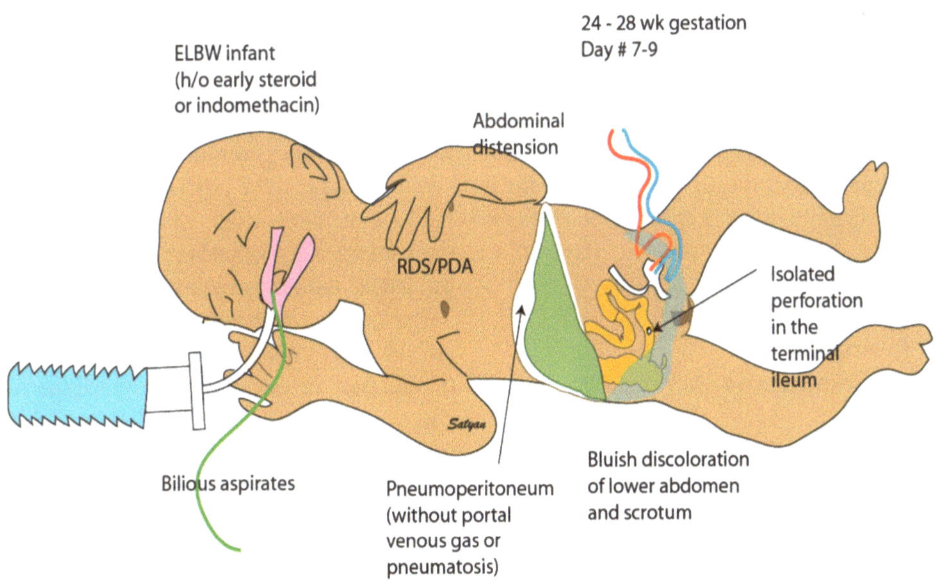

Fig. 13.7 A typical patient with spontaneous intestinal perforation (SIP). These patients are of extremely low gestational age (median—26 weeks), presenting often with asymptomatic pneumoperitoneum by days 7–9. Some patients may present with bluish discoloration of the abdomen. There is no evidence of pneumatosis or portal venous air. Many of these infants are still on respiratory support for RDS and/or PDA and may have umbilical lines from birth. Pathology shows a perforation in the ileum without any evidence of coagulative necrosis, a finding commonly associated with NEC and ischemia

and formation of a peel on the surface of the bowel. Preoperative management consists of reducing fluid loss from the eviscerated organs and bowel. This is accomplished by administration of adequate intravenous fluids in the form of boluses of normal saline or lactated Ringer's solution to replace third space and evaporative losses. The bowel is covered with sterile, saline-soaked dressings and placed in a sterile plastic wrap. Gastric decompression is important to prevent distension of the stomach and intestines and reduce intra-abdominal pressure (IAP). Reduction of gastroschisis and primary abdominal closure is performed in the OR. This procedure may be associated with increased intra-abdominal pressure. Central venous pressure >4 mmHg, intravesical or gastric pressure >20 mmHg, and splanchnic perfusion pressure (mean arterial pressure—IAP, <44 mmHg) during primary repair are signs of decreased splanchnic and renal blood flow and the need for a staged repair [112].

In some patients when the eviscerated bowel mass is large relative to the abdominal cavity or when IAP increases during attempted primary repair, staged reduction is performed in the NICU. The intestine is covered with a prosthetic silo pouch. The pouch is subsequently reduced in stages in the NICU, allowing the abdominal cavity to gradually accommodate the increased mass without severely compromising ventilation or organ perfusion. Careful inspection of the bowel for obstructing bands, perforation, or atresia should be undertaken before placing the silo. More recent introduction of a prefabricated silo with a circular spring that can be placed into the fascial opening, without the need for sutures or general anesthesia, has made it possible to insert the silo in the delivery room or at the bedside in the NICU [112]. These procedures are performed with intravenous opioid (2–4 mcg/kg of fentanyl) and midazolam (0.1 mg/kg). A PICC line must be placed in all infants with gastroschisis for total parenteral nutrition because intestinal hypomotility and delayed initiation and advancement of oral feeds are common.

Retinopathy of Prematurity (Also See Chap. 15 Complications)

The surgical management for Retinopathy of Prematurity (ROP) may involve both laser and cryosurgery. There are numerous reports of these procedures being performed in the NICU [113] and the OR. These neonates are not usually critically ill. Hence, the risk of transporting these neonates to the OR is less than it is for very very sick neonates, although performing these procedures in the OR is believed to delay the care. This prompted the practice of evaluating and managing these infants in the NICU. In the NICU, local anesthesia and IV sedation have been used, although emergent airway management has been common. Currently, neonatologists use a local anesthetic/sedation technique and sedation/analgesia/paralysis technique with tracheal intubation or maintain their current level of respiratory support to facilitate these procedures in the NICU [81, 82].

Congenital Diaphragmatic Hernia

The management of congenital diaphragmatic hernia (CDH) now often includes NICU management with HFOV, surfactant, inhaled nitric oxide, and possibly ECMO (in up to one-third of neonates with CDH) followed by delayed surgical repair [83]. The decision to repair CDH in the NICU is often determined by the ventilatory management required to support the infant. Despite an increasing proportion of neonates undergoing corrective repair of CDH, current survival rates in a background of HFOV, iNO, and ECMO have not changed from 65 to 80 % [84]. Supporting the infant for several days allows the severity of the pulmonary hypertension to improve and vessel reactivity to wane. Although initially unstable, these infants can progressively improve resulting in better gas exchange and increased lung compliance during postnatal adaption and correct management strategies. Those infants with significant pulmonary hypoplasia (15 %) or an abnormal persistence of the pulmonary hypertension may fail to stabilize postnatally and may require ECMO. Neonates with CDH who also present with congenital heart defects (incidence ~10 %) present a heterogeneous group of heart defects that pose a daunting challenge. ECMO has been used to support these infants with survival rates for single ventricle physiology that were similar to those with CDH without a heart defect [85]. Retrospective data suggests that blood gases in the first 4 h after birth may predict outcomes in terms of ECMO requirement and mortality [86]. Those who recommend surgical repair in the NICU do so to avoid the logistical difficulties and patient safety issues associated with transferring the neonate who depends on HFOV, iNO, and/or ECMO, to the OR. If the lungs require HFOV to maintain the pCO_2 in an acceptable range and the child is scheduled for surgery in the OR, converting the ventilation mode to conventional ventilation may be considered provided the respiratory settings do not exceed those shown in Table 13.7 [61]. If the respiratory indices remain within acceptable limits after conversion to conventional ventilation, the infant may be transferred to the OR 24 h later.

A comparison of neonates after CDH surgical repair using fentanyl, pancuronium, and occasional midazolam and propofol anesthesia in the NICU and the OR demonstrated a greater mortality in the former, 33 %, compared with the latter, 7 % [61]. The NICU infants required more inhaled nitric oxide, greater mean arterial pressure, greater need for inotropic support, and a greater oxygenation index (mean airway pressure $\times FiO_2 \times 100 \div$ postductal PaO_2, usually the umbilical arterial PaO_2).

Table 13.7 Recommendations for the transition from HFOV to conventional ventilation for CDH repair

After at least 72 h since birth, with minimal inotropic support, HFOV settings should be:
$FiO_2 < 0.4$
MAP < 13 cm H_2O
Amplitude <30 cm H_2O
Oxygenation index <10
No ultrasound evidence for pulmonary hypertension
No difference in pre- and postductal saturation
Pulmonary/systemic pressure ratio <0.75
Stable with above criteria for 24 h

Cannulation for ECMO (Extracorporeal Membrane Oxygenation): ECMO is a lifesaving supportive tool that maintains gas exchange and perfusion for patients with acute reversible cardiac or respiratory failure [87]. Cardiopulmonary failure in neonates is often secondary to meconium aspiration syndrome, CDH, respiratory distress syndrome (surfactant deficiency), and pneumonia/sepsis resulting in persistent pulmonary hypertension of the newborn (PPHN). These neonates have increased pulmonary vascular resistance (PVR). They often require mechanical ventilation with high concentrations of oxygen and supportive therapy. If these measures fail to restore adequate oxygenation, inhaled nitric oxide may be used to selectively decrease pulmonary arterial pressure and improve oxygenation [114]. Neonates who are often extremely sick with hypoxemic respiratory failure, hypotension, and coagulopathy and who do not respond to conservative measures are placed on ECMO as a last resort. The CDH EURO Consortium endorsed a consensus statement for the criteria for enrolling neonates in ECMO [83].

Three different ECMO configurations are used clinically: venoarterial (VA), venovenous (VV), and double-lumen single-cannula venovenous (DLVV) bypass. Cannulation is usually performed in the NICU or PICU using high-dose fentanyl or propofol sedation. Blood pressure, heart rate and pulse oximetry, and transcutaneous PO_2 and pCO_2 monitoring are continuously performed. Fluid boluses and inotropes such as dopamine and/or epinephrine may be necessary to prevent hypotension. An activated clotting time (ACT) should be recorded before commencing the cannulation. Heparin is administered after the surgeon makes a transverse cervical incision and exposes the common carotid artery and internal jugular vein. The artery is cannulated and the tip is advanced to the junction of the innominate artery and the aorta. In preparation for the venous cannulation, the lungs should continue to be ventilated and the neonate should be paralyzed pharmacologically to prevent spontaneous respiration and aspiration of air. The venous cannula is advanced to the inferior aspect of the right atrium (VA). The cannula positions are confirmed by chest radiograph. The double-lumen venous catheter (DLVV) is placed with the tip in the mid-right atrium so that the oxygenated blood flow is directed toward the tricuspid valve. The catheters are then connected to the ECMO circuit.

The sedation practices during ECMO vary widely among institutions. With concerns of hypotension during cannulation, most sedate the neonates with fentanyl or sufentanil infusion and midazolam and only paralyze the infant for the cannulation.

As the infant's medical problems improve, the flow in the ECMO circuit may be gradually weaned. On moderate ventilator settings, the cannulae are clamped with the circuit bypassing the infant via the bridge. If the infant remains stable for 2–4 h, decannulation may be performed. Under sterile conditions, the infant is placed in Trendelenburg position and muscle relaxants are administered. The venous catheter is removed first and the vessel is ligated. The arterial catheter is then removed and the carotid artery is either ligated or repaired. Many infants require a gradual weaning from opioids after ECMO.

Anesthesia for Neonates on ECMO in the NICU

ECMO has become part of the strategy to stabilize high-risk infants with CDH [88]. There are several important features of this procedure with which the anesthesiologist needs to be familiar. The ECMO circuit is managed by an ECMO technician under the direction of the ICU/ECMO attending. Although the ECMO circuit is similar to the cardiopulmonary bypass circuit in cardiac surgery, it is different because the ECMO circuit has no reservoir, and without an adequate filling pressure (gravity and CVP), flow into the ECMO pump will be inadequate. Two types of pumps are used in ECMO: roller pumps for children generally >10 kg and centrifugal pumps for those <10 kg. Venous arterial ECMO, which is commonly used for CDH, can provide full cardiac and pulmonary support, with the ventilation strategy usually required to maintain adequate lung inflation. However depending on the flow in the ECMO circuit (as a percentage of cardiac output), blood can pass through the lungs so that the oxygen saturation may be less than that from the arterial cannula. This is usually associated with an arterial waveform that demonstrates systolic and diastolic features. Hence, it is possible for the saturation to decrease during the procedure if the ECMO flows are changed or interrupted. In such a case, ventilation may have to be manipulated. Furthermore, if the preload decreases too much, the ECMO pump will "cut off," and pump flow will not resume until the preload is reestablished. Blood products and medications can be easily and reliably administered through the ECMO circuit.

As with any patient who is anticoagulated, the risks of bleeding complications are substantial during ECMO. However, several strategies have been developed to limit this risk. The degree of anticoagulation is usually reduced, with

ACT times limited to between 140 and 160 s during ECMO rather than the 180–200 s used for the ECMO run [89].

The antifibrinolytic agent epsilon-aminocaproic acid (EACA) is also frequently used to reduce surgical bleeding and intracranial hemorrhage [90]. EACA should be administered as a bolus dose of 100 mg/kg IV over 20 min followed by an IV infusion of 25–33 mg/kg/h for 72 h postoperatively [91]. To date, there is only one report of a thrombotic event either in the neonate or the ECMO circuit related to EACA use [92]. Platelet count should be maintained greater than 100,000/mm^3 during ECMO. Other strategies to reduce bleeding include ECMO without heparinization, heparin-bonded ECMO circuits (Carmeda® BioActive Surface), and recombinant factor VII [88].

The optimal time to repair CDH in a neonate on ECMO remains unclear [93]. Initial studies indicated that when CDH repair was performed before decannulation from ECMO, the mortality rate was greater than when it was done after decannulation. The association of the mortality rate after CDH repair and ECMO is related in part, to the overall incidence of bleeding complications [94]. Neonates who died after CDH on ECMO had a significantly greater incidence of surgical site, CNS, and pulmonary and gastrointestinal hemorrhages. In fact, a validated score [94] for predicting outcome for ECMO CDH patients includes hemorrhage, as well as other ECMO complications and pre-ECMO parameters as components of an ECMO CDH mortality prediction score.

Recently a report of early CDH surgical repair within the first 2 days of ECMO has reported outcomes similar to those published for post-ECMO surgery, without increased risk of surgical hemorrhage [90]. Proposed benefits of this early surgery included surgery before the neonate had developed significant anasarca as well as the use the post-repair ECMO time to allow the pulmonary vascular resistance to decrease and the lungs to heal.

When providing anesthesia for these patients in the NICU, a very close liaison with the neonatologist as well as the perfusionist is required. These infants do not have the same degree of safety net as a full cardiopulmonary bypass patient. Coagulation abnormalities should be corrected aggressively. The infants may need vasopressors during the procedure to maintain an adequate mean arterial blood pressure, and careful observation of the venous filling pressures is important.

Sedation for Imaging Procedures (MRI/CT)

Sedation is often required for neonatal patients requiring radiological procedures such as MRI or CT scan [95]. Standard anesthesia monitors that are compatible with both MRI and CT equipment are available and should be used. However, temperature monitoring during MRI scans is not available. All monitoring wires should be straight (not coiled) and probes placed as far from the magnetic coil as possible to diminish the possibility of thermal injury. Medications and/or procedures used for sedation depend on the age and cardiorespiratory status of the infant. Many infants less than 3 months of age without any cardiorespiratory compromise can be fed and wrapped snugly for a MRI and CT without sedation [101]. Older infants may be given chloral hydrate or midazolam for sedation [96], although general anesthesia is more frequently required with appropriate airway management as an alternative to the complications associated with chloral hydrate sedation in young infants [102, 97]. Full-term neonates may be sedated for CT scan after standard monitors are applied by simply inducing anesthesia with 8 % sevoflurane, applying nasal prongs with 2 l/min oxygen, placing a roll under their shoulders, and allowing the scan to proceed while the neonate breathes spontaneously. Current CT scan imaging is so rapid that neonates often do not recover from the inhalational induction before the scan is completed. These same neonates may also require MRI, which usually lasts 1–2 h. The approach to anesthesia in the neonate for an MRI scan begins with an inhalational induction with sevoflurane and nitrous oxide, followed by IV cannulation and discontinuation of the nitrous oxide. Most neonates with normal craniofacial anatomy and airways can be sedated for the scan using a continuous propofol infusion. The neonate is positioned supine with a small roll under the shoulders and the neck extended. Nasal cannulae are applied while the child breathes spontaneously and anesthesia maintained with a propofol infusion. Neonates and those who are cognitively impaired may require greater infusion rates of propofol than toddlers (who usually require 250–300 μg/kg/min) to stop moving during scan. Propofol infusion rates in neonates are greater than in older children, reaching 400 μg/kg/min at the beginning to transition from the sevoflurane induction and prevent movement during the initial scan. Thereafter, the infusion rate of propofol may be tapered to 250–300 μg/kg/min. Respiration is monitored using the baffled nasal cannula with a CO_2 sample line and pulse oximetry. Dexmedetomidine has been used for sedation for MRI scans in infants and children with non-instrumented airways using very large doses of 3 mcg/kg loading followed by 2 mcg/kg/h infusion [98], whereas we have shown that a small dose of IV midazolam (0.1 mg/kg) given at the beginning of the sedation allows for much smaller infusion rates of dexmedetomidine, 1 mcg/kg loading dose followed by 0.5 mcg/kg/min [115]. There are no data regarding dosing of dexmedetomidine for sedation in neonates, although pharmacokinetic data suggests that the clearance of dexmedetomidine in neonates is one-third than in adults, which might mean that the infusion rate could be reduced [100]. In those with craniofacial and airway anomalies and in ex-premature infants (<60 weeks postconceptional age), tracheal intubation (or an LMA) may be indicated to complete the scan.

Cardiac MRI

There is a growing use of cardiac MRI scans to diagnose cardiac disease in infants, including those in the NICU [133]. Cardiac MRIs are capable of imaging all of the thoracic organs, the respiratory anatomy, as well as cardiac function and anatomy in a single technique, without radiation exposure. In the critically ill neonate, monitoring both the arterial and venous pressures is important to titrate the dose of anesthesia and volume of fluids. Although cardiac MRI scans often require prolonged anesthesia, their duration is similar to that of diagnostic catheter procedures. Additional challenges during MRI in neonates include the limited access to the neonate while within the scanner, the need for an MRI-compatible anesthetic workstation, borderline reliable MRI-compatible neonatal monitors, and temperature control. The low ambient temperature required to cool the magnet combined with the neonate's inability to maintain normothermia and the lack of MRI-compatible effective warming devices increase the risk for perianesthetic hypothermia in neonates in the scanner. Consequently, neonates must be cocooned in warm blankets.

Equipment challenges present a daunting financial obstacle if anesthetic services were included in the design of MRI units, although the capital cost of MRI-compatible anesthetic equipment is a very small fraction of the total cost of the MRI unit. MRI-compatible anesthesia workstations are available for use within the MRI scanner room. If an MRI-compatible workstation is not available, then the workstation must remain beyond the perimeter of the scanner, and long breathing circuit tubing must be fed through the copper hole in the wall to ventilate the neonate during a general anesthetic. Reliable monitoring is essential for all patients who require anesthesia for MRI. This is a particular challenge for infants as the monitors are often not optimized for very small patients. One of the more problematic monitors is the pulse oximeter, which often dislodges from the digit on which it was applied in neonates. In addition, there is often a limited choice of sizes of blood pressure cuff. Additional risks from the MRI environment include ferromagnetic projectiles that may kill the child within the scanner.

Cardiac Catheterization Laboratory

One of the most common areas outside of the NICU and operating room where neonates require sedation and anesthesia is the cardiac catheterization laboratory. Transthoracic echocardiography in infants has a very good image window so that most cardiac diagnoses can be undertaken using noninvasive echocardiography. However, infants with complex cardiac abnormalities may require a diagnostic cardiac catheterization procedure to accurately determine the nature of the anatomy, function, and physiology as well as for cardiac interventions, often to increase pulmonary and aortic blood flows. This is more likely to be a concern in those infants who are critically ill in the NICU and may require the services of the pediatric anesthesiologist. In addition, MRI of the heart and lengthy electrophysiologic procedures such as radiofrequency ablation of aberrant conduction pathways, pacemaker insertion, and automatic implantable cardioverter defibrillator placements in infants have required the services of a skilled anesthesiologist knowledgeable in cardiac anesthesia for infants [103].

Several common cardiac diagnoses that may require intervention are presented (Table 13.8).

Table 13.8 Diagnosis requiring cardiac intervention

Balloon atrial septostomy—infants <8 weeks age for:
TGA – before switch procedure if hemodynamically unstable
TAPVR with restrictive ASD
Tricuspid atresia with restrictive ASD
PV atresia with intraventricular septum
Hypoplastic left heart partially reduces gradient across atrial septum
Blade atrial septostomy > older than 8 weeks age:
Same as per balloon septostomy
Balloon dilation of cardiac valves for:
Pulmonary valve stenosis
Aortic valve stenosis
Coarctation (NB., surgery is still the preferred treatment in neonate and infants (post-dilation aneurysm risk is greater))

TGA transposition of the great arteries; TAPVR total anomalous pulmonary venous return, ASD atrial septal defect, PV pulmonary valve

There are several aspects of the sedation or anesthesia in neonates that must be considered in the cardiac catheterization lab. First, the cardiologists require physiologic variables as close to the normal values for the neonate as possible in order to make correct diagnoses regarding the heart defect. As a result, it is important that we provide enough anesthesia for the neonate for the investigation but not too much anesthesia to depress the myocardium. That anesthetics generally decrease cardiac contractility and disturb the balance of shunts in a dose-dependent manner should provide a metric for the amount of anesthetic that should be administered. Hemodynamic measurements recorded during a diagnostic cardiac cath under general anesthesia may be discrepant from those estimated by the awake echocardiogram if excessive doses of anesthetics that depress the myocardium and vasodilate the peripheral vasculature are administered. Second, the anesthetics may alter the balance of SVR and PVR, thereby changing the amount and direction of shunted blood resulting in changes in the shunt fraction. This may be reflected in both the cardiac cath images as well as the oxygen saturation measurements used to estimate the size of the shunt. Third, the anesthetics may decrease cardiac contractility or vasodilate the peripheral vasculature altering the pressure gradient across a narrowed cardiac valve or outflow tract, thereby raising doubts about whether or not to dilate the restricted orifice. If a balloon procedure is undertaken, significant changes in cardiac function may occur resulting in redistribution of blood flow that can cause complications especially in a critically ill neonate with limited cardiopulmonary reserve [104]. Most importantly, in the cardiac catheterization laboratory, access to the neonate is restricted by the presence of bulky radiological equipment requiring remote access to the IV injection ports and possibly obstructed views of the monitors by equipment and the dark lighting. Furthermore, if the anesthesiologist does not work in the cath lab frequently, the environment is unfamiliar and the nursing assistance may be variable. None of these issues may become important until an acute crisis occurs.

Blood loss is infrequent during cardiac catheterizations (4–7 %), but when procedures such as balloon dilatation are involved, the blood loss could be catastrophic [137]. In most centers, routine cardiac catheterizations do not involve much blood loss as the only vascular access occurs at the site of venous or arterial cannulation. Most cardiologists pay meticulous attention to stopping all bleeding once their catheters are positioned, but a minority does not. When the latter cardiologists are involved, 1–2 units of packed red blood cells should be present in the cath lab before commencing the procedure. Blood must always be present for balloon dilatations as a ruptured major vessel or dissection of a vessel may occur. The transfusion rate for interventional cases in one multicenter study (all-age children) was 14 % [137]. It is wise to check the units to be certain the bags have been assigned to the neonate under your care, although most blood release for this purpose is type O negative.

Preanesthetic Assessment of the Neonate in the Cath Lab

The preanesthetic assessment of the neonate who is scheduled for cardiac cath lab procedures is exceedingly important in neonates. The history and physical examination should focus on the heart defect identifying limitations such as heart failure denoted by tachypnea, poor feeding, and recurrent URTI, which also may be due to excess pulmonary blood flow. Details of every previous anesthetic and previous cardiac surgery and interventions are important to document. For example, the presence of a subclavian flap for coarctation repair requires that the NIBP and pulse oximetry probe should be sited on another extremity. These neonates often have a history of multiple previous admissions and procedures, which may make it difficult to establish IV access. Although drug allergies are infrequent in neonates, family history of reactions to anesthetics and polymorphisms in enzyme systems should be documented. The preoperative hematocrit may reflect systemic problems such as nutritional deficiency, feeding difficulties, chronic illness or chronic hypoxia, and repeated blood draws. If the HCT exceeds 65 %, hyperviscosity may present difficulties and may require phlebotomy before commencing the procedure.

Anesthetic Technique

There is a host of different sedation and anesthesia regimens (Table 13.9) that have been used in neonates in the cath lab [104, 105, 116–122]. In many institutions, cardiac catheterization was historically performed using an oral [105] or intramuscular sedation. Deep sedation with oral medications is unreliable both in onset, efficacy, and duration. As a result, IM cocktails such as CM3 (meperidine, promethazine, and chlorpromazine) were more commonly used. However, this form of IM deep sedation is now rare due to the unpredictable nature of sedation, the slow emergence, and the risk of sterile abscess. More importantly, published reports [116, 117] of respiratory compromise and cardiac decompensation led to recommendations from the APA [118] against their use.

Neonates whose airways are already intubated are often sedated and ventilated by the NICU team using intermittent doses of midazolam and fentanyl and neuromuscular blocking agents. Although there are several theoretical benefits from maintaining spontaneous respiration during a diagnostic catheterization such as avoiding circulatory depression and avoiding the physiologic consequences of positive pressures within the chest but mostly we ventilate the lungs. However, the risks of hypoventilation, atelectasis and desaturation, hypoxia, and cardiac arrest in critically ill neonates are too great to recommend this approach in most neonates.

General inhalational anesthesia with tracheal intubation and paralysis (if needed) remains the most common anesthetic regimen for many neonates (Table 13.9). The incidence of respiratory and/or cardiac complications secondary to IV sedation in infants whose airways are not intubated is 5 %. These adverse events during cardiac catheterization are more likely to occur in those infants with complex or cyanotic heart disease, young age, and reduced body weight. The incidence of airway complications is more likely in several subgroups of infants as listed in Table 13.10.

Table 13.9 Sedation techniques

1. Inhalational anesthesia (a) Sevoflurane (b) Isoflurane (c) Desflurane
2. TIVA (a) Propofol (b) Ketamine (c) Remifentanil (d) Dexmedetomidine
3. Regional anesthesia: caudal/epidural or spinal

Table 13.10 Risk factors for airway events

Sedation
Airway abnormalities
GERD (gastroesophageal reflux disease)
High PVR
IJ/SCV access
Prostaglandin infusion
Down syndrome

Intravenous sedation with propofol has been used for cardiac catheterization, although hypotension may present a concern at induction of anesthesia in premature infants who are hypovolemic. Ketamine is also a popular anesthetic because it maintains cardiac function (often despite hypovolemia) and side effects such as behavior problems do not occur in neonates [120, 121]. Its use is often combined with midazolam [105]. Pulmonary hypertension is associated with significant perioperative risk for complications in infants because it may cause a pulmonary hypertensive crisis and cardiac arrest. In adults, there is evidence that ketamine increases pulmonary artery pressures, although recent studies have disputed this notion [120, 122].

High-dose opioid anesthesia is considered the safest anesthetic technique for neonates with cardiac disease, but it may preclude tracheal extubation at the conclusion of the procedure. This is true for opioids such as fentanyl and sufentanil because of their prolonged half-lives. However, if the high-dose opioid technique were based on remifentanil, an opioid with a context-sensitive half-life of less than 5 min in neonates, then recovery will occur within minutes after terminating the remifentanil infusion and the airway could be extubated immediately. Interestingly, some have maintained spontaneous respiration during remifentanil sedation (0.1–0.2 mcg/kg min) in infants for cardiac cath, although the dose required was quite variable and the need for supplemental sedation increased the risk of apnea [123, 124]. Remifentanil has also been administered in combination with an inhalational-based anesthetic in the cardiac cath lab [125], although the only pain that occurs is at the initial vascular access and if balloon dilatation is performed. In this situation, remifentanil may be used more for its sedative rather than analgesic effect. Interestingly, glycopyrrolate was needed to prevent bradycardia in these infants.

Dexmedetomidine, an alpha-2 agonist, has been advocated for cardiac catheterization both as a solo anesthetic [126] and as an adjunct to inhalational or IV sedation regimen [127]. It has been used safely in neonates when combined with sevoflurane for surgical procedures [128]. Although dexmedetomidine may transiently increase systemic blood pressure and systemic vascular resistance (the loading dose) in those with pulmonary hypertension, pulmonary vascular resistance remained unchanged [129].

Some have advocated spinal anesthesia with hyperbaric 0.5 % bupivacaine 1 mg/kg for infants undergoing cardiac catheterization [119], although the failure rate was 25 %, and supplemental IV sedation was required in 50 % of the infants. The potential benefits of this technique include stable hemodynamics, a reduced BIS without adding sedatives and avoiding the need to intubate the trachea in infants who could be at increased risk for extubation failure, and prolonged post-procedural ventilation due to chronic respiratory disease [106, 107]. However, if a spinal technique were selected to prevent postoperative apneas in an ex-premature infant undergoing cardiac cath, the frequent need of adjunctive sedatives would result in an incidence of apnea no different from that of a general anesthetic [107].

Although EP studies in neonates are infrequent, they may be performed for pharmacologically resistant tachyarrhythmias [130]. As a result of the complex nature of these procedures and the concern regarding the safety of prolonged deep sedation, general anesthesia is often required. A study of EP cases in adults questioned the safety of deep sedation because of the substantial (40 %) risk of airway complications [131]; however, comparable data in neonates have not been forthcoming.

Several anesthetic regimens may be used to anesthetize neonates for EP cases [132]. However, it is best to avoid anesthetics that inhibit the sympathetic nervous system, such as dexmedetomidine, to minimize the risk of interfering with the detection and treatment of the arrhythmias. Total intravenous anesthesia with continuous infusions of propofol and remifentanil has been effective in this situation. Inhalational anesthetic may also be used; however, a rapid increase in the inspired concentration of desflurane in the absence of a background of opioids may induce paroxysmal sympathetic stimulation, although this has never been documented in a neonate. Sevoflurane maintains a stable heart rate and myocardial contractility in children with congenital heart defects [108]. All three inhalational anesthetics, isoflurane, desflurane, and sevoflurane, prolonged the QT interval without increasing the dispersion of repolarization and, therefore, without increasing the risk of torsades. The clinical significance of this last effect in the presence of an intrinsic myocardial conduction defect remains unclear. In cases in which the neonate is hemodynamically unstable or the arrhythmias are potentially life-threatening, invasive arterial pressure monitoring may be indicated.

Complications

Complications from cardiac catheter procedures have been reviewed in some detail in the literature [130, 131, 134–139]. The overall incidence of all complications during interventional procedures (10 %) was almost twice that for diagnostic procedures [134] with airway complications comprising 3 % of the complications. When the risk of complications after cardiac cath was stratified by age, the risk in infants was twice that in older children [137, 138]. Other risk factors included low weight and cyanotic or complex congenital heart disease [136].

Interventional procedures have additional potential complications related to the anatomy and the procedure. Complications from balloon atrial septostomy include transient arrhythmias with premature ventricular contractions, supraventricular tachycardia and atrial fibrillation the most common. Partial/complete heart block and ventricular tachycardia may also occur. Failure to create an adequately sized atrial communication, perforation, or damage to the intracardiac valve has also been reported. Balloon dilation of the pulmonary valve is one of the most common interventional cardiac catheter procedures in infants, indicated for a pulmonary valve gradient >50 mmHg. These infants are usually receiving prostaglandin E1 infusions to maintain ductal patency. As a result of the respiratory depressant effects of the PGE1, these infants often require tracheal intubation. Aortic valve dilation has similar but greater risks than pulmonary valve dilation, most notably attributed to the risk of ventricular fibrillation from which resuscitation may be a challenge. Young infants may be at greater risk for complications from catheter-based therapies [138], although the risk is probably less than that of the surgical approach. In some cases, this allows a palliative procedure to be performed before a safer definitive repair can be undertaken, when the child has grown.

Pulmonary arterial hypertension (PAH) can lead to significant cardiac dysfunction and is known to place the infant at an increased risk of perioperative cardiovascular complications. Baseline suprasystemic PAH is a significant predictor of major complications [139]. Children with suprasystemic PAH have a significant risk of major perioperative complications, including cardiac arrest and pulmonary hypertensive crisis.

Rarely, the wire or catheter perforates a wall in the heart or a major blood vessel or the balloon ruptures a major valve or artery during a controlled dilatation. This potential disaster is best managed by increasing the inspired oxygen concentration to 100 %, calling the cardiac surgery team for possible emergency bypass, stopping the procedure, and leaving the perforating wire/catheter in place or the balloon inflated. Blood should be available in the room to transfuse if bleeding persists. If the femoral venous catheter is involved in the perforation, a second large bore IV should be accessed for transfusion of blood products. A blood warmer should be placed inline to warm the blood during transfusion. If surgery is required, additional blood should be ordered and a transport monitor and stretcher prepared for the rapid transfer to the operating room. The severity of the perforation or accumulation of pericardial blood should be assessed using transthoracic echocardiography before transfer. If a hemopericardium is forming, pericardiocentesis should be performed immediately to preclude a cardiac tamponade.

Conclusion

The provision of anesthesia in the NICU and in medical units for neonates can be a daunting challenge. These infants are usually among the most critically ill neonates we are asked to anesthetize, often requiring major surgery and with substantive mortality rates. Practicing in an unfamiliar environment without access to the usual anesthesia equipment requires that the anesthesiologist be proactive in deciding what is required to successfully manage the infant. Furthermore, the NICU is often remote from the OR, rendering the anesthesiologist a virtual "solo" practitioner as assistance from other anesthesiologists and anesthesia technicians may be delayed or completely unavailable, such as at night. Restricted access to the infant and the use of unfamiliar ventilation modes and monitors also make care more difficult. The anesthetic prescription is usually relatively straightforward with most reports using an opioid-relaxant technique. It is very important to establish excellent communication between all the physicians and healthcare staff involved in the case. The anesthesiologist should use the knowledge and skills of the NICU staff including the physicians, nurses, and respiratory therapists to ensure the anesthetic proceeds smoothly. This will help to overcome potential difficulties that can arise during anesthesia in remote and unfamiliar locations. Teamwork and planning are of paramount importance in order to deliver safe, optimal care for these very ill neonates.

References

1. Davis JM, Auten RL. Maturation of the antioxidant system and the effects on preterm birth. Semin Fetal Neonatal Med. 2010;15(4):191–5.
2. Saugstad OD, Sejersted Y, Solberg R, et al. Oxygenation of the newborn: a molecular approach. Neonatology. 2012;101:315–25.
3. Carlo WA, Finer NN, Walsh MC, Rich W, Gantz MG, Laptook AR, et al. Target ranges of oxygen saturation in extremely preterm infants. N Engl J Med. 2010;362(21):1959–69.
4. Finer NN, Carlo WA, Walsh MC, Rich W, Gantz MG, Laptook AR, et al. Early CPAP versus surfactant in extremely preterm infants. N Engl J Med. 2010;362(21):1970–9.
5. Stenson BJ, Tarnow-Mordi WO, Darlow BA, et al. Oxygen saturation and outcomes in preterm infants. NEJM. 2013;368: 2094–104.
6. Schmidt B, Whyte RK, Asztalos EV, et al. Effects of targeting higher vs lower arterial oxygen saturations on death or disability in extremely preterm infants: a randomized clinical trial. JAMA. 2013;309:2111–20.
7. Askie LM, Henderson-Smart DJ, Ko H. Restricted versus liberal oxygen exposure for preventing morbidity and mortality in

preterm or low birth weight infants. Cochrane Database Syst Rev 2009:CD001077.
8. Lakshminrusimha S, Russell JA, Steinhorn RH, Ryan RM, Gugino SF, Morin 3rd FC, et al. Pulmonary arterial contractility in neonatal lambs increases with 100 % oxygen resuscitation. Pediatr Res. 2006;59(1):137–41.
9. Vento M, Asensi M, Sastre J, Garcia-Sala F, Pallardo FV, Vina J. Resuscitation with room air instead of 100 % oxygen prevents oxidative stress in moderately asphyxiated term neonates. Pediatrics. 2001;107(4):642–7.
10. Naumburg E. Results of recent research on perinatal risk factors: resuscitation using oxygen increases the risk of childhood leukemia. Lakartidningen. 2002;99(24):2745–7.
11. Short JA, van der Walt JH. Oxygen in neonatal and infant anesthesia–current practice in the UK. Paediatr Anaesth. 2008;18(5):378–87.
12. de Graaff JC, Bijker JB, Kappen TH, et al. Incidence of intraoperative hypoxemia in children in relation to age. Anesth Analg. 2013;117:169–75.
13. Hardman JG, Wills JS. The development of hypoxaemia during apnoea in children: a computational modelling investigation. Br J Anaesth. 2006;97(4):564–70.
14. Mort TC. Preoxygenation in critically ill patients requiring emergency tracheal intubation. Crit Care Med. 2005;33(11): 2672–5.
15. Burri PH. Fetal and postnatal development of the lung. Annu Rev Physiol. 1984;46:617–28.
16. Cote CJ, Zaslavsky A, Downes JJ, Kurth CD, Welborn LG, Warner LO, et al. Postoperative apnea in former preterm infants after inguinal herniorrhaphy. A combined analysis. Anesthesiology. 1995;82(4):809–22.
17. Miller MJ, Martin RJ, Carlo WA, Fouke JM, Strohl KP, Fanaroff AA. Oral breathing in newborn infants. J Pediatr. 1985;107(3): 465–9.
18. Miller MJ, Carlo WA, Strohl KP, Fanaroff AA, Martin RJ. Effect of maturation on oral breathing in sleeping premature infants. J Pediatr. 1986;109(3):515–19.
19. Knauth A, Baumgart S. Accurate, noninvasive quantitation of expiratory gas leak from uncuffed infant endotracheal tubes. Pediatr Pulmonol. 1990;9(1):55–60.
20. Litman RS, Maxwell LG. Cuffed versus uncuffed endotracheal tubes in pediatric anesthesia: the debate should finally end. Anesthesiology. 2013;118:500–1.
21. Weiss M, Dullenkopf A, Fischer JE, Keller C, Gerber AC, et al. Prospective randomized controlled multi-center trial of cuffed or uncuffed endotracheal tubes in small children. Br J Anaesth. 2009;103:867–73.
22. Sathyamoorthy M, Lerman J, Lakshminrusimha S, Feldman D. Inspiratory stridor after tracheal intubation with a MicroCuff® tracheal tube in three young infants. Anesthesiology. 2013; 118:748–50.
23. Sathyamoorthy M, Lerman J, Asariparampil R, Lakshminrusimha S. Incidence of Stridor in a neonatal intensive care unit (NICU) after the use of uncuffed and MicroCuff® tracheal tubes: a retrospective review. Anesthesiology Abstracts San Francisco, 2013;A1199.
24. Kumar VH, Hutchison AA, Lakshminrusimha S, Morin 3rd FC, Wynn RJ, Ryan RM. Characteristics of pulmonary hypertension in preterm neonates. J Perinatol. 2007;27(4):214–19.
25. Lakshminrusimha S, Steinhorn RH. Pulmonary vascular biology during neonatal transition. Clin Perinatol. 1999;26(3):601–19.
26. Shankaran S, Langer JC, Kazzi SN, Laptook AR, Walsh M. Cumulative index of exposure to hypocarbia and hyperoxia as risk factors for periventricular leukomalacia in low birth weight infants. Pediatrics. 2006;118(4):1654–9.
27. Miranda P. Intraventricular hemorrhage and posthemorrhagic hydrocephalus in the preterm infant. Minerva Pediatr. 2010;62(1): 79–89.
28. Noori S, Stavroudis TA, Seri I. Systemic and cerebral hemodynamics during the transitional period after premature birth. Clin Perinatol. 2009;36:723–36.
29. McKee LA, Fabres J, Howard G, Peralta-Carcelen M, Carlo WA, Ambalavanan N. PaCO2 and neurodevelopment in extremely low birth weight infants. J Pediatr. 2009;155(2):217–21 e1.
30. Sheard NF, Kleinman RE. TPN cholestasis in premature infants: the role of parenteral nutrition solutions. Pediatr Ann. 1987;16(3):243, 6, 8, 50 & 52.
31. Martin RJ, Fanaroff AA, Walsh MC, editors. Fanaroff and Martin's Neonatal Perinatal Medicine – Diseases of the fetus and infant. 9th ed. St. Louis: Elsevier Mosby; 2011.
32. Greer FR. Osteopenia of prematurity. Annu Rev Nutr. 1994; 14:169–85.
33. Mitchell SM, Rogers SP, Hicks PD, Hawthorne KM, Parker BR, Abrams SA. High frequencies of elevated alkaline phosphatase activity and rickets exist in extremely low birth weight infants despite current nutritional support. BMC Pediatr. 2009;9:47.
34. Bachiller PR, Chou JH, Romanelli TM, Roberts Jr JD. Neonatal emergencies. In: Coté CJ, Lerman J, Anderson BA, editors. A practice of anesthesia for infants and children. Philadelphia: Saunders Elsevier; 2013. Chap. 36.
35. Frawley G, Bayley G, Chondros P. Laparotomy for necrotizing enterocolitis: intensive care nursery compared with operating theatre. J Paediatr Child Health. 1999;35(3):291–5.
36. McKee M. Operating on critically ill neonates: the OR or the NICU. Semin Perinatol. 2004;28(3):234–9.
37. Mallick MS, Jado AM, Al-Bassam AR. Surgical procedures performed in the neonatal intensive care unit on critically ill neonates: feasibility and safety. Ann Saudi Med. 2008;28(2): 105–8.
38. Rees CM, Hall NJ, Eaton S, Pierro A. Surgical strategies for necrotising enterocolitis: a survey of practice in the United Kingdom. Arch Dis Child Fetal Neonatal Ed. 2005;90(2):F152–5.
39. Parente A, Canizo A, Huerga A, Lain A, Fanjul M, Carrera N, et al. Is it correct to use neonatal intensive care units as operating rooms? Cir Pediatr. 2009;22(2):61–4.
40. Laptook A, Tyson J, Shankaran S, McDonald S, Ehrenkranz R, Fanaroff A, et al. Elevated temperature after hypoxic-ischemic encephalopathy: risk factor for adverse outcomes. Pediatrics. 2008;122(3):491–9.
41. John T, Colvin R, Ferrall B. Improving the management and delivery of bedside patent ductus arteriosus ligation. AORN J. 2007;86(2):231–8.
42. Wortham BM, Rais-Bahrami K. Umbilical vein catheterization. In: MacDonald MG, Ramasethu J, editors. Atlas of procedures in neonatology. 4th ed. Philadelphia: Lippincott Willimas & Wilkins; 2007. p. 177.
43. Wortham BM, Gaitatzes CG, Rais-Bahrami K. Umbilical artery catheterization. In: MacDonald MG, Ramasethu J, editors. Atlas of procedures in neonatology. 4th ed. Philadelphia: Lippincott Willimas & Wilkins; 2007. p. 157.
44. Massaro AN, Rais-Bahrami K, Eichelberger MR. Peripheral arterial cannulation. In: MacDonald MG, Ramasethu J, editors. Atlas of procedures in Neonatology. 4th ed. Philadelphia: Lippincott Willimas & Wilkins; 2007. p. 186.
45. Schindler E, Kowald B, Suess H, et al. Catheterization of the radial or brachial artery in neonates and infants. Pediatr Anesth. 2005;15:677–82.
46. Morray JP, Brandford HG, Barnes LF, Oh SM, Furman EB. Doppler-assisted radial artery cannulation in infants and children. Anesth Analg. 1984;63(3):346–8.

47. Lerman J, Coté CJ, Steward DJ. Manual of pediatric anesthesia; with an index of pediatric syndromes. 6th ed. 2009.
48. Bhananker SM, Liau DW, Kooner PK, et al. Liability related to peripheral venous and arterial catheterization: a closed claims analysis. Anesth Analg. 2009;109:124–9.
49. Morray J, Todd S. A hazard of continuous flush systems for vascular pressure monitoring in infants. Anesthesiology. 1983;58: 187–9.
50. Rorke JM, Ramasethu J, Chahine AA. Central venous catheterization. In: MacDonald MG, Ramasethu J, editors. Atlas of procedures in neonatology. 4th ed. Philadelphia: Lippincott Willimas & Wilkins; 2007. p. 199.
51. Meyer S, Sander J, Graber S, et al. Agreement of invasive versus non-invasive blood pressure in preterm neonates is not dependent on birth weight or gestational age. J Paediatr Child Health. 2010;46:249–54.
52. Konig K, Casalaz DM, Burke EJ, et al. Accuracy of non-invasive blood pressure monitoring in very preterm infants. Intensive Care Med. 2012;38:670–6.
53. Pejovic B, Peco-Antic A, Marinkovic-Eric J. Blood pressure in non-critically ill preterm and full-term neonates. Pediatr Nephrol. 2007;22:249–57.
54. Tingay DG, Mun KS, Perkins EJ. End tidal carbon dioxide is as reliable as transcutaneous monitoring in ventilated postsurgical neonates. Arch Dis Child Fetal Neonatal Ed. 2013;98:F161–4.
55. Singh BS, Gilbert U, Singh S, et al. Sidestream microstream end tidal carbon dioxide measurements and blood gas correlations in neonatal intensive care unit. Pediatr Pulmonol. 2013;48: 250–6.
56. Cassey JG, King RA, Armstrong P. Is there thermal benefit from preoperative warming in children? Paediatr Anaesth. 2010;20(1): 63–71.
57. Kent AL, Williams J. Increasing ambient operating theatre temperature and wrapping in polyethylene improves admission temperature in premature infants. J Paediatr Child Health. 2008;44(6):325–31.
58. Buisson P, Bach V, Elabbassi EB, Chardon K, Delanaud S, Canarelli JP, et al. Assessment of the efficiency of warming devices during neonatal surgery. Eur J Appl Physiol. 2004; 92(6):694–7.
59. Tander B, Baris S, Karakaya D, Ariturk E, Rizalar R, Bernay F. Risk factors influencing inadvertent hypothermia in infants and neonates during anesthesia. Paediatr Anaesth. 2005;15(7): 574–9.
60. Lago P, Meneghini L, Chiandetti L, Tormena F, Metrangolo S, Gamba P. Congenital diaphragmatic hernia: intensive care unit or operating room? Am J Perinatol. 2005;22(4):189–97.
61. Finer NN, Woo BC, Hayashi A, Hayes B. Neonatal surgery: intensive care unit versus operating room. J Pediatr Surg. 1993;28(5):645–9.
62. Carbajal R, Rousset A, Danan C, Coquery S, Nolent P, Ducrocq S, et al. Epidemiology and treatment of painful procedures in neonates in intensive care units. JAMA. 2008;300(1):60–70.
63. Anand KJ, Hall RW. Controversies in neonatal pain: an introduction. Semin Perinatol. 2007;31(5):273–4.
64. Hall RW, Boyle E, Young T. Do ventilated neonates require pain management? Semin Perinatol. 2007;31(5):289–97.
65. Kumar P, Denson SE, Mancuso TJ. Premedication for nonemergency endotracheal intubation in the neonate. Pediatrics. 2010;125(3):608–15.
66. Bouchut JC, Godard J, Claris O. High-frequency oscillatory ventilation. Anesthesiology. 2004;100(4):1007–12.
67. Goldsmith J, Karotkin E. Assisted ventilation of the neonate. 5th ed. Philadelphia: Saunders; 2010.
68. Bowen SL. Transport of the mechanically ventilated neonate. Respir Care Clin N Am. 2002;8(1):67–82.
69. Schily M, Koumoukalis H, Lerman J, et al. Can pediatric anesthesiologists detect an occluded tracheal tube in neonates? Anesth Analg. 2001;93:66–70.
70. Moore GP, Lawrence SL, Maharajh G, et al. Therapeutic strategies, including a high surgical ligation rate, for patent ductus arteriosus closure in extremely premature infants in a North American centre. Paediatr Child Health. 2012;17:e26–31.
71. Malviya MN, Ohlsson A, Shah SS. Surgical versus medical treatment with cyclooxygenase inhibitors for symptomatic patent ductus arteriosus in preterm infants. Cochrane Database Syst Rev. 2013;28(3), CD003951. pub 3.
72. Hazeem AAA, Gillespie MJ, Thun J, et al. Percutaneous closure of patent ductus arteriosus in small infants with significant lung disease may offer faster recovery of respiratory function when compared to surgical ligation. Catheter Cardiovasc Interv. 2013;82:526–33.
73. Ko YC, Chang CI, Chiu IS, Chen YS, Huang SC, Hsieh WS. Surgical ligation of patent ductus arteriosus in very-low-birth-weight premature infants in the neonatal intensive care unit. J Formos Med Assoc. 2009;108(1):69–71.
74. Raval MV, Laughon MM, Bose CL, Phillips JD. Patent ductus arteriosus ligation in premature infants: who really benefits, and at what cost? J Pediatr Surg. 2007;42(1):69–75.
75. Gould DS, Montenegro LM, Gaynor JW, Lacy SP, Ittenbach R, Stephens P, et al. A comparison of on-site and off-site patent ductus arteriosus ligation in premature infants. Pediatrics. 2003;112(6 Pt 1):1298–301.
76. Srinivasan PS, Brandler MD, D'Souza A. Necrotizing enterocolitis. Clin Perinatol. 2008;35(1):251–72.
77. Spaeth JP, Kurth CD. The extremely premature infant (micropremie). In: Cote CJ, Lerman J, Todres ID, editors. A practice of anesthesia for infants and children. 5th ed. Philadelphia: Saunders Elsevier; 2013. p. 735–46.
78. Attridge JT, Herman AC, Gurka MJ, Griffin MP, McGahren ED, Gordon PV. Discharge outcomes of extremely low birth weight infants with spontaneous intestinal perforations. J Perinatol. 2006;26(1):49–54.
79. Gordon PV, Attridge JT. Understanding clinical literature relevant to spontaneous intestinal perforations. Am J Perinatol. 2009; 26(4):309–16.
80. Klein KS, Aucott S, Donohue P, Repka M. Anesthetic and airway management during laser treatment for retinopathy of prematurity: a survey of US ophthalmologists and neonatologists. J AAPOS. 2013;17:221–2.
81. Orge FH, Lee TJ, Walsh M, et al. Comparison of fentanyl and morphine in laser surgery for retinopathy of prematurity. J AAPOS. 2013;17:135–9.
82. Haroon J, Chamberlain RS. An evidence-based review of the current treatment of congenital diaphragmatic hernia. Clin Pediatr. 2013;52:115–24.
83. Garriboli M, Duess JW, Ruttenstock E, et al. Trends in the treatment and outcome of congenital diaphragmatic hernia over the last decade. Pediatr Surg Int. 2012;28:1177–81.
84. Dyamenahalli U, Morris M, Rycus P, et al. Short-term outcome of neonates with congenital heart disease and diaphragmatic hernia treated with extracorporeal membrane oxygenation. Ann Thorac Surg. 2013;95:1373–6.
85. Park HW, Lee BS, Lim G, et al. A simplified formula using early blood gas analysis can predict survival outcomes and the requirements for extracorporeal membrane oxygenation in congenital diaphragmatic hernia. J Korean Med Sci. 2013;28: 924–8.
86. Frischer JS, Stolar CJH. Extracorporeal membrane oxygenation. In: Holcomb III GW, Murphy JP, Ostlie DJ, editors. Ashcraft's pediatric surgery. 5th ed. Philadelphia: Saunders Elsevier; 2010. p. 74–86.

87. Tsao K, Lally KP. Surgical management of the newborn with congenital diaphragmatic hernia. Fetal Diagn Ther. 2011;29:46–54.
88. Fallon SC, Cass DL, Olutoye OO, Zamora IJ, Lazar DA, Larimer EL, Welty SE, Moise AA, Demny AB, Lee TC. Repair of congenital diaphragmatic hernias on extracorporeal membrane oxygenation (ECMO): Does early repair improve patient survival? J Pediatr Surg. 2013;48:1172–6.
89. Dassinger MS, Copeland DR, Gossett J, Little DC, Jackson RJ, Smith SD. Early repair of congenital diaphragmatic hernia on extracorporeal membrane oxygenation. J Pediatr Surg. 2010;45(4):693–7.
90. Horwitz JR, Cofer BR, Warner BW, et al. A multicenter trial of 6-aminocaproic acid (Amicar) in the prevention of bleeding in infants on ECMO. J Pediatr Surg. 1998;33:1610–13.
91. Hocker JR, Saving KL. Fatal aortic thrombosis in a neonate during infusion of epsilon-aminocaproic acid. J Pediatr Surg. 1995;30:1490–2.
92. Bryner BS, West BT, Hirschl RB, Drongowski RA, Lally KP, Lally P, et al. Congenital diaphragmatic hernia requiring extracorporeal membrane oxygenation: does timing of repair matter? J Pediatr Surg. 2009;44(6):1165–72.
93. Haricharan RN, Barnhart DC, Cheng H, Delzell E. Identifying neonates at a very high risk for mortality among children with congenital diaphragmatic hernia managed with extracorporeal membrane oxygenation. J Pediatr Surg. 2009;44(1):87–93.
94. Cote CJ, Wilson S. Guidelines for monitoring and management of pediatric patients during and after sedation for diagnostic and therapeutic procedures: an update. Paediatr Anaesth. 2008;18(1):9–10.
95. Smevik B, Borthne A. Magnetic tomography–new imaging techniques and future perspectives. Tidsskr Nor Laegeforen. 2000;120(13):1557–61.
96. Litman RS, Soin K, Salam A. Chloral hydrate sedation in term and preterm infants: an analysis of efficacy and complications. Anesth Analg. 2010;110:739–46.
97. Mason KP, Zurakowski D, Zgleszewski SE, et al. High dose dexmedetomidine as the sole sedative for pediatric MRI. Pediatr Anesth. 2008;18:403–11.
98. Trevisanuto D, Giuliotto S, Cavallin F, et al. End-tidal carbon dioxide monitoring in very low birth weight infants: correlation and agreement with arterial carbon dioxide. Pediatr Pulmonol. 2013;47:367–72.
99. Potts AL, Warman GR, Anderson BJ. Dexmedetomidine disposition in children: a population analysis. Paediatr Anesth. 2008;18:722–30.
100. Kammer B, Helmberger H, Keser CM, Coppenrath E, Schneider K. Magnetic resonance imaging of pediatric patients. In: Reimer P, Parizel PM, Meaney JFM, Stichnoth FA, editors. Clinical MR imaging. New York: Springer; 2010. p. 611–762.
101. Schulte-Uentrop L, Goepfert MS. Anaesthesia or sedation for MRI in children. Curr Opin Anaesthesiol. 2010;23(4):513–17.
102. Andropoulos DB, Stayer SA. An Anesthesiologist for all pediatric cardiac catheterizations: Luxury or necessity? J Cardiothorac Vasc Anesth. 2003;17(6):683–5.
103. Malviya S, Burrows FA, Johnston AE, Benson LN. Anaesthetic experience with paediatric interventional cardiology. Can J Anaesth. 1989;36(3):320–4.
104. Auden SM, Sobczyk WL, Solinger RE, Goldsmith LJ. Oral ketamine/midazolam is superior to intramuscular meperidine, promethazine, and chlorpromazine for pediatric cardiac catheterization. Anesth Analg. 2000;90(2):299–305.
105. Hermanns H, Stevens MF, Werdehausean R, et al. Sedation during spinal anaesthesia in infants. Br J Anaesth. 2006;97:380–4.
106. Welborn LG, Rice LJ, Hannallah RS, et al. Postoperative apnea in former preterm infants: prospective comparison of spinal and general anesthesia. Anesthesiology. 1990;72:838–42.
107. Russell IA, Miller Hance WC, Gregory G, et al. The safety and efficacy of sevoflurane anesthesia in infants and children with congenital heart disease. Anesth Analg. 2001;92:1152–8.
108. de Souza JC, Fraga JC. Is mortality rate influenced by the site of involvement in neonates undergoing laparotomy for necrotizing enterocolitis? J Pediatr Surg. 2009;44(8):1534–9.
109. Attridge JT, Clark R, Gordon PV. New insights into spontaneous intestinal perforation using a national data set (3): antenatal steroids have no adverse association with spontaneous intestinal perforation. J Perinatol. 2006;26(11):667–70.
110. Attridge JT, Clark R, Walker MW, Gordon PV. New insights into spontaneous intestinal perforation using a national data set: (1) SIP is associated with early indomethacin exposure. J Perinatol. 2006;26(2):93–9.
111. Kelleher C, Langer JC. Congenital abdominal wall defects. In: Holcomb III GW, Murphy JP, Ostlie DJ, editors. Ashcraft's pediatric surgery. 5th ed. Philadelphia: Saunders Elsevier; 2010.
112. Anand D, Etuwewe B, Clark D, Yoxall CW. Anaesthesia for treatment of retinopathy of prematurity. Arch Dis Child Fetal Neonatal Ed. 2007;92(2):F154–5.
113. Konduri GG, Kim UO. Advances in the diagnosis and management of persistent pulmonary hypertension of the newborn. Pediatr Clin North Am. 2009;56(3):579–600.
114. Heard C, Burrows F, Johnson K, et al. A comparison of dexmedetomidine-midazolam with propofol for maintenance of anesthesia in children undergoing magnetic resonance imaging. Anesth ANalg. 2008;107:1832–9.
115. Nahata MC, Ootz MA, Krogg EA. Adverse effects of meperidine, promethazine, and chlorpromazine for sedation in pediatric patients. Clinical Pediatr. 1985;24:558–60.
116. Brown ET, Corbett SW, Green SM. Iatrogenic cardiopulmonary arrest during pediatric sedation with meperidine, promethazine, and chlorpromazine. Pediatr Emerg Care. 2001;17(5):351–3.
117. Parks BR, Snodgrass SR. Reappraisal of lytic cocktail/demerol, phenergan, and thorazine (DPT) for the sedation of children. Pediatrics. 1996;97(5):779–80.
118. Katznelson R, Mishaly D, Hegesh T, Perel A, Keidan I. Spinal anesthesia for diagnostic cardiac catheterization in high-risk infants. Pediatr Anesth. 2005;15:50–3.
119. Oklu E, Bulutcu FS, Yalcin Y, Ozbek U, Cakali E, Bayindir O. Which anesthetic agent alters the hemodynamic status during pediatric catheterization? Comparison of propofol versus ketamine. J Cardiothorac Vasc Anesth. 2003;17(6):686–90.
120. Abbas SM, Rashid A, Latif H. Sedation for children undergoing cardiac catheterization: a review of literature. J Pak Med Assoc. 2012;62(2):159–63.
121. Williams GD, Maan H, Ramamoorthy C, Kamra K, Bratton SL, Bair E, Kuan CC, Hammer GB, Feinstein JA. Perioperative complications in children with pulmonary hypertension undergoing general anesthesia with ketamine. Pediatr Anesth. 2010;20:28–37.
122. Kaynar A, Kelsaka E, Karakaya D, Sungur M, Baris S, Demirkaya M, Sarıhasan B, Baysal K. Effects of different doses of remifentanil infusion on hemodynamics and recovery in children undergoing pediatric diagnostic cardiac catheterization. J Cardiothorac Vasc Anesth. 2011;25(4):660–4.
123. Dönmez A, Kizilkan A, Berksun H, Varan B, Tokel K. One center's experience with remifentanil infusions for pediatric cardiac catheterization. J Cardiothorac Vasc Anesth. 2001;15(6):736–9.
124. Foubert L, Reyntjens K, de Wolf D, Suys B, Moerman A, Mortier E. Remifentanil infusion for cardiac catheterization in children

with congenital heart disease. Acta Anaesthesiol Scand. 2002;46:355–60.
125. Kunisawa T, Kurosawa A, Oikawa M, Mizobuchi M, Hayashi D, Iwasaki H. A high dose of dexmedetomidine using the BIS monitor™ for diagnostic and interventional cardiac catheterization in a toddler with congenital heart disease. J Anesth. 2012;26(2):254–8.
126. Ülgey A, Aksu R, Bicer C, Akin A, Altuntaş R, Esmaoğlu A, Baykan A, Boyaci A. Is the addition of dexmedetomidine to a ketamine-propofol combination in pediatric cardiac catheterization sedation useful? Pediatr Cardiol. 2012;33(5):770–4.
127. Ozcengiz D, Gunes Y, Atci M. Preliminary experience with dexmedetomidine in neonatal anesthesia. J Anaesth Clin Pharmacol. 2011;27(1):17–22.
128. Friesen RH, Nichols CS, Twite MD, Cardwell KA, Pan Z, Pietra B, Miyamoto SD, Auerbach SR, Darst JR, Ivy DD. The hemodynamic response to dexmedetomidine loading dose in children with and without pulmonary hypertension. Anesth Analg. 2013;117(4):953–9.
129. Turner CJ, Lau KC, Sholler GF. Outcomes of interventional electrophysiology in children under 2 years of age. Cardiol Young. 2012;22(5):499–506.
130. Trentman TL, Fassett SL, Mueller JT, Altemose GT. Airway interventions in the cardiac electrophysiology laboratory: a retrospective review. J Cardiothorac Vasc Anesth. 2009;23(6):841–5.
131. Lu F, Lin J, Benditt DG. Conscious sedation and anesthesia in the cardiac electrophysiology laboratory. J Cardiovasc Electrophysiol. 2013;24(2):237–45.
132. Odegard KC, Dinardo JA, Tsai-Goodman B, Powell AJ, Geva T, Laussen PC. Anaesthesia considerations for cardiac MRI in infants and small children. Pediatr Anesth. 2004;14:471–6.
133. Yılmazer MM, Üstyol A, Güven B, Öner T, et al. Complications of cardiac catheterization in pediatric patients: a single center experience. Turk J Pediatr. 2012;54:478–85.
134. Bennett D, Marcus R, Stokes M. Incidents and complications during pediatric cardiac catheterization. Pediatr Anesth. 2005;15:1083–8.
135. Huang Y-C, Chang J-S, Lai Y-C, Li P-C. Importance of prevention and early intervention of adverse events in pediatric cardiac catheterization: a review of three years of experience. Pediatr Neonatol. 2009;50(6):280–6.
136. Bergersen L, Marshall A, Gauvreau K, Beekman R, Hirsch R, et al. Adverse event rates in congenital cardiac catheterization – a multicenter experience. Catheter Cardiovasc Interv. 2010;75:389–400.
137. Schneider DJ, Moore JW. Interventional cardiac catheterization in very small infants. Progr Pediatr Cardiol. 2001;14:27–33.
138. Carmosino MJ, Friesen RH, Doran A, Ivy DD. Perioperative complications in children with pulmonary hypertension undergoing noncardiac surgery or cardiac catheterization. Anesth Analg. 2007;104(3):521–7.

Pain Assessment and Management

14

Richard F. Howard

Introduction

The neonate shows unique responses to nociceptive inputs that are a result of immature sensory and motor systems. In addition, physical development and the maturation of drug metabolism and elimination pathways can profoundly impact the efficacy, toxicity, and side effects of analgesics. Important functional differences in pain processing mechanisms are present at the site of pain and in the CNS that lead to profound differences in pain signaling in the neonate compared with the adult. Immature and uncoordinated motor systems change and restrict the range of possible behavioral responses to pain, and postnatal changes in the expression, distribution, and function of transmitters and receptors involved in the actions of analgesics influence their effects. The neonatal period is characterized by profound neuroplasticity and it appears that as a consequence both painful events and exposure to certain compounds, notably some analgesics, have the potential to cause long-term adverse effects in this age group that would not occur at older ages. Therefore, the planning and implementation of safe and effective analgesia for neonates cannot simply be extrapolated from scaled-down versions of techniques used in older children and adults. Rather, they must be carefully constructed and implemented on the basis of a clear understanding of developmental neurobiology and pharmacology.

In this chapter, the development of nociception, the assessment of pain in the preterm and term infant and the principles of perioperative and procedure-related pain management will be discussed.

R.F. Howard, BSc, MB, ChB, FRCA, FFPM (✉)
Department of Anesthesia and Pain Medicine,
Great Ormond Street Hospital for Children,
NHS Foundation Trust, London WC1N3JH, UK
e-mail: R.Howard@ich.ucl.ac.uk

The Development of Nociceptive Systems

The neonate is known to be relatively much more sensitive to nociceptive pain, i.e., potentially tissue-damaging or noxious sensory inputs than are older children and adults. Evidence indicates that premature infants from 24 weeks gestation manifest a full range of neurohumoral and metabolic responses to painful stimulation [1]. Whether the premature infant recognizes the nociception as pain as in adults and distinguishes it from other conditions remains unclear. Nociceptive thresholds are lower at birth but increase as a function of developmental age throughout infancy and childhood [2]. Studies of thresholds to mechanical stimuli (touch, pressure) in infants from preterm to 3 months of age show a clear linear relationship between the mechanical forces needed to trigger a reflex withdrawal response and chronological age [1, 3]. This increase in sensitivity is important; the physiological consequences of unmodified painful tissue-damaging inputs at this age were first clearly demonstrated in human studies that measured the "stress" response to major surgery in neonates who received "light" general anesthesia. The results included a massive, robust, and potentially harmful neuroendocrine stress response to pain, prevented by stronger anesthesia and analgesia, that occurred in neonates and infants at the youngest ages [4, 5]. In addition, pain relief during and after surgery improved important associated postoperative physiological outcomes such as respiratory function, highlighting the importance of analgesia in overall management strategies [5]. Many aspects of maturation are subject to activity-dependent developmental control. For example, there is concern that abnormal events during the neonatal period such as severe pain may alter normal development and lead to adverse long-term consequences to sensory processing mechanisms. In fact, surgery or injury in the neonatal period has been shown to change nociceptive thresholds and the response to subsequent pain months or even years later, although the precise mechanisms involved and the exact roles of pain intensity and analgesia are still not

J. Lerman (ed.), *Neonatal Anesthesia*, DOI 10.1007/978-1-4419-6041-2_14,

fully understood [6–8]. In order to fully appreciate the actual and potential consequences of pain in the neonate, it is necessary to understand how the infant processes nociceptive information and how these inputs are capable of altering CNS development.

Pain Processing Mechanisms

Nociceptors and sensory pathways are present from embryonic stages of development, but they undergo considerable postnatal reorganization and functional change. Refinement of sensory-motor coordination and the development of complex integrative central processing functions, particularly in the brain, take place throughout infancy, childhood, and adolescence although some of the most important, rapid and profound changes occur during the neonatal period.

CNS plasticity, or the capacity for change and adaptation in the central nervous system, is probably never greater than during this period. In fact, such plasticity is essential for neural development, and "normal" level of activity in nociceptive pathways is one mechanism by which this process is controlled. Conversely, unmodified abnormally high levels of activity such as during surgery without anesthesia or severe pain without analgesia may be contributors to some of the long-term changes in pain perception.

Basic Nociception

Neonates exhibit reduced response thresholds to touch, heat and pain that gradually increase as the nervous system matures. These changes are mediated by alterations in the central connections and function of nociceptors and activity in modulatory pathways; they are briefly summarized in Table 14.1. Painful mechanical, thermal, and chemical stimuli are normally detected by polymodal slow conducting C and fast A-delta fiber nociceptors, whose cell bodies are located in the dorsal root ganglion (DRG) and whose central terminals are mostly found in nociceptive specific areas of the superficial dorsal horn of the spinal cord (laminae I and II, Fig 14.1a). A-delta fibers terminate directly on ascending "projection" neurons in lamina I, whereas C-fibers generally terminate on interneurons located in lamina II. Fast-conducting A-beta fibers mostly detecting innocuous touch and pressure terminate in deeper laminae of the cord.

In early development, these central terminals are relatively less well localized, and those of low-threshold A-fibers overlap with C-fiber terminals in lamina II (Fig 14.1b), thereby potentially activating nociceptive projection neurons when stimulated. A reduction in specificity due to this structural difference is augmented by lack of myelination and immature ion channel kinetics that alter neuronal conduction times and synaptic strength leading to a more diffuse central response to peripheral stimuli. Intrinsic spinal cord and descending inhibitory controls are also less well organized and reduced in strength. In contrast to the adult, contralateral cutaneous inhibitory receptive fields are not matched to their corresponding excitatory fields [6]. Cutaneous receptive fields, the area of skin that excites an individual sensory neuron when stimulated, are relatively larger and more overlapping at birth such that each stimulus is cable of inducing a response in many more neurons at this time [9]. This lack of specificity, organization, and control is mirrored in motor circuits such that output responses are also more diffuse and less well integrated spatially and temporally [6]. Although little is currently known about nociceptive processing in higher centers of the brain, physiological studies in premature neonates have demonstrated that painful inputs are capable of producing measurable responses from at least 24 weeks postconception [10].

Sensitization, Inflammatory and Neuropathic Pain

The decrease in sensory thresholds that develop at the site of an injury is known as primary hyperalgesia; it is accompanied by a temporary reduction in thresholds both in the surrounding non-injured tissue and at distant sites known as secondary hyperalgesia. These post injury changes in sensitivity are characteristic of inflammatory pain, a normal part of the healing process. This pain responds fairly well to analgesics and will usually resolve spontaneously as the injury resolves. The processes responsible are known as sensitization, a phenomenon that involves many different mechanisms both in the periphery and CNS [11]. If damage occurs to nerves or nervous tissue, a state of more prolonged pain that is known as neuropathic pain may follow. Although neuropathic pain also

Table 14.1 Factors contributing to augmented pain responses in the neonate compared with the adult

Factor	Effect
Low-threshold A-fiber mechanoreceptors terminate centrally on nociceptive relay pathways	Weaker stimuli activate pain specific pathways
Weak intrinsic inhibitory mechanisms in spinal cord	Relative augmentation of pain signal
Reduced descending inhibition	Relative augmentation of pain signal
Large and overlapping cutaneous receptive fields	Amplification of stimulus effect due to increased numbers of neurons activated
Poorly localized and diffuse sensory-motor connexions	Less anatomically specific and more generalized motor responses

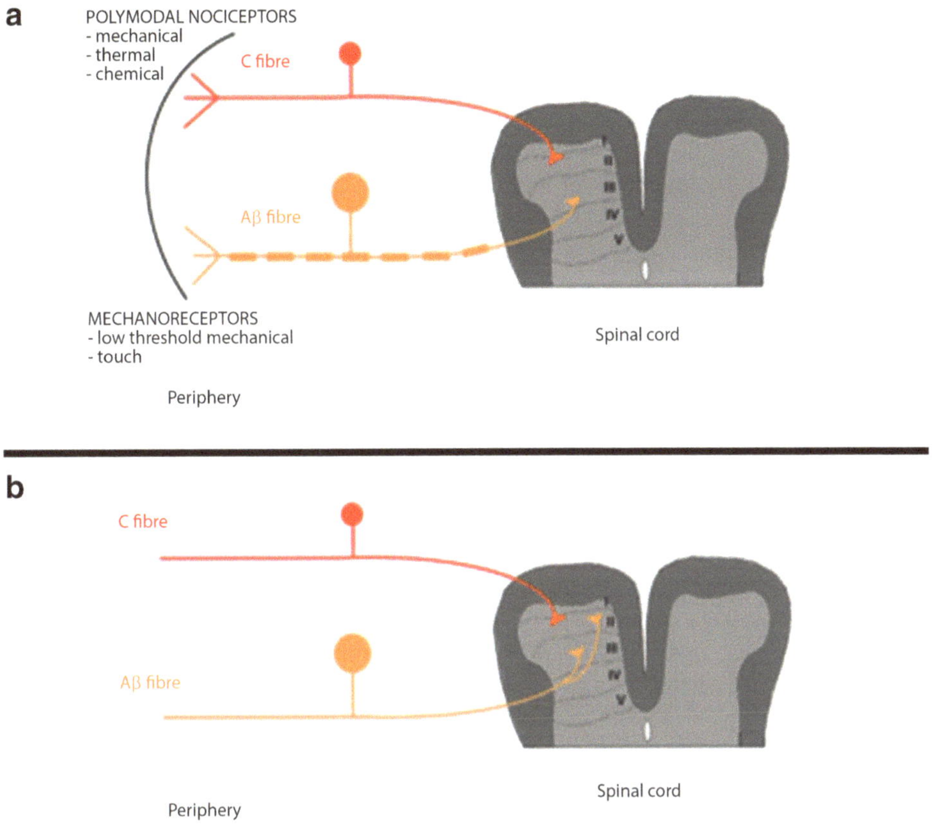

Fig 14.1 (**a**) Adult sensory inputs. (**b**) Neonatal sensory inputs

involves sensitization, unlike inflammatory pain, it often does not resolve spontaneously and is often difficult to treat. Neuropathic pain is a component of many chronically painful conditions such as phantom limb pain, diabetic neuropathy, trigeminal neuralgia, complex regional pain syndrome (CRPS) and many others. Both sensitization and the mechanisms underlying neuropathic pain are under intense research scrutiny with the aim of finding more effective analgesics [12].

These responses are different in neonates. Primary hyperalgesia at the site of an injury is known to occur from birth. Although recovery seems to be more rapid in neonates, a more prolonged inflammatory hyperalgesia has also been demonstrated after repetitive injury [13]. Secondary hyperalgesia appears to be less prominent at younger ages and is slower to develop [14]. Neuropathic pain has not been reported in neonates or infants, even after severe nerve injuries that represent a potent cause of pain in adults, such as brachial plexus damage [15]. Laboratory investigations have confirmed that nerve damage does not produce signs of neuropathic pain in either the neonatal or infant period. Recent studies have suggested that this may be due to immaturity of immune responses in the spinal cord involving microglia and peripheral cellular immunity known to maintain neuropathic pain in adults [16–18].

Long-Term Effects of Pain and Analgesia in the Neonatal Period

There is also evidence that pain in the neonatal period can lead to augmented responses to pain some time later. Boys who underwent neonatal circumcision without analgesia showed an enhanced response to pain at 3 months during immunization in comparison with those who did receive analgesia or were not circumcised [19]. Infants who had abdominal surgery repeated in the same dermatome as a previous operation before 3 months of age showed increased pain responses and analgesic requirements compared with controls [7]. Even more “minor” events such as heel stick blood sampling are a significant cause of pain in the neonate [20]. They too can lead to augmentation of the response to subsequent pain or may even be associated with more serious morbidity and poorer outcomes, especially when repeated frequently, e.g., in ICU [13, 21]. More complex and subtle effects have also been shown in cohorts of children who had neonatal surgery and ICU admission. A relative increase in temperature and touch thresholds near the site of surgery has been observed, but some children also have a more generalized decrease in temperature threshold [8, 22, 23]. Although the precise mechanisms behind these observations are not known, it is clear that sensory development depends on a normal balance of sensory activity, and if this is disrupted, then abnormal patterns or even failure of normal maturation can occur. In the laboratory, maturation of nociceptive reflexes can be delayed or abolished by blocking sensory inputs with local anesthesia for long periods [24]. NMDA receptor activity has been shown to be important for normal sensory development in rat pups as chronic NMDA receptor blockade prevents the normal withdrawal of A-fibers from lamina II described above and a consequent persistence of low sensory thresholds [25].

A panoply of other physiologic sequelae have been reported after painful stimulation in premature infants. During the early brain growth period in premature infants, repetitive painful procedures have been shown to reduce both white matter and subcortical gray matter, leading to impaired brain development [26]. A growing body of evidence has associated repetitive painful procedures in the early postnatal period in premature infants with reduced weight gain and increased head circumference in the early postnatal period [27].

A number of drugs and chemical compounds may also cause long-term adverse effects when administered in the neonatal period over and above altered pharmacokinetic or pharmacodynamic responses due to immaturity. Neuroapoptosis, or programmed cell death, is a component of normal maturation in which cells that do not form functional connexions are eliminated. Drugs that are NMDA antagonists and/or GABA agonists in particular have the potential to markedly increase apoptosis to such an extent that neural development is damaged leading to deficits in, e.g., memory and learning. Although these effects have only been demonstrated in animal models to date, many general anesthetics have been implicated including ketamine (see below), a potent non specific NMDA antagonist that is also used as an analgesic.

These many factors impact the assessment, measurement and management of neonatal pain such that considerable specialist knowledge and skills are needed in order to deliver developmentally appropriate care.

Assessment of Pain

Frequent assessment of pain is an essential component of good pain management; however, this can be problematic in immature, preverbal infants. Accurate assessment including measurement of pain intensity contributes to the prevention or early recognition of pain, as well as for monitoring the effectiveness of analgesia [28]. Overall there are three fundamental approaches to pain assessment in children:

- Self-report: an individual's personal description of pain and rating of intensity
- Behavioral: observation of changes in facial expression and body posture due to pain
- Physiological: measurement of changes in physiological arousal consequent to pain

Obviously, self-report is impossible in neonates, and therefore one of the indirect measures of pain must be used. This is associated with disadvantages; perceived pain intensity is known to depend on many subjective influences apart from the degree of injury and tissue damage. Stress, anxiety, attention, and expectation, which are modulated by context, mood, previous experience, and underlying personality traits all contribute to the degree of unpleasantness of pain; the extent to which such factors can influence pain perception in the neonate is largely therefore a matter of speculation.

Nevertheless, in neonates, the observation of behaviors such as facial expression, cry, and posture and measurements of physiological variables such as heart rate and blood pressure have been used to assess pain and gauge its intensity in the absence of viable more objective alternatives. These observations and measures are subject to many external and internal influences aside from pain, which leads to difficulties in interpretation. For physiological variables in particular, a reduction in their reliability tends to occur over time due to homeostatic controls. In an attempt to improve accuracy, observations and measurements have been frequently incorporated into multidimensional pain measurement "tools" or "instruments" that are generally presented as checklists or scoring systems; the range of such observations and their validity and usability have been reviewed recently [29–32].

Pain Measurement Tools

A bewilderingly large number of pain assessment tools or scales have been designed for use in the neonate, some examples are given in Table 14.2 [1]. There is a considerable research literature on the subject, and it is now agreed that in order to be "fit for purpose", a pain assessment tool should have undergone a rigorous process of development.

To be considered reliable, an individual tool must be validated in the patient population and the clinical context and type of pain (e.g., postoperative or procedural) for which it is to be used. Despite the proliferation and availability of tools, they have not always adequately completed this process nor been used consistently or well; inconsistencies have been identified between reported assessment practice and documented practice [46–48]. Several factors may be responsible for this situation including the large number of scales that are available, limitations to individual scales that mean no single one can be universally recommended for use in all neonates in every situation, and "usability" factors that lead to individual user preferences that might not be scientifically appropriate.

Given the difficulty in finding the "Holy Grail" of behavioral pain scales for neonates, investigators have begun to pursue objective physiologic tools [1]. These pursuits have

Table 14.2 Pain measurement tools

BPS [33], behavioral pain score
CHIPPS [34], children and infants postoperative pain scale
COMFORT [35, 36]
CRIES [37]
CSS [38], clinical scoring system
DSVNI [39], distress scale for ventilated newborn infants
LIDS [40], Liverpool infant distress scale
NFCS [41], neonatal facial coding system
NIPS [42], neonatal infant pain scale
PAT [43], pain assessment tool
PIPP [44], premature infant pain profile
SUN [45], scale for use in newborns

included regional oxygen saturation in the brain (as in near-infrared spectroscopy), EEG, heart rate variability, skin conductance and neurohumoral responses. Although each appears to be an objective metric that may reflect the neonate's response to a painful stimulus, some of the metrics under investigation are invasive, others reflect a time course that may not correspond to the level of stimulation, and others remain imprecise. This remains an active work in progress that may require an aggregate of different measurements to provide a reliable and consistent metric of pain in the neonate.

Selecting an Appropriate Pain Assessment Tool

Recommendations and guidelines have been produced by a number of professional bodies outlining the currently available tools and advising on their suitability for different circumstances [29, 31, 32]. Training and support are required for successful implementation of the best validated tools, and this should be combined with ongoing monitoring and audits of practice. Three of the most widely endorsed tools are the PIPP [44], CRIES [37], and COMFORT [35] scales. The PIPP (Table 14.3) creates a score from 18 to 21 depending on gestational age and behavioral state, with 0–6 reflecting no pain, 6–12 reflecting mild to moderate pain and above 12 indicating severe pain; it is suitable for procedural pain and ongoing postoperative pain. CRIES includes similar indicators to PIPP: crying, oxygen requirements, increases in heart rate or blood pressure, facial expression and sleep behavior. CRIES creates a score from 0 to 10, similar to most self-report or observational measures of pain. The COMFORT [36] tool is more complex, originally developed in 1992 as an assessment of global comfort in pediatric intensive care. Since that time it has undergone a number of validation studies for both procedural and ongoing postoperative pain in intensive care. It is frequently chosen for use in the sickest neonates, e.g., after cardiac surgery.

Table 14.3 The PIPP [44] pain assessment tool

Gestational age	
≥36 weeks	0
32 weeks to 35 weeks 6 days	1
28 weeks to 31 weeks 6 days	2
<28 weeks	3
Behavioral state	
Active/awake eyes open facial movements	0
Quiet/awake eyes open no facial movements	1
Active/sleep eyes closed facial movements	2
Quiet/sleep eyes closed no facial movements	3
Heart rate maximum	
0–4 beats per minute increase	0
5–14 beats per minute increase	1
15–24 beats per minute increase	2
≥25 beats per minute increase	3
Oxygen saturation minimum	
0–2.4 % decrease	0
2.5–4.9 % decrease	1
5.0–7.4 % decrease	2
7.5 % decrease or more	3
Brow bulge	
None (≤9 % of time)	0
Minimum (10–39 % of time)	1
Moderate (40–69 % of time)	2
Maximum (>=70 % of time)	3
Eye squeeze	
None (≤ 9 % of time)	0
Minimum (10–39 % of time)	1
Moderate (40–69 % of time)	2
Maximum ≥70 % of time)	3
Nasolabial furrow	
None (≤9 % of time)	0
Minimum (10–39 % of time)	1
Moderate (40–69 % of time)	2
Maximum (≥70 % of time)	3
Score total (0–21)	

Planning and Organizing Pain Management

Multimodal or Balanced Analgesia

Current strategies for the treatment of acute pain are centered on the concept of multimodal analgesia, which was first proposed in order to increase the efficacy of analgesics while reducing their adverse effects [49]. The supporting rationale is that the major pharmacological groups of analgesics act on different components of pain pathways and as such their effects are likely to be complementary. This is also likely to be true in the neonate, but developmental factors influencing the effects and therefore appropriateness of many analgesics must also be considered. It is logical to use combinations of analgesics, such as acetaminophen, opioids, and local anesthetics in conjunction in order to achieve the optimum effect while keeping the dose of each, and therefore side effects, at a moderate level. Sucrose and non-pharmacological pain management strategies such as nonnutritive sucking (NNS), swaddling, massage, etc. also have an important place in neonatal pain management, particularly for procedural pain, and should therefore be included in a multimodal regimen where it is appropriate.

Information and Protocols: Pain Management Plans

The provision of training and education for healthcare workers and availability of written and verbal information for families and carers are pivotal for successful pain management. Analgesic regimens should be pre-planned wherever possible and implemented with supporting educational programs, provision and maintenance of necessary equipment and clear developmentally appropriate management protocols. Pain management protocols must be sufficiently flexible to allow for differences in analgesic requirements due to developmental age and other factors; they should include a pain assessment and reassessment plan, encompass management of background and incident (breakthrough) pain and stipulate monitoring and management of adverse effects.

A well-designed protocol will therefore ensure efficacy and uniformity of treatment and facilitate ongoing evaluation of effectiveness. Protocols for pain management should also be designed in conjunction with ongoing global management strategies such as family-centered and developmental care [50, 51]. The implementation of family-centered care involves the establishment of a partnership between parents or carers and nursing staff and other healthcare workers that substantially increases parents' role in their child's in-hospital care. Developmental care in NICU is an increasingly popular strategy for reducing stress-related morbidity in premature neonates; stressful and painful inputs are reduced by observing responses on an individualised basis and carefully reorganizing and planning care [52].

Developmental Pharmacology of Analgesics

Relatively few analgesics have a clearly established role in neonatal pain management. Detailed analgesic clinical pharmacology is discussed in other chapters.

Acetaminophen (Paracetamol)

Acetaminophen is an antipyretic and mild analgesic that has been widely used for all ages, including premature neonates. Acetaminophen is used for the management of pain of mild to moderate severity; more severe pain is not controlled by acetaminophen alone. It is often combined with more potent analgesics for postoperative pain after major surgery in neonates, with conflicting results: one study showed significant morphine-sparing effect of intravenous paracetamol [53], whereas another showed no additional effect of rectal acetaminophen when combined with morphine [54].

The precise mechanism of action of acetaminophen is unknown, but central cyclooxygenase (COX) inhibition is probably important; other mechanisms have also been proposed including NMDA and serotonin antagonism and a possible action on cannabinoid receptors [55–57]. Alterations in the pharmacokinetic handling of acetaminophen have significant implications for safe dosing in neonates. Gastrointestinal absorption is delayed in premature neonates, whereas rectal bioavailability is initially greater in the premature and then decreases toward the usual value of 0.5 with increasing age [58]. The volume of distribution decreases and clearance increases from 28 weeks postconceptional age, resulting in a gradual decrease in the elimination half-life.

Acetaminophen is metabolized via both sulfation and glucuronidation, and the increased maturity of the sulfation pathway early in development and relatively high levels of glutathione at this time may provide some "protection" against toxicity in neonates [59]. However, as many kinetic studies have investigated single-dose administration only, caution is warranted with repeated dosing for more than two or three days [59]. Increased production of the reactive product N-acetyl-p-benzoquinoneimine occurs leading to liver toxicity if the usual metabolic enzyme systems become saturated due to overdose or if glutathione is depleted (e.g., with prolonged fasting).

Dose guidelines based on formulation, route of administration, weight and developmental age have been determined by pooled population analysis (Tables 14.4 and 14.5). Antipyretic plasma levels are 10–20 mg/l, levels required for analgesia are thought to be similar, and so most dosing regimens aim to maintain trough plasma concentrations of 10 mg/l [61]. A greater initial dose followed by maintenance doses not exceeding recommended maximum daily doses is generally recommended. Peak plasma levels are rapidly achieved after oral ingestion, but there is a 1–2 h lag before the maximum therapeutic effect; the onset of analgesia after IV administration may be much faster [62]. As rectal bioavailability is much reduced and more variable than oral bioavailability, greater initial doses are recommended when this route is used except in the premature infant. Two intravenous preparations of acetaminophen are available: IV acetaminophen and propacetamol. Propacetamol is a prodrug, which is hydrolyzed to 50 % acetaminophen and is therefore administered in twice the dose of the native drug, i.e., 1 g propacetamol is equivalent to 500 mg acetaminophen. This is a

Table 14.4 Acetaminophen dosing guide—oral and rectal administration

Age	Route	Loading dose	Maintenance dose	Interval	Maximum daily dose	Duration at maximum dose
28–32 weeks PCA	Oral	20 mg/kg	10–15 mg/kg	8–12 h	30 mg/kg	48 h
	Rectal	20 mg/kg	15 mg/kg	12 h		
32–52 weeks PCA	Oral	20 mg/kg	10–15 mg/kg	6–8 h	60 mg/kg	48 h
	Rectal	30 mg/kg	20 mg/kg	8 h		
>3 months	Oral	20 mg/kg	15 mg/kg	4 h	90 mg/kg	72 h
	Rectal	40 mg/kg	20 mg/kg	6 h		

PCA post-conceptual age

Table 14.5 Intravenous acetaminophen/propacetamol dosing guide[a]

Age	Drug	Loading dose (mg/kg)	Maintenance dose (mg/kg)	Dose interval	Maximum daily dose (mg/kg)
<32 weeks PCA	Propacetamol	40	20	12 h	60
	Acetaminophen	20	10	12 h	30
32–36 weeks PCA	Propacetamol	40	20	8 h	80
	Acetaminophen	20	10	8 h	40
36–52 weeks PCA	Propacetamol	40	20	6 h	100
	Acetaminophen	20	10	6 h	50
>1month	Propacetamol	30	30	6 h	120
	Acetaminophen	15	15	6 h	60

[a]Adapted from Allegaert et al. [60]

potential source of confusion and error [60]. The clearance of propacetamol is reduced in infants less than 1 year of age, thus reducing the maintenance doses [63]. Histamine release, pain on injection and contact dermatitis in healthcare workers have been reported with propacetamol. Additionally, mild platelet dysfunction has been reported [64, 65]. Intravenous acetaminophen appears to be devoid of these drawbacks, and therefore it has gained widespread acceptance in pediatric practice.

Several cases of massive overdose of IV paracetamol have been reported in preterm neonates and young infants to date [66–68]. In all instances, full recovery occurred without long-term sequelae. These did not appear to be the result of confusion of paracetamol with propacetamol. Recognizing the risk for potential liver failure or death from an iatrogenic overdose of acetaminophen in a neonate should prompt every institution to implement very tight controls on the dose of paracetamol when it is prescribed for neonates.

Nonsteroidal Anti-inflammatory Drugs

Nonsteroidal Anti-inflammatory Drugs (NSAIDs) are not currently used in neonates for analgesia due to the uncertainty regarding their efficacy, and potential for adverse effects results in an unfavorable benefit-risk ratio. They act by inhibition of cyclooxygenase, enzymes that regulate many cellular functions by the production of prostaglandins and other substances. Prostaglandins have multiple roles in early development, and inhibition of their synthesis with NSAIDs may potentially result in the disruption of the sleep cycle, an increased risk of pulmonary hypertension, alterations in cerebral blood flow, decreased organ perfusion and renal function and disrupted thermoregulation [69].

In premature neonates in intensive care, prophylactic intravenous indomethacin reduces both the need for surgical ligation of patent ductus arteriosus and the incidence of grades 3 and 4 intraventricular hemorrhage. Reductions in cerebral, renal, and mesenteric blood flow velocity occur for 2 h after bolus indomethacin, but can be minimized by continuous infusion. Renal effects are also less with the use of ibuprofen compared with indomethacin. There is therefore a potential to reduce NSAID-related adverse effects. However, laboratory studies have shown a reduced efficacy of NSAIDs in young rodents, casting doubt on their value as analgesics in infants [70].

Opioids

Morphine is the prototypic opioid, having been extensively investigated in the neonate and used to treat severe acute pain after surgery and in the ICU. Dose requirements and clinical responses to opioid agents differ markedly between premature and term neonates and infants and children. Multiple factors contribute to these differences including age-dependent alteration in body composition and organ function influencing opioid pharmacokinetics and genetic and developmental factors that change opioid pharmacodynamics. Therefore, regular pain assessment with individual titration and adjustment of doses according to response is required to achieve analgesia and minimize adverse effects. Tolerance leading to dose escalation and subsequent physical withdrawal response if opioid infusion rates are reduced too rapidly are distressingly frequent problems after medium- to long-term use in intensive care [71]. Other more lipophilic opioids such as hydromorphone, fentanyl, and remifentanil are also sometimes chosen for acute pain management in neonates and are therefore discussed below along with tramadol and the morphine prodrug, codeine.

Morphine

Morphine can be given orally or parenterally. Morphine solutions are generally well absorbed orally, but the pharmacokinetics and efficacy of oral opioids have not been clearly established in neonates. Oral morphine can be give at a dose of 0.2 mg/kg every 4 to 6 h in monitored non-ventilated neonates (Table 14.6). Parenteral morphine is usually given intravenously either by intermittent dosing, continuous infusion or in a nurse-controlled analgesia (NCA) regimen (Tables 14.5 and 14.6) [72]. Subcutaneous morphine is also used. The pharmacokinetics and clinical use of morphine in neonates have been reviewed extensively [73–76]. The pharmacokinetics of IV morphine are developmentally regulated. In the neonatal period, the pharmacokinetics are characterized by high inter-patient variability and reduced clearance, rendering the clinical effects of morphine less predictable than in older children. In neonates 1–7 days of age, the clearance of morphine is markedly diminished, being 30 % of that of older infants and children. As a result, the elimination half-life is approximately 1.7-fold greater than in older children [76, 77]. Infusion rates and dose intervals must therefore be adjusted according to both age and weight of the neonate, to avoid accumulation. Although the plasma levels associated with analgesia are not well defined, a mean steady-state plasma concentration of 10 ng ml^{-1} is a reasonable target in the neonate. This level may be achieved in children in intensive care after noncardiac surgery with a morphine hydrochloride infusion of 5 mcg h^{-1} kg^{-1} at birth (term neonates), 8.5 mcg h^{-1} kg^{-1} at 1 month, 13.5 mcg h^{-1} kg^{-1} at 3 months, 18 mcg h^{-1} kg^{-1} at 1 year and 16 mcg h^{-1} kg^{-1} for 1- to 3-years-old children [75]. A recent retrospective audit of morphine consumption over a wide age range by the same investigators indicated that morphine infusion rates of 10 mcg h^{-1} kg^{-1} appear appropriate for neonates and infants 1–6 months of age, but given the interindividual variability in responses, the rate should be adjusted to the infant's pain level, concomitant medications, and physiological responses [78]. Conversely, a common threshold for respiratory depression in neonates, infants, and children has been defined as 20 ng ml^{-1} [79]. Any differences in efficacy observed between continuous infusion and intermittent boluses of morphine probably relate more to the age appropriate total dose of drug received, rather than the route of administration [80, 81] Sedation and respiratory depression are the most frequently reported adverse events after morphine (and other opioids) [82] administration. Adverse effects of morphine can be reversed by administering the opioid antagonist naloxone A timely administration of naloxone should facilitate complete recovery from the adverse effects.

Table 14.6 Morphine dosing and morphine infusion

Morphine dosing	
Preparation	
Oral solution	200 mcg/kg, 4–6 hourly
Intravenous	25–50 mcg/kg initial dose (titrated according to response)
	25 mcg/kg every 30 min–1h
Morphine infusion	
Preparation	Morphine sulfate 1 mg/kg in 50 ml solution
Concentration	20 mcg/kg/ml (0.02 mg/kg/ml)
Initial dose	0.5–2.5 ml (0.01–0.05 mg/kg)
Infusion rate	0.1–0.6 ml/h (2–12mcg/kg/h)

Box 1 Nurse-Controlled Analgesia (NCA)

NCA is a demand-led alternative for patients who are too young or unable to use PCA (patient-controlled analgesia). It is designed to provide safe, potent, flexible and convenient pain control by combining the possibility of a continuous opioid analgesic infusion with on-demand bolus doses of analgesia administered according to predetermined limits. NCA was first developed for infants and those children and adults who were unable to operate the PCA handset and was subsequently adapted for neonates [72]. The protocol for the initial infusion of NCA in a postsurgical neonate is shown in Table 14.7.

Table 14.7 NCA (morphine) protocol for neonates and infants

NCA[a] for neonatal use	
Preparation	Morphine sulfate 1 mg/kg in 50 ml solution
Concentration	0.02 mg/kg/ml
Initial dose	0.5–2.5 ml (0.01–0.05 mg/kg)
Pump programming	
Background infusion	0–0.5 ml (0–0.01 mg/kg/h)
NCA dose	0.5–1.0 ml (0.01–0.02 mg/kg)
Lockout interval	20 or 30 min

[a]NCA is a demand-led, flexible morphine infusion system using a PCA infusion pump [72]. It is suitable for neonates not receiving respiratory support provided they are closely monitored by appropriately trained staff

Fentanyl

Fentanyl is a synthetic, high-potency (100x morphine) lipid-soluble opioid; its main use is for intraoperative analgesia where its rapid onset, short initial half-life, and cardiovascular stability at larger doses are an advantage. Fentanyl is also used by infusion in ICU, and it has some advantages for procedural pain owing to its rapid onset. Unfortunately it also creates the potential to more rapidly develop tolerance after prolonged use and may cause opioid withdrawal syndromes.

After a single intravenous dose, the duration of action of fentanyl is 30–45 min. Given its high lipid solubility, the pharmacokinetic profile of fentanyl is context sensitive, such that its half-life progressively increases with the duration of the infusion [83]. High-dose fentanyl has been associated with chest wall rigidity and subsequent difficulty in ventilation. Accordingly, large doses are usually given only when respiration is controlled [84]. Fentanyl can also be given neuraxially; in the epidural space, it is used alone or in combination with an infusion of local anesthetic after major surgery [85, 86]. Alfentanil and sufentanil are fentanyl analogs with different potencies and durations of effect. Their principal use is during anesthesia, but they have also been used for postoperative pain and pain due to brief procedures particularly in the ICU [87, 88]. Sufentanil is more potent, but otherwise very similar to fentanyl in its clinical effect. It has been administered by infusion in the ICU, but probably does not offer significant advantage. Alfentanil is less potent than fentanyl. Its pharmacokinetics have been studied in the neonate. Its duration of action after a single dose is relatively brief, making it suitable for use during tracheal intubation [78]. However like fentanyl, doses effective for painful procedures can lead to chest wall rigidity in neonates and therefore should probably only be used if ventilation is controlled [89].

Remifentanil

Remifentanil is an ultrashort-acting fentanyl analog that is metabolized by the ubiquitous tissue and plasma esterases. Consequently, its elimination is rapid and fixed and independent of liver and renal function. The context sensitive half-life of remifentanil remains in the order of a few minutes even after several hours of infusion, a product of its rapid degradation by esterases. This characteristic has obvious advantages in anesthesia and sedation practice. Indeed, the role of remifentanil in pediatric anesthesia and intensive care has been reviewed recently [90].

Although remifentanil has been used during surgery and in ventilated neonates in ICU, the rapid development of tolerance and possibility of opioid-induced hyperalgesia are potential problems. If remifentanil is used during anesthesia, then longer acting opioids are usually introduced immediately before or after awakening to prevent severe pain from developing in the early postoperative period [91].

Hydromorphone

Hydromorphone is a potent semisynthetic morphine derivative that is popular in pediatric practice having been used extensively in PCA and epidural analgesia regimens in older children. Hydromorphone is approximately 4 or 5 times more potent than morphine and has a lipid solubility intermediate between morphine and fentanyl. It has no active metabolites which is potentially an advantage in the neonates, although it has not been well described or studied in this age group.

Codeine

Codeine is a low-potency opioid that has been popular in pediatric practice. Its primary indication is for mild to moderately severe pain. Traditionally codeine has been chosen where respiratory depression, sedation, or other opioid-related side effects are a particular concern, e.g., in the neonate and after neurosurgery, although the use of codeine for these indications has been challenged because of uncertainties regarding its efficacy and safety [92].

Codeine is a morphine prodrug; about 10–15 % of each dose of codeine is metabolized to morphine by the cytochrome P450 enzyme CYP2D6, and this metabolite is thought to be responsible for its analgesic effect as analgesia cannot be demonstrated in human volunteers in whom the pathway is pharmacologically blocked. CYP2D6 activity is genetically regulated, with 5–40 % of individuals in some populations having reduced, little, or no activity ("slow and intermediate metabolizers"), and consequently is less able to produce morphine from codeine. This has led to widespread unpredictability in its analgesic effects [93]. Conversely "ultrarapid metabolizers" may experience adverse effects in the form of respiratory depression from the rapid conversion of codeine to morphine [92]. CYP2D6 activity is also developmentally regulated, with reduced activity in the very young [94]. Codeine should be avoided when pain assessment is difficult or impossible and in individuals with known polymorphisms of CYP2D6. In general, we do not recommend codeine for the management of pain in neonates.

Tramadol

Tramadol is a synthetic opioid analgesic that also inhibits serotonin and norepinephrine reuptake [95]. Its clinical pharmacology has been reviewed recently. It is used widely for acute and chronic pain in children, and there is an extensive body of literature describing its efficacy and indications. The pharmacokinetics of tramadol in neonates and infants have been investigated. Clearance is reduced in the neonate, but reaches 80 % of adult values by 1 month of age [96, 97].

No relationship has been established between postmenstrual age and O-desmethyltramadol production (see below).

As in the case of codeine, tramadol is metabolized by the cytochrome enzyme CYP2D6 to its major active metabolite

O-desmethyltramadol, which has a 200× greater affinity for the mu opioid receptor than the parent compound. CYP2D6 is genetically and developmentally regulated (see codeine metabolism above), which may hold implications for its use in very young patients. The effect of CYP2D6 polymorphism on the efficacy and disposition of tramadol at this time is unknown.

Opioid side effects have been reported to be less prominent with tramadol in neonates, although this has not been confirmed when equi analgesic doses were used [95, 98].

Novel Non-opioid Analgesics

Clonidine and Dexmedetomidine

Clonidine and dexmedetomidine are alpha$_2$ adrenergic agonists capable of producing analgesia both systemically and neuraxially. Clonidine has been more widely used and studied than dexmedetomidine to date. Clonidine has analgesic, sedative and antiemetic properties; it can also cause hypotension and bradycardia. It has been used as a sedative infusion in ICU areas and for the symptomatic treatment of effects due to the rapid withdrawal from opioids [99].

Pharmacokinetic data regarding alpha$_2$ agonists in neonates do not exist and in children are limited. After systemic administration, plasma concentrations of clonidine within the range 0.2–2.0 ng/ml are thought to be clinically effective [100]. The pharmacokinetics of epidural clonidine in 1–9-year-olds was similar to that in adults [101]. Dose-dependent sedation, hypotension, and bradycardia occur after systemic clonidine. Neonates appear to be more susceptible to both the effects and side effects of clonidine. Since the reporting of a case of severe delayed respiratory depression in a neonate who was given 2 mcg/kg caudal epidural clonidine, a number of similar reports have appeared in the literature that have resulted in an advisory to use caution when considering the use of clonidine by any route in this age group [102–105]. Epidural dexmedetomidine analgesia was also found to be developmentally regulated and relatively greater in neonates in a laboratory model. These data suggest that dexmedetomidine may be better tolerated than clonidine in neonates [106].

Ketamine

Ketamine is a glutamate NMDA receptor antagonist that has been used for many years as an intravenous general anesthetic. Its principal advantages include profound analgesia, relative preservation of respiration and respiratory reflexes and cardiovascular stimulation. Ketamine produces a state of "dissociative" anesthesia that has the disadvantage that emergence phenomena may occur including hallucinations and unpleasant dreams. After small doses (<1 mg/kg), ketamine is an effective analgesic. In particular, it reduces the hypersensitivity due to central sensitization after injury or surgery in both inflammatory and neuropathic conditions. Although there are numerous publications concerning the analgesic effects of ketamine, a recent systematic review concluded that its role in the management of postoperative pain in the adult remains unclear [107].

The NMDA receptor undergoes developmental changes in distribution, structure, and function. It is thought to play an important role in regulating neuronal plasticity during the developmental period [108]. The precise impact of these changes on the efficacy or toxicity of ketamine (or other NMDA antagonists) during the neonatal period remains incompletely understood. The principal uses of ketamine in neonatal practice have been as an intravenous induction agent in high-risk patients with cardiovascular disease and for procedural sedation. The potential for neurotoxicity from systemically or spinally administered NMDA antagonists is also a concern and has been the subject of considerable and ongoing debate [109]. Systemically administered ketamine, and a number of other substances including some sedatives and anesthetic agents, can produce damaging neurodegeneration in the rodent brain if exposure occurs during a critical period of early postnatal development [110]. The significance of these findings in humans and implications for clinical practice remain unknown at this time [111]. Early studies in primates indicate that similar histological damage is possible, but critically depends on the age at exposure, drug dose and duration of treatment, with the greatest risks being conferred inter-utero and in the first few days of life [112]. Spinally (epidural) administered preservative-free ketamine has not been clinically implicated in causing neurotoxicity, although recent research in rodents has led to the conclusion that the benefit-risk ratio is unlikely to be favorable in neonates and young children, and so it should be avoided [102, 113].

Local Anesthetics

Local anesthesia (LA) is very important in infant acute pain management, particularly during and after surgery and for procedural pain where opioid requirements and opioid-induced side effects such as depression of respiration can be reduced or avoided. Topical LA, LA infiltration, and peripheral and central regional analgesia are all used extensively to prevent or treat acute pain in neonates. The detailed pharmacology of local anesthetics is discussed elsewhere.

Lidocaine, Bupivacaine, Levobupivacaine and Ropivacaine

The amide-type LAs lidocaine and bupivacaine have been the most commonly used in neonates for several decades, and there is considerable clinical experience of their efficacy and safety at all ages. Lidocaine has a rapid onset and is of short to intermediate duration; it is used for local infiltration and regional nerve blocks, particularly where a rapid response is required. EMLA (eutectic mixture of local anesthetics) is a combination of lidocaine and prilocaine for topical analgesia—see below for a detailed description. Bupivacaine has a slower onset and long duration, 4 h analgesia or longer can be expected after single-dose central nerve blocks, and consequently it has been the first choice for postoperative analgesia. Their pharmacology and pharmacokinetics have been well investigated and were reviewed recently [114]. Bupivacaine is a racemic mixture. The S(+) enantiomer, levobupivacaine, has a slightly improved in vivo and in vitro safety profile compared with bupivacaine, but is otherwise similar [115, 116]. Ropivacaine is also a levo-enantiomer amide LA with similar clinical properties to bupivacaine except that motor block is slower in onset, less intense and shorter in duration [102]. Ropivacaine may have theoretical advantages during prolonged infusion in neonates and infants, when compared with bupivacaine, as the former's context sensitive half-life does not increase with the duration of infusion [102].

Toxicity of LAs depends on the age of the patient, the drug, absolute dose, and route of administration. Neurotoxicity and cardiotoxicity have been reported in neonates who may have a reduced threshold for toxicity, although toxic events are quite rare provided dosage recommendations are followed [117]. LAs are extensively protein bound (>90 %), with the free, unbound fraction being the pharmacologically active fraction. AAG (alpha-acid glycoprotein) and albumin are the most important plasma proteins that bind drug; AAG levels in blood are reduced in the neonate resulting in increased unbound fractions of lidocaine and bupivacaine [118, 119]. Plasma bupivacaine concentrations >3mcg/ml are associated with neurotoxicity in the awake adult, cardiotoxicity with levels >4mcg/ml. Equivalent blood concentrations in neonates are not known, but toxicity has been reported after epidural bupivacaine infusion at doses greater than 0.3 mg/kg/h, leading to a reduction in the recommended infusion rate in neonates to 0.2 mg/kg/h or less [120, 121] and duration of infusion of 48 h [122]. In contrast to levels after epidural bupivacaine, the plasma levels after epidural ropivacaine infusion in infants <1 year of age did not continue to increase with the duration of the infusion, although the absolute levels and free fraction were similarly increased at younger ages [123].

EMLA, Amethocaine Gel, and Other Topical LA Preparations

Topical local anesthesia has revolutionized the practice of minor needle-related procedures such as venipuncture, venous cannulation and lumbar puncture [124]. A number of preparations are available, the most frequently studied and used being EMLA and Ametop (amethocaine or tetracaine gel).

EMLA is a eutectic mixture of lidocaine and prilocaine such that the combination has a melting point that is less than either of the constituents. This mixture, formulated as a cream, effects local anesthesia when applied to intact skin for approximately 60 min under an occlusive dressing, with a duration of analgesia that may last several hours. If applied to the mucosa, however, the absorption of the local anesthetic is much more rapid and extensive and may cause methemoglobinemia and seizures [125]. EMLA is suitable for use in the neonate in single doses; multiple doses should be limited to a maximum of 4 applications per day and under close supervision to avoid methemoglobinemia. Measurement of blood methemoglobin levels has been advised if multiple applications or large doses of EMLA are applied [126, 127]. Prilocaine causes methemoglobinemia indirectly via its primary metabolite, o-toluidine. Methemoglobin is an oxidized form of hemoglobin that has a reduced oxygen-carrying capacity. Methemoglobin reductase, the enzyme that catalyzes reduction to hemoglobin, is also developmentally regulated, rendering neonates susceptible to methemoglobinemia because fetal hemoglobin is more easily oxidized [128]. Minor side effects of transient paleness, or redness, and edema of the skin may occur after the application of EMLA.

Tetracaine, the essential ingredient in Ametop, is a potent ester-type local anesthetic. Given its systemic toxicity, its clinical use is limited to intrathecal and surface anesthesia. Four percent tetracaine gel (Ametop) produces surface anesthesia in about 30 min and has an absorption and elimination half-life of about 75 min and a duration of analgesia of 4–6 h. Only 15 % of topically applied tetracaine is bioavailable. Tetracaine produces a more rapid onset and longer lasting duration of effect than EMLA. It has been shown to be effective in the neonate [129, 130], although it may not be effective for all procedures [131]. Mild erythema at the site of application is frequently observed but of little consequence; edema of the skin, itching, and even blistering have been reported in older children but are rare in the neonate.

Sucrose

Sucrose solutions reduce physiological and behavioral signs of pain in neonates during brief painful procedures such as heel lance blood sampling [132]. This effect may be mediated by activation of descending modulatory pathways by activation of intrinsic opioid systems in response to the sweet taste [133]. The prescription for sucrose analgesia is 0.5–2.0 ml of a 24 % solution of sucrose administered 1–2 min before the painful stimulus [134]. Although studies have found that dosing ranges between 0.05 and 2.0 ml of 12–24 % solutions are effective [135], it can also be given using a pacifier or dripped directly onto the tongue using a syringe. The number of drops that should be used should be gauged by the infant's response to pain. However, there is no actual known analgesic dose. Coughing, choking, gagging and transient oxygen desaturation can occur. The safety of multiple administrations in very small preterm infants has been questioned as changes in neurobehavioral responses were observed after repeated sucrose administration in this age group [136, 137].

Postoperative Pain Management

Postoperative pain management should always be planned before undertaking surgery [138]. Initiation of postoperative pain relief is usually considered to be part of the plan of anesthesia; patients should not normally be discharged from the PACU (postanesthesia recovery unit) or returned to the ICU until they are comfortable and an ongoing pain management plan is established. Pain management protocols should include pain assessment, monitoring, criteria for additional analgesia, management of side effects, and criteria for transition to simpler, usually oral, analgesia when appropriate. The range of surgical complexity and thus the range of postoperative pain in neonatal surgery cover the spectrum from relatively minor, as in the case of circumcision or uncomplicated inguinal hernia repair on otherwise well neonates, to major interventions in life-threatening circumstances carried out on very sick infants. Appropriate analgesia depends on the exact prevailing circumstances that would depend on the type of surgery, physical state of the child and available facilities for postoperative care and level of staff training. Some of the more commonly encountered procedures, divided into three groups of increasing complexity, are given in Table 14.8. Conventionally, analgesia is commenced intraoperatively as part of the plan of anesthesia using combinations of local anesthetics, opioids, and acetaminophen and suitable ongoing analgesia administered orally, rectally or parenterally as indicated.

Table 14.8 Common surgical procedures

Neonatal surgery
Group 1
Inguinal hernia repair
Pyloromyotomy
Orchidopexy, orchidectomy
Group 2
Duodenal atresia
Intestinal malrotation
Colostomy formation
Urogenital malformations
Group 3
Bowel resections NEC
Esophageal atresia
Congenital diaphragmatic hernia
PDA repair
Congenital heart surgery

Group 1: Inguinal Hernia Repair, Circumcision, Pyloromyotomy, etc

Neonates presenting for this type of surgery are usually healthy; the procedures are relatively brief and are sometimes performed using minimally invasive laparoscopic techniques:

(a) Local anesthesia: Caudal epidural analgesia or simple local anesthetic nerve blocks such as ilioinguinal block and penile block are often effective. If these techniques are not suitable, then subcutaneous infiltration at the surgical incision or laparoscope port sites with a relatively long-acting local anesthetic such as levobupivacaine is an option.
(b) Opioid analgesia: Fentanyl or other suitable opioid administered as part of anesthesia can be continued into the postoperative period if necessary using oral morphine solution as oral intake is usually rapidly resumed. Oral morphine can be given every 4 h if necessary, but it is unusual for neonates to require more than one or two doses after these procedures.
(c) Acetaminophen: A loading dose should be administered during surgery, preferably intravenously. Oral and rectal dosing are options; the first dose can be given before surgery, but rectal absorption is less predictable in neonates. Acetaminophen can be continued orally at appropriate doses for 2 or 3 days as necessary.

Group 2: Major Gastrointestinal or Genitourinary Surgery

Although surgery can be quite prolonged and relatively invasive, the majority of neonates presenting for these procedures are healthy and can be expected to recover rapidly. A potential problem is that large doses of intraoperative opioids may be required to obtund physiological responses to surgery, which may result in delayed recovery and possibly necessitating postoperative respiratory support:

(a) Local anesthesia: Continuous epidural analgesia should be considered for this group as it allows early postoperative extubation and reduces the need for ongoing respiratory support.
(b) Opioid: High-potency analgesics such as parenteral opioids or local anesthetic infusions may be needed as part of a "balanced analgesia" approach. Intravenous opioid infusion may be needed postoperatively, and NCA (see above) should be considered because it is easier to adapt dose requirements to individual patients and circumstances.
(c) Acetaminophen: Intravenous paracetamol has been shown to reduce the postoperative morphine requirements in neonates and infants after major abdominal and

thoracic surgery [53]. Rectal acetaminophen failed to reduce morphine requirements in neonates after major abdominal surgery [54]. But as rectal absorption is unreliable and pain assessment difficult in these infants, further study is indicated before this strategy is abandoned. Acetaminophen, and particularly intravenous acetaminophen, should not be given at full dose for more than a few days because of potential toxicity. Therefore it may be prudent to delay its use until epidural or IV opioid infusions are being withdrawn on postoperative days 2 and 3.

Group 3: Cardiothoracic Surgery or Complex Gastrointestinal/Genitourinary Surgery

These infants are frequently unwell, in poor clinical condition or critically ill. Sepsis, cardiorespiratory insufficiency and significant blood loss can complicate the perioperative period. Few of these neonates are extubated within the first postoperative day. Premature neonates with necrotizing enterocolitis who need GI surgery or ventilator-dependent neonates with PDA are often too immature or too unwell to tolerate procedures such as epidural placement unless strongly indicated. Potent intravenous opioid analgesia by continuous infusion or NCA with or without acetaminophen is the mainstay of analgesia in this group. Postoperative pain management after cardiac surgery in neonates has been reviewed recently [139].

Analgesia for Neonates in ICU

Neonates who have undergone surgery require analgesia; this is usually given in the form of opioid infusions in ICU settings. Premature and other neonates in ICU who need respiratory support may also require pain relief, but there is ongoing and currently unresolved debate regarding whether the use of opioid infusions in neonates who are ventilated in ICU should be routine. Typically these infants undergo numerous painful medical procedures such as heel lance blood sampling, insertion of arterial lines, lumbar puncture and many others. Sedation and analgesia are often provided for laryngoscopy and insertion of the tracheal tube in the neonate, although maintaining the tube in the trachea may itself be painful. Aside from humanitarian and ethical reasons for giving analgesia, routine use of morphine infusions may improve cardiorespiratory stability in ventilated neonates. A pilot study has also suggested that the use of opioids may improve neurological outcome [140]. This benefit was not confirmed in a subsequent large study, which initially reported an association between bolus morphine administration and worse outcome [141]. Subsequent reanalysis of the data has revealed that poor neurological outcomes were related to pre existing hypotension and that morphine therapy was not a contributory factor [142]. However, morphine infusions can produce hypotension, and the safety, efficacy, and long-term outcomes of analgesia and sedation in ventilated neonates require further evaluation. Although evidence suggested that the use of morphine in neonatal animals confers possible long-term neurocognitive, neurobehavioral and neuroanatomical changes, two recent studies of ventilated premature neonates who were randomized to receive either morphine (10 μg/kg/h) or no morphine in the early postnatal period failed to show any serious long-term neurocognitive or neurobehavioral consequences in the morphine-treated group after 5 and then 8–9 years [143]. In contrast, midazolam, a sedative frequently used in older patients in intensive care, has been strongly associated with an increased incidence of poor neurological outcome in neonates [140]. Hence, the use of such drugs requires a careful benefit to risk analysis. Although there is currently insufficient evidence to support routine opioid infusions in ventilated neonates, morphine appears safer than midazolam as a sedative in this age group. As the risks involved are often subtle, difficult to measure, and their mechanisms poorly understood, the selective use of opioids based on the assessment of pain, clinical judgment, and the current best available evidence has been recommended [144, 145].

Procedural Pain

A number of documents including reviews, guidelines and policy statements have been published recently on the subject of procedural pain management in the neonate [146–148]. Analgesia for neonatal procedural pain has been relatively well studied, yet it is clear that many procedures are often poorly managed [20]. Painful procedures include blood sampling, insertion of intravenous and intra-arterial catheters, retinal laser treatment, insertion and removal of chest tubes, and tracheal intubation, among others. In some cases, procedures are performed on neonates that would always entail general anesthesia in older children and adults. This is not consistent with evidence that the neonate has increased sensitivity to nociceptive pain (see above). General considerations regarding procedural pain management are given in Table 14.9. Procedural pain management should include both pharmacological and non-pharmacological strategies whenever possible. For example, if feasible, breast-feeding mothers should be encouraged to breast-feed during the procedure [149–151]. Nonnutritive sucking, sucrose, or other sweet solutions are effective in term and premature infants, and tactile stimulation or kangaroo care (skin to skin contact) are

Table 14.9 Procedural pain management[a]

1. Consider if the planned procedure is necessary and how the information it will provide might influence care
2. Are available analgesics and pain management strategies likely to provide adequate pain relief? Is sedation or general anesthesia indicated?
3. Avoid multiple procedures if possible. Cohorting several procedures may be less stressful as long as effective analgesia is provided
4. Consider if the modification of the procedure (e.g., venipuncture is less painful than heel lance) would reduce pain
5. Allow sufficient time for analgesic drugs and other analgesic measures to be effective
6. Ensure that appropriate personnel are available, and enlist experienced help when necessary
7. Formulate a clear plan of action should the procedure fail or pain become unmanageable using the techniques selected

[a]Adapted from [138]. A guideline from the Association of Paediatric Anaesthetists of Great Britain and Ireland

useful strategies for brief procedures in the premature infant [152–154]. Published guidelines have reviewed the evidence for the effectiveness of pharmacological treatments for specific procedures, e.g., local anesthesia or opioids, and they should be consulted to inform locally developed protocols [147, 148, 154].

References

1. Maxwell LG, Malavolta CP, Fraga MV. Pain management in the peripartum period assessment of pain in the neonate. Clin Perinatol. 2013;40:457–69.
2. Fitzgerald M, Howard RF. The neurobiologic basis of paediatric pain. In: Schechter NL, Berde CB, Yaster M, editors. Second Edition. Philadelphia, PA: Lippincott Williams and Wilkins; 2003. p. 19–42.
3. Andrews K, Desai D, Dhillon H, Wilcox D, Fitzgerald M. Abdominal sensitivity in the first year of life: comparison of infants with and without prenatally diagnosed unilateral hydronephrosis. Pain. 2002;100:35–46.
4. Anand K, Hansen D, Hickey P. Hormonal-metabolic stress responses in neonates undergoing cardiac surgery. Anaesthesiology. 1990;73(4):661–70.
5. Anand K, Hickey P. Halothane-morphine compared with high-dose sufentanil for anaesthesia and postoperative analgesia in neonatal cardiac surgery. N Engl J Med. 1992;326(1):1–9.
6. Fitzgerald M, Walker SM. Infant pain management: a developmental neurobiological approach. Nat Clin Pract Neurol. 2009; 5(1):35–50.
7. Peters J, Schouw R, Anand K, van Dijk M, Duivenvoorden H, Tibboel D. Does neonatal surgery lead to increased pain sensitivity in later childhood? Pain. 2005;114(3):444–54.
8. Walker SM, Franck LS, Fitzgerald M, Myles J, Stocks J, Marlow N. Long-term impact of neonatal intensive care and surgery on somatosensory perception in children born extremely preterm. Pain. 2009;141(1–2):79–87.
9. Fitzgerald M. The post-natal development of cutaneous afferent fiber input and receptive field organization in the rat dorsal horn. J Physiol. 1985;364:1–18.
10. Slater R, Worley A, Fabrizi L, et al. Evoked potentials generated by noxious stimulation in the human infant brain. Eur J Pain. 2010;14(3):321–6.
11. Woolf CJ. Central sensitization: implications for the diagnosis and treatment of pain. Pain. 2011;152(3):S2–15.
12. Campbell JN, Meyer RA. Mechanisms of neuropathic pain. Neuron. 2006;52(1):77–92.
13. Taddio A, Shah V, Gilbert-MacLeod C, Katz J. Conditioning and hyperalgesia in newborns exposed to repeated heel lances. JAMA. 2002;288:857–61.
14. Walker SM, Meredith-Middleton J, Lickiss T, Moss A, Fitzgerald M. Primary and secondary hyperalgesia can be differentiated by postnatal age and ERK activation in the spinal dorsal horn of the rat pup. Pain. 2007;128(1–2):157–68.
15. Anand P, Birch R. Restoration of sensory function and lack of long-term chronic pain syndromes after brachial plexus injury in human neonates. Brain. 2002;125(Pt 1):113–22.
16. Howard RF, Walker SM, Mota PM, Fitzgerald M. The ontogeny of neuropathic pain: postnatal onset of mechanical allodynia in rat spared nerve injury (SNI) and chronic constriction injury (CCI) models. Pain. 2005;115(3):382–9.
17. Moss A, Beggs S, Vega-Avelaira D, et al. Spinal microglia and neuropathic pain in young rats. Pain. 2007;128(3):215–24.
18. Costigan M, Moss A, Latremoliere A, et al. T-cell infiltration and signaling in the adult dorsal spinal cord is a major contributor to neuropathic pain-like hypersensitivity. J Neurosci. 2009;29(46): 14415–22.
19. Taddio A, Katz J, Ilersich A, Koren G. Effect of neonatal circumcision on pain response during subsequent routine vaccination [see comments]. Lancet. 1997;349(9052):599–603.
20. Carbajal R, Rousset A, Danan C, et al. Epidemiology and treatment of painful procedures in neonates in intensive care units. JAMA. 2008;300(1):60–70.
21. Anand K, Scalzo F. Can adverse neonatal experiences alter brain development and subsequent behavior? Biol Neonate. 2000;77: 69–82.
22. Schmelzle-Lubiecki BM, Campbell KA, Howard RH, Franck L, Fitzgerald M. Long-term consequences of early infant injury and trauma upon somatosensory processing. Eur J Pain. 2007;11(7): 799–809.
23. Hermann C, Hohmeister J, Demirakca S, Zohsel K, Flor H. Long-term alteration of pain sensitivity in school-aged children with early pain experiences. Pain. 2006;125(3):278–85.
24. Waldenstrom A, Thelin J, Thimansson E, Levinsson A, Schouenborg J. Developmental learning in a pain-related system: evidence for a cross-modality mechanism. J Neurosci. 2003; 23(20):7719–25.
25. Beggs S, Torsney C, Drew L, Fitzgerald M. The postnatal reorganization of primary afferent input and dorsal horn cell receptive fields in the rat spinal cord is an activity-dependent process. Eur J Neurosci. 2002;16(7):1249–58.
26. Brummelte S, Grunau RE, Chau V, et al. Procedural pain and brain development in premature newborns. Ann Neurol. 2012;71: 385–96.
27. Vinall J, Miller SP, Chau V, et al. Neonatal pain in relation to postnatal growth in infants born very preterm. Pain. 2012;153:1374–81.
28. Finley GA, Franck L, Grunau R, von Baeyer CL. Why Children's Pain Matters. Pain – Clinical Updates. 2005;13(4):1–6.
29. Hummel P, van Dijk M. Pain assessment: current status and challenges. Semin Fetal Neonatal Med. 2006;11(4):237–45.
30. Franck L, Greenberg C, Stevens B. Pain assessment in infants and children. Paediatr Clin North Am. 2000;47(3):487–512.

31. Clinical Guidelines for the Recognition and Assessment of Acute Pain in Children. 2009. http://www.rcn.org.uk/__data/assets/pdf_file/0004/269185/003542.pdf. Accessed Sep 2013)
32. Howard R, Carter B, Curry J, et al. Good practice in postoperative and procedural pain management: **guidelines** from the Association of Paediatric Anaesthetists. Paediatr Anaesth. 2008;18(1):1–81.
33. Pokela M. Pain relief can reduce hypoxaemia in distressed neonates during routine treatment procedures. Paediatrics. 1994;93:379.
34. Buttner W, Fincke W. Analysis of behavioural and physiological parameters for the assessment of postoperative analgesic demand in newborns, infants and young children. Paediatr Anaesth. 2000;10:303–18.
35. van Dijk M, de Boer J, Koot H, Tibboel D, Passchier J, Duivenvoorden H. The reliability and validity of the COMFORT scale as a postoperative pain instrument in 0 to 3-year-old infants. Pain. 2000;84(2–3):367–77.
36. Ambuel B, Hamlett K, Marx C, Blumer J. Assessing distress in paediatric intensive care environments: the COMFORT scale. J Paediatr Psychol. 1992;17(1):95–109.
37. Krechel SW, Bildner J. CRIES: a new neonatal postoperative pain measurement score. Initial testing of validity and reliability. Paediatr Anaesth. 1995;5(1):53–61.
38. Barrier G, Attia J, Mayer M, Amiel-Tilson C. Measurement of postoperative pain and narcotic administration in infants usind a new clinical scoring system. Intensive Care Med. 1989; 15S:37–9.
39. Sparshott M. The development of a clinical distresss scale for ventilated newborn infants: Identification of pain and distress based on validated behaivoural scores. J Neonatal Nurs. 1996;2:5.
40. Horgan M, Choonara I. Measuring pain in neonates: an objective score. J Paediatr Nurs. 1996;8:24–8.
41. Grunau R, Craig K. Pain expression in neonates: facial action and cry. Pain. 1987;28(3):395–410.
42. Lawrence J, Alcock D, McGrath P. The development of a tool to assess neonatal pain. Neonatal Netw. 1993;12:59–66.
43. Hodgkinson K, Bear M, Thorn J. Measuring pain in neonates: evaluating an instrument and developing a common language. Aust J Adv Nurs. 1994;12:17–22.
44. Ballantyne M, Stevens B, McAllister M, Dionne K, Jack A. Validation of the premature infant pain profile in the clinical setting. Clin J Pain. 1999;15(4):297–303.
45. Blauer T, Gerstmann D. A simultaneous comparion of three neonatal pain scales during common NICU procedures. Clin J Pain. 1988;14:39–47.
46. Karling M. RenstrC6m M, Ljungman G. Acute and postoperative pain in children: A Swedish nationwide survey. Acta Paediatrica. 2002;91(6):660–6.
47. Broome ME, Richtsmeier A, Maikler V, Alexander M. Paediatric pain practices: A national survey of health professionals. J Pain Symptom Manage. 1996;11.
48. Simons J, MacDonald LM. Changing practice: implementing validated paediatric pain assessment tools. J Child Health Care. 2006;10:160–76.
49. Kehlet H, Dahl JB. The value of "multimodal" or "balanced analgesia" in postoperative pain treatment. Anaesth Analg. 1993;77(5):1048–56.
50. McAnulty GB, Duffy FH, Butler SC, Bernstein JH, Zurakowski D, Als H. Effects of the Newborn Individualized Developmental Care and Assessment Program (NIDCAP) at age 8 years: preliminary data. Clin Paediatr (Phila). 2010;49(3):258–70.
51. McAnulty G, Duffy FH, Butler S, et al. Individualized developmental care for a large sample of very preterm infants: health, neurobehaviour and neurophysiology. Acta Paediatr. 2009;98(12): 1920–6.
52. Symington A, Pinelli J. Developmental care for promoting development and preventing morbidity in preterm infants. Cochrane Database Syst Rev. 2006;19(2):CD001814. Online.
53. Ceelie I, de Wildt SN, van Dijk M, et al. Effect of intravenous paracetamol on postoperative morphine requirements in neonates and infants undergoing major noncardiac surgery. JAMA. 2013;309:149–54.
54. van der Marel CD, Peters JW, Bouwmeester NJ, Jacqz-Aigrain E, van den Anker JN, Tibboel D. Rectal acetaminophen does not reduce morphine consumption after major surgery in young infants. Br J Anaesth. 2007;98(3):372–9.
55. Koppert W, Wehrfritz A, Korber N, et al. The cyclooxygenase isozyme inhibitors parecoxib and paracetamol reduce central hyperalgesia in humans. Pain. 2004;108(1–2):148–53.
56. Anderson B. What we don't know about paracetamol in children. Paediatr Anaesth. 1998;8(6):451–60.
57. Ottani A, Leone S, Sandrini M, Ferrari A, Bertolini A. The analgesic activity of paracetamol is prevented by the blockade of cannabinoid CB1 receptors. Eur J Pharmacol. 2006;531(1–3):280–1.
58. Anderson B, van Lingen R, Hansen T, Lin Y, Holford N. Acetaminophen developmental pharmacokinetics in premature neonates and infants: a pooled population analysis. Anaesthesiology. 2002;96(6):1336–45.
59. Cuzzolin L, Antonucci R, Fanos V. Paracetamol (acetaminophen) efficacy and safety in the newborn. Curr Drug Metab. 2013;14:178–81.
60. Allegaert K, Murat I, Anderson BJ. Not all intravenous paracetamol formulations are created equal. Paediatr Anaesth. 2007;17(8):811–2.
61. Anderson B, Woollard G, Holford N. Acetaminophen analgesia in children: placebo effect and pain resolution after tonsillectomy. Eur J Clin Pharmacol. 2001;57:559–69.
62. Murat I, Baujard C, Foussat C, et al. Tolerance and analgesic efficacy of a new i.v. paracetamol solution in children after inguinal hernia repair. Paediatr Anaesth. 2005;15(8):663–70.
63. Anderson B, Pons G, Autret-Leca E, Allegaert K, Boccard E. Paediatric intravenous paracetamol (propacetamol) pharmacokinetics: a population analysis. Paediatr Anaesth. 2005;15(4):282–92.
64. Barbaud A, Reichert-Penetrat S, Trechot P, Cuny J, Weber M, Schmutz J. Occupational contact dermatitis to propacetamol. Allergological and chemical investigations in two new cases. Dermatology. 1997;195(4):329–31.
65. Niemi T, Backman J, Syrjala M, Viinikka L, Rosenberg P. Platelet dysfunction after intravenous ketorolac or propacetamol. Acta Anaesthesiol Scand. 2000;44(1):69–74.
66. de la Pinitiere A, Beuchée A, Bétrémieux PE. Intravenous propacetamol overdose in a term newborn. Arch Dis Child Fetal Neonatal Ed. 2003;88:F351–266.
67. Niven DG, Shung J. Intravenous paracetamol overdose in a preterm infant during anaesthesia. Paediatr Anaesth. 2010;20:105–7.
68. Beringer RM, Thompson JP, Parry S, Stoddart PA. Intravenous paracetamol overdose: two case reports and a change to national treatment guidelines. Arch Dis Child. 2011;96:307–8.
69. Morris JL, Rosen DA, Rosen KR. Nonsteroidal anti-inflammatory agents in neonates. Paediatr Drugs. 2003;5(6):385–405.
70. Ririe D, Prout H, Barclay D, Tong C, Lin M, Eisenach J. Developmental differences in spinal cyclooxygenase 1 expression after surgical incision. Anaesthesiology. 2006;104(3):426–31.
71. Ista E, van Dijk M, Gamel C, Tibboel D, de Hoog M. Withdrawal symptoms in children after long-term administration of sedatives and/or analgesics: a literature review. "Assessment remains troublesome". Intensive Care Med. 2007;33(8):1396–406.
72. Howard RF, Lloyd-Thomas A, Thomas M, et al. Nurse-controlled analgesia (NCA) following major surgery in 10,000 patients in a children's hospital. Paediatr Anaesth. 2010;20(2):126–34.

73. Kart T, Christrup L, Rasmussen M. Recommended use of morphine in neonates, infants and children based on a literature review: part 1–Pharmacokinetics. Paediatr Anaesth. 1997;7(1):5–11.
74. Kart T, Christrup L, Rasmussen M. Recommended use of morphine in neonates, infants and children based on a literature review: part 2–Clinical use. Paediatr Anaesth. 1997;7(2):93–101.
75. Bouwmeester N, Anderson B, Tibboel D, Holford N. Developmental pharmacokinetics of morphine and its metabolites in neonates, infants and young children. Br J Anaesth. 2004;92(2):208–17.
76. Berde CB, Sethna NF. Analgesics for the treatment of pain in children. N Engl J Med. 2002;347(14):1094–103.
77. Anderson BJ, Meakin GH. Scaling for size: some implications for paediatric anaesthesia dosing. Paediatr Anaesth. 2002;12:205–19.
78. Taylor J, Liley A, Anderson BJ. The relationship between age and morphine infusion rate in children. Paediatr Anaesth. 2013;23:40–4.
79. Lynn A, Nespeca M, Opheim K, Slattery J. Respiratory effects of intravenous morphine infusions in neonates, infants, and children after cardiac surgery. Anaesth Analg. 1993;77(4):695–701.
80. Lynn A, Nespeca M, Bratton S, Shen D. Intravenous morphine in postoperative infants: intermittent bolus dosing versus targeted continuous infusions. Pain. 2000;88(1):89–95.
81. van Dijk M, Bouwmeester N, Duivenvoorden H, et al. Efficacy of continuous versus intermittent morphine administration after major surgery in 0-3-year-old infants; a double-blind randomized controlled trial. Pain. 2002;98(3):305–13.
82. Niesters M, Overdyk F, Smith T, Aarts L, Dahan A. Opioid-induced respiratory depression in paediatrics: a review of case reports. Br J Anaesth. 2013;110:175–82.
83. Ginsberg B, Howell S, Glass PS, et al. Pharmacokinetic model-driven infusion of fentanyl in children. Anaesthesiology. 1996;85(6):1268–75.
84. Fahnenstich H, Steffan J, Kau N, Bartmann P. Fentanyl-induced chest wall rigidity and laryngospasm in preterm and term infants. Crit Care Med. 2000;28:836–9.
85. Murrell D, Gibson P, Cohen R. Continuous epidural analgesia in newborn infants undergoing major surgery. J Paediatr Surg. 1993;28(4):548–52. discussion 552-543.
86. Lejus C, Surbled M, Schwoerer D, et al. Postoperative epidural analgesia with bupivacaine and fentanyl: hourly pain assessment in 348 paediatric cases. Paediatr Anaesth. 2001;11:327–32.
87. Tibboel D, Anand KJS, van den Anker JN. The pharmacological treatment of neonatal pain. Semin Fetal Neonatal Med. 2005;10(2):195–205.
88. Anand KJ, Hall RW. Pharmacological therapy for analgesia and sedation in the newborn. Arch Dis Child Fetal Neonatal Ed. 2006;91(6):F448–453.
89. Saarenmaa E, Huttunen P, Leppaluoto J, Fellman V. Alfentanil as procedural pain relief in newborn infants. Arch Dis Child Fetal Neonatal Ed. 1996;75(2):F103–107.
90. Penido MG, Garra R, Sammartino M, Pereira e Silva Y. Remifentanil in neonatal intensive care and anaesthesia practice. Acta Paediatr. 2010;99(10):1454–63.
91. Steinmetz J, Holm-Knudsen R, Sorensen MK, Eriksen K, Rasmussen LS. Hemodynamic differences between propofol-remifentanil and sevoflurane anaesthesia for repair of cleft lip and palate in infants. Paediatr Anaesth. 2007;17(1):32–7.
92. Williams D, Hatch D, Howard R. Codeine phosphate in paediatric medicine. Br J Anaesth. 2001;86:421–7.
93. Williams D, Patel A, Howard R. Pharmacogenetics of codeine metabolism in an urban population of children and its implications for analgesic reliability. Br J Anaesth. 2002;89:839–45.
94. Williams D, Dickenson A, Fitzgerald M, Howard R. Developmental regulation of codeine analgesia in the rat. Anaesthesiology. 2004;100(1):92–7.
95. Grond S, Sablotzki A. Clinical pharmacology of tramadol. Clin Pharmacokinet. 2004;43(13):879–923.
96. Allegaert K, Anderson B, Verbesselt R, et al. Tramadol disposition in the very young: an attempt to assess in vivo cytochrome P-450 2D6 activity. Br J Anaesth. 2005;95(2):231–9.
97. Allegaert K, Van den Anker J, Verbesselt R, et al. O-demethylation of tramadol in the first months of life. Eur J Clin Pharmacol. 2005;61(11):837–42.
98. Ozalevli M, Unlugenc H, Tuncer U, Gunes Y, Ozcengiz D. Comparison of morphine and tramadol by patient-controlled analgesia for postoperative analgesia after tonsillectomy in children. Paediatr Anaesth. 2005;15(11):979–84.
99. Suresh S, Anand K. Opioid tolerance in neonates: mechanisms, diagnosis, assessment, and management. Semin Perinatol. 1998;22:425–33.
100. Lonnqvist PA, Bergendahl HT, Eksborg S. Pharmacokinetics of clonidine after rectal administration in children. Anaesthesiology. 1994;81(5):1097–101.
101. Ivani G, Bergendahl H, Lampugnani E, et al. Plasma levels of clonidine following epidural bolus injection in children. Acta Anaesthesiol Scand. 1998;42(3):306–11.
102. Dalens B. Some current controversies in paediatric regional anaesthesia. Curr Opin Anaesthesiol. 2006;19(3):301–8.
103. Breschan C, Krumpholz R, Likar R, Kraschl R, Schalk H. Can a dose of 2microg.kg(-1) caudal clonidine cause respiratory depression in neonates? Paediatr Anaesth. 1999;9(1):81–3.
104. Breschan C, Jost R, Krumpholz R, et al. A prospective study comparing the analgesic efficacy of levobupivacaine, ropivacaine and bupivacaine in paediatric patients undergoing caudal blockade. Paediatr Anaesth. 2005;15(4):301–6.
105. Peutrell JM, Lonnqvist PA. Neuraxial blocks for anaesthesia and analgesia in children. Curr Opin Anaesthesiol. 2003;16(5):461–70.
106. Walker S, Howard R, Keay K, Fitzgerald M. Developmental age influences the effect of epidural dexmedetomidine on inflammatory hyperalgesia in rat pups. Anaesthesiology. 2005;102(6):1226–34.
107. Elia N, Tramer M. Ketamine and postoperative pain–a quantitative systematic review of randomised trials. Pain. 2005;113(1–2):61–70.
108. Fitzgerald M. The development of nociceptive circuits. Nat Rev Neurosci. 2005;6(7):507–20.
109. Haberny KA, Paule MG, Scallet AC, et al. Ontogeny of the N-methyl-D-aspartate (NMDA) receptor system and susceptibility to neurotoxicity. Toxicol Sci. 2002;68(1):9–17.
110. Young C, Jevtovic-Todorovic V, Qin Y, et al. Potential of ketamine and midazolam, individually or in combination, to induce apoptotic neurodegeneration in the infant mouse brain. Br J Pharmacol. 2005;146(2):189–97.
111. Mellon RD, Simone AF, Rappaport BA. Use of anaesthetic agents in neonates and young children. Anaesth Analg. 2007;104(3):509–20.
112. Slikker Jr W, Zou X, Hotchkiss CE, et al. Ketamine-induced neuronal cell death in the perinatal rhesus monkey. Toxicol Sci. 2007;98(1):145–58.
113. Walker SM, Westin BD, Deumens R, Grafe M, Yaksh TL. Effects of intrathecal ketamine in the neonatal rat: evaluation of apoptosis and long-term functional outcome. Anaesthesiology. 2010;113(1):147–59.
114. Mazoit J, Dalens B. Pharmacokinetics of local anaesthetics in infants and children. Clin Pharmacokinet. 2004;43(1):17–32.

115. Foster R, Markham A. Levobupivacaine: a review of its pharmacology and use as a local anaesthetic [In Process Citation]. Drugs. 2000;59(3):551–79.
116. Morrison S, Dominguez J, Frascarolo P, Reiz S. A comparison of the electrocardiographic cardiotoxic effects of racemic bupivacaine, levobupivacaine, and ropivacaine in anaesthetized swine [In Process Citation]. Anaesth Analg. 2000;90(6):1308–14.
117. Dalens B, Mazoit J. Adverse effects of regional anaesthesia in children. Drug Saf. 1998;19(4):251–68.
118. Luz G, Wieser C, Innerhofer P, Frischhut B, Ulmer H, Benzer A. Free and total bupivacaine plasma concentrations after continuous epidural anaesthesia in infants and children. Paediatr Anaesth. 1998;8(6):473–8.
119. Lerman J, Strong HA, Ledez KM, Swartz J, Reider MJ, Burrows FA. Effects of age on the serum concentrations of $alpha_1$ acid glycoprotein and the binding of lidocaine in paediatric patients. Clin Pharmacol Ther. 1989;46:219–25.
120. Mevorach D, Perkins F, Isaacson S. Bupivacaine toxicity secondary to continuous caudal epidural infusion in children [letter; comment]. Anaesth Analg. 1993;77(6):1305–6.
121. Berde CB. Convulsions associated with paediatric regional anaesthesia. Anaesth Analg. 1992;75:164–6.
122. Larsson BA, Lonnqvist PA, Olsson GL. Plasma concentrations of bupivacaine in neonates after continuous epidural infusion. Anaesth Analg. 1997;84:501–5.
123. Bosenberg AT, Thomas J, Cronje L, et al. Pharmacokinetics and efficacy of ropivacaine for continuous epidural infusion in neonates and infants. Paediatr Anaesth. 2005;15(9):739–49.
124. Eidelman A, Weiss JM, Lau J, Carr DB. Topical anaesthetics for dermal instrumentation: a systematic review of randomized, controlled trials. Ann Emerg Med. 2005;46(4):343–51.
125. Larson A, Stidman T, Banerji S, et al. Seizures and methemoglobinemia in an infant after excessive EMLA application. Paediatr Emerg Care. 2013;29:377–9.
126. Essink-Tjebbes C, Hekster Y, Liem K, van Dongen R. Topical use of local anaesthetics in neonates. Pharm World Sci. 1999;21(4):173–6.
127. Taddio A, Ohlsson A, Einarson TR, Stevens B, Koren G. A systematic review of lidocaine-prilocaine cream (EMLA) in the treatment of acute pain in neonates. Paediatrics. 1998;101(2):E1.
128. Nilsson A, Engberg G, Henneberg S, Danielson K, De Verdier C. Inverse relationship between age-dependent erythrocyte activity of methemoglobin reductase and prilocaine-induced methemoglobinaemia during infancy. Br J Anaesth. 1990;64(1):72–6.
129. Jain A, Rutter N. Does topical amethocaine gel reduce the pain of venepuncture in newborn infants? A randomised double blind controlled trial. Arch Dis Child Fetal Neonatal Ed. 2000;83(3):F207–210.
130. Long CP, McCafferty DF, Sittlington NM, et al. Randomized trail of novel tetracaine patch to provide local anaesthesia in enonates undergoing venepuncture. Br J Anaesth. 2003;91:514–8.
131. Patel A, Czemiawski B, Gray S, Lui E. Does topical amethocaine gel reduce pain from heel prick blood sampling in premature infants? A randomized double-blind cross-over controlled study. Paediatr Child Health. 2003;8:222–5.
132. Stevens B, Yamada J, Ohlsson A. Sucrose for analgesia in newborn infants undergoing painful procedures. Cochrane Database Syst Rev (Online). 2010; (1):CD001069 (pub 3).
133. Anseloni VC, Ren K, Dubner R, Ennis M. A brainstem substrate for analgesia elicited by intraoral sucrose. Neuroscience. 2005;133(1):231–43.
134. Lefrak L, Burch K, Caravantes R, et al. Sucrose analgesia: identifying potentially better practices. Paediatrics. 2006;118(2):S197–202.
135. Stevens B, Yamada J, Lee GY, Ohlsson A. Sucrose for analgesia in newborn infants undergoing painful procedures.[update of Cochrane Database Syst Rev. 2013;(Jan 31 (1):CD001069; PMID: 23440783). Cochrane Database Syst Rev. 2010;1, CD001069.
136. Johnston CC, Filion F, Snider L, et al. How much sucrose is too much sucrose? Paediatrics. 2007;119(1):226.
137. Johnston CCFF, Snider L, Majnamer A, Limperopoulos C, Walker CD, Veilleux A, Pelausa E, Cake H, Stone S, Sherrard A, Boyer K. Routine sucrose analgesia during the first week of life in neonates younger than 31 weeks post conceptual age. Paediatrics. 2002;110(3):523–8.
138. A guideline from the Association of Paediatric Anaesthetists of Great Britain and Ireland. Good Practice in Postoperative and Procedural Pain Management. 2nd Edition. Paediatr Anaesth. 2012;22(1):1–79.
139. Hammer GB, Golianu B. Opioid analgesia in neonates following cardiac surgery. Semin Cardiothorac Vasc Anaesth. 2007; 11(1):47–58.
140. Anand KJ, Barton BA, McIntosh N, et al. Analgesia and sedation in preterm neonates who require ventilatory support: results from the NOPAIN trial. Neonatal Outcome and Prolonged Analgesia in Neonates. Arch Paediatr Adolesc Med. 1999;153(4):331–8.
141. Anand KJ, Hall RW, Desai N, et al. Effects of morphine analgesia in ventilated preterm neonates: primary outcomes from the NEOPAIN randomised trial. Lancet. 2004;363(9422): 1673–82.
142. Hall RW, Kronsberg SS, Barton BA, Kaiser JR, Anand KJ. Morphine, hypotension, and adverse outcomes among preterm neonates: who's to blame? Secondary results from the NEOPAIN trial. Paediatrics. 2005;115(5):1351–9.
143. de Graaf J, van Lingen RA, Valkenburg AJ, et al. Does neonatal morphine use affect neuropsychological outcomes at 8 to 9 years of age? Pain. 2013;154:449–58.
144. de Graaf J, van Lingen RA, Simons SH, et al. Long-term effects of routine morphine infusion in mechanically ventilated neonates on children's functioning: Five-year follow-up of a randomized controlled trial. Pain. 2011;152:1391–7.
145. Ng E, Taddio A, Ohlsson A. Intravenous midazolam infusion for sedation of infants in the neonatal intensive care unit. Cochrane Database Syst Rev. 2003;1, CD002052.
146. Bellu R, de Waal KA, Zanini R. Opioids for neonates receiving mechanical ventilation. Cochrane Database Syst Rev. 2008;1: CD004212. pub 3.
147. Anand KJ, Johnston CC, Oberlander TF, Taddio A, Lehr VT, Walco GA. Analgesia and local anaesthesia during invasive procedures in the neonate. Clin Ther. 2005;27(6):844–76.
148. Lago P, Garetti E, Merazzi D, et al. Guidelines for procedural pain in the newborn. Acta Paediatr. 2009;98(6):932–9.
149. Carbajal R, Veerapen S, Couderc S, Jugie M, Ville Y. Analgesic effect of breast feeding in term neonates: randomised controlled trial. BMJ. 2003;326(7379):13.
150. Shah PS, Herbozo C, Aliwalas LL, Shah VS. Breastfeeding or breast milk for procedural pain in neonates. Cochrane Database Syst Rev. 2012;12:CD004950. pub3.
151. Shah V, Taddio A, Rieder MJ. Effectiveness and tolerability of pharmacologic and combined interventions for reducing injection pain during routine childhood immunizations: systematic review and meta-analyses. Clin Ther. 2009;31(2):S104–151.
152. Johnston CC, Filion F, Campbell-Yeo M, et al. Enhanced kangaroo mother care for heel lance in preterm neonates: a crossover trial. J Perinatol. 2009;29(1):51–6.
153. Harrison D, Yamada J, Stevens B. Strategies for the prevention and management of neonatal and infant pain. Curr Pain Headache Rep. 2010;14(2):113–23.
154. Mackenzie A, Acworth J, Norden M, Jeffery H, Dalziel S, Munro J. Guideline Statement: Management of Procedure-related Pain in Neonates. Paediatrics and Child Health Division RACP: Sydney, NSW, Australia; 2005.

Regional Anesthesia

15

Adrian Bosenberg

Regional anesthesia, although technically challenging in neonates, has wide ranging benefits. Effective pain relief after surgery plays a significant role in the surgical outcome. Most major surgery is performed within the first few days of life—a time when critical physiological transitions are taking place. The challenge is to provide safe and effective analgesia [1, 2].

Although it may not be possible to completely eliminate postoperative pain, particularly in spontaneously breathing neonates, much can be done to reduce the intensity of pain. Traditionally intravenous morphine or other opioids are used, but these mandate ventilatory support and close monitoring in a neonatal intensive or similar high care unit. In contrast, regional anesthesia comes closest to achieving complete analgesia in both ventilated and spontaneously breathing neonates [1–4].

Most regional blocks are placed during general anesthesia to ensure an immobile patient [5]. In certain situations, however, spinals [6], epidurals [7], caudal catheters [8, 9] and peripheral nerve blocks [10, 11] have been placed in "awake" neonates. However sedation or conversion to general anesthesia is generally required for major abdominal surgery [7, 8, 12].

Specialized equipment is required to perform regional anesthesia in neonates [2, 13]. Portable high-frequency ultrasound has improved our ability to place epidurals and peripheral nerve blocks safely. Neonates are ideal subjects for ultrasound-guided blocks [14, 15] given that most peripheral nerves are superficial and the nerves and surrounding structures can be readily defined. Even the spinal cord can be visualized in neonates, since the ossification of the vertebrae is limited [14, 15]. Despite these innovations, overall experience with major blocks in neonates remains relatively limited (Table 15.1).

A. Bosenberg, MB, ChB, FFA, (SA) (✉)
Department Anesthesiology and Pain Management, Seattle Children's Hospital, 4800 Sandpoint Way NE, Seattle, WA 98105, USA
e-mail: adrian.bosenberg@seattlechildrens.org

Risks and Benefits

Before implementing any new pain management strategy, the risks and benefits must be carefully evaluated to avoid putting the neonate at increased risk [1, 2]. Potential benefits of regional anesthesia must be weighed against the individual practitioner's ability to perform the technique successfully as well as the ability of the healthcare staff on the ward or in the intensive care unit to manage continuous infusions of local anesthetics and/or opioids safely.

Benefits: Surgically induced pain causes a spectrum of autonomic, hormonal metabolic, immunologic/inflammatory and neurobehavioral sequelae, many of which have associated detrimental effects [2, 16–22]. Acute pain can also have negative physiological consequences that include impairment of respiratory effort and systemic and pulmonary vasoconstriction that negatively influences compromised organ function [2, 15–19, 23].

In the late 1980s, Anand et al. first demonstrated that neonates, including preterm infants, are capable of mounting both hormonal and metabolic stresses in response to surgery [16]. They demonstrated that opioids inhibit the stress response to surgery. The stress response varies directly with the degree of surgical stress [2, 16], even after minor surgery. Moreover, severe stress may be pathological and could contribute to increased postoperative morbidity and mortality. Extreme catecholamine responses are associated with the worst outcome [2, 17]. Regional anesthesia appears to inhibit the hormonal stress response more effectively than opioids [18, 20, 21].

Neonates, and in particular preterm infants, exposed to the deleterious effects of pain are also at risk of impaired neurodevelopment and altered pain sensitivity [24–29]. Long-term effects may include emotional, behavioral and learning disabilities. In theory, regional anesthesia may avoid or, when used in combination with anesthesia, reduce the neurotoxicity associated with general anesthetics in neonates and young infants [26–30].

J. Lerman (ed.), *Neonatal Anesthesia*, DOI 10.1007/978-1-4419-6041-2_15,

Table 15.1 Neonatal epidural risk based on data accumulated from publications worldwide

Author	Number of institutions	Number cases	Complications	References
Murrell (1992)	Sydney, Australia 1	20	0	[33]
Van Niekerk (1990)	Utrecht, Netherlands 1	20	V 1	[146]
Bosenberg (1998, 2005)	South Africa 2	240,11,35	DP 1,C 1, V 1	[32, 41, 83]
ADARPEF (1994)	France, Belgium, Italy 38	43	0	[60]
Yamashita (1992–2002)	Japan 1	950	DP 7	[62]
Webster (1993)	Ontario, Canada1	18	V 2	[175]
Williams (1995)	Vermont 1	17 with spinal	0	[34]
Courreges (1996)	France 1	45	0	[67]
Tobias (1996)	Columbia, USA 1	25	0	[89]
Hasan (1994)	London 1	12	0	[65]
Vas (1999, 2001,2003)	Bombay 1	20	0	[66]
National UK audit (2010)	UK 21	529	C 1 DE 3	[58]
Frawley (2000)	Melbourne, Australia 1	50 with spinal	0	[233]
Somri (2007)	Israel 1	24 with spinal	0	[8]
Valairucha (2002)	Boston 1	115 caudal cath	A-1	[149]
Krishnan (2006)	Birmingham 1	20	0	[49]
Willschke (2007)	South Africa 1	85,20	0	[14]
Raghavan (2008)	Birmingham 1	22	0	[43]
Schenkman (2009)	Israel 1	44	V 5M1	[50]
Kost-Byerly (2002–2007)	Baltimore, USA 1	23	0	[152]
Bailey (2001–2002)	Philadelphia, USA 1	28 caudal cath	0	[183]
PRAN (2007–2010)	USA 8	72	DP 2	[5]
ADARPEF (2010)	France, Tunis, Quebec, Swiss, Belgium 45	46	DP 1	[60]
Willschke et al (2011)	Vienna 1	20	0	[7]
Total	~99 institutions	2594	DP11 DE 3 C2 V 9M 1	

Caudal catheters are included

DP dural puncture, *V* intravascular, *S* total spinal, *B* bloody tap, *DE* drug error, *H* hypotension, *C* convulsion, *M* meningitis, *A* aberrant presacral placement

There are additional advantages to combining regional with general anesthesia [2, 4, 14, 31, 32]. Neonates, as a group, are at greater risk for adverse sequelae under general anesthesia given their immature organ systems (cardiovascular, central nervous, and respiratory) that are sensitive to the depressant effects of anesthetic agents. Neonatal myocardial function is particularly sensitive to both inhaled and intravenous anesthetics. When combined with general anesthesia, regional anesthesia provides profound analgesia with minimal hemodynamic effects, even in those with congenital heart disease [3, 32, 34–44]. A successful block allows reduced concentrations of inhalational agents to be used [3, 4, 32], thereby attenuating the severity of cardiovascular and respiratory depression [3] and may facilitate a faster recovery. Furthermore, inhalational agents have a reciprocal protective effect in that they increase the threshold of local anesthetic toxicity [45].

Regional anesthesia also reduces the requirement for muscle relaxants by providing motor relaxation. Neuraxial blockade facilitates the reduction of gastroschisis [43], omphalocele and diaphragmatic hernia [32, 41] by providing analgesia and relaxation of the abdominal musculature independent of the mode of ventilation [4, 6, 32, 34]. Caudal blocks have been used to reduce incarcerated inguinal herniae before surgery [40].

Neuraxial anesthesia may stimulate respiration and alter respiratory mechanics [46, 47]. The effects of neuraxial blockade on ventilation depend on the level and intensity of the block, as well as the clinical scenario. Neuraxial blockade may diminish abdominal and intercostal muscle activity, particularly in the compliant chest wall of neonates. On the other hand, it may improve diaphragmatic activity and excursion, thus offsetting a loss of accessory muscle function [33–35, 37]. The ventilatory response to CO_2 is also improved, resulting in more efficient ventilation and maintenance of normocarbia [46, 47, 50, 51]. The pain relief provided by epidural analgesia improves ventilatory mechanics [34, 43, 47] and reduces the need for and duration of assisted or controlled ventilation after major abdominal or thoracic surgery [4, 34, 48–51]. As a consequence, ventilator-associated morbidity and mortality is reduced [41, 48–51].

Spinal anesthesia was reintroduced into pediatric anesthetic in the mid-1980s in an effort to reduce the respiratory complications, especially apnea, after surgery in preterm and ex-preterm infants. The impact on the outcomes from anesthesia was significant [6, 35, 52, 53]. As a result, spinal anesthesia and, more recently, caudal epidural analgesia have been advocated for high-risk neonates at risk for perioperative apnea after surgery [1, 3, 52]. The ex-preterm infants of today differ from those of the 1980s. Improvements in neonatal intensive care and ventilation strategies as well as surfactant have reduced the incidence and severity of bronchopulmonary dysplasia. Recent evidence investigating the perioperative risk of apnea in preterm infants anesthetized with the current inhalational agents (sevoflurane, desflurane) and remifentanil or receiving regional anesthesia for surgery failed to establish the superiority of one technique over the other [52, 54].

Regional anesthesia may have salutary effects on gastrointestinal function. It enhances the early return of gastrointestinal motility [44, 55, 56], particularly after gastroschisis repair [21, 43]. In necrotizing enterocolitis, the vasodilatory effects of autonomic blockade may improve splanchnic perfusion [32, 55], while opioids increase intestinal smooth muscle tone that may increase the risk of anastomotic leaks [55]. Lastly, oral feeding may resume earlier and speed recovery after minor surgery in the presence of a regional block [6, 34, 52, 53].

The immunosuppressive effect of regional anesthesia is attenuated compared with that reported with opioids [20, 21, 56]. Local anesthetics, but not opioids, stimulate natural killer cells, which play an important role in nonspecific cellular mediated and antitumor immunity [22, 56]. Local anesthetics (bupivacaine) also confer antimicrobial action and inhibit bacterial growth [56].

Lastly, the economic benefits of regional anesthesia include a reduction in the anesthetic costs, fewer days in the neonatal intensive care, earlier discharge, and more efficient use of the ward nurse's time. However, to realize these benefits, the staff must be trained to care for neonates with epidural infusions and other regional blocks.

Risks: The efficacy of regional anesthesia in neonates is not in dispute, but where opinions differ is in the ability to safely perform regional anesthesia in neonates [31]. Some consider the risks of regional anesthesia too great for routine use by individuals who do not have the requisite expertise [31, 44]. Although the risks associated with opioid and epidural analgesia in children are similar [57, 58], the risks associated with epidural analgesia and peripheral nerve blocks in neonates are less clear. The numbers of neonates in published surveys are relatively small in comparison with the numbers of children and adults [58–67]. The aggregate of published series from approximately 99 institutions yielded only one serious complication, meningitis, in the 2,594 published cases [50] (Table 15.1). Complications, as rare as they are, usually occur early "at the end of the needle," i.e., when the anesthesiologist is still present. For example, the risk of a dural puncture is approximately 1:250, and convulsions 1:1,250 in neonates (Table 15.1). Every effort should be made to eliminate drug errors, a feature in the UK audit [58]. Anecdotal reports of spinal cord injuries bear testimony that these unfortunate disasters can occur, although infrequently [68]. It is generally recommended that neonatal epidural blocks should only be performed by those with the technical expertise despite the advent of ultrasound that may further reduce the risks [69].

Anatomical Considerations (Table 15.2)

Recent ultrasound studies have demonstrated that the conus medullaris (terminal end of the spinal cord) lies between L1 and L2 in the majority of neonates including preterm infants [14, 72]. The conus is not fixed but moves with changes in body position [73], although rarely does it extend beyond L3. A conus that extends caudally beyond L3 suggests a tethered cord [14, 72–75]. The dural sac usually terminates between S2 and S4, but maybe lie within millimeters of the sacral hiatus [14, 75].

The shape of the vertebral column develops over the first year of postnatal life. At birth, the vertebral column has a single shallow anteriorly concave curve extending from the C1 to L5. A secondary cervical curve appears when head control is achieved, usually by 6 months, and the lumbar curve develops with weight bearing, by ~1 year. In neonates, the spinous processes are parallel and horizontal facilitating a midline approach to the epidural space at all levels. The largest intervertebral spaces are found between T12–L1 and L5–S1, respectively.

The sacrum is narrower and flatter, ossification is incomplete, and the vertebrae are separate facilitating sacral intervertebral epidural blocks. Sacral dimples or pits may reflect an occult spina bifida, which should be excluded using ultrasound, CT or MRI before attempting a neuraxial block.

A posterior midline approach to the epidural space in neonates is regarded as the safest approach for several reasons. With a triangular spinal canal, the widest aspect of the epidural space is the midline where the epidural veins and arteries are less dense [75]. The epidural space is narrow (0.9–2.4 mm; median 1.5 mm) [14, 76] and less compliant, while the ligamentum flavum is thinner, is less dense and offers less resistance to the advancing epidural needle than in adults. Pressures generated during the passage of an epidural needle through the ligamentum flavum range from 35 to 105 mmHg (mean 70 mm) and the epidural pressures range from 1 to 10 mmHg [77].

Epidural fat consists of spongy gelatinous lobules with distinct spaces and offers minimal resistance to the passage

Table 15.2 Important anatomical and physiological similarities and differences between neonate and adolescents (adults)

Anatomy	Neonate	Adolescents (adult)
Conus medullaris	L1–L2	L1
Dural sac	S2–S4	S2–S4
Intercristal line	L4	L4
Vertebral column	Concave C1–L5	Secondary curves
	Mainly cartilaginous	Ossified
Spinous processes	Lumbar more horizontal, parallel Orientation T10–T12 similar to lumbar Midline approach easy	Lumbar angled caudad All thoracic spines angled caudad
Intervertebral space	Largest T12–L1; L5–S1	
Ligamentum flavum	Thinner, less dense	Thicker, fibrous
Epidural space	1–2 mm; less compliant Spongy gelatinous fat lobules	Compliant Densely packed lobules fibrous strands
Sacrum	Flatter; less ossified	Fully ossified by 30 years
Nerves	Thinner less myelination	
CSF volume	4 ml/kg	2 ml/kg
Physiology		
Blood pressure	Stable	Hypotension
Pulse rate	Stable	Bradycardia
Respiratory	Diaphragmatic function improved, ventilatory response CO_2 enhanced	Similar
CNS	Cortical arousal reduced Lower BIS	Similar
Endocrine	Inhibition stress response	Similar
GIT function	Earlier return	Similar

GIT is gastrointestinal track

of local anesthetic and an epidural catheter. The epidural veins have no valves and connect directly with intracranial veins. As a consequence, foreign material such as air or drugs inadvertently injected into the epidural veins can reach the brain without impediment.

The effective concentration of local anesthetics in neonates is less than in older children as the nerves in the former are thinner and less myelinated than those in the latter. The nerve trunks to the lower limbs are not fully myelinated until the second year of life. The degree of myelination influences the pharmacodynamic effects of local anesthetics.

The CSF volume in neonates <1.5 kg, 4 ml/kg, is relatively large compared with that in adults and older children, 2 ml/kg. CSF production in neonates, 0.35 ml/min, is also greater than that in adults. This explains, in part, why neonates require proportionately larger doses of local anesthetic for spinal block than older children.

In terms of peripheral nerve blocks in neonates, it is important to appreciate that the muscle layers of the thoracic and abdominal wall are thinner, less well defined, and more compliant than in older children. The sciatic nerve divides within the popliteal fossa [78], the ilioinguinal and iliohypogastric nerves lie 3–5 mm medial to the anterior superior iliac spine [79], and the musculocutaneous nerve is easily included in an axillary block because of its proximity to the divisions [80] (Fig. 15.1).

Pharmacological Differences

The pharmacological differences in neonates vary with gestational age-related changes in body fluid compartments, plasma protein concentrations, distribution of cardiac output and the functional maturity of liver and kidneys [81]. Other contributing factors include less body fat (15 % body weight) and skeletal mass (25 % body weight), a proportionally larger brain and liver and greater cardiac output and regional blood flow to vessel-rich organs resulting in more rapid uptake of drugs.

Neonates are at greater risk of drug toxicity than older children [2, 82]. Albumen and α_1-acid glycoprotein concentrations in neonates are less than those in children [82–90], thus increasing the free fraction of the circulating drugs. Since local anesthetics are basic drugs, the reduced concentration of α_1-acid glycoprotein increases the free fraction of local anesthetics in blood. However, α_1-acid glycoprotein is an acute phase protein and, as such, increases during acute illnesses and with surgical stress [83, 86]. This latter effect offsets the reduced concentration of α_1-acid glycoprotein in neonates, offering some protective effect by attenuating the free fraction of the local anesthetic. In addition, a greater fraction of local anesthetic is excreted unchanged in the urine because of the reduced hepatic blood flow and immature

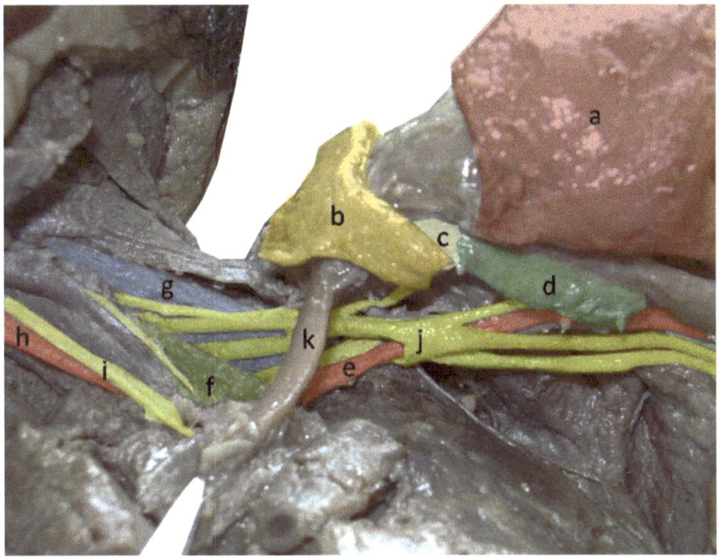

Fig. 15.1 Anatomical dissection of the axilla of a neonatal cadaver demonstrating the close relationship of the axillary artery and the cords and branches of the brachial plexus. The musculocutaneous branch is easily included even with small volumes of local anesthetic. Brachial plexus (**j**) and related structures within the axilla and at the root of the neck. Structures include the: (**a**) pectoralis major and (**b**) pectoralis minor muscles, (**c**) coracoid process, (**d**) coracobrachialis muscle, (**e**) axillary artery, (**f**) anterior and (**g**) middle scalene muscles, (**h**) common carotid artery, (**i**) vagus nerve, (**k**) clavicle

cytochrome P450 (CYP) enzyme system [83, 88]. Plasma cholinesterase activity in neonates is 50 % that in adults, slowing the clearance of ester local anesthetics such as chloroprocaine, from the blood. On balance, chloroprocaine is viewed as a safer local anesthetic in neonates than the amide anesthetics because its metabolism depends on only one enzyme [2, 35, 89].

Vascularity of the injection site and regional blood flow influence the rate of uptake of local anesthetics. The rate of absorption and therefore the peak blood concentration is reduced by the addition of a vasoconstrictor. Epinephrine prolongs the duration of action of local anesthetics [91, 92] by up to 50 % in neonates [6, 91–93]. In the author's experience the duration of caudal bupivacaine is virtually doubled by the addition of epinephrine 1:400,000 (unpublished data). However, during continuous epidural infusions, the initial effect of epinephrine to prolong the duration of the block is minimal after 3 h [94]. Hence, epinephrine is recommended for one-shot caudal epidural blocks and not for continuous infusions.

Lung function also plays an important role in modulating the duration of action of local anesthetics. Approximately 60–80 % of an intravenous bolus of lidocaine is absorbed on the first pass through the lungs. However, in neonates with right to left intracardiac shunts, the reduced uptake of local anesthetic by the lungs may increase the peak blood concentration by 100 % and, with it, the risk of local anesthetic toxicity [95].

Little is known about the pharmacokinetics of longer-acting local anesthetics in neonates [2, 83–85, 88, 96]. Using anecdotal reports of toxicity after bupivacaine, the recommended caudal/epidural infusion rates for bupivacaine for postoperative analgesia is 0.2 mg/kg/h for neonates and infants less than 6 months of age and up to 0.4 mg/kg/h for infants >6 months of age. The plasma concentrations recorded in neonates were greater than those in infants, although the concentrations in both age groups were <2–3 μg/ml the purported threshold for toxicity in humans [83, 88, 96]. The plasma concentrations of bound bupivacaine accumulate after a 48 h infusion in neonates and infants [96], whereas the concentrations of bound ropivacaine do not accumulate after infusions up to 72 h in duration [83]. Thus, ropivacaine appears to be the safer local anesthetic for epidural infusions lasting 48–72 h in neonates [88, 89, 96].

Neuraxial Blockade

Spinal

Bainbridge described the first spinal anesthetic performed on an infant in 1899, and early in the twentieth century, Lord H Tyrell Gray suggested that spinal anesthesia "would occupy an important place in the surgery of children in the future." Although the popularity of spinal anesthesia waned as the safety of general anesthesia improved, these prophetic words may still be realized considering the current controversy regarding the neurotoxicity of general anesthetics in neonates. The popularity of spinal anesthesia was rekindled in the early 1980s when Abaijan proposed its use for ex-preterm infants undergoing inguinal hernia repair [6]. Currently, spinal anesthesia remains limited to selected high-risk infants in whom general anesthesia may pose a major risk [97].

Spinal anesthesia has been used alone or in combination with an epidural for a wide variety of surgeries including inguinal hernia repair, ligation of patent ductus arteriosus, pyloromyotomy, gastrostomy, gastroschisis [98], omphalocele, exploratory laparotomy, lower abdominal surgery (colostomy, anoplasty, rectal biopsy, circumcision) meningomyelocele repair or orthopedic surgery [6, 99, 100].

The duration of action of spinal anesthesia in neonates is much less than it is in adults, despite the relatively larger doses used in the former. The duration of action appears to depend directly on age [93, 101, 102]. For practical purposes, an effective plane of surgical anesthesia after spinal block lasts up to ~40–60 min with bupivacaine, levobupivacaine [103, 104], and ropivacaine [104, 105]; up to 1.5 h with tetracaine plain, or 2 h with tetracaine with epinephrine [6, 93]; and up to 1 h after lidocaine 3 mg/kg with epinephrine [93]. Spinal anesthesia can be used to facilitate placement of an epidural block [8] in order to prolong the duration [8, 9]. Intrathecal clonidine (1 μg/kg) may also be used to perform surgery, although it is associated with more sedation and apnea than the local anesthetics [101, 103].

Spinal anesthesia rarely produces significant changes in heart rate or blood pressure in neonates, even with blockade to thoracic levels [6, 100]. Reduced cortical arousal caused by peripheral deafferentation [44, 106] or a decrease in cerebral blood flow [107] should be born in mind when additional sedatives are used [106]. The incidence of postoperative apnea in preterm neonates who received spinal anesthesia was less than that after general anesthesia, provided sedatives (e.g., midazolam 0.2 mg/kg, propofol 1 mg/kg) were avoided [6, 100, 108, 109].

Complications: Based on two large series [6, 100], the incidence of serious complications (nerve injury, meningitis, arachnoiditis) [110, 111] after spinal anesthesia is rare in neonates, but greater in neonates than older infants and children [109]. Failure rates for effective spinal anesthesia in neonates range from 5 % (in experienced hands) [6] to 17 % (trainees) [6, 31, 108] with a bloody tap rate of 10 % [101]. Bradycardia (<100 bpm) and apnea can be treated with tactile stimulation, atropine 0.1 mg/kg, or ventilatory support as indicated. The incidence of bradycardia ranges from 1.2 to 1.8 % [6, 100]. The incidence of high spinal blockade (0.1–0.6 %), heralded by apnea but usually not associated with hypotension or bradycardia, has been associated with the administration of large doses of local anesthetics and early elevation of the legs when applying the electrocautery pad to the back or "top-ups" when the level is inadequate. Unilateral spinal blockade in neonates has also been described [112]. Blood plasma concentrations of bupivacaine after spinal administration are small (0.2–0.3 mcg/ml) and unaffected by the addition of epinephrine [113].

Technique: Using a sterile technique, a spinal anesthetic may be placed using a 25 ga or styletted 22 ga 1.5 in. spinal needle in the sitting or lateral decubitus position. Chlorhexidine in 70 % alcohol is currently recommended for skin preparation. The antiseptic should completely dry before inserting the spinal needle to preclude transfer of alcohol to the subarachnoid space. Spinal anesthesia is usually placed at L3–L4 or L4–L5. A prior ultrasound scan is useful to determine the exact location of the dural sac and to exclude any central nervous system or bony anomalies. Once free flow of CSF is obtained through the spinal needle, the local anesthetic can be administered using a 1 ml syringe. The onset of the block is reflected by profound motor block in the lower extremities within seconds of completing the delivery of local anesthetic. Care should be taken to avoid positioning the infant head down, i.e., when applying the electrocautery pad on the back, before the block height has been set to avoid a high spinal block. Instead, the neonate should be logrolled to apply monitors and other devices.

If the neonates requires placating gentle stroking, soothing or dextrose water on a pacifier is effective [114]. Intravenous sedation may be necessary in ~25 % of cases [6, 100], but it does increase the risk of perioperative apnea [100].

Dose Guidelines

Hyperbaric tetracaine 0.5 %; 0.6–1 mg/kg
Isobaric bupivacaine or ropivacaine 0.5 %; 0.6–1 mg/kg
Hyperbaric lidocaine 3 mg/kg

Adjuvants

Epinephrine 5–10 mcg/kg prolongs the duration of action.
Clonidine 1 mcg/kg prolongs analgesia [102].

Caudal Block

Caudal analgesia is frequently used to provide analgesia for surgery below the umbilicus [39, 70, 71, 115]. The popularity of caudal blockade stems from its simplicity, safety and efficacy and is usually performed in combination with general anesthesia [5]. Larger doses are required for upper abdominal surgery [116], but achieving this level of blockade is less predictable unless a caudal catheter is introduced. Caudal blocks are effective as the sole anesthetic, particularly for ex-preterm infants undergoing inguinal hernia repair [117]. They have also been used to reduce incarcerated inguinal herniae [40], to improve compromised perfusion

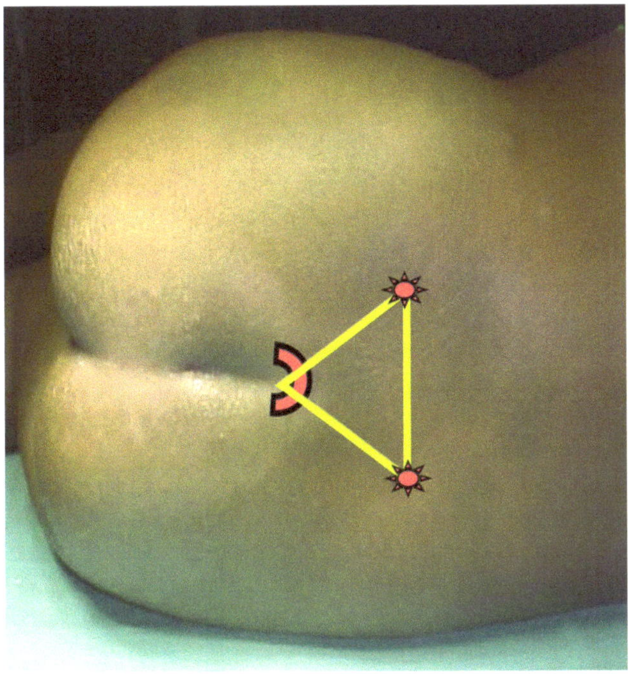

Fig. 15.2 Caudal block. The sacral hiatus lies at the apex of an equilateral triangle with the line drawn between the posterior superior iliac spines as the base

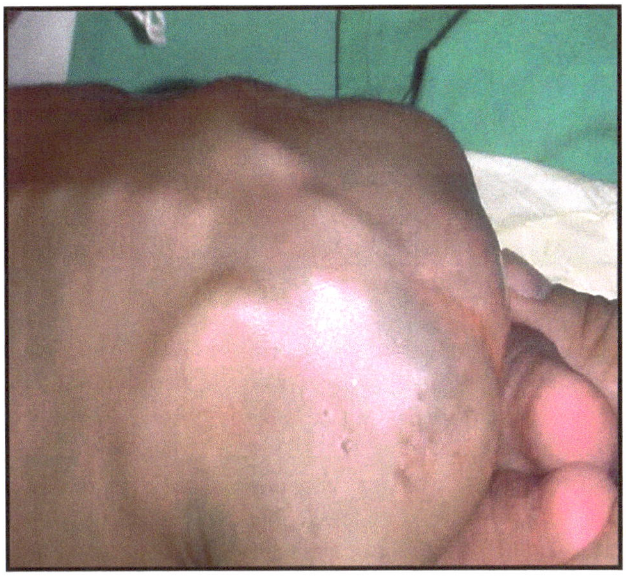

Fig. 15.3 Caudal block. The knee-chest position may be used to facilitate placement of the caudal in awake neonates

after umbilical catheterization [118] and penile block [119] and to facilitate PICC line placement in extreme preterm infants [120].

Anatomy: The sacral hiatus is between the sacral cornu, two prominences that represent the remnants of the fifth sacral arch, and extends to the fused arch of the fourth sacral vertebra. The sacrococcygeal membrane, an extension of the ligamentum flavum, covers the sacral hiatus separating the caudal space from the subcutaneous tissue. Considerable variation in the sacral hiatal anatomy exists mainly due to incomplete posterior fusion of other sacral vertebrae. However, a few important surface landmarks can be used to enhance successful placement in both normal and abnormal sacra. The sacral hiatus virtually always lies at the apex of an inverted equilateral triangle whose base is a line between the posterior superior iliac spines (Figs. 15.2 and 15.3). The intersection of a line drawn from the patella through the greater trochanter (with the hips flexed at 90°) with a line drawn down the vertebral column is another useful landmark (Fig. 15.3).

Technique: Caudal block can be performed in the lateral decubitus position or prone knee-chest position—a useful position for an "awake" caudal block [121] (Fig. 15.2). Under sterile conditions a short-beveled needle, held between the thumb and index finger, is introduced at approximately 30–45° to the skin (i.e., with the bevel parallel to the skin) with the skin between the sacral cornua held taut by the thumb and index finger of the opposite hand. The needle is then advanced until it pierces the sacrococcygeal ligament [122] and a "give" is felt. The needle is now in the caudal space, which can be confirmed by a loss of resistance. If the needle tip is extremely sharp, a "give" may not be felt; hence, most prefer to use a needle that is not extremely sharp. Penetration of the sacrococcygeal membrane just above a line between the sacral cornua carries a smaller incidence of bloody tap in the author's experience. The dural sac lies within 5–10 mm of the sacral hiatus in the majority of neonates [14], and thus changing the angle and advancing the needle, as described in adults, is unnecessary as it may result in a dural puncture or bloody tap [38]. Using a 22 g IV cannula is popular [38, 123], but in the author's experience, it carries a greater incidence of failure (subcutaneous injection) and bloody taps (see below).

After negative aspiration for blood and CSF, the required volume of local anesthetic can be injected. Aspiration should be gentle since strong negative pressure may cause the low-pressure epidural vessels to collapse before a positive aspiration test can be elicited [38]. In the event of a "bloody tap," the needle should be redirected or removed and reinserted more cephalad. Local anesthetic injection should proceed with caution after a bloody tap considering the greater risk of an intravascular injection under these circumstances [124]. Ultrasound can be used to "visualize" the spread within the caudal epidural space [125].

To provide a diverging opinion, the editor has always used a 22 g IV cannula for caudal block in neonates. In this approach, the skin is nicked with a "dull" needle down to the level of the subcutaneous tissue to introduce the IV catheter/needle into the subcutaneous tissue. This should minimize the risk of translocating epidermal tissue to the caudal space when the catheter/needle is advanced through an intact epidermis (see Complications below). The IV catheter/needle is then advanced through the nick. When the sacrococcygeal ligament is pierced, the catheter/needle is advanced 2–3 mm further, and the needle is transfixed while the catheter is slid off into the caudal canal. If the needle had inadvertently pierced the bone of the sacrum during insertion, the catheter would accordion rather than thread smoothly when it was advanced. This should ensure an inadvertent osseous cannulation did not occur. Once the needle is withdrawn, the remaining catheter is observed for either blood or clear CSF flashback. The editor does not aspirate the catheter at any time because if the catheter had pierced a vein, the vein would collapse when the catheter was aspirated and no blood will be collected. If the catheter were in the bone, again nothing will be returned during aspiration. Lastly, if the catheter were in the subarachnoid space and the sac punctured, CSF will flow back immediately upon withdrawal of the needle, before the catheter was aspirated. To ensure local anesthetic is injected into the caudal space and not subcutaneously, as the operator begins to inject local anesthetic into the catheter, the index finger of the free hand is gently placed over the sacrococcygeal ligament to detect a subcutaneous injection [99]. Although much debate has occurred with regard to the use of a test dose of drug and the determination of the location of the tip of the catheter, the editor treats the entire dose of local anesthetic to be administered (usually 1 mL/kg of 0.125 % bupivacaine) as a test dose, infusing 1 mL at a time while monitoring the ECG for 30–60 s before continuing.

Complications: The incidence of all complications after caudal/epidural blocks in neonates is threefold greater than in infants and eightfold greater than in children [126]. The two most common complications reported were a local skin infection and drug error [127]. Dural puncture and subsequent injection may lead to a total spinal and respiratory arrest (apnea). Systemic toxicity may be heralded by EKG (ST segment elevation and peaked T waves) changes, arrhythmia, cardiovascular collapse or convulsions after accidental intravascular or sacral intraosseous injection (incidence 0.4 %) [128]. Intrapelvic, intraosseous, and intravascular injections [129, 130] are very rare with proper technique. Urinary retention is not a substantive concern in neonates. Nerve injury and neurological deficits have not been reported in neonates. Inclusion dermoid tumors have been reported, but only anecdotally. The risk of introducing nucleated epidermal cells from stratum spinosum during caudal block is small and is similar with 22 g hollow needles and styletted 22 g caudal block needles [131–133].

Dosage: Many formulae have been proposed for the volume of local anesthetic required for a caudal block based on the neonate's weight, age, and length [115, 124, 134–137]. The most practical is that suggested by Armitage [124]:

0.5 ml/kg of local anesthetic for sacrolumbar dermatomes
1.0 ml/kg for lumbar thoracic dermatomes (subumbilical)
1.25 ml/kg for mid-thoracic dermatomes (upper abdominal)

Bupivacaine 0.125–0.25 % [138], ropivacaine 0.1–0.2 % [139–143], levobupivacaine 0.25 % [142], and chloroprocaine 3 % [35, 89] are effective. The duration of analgesia depends upon the dose and specific local anesthetic administered, the use of epinephrine, the site of surgery and whether a continuous catheter is used [35, 71]. Increasing the concentration of local anesthetic does not offer additional advantage but may increase the incidence of side effects (e.g., motor blockade) and/or complications. Clonidine (1 μg/kg) has been used to prolong the duration of analgesia about several hours [144] but is associated with an increased risk of sedation and apnea, particularly with a dose of 2 μg/kg [145].

Caudal Catheter Techniques

A catheter can be introduced via the sacral hiatus in neonates to prolong the duration of caudal block [9, 35] and to access the sacral, lumbar, or thoracic nerve roots [4, 146–160]. This technique was developed before the introduction of pediatric epidural needles. Specialized equipment is not required [4], and the risk of dural puncture or spinal cord injury may be less than with lumbar epidural placement in less-experienced hands [4, 147].

Technique: An 18 or 20G IV cannula, Crawford needle or specifically designed kits [147, 148] can be used to access the caudal space. A 20–24G epidural catheter that passes easily through the cannula is measured against the neonate's back to the dermatome level of the planned surgical incision. This predetermined length can then be introduced gently into the caudal/epidural space (Fig. 15.4). Flexion or extension of the infant's spine [4, 50], flushing the catheter with saline [4, 147] or twisting/rolling the catheter in the operator's fingers [4, 50] can be used to advance the catheter. Thin (24G) flexible catheters may curl in the sacrolumbar epidural space and fail to reach their target dermatome. This problem can be overcome by using styletted catheters, although they can be expensive [152, 154, 155]. Attempts to feed the catheter against resistance are potentially harmful. It is important not to force the catheter should resistance be encountered, as the catheter tip may impinge on a nerve root or puncture a blood vessel rather than advance. It may also puncture the dura and pass up the subdural or subarachnoid space. Instead of

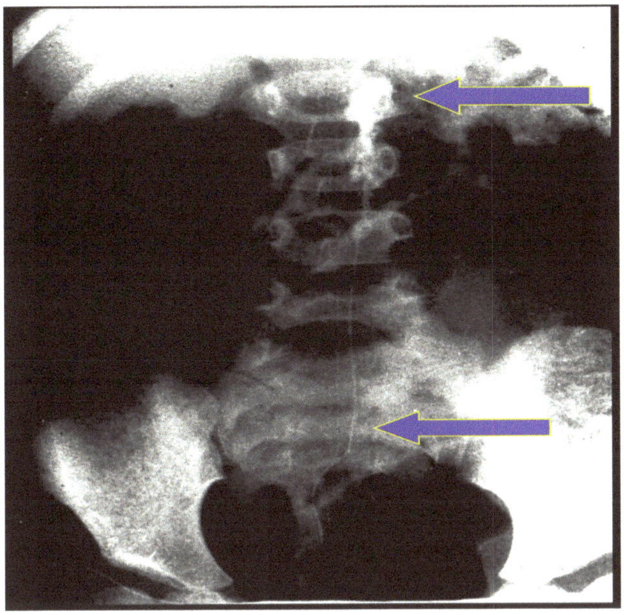

Fig. 15.4 A predetermined length of catheter can be introduced into the epidural space to the desired level via the sacral hiatus. An epidurogram or ultrasound can be used to confirm placement. In this epidurogram, contrast filled the caudal catheter, which was introduced at the sacral hiatus (*lower arrow*), and threaded up to the L1 level (*upper arrow*)

forcing a catheter to advance, it may be necessary to administer larger volumes of local anesthetic to achieve the desired level of blockade. The choice between single- and multi-orifice catheters is moot, since the latter function as single orifice catheters (perfusing the proximal orifice in all instances) at the small infusion rates used in epidural infusions [156].

Accurate placement of epidural catheters depends on the facilities available. Several techniques including epidurography [4, 146, 149, 161], fluoroscopy, electrocardiography [154, 155, 162], nerve stimulation [159, 160], and ultrasonography [125, 150, 157, 163] may be used. Electrical stimulation with wired epidural catheters allows real-time adjustment of the catheter level but requires specifically designed equipment. In the author's experience of more than 500 infants, 20 g nylon catheters (Portex®) may be threaded to within one vertebral body of the preselected level in the epidural space. Difficulties have been described reaching the desired dermatome level in preterm infants and when a Tuohy needle is used [9, 146]. The curve of a Tuohy needle may cause the catheter to curl if the lumen is not properly aligned within the caudal space.

Complications: These include failure to position the catheter at the desired level, dural puncture, intravascular placement [50, 153], bacterial colonization of the catheter tip (20–30 %) [99, 164, 165], and one reported case of meningitis [50]. Careful aseptic technique with chlorhexidine, rather than Proviodine, for all catheter techniques carries a lower risk of colonization [166]. However, colonization has not been shown to progress to abscess formation in the central nervous system. Tunneling catheters subcutaneously away from the diaper area may further reduce the risk of prolonged infusions [164, 165].

Dosage: For single dosing, 0.5–0.75 ml/kg 0.25 % bupivacaine or 0.2 % ropivacaine depending on the number of dermatomes required to be blocked [4].

Since neonates are not ambulatory, these concentrations will not impair discharge because of lower extremity weakness. Previous studies in children demonstrated that for 0.175 % bupivacaine with epinephrine, 0.7–1.3 ml/kg provided similar analgesia and discharge times after inguinal hernia surgery [167]. For ropivacaine, 1 ml/kg of a 0.25 % solution achieved a block to T11 with a time to first analgesia of 6 h. However, a 0.15 % solution of ropivacaine in a volume of 1.5 ml/kg achieved a block to T7 and time to first analgesia of 9 h [168].

For continuous epidural infusions for postoperative pain, 0.2–0.25 mg/kg/h bupivacaine is recommended to prevent toxic blood concentrations for 48 h [96]. This may be administered as 0.2 ml/kg/h of a 0.1 % bupivacaine solution. Ropivacaine dosing should be 0.2 mg/kg/h of a 0.1 % solution. In contrast to bupivacaine, ropivacaine does not accumulate as the duration of infusion increases [23].

Lumbar and Thoracic Epidural

Lumbar epidural is indicated for lower abdominal, pelvic and lower limb surgery, whereas a thoracic epidural is indicated for upper abdominal or thoracic surgery [169], particularly in poor-risk patients with respiratory disabilities [170]. Experience with these epidural techniques in neonates is limited [32, 50, 51, 58, 83, 171]. Few dermatomes are involved in the transverse abdominal incision favored by pediatric surgeons and thus can be easily covered by an accurately placed epidural. Epidural placement is usually performed in an anesthetized child, although it can also be performed with sedation [7] or after initial spinal blockade when indicated [8]. In view of the potential risk of spinal cord trauma, thoracic epidurals should only be performed by experienced providers familiar with epidurals in neonates.

Technique: Using a sterile technique, the skin should be punctured to facilitate smooth insertion of a 19 or 20 g Tuohy needle. A midline approach is preferred since the epidural space is widest at this point and the epidural vessels less dense. The interspace chosen should be as close to the dermatome of the surgical incision as possible.

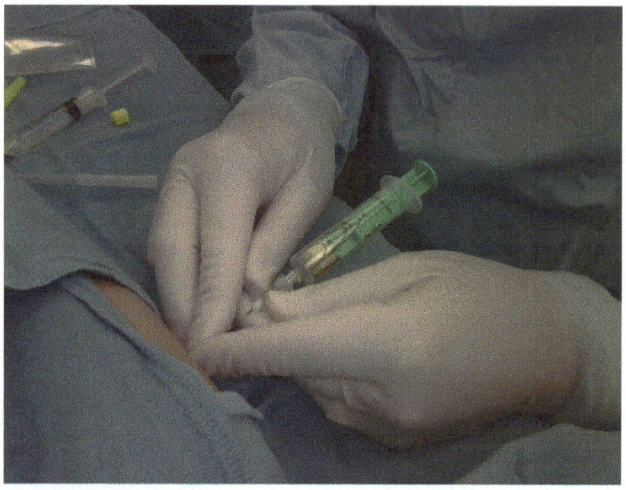

Fig. 15.5 The epidural needle can be introduced almost vertically to the skin in neonates when the back is flexed in the lateral decubitus position. Loss of resistance to air is considered more sensitive for detecting the 1–2 mm wide epidural space

The needle angulation depends on the level of epidural puncture and is greatest in the mid-thoracic region. Below this level, a more perpendicular approach can be used since the spinous processes in the lumbar region are almost horizontal when the back is flexed [172, 173] (Fig. 15.5). T12–L1 and L1–L2 interspaces are the largest and most easily palpable. The skin-epidural distance ranges from 5 to 12 mm depending on the gestational age and weight [32]. Ultrasound can be used to measure this distance [14].

Both air and saline have been advocated for the loss of resistance test to identify the epidural space [173, 174]. Saline is more popular according to a recent survey [174], although air is perhaps more sensitive [32, 172]. Using air for loss of resistance often results in the injection of air into the epidural space, and this maneuvre could cause an air embolus or rarely intra-arterial air embolus, specifically in the artery of Adamkiewicz, leading to paralysis. A "drip and tube" method has also been used successfully [62].

A catheter should be introduced at least 2 cm into the epidural space for continuous infusion or intermittent "top-ups" depending on whether an open tip or closed tip catheter is used [156]. This is best done after the "test dose" has "opened" the epidural space to facilitate the passage of the catheter [4, 147]. The length of catheter introduced into the epidural space is important: too much length increases the risk of a unilateral blockade, whereas too little could cause a failed block or increased local anesthetic leakage. Ultrasound can confirm correct catheter placement [157].

Complications: No serious complications, except dural puncture, have been reported in large published series [23, 32, 50, 51, 58, 83, 171, 175] (Table 15.1) Anecdotal case reports of spinal cord injury and air embolism bear testimony to the potential for disaster [176].

Dosing Guidelines: An initial bolus dose of 0.5 ml/kg followed by an infusion of 0.1 ml/kg/h 0.2 % ropivacaine or bupivacaine provided satisfactory analgesia [32, 83, 177]. One study recommended 0.6 ml/kg as the optimal bolus dose for abdominal surgery [178]. A smaller initial bolus of 0.33 ml/kg 0.25 % bupivacaine or 0.2 % ropivacaine is required for thoracic epidurals [179]. In the author's experience, larger volumes of up to 0.5 ml/kg may be required in small infants. *Top-up* doses should be half the original volume.

Sacral Epidural Block

Busoni described two approaches to the sacral epidural space [180, 181]. The *sacral intervertebral block* [169, 182] is possible in neonates since the sacral vertebrae are not fused. This block is particularly useful in neonates in whom the sacral hiatus cannot be identified and thus a caudal approach is not possible, e.g., obese neonates or high anorectal malformations with associated sacral abnormalities [182]. The *modified Taylor approach* [151, 181] between L5 and S1 is possible because of the large space between spinous process of the fifth lumbar vertebra and the rudimentary spinous process of the first sacral vertebra. These approaches have less risk of spinal cord damage or dural puncture [14, 75]. Furthermore, indwelling catheters with continuous infusions at these sites are less likely to become contaminated because of the greater distance from the anus [181].

Technique: The posterior superior iliac spines are identified with the neonate in the lateral decubitus position and with the hips flexed. A line between the posterior superior iliac spines bisects the second sacral vertebral arch (S2). The largest sacral intervertebral space (S2–S3) is easily identified 0.5–1.0 cm caudad to this line. The L5–S1 interspace is located 0.5–1.0 cm cephalad of this line and is also easily palpable provided the overlying sacral fat pad is not thick. In this case, an epidural needle can be introduced to contact bone and then "walked" cephalad or caudad on the sacral vertebra till the interspace is identified.

After skin preparation, the skin should be punctured to facilitate insertion of the 19 or 20 g Tuohy needle. No flexion is required since the spinous processes of the sacrum are rudimentary. The epidural space can be identified using a "loss of resistance" technique. The Tuohy needle can then be inclined to facilitate threading the catheter.

Dosing Guidelines: These are the same as those described for caudal block.

Table 15.3 Regimens for continuous epidural infusions used in neonates

Drug	Dose (mg kg h)	Additive	Ages	Site	Author	References
Bupivacaine	0.2		Neonate		Berde	[186]
Bupiv 0.2 %	0.1		Neonate	L,T	Bosenberg	[32, 48]
Bupiv 0.2 %	0.1		Neonate		Larsson	[96]
Bupiv 0.1 %	0.2	F 1 μg ml	Neonate, infant	L	Murrell	[33]
Bupiv 0.125 %	0.2–0.3		Neonate–4 m	L	Wolf	[138]
Bupiv 0.125–0.25 %	0.25		Neonate–6 year	L,T	Luz	
Bupiv 0.2 %	0.2		Neonate infant	L	Meignier	
Bupiv 0.2 %	0.2		Neonate infant	L	Schenkman	[50]
Ropivacaine 0.2 %	0.1–0.2		Neonate–1 year	L,T	Bosenberg	[83]

L Lumbar epidural, *T* thoracic epidural, *F* fentanyl

Continuous Epidural Infusions

Postoperative analgesia can be maintained using intermittent "top-ups" [4, 32] or continuous infusions of local anesthetic [32, 33, 35, 83, 88, 89, 96, 142, 183, 186]. As significant hypotension is unlikely, swings in blood pressure—a problem in adults—are not a feature in neonates. Intermittent "top-ups" are therefore a useful alternative when infusion pumps cannot deliver small hourly volumes of local anesthetics accurately.

A recent survey failed to reach a consensus on the selection of local anesthetic agent or concentration in clinical practice [184, 185]. Dosage guidelines suggested by Berde for racemic bupivacaine (i.e., 0.2 mg/kg/h for neonates and infants under 3 months) have proven to be safe and effective for both ropivacaine and bupivacaine [58, 83, 88, 96, 186]. Berde reported no complications with this dosing guideline in more than 1,400 children [186]. No complications were recorded in over 500 neonates, ranging from 0.5 to 5 kg, in this author's unpublished experience.

Desparmet used a smaller loading dose 0.5 ml/kg 0.25 % bupivacaine followed 30 min later by a similar infusion dose of 0.08 ml/kg/h using a volumetric infusion pump [187] (Table 15.3). For simplification, ease of calculation and an adequate volume to ensure a complete block, an infusion of 0.1 ml/kg/h, works well in the author's experience provided the catheter tip lies close to the dermatome of the surgical incision. Meignier used a smaller infusion rate 0.06 ml/kg/h for thoracic epidurals [188] (Table 15.3). For neonates <2 kg, the author reduces the concentration of local anesthetic, i.e., 0.1 % ropivacaine or bupivacaine.

For practical purposes once a particular infusion rate has been selected, regular assessment of the level of blockade, as well as an assessment of the degree of motor blockade should be performed. Adjustments to the infusion rate should be made as necessary (Table 15.3). If the maximal infusion rate is reached and the child still remains agitated, a manual "top-up" with lidocaine (avoiding toxic doses of local anesthetic) is an option to determine whether the caudal/epidural block can be salvaged. If the block remains inadequate, then a systemic opioid or epidural adjuvants can be considered. A check of the insertion site for signs of infection should also be included in the regular assessment.

Epidural Adjuvants

Few adjuvants have been used extensively in neonates despite the variety used in older children [183, 189, 190]. Most of these additives have been investigated in inguinal surgery as the model to evaluate their efficacy and risk/benefit ratio. Whether these findings can be extrapolated to major abdominal or thoracic surgery is debatable. The potential risk seems unjustified for relatively minor surgery since oral or rectal analgesia with less risk appear equally effective.

Epidural fentanyl carries a significant dose-dependent risk of respiratory depression without substantial analgesic benefit [183]. Moreover, it causes urinary retention, pruritus and ileus. Nausea, vomiting, and pruritus are difficult to assess in neonates and preterm infants but may be expressed as irritability and being fussy and "unsettled." When administered via a thoracic epidural, fentanyl is absorbed systemically and acts on the central nervous system. In the lumbar region, fentanyl probably acts locally as well as systemically. Clonidine has been used as an adjuvant for caudal or epidural infusions in neonates. At the recommended bolus dose (0.5–1 mcg/kg) or infusion rate (<0.1 mcg/kg/h), the hemodynamic effects are limited. Clonidine provides synergistic analgesia and, unlike epidural opioids, produces little or no ileus, nausea and vomiting, pruritus, or urinary retention. Even at doses that cause sedation, the respiratory drive with clonidine is better preserved than with opioids.

Ultrasound Imaging of Spinal Cord

Incomplete ossification of the posterior elements of the spinal canal in neonates allows accurate ultrasound evaluation of spinal cord structures using high frequency 7–12 MHz linear array transducer probes [74, 75, 158, 159, 191, 192]. The best acoustic views are obtained in preterm infants.

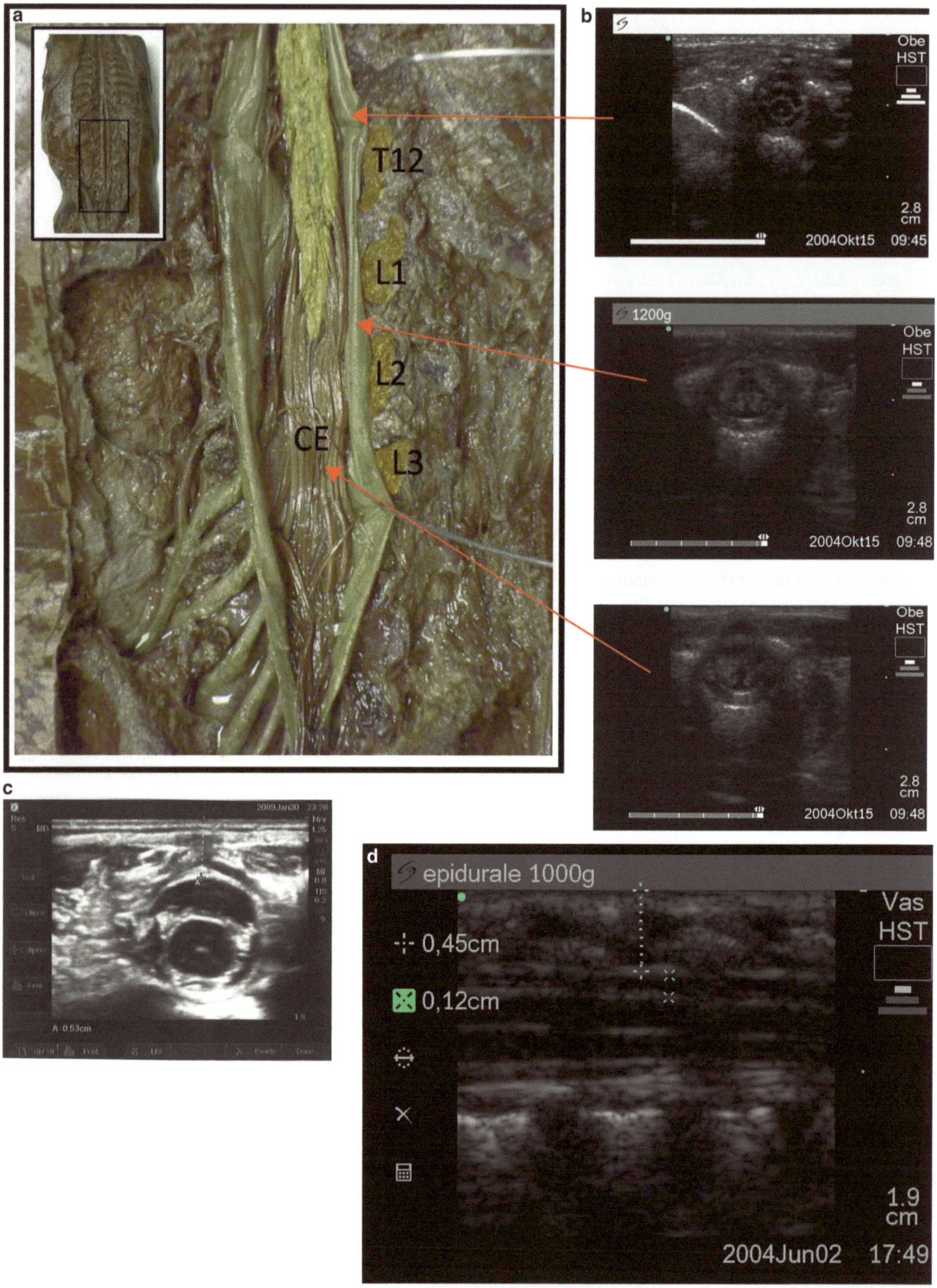
a
T12
L1
L2
CE
L3
b
Obe
HST
2.8 cm
2004Okt15 09:45
1200g
Obe
HST
2.8 cm
2004Okt15 09:48
Obe
HST
2.8 cm
2004Okt15 09:48
c
A 0.53cm
d
epidurale 1000g
Vas
HST
0,45cm
0,12cm
1.9 cm
2004Jun02 17:49

Information about the anatomical relationships of the spinal cord, dura mater, and epidural space (size, depth) can be applied effectively [74, 75, 193]. The skin-epidural depth can be measured and serve as a guide at which loss of resistance can be expected. The exact location of the conus can also be determined [74, 193].

In axial scans (Fig. 15.6a), the spinal cord is a hypoechoic (black) oval structure with a central hyperechoic (white) area representing the base of the invaginated paramedian sulcus. The hypoechoic spinal cord tapers to the conus medullaris. At this level, the rest of the vertebral canal is filled with multiple small rounded hyperechoic structures representing the cauda equina seen in cross section. The dura mater forms a hyperechoic (white) ring bordering the spinal canal; the pia mater is a hyperechoic ring surrounding the spinal cord. The cerebrospinal fluid is hypoechoic. The paraspinous muscles appear as an ovoid hypoechoic structures either side of the midline.

In sagittal longitudinal scans (Fig. 15.6b) the spinal cord elements are bounded by the pia appearing as hyperechoic parallel lines that converge at the conus. The cord is homogeneously hypoechoic with a central hyperechoic line (central sulcus). The dura mater is the hyperechoic line closely applied to the bony elements. The spinous processes can be identified by the "sawtooth" effect at regular intervals above the spinal canal and its contents.

Using real-time imaging, ultrasound can be used to verify the correct placement of a Tuohy needle, the injection of local anesthetic and the position of the catheter within the epidural space [157, 191, 193]. The epidural space in neonates ranges from 1 to 3 mm in depth [14]. The lengths of the 19G (Portex®) or 20G (Arrow®) Tuohy needle orifices are 2 and 3 mm, respectively. This suggests that dural tenting must occur at the time of either needle placement or epidural catheter insertion when epidurals are placed in neonates and infants. Ultrasound can also be used to determine the position of the catheter tip introduced via the sacral hiatus [157, 191].

Anatomical abnormalities [192, 195], particularly in those neonates with vertebral anomalies, unusual pits (Fig. 15.7) or tufts of hair suggesting an underlying spina bifida, can be identified using ultrasound. Anatomical abnormalities of the spinal cord (e.g., syrinx, diastematomyelia) can also be identified using ultrasound [192, 195].

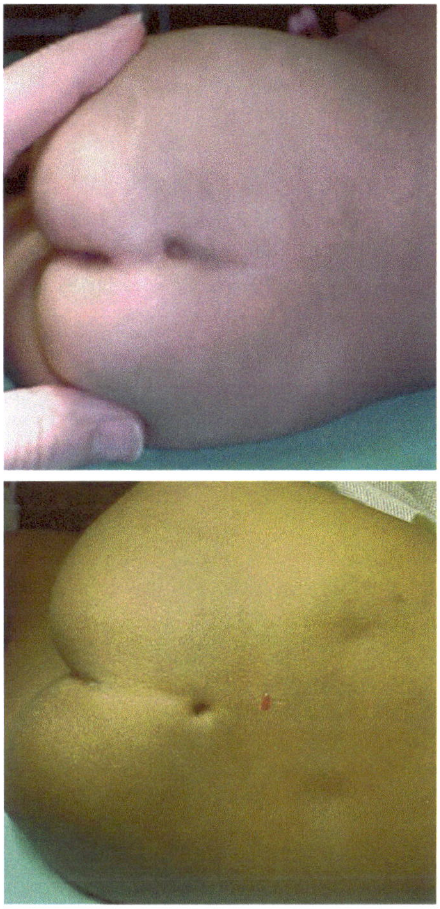

Fig. 15.7 Skin dimples or pits may indicate underlying spina bifida or cord abnormalities. Ultrasonography can be used to exclude these anomalies prior to caudal or epidural placement

Peripheral Nerve Blocks

Every peripheral nerve block can be performed in neonates [10, 11, 194, 196–204] to provide analgesia postsurgery and for sympathetic blockade to facilitate PICC line placement [10, 11, 201] or as part of the management of vascular complications [10, 11, 194, 198, 203, 204]. Nerve blocks can been placed using anatomical landmarks, a nerve stimulator [200], or ultrasound guidance [15, 197, 200] and are almost always placed during anesthesia, or awake, in selected cases. Ultrasound guidance is most accurate particularly

Fig. 15.6 (**a**) Cadaveric dissection of lumbar spine with four vertebrae identified: Thoracic 12, and Lumbar 1, 2 and 3, dura opened and CE identifying cauda equina. Note conus medullaris ending at L2 (Photo and dissection by A van Schoor, Ph.D). (**b**) Axial ultrasound images of the spine corresponding to three levels of the spinal cord in the dissection. From top to bottom: thoracic spine, conus medullaris and cauda equina as depicted by arrows. (**c** & **d**) The depth of the epidural space can be measured prior to placement. Abnormalities and normal variants of relevant anatomy can be excluded prior to epidural placement. (**d**) Sagittal longitudinal ultrasound image of spinal cord in a 1kg neonate. The distance from the skin to epidural space is shown as 4.5mm and the CSF depth to spinal cord is 1.2mm

when purely sensory nerves are blocked [200]. Peripheral nerves in neonates are less myelinated and thus reduced local anesthetic concentrations can be used successfully. For practical purposes a dose 0.1–0.2 ml/kg is sufficient to block most peripheral nerves.

Axillary blocks have been used to provide vasodilatation to facilitate PICC line placement [10, 11, 201] or for limb salvage after misadventures with arterial catheterization [198, 202]. Greater concentrations speed the onset of blockade and provide motor block useful for PICC line placement in awake neonates [11], whereas reduced concentrations are suitable for sympathectomy and analgesia. Dose guidelines: 0.5–1.0 ml 0.125–0.5 % bupivacaine depending on the aim. A *stellate ganglion block*, using a paratracheal approach onto Chassaignac's tubercle at the cricoid level, has also been used for this purpose [203, 204].

Femoral nerve blocks have been used for PICC line placement in the lower limbs, muscle biopsy [196], skin graft and clubfoot repair in infants [199]. Successful placement of local anesthetic just lateral to the femoral arterial pulse can be achieved using anatomical landmarks, nerve stimulation or ultrasound guidance. This block is relatively free of complications, but the hip's joint capsule deep to the artery may be entered.

Infraorbital Nerve Block: Although neonatal cleft lip repair (cheiloplasty) remains controversial (and is no longer performed in many institutions because the cosmetic result is not as good as originally thought) [194], an infraorbital nerve block can provide excellent analgesia without respiratory depression [194, 205, 206]. This block may be particularly useful in infants in infants with airway anomalies airway anomalies that could be compromised if opiates are used for cleft lip repair [206].

The infraorbital foramen is difficult to palpate in neonates and small infants. Two approaches have been described—a transcutaneous and an intraoral transmucosal approach. The nerve exits the infraorbital foramen, which is midway (15–17 mm) along a (30–34 mm) line drawn from the angle of the mouth to the midpoint of the palpebral fissure, approximately 7–8 mm from the ala nasi [194]. The nerve can be blocked using a 27–30 g needle that is introduced perpendicular to the skin down and passed through tissue to the bone, but not into the foramen. The intraoral approach relies on the ability to palpate the foramen. A needle may be introduced through the alveolar mucosal margin beneath the palpating finger. Both approaches provide analgesia with minimal risk of respiratory depression compared to fentanyl [205, 206]. *Dosage*: 0.5–1 ml 0.25–0.5 % bupivacaine [194, 205], or ropivacaine, with 1:200,000 epinephrine.

Ilioinguinal Nerve Block: can provide analgesia comparable to caudal blockade for inguinal herniotomy or orchidopexy [207, 208]. The ilioinguinal and iliohypogastric nerves lie between the transversus abdominis and internal oblique muscles, the former 2.2 mm and the latter 3.8 mm medial to the anterior superior iliac spine [80, 209]. Under sterile conditions, a needle can be introduced under ultrasound guidance in a medial to lateral direction, i.e., toward the iliac muscle and bone. In the absence of an ultrasound guide, the needle insertion distance (mm) is 0.6 × weight (kg) + 1.8 [209]. The muscle layers in neonates are thin and compliant. The risk of penetrating the peritoneal cavity is much greater than in children if the needle is not advanced with caution [210].

When ultrasound is not available, the identification of the "pop" as a short-beveled needle penetrates the external oblique aponeurosis. This "pop" can be facilitated by introducing the needle at an angle—the greater the angle the "thicker" the aponeurosis becomes. High plasma concentrations of local anesthetics have been reported [207, 210], although this block is relatively free of complications. *Transient femoral nerve block* [211, 212] and *colonic perforation* have been described [213]. *Dosage*: 0.1–0.2 ml/kg 0.25–0.5 % bupivacaine or 0.2–0.5 % ropivacaine.

Transabdominal Plane (TAP): block is becoming an increasingly popular alternative for intraoperative and early postoperative analgesia for selected upper (ileostomy closure) [214] or mid-abdominal procedures (colostomy) [215] involving the abdominal wall [214–219]. Under sterile conditions and using "in plane" ultrasound guidance, the lateral branch of the intercostal nerves can be blocked in the tissue plane between the internal oblique and transversus abdominis provided the spread of local anesthetic extends posterior to the midaxillary line. Hydrodissection of this tissue plane confirms correct placement of a short-beveled needle introduced subcostally or above the iliac crest. The muscle layers are thin and compliant, and the risk of penetrating the peritoneal cavity, liver, or spleen is substantial if the needle is not advanced with caution (see Fig. 15.8). *Dose*: 0.2–0.5 ml/kg 0.25 bupivacaine or 0.2 % ropivacaine.

Intercostal Nerves: can be blocked under direct vision at surgery or using ultrasound guidance to provide analgesia after thoracotomy or chest tube placement in both cyanotic and acyanotic neonates. *Dosage*: 0.6 ml/kg (1.5 mg/kg) 0.25 % bupivacaine with epinephrine [220]. Blood concentrations using this dose are variable, but no adverse events were noted [220]. Note that the uptake of local anesthetic from an intercostal block is the fastest of any site for regional anesthesia and the most likely to produce toxic blood concentrations of local anesthetic and briefest block. To prevent these effects, epinephrine should be used as an adjunct to the local anesthetic.

Paravertebral Block: Direct placement of a catheter for continuous paravertebral block is technically difficult in neonates [222, 223]. Extrapleural paravertebral placement

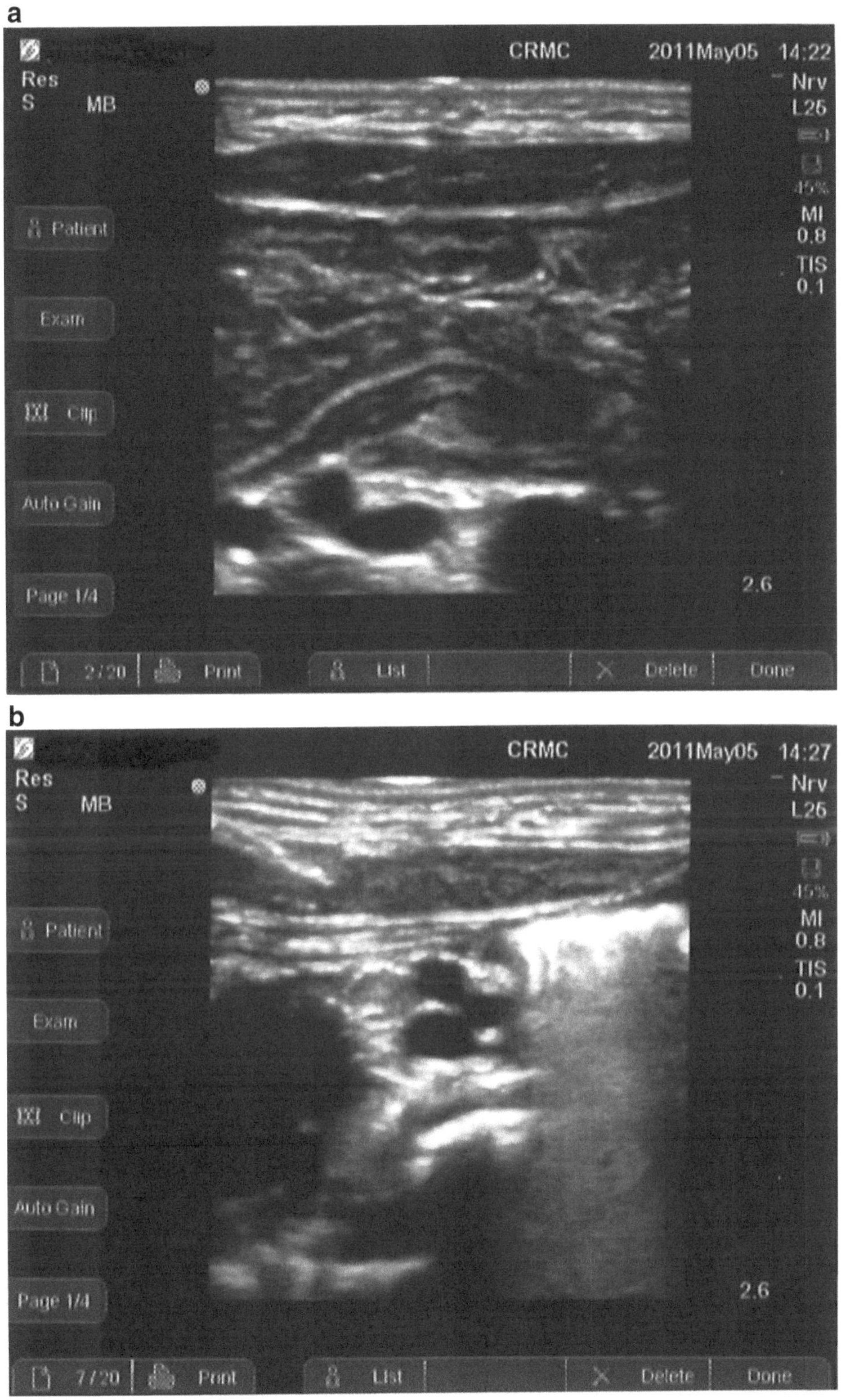

Fig. 15.8 Ultrasound images of the rectus sheath block through a compliant abdominal wall. (**a**) Prior to application of any pressure with the probe or needle. (**b**) With minimal pressure during needle insertion, the abdominal wall and rectus muscles can be pushed dangerously close to the aorta and inferior vena cava

under direct vision immediately before chest closure is a viable alternative for management of post thoracotomy pain. After an initial bolus of 0.5 ml/kg 0.25 % bupivacaine, a continuous infusion of 0.2 ml/kg/h 0.125–0.25 % bupivacaine with epinephrine provides satisfactory analgesia.

Topical Anesthesia: During the past two decades, there has been a substantial increase in the number and types of topical anesthetics [221]. Options for the prevention of neonatal pain associated with skin-breaking procedures were previously limited to injections of lidocaine. Topical anesthetics are now available as creams, gels, and a heat-activated patch system [221]. The onset time varies for each modality and careful planning is needed to coincide with the peak effect. Indications range from peripheral IV placement, lumbar puncture, circumcision, and heel sticks.

Management of Local Anesthetic Toxicity

Neonates are more susceptible to local anesthetic toxicity because their blood concentration of alpha1 acid glycoprotein is less than that in older children, the elimination of local anesthetics is slower and the volume of local anesthetic required is greater [224, 225, 227]. Prevention is therefore better than cure since the management of local anesthetic toxicity in neonates may be difficult. A variety of drugs have been used with limited success in the past [226], although recent reports of successful management using 20 % lipid emulsion are encouraging [227, 228].

Initial resuscitation should always proceed according to PALS guidelines, aiming at securing the airway, hyperventilation (to reduce the free fraction by inducing respiratory alkalosis) and circulatory support. Lipid emulsion (20 % Intralipid®) should be given as soon as possible [228, 229, 230]. An initial bolus of 1 ml/kg IV Intralipid® should be given over 1 min followed by up to two repeated boluses at 3–5min intervals (for a total dose of 3 ml/kg), observing the electrocardiogram for a return to normal sinus rhythm. After 3 ml/kg Intralipid® have been administered or cardiovascular stability restored, the infusion rate should be reduced to 0.25 ml/kg/h infusion . Propofol or etomidate, formulated in lipid emulsion, is not an appropriate substitute for Intralipid® particularly in the presence of cardiovascular collapse [230].

Conclusion

The benefits of regional anesthesia are significant, but safety should remain our primary concern particularly with today's high expectations and zero tolerance for morbidity after anesthesia. While most regional anesthetic technique are simple to perform, they should never be considered routine because of the risks involved [231]. Careful consideration of the indications and contraindications together with the setting (day case or hospital) should influence the decision. Continuous infusions and nerve blocks have limited duration. It is prudent to plan subsequent analgesia as part of a multimodal approach [232]. In general, the more peripheral the block, the lower the risk. Epidural anesthesia should be performed by, or under the guidance of, an experienced practitioner.

References

1. Prevention and management of pain in neonates: an update AAP and Canadian Pediatric Society. Pediatrics 2006; 118: 2231–4. Re-affirmed May 2010.
2. Berde CB, Jaksic T, Lynn AM, Maxwell LG, Soriano SG, Tibboel D. Anesthesia and analgesia during and after surgery in neonates. Clin Ther. 2005;27:900–21.
3. Moriarty A. In praise of the epidural space. Pediatr Anesth. 2002;12:836–7.
4. Bosenberg AT, Bland BAR, Schulte-Steinberg O, Downing J. Thoracic epidural via the caudal route in infants. Anesthesiology. 1988;69:265–9.
5. Polaner DM, Taenzer AH, Walker BJ, et al. Pediatric regional anesthesia network (PRAN): a multi-institutional study of the use and incidence of complications of pediatric regional anesthesia. Anesth Analg. 2012;115:1353–6.
6. Williams RK, Adams DC, Aladjem EV, Kreutz JM, Sartorelli KH, Vane DW, Abajian JC. The safety and efficacy of spinal anesthesia for surgery in infants: vermont infant spinal registry. Anesth Analg. 2006;102:67–71.
7. Willschke H, Machata AM, Rebhandl W, Benkoe T, Kettner SC, Brenner L, Marhofer P. Management of hypertrophic pyloric stenosis with ultrasound guided single shot epidural anesthesia – a retrospective analysis of 20 cases. Pediatr Anesth. 2011;21: 110–5.
8. Somri M, Tome R, Yanovski B, et al. Combined spinal-epidural anesthesia in major abdominal surgery in high-risk neonates and infants. Paediatr Anaesth. 2007;17:1059–65.
9. Peutrell JM, Hughes DG. Epidural anaesthesia through caudal catheters for inguinal herniotomies in awake ex-premature babies. Anaesthesia. 1993;48:128–31.
10. Messeri A, Calamandrei M. Percutaneous central venous catheterization in small infants: axillary block can facilitate the insertion rate. Paediatr Anaesth. 2000;10(5):527–30.
11. Keech K, Bosenberg A. Axillary block for PICC Lines in critically ill neonates. Abstract Society Pediatric Anesthesia (SPA) Annual meeting 2010 San Antonio.
12. Bosenberg AT, Lonnqvist PA. The potential future or just a way of trespassing the safety limits of pediatric regional anesthesia? Pediatr Anesth. 2011;21:95–7.
13. Sethna NF, Berde CB. Pediatric regional anesthesia equipment. Int Anesthesiol Clin. 1992;30:163–76.
14. Willschke H, Bosenberg A, Marhofer P, et al. Epidural catheter placement in neonates: sonoanatomy and feasibility of ultrasonographic guidance in term and preterm neonates. Reg Anesth Pain Med. 2007;32:34–40.
15. Marhofer P, Willschke H, Kettner S. Imaging techniques for regional nerve blockade and vascular cannulation in children. Curr Opin Anaesthesiol. 2006;19:293–300.
16. Anand KJ, Sippell WG, Aynsley-Green A. Randomised trial of fentanyl anaesthesia in preterm babies undergoing surgery: effects on the stress response. Lancet. 1987;1:62–6.

17. Barker DP, Rutter N. Stress severity illness and outcome in ventilated preterm infants. Arch Dis Child. 1996;75:F187–90.
18. Wolf AR, Doyle E, Thomas E. Modifying the stress responses to major surgery: spinal vs extradural vs opioid analgesia. Pediatr Anesth. 1998;8:305–11.
19. Humphreys N, Bays S, Parry AJ, et al. Spinal anesthesia with an indwelling catheter reduces the stress response in pediatric open-heart surgery. Anesthesiology. 2005;103:113–1120.
20. Hollmann MW, Durieux ME. Local anesthetics and the inflammatory response. Anesthesiology. 2000;93:858–75.
21. Holmann MW, Durieux ME, Graf BM. Novel local anaesthetics and novel indications for local anaesthetics. Curr Opin Anaesthesiol. 2001;14:741–49.
22. de Forget P, Kock M. Could anesthesia, analgesia and sympathetic modulation affect neoplastic recurrence after surgery? A systematic review centered over the modulation of natural killer cells activity. Ann Fr Anesth Reanim. 2009;109:1464–9.
23. Bosenberg AT, Johr M, Wolf AR. Pro con debate: the use of regional vs systemic analgesia for neonatal surgery. Pediatr Anesth. 2011;21:1247–58.
24. Sanders RD, Davidson A. Anesthetic induced neurotoxicity of the neonate: time for clinical guidelines? Pediatr Anesth. 2009;19: 1141–6.
25. Perouansky M, Hemmings HC. Neurotoxicity of general anesthetics. Anesthesiology. 2009;11:1365–71.
26. Wang C, Slikker Jr W. Strategies and experimental models for evaluating anesthetics: effects on the developing nervous system. Anesth Analg. 2008;106:1643–58.
27. Slikker Jr W, Zou X, Hotchkiss CE, et al. Ketamine-induced neuronal cell death in the perinatal rhesus monkey. Toxicol Sci. 2007;98:145–58.
28. Davidson A, Soriano SG. Does anaesthesia harm the developing brain –evidence or speculation? Pediatr Anaesth. 2004;14: 199–200.
29. Istaphanous GK, Loepke AW. General anesthetics and the developing brain. Curr Opin Anaesthesiol. 2009;22:368–73.
30. Yaholam B, Athiraman U, Soriano SG, et al. Spinal anesthesia in infant rats: development of a model and assessment of neurologic outcomes. Anesthesiology. 2011;114:1325–35.
31. Jöhr M, Berger TM. Regional anaesthetic techniques for neonatal surgery: indications and selection of techniques. Best Pract Res Clin Anaesthesiol. 2004;18:357–75.
32. Bösenberg AT. Epidural analgesia for major neonatal surgery. Paediatr Anaesth. 1998;8:479–83.
33. Murrell D, Gibson PR, Cohen RC. Continuous epidural analgesia in newborn infants undergoing major surgery. J Pediatr Surg. 1993;28:548–53.
34. Williams RK, McBride WJ, Abajian JC. Combined spinal and epidural anaesthesia for major abdominal surgery in infants. Can J Anaesth. 1997;44:511–4.
35. Henderson K, Sethna NF, Berde CB. Continuous caudal anesthesia for inguinal hernia repair in former preterm infants. J Clin Anesth. 1993;5:129–33.
36. Monsel A, Salvat-Toussaint A, Durand P, Haas V, Baujard C, Rouleau P, El Aouadi S, Benhamou D, Asehnoune K. The transesophageal Doppler and hemodynamic effects of epidural anesthesia in infants anesthetized with sevoflurane and sufentanil. Anesth Analg. 2007;105:46–50.
37. Oberlander TF, Berde CB, Lam KH, et al. Infants tolerate spinal anesthesia with minimal overall autonomic changes: analysis of heart rate variability in former premature infants undergoing hernia repair. Anesth Analg. 1995;80:20–7.
38. Bosenberg A, Ivani G. Regional anaesthesia - children are different. Pediatr Anesth. 1998;8:447–50.
39. Lerman J. Local anesthetics belong in the caudal/epidural space, not in the veins! Can J Anaesth. 1997;44:582–6.
40. Brindley N, Taylor R, Brown S. Reduction of incarcerated inguinal hernia in infants using caudal epidural anaesthesia. Pediatr Surg Int. 2005;21:715–17.
41. Hodgson RE, Bösenberg AT, Hadley LG. Congenital diaphragmatic hernia repair–impact of delayed surgery and epidural analgesia. S Afr J Surg. 2000;38:31–4.
42. Terrier G, Lansade A, Ugazzi M, Favereau JP, Longis B, Alain JL. Contribution of continuous peridural analgesia to neonatal surgery. Chir Pediatr. 1990;31:217–8.
43. Raghavan M, Montgomerie J. Anesthetic management of gastroschisis–a review of our practice over the past 5 years. Paediatr Anaesth. 2008;18:1055–9.
44. Jöhr M. Regional anesthesia in newborn infants, infants and children–what prerequisites must be met? Anaesthesiol Reanim. 2003;28:69–73.
45. Murat I. Chapter 3 Pharmacology In: Regional anesthesia in infants children and adolescents. Dalens BJ, editor. Baltimore: Williams & Wilkins; 1995.
46. Hatch DJ, Hulse MG, Lindahl SGE. Caudal analgesia in children: influence of ventilatory efficiency during halothane anaesthesia. Anaesthesia. 1984;39:873–8.
47. von Ungern-Sternberg BS, Regli A, Frei FJ, Hammer J, Schibler A, Erb TO. The effect of caudal block on functional residual capacity and ventilation homogeneity in healthy children. Anaesthesia. 2006;61:758–63.
48. Bosenberg AT, Hadley GP, Wiersma R, et al. Oesophageal atresia: caudothoracic epidural anaesthesia reduces the need for postoperative ventilatory support. Pediatr Surg Int. 1992;7:289–91.
49. Krishnan K, Marcus R. Epidural analgesia for tracheo-oesophageal fistula repair. Abstract APAGBI Scientific meeting Cardiff; 2006
50. Shenkman Z, Hoppenstein D, Erez I, Dolfin T, Freud E. Continuous lumbar/thoracic epidural analgesia in low-weight paediatric surgical patients: practical aspects and pitfalls. Pediatr Surg Int. 2009;25:623–34.
51. Aspirot A, Pulingandla PS, Bouchard S, Su W. A contemporary evaluation of surgical outcome in neonate and infants undergoing lung resection. J Pediatr Surg. 2008;43:508–12.
52. Craven PD, Badawi N, Henderson-Smart DJ, O'Brien M. Regional (spinal, epidural, caudal) versus general anaesthesia in preterm infants undergoing inguinal herniorrhaphy in early infancy. Cochrane Database Syst Rev. 2003;3, CD003669.
53. Gerber AC, Weiss M. Awake spinal or caudal anaesthesia in preterms for herniotomies: what is the evidence based benefit compared with general anaesthesia? Curr Opin Anaesthesiol. 2003;16:315–20.
54. Sale SM, Read JA, Stoddart PA, Wolf AR. Prospective comparison of sevoflurane and desflurane in formerly premature infants undergoing inguinal herniotomy. Br J Anaesth. 2006;96: 774–8.
55. Hoehn T, Jetzek-Zader M, Blohm M, Mayatepek E. Early peristalsis following epidural analgesia during abdominal surgery in an extremely low birth weight infant. Paediatr Anaesth. 2007;17:176–9.
56. Borgeat A, Aguirre J. Update on local anaesthetics. Curr Opin Anaesthesiol. 2010;23:466–71.
57. Morton NS, Errera A. APA national audit of pediatric opioid infusions. Pediatr Anesth. 2010;20:119–25.
58. Llewellyn N, Moriarty A. The national paediatric epidural audit. Pediatr Anesth. 2007;17:520–32.
59. Giaufre E, Dalens B, Gombert A. Epidemiology and morbidity of regional anesthesia in children: a one-year prospective survey of the French-language society of pediatric anesthesiologists. Anesth Analg. 1996;83:904–12.
60. Ecoffey C, Lacroix F, Giaufre E, et al. Epidemiology and morbidity of regional anesthesia in children: a follow-up one year prospective survey of the French-language society of paediatric anaesthesiologists (ADARPEF). Pediatr Anesth. 2010;20:1061–69.

61. Rochette A, Dadure C, Raux O, Troncin R, Mailheé P, Capdevila X. A review of pediatric regional anesthesia practice during a 17-year period in a single institution. Pediatr Anesth. 2007;17:874–80.
62. Osaka Y, Yamashita M. Intervertebral epidural anesthesia in 2,050 infants and children using the drip and tube method. Reg Anesth Pain Med. 2003;28:103–7.
63. Yamashita M, Osaka Y. Some hints to make neonatal epidural anaesthesia less difficult. Paediatr Anaesth. 2000;10:110–1.
64. Yamashita M, Tsuji M. Identification of the epidural space in children. The application of micro-drip infusion set. Anaesthesia. 1991;46:872–4.
65. Hasan MA, Howard RF, Lloyd-Thomas AR. Depth of epidural space in children. Anaesthesia. 1994;49:1085–7.
66. Vas L, Naregal P, Sanegiri S, Negri A. Some vagaries of neonatal lumbar epidural anaesthesia. Pediatr Anaesth. 1999;9:217–23.
67. Courrèges P, Lecoutre D, Poddevin F, Bayart R. Epidural anesthesia in children under 3 months of age. Apropos of 49 cases. Cah Anesthesiol. 1996;44(5):403–8.
68. Breschan C, Krumpholz R, Jost R, Likar R. Intraspinal haematoma following lumbar epidural anaesthesia in a neonate. Pediatr Anesth. 2001;11:105–8.
69. Rubin K, Sullivan S, Sadhasivan S. Are peripheral and neuraxial block with ultrasound guidance more effective and safer in children? Pediatr Anesth. 2009;19:92–6.
70. Busoni P. Anatomy. In: Saint-Maurice C, Schulte-Steinberg O, editors. Regional anaesthesia in children. Fribourg: Mediglobe; 1990. p. 16–25.
71. Dalens B. Regional anaesthesia in children. Anesth Analg. 1989;68:654–72.
72. Rowland-Hill CA, Gibson PJ. Ultrasound determination of the normal location of the conus medullaris in neonates. Am J Neuroradiol. 1995;16:469–72.
73. Hamid M, Fallet-Bianco C, Delmas V, Plaisant O. The human epidural anterior epidural space: morphological comparison in adult and fetal specimens. Surg Radiol Anat. 2002;24:194–200.
74. Koo BN, Hong JY, Kim JE, Kil HK. The effect of flexion on the level of termination of the dural sac in paediatric patients. Anaesthesia. 2009;64:1072–6.
75. Shin SK, Hong JY, Kim WO, Koo BN, Kim JE, Kil HK. Ultrasound evaluation of the sacral area and comparison of sacral interspinous and hiatal approach for caudal block in children. Anesthesiology. 2009;111:1135–40.
76. Kil HK, Koo BN, Kim WO. To make epidural catheterisation less difficult in infants. Pediatr Anesth. 2006;16:1196–7.
77. Vas L, Raghavendran S, Hosalkar H, Patil B. A study of epidural pressures in infants. Pediatr Anesth. 2001;11:575–83.
78. Schabort D. Anatomy relevant to lower limb blocks in newborn infants. MSc (Anatomy) Thesis Univ Pretoria; 2005.
79. Van Schoor AN. Paediatric regional anaesthesia – a clinical anatomical study. PhD Thesis Univ Pretoria; 2010.
80. Van Schoor AN, Boon JM, Bosenberg AT, Abrahams PH, Meiring JH. Anatomical considerations of the pediatric ilioinguinal/iliohypogastric nerve block. Pediatr Anesth. 2005;15:371–7.
81. Röper A, Lauven PM. Pharmacokinetics in newborns and infants. Anasthesiol Intensivmed Notfallmed Schmerzther. 1999;34:616–25.
82. Le Dez KM, Swartz J, Strong A, Burrows FA, Lerman J. The effect of age on serum concentration of α acid glycoprotein in newborns infants and children. Anesthesiology. 1986;65:3 A421.
83. Bosenberg AT, Thomas J, Cronje L, Lopez T, Crean PM, Gustafsson U, Huledal G, Larsson LE. Pharmacokinetics and efficacy of ropivacaine for continuous epidural infusion in neonates and infants. Paediatr Anaesth. 2005;15:739–49.
84. Rapp HJ, Molnar V, Austin S, Krohn S, Gadeke V, Motsch J, Boos K, Williams DG, Gustafsson U, Huledal G, Larsson L. Ropivacaine kinetics in neonates and infants: a population pharmacokinetic evaluation following single shot caudal block. Pediatr Anesth. 2001;14:724–32.
85. Hansen TG, Ilett KF, Reid C, Lim SI, Hackett LP, Bergesio R. Caudal ropivacaine in infants: population pharmacokinetics and plasma concentrations. Anesthesiology. 2001;94:579–84.
86. Booker PD, Taylor C, Saba G. Perioperative changes in alpha 1-acid glycoprotein concentrations in infants undergoing major surgery. Br J Anaesth. 1996;76:365–8.
87. Mather LE, Longe GT, Thomas J. The binding of bupivacaine to maternal and foetal plasma proteins. J Pharm Pharmacol. 1971;23:359.
88. Berde CB, Yaster M, Meretoja O, McCann ME, Huledal G, Gustafsson U, Larsson LE. Stable plasma concentrations of unbound ropivacaine during postoperative epidural infusion for 24–72 hours in children. Eur J Anaesthesiol. 2008;25:410–7.
89. Tobias JD, Rasmussen GE, Holcomb GW, et al. Continuous caudal anaesthesia with chloroprocaine as an adjunct to general anaesthesia in neonates. Can J Anaesth. 1996;43:69–72.
90. Mazoit JX, Denson DD, Samii K. Pharmacokinetics of bupivacaine in infants after caudal anaesthesia. Anesthesiology. 1988;68:387–91.
91. Murat I, Delleur MM, Esteve C, Egu JF, Raynaud P, Saint-Maurice C. Continuous extradural anaesthesia in children. Clinical and hemodynamic implications. Br J Anaesth. 1987;59:1441–50.
92. Warner MA, Kunkel SE, Offord KO, Atchison SR, Dawson B. The effects of age, epinephrine and operative site on duration of caudal analgesia in pediatric patients. Anesth Analg. 1987;66:995–8.
93. Rice L, DeMars P, Whalen T, Crooms JC, Parkinson SK. Duration of spinal anesthesia in infants less than one year of age. Reg Anesth. 1994;19:325–29.
94. Miyabe M, Kakiuchi Y, Inomata S, Ohsaka Y, Kohda Y, Toyooka H. Epinephrine does not reduce the plasma concentration of lidocaine during continuous epidural infusion in children. Can J Anaesth. 2002;49:706–10.
95. Bokesch P, Castaneda AR, Ziemer G, Wilson JM. The influence of a right-to-left cardiac shunt on lidocaine pharmacokinetics. Anesthesiology. 1987;67:739–44.
96. Larsson BA, Lönnqvist PA, Olsson GL. Plasma concentrations of bupivacaine in neonates after continuous epidural infusion. Anesth Analg. 1997;84:501–5.
97. Suresh S, Hall SC. Spinal anesthesia in infants: is the impractical practical? Anesth Analg. 2006;102:65–6.
98. Vane DW, Abajian JC, Hong AR. Spinal anesthesia for primary repair of gastroschisis: a new and safe technique for selected patients. J Pediatr Surg. 1994;29:1234–5.
99. Bosenberg A, Flick RP. Regional anesthesia in neonates and infants. Clin Perinatol. 2013;40:525–38.
100. Kachko L, Simhi E, Tzeitlin E, Efrat R, Tarabikin E, Peled E, Metzner I, Katz J. Spinal anesthesia in neonates and infants – a single-center experience of 505 cases. Pediatr Anesth. 2007;17:647–53.
101. Rochette A, Raux O, Troncin R, Dadure C, Verdier R, Capdevilla X. Clonidine prolongs spinal anesthesia in newborns: a prospective dose-ranging study. Anesth Analg. 2004;98:56–9.
102. Rochette A, Troncin R, Raux O, Dadure C, Lubrano JF, Barbotte E, Capdevilla X. Clonidine added to bupivacaine in neonatal spinal anesthesia: a prospective comparison in 124 preterm and term infants. Paediatr Anaesth. 2005;15:1072–7.
103. Frawley GP, Farrell T, Smith S. Levobupivacaine spinal anesthesia in neonates: a dose range finding study. Pediatr Anesth. 2004;14:838–44.
104. Frawley G, Smith KR, Ingelmo P. Relative potencies of bupivacaine, levobupivacaine, and ropivacaine for neonatal spinal anaesthesia. Br J Anaesth. 2009;103:731–8.

105. Frawley G, Skinner A, Thomas J, Smith S. Ropivacaine spinal anesthesia in neonates: a dose range finding study. Paediatr Anaesth. 2007;17:126–32.
106. Hermanns H, Stevens MF, Werdehausen R, Braun S, Lipfert P, Jetzek-Zader M. Sedation during spinal anaesthesia in infants. Br J Anaesth. 2006;97:380–4.
107. Bonnet MP, Larousse E, Asehnoune K, Benhamou D. Spinal anesthesia with bupivacaine decreases cerebral blood flow in former preterm infants. Anesth Analg. 2004;98:1280–3.
108. Kim J, Thornton J, Eipe N. Spinal anesthesia for the premature infant: is this really the answer to avoiding postoperative apnea? Pediatr Anesth. 2009;19:54–72.
109. Walker SM, Yaksh TL. Neuraxial analgesia in neonates and infants: a review of clinical and preclinical strategies for the development of safety and efficacy data. Anesth Analg. 2012;115:638–62.
110. Easley RB, George R, Connors D, Tobias JD. Aseptic meningitis after spinal anesthesia in an infant. Anesthesiology. 1999; 91:305–7.
111. Luz G, Buchele H, Innerhofer P, Maurer H. Spinal anaesthesia and meningitis in former preterm infants: cause- effect? Pediatr Anesth. 1999;9:262–4.
112. Chabás E, Sala X, Nalda MA. Unilateral spinal analgesia in a neonate. Anaesthesia. 1995;50:182.
113. Beauvoir C, Rochette A, Desch G, D'Athis F. Spinal anaesthesia in newborns: total and free bupivacaine plasma concentration. Paediatr Anaesth. 1996;6:195–9.
114. Hoyle Jr JD, Rogers AJ, Reischman DE, Powell ED, Borgialli DA, Mahajan PV, Trytko JA, Stanley RM. Pain intervention for infant lumbar puncture in the emergency department: physician practice and beliefs. Acad Emerg Med. 2011;18:140–4.
115. Yaster M, Maxwell LG. Pediatric regional anaesthesia. Anesthesiology. 1989;70:324–38.
116. Moyao-García D, Garza-Leyva M, Velázquez-Armenta EY, Nava-Ocampo AA. Caudal block with 4 mg x kg-1 (1.6 ml x kg-1) of bupivacaine 0.25 % in children undergoing surgical correction of congenital pyloric stenosis. Paediatr Anaesth. 2002;12:404–10.
117. Hoelzle M, Weiss M, Dillier C, Gerber A. Comparison of awake spinal with awake caudal anesthesia in preterm and ex-preterm infants for heriotomy[1]. Pediatr Anesth. 2010;20:620–4.
118. Hargreaves DM, Spargo PM, Wheeler RA. Caudal blockade in the management of aortic thrombosis following umbilical artery catheterisation. Anaesthesia. 1992;47:493–5.
119. Berens R, Pontus Jr SP. A complication associated with dorsal penile nerve block. Reg Anesth. 1990;15:309–10.
120. Abouleish AE, Chung DH, Cohen M. Caudal anesthesia for vascular access procedures in two extremely small premature neonates. Pediatr Surg Int. 2005;21:749–51.
121. Johr M, Seiler SJ, Berger TM. Caudal anesthesia with ropivacaine in an awake 1,090-g baby. Anesthesiology. 2000;93:593.
122. Park JH, Koo BN, Kim JY, Cho JE, Kim WO, Kil HK. Determination of the optimal angle for needle insertion during caudal block in children using ultrasound imaging. Anaesthesia. 2006;61:946–9.
123. Menzies R, Congreve K, Herodes V, Berg S, Mason DG. A survey of pediatric caudal extradural anesthesia practice. Paediatr Anaesth. 2009;19:829–36.
124. Armitage EN. Regional anaesthesia. In: Sumner E, Hatch DJ, editors. Textbook of pediatric anaesthesia practice. London: WB Saunders; 1989. p. 221.
125. Roberts SA, Guruswamy V, Galvez I. Caudal injectate can be reliably imaged using portable ultrasound–a preliminary study. Paediatr Anaesth. 2005;15:948–52.
126. Wong GK, Arab AA, Chew SC, Naser B, Crawford MW. Major complications related to epidural analgesia in children: a 15-year audit of 3,152 epidurals. Can J Anesth. 2013;60:355–63.
127. Wong GK, Can J Anesth 2013 above. Hubler M, Gabler R, Ehm B, Oertel R, Gama de Abreu M, Koch T. Successful resuscitation following ropivacaine-induced systemic toxicity in a neonates. Anaesthesia 2010:65;1137–40.
128. Dalens B, Hasnaoui A. Caudal anesthesia in pediatric surgery: success rate and adverse effects in 750 consecutive patients. Anesth Analg. 1989;68:83–9.
129. Wittum S, Hofer CK, Rolli U, Suhner M, et al. Sacral osteomyelitis after single-shot epidural anesthesia via the caudal approach in a child. Anesthesiology. 2003;99:503–5.
130. Emmanuel ER. Post-sacral extradural catheter abscess in a child. Br J Anaesth. 1994;73:548–9.
131. Tabaddor K, Lamorgese JR. Lumbar epidermoid cyst following single puncture. J Bone Joint Surg Am. 1975;8:1168–9.
132. Baris S, Guldogus F, Baris YS, Karakaya D, Kelsaka E. Is tissue coring a real problem after caudal injection in children. Pediatr Anesth. 2004;14:755–8.
133. Goldschneider KR, Brandom BW. The incidence of tissue coring during the performance of caudal injection in children. Reg Anesth Pain Med. 1999;24:553–6.
134. McCaul K. Caudal blockade. In: Cousins MJ, Bridenbaugh PO, editors. Neural blockade in clinical anaesthesia and management of pain. Philadelphia: JB Lippincott; 1980. p. 275.
135. Schulte-Steinberg O, Rahlfs VW. Spread of extradural analgesia following caudal injection in children - a statistical study. Br J Anaesth. 1977;49:1027–34.
136. Takasaki M, Dohi S, Kawabata Y, Takayashi T. Dosage of lidocaine for caudal anaesthesia in infants and children. Anesthesiology. 1977;47:527–9.
137. Busoni P, Andreucetti T. The spread of caudal analgesia in children: a mathematical model. Anaesth Intensive Care. 1986; 14:140–4.
138. Wolf AR, Valley RD, Fear DW, Roy WL, Lerman J. Bupivacaine for caudal analgesia in infants and children. The optimal effective concentration. Anesthesiology. 1988;69:102–6.
139. Bosenberg AT, Thomas J, Lopez T, Lybeck A, Huizar K, Larrson LE. Efficacy of caudal ropivacaine 1, 2 or 3 mg.ml for postoperative analgesia in children. Pediatr Anaesth. 2002;12:53–8.
140. Ingelmo P, Frawley G, Astuto M, Duffy C, Donath S, Disma N, Rosano G, Fumagalli R, Gullo A. Relative analgesic potencies of levobupivacaine and ropivacaine for caudal anesthesia in children. Anesth Analg. 2009;108:805–13.
141. Karmakar MK, Aun CST, Wong ELY, Wong ASY, Chan SKC, Yeung CK. Ropivacaine undergoes slower systemic absorption from the caudal epidural space in children than bupivacaine. Anesth Analg. 2002;94:259–65.
142. Chalkiadis GA, Anderson BJ, Tay M, Bjorksten A, Kelly JJ. Pharmacokinetics of levobupivacaine after caudal epidural administration in infants less than 3months of age. Br J Anaesth. 2005;95:524–9.
143. Rapp HJ, Molnár V, Austin S, Krohn S, Gädeke V, Motsch J, Boos K, Williams DG, Gustafsson U, Huledal G, Larsson LE. Ropivacaine in neonates and infants: a population pharmacokinetic evaluation following single caudal block. Paediatr Anaesth. 2004;14:724–32.
144. El-Hennawy AM, Abd-Elwahab AM, Abd-Elmaksoud AM, El-Ozairy HS, Boulis SR. Addition of clonidine or dexmedetomidine to bupivacaine prolongs caudal analgesia in children. Br J Anaesth. 2009;103:268–74.
145. Breschan C, Krumpholz R, Likar R, Kraschl R, Schalk HV. Can a dose of 2micro.kg(−1) caudal clonidine cause respiratory depression in neonates? Pediatr Anesth. 1999;9:81–3.
146. van Niekerk J, Bax-Vermeire BM, Geurts JW, Kramer PP. Epidurography in premature infants. Anaesthesia. 1990;45:722–5.

147. Rasch DK, Webster DE, Pollard TG, Gurkowski MA. Lumbar and thoracic epidural analgesia via the caudal approach for postoperative pain relief in infants and children. Can J Anaesth. 1990;37:359–62.
148. Bhandal N, Rogers R, Berg S, Mason DG. Paediatric caudal extradural catheterisation: an evaluation of a purpose designed equipment set. Anaesthesia. 2006;61(3):277–81.
149. Valairucha S, Seefelder C, Houck CS. Thoracic epidural catheters placed by the caudal route in infants: the importance of radiographic confirmation. Paediatr Anaesth. 2002;12:424–8.
150. Schwartz D, King A. Caudally threaded thoracic epidural catheter as the sole anesthetic in a premature infant and ultrasound confirmation of the catheter tip. Paediatr Anaesth. 2009;19:808–10.
151. Gunter JB. Thoracic epidural anesthesia via the modified Taylor approach in infants. Reg Anesth Pain Med. 2000;25:561–5.
152. Kost-Byerly S, Jackson EV, Yaster M, Kozlowski LJ, Mathews RI, Gearhart JP. Perioperative anesthetic and analgesic management of newborn bladder exstrophy repair. J Pediatr Urol. 2008;4:280–5.
153. Mancuso TJ, Bacsik J, Overbey E. Positive test dose in a neonate with a caudally placed epidural catheter. Pediatr Anesth. 2000;10:565–6.
154. Tsui BC. Thoracic epidural catheter placement in infants via the caudal approach under electrocardiographic guidance: simplification of the original technique. Anesth Analg. 2004;98:273.
155. Tsui BC, Seal R, Koller J. Thoracic epidural catheter placement via the caudal approach in infants by using electrocardiographic guidance. Anesth Analg. 2002;95:326–30.
156. Fegley AJ, Lerman J, Wissler R. Epidural multiorifice catheters function as single orifice catheters: an in vitro study. Anesth Analg. 2008;107:1079–81.
157. Chawathe MS, Jones RM, Gildersleve CD, Harrison SK, Morris SJ, Eickmann C. Detection of epidural catheters with ultrasound in children. Pediatr Anesth. 2003;13:681–4.
158. Rapp HJ, Folger A, Grau T. Ultrasound-guided epidural catheter insertion in children. Anesth Analg. 2005;101:333–9.
159. Goobie SM, Montgomery CJ, Basu R, McFadzean J, O'Connor GJ, Poskitt K, Tsui B. Confirmation of direct epidural placement using nerve stimulation in pediatric anesthesia. Anesth Analg. 2003;97:984–8.
160. Tsui BC, Wagner A, Cave D, Kearney R. Thoracic and lumbar epidural analgesia via a caudal approach using electrical stimulation guidance in pediatric patients: a review of 289 patients. Anesthesiology. 2004;100:683–9.
161. Taenzer AH, Clark C 5th, Kovarik WD. Experience with 724 epidurograms for epidural catheter placement in pediatric anesthesia. Reg Anesth Pain Med. 2010:35;432–5.
162. Tsui BC. Innovative approaches to neuraxial blockade in children: the introduction of epidural nerve root stimulation and ultrasound guidance for epidural catheter placement. Pain Res Manag. 2006;11:173–80.
163. Tsui BC, Pain Res Manag 2006 above. Roberts SA, Galvez I. Ultrasound assessment of caudal catheter position in infants. Pediatr Anesth. 2005:15;429–32.
164. Kost-Byerly S, Tobin JR, Greenberg RS, Billett C, Zahurak M, Yaster M. Bacterial colonization and infection rate of continuous epidural catheters in children. Anesth Analg. 1998;86:712–6.
165. Bubeck J, Boos K, Krause H, Thies KC. Subcutaneous tunneling of caudal catheters reduces the rate of bacterial colonization to that of lumbar epidural catheters. Anesth Analg. 2004;99: 689–93.
166. Kinirons B, Mimoz O, Lafendi L, Naas T, Meunier J, Nordmann P. Chlorhexidine versus povidone iodine in preventing colonization of continuous epidural catheters in children: a randomized, controlled trial. Anesthesiology. 2001;94:239–44.
167. Schrock CR, Jones MB. The dose of caudal epidural analgesia and duration of postoperative analgesia. Paediatr Anesth. 2003;13:403–8.
168. Hong JY, Han SW, Kim WO, et al. A comparison of high volume low concentration ropivacaine in caudal analgesia for pediatric orchidopexy. Anesth Analg. 2009;109:1073.
169. Nishiyama T, Hanaoka K, Ochiai Y. The median approach to transsacral epidural block. Anesth Analg. 2002;95:1067–70.
170. Ballantyne JC, Carr DB, de Ferranti S. The comparative effects of postoperative analgesic therapies on pulmonary outcome: cumulative meta-analyses of randomized, controlled trials. Anesth Analg. 1998;86:598–612.
171. Ecoffey C, Lacroix F, Giaufre E, Orliaguet G, et al. Epidemiology and morbidity of regional anesthesia in children: a follow-up one-year prospective survey of the French-language society of pediatric anesthesiologists (ADARPEF). Pediatr Anesth. 2010;20:1061–89.
172. Ecoffey C, Dubousset AM, Samii K. Lumbar and thoracic epidural anaesthesia in infants and children. Anesthesiology. 1986;65:87–90.
173. Dalens BJ, editor. Pediatric regional anaesthesia. CRC: Florida; 1990. p. 375–415.
174. Ames WA, Hayes JA, Petroz GC, Roy WL. Loss of resistance to normal saline is preferred to identify the epidural space: a survey of Canadian pediatric anesthesiologists. Can J Anaesth. 2005;52:607–12.
175. Webster AC, McKishnie JD, Watson JT, Reid WD. Lumbar epidural anaesthesia for inguinal hernis in low birth weight infants. Can J Anaesth. 1993;40:670–5.
176. Kasai T, Yaegashi K, Hirose M, Tanaka Y. Spinal cord injury in a child caused by an accidental dural puncture with a single-shot thoracic epidural needle. Anesth Analg. 2003;96:65–7.
177. Aarons L, Sadler B, Pitsiu M, et al. Population pharmacokinetics analysis of ropivacaine and its metabolite 2',6'-pipecoloxylidide from pooled data in neonates, infants, and children. Br J Anaesth. 2011;107:409–24.
178. Ingelmo P, Locatelli BG, Frawley G, Knottenbelt G, Favarato M, Spotti A, Fumagalli R. The optimum initial pediatric epidural bolus: a comparison of four local anesthetic solutions. Pediatr Anesth. 2007;17:1166–75.
179. Busoni P. Single shot thoracic epidural block. In: Saint-Maurice C, Schulte-Steinberg O, editors. Regional anaesthesia in children. Switzerland: Mediglobe SA; 1990. p. 110–2.
180. Busoni P, Sarti A. Sacral intervertebral epidural block. Anesthesiology. 1987;67:993–5.
181. Busoni P, Messeri A, Sarti A. The lumbosacral epidural block: a modified Taylor approach for abdominal urologic surgery in children. Anaesth Intensive Care. 1991;19:325–8.
182. Cooper MG, Sethna NF. Epidural analgesia in patients with congenital lumbosacral spinal anomalies. Anesthesiology. 1991;75:370–4.
183. Bailey PD, Rose JB, Keswani SG, Adzick NS, Galinkin JL. Does the use of fentanyl in epidural solutions for postthoracotomy pain management in neonates affect surgical outcome? J Pediatr Surg. 2005;40:1118–21.
184. Ivani G, Mossetti V. Regional anesthesia for postoperative pain control in children: focus on continuous central and perineural infusions. Paediatr Drugs. 2008;10:107–14.
185. Dobereiner EF, Cox RG, Ewen A, Lardner DR. Evidence-based clinical update: which local anesthetic drug for pediatric caudal block provides optimal efficacy with the fewest side effects? Can J Anaesth. 2010;57:1102–10.
186. Berde CB. Convulsions associated with pediatric regional anaesthesia. Anesth Analg. 1992;75:164–6.
187. Desparmet J, Meistelman Barre J, Saint MC. Continuous epidural infusion of bupivacaine for postoperative pain relief in children. Anesthesiology. 1987;67:108.

188. Meignier M, Souron R, Le Neel JC. Postoperative dorsal analgesia in the child with respiratory disabilities. Anesthesiology. 1983;59:473–5.
189. Lonnqvist PA, Ivani G, Moriarty T. Use of caudal-epidural opioids in children: still state of the art or the beginning of the end? Pediatr Anesth. 2002;12:747–9.
190. Lonnqvist PA. Adjuncts to caudal block in children–Quo vadis? Br J Anaesth. 2005;95:431–3.
191. Willschke H, Marhofer P, Bosenberg A, Johnston S, et al. Epidural catheter placement in children: comparing a novel approach using ultrasound with the standard loss of resistance technique. Br J Anaesth. 2006;97:200–7.
192. Lowe LH, Johanek AJ, Moore CW. Sonography of the neonatal spine. Part 1 Normal anatomy, imaging pitfalls and variations that may simulate disorders. AJR. 2007;188:733–38.
193. Marhofer P, Bosenberg A, Sitzwohl C, et al. Pilot study of neuraxial imaging by ultrasound in infants and children. Pediatr Anesth. 2005;15:671–6.
194. Bosenberg AT, Kimble FW. Infraorbital nerve block in neonates for cleft lip repair. Anatomical study and clinical application. Br J Anaesth. 1995;74:506–8.
195. Schenk J-P, Herweh C, Gunther P, et al. Imaging of congenital anomalies and variations of the caudal spine and back of neonates and small infants. Eur J Radiol. 2006;58:3–14.
196. Sethuraman M, Neema PK, Rathod RC. Combined monitored anesthesia care and femoral nerve block for muscle biopsy in children with myopathies. Paediatr Anaesth. 2008;18:691.
197. Oberndorfer U, Marhofer P, Bösenberg A, Willschke H, Felfernig M, Weintraud M, Kapral S, Kettner SC. Ultrasonographic guidance for sciatic and femoral nerve blocks in children. Br J Anaesth. 2007;98:797–801.
198. Hack WW, Vos A, Okken A. Incidence of forearm and hand ischaemia related to radial artery cannulation in newborn infants. Intensive Care Med. 1990;16:50–3.
199. Bösenberg AT. Lower limb nerve blocks in children using unsheathed needles and a nerve stimulator. Anaesthesia. 1995; 50:206–10.
200. Willschke H, Bosenberg A, Marhofer P, Johnston S, Kettner S, Eichenberger U, Wanzel O, Kapral S. Ultrasonographic-guided ilioinguinal/iliohypogastric nerve block in pediatric anesthesia: what is the optimal volume. Anesth Analg. 2006;102: 1680–4.
201. Messeri A, Calamandrei M, Agostino MR, Busoni P. The use of brachial plexus block for venous catheterization in low and very low birthweight infants. Anesthesiology. 1998;88:837.
202. Breschan C, Kraschl R, Jost R, Marhofer P, Likar R. Axillary brachial plexus block for treatment of severe forearm ischemia after arterial cannulation in an extremely low birth-weight infant. Paediatr Anaesth. 2004;14:681–4.
203. Lagade MR, Poppers PJ. Stellate ganglion block: a therapeutic modality for arterial insufficiency of the arm in premature infants. Anesthesiology. 1984;61(2):203–4.
204. Elias M. Continuous cervico-thoracic sympathetic ganglion block: therapeutic modality for arterial insufficiency of the arm of a neonate. Middle East J Anesthesiol. 2001;16:359–63.
205. Simion C, Corcoran J, Iyer A, Suresh S. Postoperative pain control for primary cleft lip repair in infants: is there an advantage in performing peripheral nerve blocks? Paediatr Anaesth. 2008; 18:1060–5.
206. Mayer MN, Bennaceur S, Barrier G, Couly G. Infra-orbital nerve block in early primary cheiloplasty. Rev Stomatol Chir Maxillofac. 1997;98:246–7.
207. Shandling B, Steward D. Regional analgesia for postoperative pain in pediatric outpatient surgery. J Pediatr Surg. 1980;15: 477–80.
208. Smith T, Moratin P, Wulf H. Smaller children have greater bupivacaine plasma concentrations after ilioinguinal block. Br J Anaesth. 1996;76:452–5.
209. van Schoor AN, Bosmann MC, Bosenberg AT. Revisiting the anatomy of the ilioinguinal/iliohypogastric nerve block. Pediatr Anesth. 2013;23:390–4.
210. Weintraud M, Marhofer P, Bösenberg A, Kapral S, Willschke H, Felfernig M, Kettner SC. Ilioinguinal/iliohypogastric blocks in children: where do we administer the local anesthetic without direct visualisation? Anesth Analg. 2008;106:89–93.
211. Derrick J, Aun C. Transient femoral nerve palsy after ilioinguinal nerve block. Anaesth Intensive Care. 1996;24:115.
212. Rosario DJ, Skinner PP, Rafferty AT. Transient femoral nerve palsy complicating preoperative ilioinguinal nerve block for inguinal herniorrhaphy. Br J Surg. 1994;81:897.
213. Johr M, Sossai R. Colonic perforation puncture during ilioinguinal nerve block in a child. Anesth Analg. 1999;88:1051–2.
214. Jacobs A, Thies KC. Ultrasound-guided transversus abdominis plane block for reversal of ileostomy in a 2-kg premature neonate. Paediatr Anaesth. 2009;19:1237–8.
215. Bielsky A, Efrat R, Suresh S. Postoperative analgesia in neonates after major abdominal surgery: 'TAP' our way to success! Paediatr Anaesth. 2009;19:541–2.
216. Fredrickson MJ, Seal P. Ultrasound-guided transversus abdominis plane block for neonatal abdominal surgery. Anaesth Intensive Care. 2009;37:469–72.
217. Hardy CA. Transverse abdominis plane block in neonates: is it a good alternative to caudal anesthesia for postoperative analgesia following abdominal surgery? Paediatr Anaesth. 2009;19:56.
218. Mai CL, Young MJ, Quraishi SA. Clinical implications of the transversus abdominis plane block in pediatric anesthesia. Pediatr Anesth. 2012;22:831–40.
219. Jacobs A, Bergmans E, Arul GS, This KC. The transversus abdominis plane (TAP) block in neonates and infants – results of an audit. Pediatr Anesth. 2011;21:1078–80.
220. Brickler SRW, Telford RJ, Booker PD. Pharmacokinetics of bupivacaine following intraoperative intercostal nerve block in neonates and in infants aged less than 6 months. Anesthesiology. 1989;70:942–7.
221. Lehr VT, Taddio A. Topical anesthesia in neonates: clinical practices and practical considerations. Semin Perinatol. 2007;31: 323–9.
222. Karmakar MK, Booker PD, Franks R, Pozzi M. Continuous extrapleural paravertebral infusion of bupivacaine for post-thoracotomy analgesia in young infants. Br J Anaesth. 1996;76:811–5.
223. Cheung SL, Booker PD, Franks R, Pozzi M. Serum concentrations of bupivacaine during prolonged continuous paravertebral infusion in young infants. Br J Anaesth. 1997;79(1):9–13.
224. Gunter JB. Benefits and risks of local anesthetics in infants and children. Paediatr Drugs 2002:4;649–72.
225. Berde CB. Toxicity of local anesthetics in infants and children. J.Pediatr. 1993;122: Pt 2:S14–20.
226. Lin EP, Aronson LA. Successful resuscitation of bupivacaine-induced cardiotoxicity in a neonate. Paediatr Anaesth. 2010;20: 955–7.
227. Shah S, Gopalakrishnan S, Apuya J, Shah S, Martin T. Use of Intralipid in an infant with impending cardiovascular collapse due to local anesthetic toxicity. J Anesth. 2009;23:439–41.
228. Neal JM, Bernards CM, Butterworth 4th JF, Di Gregorio G, Drasner K, Hejtmanek MR, Mulroy MF, Rosenquist RW, Weinberg GL. ASRA practice advisory on local anesthetic systemic toxicity. Reg Anesth Pain Med. 2010;35:152–6.
229. Picard J, Meek T. Lipid emulsion to treat overdose of local anaesthetic: the gift of the glob. Anaesthesia. 2006;61:107–9.

230. Weinberg GL. Lipid not propofol treats bupivacaine overdose. Reg Anesth Pain Med. 2006;31:296–303.
231. Polaner DM, Drescher J. Pediatric regional anesthesia: what is the current safety record. Paediatr Anaesth. 2011;21: 737–42.
232. Yamada J, Stinson J, Lamba J, Dickson A, McGrath PJ, Stevens B. A review of systematic reviews on pain interventions in hospitalized infants. Pain Res Manag. 2008;13:413–20.
233. Frawley G, Ragg P, Hack H. Plasma concentrations of bupivacaine after combined spinal epidural anaesthesia in infants and neonates. Paediatr Anaesth 2000;10:619–25.

Anesthetic Complications in the Neonate

16

Pete G. Kovatsis and Monica Kleinman

Introduction

The neonate is at risk for increased perianesthetic complications attributed, in part, to such factors as the transitional circulation and the immaturity of many organ systems and metabolic processes. In the preterm neonate, incomplete maturation of all organ systems, in particular the pulmonary and cardiovascular systems, further magnifies the risks in the perioperative period. Neonatal surgical or interventional procedures, such as repair or palliation of major congenital anomalies or management of life-threatening complications of prematurity, are rarely elective. Excellent communication and collaboration among the neonatal, anesthesia, and surgical teams are essential to optimize the outcome. Despite best intentions, preparation, and experience, perianesthetic adverse events confront all practitioners. The discussion of complications and risks for all procedures and therapeutic options is beyond the scope of this chapter; therefore, the focus here is to provide an overview of the adverse events to which neonates are particularly vulnerable and of the potential risks from anesthetic agents.

Perianesthetic Mortality and Adverse Events

The first reviews of perioperative morbidity and mortality in infants and children, which date back to the 1950s, reported the incidence of adverse events in infants and children to be greater than it was in adults [1, 2]. In 1961, the difference in the incidence of perioperative cardiac arrest between adults and children was attributed primarily to the greater incidence of cardiac arrest in infants [3]. In 1959, investigators concluded that greater than one-third of the deaths in children under 10 years of age occurred in neonates during the first week of life [4]. In 1964, the Baltimore Anesthesia Study Committee estimated an anesthesia-related mortality rate of 3.3 per 10,000 children under 15 years old, with the neonate accounting for a staggering 20.4 % of these deaths [5].

A recent study demonstrated that death within the first 24 h after anesthesia is uncommon in pediatric patients. In a review of >100,000 anesthetics over a 5½-year period from the Royal Children's Hospital in Melbourne, the 24-h mortality from any cause was 13.4/10,000 anesthetics, with a significantly greater (15-fold) rate in neonates (180.1/10,000) [6]. Analysis of all deaths suggested that the death rate attributable to anesthesia-related factors was small, ~1/10,000, with only one neonatal death in this category.

Studies continue to show that adverse events occur more commonly in infants than in older children [3, 7–24]. Most publications included neonates in infants category while relying on self-reporting of incidents and do not specifically detail adverse events in the neonate. Underreporting is a common problem with self-reported events, which underestimates the true incidence of perianesthetic adverse events compared with what has been published [25–28]. Some epidemiologic studies relied on reporting critical incidents to a national database or reviewed closed claims. However, because these reports do not include a denominator, the frequency of critical events cannot be determined. Additionally, adverse event studies can suffer from nonuniform definitions of clinical complications, difficulty in achieving statistical power, inability to control for or identify confounding variables, and regional differences in clinical practice. These factors limit the value of the individual studies themselves and prohibit direct comparisons of studies. As Derrington and Smith stated: "In addition, there is probably an unknown and unquantifiable number of errors which may or may not be involved in a chain of events resulting

P.G. Kovatsis, MD (✉)
Department is Anesthesia, Perioperative and Pain Medicine.
The Division is Critical Care, Boston Children's Hospital, Harvard Medical School, 300 Longwood Avenue, Boston, MA 02115, USA
e-mail: pete.kovatsis@childrens.harvard.edu

M. Kleinman, MD
Department is Anesthesia, Perioperative and Pain Medicine,
The Division is Critical Care, Boston Children's Hospital,
300 Longwood Avenue, Boston, MA 02115, USA

J. Lerman (ed.), *Neonatal Anesthesia*, DOI 10.1007/978-1-4419-6041-2_16,

in morbidity or mortality, but which go unnoticed and therefore unreported" [29].

In the first published prospective survey of pediatric anesthesia-related morbidity and mortality, 27 major complications were defined as fatal, life threatening, or resulting in severe sequelae through the first 24 h after an anesthetic from a sample of 40,240 anesthetics in children younger than 15 years drawn from 440 randomly chosen institutions in France between 1978 and 1982 [23]. The observed incidence of morbidity was 7 per 10,000 anesthetics with a mortality rate of 1 in 40,000. The risks were greater in infants (43 per 10,000 if <1 year old) than in children (5 per 10,000). Neonates were not distinguished as a group distinct from the infant group. Respiratory failure was the most common cause of major complications in the infants, whereas respiratory failure and cardiac failure were equally responsible for major complications in children. Greater ASA physical status, coexisting diseases, previous anesthesia, and emergency surgery were all associated with an increased risk of complications.

In a retrospective review of anesthetic morbidity and mortality data from a single pediatric hospital in Canada [9], adverse events were collected for up to 3 days postoperatively in children less than 16 years old between 1982 and 1987. These events were those that required an intervention intraoperatively by the anesthesiologists, selected events in the recovery room reported by the recovery room nurse, and any additional occurrences noted on chart review within 72 h of the procedure (without distinguishing if the events were related to the surgical procedure or the anesthetic). Of the 29,220 anesthetics that were reviewed in this series, only 361 anesthetics involved neonates. Rare events that occur in such a small number of cases may skew the results and the interpretation. The incidence of adverse events was greatest in neonates (1,468 intraoperative, 1,662 early postoperative, and 3,815 postoperative per 10,000) including mortality (83 intraoperative and 148 postoperative per 10,000). Neonates with complications were more likely to be physical status III or greater and scheduled for more major surgical procedures. In neonates, respiratory complications accounted for the vast majority of intraoperative events (54 %), whereas blood pressure derangements (44 %) and respiratory events (38 %) accounted for the majority of the postoperative period. Some events occurred more than once and/or multiple events were observed in the same patient. No information was provided to indicate whether the same neonates who had intraoperative respiratory or cardiovascular events maintained instability into the postoperative period or what fraction of postoperative events occurred in different neonates. The researchers identified increased risks of hypothermia and cardiovascular instability during transport from the NICU to the operating rooms in neonates weighing <1 kg and modified their practice to perform selected procedures in the NICU.

Despite differences in study design, data sets, and analysis, additional studies [8, 11, 13–17, 19, 22, 24] paralleled the general findings of these early studies, concluding that the risks are greater in infants and more specifically in neonates; respiratory and airway the leading category of adverse events; and other factors such as ASA physical status III–V, emergency surgery, and comorbidities increasing the risk in the perioperative period. When adverse events between operating room and nonoperating room venues were compared, the incidence of events in neonates and infants was greater irrespective of the location, and once again, respiratory events were most common [12].

Cardiac arrest during anesthesia is a rare but sentinel event with a reported incidence of 1.4 to 4.6 per 10,000 anesthetics and a mortality rate ranging from 7.5 to 28 % [7, 18, 30, 31]. The Pediatric Perioperative Cardiac Arrest (POCA) registry, a voluntary reporting system of intraoperative cardiac arrests, reported the number of cardiac arrests in children with and without heart disease (congenital or acquired) [31]. Children with cardiac disease were more likely to experience an arrest from a cardiac cause (50 % vs. 38 %). Of note, cardiac arrest in those with heart disease was more likely to occur in the general operating room (54 %) than in the cardiac OR (26 %) or catheterization laboratory (17 %). There were no data specific to neonates, although a significant number of events did occur in infants <6 months of age (47 % and 39 % of the those with and without cardiac disease, respectively). In another study of infants with congenital heart disease who suffered perioperative cardiac arrest during cardiac surgery, the risk of anesthesia-related cardiac arrest was greater than reported in the general pediatric population [30]. Among the congenital heart disease patients, neonates had a greater incidence of anesthesia-related cardiac arrest than older children.

Postoperative cardiac arrest is a significant risk factor for mortality among many subgroups including neonates. When cardiac arrest occurs after complex cardiac surgery, mortality is almost twofold greater in LBW infants (defined as <2.5 kg) than it is in the total population of neonates (6.8 vs. 12.1 %) [32]. There is scant literature on the rate of postoperative cardiac arrest in the neonatal intensive care unit. In a large series of pediatric intensive care unit patients who suffered cardiac arrest, survival to discharge for neonates was 27 % [33].

Respiratory and Airway Complications

That respiratory complications and loss of the airway are the most common adverse events in neonates and infants after anesthesia is not surprising [34]. Studies have consistently demonstrated that airway and respiratory events are among the most common complications during pediatric anesthesia, with laryngospasm and/or "airway obstruction" occurring most frequently [11, 12, 19, 22, 24, 31]. Laryngospasm is the leading cause of cardiac arrest in the respiratory subgroup from the POCA registry [7, 18]. A study of the incidence of laryngospasm in all ages reported that infants 1–3 months of age carried the greatest risk [20].

In neonates and young infants, the combination of pronounced airway protective reflexes, smaller airway caliber, and a more cartilaginous chest wall results in an increased risk of obstruction during inspiration. Even during "normal breathing," the compliant chest wall of neonates and infants leads to lower transpulmonary pressures and lung volumes that contribute to an increased tendency for airway collapse. Because of this propensity for obstruction at static functional residual capacity (FRC), infants (and neonates in particular) need to maintain a dynamic FRC. Early diaphragmatic contraction and laryngeal "braking" (vocal cord adduction) during expiration generate dynamic FRC by supporting a greater lung volume during the respiratory cycle. Sedatives and anesthetics impair or ablate the neonate's capacity to sustain these respiratory adaptations. During the delivery of anesthesia, the provider can compensate by using continuous positive airway pressure (CPAP), assisted ventilation, or controlled ventilation with positive end-expiratory pressure (PEEP) to avoid respiratory compromise. These developmental mechanical properties, coupled with high oxygen consumption and high oxygen affinity of fetal hemoglobin in the neonate, increase the risk of perioperative hypoxemia and hypercapnia and postoperative respiratory events [9].

Respiratory control in the neonate is characterized by blunted responses to CO_2 and hypoxia. The response to an increase in CO_2, which is mediated through central chemoreceptors, is blunted in neonates, at both early postconceptional and postnatal ages. The hypoxic response is biphasic with the initial response being hyperventilation followed by hypoventilation, bradycardia, and apnea if the hypoxia is not remedied quickly. Residual trace concentrations of inhalational anesthetics may abolish the initial hyperventilatory response to hypoxia in the neonate. These responses are all exaggerated in preterm infants, and in particular the risk of perioperative apnea is increased when anemia, hypothermia, metabolic derangements, sepsis, lung disease, and residual anesthetics are also present. In fact, all of these responses are further blunted in the perioperative period, increasing the risk of respiratory complications in the form of apnea and hypoxemia.

Many neonates exhibit periodic breathing, relative tachypnea with interspersed periods of apnea not associated with bradycardia and/or significant hypoxemia [35, 36]. Significant or pathologic apnea is defined by the cessation of breathing in excess of 15 s or for any duration when the apnea is accompanied by bradycardia, cyanosis, or pallor. This is particularly common in preterm neonates [36, 37]. Postoperative apnea in the preterm neonate and infant may also exhibit an obstructive component since anesthetic agents blunt the respiratory drive and depress upper airway muscle tone as well as the respiratory coordination needed to maintain the upper airway [38]. Neonates are also more prone to upper airway obstruction related to head and neck position, which is more likely to occur with residual sedatives or analgesics.

In 1982, a retrospective analysis of the risk of perioperative apnea after hernia surgery in preterm and full-term neonates and infants reported a 20 % incidence of perioperative apnea in preterm neonates compared with a zero incidence in full-term neonates [39]. This prompted at least four prospective trials that culminated in a combined analysis in 1995 that determined that "apnea was strongly and inversely related to both gestational age and postconceptual age" with associated risk factors of ongoing preoperative apnea and anemia [40]. The authors concluded that the incidence of apnea decreases to less than 1 % beyond a postconceptional age of 54–56 weeks, but the validity of their conclusion has been questioned [41]. It is well established that neonates, premature neonates, and ex-premature infants require postoperative monitoring for apnea and bradycardia. In those free of significant comorbidites such as continued pathologic apnea and major organ disease (e.g., intraventricular hemorrhage), a conservative upper limit for admission of 60 weeks postconceptional age with a minimum of 12 h observation during which the child has no apnea has been widely adopted.

Regional anesthesia (spinal, caudal, or spinal and caudal without additives to the local anesthetic other than epinephrine) in ex-premature infants is an alternative technique that should not increase the incidence of perioperative apnea. However, if any sedation is administered, the incidence of perioperative apnea will be similar to that after a general anesthetic [42–45]. In a direct comparison of spinal and general anesthesia, spinal anesthesia did not reduce the risk of central apnea in premature infants, although there was less desaturation and bradycardia in the perioperative period [46]. Spinal anesthesia requiring supplemental sedatives, or a partially failed spinal requiring general anesthesia, may be associated with a high risk of postoperative apnea [47, 48]. These authors also postulated that infants with a postconceptional age of approximately 41 weeks or less have an increased risk of delayed postoperative apnea, particularly when comorbidities are present. The least-soluble potent inhalation agent, desflurane, facilitates a rapid emergence from anesthesia and may decrease the risk of postoperative apnea when combined with a regional technique [49–51], although there is insufficient evidence to support such a claim at this time [52]. However, given the failure rate and the relative stress of awake regional techniques, the authors propose that a prospective study comparing sevoflurane/desflurane with a regional technique to an awake regional technique is warranted.

In a prospective study of general (GA) versus combined spinal-epidural anesthesia (CSEA) in 50 term or mildly premature infants at a mean age of approximately 6 weeks and postconceptional age of 48.5 (GA) and 46.1 (CSEA) for gastrointestinal surgery, the incidence of adverse cardiorespiratory events in the first eight postoperative days in the GA group was significantly greater than in the group receiving CSEA [53]. Of note, the infants who received GA were treated with a fentanyl infusion for postoperative analgesia, whereas the CSEA group received a continuous infusion of bupivacaine via the thoracic epidural catheter. The postoperative analgesic regimen may have contributed to the increased incidence of adverse cardiorespiratory events in the general anesthesia group.

Methylxanthines such as caffeine reduce but do not eliminate the risk of postoperative apnea in preterm infants. They may be administered when neonates present to the operating room with continued apnea or have apnea postoperatively [54, 55]. Methylxanthines also reduce the extubation failure rate in preterm infants in the NICU but not specifically in the postanesthetic period [56]. Recent evidence suggests that polymorphisms in the adenosine1 receptor gene may explain interindividual variability in response to caffeine: infants >28 weeks gestation who responded to caffeine carried the rs16851030 C/C A1 genotype [57]. Further studies are warranted to explore the role of adenosine polymorphisms in a larger population of premature infants.

That the incidence of apnea of prematurity is inversely related to hematocrit has generated much interest. Although a number of studies have explored this relationship, what remains unclear is whether the oxygen-carrying capacity or the blood volume is the trigger for the apnea. In a computer-monitored setting of 67 spontaneously breathing, very low birth weight infants who received blood transfusions, the transfusions decreased the incidence of apnea of prematurity [58]. Furthermore, the risk of an apnea during the subsequent 12 h was also reduced suggesting that the mechanism by which blood transfusions reduce the risk of apnea is by increasing the oxygen-carrying capacity of the blood rather than by expanding the blood volume.

Neonates can develop stridor after tracheal extubation, although the incidence is not well documented. Systematic reviews, including neonatal studies, have consistently shown that neither IV steroids nor nebulized racemic epinephrine prevents post-extubation stridor [59–62].

Acquired subglottic stenosis is a known complication of prolonged tracheal intubation in the neonate. The incidence of subglottic stenosis after tracheal intubation in the neonatal period ranges from 1 to 8 % [63–65], but it has decreased over time [66, 67]. Prolonged duration of intubation and reduced birth weight are associated with a greater risk for subglottic stenosis [63, 68]. In a large series of pediatric patients undergoing cardiac surgery, the incidence of subglottic stenosis was 2.3 % in infants less than 1 year of age [69]. A duration of intubation of greater than 96 h was an associated risk factor for sublgottic stenosis, although there was no difference in the incidence between those whose airways were intubated with cuffed versus uncuffed endotracheal tubes.

Oral or airway stimulation may lead to mild or severe bradycardia and even potentially asystole and apnea. These cardiorespiratory reflexes are mediated by the vagus nerve. Pretreating neonates, the age group at greatest risk for bradycardia, with an anticholinergic before induction of anesthesia or intubation prevents or minimizes this reflex. Clinical reports support the impression that intraoperative bradycardia in infants has decreased from pre-2000 (127 per 10,000 anesthetics [13]) to post-2000 (33 per 10,000 anesthetics [18]). The transition from halothane to sevoflurane may account in part for this observation, but determining causality is difficult based on the available data.

Aspiration of gastric contents in the perianesthetic period is another rare, but potentially fatal complication that may occur. The reported incidence of aspiration in infants ranges from 3.6 to 10.2 per 10,000 [8, 19, 23, 70, 71]. One study reported that the incidence of pulmonary aspiration during emergency procedures exceeded that during nonemergent ones, with the majority occurring at induction of anesthesia [71]. In contrast, an analysis of over 50,000 anesthetics demonstrated that although the risk of aspiration was marginally increased under emergency conditions, it best correlated with ASA physical status [70]. Both of these studies found no instances of aspiration in neonates. In neither study did any of the patients who aspirated have serious morbidity, although a few did require prolonged postaspiration ventilator support. While severe morbidity and mortality is unlikely after aspiration, closed claims analysis and national databases revealed that aspiration is one of the causes of these serious untoward complications [11, 17, 72].

Location of Operative Procedures

Transporting neonates, particularly critically ill neonates, between hospital locations has many potential dangers (See Chap. 13, Anesthesia outside the operating room). During transport beyond the relatively safe environment of the neonatal ICU or operating room, the critically ill neonate is vulnerable to a variety of mishaps, including equipment failure, disconnections from drug infusions and equipment, temperature instability, and even provider distraction. Sophisticated neonatal ICU ventilators are often unavailable, leaving the critically ill patient with less than ideal ventilation techniques during transport. Vieira et al. reported the incidence of complications after 1,197 intrahospital neonatal transports, of which 22.6 % involved transfer for surgical procedures [73].

Complications occurred in 27 % of transports, with an odds ratio of 4.0 for patients traveling to the operating room.

While the traditional location for providing anesthesia and performing major surgical procedures has been the operating room, over the past two decades, the practice of bringing resources to the patient has gained favor to mitigate risk, especially for preterm infants. In many institutions surgical procedures are either routinely performed in the NICU or the option to perform on-site exists if the risk of transporting the patient outside of the NICU is determined to be excessive. A 1993 report described the characteristics and outcomes of 193 neonates who underwent surgery either in the NICU or in the OR [74]. Not unexpectedly, infants whose surgery was performed in the NICU had a higher acuity of illness as evidenced by preoperative requirement for mechanical ventilation. Likewise, surgical procedures performed in the NICU as opposed to the OR involved patients with reduced birth weights and gestational age. Overall mortality was greater in the NICU surgery group (14 vs. 2 %). No differences were observed in the rate of postsurgical sepsis. Of note, neonates were more likely to become *hyper*thermic ($T>37.5$) in the OR than in the NICU setting. In two reviews comprising >80 neonates who underwent a range of surgeries in the NICU, there were no anesthesia-related deaths [74, 75].

Major surgeries have also been performed in the NICU including ligation of the ductus arteriosus. In >120 neonates who underwent ligation of the patent ductus in the NICU, one center reported a surgical complication rate of 17 % [76], although overall, there were no deaths [77]. In another series of 42 neonates with congenital diaphragmatic hernia who required HFOV, surgical repair performed in the NICU rather than the OR resulted in more infectious complications in the NICU surgical group but no difference in mortality [78]. In a retrospective analysis of 233 neonates who required laparotomy for necrotizing enterocolitis, the mortality in infants <1,500 g who were operated on in the NICU because they were judged to have significant risk of transport to the OR was no different from those who were operated on in the OR [79]. The reason for this apparent lack of difference in mortality may be due to either the reduced mortality in the more critically-ill neonates who had surgery in the NICU or the increased mortality in less critically-ill neonates who were transferred to the OR for surgery. Other procedures that have been performed in the NICU include cryotherapy for retinopathy of prematurity [80], cannulation for extracorporeal membrane oxygenation (ECMO), balloon atrial septostomy [81], and less commonly, ventriculosubgaleal shunts for posthemorrhagic hydrocephalus [82].

Before traveling between the ICU and a procedural area, providers should ascertain that the appropriate equipment and supplies are present and functional, including an adequate supply of supplemental oxygen. The transport team should review their roles and plans for potential adverse events. Physiologic monitoring should be maintained at a level similar to that in the ICU/OR environment to facilitate early detection of any changes in vital signs. The use of a transport incubator supports thermoregulation but may impair the team's ability to visualize the infant and to access tubes and lines. Given these risks, in the case of extremely ill neonates, the providers involved should discuss whether and where (i.e., NICU vs. operating room) surgical procedures can be accomplished most safely.

Specific Complications

Transfusions

Transfusions are frequently required for critically ill neonates undergoing anesthesia for surgical conditions. In a large series of VLBW neonates, mortality increased in those who received more than one transfusion [83]. These infants are particularly vulnerable to transfusion-related complications including hyperkalemia, citrate-induced electrolyte alterations (ionized hypocalcemia and hypomagnesemia), and hypothermia.

Hyperkalemia has been a leading cause of cardiac arrest under cardiovascular causes in the latest publication from the POCA registry [7]. Hyperkalemia accumulates in the acellular fraction of packed red blood cell units (CPD and CPDA-1) as it leaks from red blood cells that have been stored for a prolonged period, increasing linearly with the number of days of storage. Hyperkalemia may also be present in plasma if the blood was stored as whole blood for a prolonged period and then separated into components immediately before administration. The leak of potassium from red blood cells is accelerated by storing the blood in cool temperatures and by irradiation. The risk of hyperkalemia in the neonate is directly related to the speed of the transfusion of the red blood cells, especially if the rate exceeds 1 ml/kg/min [84]. With the volume of the right atrium approximately 5–10 ml, the rapid administration of cold hyperkalemic red blood cells through a central line directly into the right atrium may cause the atrium to become irritable and trigger atrial and then ventricular arrhythmias or cardiac arrest [85]. Risk factors for hyperkalemia in the neonate include the transfusion of old, cold blood, rapid and/or massive transfusion, hypocalcemia, irradiation, renal dysfunction, and transfusion through central venous access [85–87]. The use of fresh units of blood and blood that has been stored for the least time since irradiation minimizes the concentration of potassium that may accumulate in the unit of blood. Washing and warming the blood can minimize transfusion-induced hyperkalemia and the associated risk of cardiac arrhythmias, particularly if the blood had been stored for a prolonged period. However, the greater the interval between washing and administering the RBCs, the more potassium will leak out of cells. Other strategies include the use of peripheral access for the transfusion, avoiding old whole blood and maintaining ionized calcium concentrations in blood [84–86].

Citrate is used as anticoagulant in most transfused products and binds calcium and magnesium. Frozen plasma, whole blood, and platelets have the greatest quantities of citrate followed by red blood cell units and cryoprecipitate. Washing the units of blood removes the citrated plasma from the red blood cell units. The metabolism of citrate is diminished in neonates, rendering them prone to the prolonged effects of circulating citrate compared with older children and adults [84]. Clinically, the rapid administration of citrate-containing blood products binds ionized calcium and causes bradycardia and hypotension that are magnified in the neonatal myocardium (See Chap. 2, Physiology and Development of the Term and Preterm Neonate). Slow intravenous administration of calcium prevents or reverses these derangements. Exposure to large volumes of citrate through a massive transfusion may also lead to metabolic alkalosis from the accumulation of citrate.

Vascular Access

Reliable vascular access is vital to the management of critically ill neonates, but can also be a significant challenge to secure and maintain. Vascular access is associated with a wide variety of complications and requires constant surveillance to diagnosis and minimizes the potential for harm. Common peripheral access issues include infections, disconnections, phlebitis, and extravasations. Extravasations can lead to significant complications including tissue necrosis and compartment syndrome. Less common complications include nerve damage, thrombosis, and embolism. Arterial lines have the added concerns of ischemic injury, emboli, formation of an arteriovenous fistula, and inadvertent injection of IV drugs [88]. Proper labeling of lines and access ports should minimize the chance of intra-arterial administration of a medication. During the perioperative period, the incidence of thrombophlebitis and adverse events after arterial line cannulation in neonates was 185 and 148 in 10,000, respectively, whereas the incidence in infants, the group closest to neonates for these complications, was 20 and 49 in 10,000 respectively [9].

Central venous access is essential for many critically ill neonates, yet introduces a wide range of potential complications [89, 90]. Large vessel or atrial perforation may occur either during attempts to place the line or after the line is placed due to erosion by the catheter. Emergent and potentially life-threatening conditions associated with central venous catheters include pneumothorax, hemothorax, and cardiac tamponade. These must be considered in any neonate who suddenly develops cardiopulmonary instability. Other reported complications include thrombosis (vessel and/or line), embolism, infection, hydrothorax, chylothorax, and unplanned displacement. In a retrospective review of 587 central venous catheters in neonates and infants, the complication rate was 28 % (dislodgement 11.6 %, perforation 5.3 %, obstruction 5 %, infection 4 %, thrombosis 1 %), with two deaths due to cardiac tamponade [91]. The combination of an underdeveloped coagulation system, small caliber vessels, and underlying critical illness places the neonate at risk for thromboembolic events. A Canadian, multi-institutional registry [92] reported that thrombosis occurred very infrequently in neonates (97 cases over more than 3 years from 64 centers), but when it did occur, it occurred with indwelling catheters (89 %) and/or in the presence of systemic infection (29 %). The registry also concluded that the greatest mortality occurred in neonates with an aortic, right atrial, or SVC thrombosis.

In addition to the common complications associated with chronic indwelling vascular catheters such as infection and thrombosis [93, 94], peripherally inserted central catheters (PICC) introduce a unique complication: rupture and potential embolization of the catheter fragment. In a series of 1650 PICC, 11 fractures (0.67 %) occurred, requiring invasive retrieval of fragments via a percutaneous intravascular approach [95]. Factors that were associated with fracture of the catheter included the duration of placement, line occlusion, and leaking at the insertion site [96]. Only 10 ml or larger syringes are recommended for injections into PICC to avoid application of excessive intraluminal pressure in these catheters.

Oxygen Toxicity

The relationship between oxygen therapy and injury to the premature infant's organs has been well known for decades. Exposure to increased concentrations of oxygen in the first few weeks after birth is associated with an increase in risk of retinopathy of prematurity and bronchopulmonary dysplasia [96–98]. If restricting the inspired concentration of oxygen could reduce these retinal and pulmonary sequelae, then it was equally reasonable to question whether there was any risk associated with reduced inspired concentrations of oxygen in very low birth weight and preterm/full-term neonates? Two randomized trials of high (91–95 %) versus low (85–89 %) oxygen saturations in preterm infants between 24 and 27 weeks' gestation reported an increased mortality in the low oxygen saturation group, albeit with less severe retinopathy of prematurity in survivors [99]. However, contradictory findings in a systematic review and a large international study suggested that oxygen saturations 85–89 % reduced ROP without increasing mortality or lung disease [100–102]. To further complicate these studies, the oximeter software during the COT and BOOST II studies was modified, the proportion of infants who were affected by the modified software differed among these studies, and the oxygen saturation ranges were not equal among the studies [103]. Furthermore, the duration of exposure to reduced oxygen saturations, the particular age at which the reduced oxygen saturations were administered, and the effects of periodic decreases in oxygen saturation below the minimum values assigned have not been analyzed to determine their potential contributions to the adverse outcomes from these large oxygen toxicity studies [103]. The optimal and target oxygen saturation for very low birth weight infants remains contentious. We do not advocate either extremely high or low oxygen saturations but based on the current contradictory evidence, advocate a moderate saturation, ~90 % to limit sequelae, recognizing that action may be needed urgently should the oxygen saturation deteriorate precipitously.

The concern for oxidative stresses on neonates led to changes in delivery room resuscitation guidelines. Two meta-analyses of randomized, controlled trials that compared the initial resuscitation with 100 % oxygen with that with room air showed greater survival with room air [104, 105]. However, the methodologies in these studies have been criticized leading to much weaker evidence of the benefit of reduced oxygen concentrations for resuscitation of the neonate [106]. In the case of the preterm neonate, best practice currently suggests using an $FiO_2 < 30$ % for the initial resuscitation of these neonates and titrating the FiO_2 thereafter to the hemoglobin oxygen saturation [107]. If the infant remains bradycardic after ventilation with room air, then transition to increasing concentrations of oxygen up to 100 % is recommended [108]. While no studies have determined the ideal oxygen concentration for use during neonatal anesthesia, recently published editorials support the avoidance of hyperoxia in neonates to minimize the risks of adverse effects [108–111].

Prevention of Adverse Events

Human Factors

Anesthesia providers are responsible for patient safety in the perianesthetic period, and thus the human dynamic in adverse events plays a significant role. As decidedly stated by Allnutt [111]:

> "...all human beings, without any exception whatsoever, make errors and that such errors are completely normal and necessary part of human cognitive function. For a … doctor to accept that he or she is as likely as anyone else to make an catastrophic error today is the first step towards prevention; whereas to claim exemption on the grounds of being a … senior professor, … or consultant [attending]…, is the first step on the road to disaster."

From a single pediatric institution, a retrospective analysis investigated the human factors in 668 reported anesthetic incidents, representing 2.4 % of total anesthetics provided [15]. The analysis found that human factors accounted for 284 (42.5 %) of the incidents with errors in judgment and failure to check (equipment, tracheal tubes, lines) as the two most common errors.

Although the following principles associated with decreased severe critical incidents (death and coma) were gathered from adult data, implementing these anesthetic management processes should have a similar impact on children: routine use of an equipment protocol and checklist, direct availability of an anesthesiologist for additional help and insight, use of full-time anesthesia team members, the presence of two anesthesia team members at emergence and transfer, and reversal of muscle relaxants at the end of an anesthetic [112]. Besides checklists, other methods to decrease human factors in adverse events include targeted feedback and updating protocols [15]. The 1989 National Confidential Enquiry into Perioperative Deaths emphasized three ideals: [114, 115]

1. Surgeons and anesthesiologists should not undertake occasional pediatric practice.
2. Anesthesiologists who care for children must keep themselves up to date and competent in pediatric anesthesia.
3. Consultant supervision of trainees needs to be kept under scrutiny.

These recommendations promoted the concept of regionalization for pediatric and in particular, neonatal surgical care in the United Kingdom, although implementation has been gradual [115]. The USA does not have any formal system of regionalization despite clustering of pediatric institutions staffed with pediatric subspecialists [116]. A survey from Japan suggested that perioperative neonatal mortality from all causes was greater in institutions that cared for less than 12 neonates per year when compared with those that cared for more [100]. This supports concepts that increased volume of cases, specialty-specific training and experience, and triaging high-risk and rare cases to specialty centers are additional strategies to decrease risk and human error [14, 18, 117–122].

Medication Errors

Another area where human factors play a pivotal role is medication errors. Despite recent advancements in neonatal pharmacokinetics, pharmacodynamics, and clinical outcome measures, significant knowledge gaps still exist [123–126]. Neonatal dosing requires dose calculation and administration of drugs from concentrations and volumes that are generally manufactured for adults. Immature organ development and metabolic processes in the neonate, amplified in the preterm neonate, together with the lack of methods to quickly and reliably measure medication effects, contribute to the complexity of determining appropriate doses and dose frequency. A variety of disease states further alter metabolism during complex and high-risk procedures that demand rapid decision-making and intervention. Given all of these significant hurdles, adverse drug events in the perianesthetic period are predictable, yet many should be avoidable.

Anesthesia providers are unique in terms of the management of medications. They prescribe, dispense, dilute, administer, and record the drugs given, frequently without the participation of other personnel. Drug calculation errors have been reported by staff and resident anesthesiologists [127–129]. The incidence of drug errors in anesthesia is 1–4 %, with untoward outcomes reported including death [127]. In 2010, the Anesthesia Patient Safety Foundation convened a summit meeting that resulted in key strategies to reduce drug errors in the operating room area [127]. Research indicates that medication errors as a percent of incidents in pediatric anesthesia have remained relatively unchanged (~2 % to 5 %) [8, 9, 12, 15, 19, 22]. A review of critical pediatric anesthetic incidents demonstrated that medication errors accounted for 4.4 %, with anaphylaxis the most common event in this category [22]. In contrast, a review of critical incidents in pediatric patients during the extended perioperative period reported to the UK National Reporting and Learning System over a 3-year period revealed that medication issues predominated (35.6 %), nearly doubling the next closest category (airway and respiration, 18.8 %) [72]. The majority of these were administration errors, including unintended additional dosing in which an anesthesiologist was one of the healthcare professionals involved but may have not made the error [72]. As this review included the hospital course, a greater overall percentage of medication errors points to increased concerns for appropriate perioperative communication between healthcare providers during the transition from the operating room to the postanesthesia care unit and intensive care unit.

Relatively fewer studies have addressed risks in neonates. However, those few studies have noted that both the adverse drug events and consequences are significantly greater in neonates than older children [130]. In both neonates and children, the incidence of drug errors is similar; however, the risk of 10–300-fold error has led to serious or potentially serious adverse sequelae, a worrisome problem considering that many drugs administered to neonates are off-label and incompletely studied [131, 132].

Adverse drug events in the NICU were included as part of a larger study in a university-affiliated pediatric hospital [133]. Adverse drug events and potential adverse drug events occurred in 19.18 and 27.4 per 1,000 hospital days, respectively, of which 14.38 adverse drug events per 1,000 hospital days were deemed preventable. Interestingly, adverse drug events in the NICU were below the average for all areas studied, with the pediatric surgical ward having a greater incidence of adverse drug events (65.01 per 1,000 hospital days).

The technique of administering bolus and continuous IV medications plays a central role in neonatal care. Undiluted or minimally diluted formulations of bolus medications result in small administration volumes (tenths of a milliliter) which can be easily lost or captured in the dead space of IV tubing, syringes, and access ports, significantly delaying or decreasing the intended drug effect. This can also lead to accidental dose stacking and its unintended complications. The administration of extra or even excessive volume may occur when less-diluted infusions are used or with the need for repeated medication flushes [134, 135]. Only preservative-free flush solutions should be used for neonates to prevent the excessive accumulation of potentially toxic preservatives such as benzyl alcohol [135, 136]. The setup of the IV and infusion lines together with the drug concentration and flow rates play an important role in the lag time to achieve steady state blood concentrations of drug and in the amount of drug in the system architecture that may be available for an inadvertent bolus [134].

The "six rights" of medication administration to avoid errors are verifying the right patient, dose, medication, time, route, and record (i.e., documentation of the medication administered and wasted) [137]. In addition to these "rights," systems must be designed and implemented to diminish the chance of errors occurring. Methods to decrease medication-related errors include stringent drug labeling on syringes and vials, barcoding all vials, color-coding by class of drugs, removing dangerous drugs from "open" anesthesia carts and drawers, and not storing similar appearing drug containers near each other [22, 138, 139]. Merry and Anderson identified the nine strategies "below for decreasing the risk of medication error in anesthesia, realizing that some of the strategies are directed towards an individual practitioner since no system has been shown to completely eliminate medications errors. Adapted from ref. [137]:

1. Systematic countermeasures should be used to decrease the number of drug administration errors in anesthesia.
2. The label on any drug ampoule or syringe should be read carefully before a drug is drawn up or injected.
3. The legibility and contents of labels on ampoules and syringes should be optimized according to agreed standards.
4. Syringes should always be labeled (or almost always: if, during the process of drawing up and administering a single medication, the syringe never leaves the practitioner's hands, a case can be made that a syringe label is not necessary, but it is probably safer simply to label all syringes).
5. Medication drawers and workspace should be formally organized, and potentially hazardous medications (e.g., epinephrine, halothane, bupivacaine) not used during routine and uneventful anesthetics should be separated from those that are (in another drawer or outside the OR).

6. An independent check: Labels should be checked with a second person or by means of a device (such as a bar-code reader linked to a computer) before any medication is drawn up or administered.
7. Errors in intravenous drug administration during anesthesia should be reported and regularly reviewed.
8. Inventory management should focus on minimizing the risk of drug error: there is a strong case for designating a pharmacist to the operating theaters, and any changes in presentation should be notified ahead of time.
9. Similar packaging and presentation of medications should be avoided where possible."

Another key strategy to prevent drug errors is to add multiple barriers to the error pathway such as standardized concentrations for continuous infusions, standardized pediatric packaging of medications (vs. relying on adult formulations), prefilled syringes, use of bar codes to verify medications prior to administration, and reengineering drug delivery systems such that intravenous, intra-arterial, and regional syringes or infusion lines cannot be interchanged [138, 139]. As with most solutions to complex problems, these steps are likely to add extra costs while still requiring the provider to remain fully engaged and diligent.

Despite decades of recognizing drug errors in anesthesia as a substantial patient safety issue, there has been minimal significant progress in medication error reduction. When institutions, industry, and governmental agencies accept and mandate standardization for the formulation, distribution, and administration of pediatric medications, coupled with individual providers to support and implement the updated standardized systems at the bedside, then adverse drug events may finally be reduced substantially.

Equipment-Related Incidents

Studies have demonstrated that equipment-related incidents in pediatric anesthesia play a small yet important role in adverse or "near-miss" events. Comparing studies is difficult as some only report critical events and others report both critical and potentially critical events. In addition, the actual definition of equipment-related incidents is not always stated or consistent between studies. Previous reviews of pediatric closed claims study in the USA [17] and the Australian Incident Monitoring Study [24] found equipment-related events in 13 % and 14 % of total claims or incidents, respectively. In the most recent pediatric closed claims analysis, equipment issues were cited in 15 % [11]. Two studies utilizing the POCA registry from 1994 to 1997 and from 1998 to 2004 show equipment-related events of 7 % and 5 % of total events, respectively, with central venous catheter complications the most frequent followed by problems with the tracheal tube or breathing circuit [7, 18]. Recent data published from the POCA registry specifically identified children with heart disease during 1994 to 2005 and reported the rate of equipment-related arrests at 9 % [31]. Again, central venous catheters were most frequently associated with equipment-related arrests, and 77.8 % of arrests attributed to central venous catheters occurred in neonates. A review of critical incidents affecting or potentially affecting the perioperative anesthetic management in children under 16 years old reported to the UK National Reporting and Learning System from 2006 to 2008 showed equipment-related incidents to be 15.7 % of the total without any deaths or reports of severe harm [72]. As this review included potential harm, the greater rate is not surprising even though venous access complications were not included in the equipment category. Equipment-related events in institutional or multi-institutional studies ranged from approximately 2 % to 10 % of total events reported [8, 15, 19, 22, 23]. Most of these involved the anesthesia machine or the breathing circuit and tracheal tube.

Addressing Risks and Adverse Events

Ideally, reconstructing the course that led to a critical incident may provide a broader overview of the processes that combined to result in an adverse event. Prospective collection of such information for adverse events is essential yet exceedingly difficult to collect particularly when the event is rare. Analysis of the contributing factors should then lead to strategies and tactics to manage and control potential safety threats, all with the goal of improving outcome. Knowing that children under the age of 3 years comprise a high-risk anesthesia population and that neonates pose the greatest risk for perioperative complications, institutions and experts that train and credential anesthesia subspecialists and those who are involved in healthcare policy development must focus on both identifying the root causes of the adverse events and developing outcomes research to appropriately implement or modify processes to prevent or reduce their occurrence [139]. Individual institutions and departments must also critically review findings addressing patient safety during anesthesia [118] by implementing new strategies or redeploying resources [113]. Optimizing patient medical management and verifying the equipment, including necessary drugs with appropriate dilutions, labels, and double checks before induction, are essential and should be done routinely except in the most emergent of situations. Setting parameter limits and alarms appropriately to aide in the prevention of adverse events by forewarning the provider is vital in such a complex environment. As anesthesia information systems, monitors, machines, and equipment advance in capacity and integration, preset alarm limits based on the age of the child and adjusted for various periods of an anesthetic can be tied into an anesthesia information management system such that as the case progresses from induction to emergence, so do appropriate alarms settings. Asking for help, either by a consultation with another pediatric anesthesiologist or having an extra team member present when needed is an excellent strategy to decrease adverse events [113]. Providers who are specifically trained for and experienced with high-risk subpopulations can decrease risk of adverse events [14, 117–120, 140]. This holds true for all areas of care, from the preoperative to the postoperative setting. Practitioners must engage in self-reflection and seek feedback, and institutions and departments must provide mechanisms and processes for feedback so that the appropriate steps may be taken to understand and prevent further mishaps. Goal-directed management has been shown to improve outcomes in adults and is showing promise in pediatrics, particularly in cardiac anesthesia with the use of cerebral oxygenation monitors and modulation of the stress response [116].

Research must continue in areas to improve patient outcomes with the goal of identifying common parameters to measure, maintaining universal definitions for parameters and their assessment, and aggregating data from multiple sources to better assess both the more common minor adverse events as well as the rare yet potentially devastating major events. Wake Up Safe, a voluntary, multi-institutional initiative organized by the Society for Pediatric Anesthesia, is attempting to achieve this ideal. Wake Up Safe is a national registry of serious adverse events that occur during the perioperative period for the purpose of quality improvement [141]. Adverse events must also be studied by utilizing multidisciplinary improvement measures that identify not only specialty-specific factors but also specialty-related and shared factors [116]. For any of these to be achievable, the development of uniform pediatric standards, central pediatric registries, appropriate benchmarks, and a robust infrastructure must occur, so that as Davis paraphrased from a contemporary politician "we can move beyond the known knowns and known unknowns to the unknown unknowns in pediatric" as well as neonatal anesthesia [142].

Anesthesia and Neurocognitive Development

For many years, analgesic and anesthetic agents were withheld from neonates due to the perceived lack of, or reduced need for, these agents during neonatal surgery. In 1987, the American Academy of Pediatrics issued a statement [143] in which they acknowledged that the increasing body of evidence indicates neonates, including preterm neonates, demonstrate appropriate physiologic responses to painful stimuli and that the extent of neonatal cortical function is far greater than previously considered [144]. The policy statement concluded that the available pharmacologic agents for the administration of anesthesia "permit relatively safe administration of anesthesia or analgesia to neonates … [and] that such administration is indicated according to the usual guidelines for the administration of anesthesia to high-risk, potentially unstable patients" [143]. In the ensuing decades, the concern regarding the safety of anesthetics administered to neonates resurfaced. This time, the concern focused directly on the risk that anesthetic agents may induce neuronal apoptosis and neurodegeneration, with effects on long-term neurodevelopment in the neonate and infant.

Early observations by researchers suggested that anesthetic agents induce neuronal cell death and neurodegeneration with possible long-term cognitive implications in neonatal rodents [145–149]. These and subsequent animal studies, including some involving subhuman primates [150], have yielded consistent neuroanatomical and neurodevelopmental sequelae after administering anesthetics to these neonatal animals that have raised concerns that similar damage may occur in human neonates and infants. In 2007, the Food and Drug Administration (FDA) reviewed the published evidence including limitations and steps taken to address concerns as follows: (i) *N*-methyl-D-aspartate-receptor antagonists and GABAergic potentiators/agonists are potentially neurotoxic to the developing brain Table 16.1; (ii) it is unclear if drug combinations increase neurotoxicity although nonclinical data suggest that combinations are more toxic than individual agents; and (iii) a lack of information prevents a determination of safety risk for available agents or combination of agents [151]. The FDA held a second hearing in March 2011 in which the regulators reiterated that an absence of properly designed studies precludes a determination of the clinical risk that anesthetic and sedative agents pose to humans [152, 153], although enigmatically they went on to declare: "…that there was insufficient information to warrant changing the practice of pediatric anesthesia, other than *to forgo elective procedures in children less than 3 years of age* [154]. Decades of clinical use have not revealed any clear clinical evidence that links anesthetic agents to harm to the developing human brain. However, we also acknowledge that prospective clinical studies on anesthetic-induced neurotoxicity have never been conducted in neonates and infants. Uncovering such associations is exceedingly difficult as there are many confounding factors that may affect the out-

Table 16.1 Effects of medications on brain apoptosis in newborn animals

Pro-apoptotic:
• Isoflurane, sevoflurane, desflurane, N_2O
• Propofol, thiopental, ketamine, midazolam, diazepam, $MgSO_4$, dexamethasone, CO_2
Anti-apoptotic:
• Lithium, melatonin, clonidine
Non-apoptotic:
• Dexmedetomidine, opioids, ± xenon
Unknown:
• Muscle relaxants

come measures, including the likely prolonged and variable period of time between exposure and effect [155]. In 2007, Anand critically assessed animal studies implicating anesthetic neurotoxicity concluding that "the limitations of the aforementioned experimental models preclude their applicability to the clinical care of infants and children" [156]. These limitations included using animals at inappropriate or incongruous neurodevelopmental stages, using anesthetics at inappropriate or incomparable doses and durations, not using comparable physiologic monitoring, and using anesthetics without appropriate surgical stimuli [156, 157]. The challenge of accounting for interspecies differences in pharmacokinetics and pharmacodynamics when extrapolating doses, duration, and time of exposure to humans is "both critical and problematic" [158, 159]. Those who exposed the issue of animal neuroapoptosis countered that doses used in animal studies were not excessive, citing studies that use subanesthetic doses in the development of neuroapoptosis, and stated that reported physiologic data in these studies are comparable with controls values. They discussed the timing of neurodevelopmental and synaptogenic periods between species and suggested a parallel can be drawn to investigations of alcohol-induced neurotoxicity in humans [160]. Even if we conceded the dosing and age differences between humans and animals, the author's own data suggest that alcohol significantly increases the severity of the neuroapoptosis only if the blood alcohol concentration exceeds 200 mg/dl for 4 h, compared with the control group [161]. This serves to underscore the time/dose dependency of anesthetic-induced neuroapoptosis as ketamine failed to increase the severity of the neuroapoptosis compared with controls in newborn subhuman primates when administered for only 3 h but did when administered for ≥9 h [150, 162]. Justification for the continued use of anesthetics for infants and children is supported from several perspectives. First, that anesthetics confer neuroprotective and anti-inflammatory effects as well as the detrimental effects of not treating pain or surgical stress [156, 157, 163, 164]. Second, that when used to treat painful stimuli, ketamine decreases neuronal degeneration compared with testing ketamine without painful stimuli [165–167]. Third, that the neurocognitive outcomes after both traumatic brain injury in adult rodents and anesthetic-induced neuroapoptosis in neonatal rodents are dramatically attenuated and possibly eliminated if the rodents were allowed to exercise and socialize with their littermates after the injury [168, 169]. Fourth, compelling evidence has demonstrated that preconditioning prevents or attenuates the severity of the apoptosis and neurocognitive dysfunction after newborn rodents were exposed to "harmful" anesthetics. Such interventions include preconditioning with a small dose of ketamine, [170] Vitamin D3, [170] a neuropeptide (NAP) [170–172], caspase-3 inhibitors (TRP-601) [173] and a single dose of erythropoietin after sevoflurane [174]. To date, the magnitude of combinations of these interventions on apoptosis and its sequelae has yet to be evaluated. These interventions may comprise the blueprint for prescribing a "safe" anesthetic for neonates.

Obtaining definitive clinical data on such a complex subject with so many confounding variables is an involved and extremely difficult task. Retrospective studies designed to assess the effects of anesthesia on neurodevelopmental outcomes reveal a concern for anesthetic-induced neurocognitive or behavioral effects [175–177]. These retrospective studies have major drawbacks, including but not limited to the difficulty in controlling for potential confounding variables including the lack of perioperative monitors, imprecise metrics, and measurement errors [175–179]. In contrast to these studies, a monozygotic concordant-discordant twin design failed to demonstrate a causal relationship between anesthesia and cognitive performance [180]. This study did not directly assess for learning disabilities, did not examine the effects of multiple anesthetics, nor did they disclose any details about the anesthetics that were administered. The authors of the study stated that children who are sick often have learning disabilities related to their underlying illness and require surgery and anesthesia due to that illness [180, 181]. A retrospective review of children whose mothers underwent obstetrical anesthesia did not reveal a detrimental effect of general anesthesia 5 years after exposure [182]. A retrospective Dutch cohort study in adolescent children who underwent inguinal hernia repair as infants compared a randomly selected, age-matched population and found no differences in their ninth grade academic scores [183]. At present, any suggestion of a causal relationship between early exposure to anesthetics and subsequent impaired cognition or psychomotor performance remains unproven and tenuous.

Two promising clinical studies may shed light on the clinical implications of anesthetics on neurodevelopment: first, a prospective randomized, multicenter trial and, second, a retrospective cohort study. The first study, the General Anesthesia Study (GAS), is a multisite, multinational, randomized, controlled study that was initiated to compare the long-term neurodevelopmental outcomes in infants who received general or regional anesthesia for hernia surgery [155, 184]. This trial is expected to be completed by 2016. The second study is the multisite Pediatric Anesthesia NeuroDevelopmental Assessment (PANDA) [185]. PANDA is a mixed epidemiologic design that retrospectively examines a cohort that underwent a single anesthetic before the age of 3 years compared with developmentally age-matched siblings without anesthetic exposure. Both groups will then undergo a prospective, direct assessment of global and specific neurodevelopmental endpoints as they mature.

The FDA, understanding that the investigation of anesthetic neurotoxicity is an overwhelming task requiring public and private intellectual and financial collaboration, has formed a public-private partnership with the acronym SAFEKIDS (Safety of Key Inhaled and IV Drugs in Pediatrics) [186]. SAFEKIDS evolved into SmartTots (Strategies for Mitigating Anesthesia Related neuroToxicity in Tots) in 2010 [187]. SmartTots (http://www.smarttots.org) is a "multi-year project designed to address major gaps in scientific information about the safe use of anesthetics and sedatives received by millions of children each year" [188]. The GAS and PANDA studies are now partnered with SmartTots.

If future clinical studies do reveal a risk of anesthetic-induced neuronal toxicity, how will this be balanced with the competing detrimental effects of untreated pain and stress? Unfortunately, the answers are neither forthcoming nor unambiguous, and it may be another generation before the complex interactions are completely understood. Regional anesthesia may play an important role by reducing the systemic administration of potential neurotoxic pharmacologic agents. Given the positive outcomes associated with early surgical intervention [158], surgery and thus anesthesia should not be postponed if clinically indicated. Practitioners must continue to focus on minimizing morbidity and mortality as our specialty awaits clarification of the actual risks associated with early anesthetic exposure in humans.

Conclusion

The incidence of perioperative morbidity and mortality is greatest in neonates and decreases thereafter with increasing age to adults. It is not surprising that neonates hold this position as they often present for emergency surgery with complicated multiorgan disease (respiratory and neurologic diseases), sepsis, and congenital heart disease. These coexisting disorders increase the perioperative risk. The complex environment and dynamics of an operating room combined with the vulnerabilities of a high-risk population converge to increase the likelihood of adverse events occurring. The ultimate goal in developing a successful anesthetic prescription is to prevent adverse events although a more realistic and achievable goal is to pursue strategies that decrease the number of adverse events and minimize their clinical consequences should they occur. Since perianesthetic systems require human interaction and decision-making, human errors are bound to occur. Continued improvements in perioperative and perianesthetic systems are essential to improve resiliency and decrease all types of errors. Through ongoing data collection and analysis using globally agreed-upon terms and definitions, continued education, innovative strategies, further standardization, and ever persistent diligence in the perianesthetic period, continued and significant improvement in safety and outcomes will be realized for our smallest and most vulnerable patient population, the neonate.

References

1. Beecher HK, Todd DP. A study of the deaths associated with anesthesia and surgery: based on a study of 599, 548 anesthesias in ten institutions 1948-1952, inclusive. Ann Surg. 1954;140:2–35.
2. Phillips OC, Frazier TM, Graff TD, Dekornfeld TJ. The Baltimore anesthesia study committee. Review of 1,024 postoperative deaths. JAMA. 1960;174:2015–9.
3. Rackow H, Salanitre E, Green LT. Frequency of cardiac arrest associated with anesthesia in infants and children. Pediatrics. 1961;28:697–704.
4. Smith RM. Anesthesia for infants and children. St. Louis: Mosby; 1959.
5. Graff TD, Phillips OC, Benson DW, Kelley E. Baltimore anesthesia study committee: factors in pediatric anesthesia mortality. Anesth Analg. 1964;43:407–14.
6. van der Griend BF, Lister NA, McKenzie IM, et al. Postoperative mortality in children after 101,885 anesthetics at a tertiary pediatric hospital. Anesth Analg. 2011;112(6):1440.
7. Bhananker SM, Ramamoorthy C, Geiduschek JM, et al. Anesthesia-related cardiac arrest in children: update from the pediatric perioperative cardiac arrest registry. Anesth Analg. 2007;105:344–50.
8. Bunchungmongkol N, Somboonviboon W, Suraseranivongse S, Vasinanukorn M, Chau-in W, Hintong T. Pediatric anesthesia adverse events: the Thai Anesthesia Incidents Study (THAI Study) database of 25,098 cases. J Med Assoc Thai. 2007;90:2072–9.
9. Cohen MM, Cameron CB, Duncan PG. Pediatric anesthesia morbidity and mortality in the perioperative period. Anesth Analg. 1990;70:160–7.
10. Flick RP, Sprung J, Harrison TE, et al. Perioperative cardiac arrests in children between 1988 and 2005 at a tertiary referral center: a study of 92,881 patients. Anesthesiology. 2007;106: 226–37. quiz 413-4.
11. Jimenez N, Posner KL, Cheney FW, Caplan RA, Lee LA, Domino KB. An update on pediatric anesthesia liability: a closed claims analysis. Anesth Analg. 2007;104:147–53.
12. Kakavouli A, Li G, Carson MP, et al. Intraoperative reported adverse events in children. Paediatr Anaesth. 2009;19:732–9.
13. Kawashima Y, Seo N, Morita K, et al. Anesthesia-related mortality and morbidity in Japan (1999). J Anesth. 2002;16:319–31.
14. Keenan RL, Shapiro JH, Kane FR, Simpson PM. Bradycardia during anesthesia in infants. An epidemiologic study. Anesthesiology. 1994;80:976–82.
15. Marcus R. Human factors in pediatric anesthesia incidents. Paediatr Anaesth. 2006;16:242–50.
16. Morita K, Kawashima Y, Irita K. Perioperative mortality and morbidity in 1999 with a special reference to age in 466 certified training hospitals of Japanese Society of Anesthesiologists–report of Committee on Operating Room Safety of Japanese Society of Anesthesiologists. Masui. 2001;50:909–21.
17. Morray JP, Geiduschek JM, Caplan RA, Posner KL, Gild WM, Cheney FW. A comparison of pediatric and adult anesthesia closed malpractice claims. Anesthesiology. 1993;78:461–7.
18. Morray JP, Geiduschek JM, Ramamoorthy C, et al. Anesthesia-related cardiac arrest in children: initial findings of the pediatric perioperative cardiac arrest (POCA) registry. Anesthesiology. 2000;93:6–14.
19. Murat I, Constant I, Maud'huy H. Perioperative anaesthetic morbidity in children: a database of 24,165 anaesthetics over a 30-month period. Paediatr Anaesth. 2004;14:158–66.
20. Olsson GL, Hallen B. Laryngospasm during anaesthesia. A computer-aided incidence study in 136,929 patients. Acta Anaesthesiol Scand. 1984;28:567–75.

21. Olsson GL, Hallen B. Cardiac arrest during anaesthesia. A computer-aided study in 250,543 anaesthetics. Acta Anaesthesiol Scand. 1988;32:653–64.
22. Tay CL, Tan GM, Ng SB. Critical incidents in paediatric anaesthesia: an audit of 10 000 anaesthetics in Singapore. Paediatr Anaesth. 2001;11:711–8.
23. Tiret L, Nivoche Y, Hatton F, Desmonts JM, Vourc'h G. Complications related to anaesthesia in infants and children. A prospective survey of 40240 anaesthetics. Br J Anaesth. 1988;61:263–9.
24. Van der Walt JH, Sweeney DB, Runciman WB, Webb RK. The Australian Incident Monitoring Study. Paediatric incidents in anaesthesia: an analysis of 2000 incident reports. Anaesth Intensive Care. 1993;21:655–8.
25. Leape LL. Error in medicine. JAMA. 1994;272:1851–7.
26. Smith AF, Goodwin D, Mort M, Pope C. Adverse events in anaesthetic practice: qualitative study of definition, discussion and reporting. Br J Anaesth. 2006;96:715–21.
27. Stanhope N, Crowley-Murphy M, Vincent C, O'Connor AM, Taylor-Adams SE. An evaluation of adverse incident reporting. J Eval Clin Pract. 1999;5:5–12.
28. Taylor JA, Brownstein D, Christakis DA, et al. Use of incident reports by physicians and nurses to document medical errors in pediatric patients. Pediatrics. 2004;114:729–35.
29. Derrington MC, Smith G. A review of studies of anaesthetic risk, morbidity and mortality. Br J Anaesth. 1987;59:815–33.
30. Odegard KC, DiNardo JA, Kussman BD, et al. The frequency of anesthesia-related cardiac arrests in patients with congenital heart disease undergoing cardiac surgery. Anesth Analg. 2007;105: 335–43.
31. Ramamoorthy C, Haberkern CM, Bhananker SM, et al. Anesthesia-related cardiac arrest in children with heart disease: data from the pediatric perioperative cardiac arrest (POCA) registry. Anesth Analg. 2010;110:1376–82.
32. Hansen G, Joffe AR, Nettel-Aguirre A, et al. Two-year survival and neurodevelopmental outcomes after cardiopulmonary resuscitation in neonatal patients after complex cardiac surgery. Resuscitation. 2011;82:313–8.
33. Meaney PA, Nadkarni VM, Cook EF, et al. Higher survival rates among younger patients after pediatric intensive care unit cardiac arrests. Pediatrics. 2006;118:2424–33.
34. Paterson N, Waterhouse P. Risk in pediatric anesthesia. Paediatr Anaesth. 2011;21:848–57.
35. Fenner A, Schalk U, Hoenicke H, Wendenburg A, Roehling T. Periodic breathing in premature and neonatal babies: incidence, breathing pattern, respiratory gas tensions, response to changes in the composition of ambient air. Pediatr Res. 1973;7:174–83.
36. Kelly DH, Stellwagen LM, Kaitz E, Shannon DC. Apnea and periodic breathing in normal full-term infants during the first twelve months. Pediatr Pulmonol. 1985;1:215–9.
37. Hoppenbrouwers T, Hodgman JE, Harper RM, Hofmann E, Sterman MB, McGinty DJ. Polygraphic studies of normal infants during the first six months of life: III. Incidence of apnea and periodic breathing. Pediatrics. 1977;60:418–25.
38. Kurth CD, LeBard SE. Association of postoperative apnea, airway obstruction, and hypoxemia in former premature infants. Anesthesiology. 1991;75:22–6.
39. Steward DJ. Preterm infants are more prone to complications following minor surgery than are term infants. Anesthesiology. 1982;56:304–6.
40. Cote CJ, Zaslavsky A, Downes JJ, et al. Postoperative apnea in former preterm infants after inguinal herniorrhaphy. A combined analysis. Anesthesiology. 1995;82:809–22.
41. Fisher DM. When is the ex-premature infant no longer at risk for apnea? Anesthesiology. 1995;82:807–8.
42. Craven PD, Badawi N, Henderson-Smart DJ, O'Brien M. Regional (spinal, epidural, caudal) versus general anaesthesia in preterm infants undergoing inguinal herniorrhaphy in early infancy. Cochrane Database Syst Rev 2003:CD003669.
43. Gerber AC, Weiss M. Awake spinal or caudal anaesthesia in preterms for herniotomies: what is the evidence based benefit compared with general anaesthesia? Curr Opin Anaesthesiol. 2003;16:315–20.
44. Frumiento C, Abajian JC, Vane DW. Spinal anesthesia for preterm infants undergoing inguinal hernia repair. Arch Surg. 2000;135:445–51.
45. Kunst G, Linderkamp O, Holle R, Motsch J, Martin E. The proportion of high risk preterm infants with postoperative apnea and bradycardia is the same after general and spinal anesthesia. Can J Anaesth. 1999;46:94–5.
46. Krane EJ, Haberkern CM, Jacobson LE. Postoperative apnea, bradycardia, and oxygen desaturation in formerly premature infants: prospective comparison of spinal and general anesthesia. Anesth Analg. 1995;80:7–13.
47. Davidson A, Frawley GP, Sheppard S, Hunt R, Hardy P. Risk factors for apnea after infant inguinal hernia repair. Paediatr Anaesth. 2009;19:402–3.
48. Kim J, Thornton J, Eipe N. Spinal anesthesia for the premature infant: is this really the answer to avoiding postoperative apnea? Paediatr Anaesth. 2009;19:56–8.
49. O'Brien K, Robinson DN, Morton NS. Induction and emergence in infants less than 60 weeks post-conceptual age: comparison of thiopental, halothane, sevoflurane and desflurane. Br J Anaesth. 1998;80:456–9.
50. Sale SM, Read JA, Stoddart PA, Wolf AR. Prospective comparison of sevoflurane and desflurane in formerly premature infants undergoing inguinal herniotomy. Br J Anaesth. 2006;96:774–8.
51. Murphy JJ, Swanson T, Ansermino M, Milner R. The frequency of apneas in premature infants after inguinal hernia repair: do they need overnight monitoring in the intensive care unit? J Pediatr Surg. 2008;43:865–8.
52. William JM, Stoddart PA, Williams SA, Wolf AR. Post-operative recovery after inguinal herniotomy in ex-premature infants: comparison between sevoflurane and spinal anaesthesia. Br J Anaesth. 2001;86:366–71.
53. Somri M, Coran AG, Mattar I, et al. The postoperative occurrence of cardio-respiratory adverse events in small infants undergoing gastrointestinal surgery: a prospective comparison of general anesthesia and combined spinal-epidural anesthesia. Pediatr Surg Int. 2011;27(11):1173–8.
54. Welborn LG, Greenspun JC. Anesthesia and apnea. Perioperative considerations in the former preterm infant. Pediatr Clin North Am. 1994;41:181–98.
55. Henderson-Smart DJ, Steer P. Prophylactic caffeine to prevent postoperative apnea following general anesthesia in preterm infants. Cochrane Database Syst Rev 2001:CD000048.
56. Henderson-Smart DJ, Davis PG. Prophylactic methylxanthines for endotracheal extubation in preterm infants. Cochrane Database Syst Rev 2010:CD000139.
57. Kumral A, Tuzun F, Vesilirmak DC, et al. Genetic basis of apnoea of prematurity and caffeine treatment response: role of adenosine receptor polymorphisms: genetic basis of apnoea of prematurity. Acta Paediatr. 2012;101:e299–303.
58. Zagol K, Lake DE, Vergales B, et al. Anemia, apnea of prematurity, and blood transfusions. J Pediatr. 2012;161:417–21.
59. Khemani RG, Randolph A, Markovitz B. Corticosteroids for the prevention and treatment of post-extubation stridor in neonates, children and adults. Cochrane Database Syst Rev 2009:CD001000 pub3.
60. Davies MW, Davis PG. Nebulized racemic epinephrine for extubation of newborn infants. Cochrane Database Syst Rev 2002:CD000506.
61. Davis PG, Henderson-Smart DJ. Intravenous dexamethasone for extubation of newborn infants. Cochrane Database Syst Rev 2001;(4):CD 000308.

62. de Cesar RG, Carvalho WB. L-epinephrine and dexamethasone in postextubation airway obstruction: a prospective, randomized, double-blind placebo-controlled study. Int J Pediatr Otorhinolaryngol. 2009;73:1639–43.
63. Dankle SK, Schuller DE, McClead RE. Risk factors for neonatal acquired subglottic stenosis. Ann Otol Rhinol Laryngol. 1986;95:626–30.
64. Jones R, Bodnar A, Roan Y, Johnson D. Subglottic stenosis in newborn intensive care unit graduates. Am J Dis Child. 1981;135:367–8.
65. Parkin JL, Stevens MH, Jung AL. Acquired and congenital subglottic stenosis in the infant. Ann Otol Rhinol Laryngol. 1976;85:573–81.
66. Walner DL, Loewen MS, Kimura RE. Neonatal subglottic stenosis–incidence and trends. Laryngoscope. 2001;111:48–51.
67. Miller JD, Carlo WA. Pulmonary complications of mechanical ventilation in neonates. Clin Perinatol. 2008;35:273–81.
68. Sherman JM, Lowitt S, Stephenson C, Ironson G. Factors influencing acquired subglottic stenosis in infants. J Pediatr. 1986;109:322–7.
69. Mossad E, Youssef G. Subglottic stenosis in children undergoing repair of congenital heart defects. J Cardiothorac Vasc Anesth. 2009;23:658–62.
70. Borland LM, Sereika SM, Woelfel SK, et al. Pulmonary aspiration in pediatric patients during general anesthesia: incidence and outcome. J Clin Anesth. 1998;10:95–102.
71. Warner MA, Warner ME, Warner DO, Warner LO, Warner EJ. Perioperative pulmonary aspiration in infants and children. Anesthesiology. 1999;90:66–71.
72. Maclennan AI, Smith AF. An analysis of critical incidents relevant to pediatric anesthesia reported to the UK National Reporting and Learning System, 2006-2008. Paediatr Anaesth. 2010;21(8):841–7.
73. Finer NN, Woo BC, Hayashi A, Hayes B. Neonatal surgery: intensive care unit versus operating room. J pediatr surg. 1993;28: 645–9.
74. Gavilanes AW, Heineman E, Herpers MJ, Blanco CE. Use of neonatal intensive care unit as a safe place for neonatal surgery. Arch Dis Child Fetal Neonatal Ed. 1997;76:F51–3.
75. Mallick MS, Jado AM, Al-Bassam AR. Surgical procedures performed in the neonatal intensive care unit on critically ill neonates: feasibility and safety. Ann Saudi Med. 2008;28:105–8.
76. Taylor RL, Grover FL, Harman PK, Escobedo MK, Ramamurthy RS, Trinkle JK. Operative closure of patent ductus arteriosus in premature infants in the neonatal intensive care unit. Am J Surg. 1986;152:704–8.
77. Gould DS, Montenegro LM, Gaynor JW, et al. A comparison of on-site and off-site patent ductus arteriosus ligation in premature infants. Pediatrics. 2003;112:1298–301.
78. Lago P, Meneghini L, Chiandetti L, Tormena F, Metrangolo S, Gamba P. Congenital diaphragmatic hernia: intensive care unit or operating room? Am J Perinatol. 2005;22:189–97.
79. Frawley G, Bayley G, Chondros P. Laparotomy for necrotizing enterocolitis: intensive care nursery compared with operating theatre. J Paediatr Child Health. 1999;35:291–5.
80. Allegaert K, Van de Velde M, Casteels I, Naulaers G, Vanhole C, Devlieger H. Cryotherapy for threshold retinopathy: perioperative management in a single center. Am J Perinatol. 2003;20:219–26.
81. Zellers TM, Dixon K, Moake L, Wright J, Ramaciotti C. Bedside balloon atrial septostomy is safe, efficacious, and cost-effective compared with septostomy performed in the cardiac catheterization laboratory. Am J Cardiol. 2002;89:613–5.
82. Karas CS, Baig MN, Elton SW. Ventriculosubgaleal shunts at Columbus Children's Hospital: Neurosurgical implant placement in the neonatal intensive care unit. J Neurosurg. 2007;107:220–3.
83. Dos Santos AM, Guinsburg R, de Almeida MF, et al. Red Blood Cell Transfusions are Independently Associated with Intra-Hospital Mortality in Very Low Birth Weight Preterm Infants. J Pediatr. 2011;159(3):371–6.
84. Barcelona SL, Thompson AA, Cote CJ. Intraoperative pediatric blood transfusion therapy: a review of common issues. Part I: hematologic and physiologic differences from adults; metabolic and infectious risks. Paediatr Anaesth. 2005;15:716–26.
85. Lee AC, Reduque LL, Luban NLC, Ness PM, Anton B, Heitmiller ES. Transfusion-associated hyperkalemic cardiac arrest in pediatric patients receiving massive transfusion. Transfusion. 2013;54(1):244–54. doi:10.1111/trf12192.
86. Sloan SR. Neonatal transfusion review. Paediatr Anaesth. 2011;21:25–30.
87. Vraets A, Lin Y, Callum JL. Transfusion-associated hyperkalemia. Transfus Med Rev. 2011;25:184–96.
88. Schindler E, Kowarld B, Suess H, et al. Catheterization of the radial or brachial artery in neonates and infants. Paediatr Anaesth. 2005;15:677–82.
89. Beluffi G, Periotti G, Silco C, Fiori P, et al. Central venous catheters in premature babies: radiological evaluation, malpositioning and complications. Pediatr Radiol. 2012;42:1000–8.
90. Jumani K, Advani S, Reich NG, et al. Risk factors for peripherally inserted central venous catheter complications in children. JAMA Pediatr. 2013;167:429–35.
91. Goutail-Flaud MF, Sfez M, Berg A, et al. Central venous catheter-related complications in newborns and infants: a 587-case survey. J Pediatr Surg. 1991;26:645–50.
92. Schmidt B, Andrew M. Neonatal thrombosis: report of a prospective Canadian and international registry. Pediatrics. 1995; 96:939–43.
93. Njere I, Islam S, Parish D, et al. Outcome of peripherally inserted central venous catheters in surgical and medical neonates. J Pediatr Surg. 2011;46:946–50.
94. Westergaard B, Classen V, Walther-Larsen S. Peripherally inserted central catheters in infants and children – indications, techniques complications, and clinical recommendations. Acta Anaesthesiol Scand. 2013;57:278–87.
95. Chow LM, Friedman JN, Macarthur C, et al. Peripherally inserted central catheter (PICC) fracture and embolization in the pediatric population. J Pediatr. 2003;142:141–4.
96. Hayes Jr D, Feola DJ, Murphy BS, Shook LA, Ballard HO. Pathogenesis of bronchopulmonary dysplasia. Respiration. 2010;79:425–36.
97. Mani V, Morton NS. Overview of total intravenous anesthesia in children. Paediatr Anaesth. 2010;20:211–22.
98. Tlucek PS, Corff KE, Bright BC, Bedwell SM, Sekar KC, Siatkowski RM. Effect of decreasing target oxygen saturation on retinopathy of prematurity. J AAPOS. 2010;14:406–11.
99. Carlo WA, Finer NN, Walsh MC, et al. Target ranges of oxygen saturation in extremely preterm infants. N Engl J Med. 2010;362:1959–69.
100. Stenson BJ, Tarnow-Mordi WO, Darlow BA, et al. Oxygen saturation and outcomes in preterm infants. N Engl J Med. 2013; 368:2094–104.
101. Askie LM, Henderson-Smart DJ, Ko H. Restricted versus liberal oxygen exposure for preventing morbidity and mortality in preterm or low birth weight infants. Cochrane Database Syst Rev 2009:CD001077.
102. Schmidt B, Whyte RK, Asztalos EV, et al. Effects of targeting higher vs lower arterial oxygen saturations on death or disability in extremely preterm infants: a randomized clinical trial. JAMA. 2013;309:2111–20.
103. Bancalari E, Claure N. Oxygenation targets and outcomes in premature infants. JAMA. 2013;309:2161–2.

104. Davis PG, Tan A, O'Donnell CP, Schulze A. Resuscitation of newborn infants with 100 % oxygen or air: a systematic review and meta-analysis. Lancet. 2004;364:1329–33.
105. Rabi Y, Rabi D, Yee W. Room air resuscitation of the depressed newborn: a systematic review and meta-analysis. Resuscitation. 2007;72:353–63.
106. Brown JVE, Moe-Byrne T, Harden M, et al. Lower versus higher oxygen concentration for delivery room stabilization of preterm neonates: systematic review. PLoS One. 2012;7(12):e52033.
107. Cernada M, Cubells E, Torres-Cuevas I, et al. Oxygen in the delivery room. Early Hum Dev. 2013;8951:S11–13.
108. Kattwinkel J, Perlman JM, Aziz K, et al. Part 15: neonatal resuscitation: 2010 American heart association guidelines for cardiopulmonary resuscitation and emergency cardiovascular care. Circulation. 2010;122:S909–19.
109. Sola A. Oxygen in neonatal anesthesia: friend or foe? Curr Opin Anaesthesiol. 2008;21:332–9.
110. Sola A, Rogido MR, Deulofeut R. Oxygen as a neonatal health hazard: call for detente in clinical practice. Acta Paediatr. 2007;96:801–12.
111. van der Walt J. Oxygen - elixir of life or Trojan horse? Part 2: oxygen and neonatal anesthesia. Paediatr Anaesth. 2006;16: 1205–12.
112. Allnutt MF. Human factors in accidents. Br J Anaesth. 1987;59:856–64.
113. Arbous MS, Meursing AE, van Kleef JW, et al. Impact of anesthesia management characteristics on severe morbidity and mortality. Anesthesiology. 2005;102:257–68. quiz 491-2.
114. Campling EA, Devlin HB, Lunn JN. The report of the national confidential enquiry into perioperative deaths 1989. London, 1990. http://www.ncepod.org.uk/pdf/1989/Full%20Report%201989.pdf.
115. Arul GS, Spicer RD. Where should paediatric surgery be performed? Arch Dis Child. 1998;79:65–70. discussion -2.
116. Hoffman GM. Outcomes of pediatric anesthesia. Semin Pediatr Surg. 2008;17:141–51.
117. Irita K, Tsuzaki K, Sawa T, et al. The state of pediatric anesthesia in Japan: an analysis of the Japanese society of anesthesiologists survey of critical incidents in the operating room. Masui. 2007;56:93–102.
118. Auroy Y, Ecoffey C, Messiah A, Rouvier B. Relationship between complications of pediatric anesthesia and volume of pediatric anesthetics. Anesth Analg. 1997;84:234–5.
119. Keenan RL, Shapiro JH, Dawson K. Frequency of anesthetic cardiac arrests in infants: effect of pediatric anesthesiologists. J Clin Anesth. 1991;3:433–7.
120. Mamie C, Habre W, Delhumeau C, Argiroffo CB, Morabia A. Incidence and risk factors of perioperative respiratory adverse events in children undergoing elective surgery. Paediatr Anaesth. 2004;14:218–24.
121. Stoddart PA, Brennan L, Hatch DJ, Bingham R. Postal survey of paediatric practice and training among consultant anaesthetists in the UK. Br J Anaesth. 1994;73:559–63.
122. Van Der Walt JH. Searching for the Holy Grail: measuring risk in paediatric anaesthesia. Paediatr Anaesth. 2001;11:637–41.
123. Anderson BJ. Developmental pharmacology; filling one knowledge gap in pediatric anesthesiology. Paediatric Anaesthesia. 2011;21:179–82.
124. Johnson TN, Rostami-Hodjegan A. Resurgence in the use of physiologically based pharmacokinetic models in pediatric clinical pharmacology: parallel shift in incorporating the knowledge of biological elements and increased applicability to drug development and clinical practice. Paediatr Anaesth. 2011;21:291–301.
125. Rigby-Jones AE, Sneyd JR. Propofol and children–what we know and what we do not know. Paediatr Anaesth. 2011;21:247–54.
126. Anderson BJ, Holford NH. Tips and traps analyzing pediatric PK data. Paediatr Anaesth. 2011;21:222–37.
127. Cooper L, Mossamann B. Medication errors in anesthesia: a review. Int Anesthesiol Clin. 2013;51:1–12.
128. De Oliveira GS, Rahmani R, Fitzgerald PC, et al. The association between frequency of self-reported medical errors and anesthesia trainee supervision: a survey of United States Anesthesiology residents-in-training. Anesth Analg. 2013;116:892–7.
129. Black S, Lerman J, Curia L, et al. Drug calculation errors in anesthesia residents and faculty. Abstract Anesthesiology. 2013;A4006.
130. Kaushal R, Bates DW, Landrigan C, et al. Medication errors and adverse drug events in pediatric inpatients. JAMA. 2001;285:2114–20.
131. Wong ICK, Ghaleb MA, Franklin BD, Barber N. Incidence and nature of dosing errors in paediatric medications: a systematic review. Drug Saf. 2004;27:661–70.
132. Muscolo S, Plevani L. Drug accountability and drug administration safety controls in the NICU. Early Hum Dev. 2012;88(2): S50–2.
133. Kunac DL, Kennedy J, Austin N, Reith D. Incidence, preventability, and impact of Adverse Drug Events (ADEs) and potential ADEs in hospitalized children in New Zealand: a prospective observational cohort study. Paediatr Drugs. 2009;11:153–60.
134. Ma H, Lovich MA, Peterfreund RA. Quantitative analysis of continuous intravenous infusions in pediatric anesthesia: safety implications of dead volume, flow rates, and fluid delivery. Paediatr Anaesth. 2011;21:78–86.
135. Zenk KE. Intravenous drug delivery in infants with limited i.v. access and fluid restriction. Am J Hosp Pharm. 1987;44: 2542–5.
136. Humma KG. Covert administration of benzyl alcohol to neonates. Pediatrics. 1982;70:509–10.
137. Merry AF, Anderson BJ. Medication errors – new approaches to prevention. Paediatric Aanesthesia. 2011;21(7):743–53.
138. Orser BA, Hyland S, U D, Sheppard I. Improving drug safety for patients undergoing anesthesia and surgery. Can J Anaesth. 2013;60:12.
139. Paterson N, Waterhouse P. Review article: risk in pediatric anesthesia. Pediatr Anesth. 2011;21(8):848–857.
140. von Ungern-Sternberg BS, Boda K, Chambers NA, et al. Risk assessment for respiratory complications in paediatric anaesthesia: a prospective cohort study. Lancet. 2010;376:773–83.
141. WAKE UP SAFE – The pediatric anesthesia quality improvement initiative. http://wakeupsafe.org/index.iphtml. Accessed 25 May 2011.
142. Davis PJ. When assessing what we know we don't know is not enough: another perspective on pediatric outcomes. Anesth Analg. 2007;105:301–3.
143. American Academy of Pediatrics. Neonatal anesthesia. Pediatrics. 1987;80:446.
144. Anand KJ, Brown MJ, Causon RC, Christofides ND, Bloom SR, Aynsley-Green A. Can the human neonate mount an endocrine and metabolic response to surgery? J Pediatr Surg. 1985; 20:41–8.
145. Fredriksson A, Archer T, Alm H, Gordh T, Eriksson P. Neurofunctional deficits and potentiated apoptosis by neonatal NMDA antagonist administration. Behav Brain Res. 2004; 153:367–76.
146. Ikonomidou C, Bittigau P, Koch C, et al. Neurotransmitters and apoptosis in the developing brain. Biochem Pharmacol. 2001;62:401–5.
147. Ikonomidou C, Bosch F, Miksa M, et al. Blockade of NMDA receptors and apoptotic neurodegeneration in the developing brain. Science. 1999;283:70–4.
148. Olney JW, Wozniak DF, Jevtovic-Todorovic V, Farber NB, Bittigau P, Ikonomidou C. Drug-induced apoptotic neurodegeneration in the developing brain. Brain Pathol. 2002;12: 488–98.

149. Jevtovic-Todorovic V, Hartman RE, Izumi Y, et al. Early exposure to common anesthetic agents causes widespread neurodegeneration in the developing rat brain and persistent learning deficits. J Neurosci. 2003;23:876–82.
150. Slikker Jr W, Zou X, Hotchkiss CE, et al. Ketamine-induced neuronal cell death in the perinatal rhesus monkey. Toxicol Sci. 2007;98:145–58.
151. Mellon RD, Simone AF, Rappaport BA. Use of anesthetic agents in neonates and young children. Anesth Analg. 2007;104: 509–20.
152. Summary Minutes for the March 10, 2011 Meeting of the Anesthetic and Life Support Drugs Advisory Committee. http://www.fda.gov/downloads/AdvisoryCommittees/CommitteesMeetingMaterials/Drugs/AnestheticAndLifeSupportDrugsAdvisoryCommittee/UCM251282.pdf. Accessed 5 May 2011.
153. Transcript for the March 10, 2011 Meeting of the Anesthetic and Life Support Drugs Advisory Committee. 2011. http://www.fda.gov/downloads/AdvisoryCommittees/CommitteesMeetingMaterials/Drugs/AnestheticAndLifeSupportDrugsAdvisoryCommittee/UCM251283.pdf. Accessed 5 May 2011
154. Rappaport B, Mellon D, Simone A, Woodcock J. Defining safe use of anesthesia in children. N Engl J Med. 2011;364: 1387–90.
155. Davidson AJ, McCann ME, Morton NS, Myles PS. Anesthesia and outcome after neonatal surgery: the role for randomized trials. Anesthesiology. 2008;109:941–4.
156. Anand KJ. Anesthetic neurotoxicity in newborns: should we change clinical practice? Anesthesiology. 2007;107:2–4.
157. Loepke AW, McGowan Jr FX, Soriano SG. CON: The toxic effects of anesthetics in the developing brain: the clinical perspective. Anesth Analg. 2008;106:1664–9.
158. McGowan Jr FX, Davis PJ. Anesthetic-related neurotoxicity in the developing infant: of mice, rats, monkeys and, possibly, humans. Anesth Analg. 2008;106:1599–602.
159. Berde C, Cairns B. Developmental pharmacology across species: promise and problems. Anesth Analg. 2000;91:1–5.
160. Jevtovic-Todorovic V, Olney JW. PRO: Anesthesia-induced developmental neuroapoptosis: status of the evidence. Anesth Analg. 2008;106:1659–63.
161. Ikonomidou C, Bittigau P, Ishimaru MJ, et al. Ethanol-induced apoptotic neurodegeneration and fetal alcohol syndrome. Science. 2000;287:1056–60.
162. Zou X, Patterson TA, Divine RL, et al. Prolonged exposure to ketamine increases neurodegeneration in the developing monkey brain. Int J Dev Neurosci. 2009;27:727–31.
163. Anand KJ. Effects of perinatal pain and stress. Prog Brain Res. 2000;122:117–29.
164. Loepke AW, Soriano SG. An assessment of the effects of general anesthetics on developing brain structure and neurocognitive function. Anesth Analg. 2008;106:1681–707.
165. Anand KJ, Garg S, Rovnaghi CR, Narsinghani U, Bhutta AT, Hall RW. Ketamine reduces the cell death following inflammatory pain in newborn rat brain. Pediatr Res. 2007;62:283–90.
166. Rovnaghi CR, Garg S, Hall RW, Bhutta AT, Anand KJ. Ketamine analgesia for inflammatory pain in neonatal rats: a factorial randomized trial examining long-term effects. Behav Brain Funct. 2008;4:35.
167. Liu J, Baek C, Han X, Athiraman U, Soriano SG. Differential regulation of survival kinases by noxious stimulation during ketamine-induced developmental neuroapoptosis. In: Pediatric anesthesiology. San Diego; 2011.
168. Itoh T, Imano M, Nishida S, et al. Exercise inhibits neuronal apoptosis and improves cerebral function following rat traumatic brain injury. J Neural Transm. 2011;118(9):1263–72.
169. Shih J, May LDV, Gonzalez HE, et al. Delayed environmental enrichment reverse sevoflurane-induced memory impairment in rats. Anesthesiology. 2012;116:586–602.
170. Turner CP, Gutierrez S, Liu C, et al. Strategies to defeat ketamine-induced neonatal brain injury. Neuroscience. 2012;210:384–92.
171. Oz S, Ivashko-Pachima Y, Gozes I. The ADNP derived peptide, NAP modulates the tubulin pool: implication for neurotrophic and neuroprotective activities. PLoS One. 2012;7(12):e51458.
172. Gozes I. Microtubules (tau) as an emerging therapeutic target: NAP (Davunetide). Curr Pharm Des. 2011;17:3413–7.
173. Chauvier D, Renolleau S, Holifanjaniaina S, et al. Targeting neonatal ischemic brain injury with a pentapeptide-based irreversible caspase inhibitor. Cell Death Dis. 2011;2:e203.
174. Pellegrini L, Bennis Y, Velly L, et al. Erythropoietin protects newborn rat against sevoflurane-induced neurotoxicity. Paediatr Anaesth. 2014;24:749–59.
175. DiMaggio C, Sun LS, Kakavouli A, Byrne MW, Li G. A retrospective cohort study of the association of anesthesia and hernia repair surgery with behavioral and developmental disorders in young children. J Neurosurg Anesthesiol. 2009;21:286–91.
176. Wilder RT, Flick RP, Sprung J, et al. Early exposure to anesthesia and learning disabilities in a population-based birth cohort. Anesthesiology. 2009;110:796–804.
177. Kalkman CJ, Peelen L, Moons KG, et al. Behavior and development in children and age at the time of first anesthetic exposure. Anesthesiology. 2009;110:805–12.
178. Kalkman CJ, Peelen L. Victorian water pumps and anesthetic neurotoxicity. J Neurosurg Anesthesiol. 2009;21:283–5.
179. DiMaggio C, Sun L, Li G. Early childhood exposure to anesthesia and risk of developmental and behavioral disorders in a sibling birth cohort. Anesth Analg. 2011;113:1143–51.
180. Bartels M, Althoff RR, Boomsma DI. Anesthesia and cognitive performance in children: no evidence for a causal relationship. Twin Res Hum Genet. 2009;12:246–53.
181. O'Brien G. Adult outcome of childhood learning disability. Dev Med Child Neurol. 2001;43:634–8.
182. Sprung J, Flick RP, Wilder RT, et al. Anesthesia for cesarean delivery and learning disabilities in a population-based birth cohort. Anesthesiology. 2009;111:302–10.
183. Hansen TG, Pedersen JK, Henneberg SW, et al. Academic performance in adolescence after inguinal hernia repair in infancy: A nationwide cohort study. Anesthesiology. 2011;114(5):1076–85.
184. A multi-site randomised controlled trial comparing regional and general anaesthesia for effects on neurodevelopmental outcome and apnoea in infants (GAS). http://www.clinicaltrials.gov 2006:NCT00756600.
185. Sun LS, Li G, Dimaggio C, et al. Anesthesia and neurodevelopment in children: time for an answer? Anesthesiology. 2008;109:757–61.
186. Durieux M, Davis PJ. The Safety of Key Inhaled and Intravenous Drugs in Pediatrics (SAFEKIDS): an update. Anesth Analg. 2010;110:1265–7.
187. SAFEKIDS Announces Name Change. 2010. http://www.smarttots.org/news.html. Accessed 22 May 3011.
188. FDA Launches SAFEKIDS Initiative with Academic and Clinical Partners: Public-Private Partnership will assess safety of anesthetics and sedatives in young children U.S. Food and Drug Administration, 2009. http://www.fda.gov/NewsEvents/Newsroom/PressAnnouncements/ucm149543.htm. Accessed 25 May 2011.

Ethical and Medicolegal Considerations

17

Thomas J. Mancuso and Jeffrey P. Burns

Ethical and medicolegal dilemmas frequently arise in the perioperative care of term and preterm neonates. This requires that pediatric anesthesiologists have a working knowledge of these ethical concerns in order to provide comprehensive care. Here we provide a concise review of common ethical challenges in the perioperative care of term and preterm neonates utilizing a widely accepted decision-making framework and then examine fundamental medicolegal concerns in neonatal care.

Reasoning About Ethical Concerns

The Four Principles Approach to Ethical Reasoning

In their landmark text *Principles of Biomedical Ethics,* bioethicists Tom Beauchamp and James Childress advocate that ethical dilemmas in clinical practice are most comprehensively considered by utilizing a framework structured upon four principles: autonomy, non-maleficence, beneficence, and justice [1]. That is, when confronting a difficult ethical dilemma in clinical practice, the four principles framework advocates that the clinician determines how to proceed by assessing the net balance of the salient concerns from the perspective of each principle. Notably for pediatric practitioners, the conceptual foundation of this framework rests on the perspective of the autonomous adult patient, and thus the four principles framework does not entirely transfer to all pediatric contexts. Nevertheless, the four principles framework is widely utilized by adult and pediatric bioethicists when resolving difficult ethical issues in the care of patients. Accordingly, it behooves the practicing pediatric anesthesiologist to be familiar with these concepts.

Limitations to the Four Principles Framework

Autonomy, from its Greek roots, literally means self-rule and is in many respects the foundation of the four principles framework. In ethics, autonomy commonly refers to an individual's freedom from control and their unconstrained ability to make profound life choices as they see fit. In the case of the neonate who has not developed the capacity to reason and make independent decisions about life choices, there can be no literal interpretation of this principle. Moreover, as mandated by legal regulations in nearly all US jurisdictions, and as supported by most pediatric ethicists, even loving parents are not free to autonomously make *any and all* medical decisions for their children, such as the refusal of blood component therapy in a life-threatening situation. Importantly, then, the foundational principle of autonomy/self-determination does not unequivocally reside even in parental decisions for their child. Parental autonomy is superseded, in part, by societal norms and standards to protect the minor as established by the supreme court of most countries.

Non-maleficence refers to the obligation of caregivers to avoid harm. While in some clinical situations, agreement on what constitutes a harm would engender little debate, for example, failing to provide any perioperative analgesia to an infant suffering from significant pain after an invasive procedure would be considered a great harm by nearly all in our society, in other cases, such as whether life-sustaining treatment is futile in a particular context, well-intended clinicians might reach opposite conclusions on whether such treatment is, or is not, a harm. The principle of *beneficence* is

T.J. Mancuso, MD, FAAP (✉)
Division of Critical Care, Boston Children's Hospital, 300 Longwood Avenue, Bader, 6th Floor, Boston, MA 02115, USA

Division of Critical Care, Boston Children's Hospital, Boston, MA, USA
e-mail: Thomas.mancuso@childrens.harvard.edu

J.P. Burns, MD, MPH
Division of Critical Care, Boston Children's Hospital, Boston, MA, USA

J. Lerman (ed.), *Neonatal Anesthesia*, DOI 10.1007/978-1-4419-6041-2_17,

on a continuum with non-maleficence, but beneficence requires more of clinicians (and others) than not causing harm. The principle of beneficence requires clinicians to take active steps to ensure a positive benefit to the patient. Beneficence includes the obligation to rescue persons from harm or harmful situations. This principle is interpreted from a translation of Hippocrates from his *Epidemics*: "As to disease, make a habit of two things, to help but at least do no harm." Yet, as with "harm," well-intended clinicians might not always agree on what constitutes a "benefit" in a particular clinical context. Again, for example, some clinicians in a given context may strenuously advocate for continuing life-sustaining treatment because they conclude that the benefits outweigh the harms, whereas others may be equally certain, after assessing the same situation, and may conclude that the harms of further treatment outweigh any potential benefit. The fourth principle, *justice*, refers to the provision of fair, equitable, and appropriate treatments to persons in light of what is owed to persons. As with the other principles, the concept of what constitutes justice is not free from differing interpretation by thoughtful clinicians or parents. In sum, while the four principles approach to reasoning about ethical dilemmas provides a framework for clinicians to think comprehensively about all of the salient features, it cannot overcome variable interpretations of each of the principles that may prevent all parties to a given case from reaching similar conclusions on how to proceed.

Perioperative Applications of the Four Principles Framework

Autonomy

The biomedical principle of autonomy mandates informed consent to medical procedures for the adult with decision-making capacity. In the ideal process, the informed consent covers the risks and benefits of the proposed procedure, the risks and benefits to alternatives to the procedure, and the risks and benefits of doing nothing. In care of the neonate, parental permission necessarily replaces direct informed consent. True informed consent requires more than a signature on a closely typed form. The parents who give permission to caregivers must themselves understand the information and the care plan and give voluntary permission without persuasion or manipulation.

The preanesthetic conversation, while often cursory, can and should be an opportunity for the pediatric anesthesiologist to inspire confidence and build rapport with the family as well as glean any important details about the infant before the procedure. Even for urgent or emergent cases, the parents have likely met and spent time with the surgeon. The pediatric anesthesiologist, however, often meets the family only immediately before the start of the procedure. This meeting may even take place in the holding area, not the ideal location or timing for an in-depth discussion of the risks, benefits, and options for anesthetic care.

The content of the informed permission conversation with the parents must be adapted to the context. In cases involving full-term neonates scheduled for relatively elective or urgent procedures such as pyloromyotomy, circumcision, or herniorrhaphy, it very well may be that the risk, small as it may be, from the provision of anesthesia is significantly greater that that posed by the surgical procedure itself. The parents may express their concern to the pediatric anesthesiologist in these situations with statements such as: "my baby is not likely to suffer from his hernia repair, I am very worried about the anesthesia." Discussion of the possible deleterious effects of various anesthetic medications on the developing central nervous system is more fully developed elsewhere. In addition to a review of this issue and other relevant anesthetic concerns, the pediatric anesthesiologist should engage in a frank and understandable exchange with the parents, asking open-ended questions and providing them with time and space to weigh all of their concerns regarding the anesthetic.

Many surgical cases involving neonates are much more significant and emergent in nature, however. In these cases, often involving preterm neonates, the risks from the condition afflicting the neonate and from the surgery itself may be quite significant reducing the anesthetic care to a resuscitation more than the provision of analgesia, unconsciousness, and vital sign stability. The question of CPR may be parts of the preanesthetic discussion. In such cases, the pediatric anesthesiologist should have a discussion with both the surgeon and neonatologist in order to appreciate the gravity of the neonate's condition and what can be expected in the operating room. It may be appropriate to have a preanesthetic discussion with the parents, the surgeon, and the NICU MDs and RNs in order to minimize the chances in this very stressful situation that the family becomes confused and unduly anxious as a result of hearing similar information but with different emphasis and language from different sources. Pinter recommends classifying surgical neonates into groups based on the chance for recovery and the quality of life the neonate will have if he/she recovers [2]. The details of the classification are not as important as ensuring that the parents are given an understanding, as much as possible, of the immediate as well as longer-term prognosis before signing the consent. For example, important differences between simple survival and direct benefits of surgery in the neonate have been highlighted [3]. In another review, the salient ethical considerations for managing preterm neonates at the extreme of viability indicated the primacy of the neonate's best interest in these difficult choices [4]. Parents are considered by all of these commentators to be the persons best suited to determine and advocate for the best interests of their neonate, underscoring the importance of the preanesthetic discussions.

Non-maleficence

The principle of non-maleficence comes into importance especially in the care of neonates at the extremes of viability and/or with such serious surgical conditions that survival is in doubt and prognosis grim. Harm, as defined by Beauchamp and Childress, means an unjustifiable setback or defeat of a person's interests [1]. They also limit their definition to physical harms. As mentioned, parents are generally, but not unequivocally, considered the prima facie authority to determine the best interests for the neonate. Yet, some have argued that the best interest standard is insufficient for severely impaired infants and advocates other viewpoints in evaluation of the care provided to these unfortunate neonates [5]. Proponents of this view argue that the suffering of infants is not given sufficient weight and propose that severely impaired infants have the right to a dignified death and supports palliative as opposed to intensive care for these unfortunate patients.

The Committee of the Fetus and Newborn (COFN) of the American Academy of Pediatrics (AAP) addressed the issue of determining an infant's best interests. In a policy statement on high-risk neonates, the committee notes, "...intensive treatment of all severely ill infants may result in the prolongation of dying accompanied by significant discomfort for the infant or survival with unacceptable quality of life...nonintensive treatment may result in increased mortality and morbidity....either approach risks undesired and unpredictable results" [6]. The COFN also notes the importance of the parents' role in decision making regarding the care of these critically ill neonates but also makes the point that the physician's first responsibility is to the patient. The committee further states that a physician is not required to provide treatment that he/she considers inappropriate or to withhold beneficial treatments [7]. In cases of honest disagreement, the COFN recommends the involvement of the hospital bioethics committee. In practice, there may be insufficient time for this to occur and the pediatric anesthesiologist must decide for himself/herself if their personal morals allow participation in the care of a particular neonate. Last, the committee's policy statement notes:

- That in cases where there is little or no chance for survival, CPR should not be begun.
- In cases where survival is possible but a good outcome is not likely, the (well informed) parental preferences should guide whether or not CPR be instituted.
- In cases where a good outcome is considered more likely, CPR and continual reevaluation of the utility of continued intensive care should be undertaken [7].

Beneficence

There are two aspects of beneficence: positive beneficence requires that clinicians act to increase the welfare of patients while utility requires clinicians to balance the benefits and burdens of an action and choose the action leading to the best overall result [1]. The utility aspect of beneficence becomes relevant to pediatric anesthesiologists in terms of assessment of the risks and benefits of appropriate anesthetic care for an operation or procedure and in the management of pain in the neonate in both intra- and postoperative periods [8]. The principle of utility serves as a useful decision-making framework in these situations since anesthetic agents have immediate deleterious cardiovascular effects as well as possibly longer-term effects on the developing central nervous system of the neonate. In the postoperative period, assessing the adequacy of analgesia can also be quite problematic. There are a variety of pain assessment tools available for the neonate for evaluation of acute, procedural, and chronic pain [9]. These tools include both physiologic and behavioral components and will be most effective only if all caregivers have ongoing training in their use. Yet, analgesics present both benefits and potential harms to the neonate. Careless use of analgesics in any neonate can lead to significant cardiopulmonary derangements. A proper balance of the benefits and harms of such essential treatment as adequate pain relief begins with clinically competent assessment of the patient and appropriate dosing of any medication.

In sum, ethical considerations of benefit and harm are inextricably linked to competent clinical care. This is particularly relevant to the provision of palliative care to infants with a life-threatening and/or terminal condition in which the unique training and expertise of the pediatric anesthesiologist can guide the development and implementation of effective treatment regimens with minimal untoward effects [10].

Justice

The concept of what constitutes justice in the context of health care is problematic as there are widely differing views in our plural society. Barnum defines benevolent injustice as an outcome in which an infant survives a difficult neonatal course but with significant morbidity such that they are dependent on significant technological support [11]. She quotes Norman Daniels' definition of justice as it applies to health care as the maintenance of normal function and then describes it as an injustice when health care fails in its primary function to maintain normal functioning of the individual neonate. Barnum elaborates that a "benevolent injustice" occurs when well-intentioned treatment leaves a neonate with significant morbidity and disabilities. Recently, outcome of perinatal care in the United States was compared with that in several other countries, including Australia, Canada, and the United Kingdom. Care in the United States differed from these other countries in providing proportionally less prenatal care but having proportionally more intensive care nursery capacity and expended significantly more resources on neonatal intensive care. Low birth weights occurred more often in the United States although the relative risk for overall neonatal mortality did not differ significantly among the four countries [12].

Case Example: In the case of the neonate born to a family of the Jehovah's Witness faith, the supreme courts in both the United States and Canada have ruled that blood products cannot be withheld if the neonate's life is believed to be in jeopardy. The tacit assumption is that the child would follow the parent's religion and hence would refuse blood even in the face of death. However, the supreme courts have ruled that this assumption may not hold true and until the neonate reaches the age of maturity to make such a decision, society must protect the child and provide the life-saving treatment.

It has been the editor's experience that in dealing with the Medical Liaison Committee of the Jehovah's Witnesses that when a face-to-face discussion takes place between the members of the committee and the parents, and the medical team, and the notion that all efforts will be made to optimize the neonate before surgery and to implement all blood-saving measures and minimize all blood loss during surgery, it becomes unnecessary to proceed to court to make the neonate a ward of the state for the period of the surgery. It has been my experience that following such discussions, although the parents may remain steadfast and refuse to consent to a blood transfusion for their neonate, they do understand and respect the efforts expended by the medical team to respect their beliefs and in most circumstances, will consent to the anesthesia and surgery.

Perioperative Do-Not-Resuscitate Orders

Neonates with existing DNR orders may require anesthesia for palliation or for placement of devices that simplify care such as a gastrostomy tube, tracheostomy, or central line. Underlying the decision to invoke a DNR order is typically the premise that the neonate has a terminal or irreversible condition and that a cardiac arrest, if it were to occur, will leave the patient in yet a worse condition, even if the resuscitation were successful. Accordingly, resuscitation in this context is not warranted. Yet, this premise does not hold in the perioperative setting because anesthetic medications inherently induce some degree of cardiorespiratory instability, which anesthesiologists expect and are present to ameliorate, if not reverse.

The American Society of Anesthesiologists (ASA) has promulgated recommendations for the care of patients with a DNR order who undergo anesthesia [13]. These recommendations strongly disagree with routine suspension of the DNR order for patients undergoing anesthesia for procedures and instead endorse a discussion among the caregivers and family members before the procedure on the overall goals of care and the extent to which resuscitation measures will be applied.

More recently, the American Academy of Pediatrics has also put forth a statement advocating a similar approach [14]. This report describes three approaches to DNR orders for children who come to the OR for anesthesia and surgery: full resuscitation, a goal-directed approach, or a procedure-directed approach. The informed consent process assumes particular importance in these cases as it is likely that neither the surgeon nor the anesthesiologist was involved in the decision to invoke the DNR order. During the preanesthetic visit, the presence of the child's primary newborn medicine physician as well as the surgeon would ensure that all members of the medical team participate in a discussion with the family to reach a congruous approach to the DNR order in the operating room.

With the procedure-directed approach to anesthetic care of these neonates, the details of intraoperative care must be carefully reviewed with the family. If the trachea is not intubated, but the procedure would generally be done with an anesthetic technique that would include tracheal intubation, this must be discussed in detail with the family. In addition, other possible eventualities that would be routinely managed in the provision of an anesthetic and that would otherwise be considered resuscitation such as stabilizing abnormal vital signs and rapid administration of IV fluids, blood, or blood products must be reviewed.

Others have advocated for a goal-directed approach to the anesthetic care of children with a DNR order in place [15]. In this approach, the medical details of perioperative care are less important than understanding and respecting the goal of the family vis-à-vis the procedure. This approach does not specify the details of anesthetic care as they are specified in the procedure-directed approach. Rather, the concept here is to utilize any techniques that are consistent with the overall goal of care that is established in the preanesthetic meeting with the family. An additional concept of great importance in this context is that whenever a DNR order is transiently altered in order to perform a procedure, whether suspended, or a procedure-directed or goal-directed approach is adopted, it is essential to clearly define a priori when these changes will commence and when they will cease. A priori agreement among the parents and caregivers on the timing for resumption of the DNR order must be respected unless all parties agree that circumstances warrant revision of the preanesthetic treatment plan. Failure to do so is a certain recipe for ethical conflict.

The Recent History of Regulatory Concerns in Perinatal Care

The Baby Doe Regulation Controversy

Few regulations have generated as much confusion and controversy as the so-called "Baby Doe" regulations [16]. Baby Doe was an infant with Down syndrome and tracheoesophageal fistula born in Bloomington, Indiana, in 1982. His parents declined corrective surgery on the grounds that he would never achieve a "minimally acceptable quality of life," and the child subsequently died. The case generated public controversy. Following a number of appeals, the final Baby Doe regulations, often referred to as the "final rule," were passed by Congress as the 1984 Amendments to the Child Abuse Prevention and Treatment Act [17]. This legislation required all states to create a regulatory system to investigate cases where medically indicated treatment is withheld from handicapped infants or risk the withholding of Federal funding for children's services. It also stipulated that "the withholding of medically indicated treatment from a disabled infant with a life-threatening condition" by parents or providers was considered medical neglect. The legislation then outlined three medical conditions that would justify withholding otherwise required treatment. According to the final rule legislation: "The term 'withholding of medically indicated treatment' means the failure to respond to the infant's life threatening conditions by providing treatment (including appropriate nutrition, hydration, and medication) which, in the treating physician's reasonable medical judgment, will be most likely to be effective in ameliorating or correcting all such conditions, except that the term does not include the failure to provide treatment (other than appropriate nutrition, hydration, or medication) to an infant when, in the treating physician's reasonable medical judgment any of the following circumstances apply:

1. The infant is chronically and irreversibly comatose;
2. The provision of such treatment would merely prolong dying, and not be effective in ameliorating or correcting the infant's life-threatening conditions, or otherwise be futile in terms of survival of the infant; or
3. The provision of such treatment would be virtually futile in terms of survival of the infant and the treatment itself under such circumstances would be inhumane" [18].

Many argued that the Baby Doe regulations are not helpful in decision making for infants because of ambiguity surrounding the term "appropriate." Regardless of how one interprets the intentions of the final rule legislation, this is not a commonly recommended framework for ethical decision making at the end-of-life in the child. The American Academy of Pediatrics (AAP) Committee on Fetus and Newborn (COFN) describes the foundations upon which difficult decisions about resuscitation rest as: clear, open communication between the health-care team and the family, active involvement of the family in decision making, continued care, when ICU care is stopped, and finally, that treatment be guided by the best interests of the child [6]. In a more recent clinical report, COFN again emphasized the importance of individualized consideration of all factors by the care team and the parents before reaching a decision about resuscitation [7]. Other commentators have noted that the literal interpretation of the regulation mandates the treatment of all critically ill neonates under all circumstances, and even possibly against the wishes of loving and informed parents, and the professional opinion of the clinicians, leading to permanent care of all infants, no matter how devastated and compromised. Few would agree that such an inflexible approach to every infant's care is wise [19].

Born-Alive Infants Protection Act

Subsequent to the Baby Doe rules, the Born-Alive Infants Protection Act (BAIPA) was passed in 2002. This law extends the definitions of "person" or "child" to include "every infant member of homo sapiens who is born alive at any stage of development" [20]. It has been suggested that the law was enacted "to repudiate the flawed notion that a child's protection of the law is dependent on whether that child's mother want him or her" [21, 22]. Later, in 2005, the Department of Health and Human Services announced that enforcement of regulations affected by that law (BAIPA) with mention of the Emergency Medical Treatment and Labor Act (EMTLA). The Emergency Medical Treatment Act requires medical practitioners and institutions to provide care to individuals with an emergency condition regardless of that individual's ability to pay. Taken together, these two acts could restrict or eliminate any practitioner or parental discretion regarding resuscitation of very low-gestational-age neonates. There is much confusion about the exact meaning of the regulations and various interpretations of the regulations that have been published. The AAP COFN, in their policy statement of Noninitiation or Withdrawal of Intensive Care for High-Risk Newborns, does not mention these regulations [6]. The AAP Neonatal Resuscitation Steering Committee commented in a letter to the editor in *Pediatrics* that BAIPA "should not, in any way affect the approach that physicians currently follow with respect to extremely premature infants" [23]. The AAP Committee on Bioethics, in their statement, Ethics and the Care of Critically Ill Children, opined that physicians may have more discretion in redirecting care of critically ill children (neonates) than is commonly realized, citing exceptions to the mandate to provide treatment except in cases where it is "futile" or "virtually futile" [7]. The AAP further supports the importance of both parental involvement in these life and death decisions along with the reasoned medical judgments of the newborn medicine physicians [6, 7]. Based on recent Senate testimony given by Eric Holder, the attorney general, the Born-Alive Infants Protection Act has not significantly affected the care provided to neonates.

Conclusions

Superb anesthetic care of neonates requires an extensive knowledge of the unique physiology of our smallest and most vulnerable patients. Yet, this alone is insufficient to ensure the provision of comprehensive care of the neonate. The pediatric anesthesiologist must equally have a working knowledge of the ethical and regulatory concerns peculiar to the neonate. In nearly all instances, clear and open communication with the parents and the neonatal clinical team will help identify ethical issues of concern and lead the way to determining the best treatment plan for each individual patient.

References

1. Beauchamp TL, Childress JF. Principles of biomedical ethics, vol. 5. New York, NY: Oxford University Press; 2001.
2. Pinter PB. End-of-life decisions before and after birth: changing ethical considerations. J Pediatr Surg. 2008;43:430–6.
3. Caniano DA. Ethical issues in the management of neonatal surgical anomalies. Semin Perinatol. 2004;28:240–5.
4. Lorenz JM. Management decisions in extremely premature infants. Semin Neonatol. 2003;8:475–82.
5. Weisleder P. Dignified death for severely impaired infants: beyond the best interest standard. J Child Neurol. 2007;22:737–40.
6. American Academy of Pediatrics Committee of Fetus and Newborn. Noninitiation or withdrawal of intensive care for the high-risk newborn. Pediatrics. 2007;119:401–3.
7. Batton DG, Committee on Fetus and Newborn. Antenatal counseling regarding resuscitation at an extremely low gestational age. Pediatrics. 2009;124:422–7.
8. Mancuso T, Burns J. Ethical concerns in the management of pain in the neonate. Pediatr Anesth. 2009;19:953–7.
9. American Academy of Pediatrics, Committee on Fetus and Newborn, Section on Surgery, Section on Anesthesiology and Pain Medicine, Canadian Paediatric Society Fetus and Newborn Committee. Prevention and management of pain in the fetus and newborn. Pediatrics. 2006;118:2231–41.
10. American Academy of Pediatrics Committee on Bioethics and Committee on Hospital Care. Palliative care for children. Pediatrics. 2000;106:351–7.
11. Barnum B. Benevolent injustice, a neonatal dilemma. Adv Neonatal Care. 2009;9:132–6.
12. Thompson L, Goodman D, Little G. Is more intensive care always better? Insights from a cross-national comparison of reproductive care. Pediatrics. 2002;109:1036–43.
13. American Society of Anesthesiologists, Committee on ethics. Ethical guidelines for the anesthesia care of patients with do-not-resuscitate orders or other directives that limit treatment. Available at http://www.asahq.org/publicationsAndServices/standards/09.pdf. Accessed 28 Feb 2010.
14. Fallat M, Deshpande J, American Academy of Pediatrics Section on Surgery, Section on Anesthesiology and Pain Medicine and Section on Bioethics. Do-Not-Resuscitate orders for pediatric patients who require anesthesia and surgery. Pediatrics. 2004;114:1686–92.
15. Truog R, Waisel D, Burns J. DNR in the OR: a goal-directed approach. Anesthesiology. 1999;90:289–95.
16. Nondiscrimination on the basis of handicap; procedures and guidelines relating to health care for the handicapped infants-HHS final rules. Federal Register 1984;49:1622–54
17. Nondiscrimination on the basis of handicap; procedures and guidelines relating to health care for the handicapped infants-HHS final rules. Federal Register 1985;50:14879–92.
18. Child Abuse Amendments of 1984, Pub. L. No. 98-457, 98 Stat. 1749 (codified as amended at 42 U.S.C. §§ 5101–5106ii (2006) and implemented in relevant part by 45 C.F.R. § 1340.15 (b) (2) (2008)
19. Koppleman L. Are the 21-year-old baby doe regulations misunderstood or mistaken? Pediatrics. 2005;115:797–803.
20. Born Alive Infant Protection Act H.R. 2175 107th Congress 2001-2002, July 23, 2002 http://www.govtrack.us/congress/billtext.xpd?bill=h107-2175
21. Sayeed S. The marginally viable newborn: legal challenges, conceptual inadequacies and reasonableness. J Law Med Ethics. 2006;600–10.
22. Sayeed S. Baby Doe redux? The department of Health and Human Services and the Born Alive Infants Protection Act: cautionary note on the normative neonatal practice. Pediatrics. 2005;116:e576–85.
23. Boyle D, Carol W, Goldsmith J, et al. Born-Alive Infants Protection Act, Public Law No. 107-207. Pediatrics. 2003;111:680–1.

Index

J. Lerman (ed.), *Neonatal Anesthesia*, DOI 10.1007/978-1-4419-6041-2,

R